AMLS ADVANCED MEDICAL LIFE SUPPORT

Ana Maria Garcia

MICP

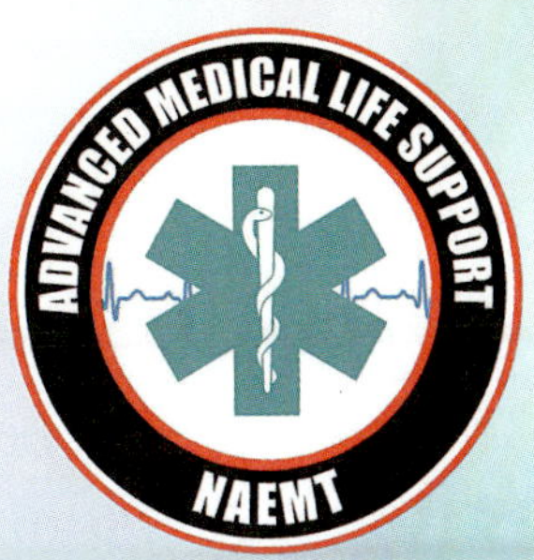

AMLS ADVANCED MEDICAL LIFE SUPPORT

An Assessment-Based Approach

Advanced Medical Life Support Committee
of The National Association of Emergency Medical Technicians

ELSEVIER
MOSBY JEMS

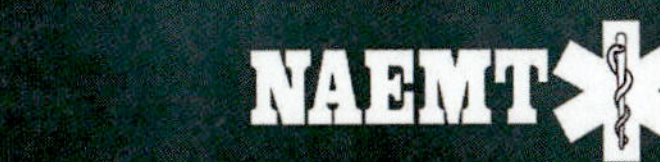

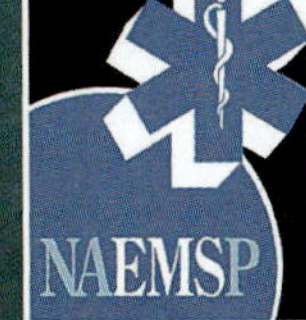

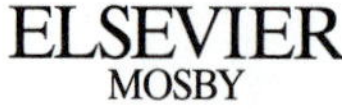

3251 Riverport Lane
St. Louis, Missouri 63043

ADVANCED MEDICAL LIFE SUPPORT
ISBN: 978-0-323-07160-4

Notices

Knowledge and best practice in this field are constantly changing. As new research and experience broaden our understanding, changes in research methods, professional practices, or medical treatment may become necessary.

Practitioners and researchers must always rely on their own experience and knowledge in evaluating and using any information, methods, compounds, or experiments described herein. In using such information or methods they should be mindful of their own safety and the safety of others, including parties for whom they have a professional responsibility.

With respect to any drug or pharmaceutical products identified, readers are advised to check the most current information provided (i) on procedures featured or (ii) by the manufacturer of each product to be administered, to verify the recommended dose or formula, the method and duration of administration, and contraindications. It is the responsibility of practitioners, relying on their own experience and knowledge of their patients, to make diagnoses, to determine dosages and the best treatment for each individual patient, and to take all appropriate safety precautions.

To the fullest extent of the law, neither the Publisher nor the authors, contributors, or editors, assume any liability for any injury and/or damage to persons or property as a matter of products liability, negligence or otherwise, or from any use or operation of any methods, products, instructions, or ideas contained in the material herein.

ISBN: 978-0-323-07160-4

Vice President and Publisher, Health Professions: Andrew Allen
Managing Editor: Laura Bayless
Publishing Services Manager: Catherine Jackson
Senior Project Manager: Carol O'Connell
Design Direction: Karen Pauls

Printed in Canada

Last digit is the print number: 9 8 7 6 5 4 3 2 1

Contributors

Editors in Chief

Linda M. Abrahamson, BA, RN, EMTP, NCEE
Committee Chair, AMLS
EMS Education Coordinator
Advocate Christ Medical Center EMS Academy
Oak Lawn, Illinois

Vince N. Mosesso, Jr, MD
Medical Director, AMLS
Associate Chief, Division of EMS
Associate Professor of Emergency Medicine
University of Pittsburgh School of Medicine
Medical Director, Prehospital Care Department
Director, Prehospital Care Rotation, Emergency Medicine Residency Program
University of Pittsburgh Medical Center
Pittsburgh, Pennsylvania

Editors

Rosemary Adam, RN, EMT-P
AMLS Committee
Nurse Instructor
The University of Iowa Hospitals
Iowa City, Iowa

Ann Bellows, RN, REMT-P, EdD
AMLS Committee
AB Training Alternatives
Eastern New Mexico University
Dona Ana Community College
Las Cruces, New Mexico

David J. Hirsch, MD, MPH
Attending Physician
Concord Emergency Medical Associates
EMS Medical Director, Department of Emergency Medicine
Concord Hospital
Concord, New Hampshire

Jeff J. Messerole, EMT-P
AMLS Committee
Clinical Instructor
Spencer Hospital
Spencer, Iowa

Contributors

Thomas L. Apelar, EMT-P
Department of Emergency Medicine
Madigan Army Medical Center
Fort Lewis, Washington

Thaddeus Bishop, EMT-P, NCEE
Division Chief/Clinical Officer
North Country EMS
Yacolt, Washington

Anthony J. Brunello, RN, BS, TNS, PHRN
Clinical Leader Cardiology Service Line & Stroke Coordinator
Provena St. Mary's Hospital
Kankakee, Illinois

Jose G. Cabanas, MD
Deputy Medical Director
Wake County EMS
Raleigh, North Carolina

Greg Clarkes, EMT-P MICP, NREMT-P
President & Education Coordinator
Canadian College of Emergency Medical Services
Edmonton, Alberta, Canada

Donna (Lowe) Cox, NREMT-P
EMS Training Officer
Designated Officer for Infection Control & Prevention
St. Louis Fire Department
St. Louis, Missouri

Jorge L. Falcon-Chevere, MD, FAAEM, FACEP
Associate Program Director
Assistant Professor
University of Puerto Rico School of Medicine
Department of Emergency Medicine
Hospital UPR Dr. Federico Trilla
Carolina, Puerto Rico

Doug Gadomski, MA, EMT-P
University of New Mexico Health Sciences Center
Albuquerque, New Mexico

Peter Laitinen, RN, BSN, NREMTP
Northeastern University
Burlington, Massachusetts

Mark D. Levine, MD, FACEP, NAEMSP
Medical Director, St. Louis Fire Department
Emergency Physician
Barnes-Jewish Hospital
Assistant Professor of Emergency Medicine
Washington University
St. Louis, Missouri

Michael Lynch, MD
Emergency Physician and Medical Toxicologist
University of Pittsburgh
Assistant Medical Director
Pittsburgh Poison Control Centers
Pittsburgh, Pennsylvania
Assistant Medical Director
West Virginia Poison Control Centers
Charleston, West Virginia

Bill McGrath, MPS, NREMT-P
EMS Department Chair
City College
Fort Lauderdale, Florida

Jeff J. Meserole, EMT-P
Clinical Instructor
Spencer Hospital
Spencer, Iowa

Brad Pierson, Firefighter, EMT-P
AMLS Committee
Peoria Fire Department
Peoria, Illinois

Frank Riboni, AAS, NREMT-P, CIC
Director, EMS Institute
St. John's University
Fresh Meadows, New York

Sarah Seiler, MSN, RN, EMT-P, CCRN, CEN
Regional Emergency Response and Recovery Coordinator
Metrolina Trauma Advisory Committee
Carolinas Medical Center
Charlotte, North Carolina

Joseph Shulman, NR/CCEMT-P, CIC
Paramedic Program Coordinator
St. John's University
Fresh Meadows, New York

G. Everett Stephens, MD, FAAEM
Assistant Clinical Professor
Department of Emergency Medicine
University of Louisville
Louisville, Kentucky

Michael Struss, NREMT-P, I/C
Emergency Medical & Rescue Institute
North Attleboro, Massachusetts

Timothy P. Toth, NREMT-P
EMS Instructor/Coordinator
Northeastern University, Institute for Emergency Medical Services
Boston, Massachusetts

Chris Weber, PhD
President
Dr. Hazmat, Inc.
Longmont, Colorado
Adjunct Instructor
Michigan State Police Emergency Management and Homeland Security Training Center
Lansing, Michigan

Kay Vonderschmidt, MPA, NREMT-P
Director of EMS Education and Research, Department of Emergency Medicine
University of Cincinnati
Cincinnati, Ohio

Katherine H. West, BSN, MSEd, CIC
Infection Control Consultant
Infection Control/Emerging Concepts, Inc.
Consultant
U.S. Public Health Service, Federal Occupational Health
Manassas, Virginia

Reviewers

Michael R. Aguilar, EMS-I, NREMT-P
University of Iowa Hospitals and Clinics Emergency Medical Services Learning Resources Center
Iowa City, Iowa

Jeffrey D. Asher, MEd, NREMT-P
Chief Paramedic Instructor
Chippewa Valley Technical College
Eau Claire, Wisconsin

Roberta "Bert" Baldus, MPAS, PA-C, RN, Paramedic Specialist, DHEd (c)
Physician Assistant Academic Coordinator
Des Moines University
Des Moines, Iowa

William A. Black, NY State CIC, NREMT-P, CCT-P
Critical Care Transport Paramedic
Transcare, Westchester Medical Center STAT transport team
Valhalla, New York

John S. Cole, MD, FACEP, EMT-P
Medical Director
STAT MedEvac
Pittsburgh, Pennsylvania

Kevin T. Collopy, BA, CCEMT-P, NREMT-P, WEMT
Flight Paramedic
Spirit Ministry Medical Transportation
Ministry Health Care
Marshfield, Wisconsin
Lead Instructor
Wilderness Medical Associates
Marshfield, Wisconsin

Jon S. Cooper, Paramedic, NCEE
Lieutenant
Baltimore City Fire Department
Baltimore, Maryland

Steven Dralle, MBA, LP
San Antonio, Texas

Bengt Eriksson, MD
Physician Consultant
Anesthetist, Anesthesia Department
Mora Hospital
Mora, Sweden

Fidel O. Garcia, EMT-P
President
Professional EMS Education, LLC
Grand Junction, Colorado

Andrew L. Guzzo, BS, NREMT-P, CCEMT-P
Instructor
Emergency Medicine Program, University of Pittsburgh School of Health and Rehabilitation Sciences
Pittsburgh, Pennsylvania

Darrin L. Hayes, NREMT-P, EMS-I
University of Iowa Hospitals and Clinics Emergency Medical Services Learning Resources Center
Iowa City, Iowa

Cathryn A. Holstein, CCEMTP
Clinical Manager
Rural/Metro Ambulance of Greater Seattle, Inc.
Seattle, Washington

Katherine Hurst, MD, MSc
Resident Physician Family Medicine
Cedar Rapids Medical Education Foundation
Cedar Rapids, Iowa

Christine C. McEachin, BSN, MBA, Paramedic/IC
Trauma Program Manager
Henry Ford Macomb Hospitals
Macomb County, Michigan

Deborah McCoy-Freeman, BS, RN, NREMT-P
EMS Education Specialist, Prehospital Care Program
University of Pittsburgh Medical Center
Pittsburgh, Pennsylvania

Jeff J. Messerole, Paramedic
Clinical Instructor
Spencer Hospital
Spencer, Iowa

Michael G. Miller, MS, BS, EMS, RN, NREMT-P
Paramedic Program Director
Creighton University
Omaha, Nebraska

Deborah L. Petty, BS, CICP, EMT-P
Paramedic Training Officer
St. Charles County Ambulance District
St. Peters, Missouri

Lynn Pierzchalski-Goldstein, RPN, BSP, PharmD
Clinical Coordinator
Penrose St. Francis Health System
Colorado Springs, Colorado

Neil Austin Plummer, NREMT-P, CCEMT-P
Flight Paramedic
Spirit Medical Transport
Marshfield, Wisconsin

Lori Reeves, BA, PS/CCP
Department Chair
Rural Health Education Partnership
Director
South Central Iowa Area Health Education Center
Indian Hills Community College
Ottumwa, Iowa

Larry Richmond, AS, NREMT-P, CCEMT-P
EMS Coordinator
Rapid City Indian Health Service Hospital
Rapid City, South Dakota

David Tauber, NREMT-P, CCEMT-P, FP-C, NCEE, I/C
Director Advanced Life Support Institute
Education Coordinator New Haven Sponsor Hospital Program
Conway, New Hampshire
New Haven, Connecticut

International Acknowledgments

Norway
Medical Director
Sindre Mellesmo

Sweden
Medical Director
Bengt Eriksson

AMLS Committee

Linda M. Abrahamson, BA, RN, EMTP, NCEE
Committee Chair, AMLS
EMS Education Coordinator
Advocate Christ Medical Center EMS Academy
Oak Lawn, Illinois

Rosemary Adam, RN, EMT-P
AMLS Committee
Nurse Instructor
The University of Iowa Hospitals
Iowa City, Iowa

Ann Bellows, RN, REMT-P, Ed D
AMLS Committee
AB Training Alternatives
Eastern New Mexico University
Dona Ana Community College
Las Cruces, New Mexico

David J. Hirsch, MD
Associate Medical Director, AMLS
EMS Fellow, Boston Emergency Medical Services
Department of Emergency Medicine, Boston Medical Center
Boston, Massachusetts

Jeff J. Messerole, EMT-P
AMLS Committee
Clinical Instructor
Spencer Hospital
Spencer, Iowa

Vince N. Mosesso, Jr, MD
Medical Director, AMLS
Associate Chief, Division of EMS
Associate Professor of Emergency Medicine
University of Pittsburgh School of Medicine
Medical Director, Prehospital Care Department
Director, Prehospital Care Rotation, Emergency Medicine Residency Program
University of Pittsburgh Medical Center
Pittsburgh, Pennsylvania

Brad Pierson, Firefighter, EMT-P
AMLS Committee
Peoria Fire Department
Peoria, Illinois

National Association of EMTs Board of Directors

Patrick F. Moore
President

Connie A. Meyer
President Elect

Donald Walsh
Secretary

Richard Ellis, NREMT-P
Treasurer

Jerry Johnston
Immediate Past President

Directors

Director Region I
Jennifer Frenette

Director Region I
James M. Slattery

Director Region II
Dennis Rowe

Director Region II
Don Lundy

Director Region III
Aimee Binning

Director Region III
Sue Jacobus

Director Region IV
Charlene Donahue

Director Region IV Director
KC Jones

Director at Large
Chuck Kearns

Acknowledgments

The Advanced Medical Life Executive Committee would like to share our gratitude to the many individuals who devoted countless hours of time in the development of the new first edition of AMLS. Perhaps Albert Schweitzer said it best: "At times our own light goes out and is rekindled by a spark from another person. Each of us has cause to think with gratitude of those who have lighted the flame within us." It is with great pleasure that the AMLS Committee, working in partnership with the National Association of Emergency Medical Technicians (NAEMT) and Mosby/Elsevier Publishing Company, have developed this textbook and instructor resources. Such collaboration has ensured that this edition remains true to the AMLS philosophy and has allowed the development of more dynamic and informative components for the book and program.

The individuals who offered contributions possess an unrelenting commitment for excellence. The hard work and fortitude of the many authors, reviewers, editors, and videographers provided the foundation for all the components of the book and program. The National Association of EMS Physicians (NAEMSP) has supported the participation of their members, Dr. Vincent Mosesso and Dr. David Hirsch. The Committee provided a conscious effort throughout the process to ensure the AMLS program maintains synergy with the NAEMT education program policies and procedures and education programs so that participants, instructors, course coordinators, and affiliate faculty find ease in teaching and dissemination of the AMLS program.

We welcomed the expertise and support of our publisher, Mosby/Elsevier. Our many thanks to Linda Honeycutt-Dickison for her guidance and to Joy Knobbe for her efforts with public relations. Our production team, headed by Carol O'Connell, worked efficiently to ensure the content was formatted, the illustrations were accurate and relevant, and the book printed on schedule.

It has been a pleasure to work with Laura Bayless, who is the person to whom we are most appreciative for answering our questions, pressuring us with deadlines, and sharing her expertise so this edition was printed on time.

It is with sincere gratitude that we thank, Corine Curd, NAEMT Education Coordinator, for her day-to-day commitment to AMLS and support of the Committee on not only this publication but for assisting in the growth of the AMLS program.

Linda M. Abrahamson, BA, RN, EMTP, NCEE
Chairperson, AMLS

Foreword

In no other aspect of emergency medical care are the skills we learned in our primary educational programs and refined over time with ongoing experience more valuable than in caring for the medical patient. These patients pose some of the greatest challenges to healthcare providers at all levels and comprise the greatest number of cases that will be dealt with, both in the field and in hospital environments.

It is while caring for the medical patient that our ability to communicate effectively with a patient and obtain a history is most important. Gathering the varied pieces of information from an ill patient and collating them into a coherent narrative to determine what led the patient to call for medical assistance requires patience, persistence, and insight to ensure that appropriate questions are asked and followed up.

Caring for the medical patient also puts our physical examination skills to the test. Physical findings in these patients are often subtle and difficult to determine in the frequently chaotic and noisy environments in which we practice.

The medical patient challenges our diagnostic capabilities as the findings are evaluated and compared to cardinal presentations, history, and physical examinations to arrive at the proper determination of potential diagnoses that will lead the provider to an appropriate course of action.

Providing the critically ill patient with the greatest opportunity for positive outcomes demands our best therapeutic decision-making and critical thinking skills. Synthesizing all the obtained data and findings while providing care and needed interventions in urgent care situations asks the utmost of a healthcare provider.

This new first edition of Advanced Medical Life Support (AMLS) creatively integrates all these crucial components into a unique, case-based approach designed to enhance the educational benefit of the program. The authors and editors have incorporated the latest evidence-based information into this text to provide the reader with the best information available regarding the care of the medical patient. They have continued to support an assessment-based approach of AMLS philosophy throughout the textbook and course. The content remains internationally compatible and includes master's level scenarios that can be utilized in the course. Components that encourage the use of simulation and online technology are newly incorporated elements.

The concept that emergency medical care is a team effort is reinforced in this text by inclusion of material about the further care of the patient that will occur in the hospital. By reading this book and participating in the AMLS course, a variety of healthcare providers, both prehospital and in-hospital, can help ensure that each and every patient will realize the greatest potential benefit and best outcome. From care initiated by the first responding members of the medical care team to providers of definitive in-hospital care, our collaborative efforts will save lives and serve our communities in ways that truly make a difference.

Peter Pons, MD

Preface

The AMLS textbook and program have been taught throughout the world since 1999, but a change in publisher has inspired a fresh start with a new first edition. This AMLS textbook and program offers continuing medical education under the auspices of the National Association of Emergency Medical Technicians (NAEMT) and Continuing Education Certifying Board for Emergency Medical Services (CECBEMS). Textbook and program content remains true to the AMLS philosophy and fosters thinking "outside the box" when assessing patients and formulating treatment plans. The case-based lecture presentations provide interactive discussion with participants. Practical application stations for each chapter provide opportunity for real-time application of textbook and lecture presentation concepts. The focus on assessment and general nonalgorithmic discussions on treatment modalities remain unique to the AMLS program. The AMLS assessment pathway emphasizes early identification of a patient's cardinal presentation. When this information is synthesized with a foundation of anatomy, physiology, pathophysiology, and efficient and thorough evaluation of historical, physical exam, and diagnostic findings, determining potential and definitive differential diagnoses is greatly enhanced. The healthcare provider's expertise in clinical reasoning and decision making are essential skills in accurately determining diagnoses and initiating treatment. All aspects of the AMLS are focused on an assessment-based approach to reduce morbidity and mortality and foster positive outcomes in medical patients.

AMLS incorporates the most current guidelines for the American Heart Association Guidelines for Cardiopulmonary Resuscitation and Emergency Cardiovascular Care and the American College of Surgeons Committee on Trauma (ACS/COT). The AMLS content and program remains an advanced course, so there is an assumption the participant in the programs has a strong foundation in anatomy, physiology, pathophysiology, and etiologies related to a variety of medical complaints. Although the textbook content and program may be challenging, emergency medical technicians (EMTs) with and without expanded scopes of practice are able to participate in courses; they are valuable members of the healthcare team.

This textbook is designed to be a required component for the AMLS programs, as well as a reference for a variety of medical emergencies. The book and the course can be informative resources for paramedic students for the medical emergency module.

The first chapter, Advanced Medical Life Support Assessment for the Medical Patient, introduces the AMLS assessment pathway and serves as a review on the components of a thorough, comprehensive assessment. To enhance the important skill of obtaining a thorough assessment, there is discussion on cardinal presentations, pattern recognition, clinical reasoning, clinical decision making, and therapeutic communication skills.

The importance of the central nervous system is covered in the second chapter, Altered Mental Status and Neurologic Disorders. Respiratory Disorders, Chapter 3, includes discussion on common respiratory complaints and reviews airway management adjuncts and strategies. Additional chapters discuss the etiology, assessment, basic and advanced diagnostic findings, and effective treatment options for shock, chest discomfort and cardiovascular disorders, endocrine/metabolic/environmental disorders, gastrointestinal/genitourinary/reproductive disorders, infectious diseases, and toxicology/hazardous materials/weapons of mass destruction diagnoses and topics.

Textbook features such as Rapid Recall Boxes, tables, and graphs are embedded throughout the book to serve as learning tools. Practical application scenarios and questions appear in each chapter to assist the reader with major chapter content review. Tables that compare and contrast common complaints appear throughout the book and serve as a quick reference for clarification and review.

NEW FEATURES

- Modifications in the format of the textbook, scenarios, and lecture presentations are intended to offer participants and instructors more streamlined navigation through the various content areas.
- Evidence-based approach for content supported by references and suggested readings
- Textbook chapters in endocrine/metabolic/environment, toxicology/hazardous materials/weapons of mass destruction, and infectious disease
- Lab values and radiograph components for diagnostic evaluation
- Laminated, folded pocket guide for use with the AMLS Assessment Pathway algorithm and 12-Lead Placement information.

- Appendices include 12-Lead Electrocardiogram Review, Normal Lab Values, Rapid Sequence Intubation, and Drug Profiles.
- Streamlined, case-based lecture presentations
- Streamlined scenario format with debriefing and explanation of diagnoses component
- A fifth complex scenario as an option in the course.
- SIM Man and MetiMan simulation scenario format for ease of use in a variety of simulation environments
- Instructor resource materials available on CD-ROM and online
- Instructor candidate monitoring within the instructor course option
- Evolve online precourse components: BLS/ALS Pretests, Simple and Complex Patient Assessment Scenario Demonstrations

The AMLS Committee and the NAEMT hope you find that the information you have read and studied in the textbook and AMLS program enhances your knowledge regarding the variety of medical emergencies your patients encounter, better preparing you to serve your EMS communities.

Linda M. Abrahamson, BA, RN, EMTP, NCEE
Chairperson, AMLS

Contents

AMLS—Past, Present, and Future

All levels of healthcare providers, both in and outside the hospital, encounter patients who present with a variety of subtle medical complaints. In the assessment process, these vague presentations offer many challenges to accurate diagnosis and optimum care. The need for additional education on medical emergencies has been identified on certification and licensure exams for prehospital healthcare providers. AMLS is designed to enhance the knowledge base for assessment and management of medical emergencies, and it does so by building on the healthcare provider's clinical background, foundation of knowledge, and skills through case-based presentations and practical applications covering a variety of etiologies that cause medical complaints. AMLS recognizes that scene safety and early identification and management in life-threatening situations are critical initial interventions that can support positive outcomes in patients.

The AMLS philosophy supports education that builds on the healthcare provider's current knowledge and scope of practice to work as a member of a team of healthcare professionals to improve patient outcomes. The combination of understanding the pathophysiology of the many medical disease processes, identifying cardinal presentations, and applying clinical reasoning skills assists the provider to perform efficient and accurate assessments. The AMLS assessment pathway is not a rigid process; rather it is a dynamic and ongoing process. It is not necessarily a critical action to alter the pathway if the patient's complaint or assessment findings necessitate doing so. The *patient* is always the priority, not the process or pathway. The order of the components of the assessment can be modified so long as all the components are evaluated.

We understand that the science and practice of medicine are in a constant state of change. However, the authors of this edition have focused on evidence-based medicine and the National Highway Traffic Safety Administration, Department of Transportation (NHTSA DOT) National Education Standards to partner primary education and standard clinical practice in today's medicine.

In next decade, we look forward to a future of growth, both domestically and abroad. AMLS is committed to providing more technology-enhanced resources in the future to encourage an interactive educational experience for course participants and faculty.

NAEMT

The NAEMT provides the administrative structure for the AMLS program. All proceeds, surcharges, royalties, and fees from the textbook and ancillary materials go directly to NAEMT. No editor or contributing author receives proceeds from these revenues. The monies received serve as an asset to NAEMT and are used for future educational projects and issues that are relevant to their membership.

International AMLS

Thanks to the success across the nation and abroad of NAEMT's inaugural continuing education program, Prehospital Trauma Life Support (PHTLS), our colleagues from around the world have easily integrated AMLS as a standard in their educational programs. Our U.S. Armed Forces have trained servicemen and women abroad serving our country in trauma response and AMLS.

To date, AMLS healthcare providers in the following countries are participating in and teaching AMLS programs: Argentina, Austria, Colombia, Canada, Germany, Hong Kong, Italy, Mexico, Sweden, Switzerland, Saudi Arabia, Norway, and Trinidad and Tobago.

AMLS and NAEMT appreciate the support of not only the AMLS programs but of the NAEMT mission. We are proud to assist in establishing education standards for healthcare providers around the globe.

Comments and Suggestions

We encourage your comments and suggestions on this first edition and for future AMLS content. We are committed to providing the most current information within an interactive, effective learning process.

Please send your comments to:

The National Association of EMTs
c/o Corine Curd, Education Coordinator
PO Box 1400
Clinton, MS 39056

You can also reach the AMLS Executive Committee via e-mail at: info@naemt.org

Visit Mosby/Elsevier, Inc. website at: www.elsevier.com

AMLS ADVANCED MEDICAL LIFE SUPPORT

CHAPTER 1

Advanced Medical Life Support Assessment for the Medical Patient

IN THIS CHAPTER, you will apply your knowledge of anatomy, physiology, pathophysiology, and epidemiology to the comprehensive, efficient AMLS assessment process, using your clinical reasoning to determine a list of differential diagnoses and formulate management strategies for a variety of medical emergencies.

Learning Objectives ***At the conclusion of this chapter, you will be able to:***

1. Discuss how to observe the scene, and describe implications the environment may have for the safety of healthcare providers and patients.
2. Discuss types of facility and situational observations, and explain their implications for safety concerns of healthcare providers and patients.
3. Identify the components of the first impression and the elements of the primary survey for patients with a variety of medical emergencies.
4. Apply the AMLS assessment pathway to rule in or out differential diagnoses, based on a patient's cardinal presentation.
5. Identify the components of the secondary survey as history (using the mnemonics OPQRST and SAMPLER), pain assessment, physical examination, and key diagnostic findings.
6. Select appropriate diagnostic assessment tools, from basic to advanced, for a variety of medical emergencies.
7. Correlate the symptoms of a patient's cardinal presentation to the appropriate body system to assess various emergent and nonemergent potential diagnoses.
8. Discuss how cultural awareness can help counter any unconscious prejudices that might impede the assessment process.
9. Compare and contrast the assessment concepts of clinical decision making, pattern recognition, and clinical reasoning.

Key Terms

Advanced Medical Life Support (AMLS) Assessment Pathway A dependable framework to support the reduction of morbidity and mortality by using an assessment-based approach to determine a differential diagnosis and effectively manage a broad range of medical emergencies

assessment-based patient management Utilizing the patient's cardinal presentation; historical, diagnostic, and physical exam findings; and one's own critical thinking skills as a healthcare professional to diagnose and treat a patient

blood pressure The tension exerted by blood on the arterial walls. Blood pressure is calculated using the following equation: Blood pressure = Flow × Resistance.

cardinal presentation The patient's primary presenting sign or symptom; often this is the patient's chief complaint, but it may be an objective finding such as unconsciousness or choking.

clinical decision making The ability to integrate assessment findings and test data with experience and evidence-based recommendations to make decisions regarding the most appropriate treatment

clinical reasoning The second conceptual component underpinning the AMLS assessment pathway, which combines good judgment with clinical experience to make accurate diagnoses and initiate proper treatment. This process assumes the provider has a strong foundation of clinical knowledge.

differential diagnosis The possible causes of the patient's cardinal presentation

pattern recognition Relating the healthcare provider's knowledge of disease pathophysiology to the patient's presenting signs and symptoms and recognizing if the patient presentation fits a particular pattern

pharmacokinetics The absorption, distribution, metabolism, and excretion of medications

primary survey The process of initially assessing the airway, breathing, circulation, and perfusion status to identify and manage life-threatening conditions and establish priorities for further assessment, treatment, and transport

pulse pressure The difference between the systolic and diastolic blood pressure; normal pulse pressure is 30 to 40 mm Hg.

secondary survey An in-depth systematic evaluation of the patient's history, physical exam, vital signs, and diagnostic information used to identify additional emergent and nonemergent conditions and modify differential diagnoses and management strategies

signs Objective evidence that a healthcare professional observes, feels, sees, hears, touches, or smells

symptoms The *S* in SAMPLER; the patient's subjective perceptions of what they feel, such as nausea, or have experienced, such as a sensation of seeing flashing lights

therapeutic communication A communication process in which the healthcare provider uses effective communication skills to obtain information about the patient and their condition, including the use of the four E's: Engagement, Empathy, Education, and Enlistment

working diagnosis The presumed cause of the patient's condition, arrived at by evaluating all assessment information thus far obtained while conducting further diagnostic testing to definitively diagnose the illness

SCENARIO

IT IS 0200 WHEN THE CALL is dispatched: "Medic 2 respond for difficulty breathing." As you pull out of the base, you turn to your partner and note, "This will be our third pulmonary edema this month." You arrive to a single story home where you find your patient in a hospital bed in the living room. By your guess, she weighs over 600 pounds (272 kg). You note she is sweating, has nasal flaring, and is clearly working hard to breathe. As you begin your assessment, your partner radios for fire department assistance and the specialized bariatric transfer ambulance. The patient is having difficulty speaking, but her daughter fills in a history of asthma, a "bad heart," and says her mom just returned from the hospital 3 days ago after gastric bypass surgery. You apply a nonrebreather oxygen mask to your patient and prepare to auscultate her breath sounds. As you ask your partner for an ETA of the additional resources you have requested, you note the dusky grey color of the patient's lips.

1 ***How will your patient assessment and care be complicated by the patient's preexisting bariatric condition?***

2 ***What conditions are you going to consider as possible diagnoses based on your findings in the primary survey?***

3 ***What additional assessments will you perform based on this patient's chief complaint and the history you have obtained?***

This chapter provides guidance for healthcare providers on how to apply their knowledge of anatomy, physiology, pathophysiology, and epidemiology to the Advanced Medical Life Support (AMLS) assessment process. An efficient AMLS assessment pathway relies not only on a provider's foundational knowledge and experience but also on therapeutic communication techniques, clinical reasoning, and decision-making skills.

In the previous scenario of difficulty breathing in a bariatric patient, would you have considered the risk for multiple medical conditions or focused solely on the respiratory system? Did you link this patient's presentation and management strategies you've experienced in difficulty breathing complaints to the recent patients who were diagnosed with pulmonary edema? Did you consider the similarities and differences in patient complaints, presentation, and management and apply that knowledge to this patient?

While doing inventory on plungers and gaskets at his hardware store, a 69-year-old former smoker with a history of high cholesterol and hypertension began to experience acute, severe back and tearing chest pain. A store clerk dialed 9-1-1. When you arrive on scene, the patient's blood pressure is elevated, and aortic regurgitation is heard on auscultation. You transport him to the emergency department (ED) of the local cardiac care hospital. Cardiac ultrasonography reveals a left-sided pericardial effusion and an aortic diameter of 34 mm. Aortic dissection is confirmed on echocardiogram.

- What does the patient's description of his pain potentially indicate?

- Based on the brief history and physical findings, would you consider this patient to be in a potentially life-threatening situation?

For this patient, a thorough assessment will guide you in investigating the respiratory, gastrointestinal (GI), and neurologic body systems for subtle associated medical emergencies other than cardiovascular.

Consider another case, and decide whether you would (1) initially rule out a respiratory or cardiovascular system dysfunction that causes these symptoms and (2) investigate the history of what medications may be involved, both prescribed and over-the-counter (OTC). Ask yourself what information at the scene may give clues to what contributed to the patient's complaint.

A 31-year-old sculptor of copper weather vanes was working on a new blue heron design in her studio when she suddenly developed left-sided chest pain and difficulty breathing. A customer who dropped by shortly thereafter to pick up his weather vane called for help. Your history taking reveals that this patient is a nonsmoker, is not overweight, and has no history of hypertension. She has a history of panic attacks, the last one having occurred more than 4 years ago. Your neurologic exam reveals that she is alert and oriented to person, place, and time, and she denies any pain or discomfort. However, she is diaphoretic (sweating profusely) and has a tachycardic heart rate and elevated blood pressure. The patient is transported to the cardiac care hospital and is found to have a left-sided pneumothorax.

- What do the skin assessment and vital signs indicate?
- What other information is consistent with a spontaneous simple pneumothorax?
- What would you expect to be revealed in your secondary survey?
- Would you determine that this patient is experiencing a life-threatening medical emergency? Or would you consider it emergent/critical but a non–life threat?

In all of the above scenarios, an organized, systematic evaluation of the patient's cardinal presentation and diagnostic, historical, and physical exam information is essential in determining the criticality of the patient, working diagnoses, and management strategies. The ability of the healthcare provider to use clinical reasoning, obtain a thorough history and physical exam, sensing clues from the environment, and apply effective communication skills emphasized in the AMLS assessment will combine to assist the provider to think outside the box and consider all possible underlying etiologies related to the presenting symptoms. This thoroughness enhances efficient interventions related to working diagnoses.

As a healthcare provider, whether you work in a healthcare facility or in the field, you know the challenges of caring for patients with medical presentations range from clear-cut to confounding. Some patients have straightforward presentations—as in the case of the aortic dissection—then there are those who have puzzling, ambiguous yet worrisome signs and symptoms that must be considered critical and emergent until proven otherwise. But even different patients experiencing an aortic dissection can have unique signs and symptoms, as in the atypical painless presentation which makes the diagnosis obscure.

Advanced Medical Life Support Assessment Pathway

Patients with nonspecific or misleading signs and symptoms may present the greatest challenge for the provider. In this chapter, we'll offer a tool designed to help you sort out these perplexing presentations. The **Advanced Medical Life Support (AMLS) Assessment Pathway** is a dependable framework for reducing morbidity and mortality by identifying early and managing effectively a broad range of medical emergencies. Determination of an accurate field or in-hospital diagnosis and initiation of a timely, effective management plan hinges on a reliable assessment process.

The success of the AMLS pathway depends on taking an efficient, comprehensive history and obtaining and correctly interpreting information from the physical examination and diagnostic assessments. Taken together, the patient's history, physical exam, risk factors, chief complaint, and cardinal presentation should begin to suggest possible diagnoses. For example, if the patient's chief complaint is low back pain, you should pursue that lead by asking follow-up questions such as:

- Have you recently sustained any injuries?
- Are you having weakness or numbness in one or both legs?
- Have you had a fever?
- Does the pain seem to move around or radiate anywhere?
- What makes it better or worse?

The presence or absence of pertinent signs and symptoms associated with the cardinal presentation are equally important. Information gleaned from the patient's answers will help you prioritize various differential diagnoses by using pattern recognition skills. In other words, conditions you've seen repeatedly have characteristic presentations compared to the current patient presentation. A healthcare provider's knowledge of the pathophysiology of disease processes combined with knowledge gained from patient care experience enhance the effectiveness of pattern recognition skills.

As you talk to the patient to obtain a history and perform a physical exam, you're looking for critical life-threatening and non–life threatening problems that must be managed within your scope of practice and with adherence to medical protocols and guidelines. You're also forming a general impression of the patient's condition. Of course, all findings should be thoroughly documented and clearly communicated to the receiving facility.

The AMLS assessment pathway supports **assessment-based patient management**. This process is not driven by rote performance skills. Instead, the AMLS pathway recognizes that although all components of the assessment process (Figure 1-1) are important to patient care, they are implemented based on the patient's unique presentation. For example, if you have a high index of suspicion that he or she has sustained an injury, performing a rapid physical exam may be a higher priority than obtaining a past medical history. The history is not omitted; it's simply given a lower priority as an assessment tool. The opposite is also true. With the medically ill patient presentation, it may be more appropriate to immediately obtain a history of the present illness and a past medical history, performing the physical exam en route to the receiving facility. The physical exam and present and past medical history are not segregated entities. They typically are evaluated in tandem with each other.

In other words, during the secondary survey, the healthcare provider should follow a dynamic, not rigid, approach during the assessment process. The assessment process should be systematic, but it should never be so rigid as to become routine. The process must remain dynamic and adaptable in order to confirm or eliminate diagnoses as more data are received and the patient's therapeutic response is noted.

Although the AMLS assessment pathway supports flexibility in deciding when to obtain specific details of a patient's history and physical exam, one important principle is that the cardinal presentation must be identified and the **primary survey** must be performed initially so that any life-threatening medical emergencies can be identified and managed without delay.

The ability to modify a systematic approach to assessment relies on clinical reasoning, pattern recognition and decision-making skills. Using the six R's can help the provider put it all together and make better judgments under pressure (Rapid Recall box). Paradoxically, by systematizing the assessment process, the AMLS pathway gives you an efficient process to apply to your own clinical reasoning and critical thinking skills—plus evidence-based principles and a dose of good ol'-fashioned common sense.

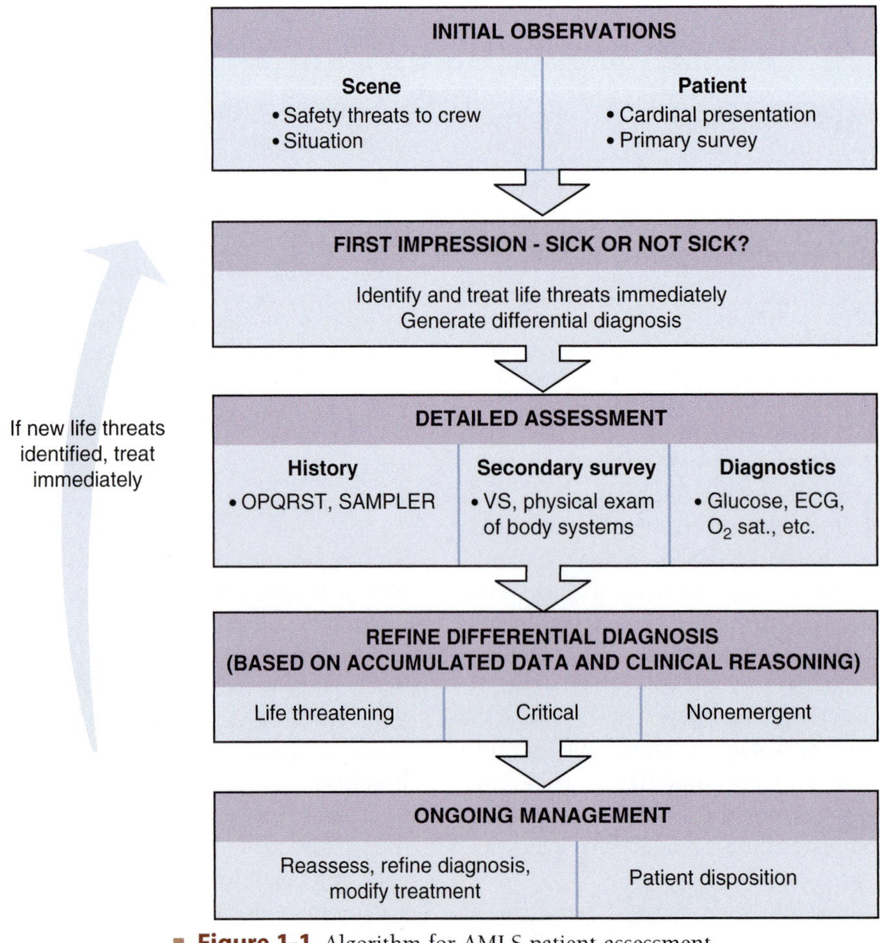
INITIAL OBSERVATIONS
Scene
• Safety threats to crew
• Situation
Patient
• Cardinal presentation
• Primary survey
FIRST IMPRESSION - SICK OR NOT SICK?
Identify and treat life threats immediately
Generate differential diagnosis
If new life threats identified, treat immediately
DETAILED ASSESSMENT
History
• OPQRST, SAMPLER
Secondary survey
• VS, physical exam of body systems
Diagnostics
• Glucose, ECG, O_2 sat., etc.
REFINE DIFFERENTIAL DIAGNOSIS
(BASED ON ACCUMULATED DATA AND CLINICAL REASONING)
Life threatening
Critical
Nonemergent
ONGOING MANAGEMENT
Reassess, refine diagnosis, modify treatment
Patient disposition

Figure 1-1 Algorithm for AMLS patient assessment.

RAPID RECALL

The Six R's

1. Read the patient – Assess the patient's condition, take his or her vital signs, treat life threats, review the chief complaint, and record your general impression.
2. Read the scene – Observe environmental conditions, safety hazards, and likely mechanisms of injury.
3. React – Manage life threats (ABCs) in the order in which they're discovered, and treat the patient based on his or her cardinal presentation.
4. Reevaluate – Reassess vital signs, and reconsider the patient's initial medical management.
5. Revise management plan – On the basis of your reevaluation and additional historical data, physical examination findings, diagnostic test results, and the patient's response to early interventions, revise your management plan to accord with the patient's new clinical picture.
6. Review performance – Critiquing your run gives you a chance to reflect on your clinical decision making and target areas in which more advanced skills or a deeper level of knowledge are needed.

It's important to understand the foundation of the AMLS assessment pathway is based on effective therapeutic communication skills, keen clinical reasoning abilities, and expert clinical decision making. Let's take a look at each of these elements in turn.

Therapeutic Communication

Obtaining a comprehensive medical history and being able to perform a thorough physical examination depend on good **therapeutic communication** techniques. To learn critical information about the patient's condition and the events that preceded it, the medical team usually speaks to the patient and his or her family or friends. Bystanders who observed the patient's accident or witnessed a collapse can offer valuable information about the acuity of the patient's condition. They can often provide clues to help identify the specific injuries sustained or to point toward a particular diagnosis.

Effective verbal communication is a dynamic process that can help gather accurate historical information, inform the patient of the risks and benefits of interventions, and obtain consent to perform a physical exam and provide medical treatment or transport. The four E's of therapeutic communication are explored in Box 1-1 and are identified as:

1. Engagement
2. Empathy
3. Education
4. Enlistment

Active Listening

When making contact with a patient and their loved ones, be sure to introduce yourself if circumstances allow. Developing a rapport with the patient assists in building their confidence in the healthcare provider and facilitates open communication.

Using active listening skills by summarizing or paraphrasing information a patient has shared is one technique that builds rapport with the patient, demonstrates what you understood him to have said, and gives him a chance to clarify any misconceptions. The LADDER mnemonic, described in the Rapid Recall box, is a tool that can help you apply active listening skills as you work with patients.

RAPID RECALL

Climbing the Assertiveness LADDER

LADDER is a six-stage process for dealing assertively with problems:

Look at your rights and what you want, and understand your feelings about the situation.

Arrange a meeting with the other person to discuss the situation.

Define the problem specifically.

Describe your feelings so the other person fully understands how you feel about the situation.

Express what you want clearly and concisely.

Reinforce the other person by explaining the mutual benefits of adopting the course of action you're recommending.

Communication Barriers

An assessment and management process can be hindered by social, linguistic, behavioral, or psychological hurdles. Recognizing communication barriers during the patient interview process can help you maximize the efficiency of the time you spend with the patient. Remember that the first barrier may be your own specialized knowledge. Avoid using medical terminology such as "tachycardia" when you could say "fast heartbeat," or "septicemia" when you could say "blood infection," for instance. Other tips for effective therapeutic communication are listed in Box 1-2.

Look for nonverbal behaviors that indicate whether the patient feels at ease. Keep in mind that patients may present with comorbid conditions that can complicate assessment and delay implementation of appropriate management strategies. Patience is essential when such a complex assessment must be made.

BOX 1-1 Key Communication Tasks: The Four E's

Communication is both a science and an art. Fortunately for those of us not blessed with natural charisma, communication skills can be learned and eventually mastered. Expending the time and effort to do so will pay off in the form of reduced likelihood of morbidity and mortality for your patients and better job satisfaction for you—plus a bit of an ego boost as your confidence and professional competence advance in tandem.

According to the Bayer Institute for Health Care Communication, EMS providers carry out four principal communication tasks: engagement, empathy, education, and enlistment.

- Engagement. Engagement is the connection between you and the patient. You must establish a comfortable rapport with the patient in order to keep him calm and elicit a thorough, accurate history. Your words and actions can convey your genuine concern about the patient or lead him to draw the opposite conclusion. Failing to introduce yourself, grilling the patient with aggressive, rapid-fire questions, and interrupting him when he's talking undermine the bond you need to develop and may cause the patient to disengage. During EMS calls, as in other situations, it's true that you don't get a second chance to make a first impression.
- Empathy. Empathy refers to your sincere identification with the patient's feelings of anxiety, pain, fear, panic, or loss. It's rooted in a sense of compassion for what the patient is going through, and it's expressed in your acknowledgment that you've seen, heard, and understood the patient and accepted her as a person, regardless of the circumstances surrounding the call. Look your patient in the eye and ask calm, open-ended questions if she is able to respond to them. Having empathy is especially important in sensitive situations such as suicide attempts, accidental drug overdoses, and cases of domestic assault.
- Education. Patient education fortifies your bond with the patient by letting him know what's happening and what you're doing about it. Begin by finding out what the patient already knows, and follow up with questions until you have all the information you need. Then inform the patient of what's happening at every stage during the rest of the call.

Take, for instance, a patient who has chest pain. Foremost in his mind is the question of what has caused it. You may not have a definitive answer for him in the field, but you can describe your treatment plan:

> Mr. Anginopolous, we're not sure whether you've had a heart attack, but until we know for certain, we're going to treat you as if you have. We're giving you aspirin, which will begin to dissolve the clot if there is one. We're going to do a few procedures, such as monitoring your heart by sticking some sensors on your chest, and we're also starting an IV in your arm in case we need to give you any more medications.

Describe tests and procedures in simple, straightforward terms. Doing so will keep the patient's anxiety in check because he'll know what to expect and what's going on around him.

- Enlistment. Enlistment means encouraging the patient to participate in her own care and treatment decisions. When soliciting the patient's consent for treatment, be sure to explain fully any possible side effects or potential adverse outcomes associated with the intervention. For example, before giving the patient a nitroglycerin tablet, explain that headaches are a frequent side effect of the medication. Be sure to offer your rationale for administering the medication or recommending the treatment despite its unwelcome side effects or dangerous risks—that is, explain that you believe the benefits of the intervention outweigh the risks.

Cultural Differences

Understanding the variances in different cultures and languages in your area will enhance your communication skills with the community of patients you serve. Investigate whether your agency or an institution in your area can provide interpreters to assist with language barriers. Bilingual family members or bystanders may be able to offer assistance. Your institution may offer assistance with sign language or multilingual interpreters.

All healthcare providers will encounter patients who have different value systems than their own. Stereotyping patients as addicts, indigents, or alcoholics, for example, can bias your approach and impair developing a rapport. Ineffective communication or miscommunication can result in the inability to obtain a thorough history, resulting in a disconnect in determining diagnoses and treatment (Figure 1-2).

Hearing Impairment

People who are hearing impaired communicate in various ways with people who can hear. They may use sign language, gestures, writing, or lip reading, any or all of which may be difficult to do when they are ill or injured. Some people with deafness have partial speech or hearing. Try to determine what the patient's abilities are, and develop your communication strategy accordingly.

The patient's family members or friends may be able to help, and interpreters for people with hearing impairments are available in many hospitals. In addition, learning how to ask a few basic questions in sign language—and interpret the answers—can be helpful. You may also be able to exchange written questions and answers with the patient, depending on his or her condition, but doing so extends the interview process.

BOX 1-2 Tips for Effective Therapeutic Communication

The patient is frustrated because you don't seem to grasp all the details of her meandering narrative. You're exasperated because she can't seem to answer a simple question without throwing in a lot of extraneous information. Heck, the two of you might as well be married.

If this is how your interaction with patients feels sometimes, making some simple adjustments in your communication technique could make a big difference. Incorporating these changes into your daily conversations takes practice, but as they say about marriage, you have to work at it. Try following these tips:

- Speak to the patient at his or her eye level and maintain good eye contact while you're talking. This is especially important with patients who are deaf if they are reading lips.
- If the patient has a hearing impairment, do not raise your voice unless the patient asks you to.
- Maintain an open, attentive body position during the interview. Try not to appear rushed or harried.
- Acknowledge your understanding of the patient by nodding and paraphrasing his or her words now and then.
- Avoid distracting mannerisms such as charting while the patient is talking, tapping or clicking a pen, or fidgeting with keys or coins in your pocket.
- Use nonverbal language to reassure the patient that you are there to help.
- Inform the patient of what you and your colleagues are doing and why. Tell her where she is being transported and what to expect when she arrives.
- Ask "what" questions, since "why" questions can sound accusatory to patients and their families.
- Show empathy by acknowledging the patient's pain, distress, anger, and other feelings. Let the patient vent if he seems able to do so in a way that doesn't threaten or cause anxiety for you or for other patients, such as other accident victims who are nearby.
- Respond to and reinforce positive behavior.
- Respect the patient's right to confidentiality by keeping your voice down as much as practicable in public or semiprivate settings, such as at the scene and in the ED.
- Protect the patient's modesty by keeping him or her covered as much as possible during the physical examination. Doing so will increase your patients' level of trust in the care you're providing and make them more willing to share pertinent health information.
- If you suspect a patient may become violent, interact with him or her in a calm, reassuring manner. Don't try to handle a violent patient alone.

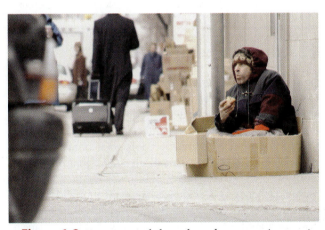

Figure 1-2 Keep in mind that a homeless person's space is his or her home. (From Aehlert BJ: Paramedic practice today: above and beyond, St Louis, 2009, Mosby.)

Safety Concerns

Domestic disputes, riots or gang activity, patients with emotional instability, hazardous materials threats, inclement weather, trapped or otherwise inaccessible patients, and the presence of other assistive resources on the scene all present safety concerns for providers and patients. Dispatch information should be considered important and relevant to scene safety issues. This information provides not only scene information but can assist in formulating initial patient impressions so you can begin a management strategy en route to the scene.

Healthcare providers should remain vigilant in assessing for and recognizing potential hazardous materials incidents and threats from weapons of mass destruction.

Be sure to follow guidelines set by your agency or institution regarding scene safety. Once the scene has been secured, remain vigilant for any potential threat.

Clinical Reasoning

Now let's explore **clinical reasoning**, the second conceptual component underpinning the AMLS assessment pathway. Most healthcare providers would agree that skills proficiency alone cannot ensure quality care. You must also be able to apply clinical reasoning—essentially, good judgment founded on a strong knowledge base seasoned by clinical experience—to make accurate diagnoses and initiate proper treatment. Clinical reasoning requires you to:

- Gather and organize relevant historical and diagnostic information.
- Filter out irrelevant or extraneous information.
- Analyze and bring to bear similar experiences you've had in assessing and treating other patients.

To do so, you must first have a broad knowledge of the anatomy, physiology, and pathophysiology of the human body. In addition, an understanding of the epidemiology of human disease processes is essential for early diagnosis, particularly when the patient's signs and symptoms do not point to an obvious cause.

Role of Clinical Reasoning

Clinical reasoning is a bridge between historical information and diagnostic test results, allowing you to draw inferences about underlying etiologies. This inductive reasoning framework helps you recognize patterns and formulate a **differential diagnosis**, a set of possible causes of the patient's condition. As assessment findings, historical information, and test results are evaluated, you can eliminate a diagnosis from consideration. Thus the differential diagnosis becomes more and more tightly focused until you arrive at a **working diagnosis**—the presumed cause of the patient's condition. The working diagnosis becomes a definitive diagnosis pending confirmation by further diagnostic tests, usually performed at the receiving facility.

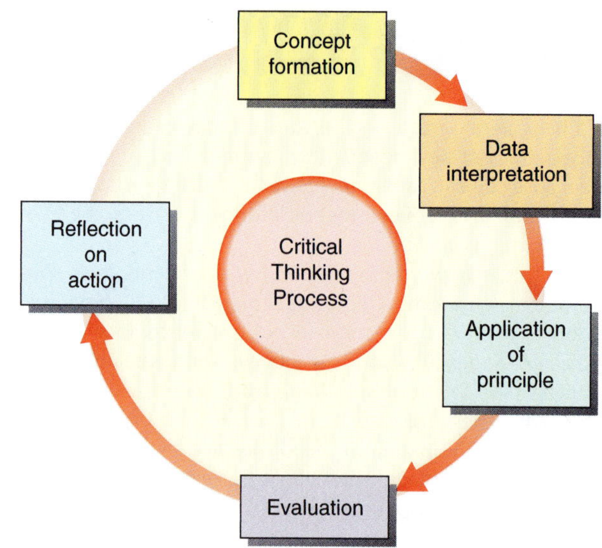

■ **Figure 1-3** Critical thinking process. (From Sanders MJ: Mosby's paramedic textbook—revised reprint, ed 3, St Louis, 2007, Mosby.)

Scope of Clinical Reasoning

Creation of a mental list of differential diagnoses is not a static process. Vital signs, lung sounds, neurologic examination findings, oxygen saturation measurements, response to interventions, laboratory and radiographic test results, and other information is used to evaluate potential diagnoses. Initial findings can be general, as in the identification of an infectious process, or specific, as in the identification of pericarditis. Your ability to efficiently assimilate data in order to determine the most plausible diagnosis hinges on adept clinical reasoning skills.

Of course, clinical reasoning is not an exact science. It's impossible in all situations to determine the correct diagnosis on the basis of the initial impression and primary survey. Barriers to doing so might include your level of medical knowledge and experience and your scope of practice, faulty learning links related to pattern recognition, the reliability of the patient's self-report, the accuracy of diagnostic test results, and the presence of multiple disease processes (comorbidities).

Yet clinical reasoning skills are essential during the entire process of assessment and treatment. During the initial assessment, you'll identify differential diagnoses on the basis of level of consciousness, airway patency, breathing patterns, adequacy of circulation/perfusion, the patient's report of his symptoms, historical data, and other information. During the secondary assessment, you'll refine these diagnoses as you analyze new diagnostic information, further historical data, and findings on physical exam. In addition, the patient's response to initial treatment assists in revising diagnoses by pinpointing any immediate medical issues.

To provide the best quality care for the patient, every provider must obtain a competent grasp of the core knowledge within his or her respective scope of practice (Figure 1-3). Book knowledge and evidence-based knowledge should be enhanced with experience and common sense, building dependable clinical reasoning skills and providing a stable footing for arriving at an accurate working diagnosis.

Clinical Decision Making

In many respects, clinical decision making overlaps with clinical reasoning. Both require a sufficient knowledge of anatomy, physiology, and pathophysiology, an ability to perform specific assessment skills, and the resourcefulness to apply complex diagnostic tools to a broad range of medical emergencies. **Clinical decision making** is the ability to integrate diagnostic data and assessment findings with experience and evidence-based recommendations to improve patient outcomes. Like clinical reasoning, medical decision making is an ongoing process that takes place at every stage of care, beginning with the creation of the differential diagnosis.

A pivotal skill necessary for effective clinical decision making is pattern recognition. You must compare the patient's presentation with similar presentations you've encountered in the past. Analyzing similar diagnoses and which strategies were effective and which were not is a useful foundation for your clinical decision making. Your clinical decision making, then, necessarily becomes more and more reliable with experience. The subtle integration of dependable clinical reasoning skills with well-honed therapeutic communication techniques makes for prudent clinical decision making, allowing you to gauge the severity of the patient's illness or injury and initiate appropriate, timely interventions.

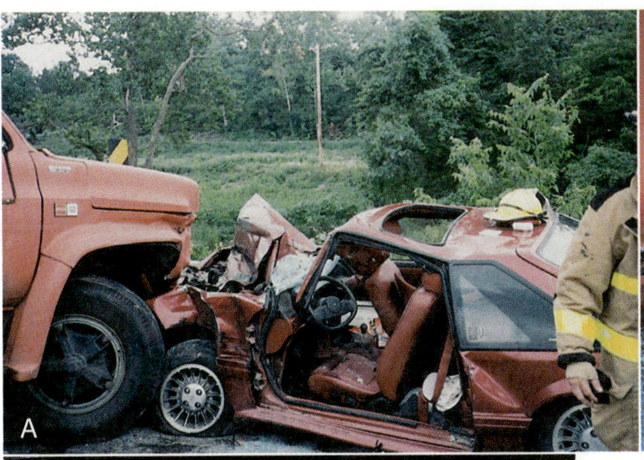

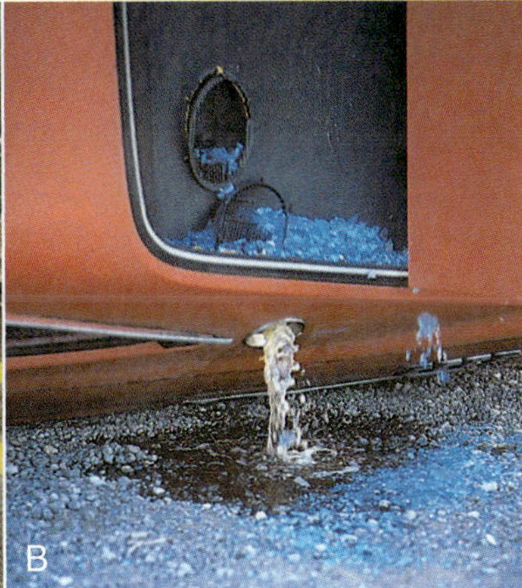

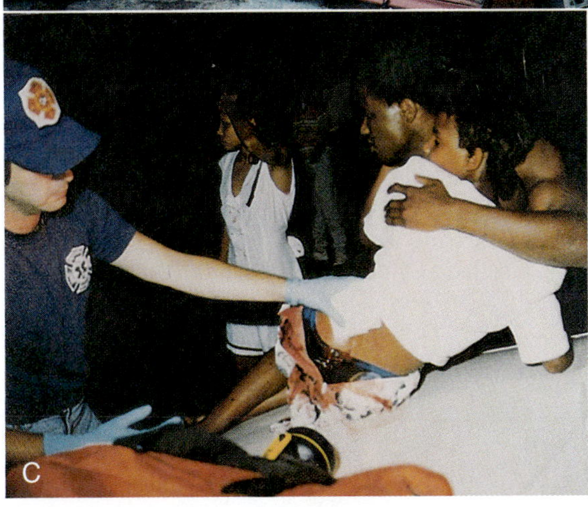

■ **Figure 1-4** A, Glass and torn metal often present safety hazards at the scene of an automobile crash. B, A gasoline leak can cause fire and explosion at a crash scene. C, Violent scenes, such as this drive-by shooting, can be especially dangerous. Be sure police have secured the scene before entering. (From Stoy WA, Platt TE, Lejeune DE: Mosby's EMT-Basic textbook—revised reprint, ed 2, St Louis, 2007, Mosby. A, Photograph by Vincent Knaus. C, Photograph by Ronald Olshwanger.)

Initial Observations

Safety Considerations

Prehospital providers reach the scene before they reach the patient. This gives you a moment to integrate what the dispatcher has told you with your own judicious observation of the scene. The scene and the potential for safety hazards or threats are continually evaluated until patient care has been transferred (Figure 1-4). Side rails left down on a patient with an altered level of consciousness is an example of an unsafe set of circumstances.

All personnel should evaluate each scene and patient situation as a potential threat to safety. Close observation of nonverbal behavior and communication with family members can lead to clues of a possibly unstable environment.

Selecting Personal Protective Equipment

As a prehospital healthcare provider, you will use information given by the dispatcher and your own survey of the scene to help select proper personal protective equipment (PPE), which includes gloves, protective eyewear, gowns, facemasks and respirators (HEPA and N-95) (Figure 1-5). In-hospital providers will use information obtained via radio communication from EMS providers on scene and the triage nurse to help determine what type of PPE is necessary for each patient. All healthcare personnel should be aware of the benefits and limitations of each. If weapons of mass destruction have been used or other

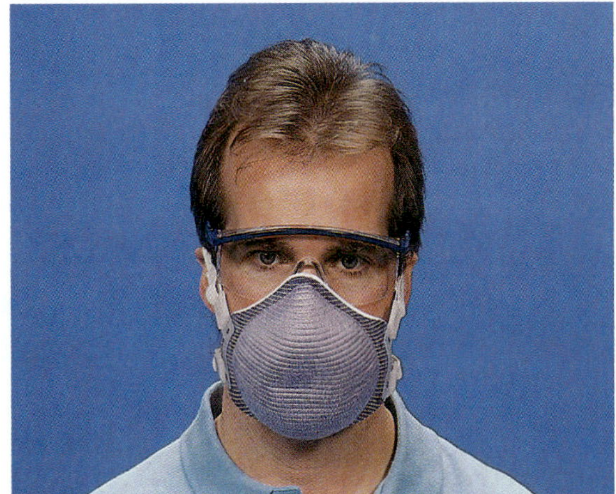

■ **Figure 1-5** The face should be shielded from the danger of splashing blood or body fluids with a HEPA filter (a product of Uvex) or N-95 particulate respirator. (From Stoy WA: Mosby's EMT-Basic textbook—revised reprint, ed 2, St Louis, 2007, Mosby.)

hazardous materials have been dispersed, a higher level of PPE may be necessary.

Standard Precautions

The Centers for Disease Control and Prevention (CDC) recommends following Standard Precautions to prevent transmission of infectious diseases such as hepatitis B and C, human immunodeficiency virus (HIV), meningitis, pneumonia, mumps, tuberculosis, chickenpox, pertussis (whooping cough), and staphylococcal infections (including methicillin-resistant *Staphylococcus aureus* (MRSA). These precautions apply to all patients in every healthcare setting, regardless of whether the patient is known to have or only suspected of having an infection. Standard Precautions include:

- Use of proper hand hygiene techniques, including handwashing before and after every patient encounter and after removal of gloves and disinfection of equipment
- Use of gloves, gown, mask, eye protection, or face shield, depending on the anticipated exposure
- Safe injection and disposal practices
- Proper cleaning and disposal of equipment and items in the patient's environment likely to have been contaminated with infectious body fluids

Standard Precautions protect not only healthcare providers but also patients by ensuring that healthcare personnel do not carry infectious agents from patient to patient on their hands or transmit them via equipment used during patient care (Figure 1-6). An exposure can occur by contact with blood or through inhalation or ingestion of respiratory secretions, airborne droplets, or saliva. Occupational Safety & Health Administration (OSHA) regulations specify training requirements, mandatory vaccinations, exposure control plans, and PPE. Levels of PPE established by the Environmental Protection Agency (EPA) are given in Box 1-3, and types of PPE used for body substance isolation are summarized in Box 1-4.

Staying Alert for Threats of Violence

Prehospital providers enter the patient's milieu, which may be a home, office, or vehicle. Anger or anxiety may be part of that environment, particularly when a stressful event such as an injury or assault has just occurred. The presence of EMS, law enforcement, or fire department personnel may make a violent person feel threatened. Behavioral red flags may precede an angry outburst or assault. During a gradual acceleration of emotion, specific behavioral clues may include pacing, gesturing, and hostile words perhaps escalating to outright threats.

Before approaching the patient, survey the environment and the patient's affect. Determine the number of patients and whether any additional resources are needed, such as more ambulances, law enforcement, and fire or hazardous materials (hazmat) assistance. Evidence of weapons, alcohol, or drug paraphernalia can be an early indicator that the situation is unsafe and law enforcement backup is needed. Ominous background noise such as

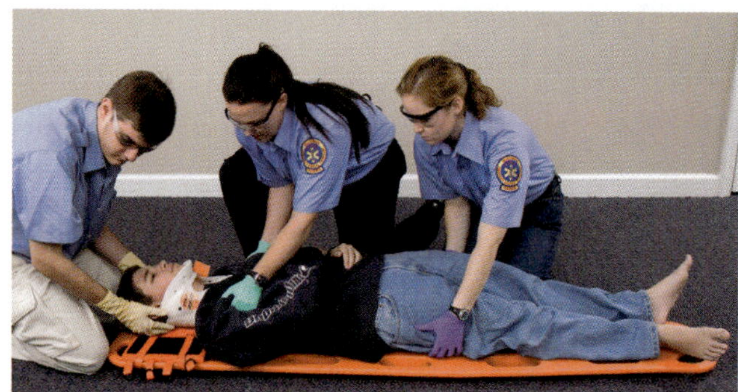

Figure 1-6 Gloved paramedics assisting a patient. (From Aehlert BJ: Paramedic practice today: above and beyond, St Louis, 2009, Mosby.)

BOX 1-3 Levels of Personal Protective Equipment

PPE is categorized by the Environmental Protection Agency (EPA) according to the level of protection it offers. Levels C, B, and A require specialized training before use. You should select a level higher than D if skin-damaging agents, such as corrosive substances, are or may be present. Emission of gases or vapors also requires a higher level of protection.

If you begin performing a different task at the same scene that brings you in closer contact with hazardous materials, you will need to upgrade your PPE accordingly. But you don't have to have a reason—if you feel uncomfortable using a lower level of protection, you should be allowed to do so on request.

A – Offers the greatest skin, eye, respiratory system, and mucous membrane protection.

B – Offers the highest level of respiratory system protection but less skin and eye protection. At least this level of protection should be selected until a reliable site analysis can be completed.

C – Used when the type and concentration of particulate matter are known, the criteria for using air-purifying respirators have been met, and skin and eye exposure are unlikely.

D – Used when no special protection from contaminants or hazards is needed; it is essentially a uniform consisting of coveralls and safety shoes or boots. It offers no protection from respiratory or skin hazards.

BOX 1-4 Types of Personal Protective Equipment for Body Substance Isolation

- Eye protection
  Used in any situation where there is the potential for contact with spitting blood or vomit. In addition, mucous membranes, especially of the eye, are common routes of exposure. Use when suctioning if the patient is vomiting or spitting blood.
- Gloves
  Wear gloves during every call. They are mandatory whenever there is a potential for contact with body fluids.
- Gown
  To protect body and clothing from being soiled
- Mask
  Needed when suctioning if the patient is vomiting, spitting blood, or is suspected of having airborne infectious disease such as influenza or TB

people arguing should cause enough concern for you to contact law enforcement to assist at the scene. Less menacing distractions such as televisions should be turned off or otherwise eliminated.

It is important to protect the integrity of the crime scene as well as the safety of the victim. Work with your colleagues to keep the scene safe. Designate one person to have contact with the patient while the other remains alert for problems, a practice followed in law enforcement. Keep your communication equipment with you. On calls involving overdose, violent crime, or potential hazardous materials exposure, stage at a reasonable distance and wait for law enforcement to advise you that the scene is safe. Listen to your instincts—if the situation doesn't feel right, leave if appropriate and call for help.

Staying Alert for Other Hazards

Assess the scene for other life-safety hazards such as downed electrical lines, fires, imminent structural collapse, and presence of hazardous materials (Figure 1-7). Animals should be secured in advance of your entry. If you do receive an animal bite, contact local animal control authorities so the animal can be confined and tested for diseases. If toxic substances are present or you can't rule out the possibility, call in the hazmat team. If you can do so at a safe distance, find out the name of the toxic substance from the Material Safety Data Sheet (MSDS) or placard numbers on containers. Networks such as WISER (Wireless Information System for Emergency Responders), from the National Library of Medicine, can provide suggestions for evacuating and information on medical toxidromes and treatments, depending on the kind of hazard present.

Safety concerns should be observed prior to patient encounters. Prehospital personnel should observe for signs of gang violence, safe access to the patient, and hostile animals or domestic disputes. Observe the environment for gang graffiti, large crowds that are gathered, hostage situations, and weapons. Maintaining the integrity of a crime scene is essential upon entry and while treating the patient (Figure 1-8).

Approaching the Patient

All practitioners must use observation techniques to read the scene and the patient on arrival, during treatment, and during transport.

Visual Observation

Healthcare providers benefit from closely observing the patient. Arriving at a prehospital scene like a residence or allied healthcare facility offers many of the same opportunities for gathering clues as you have when approaching a patient's room in an in-hospital setting (Figure 1-9).

Extrinsic clues can include body positioning, expressions of pain, and abnormal breath sounds. Decorticate or decerebrate posturing, a tripod position, or fetal body positioning in an adult are potential signs of a life-threatening condition. Moaning, cries of pain, agonal respiration, and adventitious, audible breath sounds should cause concern. Visual indications of extreme distress, such as a patient guarding his chest or abdomen or a chest pain patient holding a fist on the chest, known as *Levine's sign*, indicate an emergent situation.

Look around the room or scene for assistive devices that could indicate chronic disease processes. Walkers, canes, wheelchairs, oxygen concentrators, portable nebulizer devices, and hospital beds in private residences (Figure 1-10) are examples. Prosthetic devices and mobility aids indicate possible mobility problems that may be associated with chronic respiratory, cardiovascular, musculoskeletal, or neurologic deficits.

Body positioning can be an early indicator of "sick" or "not sick." Decorticate posturing indicates dysfunction of the cerebral cortex. In this rigid body position, the patient's elbows are bent, the arms are held close to the chest, and the fists are clenched. The toes point down, and the legs are extended (Figure 1-11, *A*).

Decorticate posturing may progress to decerebrate posturing, a grave sign indicating significant brain injury. This body position is also characterized by rigidity. The

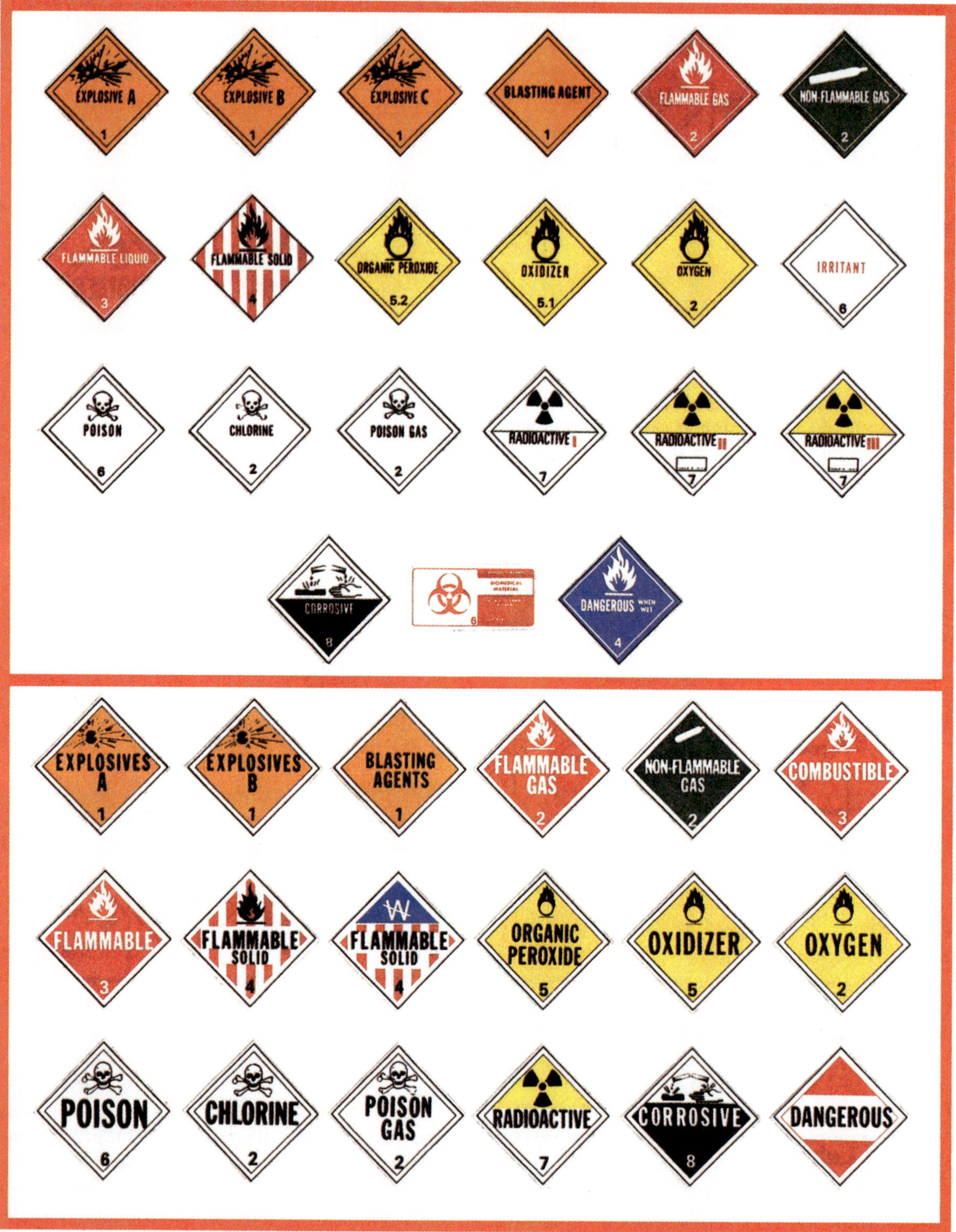

■ **Figure 1-7** Hazardous materials warning placards and labels. (From Sanders MJ: Mosby's paramedic textbook—revised reprint, ed 3, St Louis, 2007, MosbyJems.)

patient's arms and legs are extended, the toes point downward, and the head and neck are arched (Figure 1-11, *B*).

Oxygen in the home can be stored as compressed gas or liquid oxygen or may be generated with an oxygen concentrator. Oxygen may be delivered by nasal cannula, oxygen mask, tracheostomy, ventilator, continuous positive airway pressure (CPAP), or biphasic positive airway pressure (BiPAP; Figure 1-12, *B* and *C*).

The care of patients dependent on technology such as ventilators can be complicated by chronic illness and poor perfusion. Some patients may require automatic transport ventilators (ATVs). These ventilators should be identified

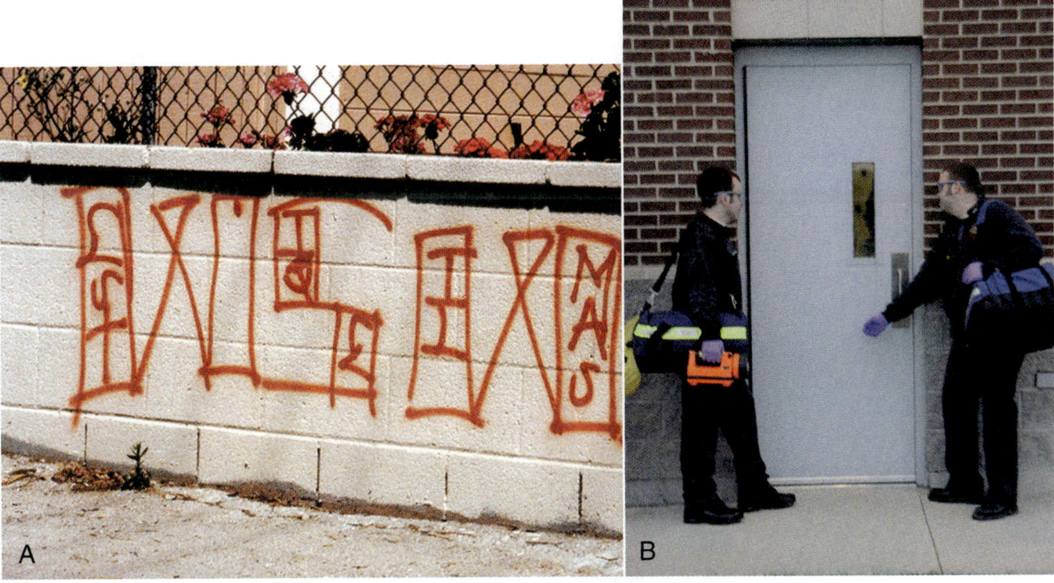

■ **Figure 1-8** Stay alert for other hazards as you approach a scene. **A**, Graffiti on a wall in Los Angeles. **B**, When knocking at a door, stand to the side. Never stand directly in front of a door or window. (**A** from Sanders MJ: Mosby's paramedic textbook, revised ed 3, St Louis, 2007, MosbyJems. **B** from Aehlert BJ: Paramedic practice today: above and beyond, St Louis, 2010, MosbyJems.)

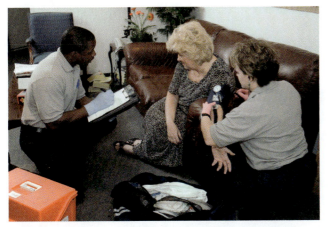

■ **Figure 1-9** Performing other tasks while conducting the interview is reasonable and efficient. (From Aehlert BJ: Paramedic practice today: above and beyond, St Louis, 2009, Mosby.)

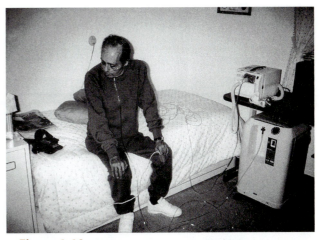

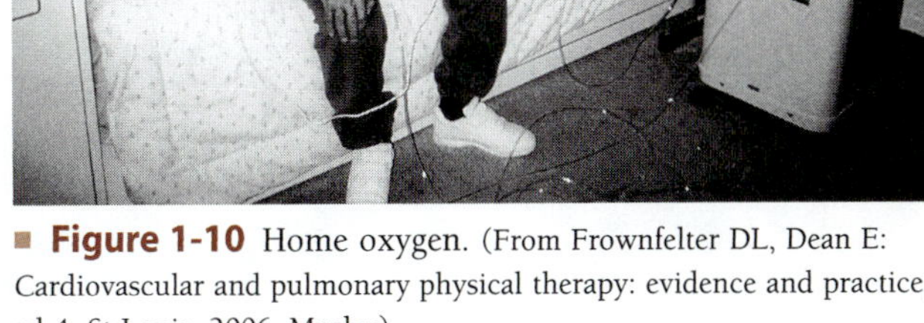

■ **Figure 1-10** Home oxygen. (From Frownfelter DL, Dean E: Cardiovascular and pulmonary physical therapy: evidence and practice, ed 4, St Louis, 2006, Mosby.)

on arrival. They are volume-cycle and rate-controlled devices. Patients are placed on these ventilators to provide extended positive-pressure ventilation. Prehospital personnel should become familiar with patients in their communities who are ventilator dependent and may require this assistive device during transport (Figure 1-13).

Olfactory Observation

Odors in the environment can also serve as warning signs of an unsafe environment even before you make contact with the patient. Evidence of gas fumes, especially with multiple patients complaining of similar distressing symptoms, indicates the need for immediate evacuation. An odor of spoiled food, mold, or insect or rodent infiltration, may indicate an unhealthy environment for the patient and family members. This type of environment may indicate failure to thrive or may be evidence of neglect or domestic abuse. This observation should be reported to the proper authorities per your local protocols and statutory requirements.

In addition to the environment, make note of unusual patient odors. Certain smells are associated with various acute or chronic disease processes, such as a fruity acetone breath odor with diabetic ketoacidosis. Observation of any excreted patient fluids such as blood, vomitus, urine, or feces may indicate dysfunction of the central nervous system (CNS). Other odors, such as a musty breath odor, can point toward chronic liver dysfunction. Significant body odor and uncleanliness may be evidence that the patient can no longer perform the activities of daily living without assistance.

Kinesthetic Observation

The sense of touch also gives us clues to the patient's condition. Patients may have skin that feels cool, cold, warm, hot, or sweaty. Excessively warm or hot skin may indicate an elevated core body temperature (Table 1-1). A hot day with high humidity can lead to hyperthermia. Intrinsic causes of hot skin include stroke, fever, and heat stroke.

Likewise, an extremely cold environment may cause hypothermia. Remember, however, that in older adult patients, hypothermia can occur even in a warm environment. These patients' immobility, inappropriate clothing, drug toxicities, and comorbid conditions cause poor perfusion and diminished compensatory mechanisms. Cool, clammy skin can also be the result of shock or compensatory mechanisms such as vasoconstriction.

Moist or wet skin is typically found in patients with heat exhaustion, exertion, or drug toxicity. Patients with

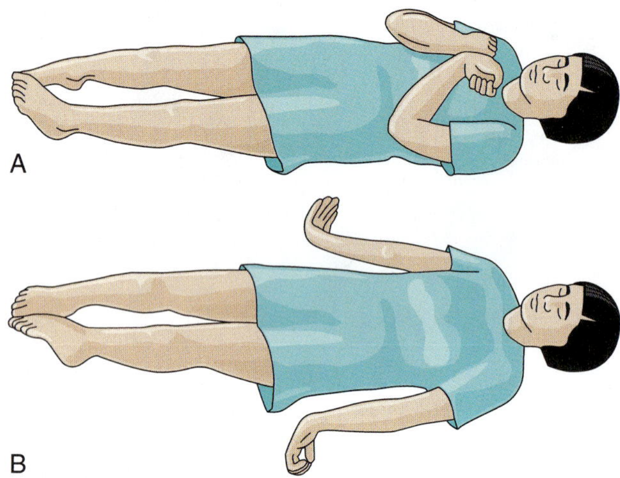

Figure 1-11 A, Decorticate posturing. B, Decerebrate posturing. (From Ignatavicius DD, Workman ML: Medical-surgical nursing: patient-centered collaborative care, ed 6, St Louis, 2010, Saunders.)

TABLE 1-1 Temperature Measurement Variances

Location	Temperature (°F)	Temperature (°C)
Actual core temperature	97.5°–100.2°	36.4°–37.9°
Esophageal probe	97.5°–100.2°	36.4°–37.9°
Rectal	97.8°–100.2°	36.6°–37.9°
Oral	95.9°–99.9°	35.5°–37.7°
Tympanic (ear)	96.3°–99.5°	35.7°–37.5°

From Aehlert BJ: Paramedic practice today: above and beyond, St Louis, 2009, Mosby.

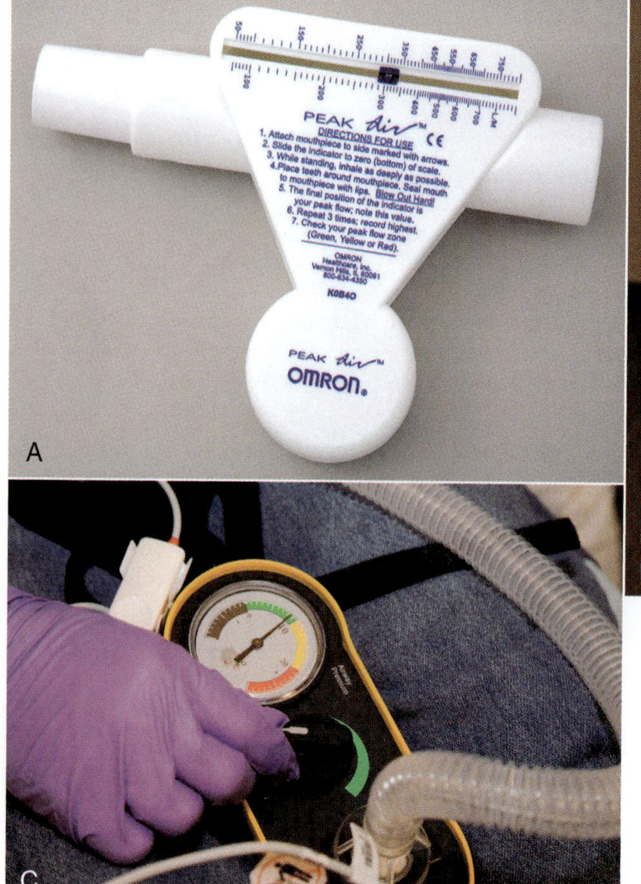

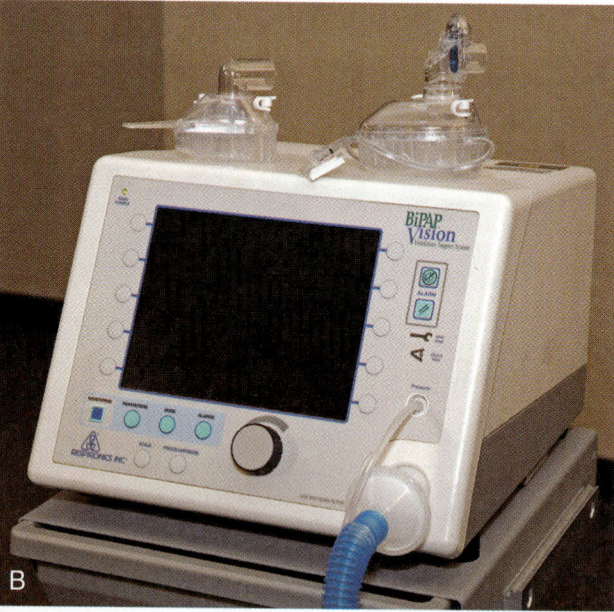

Figure 1-12 A, Peak flow meter. B, BiPAP machine. C, CPAP flow generator. (From Aehlert BJ: Paramedic practice today: above and beyond, St Louis, 2009, Mosby.)

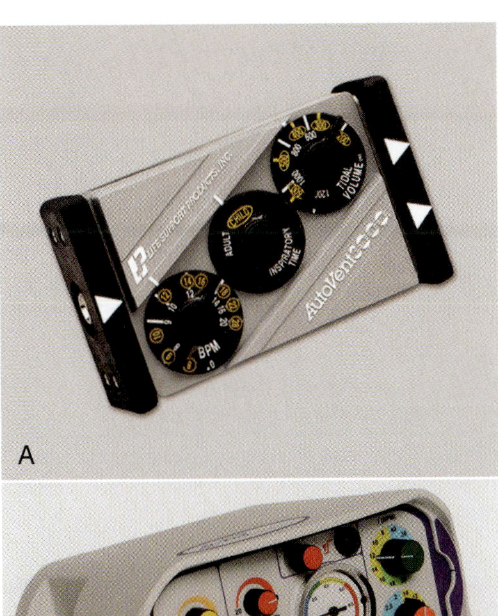

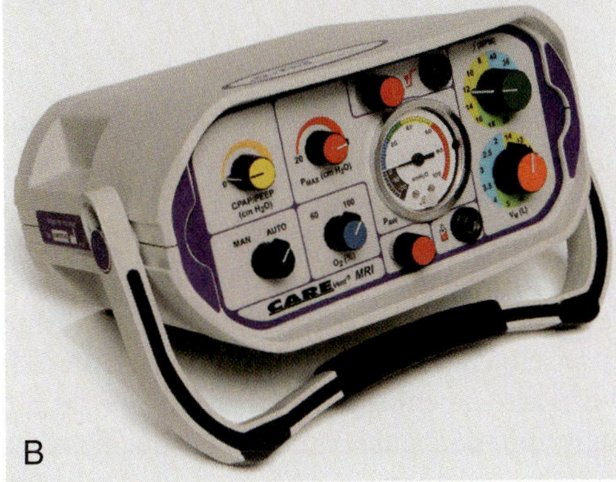

■ **Figure 1-13** Examples of automatic transport ventilators. (From Aehlert BJ: Paramedic practice today: above and beyond, St Louis, 2009, Mosby.)

cardiovascular compromise that leads to poor perfusion also present with moist skin. Patients who are dehydrated will have dry skin. Deterioration of thirst and taste mechanisms often accompany advancing age, so it is especially important to evaluate older adult patients for dry skin and dehydration.

Touch also provides essential assessment information by allowing you to feel the patient's pulse and determine the rate—too fast or too slow, weak, thready, or bounding. Touch can help identify an irregular pulse, which may indicate cardiovascular compromise.

Visual, olfactory, and kinesthetic observations at the scene will add valuable information to your knowledge of anatomy, physiology, pathophysiology, and epidemiology to help determine the patient's initial cardinal presentation.

Cardinal Presentation

In addition to obtaining information from your initial sensory observations, you should ascertain the patient's reason for asking for medical assistance. Soliciting from the patient their major complaint (e.g., area of pain, discomfort, or abnormality), their cardinal presentation, will assist you in prioritizing your approach to obtaining historical and physical exam information. The **cardinal presentation** may be symptoms—chest pain or difficulty breathing—or an observed event such as syncope. The cardinal presentation may be a compromise in airway, respiration, or circulation/perfusion, indicating that a life-threatening problem is present and requires immediate intervention (Figure 1-14). Building on dispatch information, your initial observations, and the patient's cardinal presentation, you can now begin to focus on the primary survey and continue to formulate an initial impression. The next step is to determine what underlying condition accounts for the cardinal presentation.

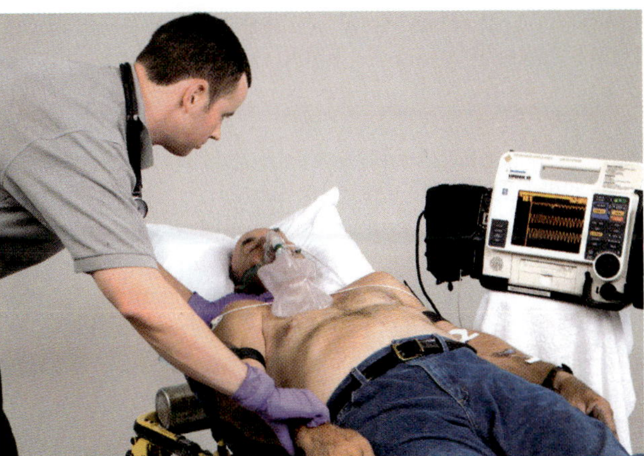

■ **Figure 1-14** Patient with a potentially life-threatening illness. (From Aehlert BJ: Paramedic practice today: above and beyond, St Louis, 2009, Mosby.)

Primary Survey

The primary survey is a key tool to identify life-threatening presentations and establish immediate management strategies. To conduct this assessment and continue to formulate an initial impression of the patient's condition, consider relevant questions you might ask:

- Is this patient likely to die now?
- What is the worst outcome this patient could experience?
- Is the patient's condition emergent (the patient is injured or ill and in need of immediate medical attention) or nonemergent (the patient is not in need of immediate medical attention)?

To determine how grave the patient's status is, you must evaluate his or her level of consciousness (LOC) and identify any airway, breathing, or circulation problems. If a life threat is identified, immediate interventions must be initiated before further assessment is performed. The remaining history taking and physical exam can be performed en route to the receiving facility.

The prehospital emergency medical team must then make transport decisions. Is the patient to be transported by ground or air? What are the implications of either mode of transportation? Which is the closest, most appropriate medical center? Should the closest facility be bypassed in favor of one that is better equipped?

If the assessment does not reveal an immediate life threat, the patient should be evaluated for critical or emergent conditions. An emergent patient is one who has a poor general impression or decreased level of consciousness, is unresponsive, shows signs and symptoms of shock, complains of severe pain, has sustained multiple injuries, or is having trouble breathing, a complicated childbirth, chest pain with a systolic blood pressure of less than 100, or uncontrolled bleeding.

At this point in the assessment process, you may not be able to pinpoint a working diagnosis, but you should begin to formulate the differential diagnosis, keeping in mind the various possible causes of the patient's signs and symptoms as further assessment data are brought to bear.

Level of Consciousness

Assessment of mental status or LOC involves evaluation of brain function. As you approach the patient, observe carefully for evidence of his LOC. For example, if the patient is conscious, note their attention span. Is it age appropriate? A patient with a fragmented attention span or who seems to be daydreaming should be assessed for hypoglycemia, dehydration, cardiovascular compromise, stroke, or head trauma.

In addition to observation, use of neurologic scoring mechanisms such as the Glasgow Coma Scale and the mnemonic AVPU (alert, verbal, pain, unresponsive) may be used to evaluate the patient. Both of these neurologic scoring tools gauge the patient's response to stimuli.

LOC is associated with the function of the reticular activating system (RAS) and the cerebral hemispheres. The RAS plays a major role of the brainstem in wakefulness and alertness. The cerebral hemispheres are responsible for awareness and understanding. Reacting to the environment occurs through the cerebral hemispheres. The RAS alerts the cerebral hemispheres so they activate a response to the stimulus, such as an emotional or physical reaction. Coma can be caused by dysfunction of the RAS or both cerebral hemispheres.

Awareness is a high-level neurologic function and demonstrates a response to person, place, and time. This is more commonly referred to as *alert and oriented × 3*, or *AO×3*. A patient who is not AO×3 might be described as drowsy, confused, or disoriented. Of course, a patient can be awake but disoriented (not aware), indicating adequate RAS function but cerebral hemisphere dysfunction.

AVPU uses stimuli (verbal commands and pain) to determine the patient's LOC. As noted earlier, the letters in the mnemonic stand for *alert* (awake), *verbal* (responds to verbal questions), *pain* (does not respond to verbal commands but responds to application of a painful stimulus), and *unresponsive* (is not alert or awake and does not respond to verbal commands or painful stimuli). Table 1-2 discusses AVPU in greater detail.

TABLE 1-2 Mental Status and AVPU

AVPU Level	Assessment Findings	
***A**lert*	Responds spontaneously; further define mental status	
	Alert and oriented × 4	Person, place, time, and event
	Alert and oriented × 3	Person, place, and time
	Alert and oriented × 2	Person and place
	Alert and oriented × 1	Person
***V**erbal*	Responds to verbal stimuli	
***P**ain*	Responds to painful stimuli	
***U**nresponsive*	Does not respond to stimuli	

From Aehlert BJ: Paramedic practice today: above and beyond, St Louis, 2009, Mosby.

The Glasgow Coma Scale (GCS) is an effective tool for assessing neurologic function (Table 1-3) and particularly important to prehospital personnel for establishing the patient's baseline level of mentation. Documented changes in the GCS assessment findings that indicate diminishing neurologic function guide in-hospital diagnostic testing and inpatient placement.

GCS evaluates the patient's response to eye opening and best verbal and motor response. The score for each of these responses should be documented (e.g., E = 3, V = 4, M = 4, for a total GCS score of 11). A score of 8 or less often indicates the need for aggressive airway management. Although 15 is the highest score possible, this does not mean the patient has full mental capacity. The GCS tool assists in determining a baseline neurologic functional status. Definitive care should not be determined on the GCS findings alone but in conjunction with other diagnostic and historical data obtained.

Assessment of LOC helps determine whether the patient's neurologic and perfusion status are stable and allows life-threatening conditions to be identified and managed early. Patients with difficulties in mentation should receive a complete neurologic examination. Neurologic assessment is discussed in detail in Chapter 2.

Airway

After assessing LOC, the patient's airway, breathing, and circulation/perfusion status must be rapidly evaluated. Airway patency must be established and maintained. A patent airway is one that allows good airflow and is free of fluids, secretions, teeth, and any other type of foreign body (e.g., food, blocks, coins, etc.) that may obstruct airflow. A patient's inability to maintain a patent airway is a life-threatening emergency and necessitates emergency interventions and immediate transport to an appropriate medical facility.

TABLE 1-3 Glasgow Coma Scale

Glasgow Coma Scale	Adult/Child	Score	Infant
***E**ye opening*	Spontaneous	4	Spontaneous
	To verbal	3	To verbal
	To pain	2	To pain
	No response	1	No response
Best ***v**erbal response*	Oriented	5	Coos, babbles
	Disoriented	4	Irritable cry
	Inappropriate words	3	Cries only to pain
	Inappropriate sounds	2	Moans to pain
	No response	1	No response
Best ***m**otor response*	Obeys commands	6	Spontaneous
	Localizes pain	5	Withdraws from touch
	Withdraws from pain	4	Withdraws from pain
	Abnormal flexion (decorticate)	3	Abnormal flexion (decorticate)
	Abnormal extension (decerebrate)	2	Abnormal extension (decerebrate)
	No response	1	No response
Total = E + V + M	3 to 15		

From Aehlert BJ: Paramedic practice today: above and beyond, St Louis, 2009, Mosby.

BOX 1-5 Basic and Advanced Life Support Airway Adjuncts

The following techniques may be used to support the airway:

- Suction
- Head tilt/chin lift maneuver
- Jaw thrust maneuver
- Insertion of an oropharyngeal airway
- Insertion of a nasopharyngeal airway
- Insertion of a supraglottic airway device such as a Combitube, Laryngeal Mask Airway, or King LT
- Intubation (oral, nasal)
- Needle percutaneous or surgical cricothyrotomy

The intervention chosen depends on what is causing the obstruction or why the airway is ineffective. Observe the patient's position or posture. Are they lying in an unnatural position on the ground or in bed? Do they seem to favor an upright position or the tripod position? In an upright position, does the patient sit upright and lean forward, with the chin slightly raised? In the tripod position, does the patient also sit upright and lean forward but is supported by their arms, with their neck slightly extended, chin projected, and mouth open? Both of these positions are used to maximize airflow. Is there head bobbing? Such movement indicates increased work of breathing and respiratory fatigue, distress, and imminent failure.

A compromised airway may require suctioning or removal of a foreign object. Open the airway, and observe the mouth and upper airway for air movement. Performing a modified jaw thrust on a trauma patient is appropriate if the potential for head, neck, or spine injury is noted. In cases of suspected trauma, manually protect the cervical spine from movement by positioning the patient in a neutral, in-line position. Look for evidence of upper airway problems, such as facial trauma, and check for the presence of vomitus and blood. Clear the airway with suction if necessary, and consider adjuncts to maintain a clear airway.

Initial basic life support (BLS) interventions can be used and, when appropriate, progress to definitive advanced life support (ALS) interventions. A thorough assessment will determine the urgency of airway management and suggest which devices are most likely to be effective. BLS and ALS adjuncts are summarized in Box 1-5.

Breathing

Breathing rate, rhythm, and effort are evaluated in the primary survey. Lung sounds may be auscultated in the primary survey if labored respirations are noted. Inefficient respiratory rates or irregular breathing patterns may require the application of supplemental oxygen devices. In the primary survey, the provider assesses for breathing that is too fast or too slow. Symmetry of the chest rise and utilization of accessory muscles should be noted. Nasal flaring, agitation, and the inability to speak several words without stopping for a breath are indications of distress and compromised air exchange (Table 1-4).

Conditions and injuries that cause a life-threatening compromise of the patient's ability to breathe include bilateral pneumothorax, tension pneumothorax, flail chest, cardiac tamponade, pulmonary embolus, or any other condition that diminishes tidal and minute volume and increases the work and effort of breathing.

TABLE 1-4 Irregular Breathing Patterns

Pattern	Description	Cause	Comments*
Tachypnea	Increased respiratory rate	Fever Respiratory distress Toxins Hypoperfusion Brain lesion Metabolic acidosis Anxiety	One of the body's coping mechanisms, but it can have a harmful effect by promoting respiratory acidosis. Because of the rapid respiratory rate, the body does not complete oxygen/carbon dioxide exchange in the alveoli. Consequently, the patient may require both oxygen and ventilatory assistance.
Bradypnea	Slower-than-normal respiratory rate	Narcotic/sedative drugs, including alcohol Metabolic disorders Hypoperfusion Fatigue Brain injury	In addition to the bradypnea, the patient may have episodes of apnea. The patient may require both oxygen and ventilatory assistance.
Cheyne-Stokes respiration	A respiratory pattern with alternating periods of increased and decreased rate and depth with brief periods of apnea	Increased intracranial pressure Congestive heart failure Renal failure Toxin Acidosis	Repeating pattern. May indicate spinal injury.
Biot's respiration	Similar to Cheyne-Stokes but with an irregular instead of a repeating pattern	Meningitis Increased intracranial pressure Neurologic emergency	Think of it as the atrial fibrillation of the respiratory system (irregularly irregular).
Kussmaul's respiration	Deep and fast breaths lacking any apneic periods	Metabolic acidosis Renal failure Diabetic ketoacidosis	Deep, labored breathing that indicates severe acidosis
Apneustic	A long, gasping inspiration followed by a very short expiration in which the breath is not completely expelled. The result is chest hyperinflation.	Brain lesion	Causes severe hypoxemia
Central neurogenic hyperventilation	A very deep, rapid respiratory rate (40-60 breaths/min)	Head injury that causes increased intracranial pressure or direct injury to the brainstem Stroke	CNS acidosis triggers rapid, deep breathing leading to systemic alkalosis.

*NOTE: Record the patient's airway status, breathing rate, rhythm, and breath sounds.

Respiratory distress can result from hypoxia, a condition in which too little oxygen is available to the body's tissues. Hypoxia can be caused by any of the aforementioned conditions or by asthma, chronic obstructive pulmonary disease (COPD), airway obstruction, or any condition that restricts normal gas exchange by the alveoli, such as pneumonia, pulmonary edema, or abnormal mucous secretions.

When the patient's cardinal presentation is respiratory distress, another possible syndrome is hyperventilation, which will lead to respiratory alkalosis. Hyperventilation may be compensating for metabolic acidosis, anxiety, fear, or CNS insult. Working diagnoses may include possible causes such as stroke and diabetic ketoacidosis.

An elevated level of carbon dioxide in the blood caused by hypoventilation is called *hypercarbia*. Hypercarbia occurs when the body cannot rid itself of carbon dioxide, causing it to build up in the bloodstream, leading to respiratory failure. Hypercarbia should be considered in every patient with decreased mental status, especially if they appear somnolent or very fatigued. In the primary survey, midaxillary lung sounds are auscultated if the patient presents with diminished level of consciousness, difficulty in breathing, or poor perfusion. Audible respiratory sounds such as wheezing are an important clinical finding. Abnormal breath sounds are summarized in Box 1-6.

Accessory muscle use and retraction can be seen at the suprasternal notch, beneath and between the ribs. If the work of breathing is increased, the patient should be monitored for respiratory distress and imminent collapse. The combination of abnormal breath sounds and accessory muscle use or retraction is a more sobering sign than abnormal breath sounds alone.

Ask pertinent questions to help determine the severity of the respiratory problem:

BOX 1-6 Abnormal Breath Sounds

- Gurgling. Whenever you hear gurgling, apply suction!
- Stridor. Stridor is a loud, high-pitched noise during inspiration that indicates the upper airway is partially blocked by infection or foreign body.
- Wheezing. Wheezing is a high-pitched musical sound that suggests the bronchi are swollen and constricted. A whistling sound is typically heard on exhalation as air moves through constricted bronchial structures. Smaller airways that are affected by diseases like asthma and anaphylaxis may present with wheezing.
- Crackles or rales. Crackles or rales are wet lung sounds heard on inspiration. It's difficult for the patient to clear this sound by coughing. Crackles and rales typically sound like rolling hair between your fingers. The wet sound is in the alveoli, which are partially filled with fluid.
- Rhonchi. Rhonchi are noisy rattling sounds generated by air flowing through mucus or around an obstruction. They can be heard on inspiration and expiration and are often due to fluid in the larger airways. Rhonchi can be a sign of chronic obstructive pulmonary disease or an infectious process such as bronchitis.

- Did the difficulty breathing come on suddenly or get worse over several days?
- Is this problem chronic or recurrent?
- Do you have any associated symptoms, such as a productive cough, chest pain, or a fever?
- Did you try to treat the condition on your own? If so, how?

The patient's respiratory rhythm should be easy, regular, and pain free. Painful or irregular breaths may indicate a medical or trauma-related emergency and should be evaluated further to determine the cause of the abnormal breathing pattern. Irregular breathing patterns are summarized in Table 1-4. Compromising breathing patterns should be identified and managed in the primary survey.

Circulation/Perfusion

The patient's pulse rate, regularity, and quality should be obtained. Palpating the radial, carotid, or femoral artery is essential. Apical pulse can be auscultated at the apex of the heart near the fifth intercostal space, a landmark known as the *point of maximum impulse* (PMI), but this does not allow assessment of pulse strength. The normal pulse rate for an adult is 60 to 100 beats per minute (bpm).

Indicators of the quality of the pulse refer to its strength and would be characterized as *absent*, *weak*, *thready*, *bounding*, or *strong*. A weak pulse may indicate poor perfusion. A bounding pulse may indicate increased pulse pressures, such as with aortic regurgitation or elevated systolic blood pressure. Factors that can decrease myocardial contractility include hypoxia, hyperkalemia, and hypercarbia. Early identification of irregular, weak, or thready pulses in the primary survey indicate poor perfusion and may prompt urgent application and interpretation of EKG findings.

The pulse should also be evaluated for its regularity. A normal pulse is regular, whereas an abnormal pulse is irregular, or arrhythmic. An irregular heartbeat may have a cardiac or respiratory cause, or it may be brought on by a toxic substance such as a drug.

Pulse pressure is calculated by subtracting diastolic blood pressure from systolic blood pressure. Normal pulse pressure is 30 to 40 mm Hg. If pulse pressure is low (less than 25% of systolic blood pressure), the cause may be low stroke volume or increased peripheral resistance. A narrowing pulse pressure may indicate shock or cardiac tamponade. Identification of pulse pressure changes are used to identify increased intracranial pressure. Observation of hypertension with a widening pulse pressure, bradycardia, and an irregular breathing pattern is a key indicator and is identified as *Cushing's triad.*

Information gathered from dispatch, your initial impression, the patient's cardinal presentation, patency of the airway and breathing, and circulation/perfusion status should suggest potential underlying diagnoses and initiate appropriate initial treatment interventions. Diagnoses and management will be continually reevaluated and modified as additional patient history, physical exam findings, and diagnostic results are obtained. The patient's response to treatment is also considered a priority in modifying ongoing treatment. Assessment and management are systematic, dynamic, and ongoing throughout the continuum of care.

Secondary Survey

Once the patient's LOC and their airway, breathing, circulation, and perfusion are determined, the **secondary survey** begins. In medical patients, vital signs are taken and a history is often obtained before a physical exam is performed. Depending on the severity of the patient's condition, the availability of healthcare personnel, and the estimated transport time to the appropriate healthcare facility, the physical exam may be performed either at the scene or en route to the receiving facility.

Also depending on the factors noted, the patient's condition may call for a focused physical examination, a rapid head-to-toe exam, or a comprehensive exam. The amount of time spent on this exam and its thoroughness will be directly related to your scope of practice as a healthcare provider, the patient's status, and the diagnostic assessment tools available (e.g., reflex hammer, otoscope, ophthalmoscope).

Vital Signs

Vital signs are the first component of the secondary survey and traditionally include pulse, respiration, body temperature, and blood pressure. You should measure these parameters frequently and continually. Even if the cardinal presentation doesn't suggest an immediate life threat, the patient's condition may deteriorate. Establishing baseline vital signs and being alert for worrisome trends during ongoing monitoring can aid in early identification of any adverse change. Even if the patient's condition remains stable and nonemergent, vital signs are indispensable to sound medical decision making. They guide establishing a specific diagnosis and formulating a treatment plan likely to be effective.

Pulse

Patients with suspected medical emergencies should be assessed for both central and peripheral pulses. The rate, regularity, and quality should be reevaluated (see Examination Techniques). Abnormal findings can lead to early application of electrocardiograph (ECG) monitoring.

Respiration

The work of breathing should be assessed for symmetry, depth, rate, and quality (Figure 1-15). For a detailed discussion of breathing, see the earlier heading.

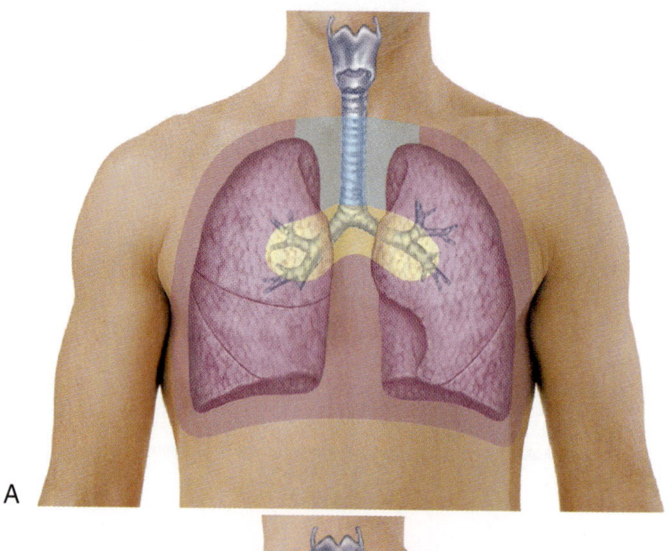

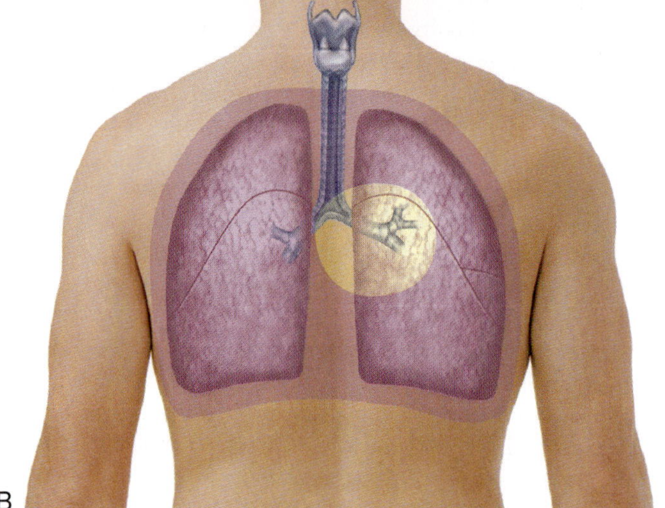

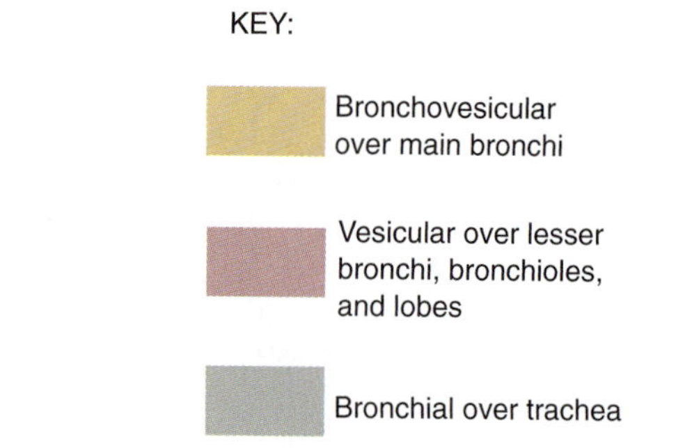

■ **Figure 1-15** Expected auscultatory sounds. **A**, Anterior view. **B**, Posterior view. (From Sanders MJ: Mosby's paramedic textbook—revised reprint, ed 3, St Louis, 2007, Mosby.)

Temperature

Oral, rectal, tympanic, or axillary temperature measurements may be taken, depending on the patient's injuries, age, and LOC. Some patients with a decreased LOC may be too agitated for an oral measurement. Facial or other injuries may also preclude use of an oral thermometer. Another way to assess temperature is simply by touching the skin (see Table 1-1).

Be sure to inspect the skin for diaphoresis (sweating) and assess the color of the skin and nail beds. The skin should be dry to the touch and feel neither cool nor hot. If the patient has anything but dry, pink, warm skin, you should look for the cause of the altered perfusion. Refer to Examination Techniques later in this chapter for details on assessing skin color and temperature.

Hyperthermia can be caused by sepsis (infection) or by medications such as antibiotics, narcotics, barbiturates, and antihistamines. Other causes of fever include heart attack, stroke, heat exhaustion, heatstroke, and burns. Hypothermia can be caused by exposure, shock, alcohol or other drug use, hypothyroidism, and in patients who are severely burned and unable to regulate their body temperature. The environment, whether too warm, cold, or humid, may affect the patient's skin temperature and should be considered when evaluating skin vital signs.

Blood Pressure

Evaluation of this vital sign provides an estimate of the patient's perfusion status and can identify pulsus paradoxus and pulse pressure. **Blood pressure** is the tension exerted by blood on the arterial walls. Blood pressure is calculated using the following equation:

$$\text{Blood pressure} = \text{Flow} \times \text{Resistance}$$

If flow or resistance is altered, blood pressure will increase or decrease. Resistance is altered when vessels narrow, increasing resistance and raising pressure, and when vessels dilate, decreasing resistance and lowering pressure.

In patients with cardiovascular disease or a life-threatening pulmonary condition, such as a pulmonary embolus or tension pneumothorax, pulsus paradoxus will be seen. *Pulsus paradoxus* is an irregularity that occurs when systolic blood pressure falls more than 10 mm Hg on inspiration. It's caused by differences in intrathoracic pressure with respiration, such as back flow of blood into the lungs as a result of heart failure.

A baseline blood pressure should be taken during initial contact with the patient. Measure blood pressure a minimum of two times while treating the patient in the prehospital environment. Ideally, the second blood pressure is taken once the patient has been secured in the ambulance or other transport vehicle. A third measurement is taken en route to the receiving facility. Initial blood pressure should be taken manually, and reassessment of blood pressure can be done using an automated device (Figure 1-16).

The vital signs should offer important information to help you formulate a more in-depth impression about the patient's status and needs. In patients with alterations in mentation, also assess the pupils and perform a mini-neurologic exam during the assessment of vital signs. Motor and sensory function, distal pulses, and capillary refill should be evaluated as well. In addition, blood glucose levels should be obtained.

Confirming or ruling out whether life threats, emergent, or nonemergent conditions exist are core considerations for initiating care at the scene, prior to packaging for transport. Modifying or establishing a new care regimen will be based on continued information gathering during the secondary survey.

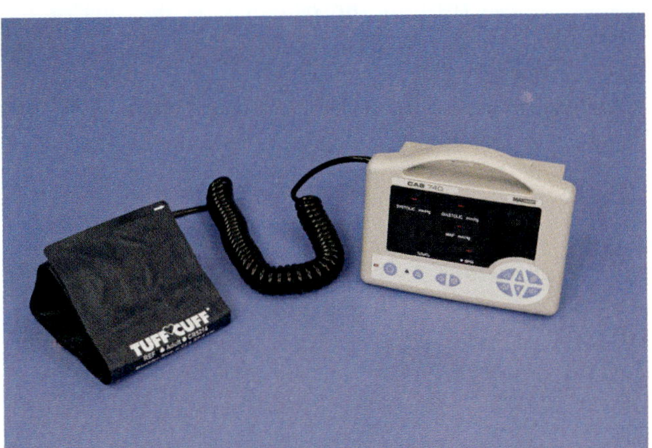

Figure 1-16 Electronic blood pressure device. (From Sanders MJ: Mosby's paramedic textbook—revised reprint, ed 3, St Louis, 2007, Mosby.)

History Taking

For patients with medical emergencies, historical information can be obtained before the physical exam is performed. Modifying the approach to obtaining historical information versus a physical exam evaluation is dependent on the patient's cardinal presentation. What is important is that a thorough assessment be performed. Many diagnostic assessments are ordered on the basis of additional information obtained during the patient interview. An efficient, systematic, comprehensive interview, then, can help you eliminate differential diagnoses, establish a working diagnosis, and determine treatment interventions.

History of the Present Illness

The history of the present illness can be obtained by using the mnemonic OPQRST, summarized in the Rapid Recall box and discussed in detail below. This tool helps define the patient's complaint by focusing on essential assessment components.

RAPID RECALL

History of the Present Illness: OPQRST

To assess the cause of a patient's injury or illness, you need to know what brought it on and when, where it hurts, and how badly. The OPQRST mnemonic will help you remember what questions to ask in order to elicit the most pertinent answers from the patient:

- **O**nset—When did the pain or discomfort begin?
- **P**alliation/provocation—Does anything make the pain better or worse?
- **Q**uality—Describe the pain (burning, sharp, dull, ache, stabbing).
- **R**adiation/referred/region—Does the pain travel or stay localized?
- **S**everity—On a scale of 0 to 10, rate your pain or discomfort.
- **T**ime/duration—How long have you been having the pain/discomfort?

Onset and Origin First, determine the time of onset and origin of the pain or discomfort (Figure 1-17). Find out what the patient was doing when symptoms began. Ask about any similar episodes the patient may have had. The following line of questioning will help elicit this information (adjust as necessary if you are unable to speak to the patient directly):

- Determine what the patient was doing when symptoms began. Pain or discomfort that occurs on exertion may have a different origin than pain or discomfort occurring at rest.

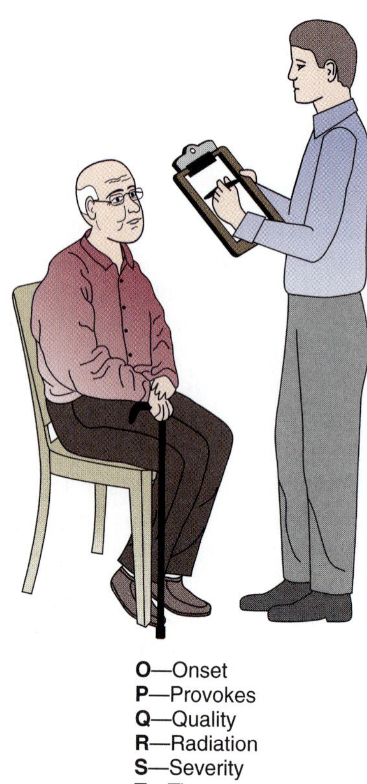

O—Onset
P—Provokes
Q—Quality
R—Radiation
S—Severity
T—Time

■ **Figure 1-17** OPQRST. (From Shade BR, Collins TE, Wertz EM, et al: Mosby's EMT-Intermediate textbook for the 1999 National Standard Curriculum, ed 3, St Louis, 2007, Mosby.)

- Find out whether the onset of symptoms was gradual or sudden.
- Identify any associated complaints, which may suggest the severity of the problem and indicate that multiple body systems are involved. Associated symptoms of importance are:
  - Trouble breathing
  - Shortness of breath
  - Pain on deep inspiration
  - Chest pain or pressure
  - Palpitations
  - Nausea or vomiting
  - Syncope (fainting)
  - Numbness or tingling
  - Indigestion (epigastric pain, abdominal pain, or bloating)
  - Confusion or disorientation
  - General feeling of illness or being out of sorts
- Evaluate any information offered by bystanders.
- Determine whether the patient has experienced similar symptoms before. Ask whether the patient is under a doctor's care, and if so, when the last visit was. Inquire about medications prescribed and other treatments given.

Palliation and Provocation *Palliation* and *provocation* refer to factors that make the patient's symptoms better (palliate them) or worse (provoke them). A patient whose chief complaint is dizziness, for instance, might say that it's better when she lies down (palliation) and worse if she tries to get out of bed suddenly (provocation).

BOX 1-7 Referred Pain

Location	Organ
Left shoulder pain	Diaphragm irritation (blood or air from rupture of other abdominal structures such as ovaries), ruptured spleen, myocardial infarction
Right shoulder pain	Liver irritation, gallbladder pain, diaphragm irritation
Right scapular pain	Liver and gallbladder
Epigastric	Stomach, lung, cardiac
Umbilical	Small intestine, appendix
Back	Aorta, stomach, and pancreas
Flanks to groin	Kidney, ureter
Perineal	Bladder
Suprapubic	Bladder, colon

Quality The patient's perception of the quality of the pain or discomfort can be an important diagnostic clue. Ask for a description of the type of pain or discomfort. Some common descriptors you may hear include "sharp," "dull," "tearing," "ripping," "crushing," "pressure," and "stabbing." The patient's description can suggest whether the pain is of visceral or somatic origin, which will help in determining the differential diagnosis. Visceral pain is from internal organs and often vague and difficult to localize, whereas somatic pain can be precisely located and more likely to be sharp or stabbing in nature. Assessing whether the discomfort is constant or occurs only intermittently, either randomly or with certain breathing patterns or movements, can be a key indicator of the body system involved and the severity of the etiology. Along with palliation and provocation, how a patient describes the quality of the pain or discomfort can also indicate the underlying body system affected. In quotation marks, document exactly how the patient describes his or her symptoms.

Radiated or Referred Pain/Region *Region, referred,* and *radiation* are all associated with the location of the pain or discomfort. Ask the patient whether he can point to where it hurts or whether the pain seems to radiate or move anywhere else (Figure 1-18 and Box 1-7). Try to ascertain whether the pain is referred, such as abdominal distention with pain in the shoulder (Kehr's sign).

Severity Ask the patient to rate the level of the pain or discomfort on a scale from 1 to 10, with 1 being the least discomfort or pain and 10 the highest. This numeric scale is commonly used by both EMS and hospital personnel. Not only will the patient's report of the severity of the pain help narrow down its source, but it might also set a useful

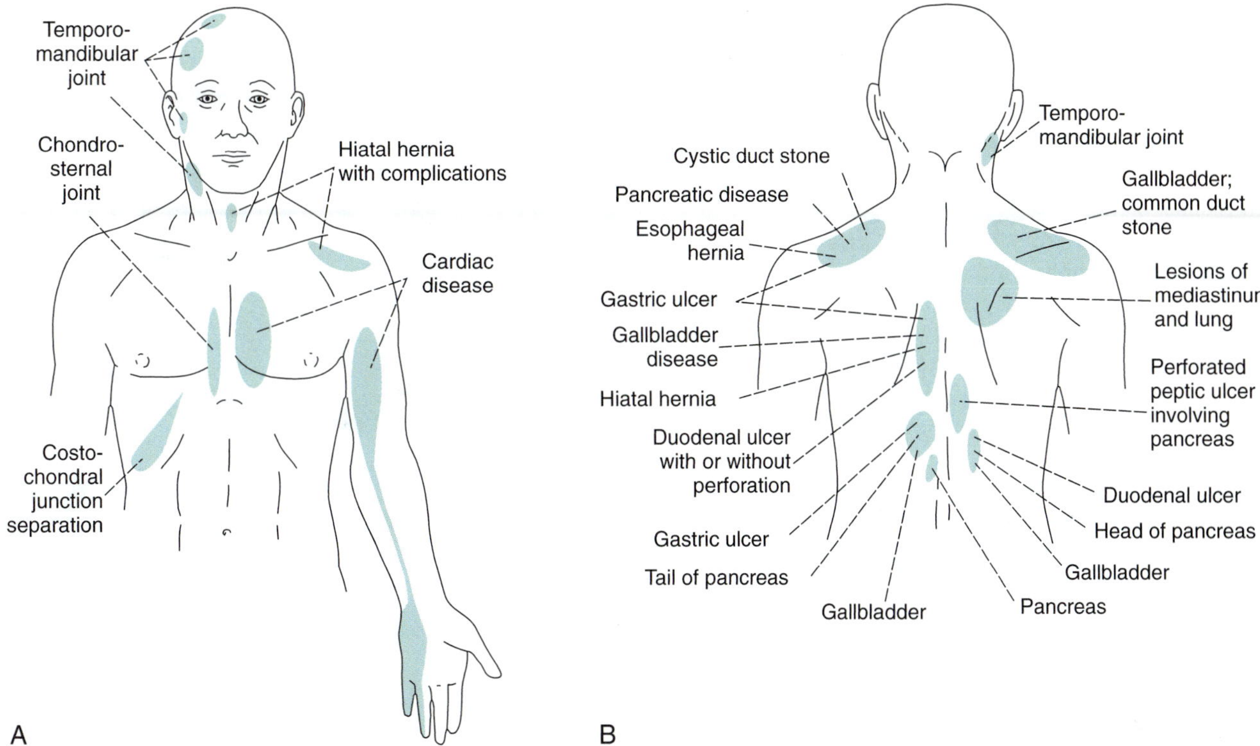

■ **Figure 1-18** Patterns of referred pain from visceral and somatic structures. **A**, Anterior distribution. **B**, Posterior distribution. (From Aehlert BJ: Paramedic practice today: above and beyond, St Louis, 2010, MosbyJems.)

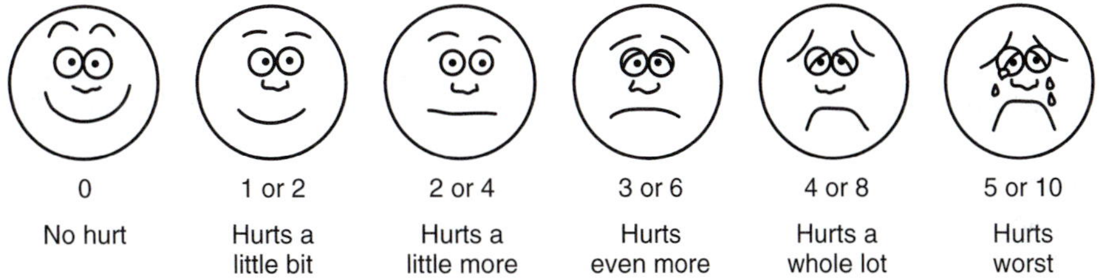

■ **Figure 1-19** Wong-Baker Faces pain rating scale. To use this scale, point to each face, and use the words to describe the pain intensity. Ask the patient to choose the face that best describes his or her own pain. Document the appropriate number. (From Hockenberry MJ, Wilson D: Wong's essentials of pediatric nursing, ed 8, St Louis, 2009, Mosby.)

baseline by which to gauge whether the patient is improving or worsening.

For patients unable to verbally communicate, the Wong-Baker FACES pain scale is a useful alternative (Figure 1-19).

Time/Duration Finally, ask the patient how long (time/duration) he has had the pain or discomfort. If the patient can't respond or isn't sure, ask his family or any bystanders to tell you exactly how long ago the patient last seemed to be normal or seemed to be feeling or acting like himself. Narrowing down the time frame may become crucial for sound medical decision making about certain conditions, such as deciding whether to administer fibrinolytic agents to a stroke patient or whether to catheterize a patient with suspected myocardial infarction (MI).

Pain Assessment The majority of patients seen by health-care providers have experienced either acute or chronic pain or discomfort. Pain and discomfort can result from infection, inflammation, and neurologic dysfunction. Injury and overuse of muscles and the skeletal system can generate acute or chronic pain. Organs in every body system can elicit pain and discomfort. Activation of nociceptive pain fibers is the root cause of both chronic and acute pain. When the fibers are stimulated, the pain impulse will travel via nerve fibers to the spinal cord to the brain.

Pain can present with very vague signs and symptoms, especially in patients who are poor historians, as in the elderly. Oftentimes, patients are taking OTC medications, self-remedies, or multiple medications. Whether OTC or prescribed, drug effects may mask the quality and severity of pain. Revealing historical information regarding pain may present differently based on the patient's cultural background and religious belief systems, making the assessment and management challenging.

Any and all complaints of pain or discomfort must be taken seriously. Exercise patience in determining the location, severity, and quality of pain. Precise patient descriptions of their experience of pain can help you differentiate pain associated with a life-threatening medical emergency from less critical pain and allow you to render appropriate pain management.

A variety of pain remedies may be encountered. Nonnarcotic analgesics that control pain or diminish the perception of pain—acetaminophen (Tylenol), nonsteroidal antiinflammatory drugs (NSAIDs) such as ibuprofen (Motrin/Advil), and naproxen (Aleve)—are typical OTC medications taken by patients. Opioid analgesics, such as morphine, hydrocodone, and oxycodone, are prescribed for acute and chronic pain.

Obtain as much information as possible on what pain medications the patient has been taking and whether self-administration of those medications has been optimal. From the additional information gathered in the present illness history, diagnoses and treatment are evaluated and modified.

Past Medical History

A sensible approach to obtaining a patient's medical history is to follow the SAMPLER mnemonic, summarized in the Rapid Recall box and detailed below.

RAPID RECALL

The SAMPLER Approach to Past Medical History

The SAMPLER mnemonic represents a sensible approach to inquiring about a patient's medical conditions:

- **S**igns/symptoms
- **A**llergies
- **M**edications
- **P**ertinent past medical history
- **L**ast oral intake (what and when)
- **E**vents preceding
- **R**isk factors

Signs and Symptoms **Symptoms**, the S in SAMPLER, are the patient's subjective perceptions of what he or she feels, such as nausea, or has experienced, such as a sensation of seeing flashing lights. **Signs** are objective data that you or another healthcare professional has observed, felt, seen, heard, touched, or smelled and usually measured, such as tachycardia. A symptom reported by the patient, such as diarrhea, becomes a sign as well when observed by a healthcare provider. All signs and symptoms should be well documented (Figure 1-20).

In awake and alert patients with no cognitive deficits, it is appropriate to use open-ended questions when asking how they are feeling. Such patients are able to process the

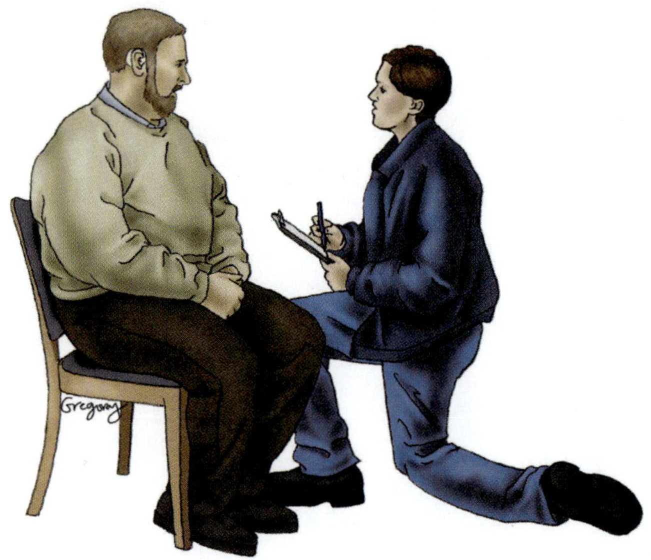

S—Signs and symptoms
A—Allergies
M—Medications
P—Pertinent past medical history
L—Last oral intake, fluid or solid
E—Events leading to the present situation
R—Risk factors

Figure 1-20 SAMPLER history. (From Shade BR, Collins TE, Wertz EM, et al: Mosby's EMT-Intermediate textbook for the 1999 National Standard Curriculum, ed 3, St Louis, 2007, Mosby.)

question and give a reply. Patients with speech, hearing, or cognitive difficulties may respond more easily to yes-or-no questions. Often a simple head nod or shake can communicate effectively enough to help you complete the history. For patients who are disabled and for older adults who are frail, use patience when obtaining information. Allowing enough time for the patient to answer the question can often be challenging. Rushing a patient's verbal response, however, will inhibit rapport, might be frustrating or intimidating, and could impede their willingness to share information. Review the earlier discussion and Box 1-2 for additional information on therapeutic communication techniques.

Allergies Many patients have allergies to prescribed or OTC medications (see the next section), animals, or food. Ask the patient about any known causes of allergic reactions and what symptoms are normally experienced, such as hives or trouble breathing. Find out how quickly the symptoms tend to develop.

Some symptoms are more worrisome than others. A patient who breaks out in a slight rash when around cats raises fewer concerns than a patient who develops stridor when a particular food is eaten. Some untoward responses are adverse reactions rather than true allergic responses. Many patients may misinterpret hypersensitivity to a food, animal, or medication as an allergy, so it becomes important to evaluate exactly how the patient responds to contact with the reported allergen or irritant. This information will help you distinguish a hypersensitivity response from an allergic or anaphylactic reaction.

Medications Include in your documentation a record of all medications the patient takes regularly, including OTC drugs and medications prescribed by all the patient's doctors. Healthcare providers may or may not know what the patient's physician may have prescribed. Drug interactions and adverse reactions must be considered in the overall medication profile.

Some patients also take OTC drugs or dietary supplements, also known as *holistic, herbal,* or *alternative medications.* Remember to ask about liquid OTC drinks and herbal teas that may have a high content of caffeine, vitamins, or other ingredients that might be causing the patient's signs and symptoms.

Pertinent Past Medical History Try to discern what medical history is pertinent to the presenting complaint. If the patient is having chest pain and had a stent placed 6 months ago, for instance, that information is pertinent to today's call for EMS. The femur fracture suffered 2 years ago is not.

In addition, a description of past surgeries, especially recent ones, is important historical information to obtain. The risk of an embolus can be identified, for example, if the patient has recently undergone surgery such as a cesarian section, hip or knee replacement, or gallstone removal.

Last Oral Intake Ask the patient when and what he last ate and drank. Be sure to document the response. A patient who has recently eaten or had something to drink may aspirate stomach contents into the lungs if he becomes unconscious and vomits or has to be anesthetized for emergency surgery and vomits while under anesthesia.

Events Preceding Find out what events led to the decision to call 9-1-1. Ask the patient, bystanders, and family the following questions: What happened today? Why did you call 9-1-1? What has made it better or worse ? This last question is appropriate when the events elapsed slowly, such as when a person has trouble breathing all night but doesn't call 9-1-1 until she also begins to have chest pain.

Risk Factors Risk factors for a given condition can be environmental, social, psychological, or familial. Is the patient living alone and at risk for falls? Does the residence contain any fall related hazards? Is the patient confined to bed and dependent on someone else to feed and care for them? Other significant risk factors for medical problems include diabetes, hypertension, gender, race, age, smoking, and obesity.

Does the patient adhere to a prescribed medication regimen? Is he able to differentiate medications and take them properly? Is there a list of medications, and is the dispensing routine clear to the patient? An often helpful suggestion for patients taking several medications is to compile a complete list and post it in a visible place for themselves and their families. Doing so can reduce the likelihood of medication error and decrease the risk of drug toxicity.

Current Health Status

The personal habits of the patient relevant to his or her overall health history can be important in determining the acuity of the current complaint. Frequent visits to their physician or emergency room for similar complaints may indicate the need for evaluation of a chronic condition and change in treatment regimens.

Alcohol or Substance Abuse and Tobacco Use Asking the patient about their use of illegal drugs (including the use of prescription drugs not prescribed), tobacco products, and alcohol may elicit important information about the potential for multiple underlying etiologies. The CAGE questionnaire can be used to help identify alcohol abuse patterns of behavior (Box 1-8). Such evaluation can indicate a chronic versus acute illness with the potential for traumatic injury. For example, a chronic alcoholic is at increased risk for subdural bleeds due to falling while intoxicated.

Immunizations Information about current screening tests and an immunization record help identify patients at risk for communicable diseases. Recent travel history outside the country is also helpful in identifying conditions that should be included in the differential diagnosis.

Family History Family history may be important if the differential diagnosis includes inherited conditions such as sickle cell disease. Asking about family members with the following diseases may indicate high risk factors for

BOX 1-8 CAGE Questionnaire

C: Have you ever been concerned about your own or someone else's drinking? Have you ever found the need to cut down on drinking?

A: Have you ever felt annoyed by criticism of your drinking?

G: Have you ever felt guilty about your drinking? Have you ever felt guilty about something you said or did while you were drinking?

E: Have you ever felt the need for a morning eye opener?

Modified from Ewing JA: Detecting alcoholism, the CAGE questionnaire, JAMA 252:1905, 1984.

the patient, aiding clinical reasoning and leading to more rapid diagnosis and treatment:

- Arthritis
- Cancer
- Headaches
- Hypertension
- Stroke
- Lung disease
- Tuberculosis
- Communicable and autoimmune diseases

Patient Advocacy You can be a patient advocate by seeking out family and friends who are supportive and may help the patient improve the safety of the home environment. Asking the patient what he or she needs to get through a difficult physical or psychological emergency is an empathetic and compassionate approach to patient care.

Patients who are able to develop a rapport with you feel more trusting in answering your questions and letting you help them make decisions about their care. Fostering an open, positive patient outlook will help limit the associated stress of an illness or injury and make it easier for you to obtain an accurate history, establish a working diagnosis, and begin prompt treatment. Review the discussion earlier in this chapter for detailed information on therapeutic communication.

Now that you have obtained additional historical information, have you considered additional underlying etiologies and diagnoses? Does the patient's response to your initial treatment warrant modification? Let's look at the information we can obtain from the physical exam.

Physical Examination

The physical examination can be a focused exam, a rapid head-to-toe exam, or a comprehensive, thorough exam. The healthcare provider must determine, based on the acuity of the patient, which exam is most appropriate. In most emergency response situations, a focused exam is appropriate in conscious patients. A rapid head-to-toe exam is necessary in patients who are unconscious or have a diminished LOC and in those whose presentation indicates possible substance abuse or toxicity. Detailed physical exams are more practical in hospital or other clinical situations, although a detailed exam may be performed by prehospital personnel if transport time allows.

The physical exam findings should augment the historical data and diagnostic assessment information already obtained to assist in ruling in or ruling out differential diagnoses. As information is gathered and critically evaluated, an appropriate treatment pathway will be identified and implemented.

Stethoscopes, otoscopes, and ophthalmoscopes are common equipment used to gather valuable information when performing a physical exam, but the tools are only as good as the examiner's observation skills. Therefore, inspection, auscultation, percussion, and palpation are critical components of the assessment process. The physical examination will help identify life threats in the primary or secondary survey. In an unconscious patient, the physical exam may be the only way to discover the cardinal presentation.

In many medical patients, historical information is obtained before the physical exam is performed. Altering the order of the components of the assessment is dependent on the severity of symptoms, criticality of the patient's status, and the cardinal presentation up to this point. The physical exam may be performed prior to the history or simultaneously with the history if enough personnel are present.

The physical exam is used to rule in or out conditions that make up the differential diagnosis constructed during the history taking. The opposite may be true of traumatic injuries. In trauma patients, a rapid physical exam may be carried out before medical information is obtained. In conscious patients, these examinations will take place simultaneously if enough healthcare personnel are available.

Examination Techniques

Inspection Inspection is the visual assessment of the patient and his or her surroundings. You begin observing visual clues to the patient's condition during the initial observation portion of the patient's exam (see earlier discussion). This preliminary inspection can reveal the implications of the environment and the severity of the patient's condition before the history is taken or the physical exam performed.

The patient's body will need to be exposed and clothing removed to conduct a proper inspection, but it is typically unnecessary to completely remove all clothing for this assessment. Environmental conditions and protection of the patient's modesty must be taken into consideration.

During the secondary survey, a focused inspection of the patient should be performed. The patient's affect and body position should be assessed for indications of the severity of the condition and the number of body systems involved. When evaluating the patient's affect, lethargy may suggest hypoxia and respiratory fatigue. At this time, the patient's hygiene, nutritional status, and nonverbal body language can be noted.

Significant injury should be identified during your visual exam. Bruising, abrasions, surgical scars (particularly evidence of previous surgeries such as cardiac surgery or lung removal, because they may be pertinent to dyspnea or other respiratory distress), and rashes should be noted. Note whether a stoma is present. Read and document any medic alert tags.

The trachea should be observed and potentially palpated to be midline. The shape of the patient's chest can offer the first clue to chronic lung disease. A barrel chest can indicate underlying COPD such as emphysema and chronic bronchitis.

A patient in a supine position with flattened neck veins may have hypovolemia. Look for any unusual neck masses, jugular venous distention (JVD), and swelling. JVD with diminished or absent breath sounds may indicate tension pneumothorax and cardiac tamponade.

Assess for the placement of vascular assistive devices (VAD) that indicate chronic disease processes and the need for nutritional support or long-term vascular access, as in the case of chemotherapy regimes or frequent blood samples.

Tracheal tugging and use of intercostal and neck muscles are a sign of distress. Asymmetry, grunting, and deep or shallow respiratory movement are abnormal. Immediate intervention should be initiated to improve oxygenation and ventilation, stabilize the work of breathing, and promote adequate perfusion.

Observation of body fluids and excretions is a key component of GI tract and genitourinary (GU) system assessment. Blood-tinged vomitus can indicate GI bleeding, ruptured esophageal varices, or long-term use of antiinflammatory medications. Hematemesis (vomiting of blood) can also occur when the patient has a bleeding peptic ulcer. Emesis (vomitus) that resembles coffee grounds indicates that digested blood is present.

Bright red blood in the stool can represent lower GI bleeding and should be considered a potential life threat. Bleeding may also occur from hemorrhoids or anal fissures. Dark, tarry, black, or dark red stool, known as *melena*, is a sign of upper GI bleeding and may also signify a life threat or critical condition.

Incontinence of urine or feces may indicate neurologic dysfunction as well as GU or GI tract dysfunction. Hematuria, or blood in the urine, is a sign of kidney dysfunction and uncontrolled hypertension.

In patients with chronic renal failure, especially those on dialysis, you may note grafts or fistulas. Patients who receive peritoneal dialysis at home will have evidence of an abdominal catheter. In addition, a gastric tube may be used in the home setting to remove fluids and gas, instill irrigation solutions or medications, or administer enteral feedings. Be alert for the possibility the patient has aspirated gastric contents, and make sure the device is working properly.

With keen observation, you'll note any kyphosis (spinal curvature), pressure ulcers, moles, abrasions, rashes, ecchymosis or hematoma, bleeding, needle or track marks, and discoloration.

Rashes Although emergent medical intervention is not required for a persistent, itchy rash (e.g., dermatitis, psoriasis), the location and color of such a rash should be noted. Any accumulation or discharge of fluid or pus should be documented. Noticeable scaling can occur from skin infections such as impetigo, which forms honey-colored crusts as it heals. Red, tender, fluctuant nodules or masses often represent abscesses.

Any skin disorder that presents with a rash or vesicles, or with lesions that leak fluid, should be considered an infectious risk to the healthcare provider. Proper body-substance isolations precautions should be observed.

Moles and Lesions Moles and lesions should be evaluated for symmetry, border irregularity, and color variation. While typically not a significant prehospital concern, such moles and lesions should raise suspicion of cutaneous melanoma, a rapidly progressing skin cancer that often metastasizes to vital organs and has a high mortality rate.

Compromised Skin Integrity Breaks in the integrity of the skin caused by open skeletal fracture indicate a risk for infection and require urgent attention. Pressure ulcers indicate the potential for diminished perfusion and a risk of sepsis.

Bruising Signs of neurologic impairment and previous injury can be observed with bruising over the eyes and mastoid process. Known as *periorbital ecchymosis* and *Battle's sign*, respectively, these markings herald a basilar skull fracture.

Dehydration Dehydration should be physically assessed by evaluating the skin in the middle of the forehead or sternum for tenting.

Body Fluids General observation of body fluids being discharged from the skin or excreted from any body orifice is important. Examples include vomitus, cerebrospinal fluid (CSF), urine or feces, and blood. Note the amount as well as its color, odor, viscosity, and location.

Auscultation **Auscultation** is the use of a stethoscope or just your ears to evaluate the presence or absence of air or fluid, heart tones, and adventitious lung sounds.

Lung Sounds The lungs initially should be auscultated in the midaxillary position. During the secondary survey, you should listen to both upper and lower lung fields, both anteriorly and posteriorly. If the patient's cardinal presentation is dyspnea or respiratory distress, lung sounds should be auscultated in the midaxillary position (Figure 1-21). Performing auscultation early in the assessment can reveal life-threatening respiratory compromise attributable to acute asthma or pulmonary edema.

Lung sounds can be auscultated in distinct areas:

- Vesicular lung sounds are auscultated over the anterior and posterior chest. Normally these sounds are soft and low pitched.
- Bronchovesicular sounds are auscultated over the main bronchi. These sounds are lower than the vesicular sounds and have a medium pitch.
- Bronchial sounds are heard over the trachea, near the manubrium of the sternum. They are typically high pitched.
- A sandpaper-like sound is an indication that the visceral and parietal pleura are rubbing together. This sign is called a *friction rub* and is associated with pulmonary diseases such as pleurisy.

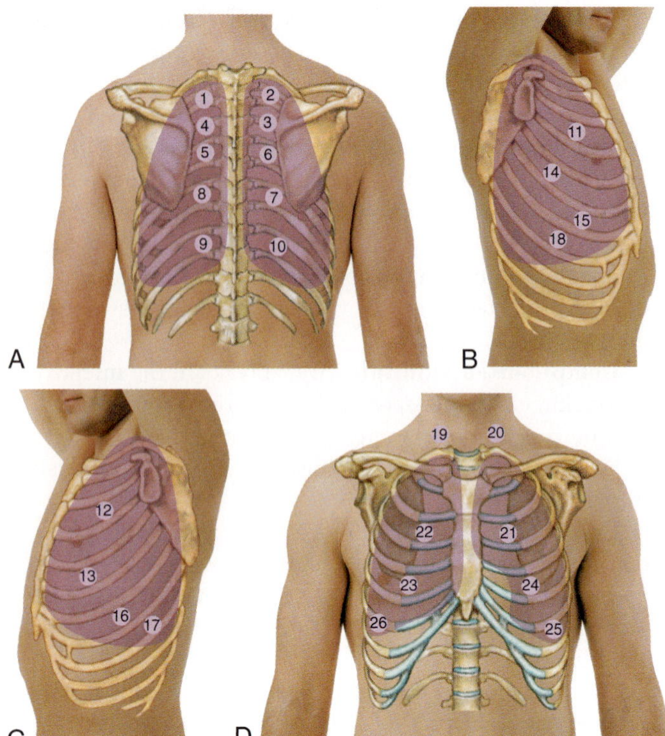

■ **Figure 1-21** When listening to lung sounds, listen to one lung and then at the same place on the other lung. Listen to at least one full inhalation and exhalation at each location. **A**, Posterior chest. **B**, Right lateral chest. **C**, Left lateral chest. **D**, Anterior chest. (From Seidel H, Ball J, Dains J, et al: Mosby's guide to physical examination, ed 6, St Louis, 2006, Mosby.)

- Adventitious lung sounds are audible sounds heard over the normal, nearly inaudible sound of breathing. They include crackles, rhonchi, and wheezing, each of which reveals valuable clues about lower airway disease (see Box 1-6).

Ask the patient to take a deep breath. Patients having acute asthma attacks tend to have more trouble exhaling than inhaling. If deep breathing causes pain or discomfort, the patient may have underlying pleurisy or a pulmonary embolism. Feel the torso for instability of bony structures. Palpate the chest for subcutaneous emphysema. Palpate the trachea for proper midline positioning. Deviation can be a late sign of pneumothorax.

Abnormal lung sounds (see Box 1-6) can result from cardiovascular compromise affecting both the cardiovascular and respiratory systems. Crackles, for example, can signal pulmonary congestion from ventricular heart failure.

Using the proper assessment tools will help you confirm or eliminate differential diagnoses related to the respiratory system. The findings of such supplemental assessments will aid your clinical reasoning and ensure that your medical decision making is well informed and accurate.

Special Circumstances As noted earlier in the chapter, some patients transported by prehospital personnel may require special transport ventilators (ATVs). They may be intubated or have other preexisting respiratory system needs that will significantly affect EMS management and prehospital care.

Heart Sounds Heart tones are auscultated for loudness (intensity), length (duration), pitch (frequency), and timing of the cardiac cycle. When listening at the fifth intercostal space, toward the apex of the heart, the normal heart sounds of S_1 and S_2 can be heard. These sounds are caused by heart muscle contraction and are best heard if the patient is leaning forward, sitting up, or in a left lateral recumbent position (and even supine). Positioning is best when the heart is closer to the left anterior chest wall. To better hear S_1, ask the patient to breathe normally then hold their breath on expiration. To better hear S_2, ask the patient to breathe normally then hold their breath on inspiration.

Abnormal heart sounds, such as murmurs, indicate a problem with the blood flow in and out of the heart. Bruits are abnormal sounds sometimes heard when the carotid arteries are auscultated; they produce high-pitched sounds that indicate blood flow obstruction in those vessels. In the case of an aneurysm, a fine tremor or vibration can be felt which can identify a blockage; these are commonly called *thrills*. Murmurs, bruits, and thrills can be benign or life threatening.

In patients with a history of heart failure, additional heart sounds can be heard. Additional heart sounds occur in the presence of ventricular disease and are often identified as S_3 and S_4. In valvular heart disease, these sounds are called *gallops*.

The S_3 sound, identified as a third heart sound, is an early clue to a diagnosis of left heart failure. Difficult to detect, it can be referred to as a *gallop,* which would sound similar to a horse's gallop. It appears approximately 0.12 to 0.16 second after the second heart sound and results from overexpansion of the ventricles as they fill with blood.

The S_4 sound occurs during the second phase of ventricular filling when the atrium contracts. This sound is thought to be caused by valvular and ventricular wall vibration. It is typically heard when there is increased resistance to ventricular filling.

Bowel Sounds Auscultation of bowel sounds, although not often performed during the prehospital evaluation, can help identify bowel obstruction. Bowel sounds should be auscultated for 30 to 60 seconds before palpation. A normal bowel makes a gurgling noise and sounds the same in each quadrant. Bowel obstructions, including air pockets, cause inconsistent, hypoactive, or absent bowel sounds in one or more quadrants. High-pitched bowel sounds in the presence of a distended abdomen may give early warning of a bowel obstruction. An obstruction or accumulation of gases can rupture the intestinal wall.

Palpation **Palpation** is the use of the hands to examine the patient by applying gentle pressure at various points on the body, such as when you feel for a pulse (Figure 1-22). The patient may feel that palpation is a form of invasion of their personal space, so be sure to ask the patient for permission before you use this technique. Palpation should be gentle and respectful. See Kinesthetic Observation earlier in this chapter for a discussion of the value of touch in patient assessment. A light touch to the outside and inside of the length of an extremity can assist with sensation status and bilateral muscle strength.

Capillary Refill Time Capillary refill time is often evaluated to determine the status of the cardiovascular system. To perform this test, pressure is applied to the nail bed until it turns white. The provider then measures the time it takes for normal color to return. A blanching time of more than 2 seconds is considered an indicator that capillary blood is being inappropriately shunted.

This test can be unreliable in adult patients for several reasons. Older adults, especially those who take many medications and those with immune system or renal disease, tend to have poor perfusion. The temperature of the environment can also reduce the accuracy of the capillary refill test. Cooler environments cause vasoconstriction as a compensatory mechanism and may give a false impression of poor perfusion status.

The abdomen should be palpated in all four quadrants. It should be soft and nontender, with no tension, swelling, or masses. Muscle guarding is an abnormal finding that

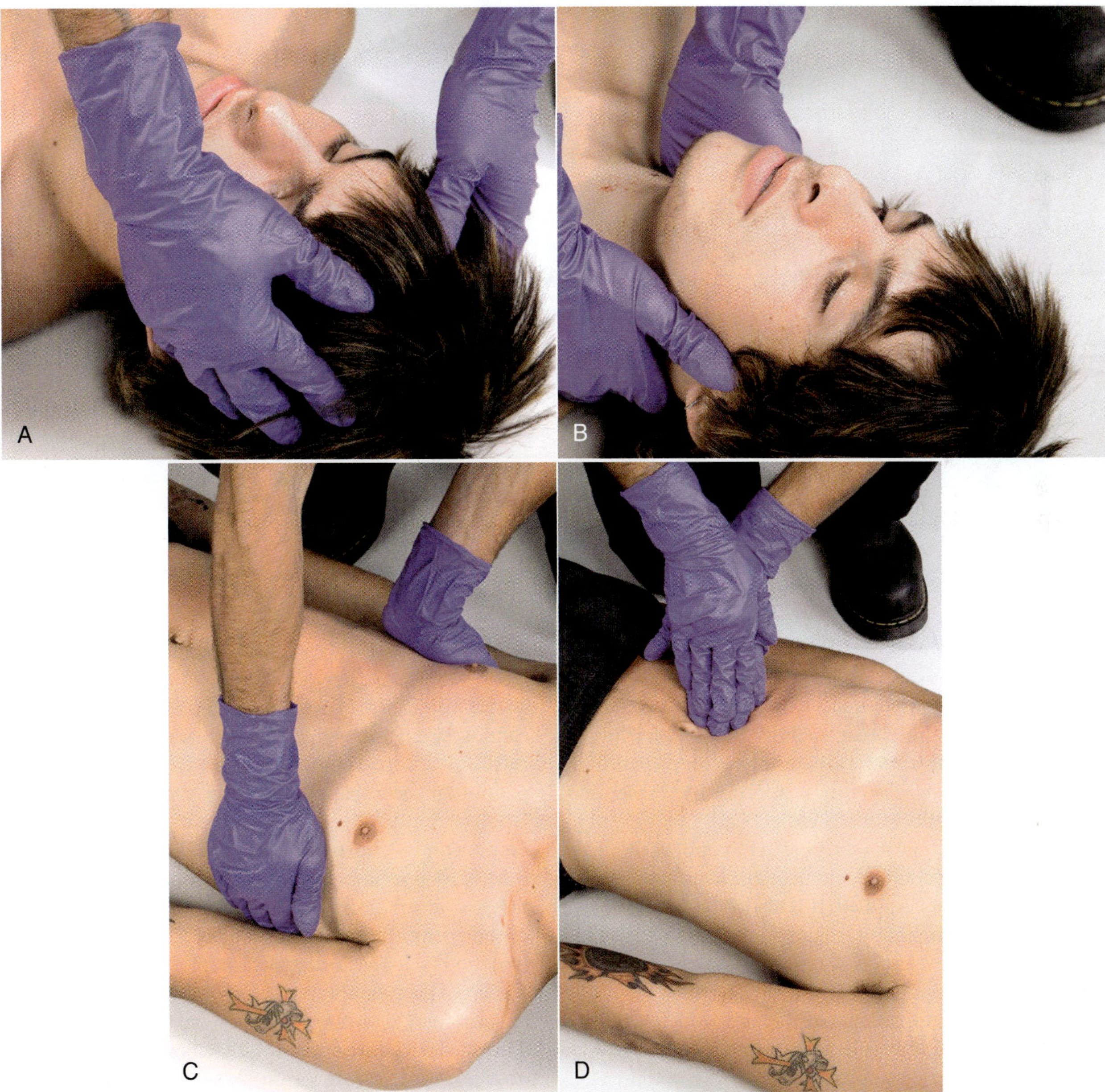

■ **Figure 1-22** A, Palpate the head for structural integrity. B, Palpate the soft tissues of the neck and each of the cervical vertebrae for tenderness. C, Evaluate the integrity of the patient's lateral chest wall by pressing your hands against the lateral rib cage. D, Palpate the abdomen.

Continued

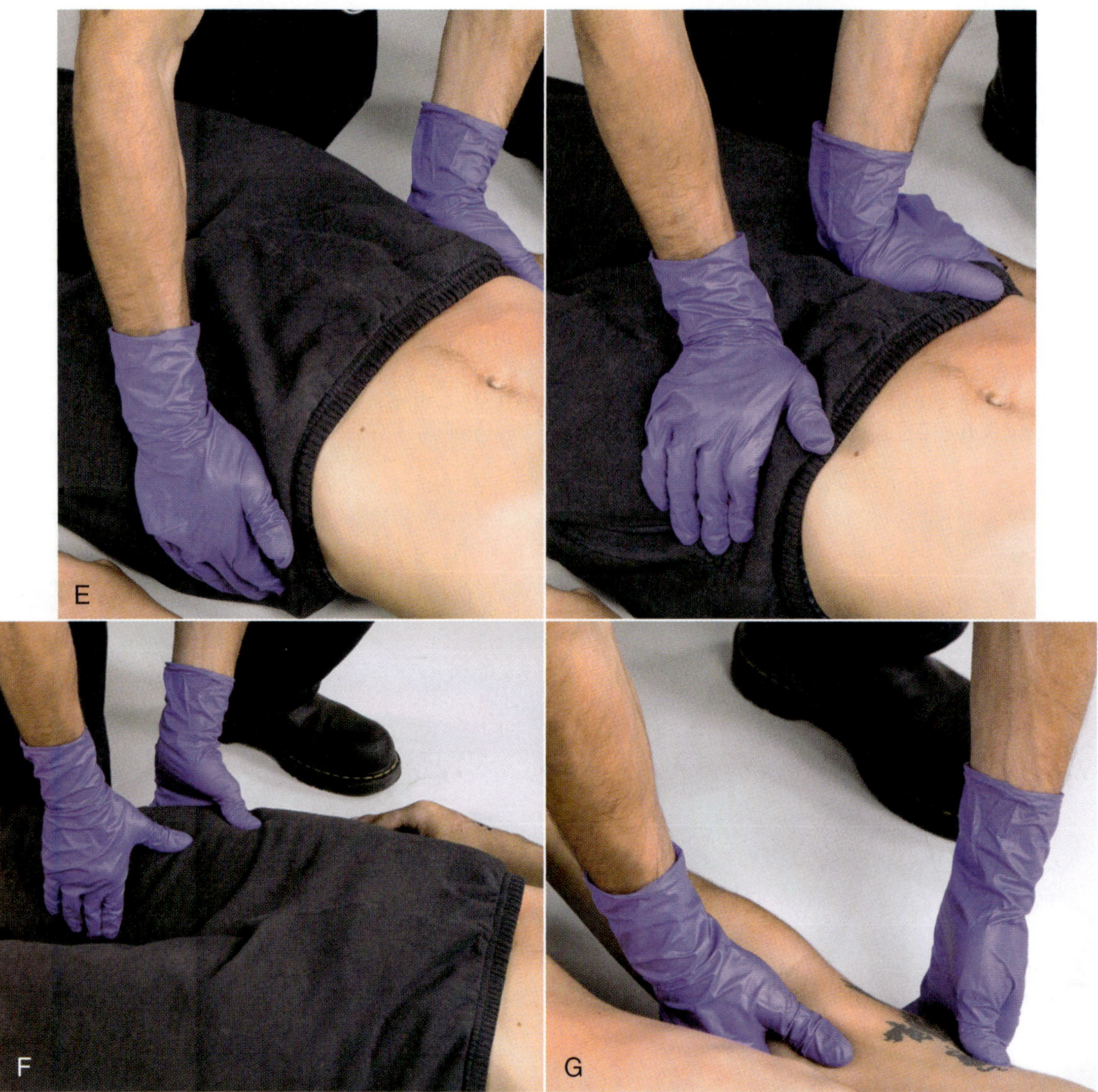

■ **Figure 1-22, Cont'd** E, Press the iliac crests medially and posteriorly. F, Palpate the femur. G, Palpate the humerus and elbow. (From Aehlert BJ: Paramedic practice today: above and beyond, St Louis, 2009, Mosby.)

indicates pain and possible underlying injury. Abdominal rigidity is a sign of a life threat, such as internal bleeding. Upper right quadrant pain that elicits a gasp on palpation, known as *Murphy's sign,* is an indication of the presence of gallstones and cholecystitis (Figure 1-23).

The quadrant with the most reported discomfort should be palpated last. Palpation should be used to evaluate pain when gentle pressure is applied. It is also a means of identifying an increase in pain on removal of gentle pressure, known as *rebound tenderness*. This sign is a red flag for peritonitis.

McBurney's point is the name of the area over the right side of the abdomen that is a third of the distance from the anterior superior iliac spine (ASIS) to the umbilicus. Localized tenderness in this area is a sign of acute appendicitis. Palpation of the left lower quadrant that elicits pain in the right lower quadrant, called *Rovsing's sign,* can also be an indicator of appendicitis. Abdominal pain that cannot be elicited on palpation can be caused by renal calculi or a urinary tract infection (UTI). Flank and back pain often accompany both of these diagnoses.

Percussion **Percussion** is used to evaluate whether air or fluid is present in body cavities. Sound waves are heard as percussion tones, which change according to the density of the tissue. The techniques of percussion and auscultation are discussed further in Chapter 3.

Percussion is not typically performed in the prehospital environment. However, this assessment provides important information regarding the abdominal cavity. If a dullness is heard during percussion, an abundance of fluid may be accumulating in this cavity, as occurs in liver failure. A hyperresonant sound may indicate that air, as opposed to fluid, is abundant (Box 1-9).

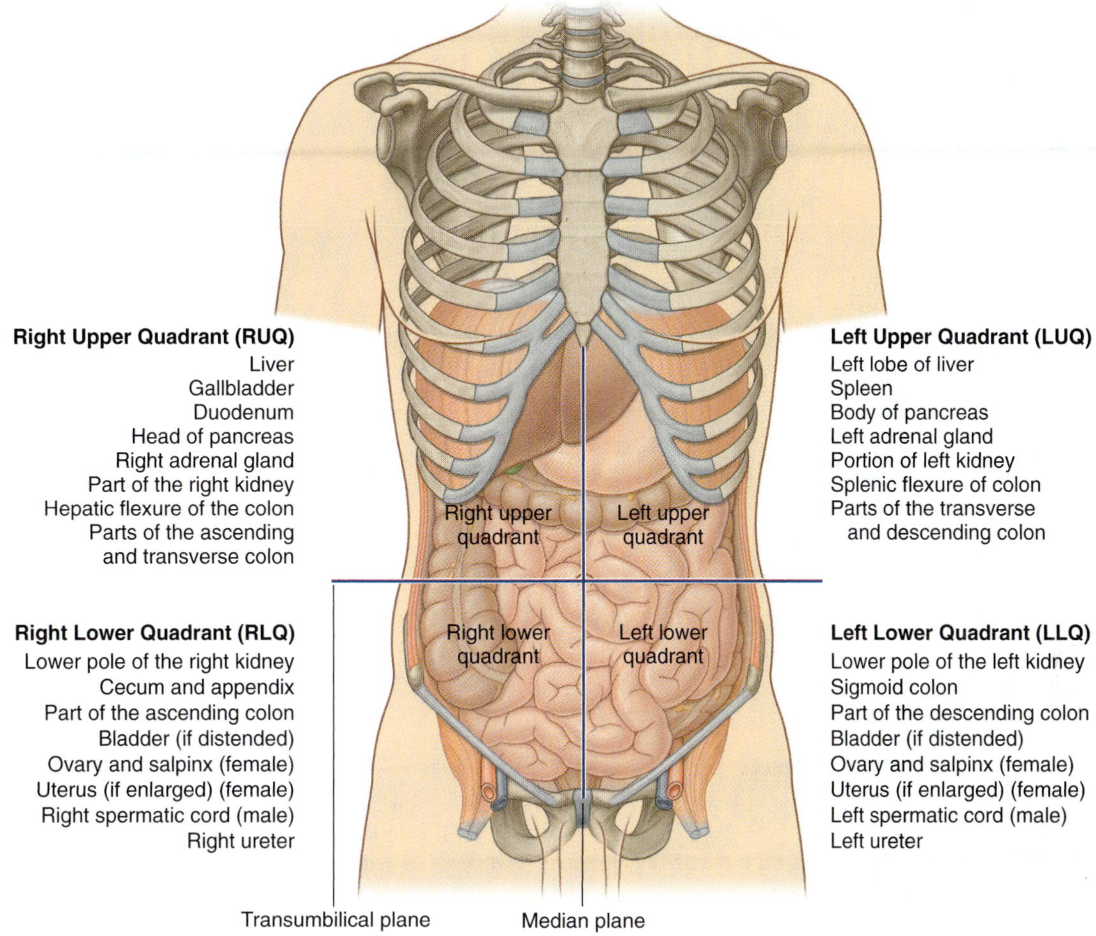

Figure 1-23 Organs contained in the four abdominal quadrants. (Modified from Drake RL, Vogl W, Mitchell AWM: Gray's anatomy for students, New York, 2005, Churchill Livingstone.)

BOX 1-9 Percussion Tones and Examples

Percussion Tone	Example
Tympany (the loudest)	Gastric bubble
Hyperresonance	Air-filled lungs (COPD, pneumothorax)
Resonance	Healthy lungs
Dullness	Liver
Flat (the quietest)	Muscle

Motor and Sensory Function

Motor and sensory function should be evaluated in all patients whether they are conscious, unconscious, or have altered mental status. If the patient is conscious, gently touch the hands and feet to determine the ability to feel light touch, indicating that distal perfusion is adequate and sensory nerve tracts are functioning properly. Withdrawal of an extremity may indicate pain or discomfort. Assessing for sensation will determine the function of the afferent sensory nerve tracts in the posterior spinal column.

The Babinski test is appropriate to use in conscious patients and in patients with altered mental status. To perform this exam, take a pen or similar dull object and run it along the lateral length of the sole of the foot. Normal reaction to this stimulation is for the toes to move downward, a response known as *plantar flexion*. This movement indicates a negative test result. A positive Babinski test is indicated by abnormal extension of the great toe and fanning of the remaining toes, a response called *dorsiflexion*. This movement suggests neurologic dysfunction (Figure 1-24).

It is important to assess the ability to feel light touch but equally important to evaluate the ability to feel pain. The patient's report of pain or response to a painful stimulus indicates that the motor nerves in the anterior spinal column are properly performing their afferent function of sending sensory messages to the central nervous system.

Motor function in all extremities should be evaluated for bilateral equality and strength (Figure 1-25). Unequal responses of left and right limbs should be considered a sign of hemiparesis (unilateral paralysis) or hemiplegia

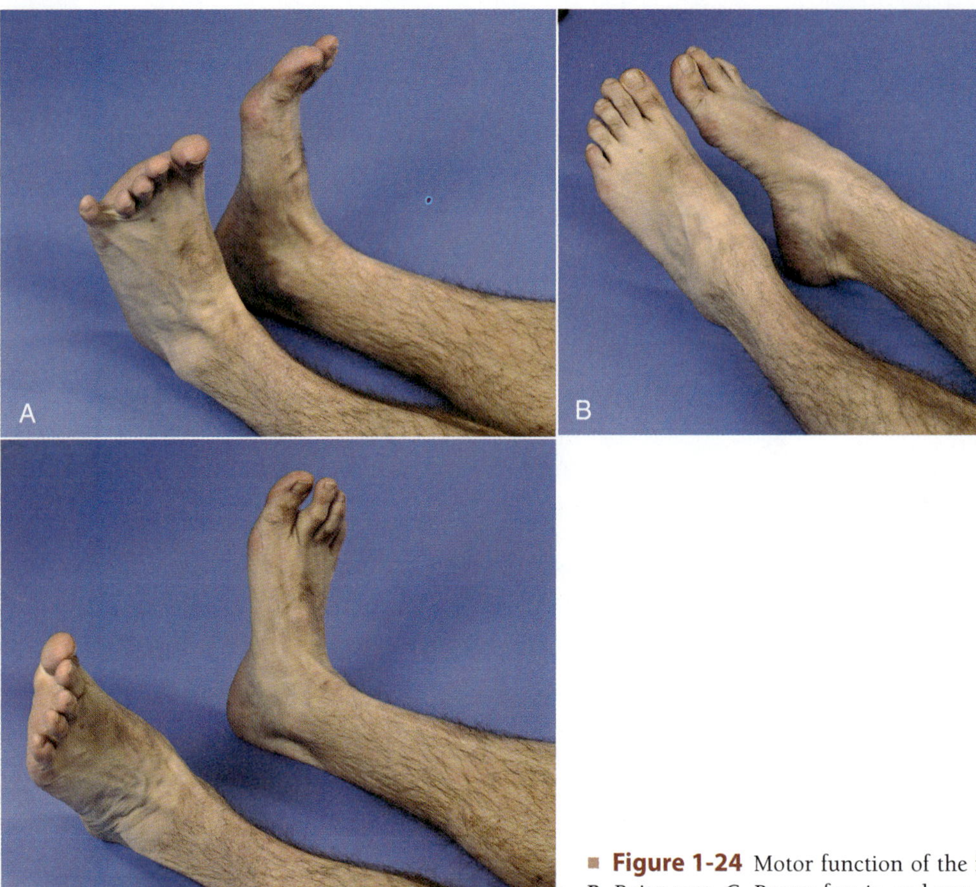

■ **Figure 1-24** Motor function of the foot and ankle. **A**, Bend toes. **B**, Point toes. **C**, Rotate feet in and out. (From Sanders MJ: Mosby's paramedic textbook—revised reprint, ed 3, St Louis, 2007, Mosby.)

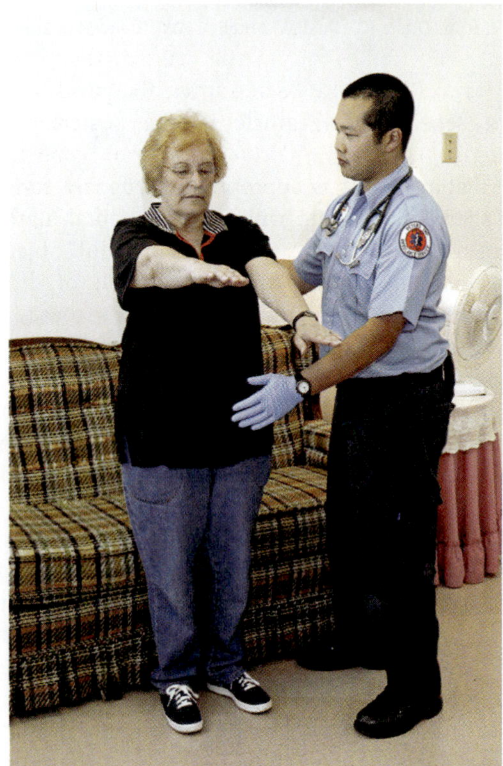

■ **Figure 1-25** Pronator drift test. (From Sanders MJ: Mosby's paramedic textbook—revised reprint, ed 3, St Louis, 2007, Mosby.)

(unilateral weakness), which can be caused by stroke, meningitis, brain tumors, or seizure activity. Bilateral upper or lower extremity weakness should raise concern for a spinal cord lesion.

Cerebellar function can be evaluated by how a patient stands and walks. Ataxia (unsteady gait) may indicate cranial nerve damage from toxicity or chronic neurologic dysfunction. A shuffling gait may indicate neurologic damage caused by Huntington's disease or Parkinson's disease. Tremors, muscle rigidity, and repetitive motion may indicate degeneration of the nervous system attributable to Alzheimer's disease or Parkinson's disease.

Patients with a variety of psychological or behavioral disorders may take antipsychotic medications that have spasmodic muscle movement as a side effect. These medications may also induce muscle dystonia, expressed as contortion of the extremities or facial tics.

Cranial Nerve Assessment All levels of healthcare providers should be proficient in performing a cranial nerve assessment as part of their physical exam. Findings identify cranial nerve impairment and glean timely information about the patient's neurologic status. The cranial nerves and their functions are summarized in Table 1-5. A mnemonic by which to remember the cranial nerves is given in the Rapid Recall box.

RAPID RECALL

Cranial Nerves Mnemonic

Oh, those confounded cranial nerves! They've confused students for generations. The mnemonic by which most of us remember them sounds like the beginning of a bad joke: A Finn and a German are sitting in a bar one night…

Of course, you could always make up your own mnemonic. Lots of people have—check out the list of cranial nerves mnemonics posted on the Internet.

On Old Olympus' Towering Top, A Finn And German Viewed Some Hops:

I Olfactory
II Optic
III Oculomotor
IV Trochlear
V Trigeminal
VI Abducens
VII Facial
VIII Acoustic (vestibulocochlear)
IX Glossopharyngeal
X Vagus
XI Spinal accessory
XII Hypoglossal

Pronator Drift The pronator drift (see Figure 1-25) is used to evaluate motor and sensory function in a suspected stroke patient. The patient is asked to close their eyes and extend their arms with palms up. Note any downward drift or drop or any inward rotation of either arm.

Head, Eyes, Ears, Nose, Throat

Physical exam of the head, eyes, ears, nose, and throat is dependent on the provider's scope of practice, patient cardinal presentation, and assessment findings. These examinations may not be necessary on every patient.

Eyes Windows to the soul or not, the eyes certainly give a useful glimpse into the patient's neurologic status. The eyes must be assessed for direction and tracking of the gaze (Figure 1-26). To do so, shine a penlight into the eye from the side of the face as the patient focuses on a distant object. In an awake and alert patient, the eyes should be open, should face in the same direction, and should move in tandem, known as a *conjugate gaze* (Figure 1-27).

Ears In patients with ataxia (unsteady gait) or diminished responsiveness to external stimuli, the ears should be assessed for discharge (clear fluid or blood), foreign bodies, and erythema of the inner ear.

An otoscope is used to evaluate the external auditory canal and check the eardrum for injury or redness representing infection or bleeding in the middle ear (Figure 1-28). This assessment tool can identify cerumen (ear wax) buildup, edema, obstructions, lesions, infections, and injury to the tympanic membrane. It can help rule out or rule in differential diagnoses that might explain pain, ataxia, or diminished response to verbal commands.

Pupils Adequately perfused pupils are equal, round, and briskly reactive to stimulation with a penlight. Pinpoint pupils suggest opiate abuse or injury to the pons. Pupil dilation indicates toxicity or diminished neurologic function (Figure 1-29).

Shining a light into the patient's eyes should cause the pupils to constrict quickly. Be sure to assess for this response in both eyes, observing whether the muscles of the eyes work synchronously so that the pupils constrict simultaneously. Unilateral dilatation in an unconscious patient may be a sign of brain herniation. Some patients may present with anisocoria, a condition characterized by pupils that are noticeably unequal in size. Pupils that

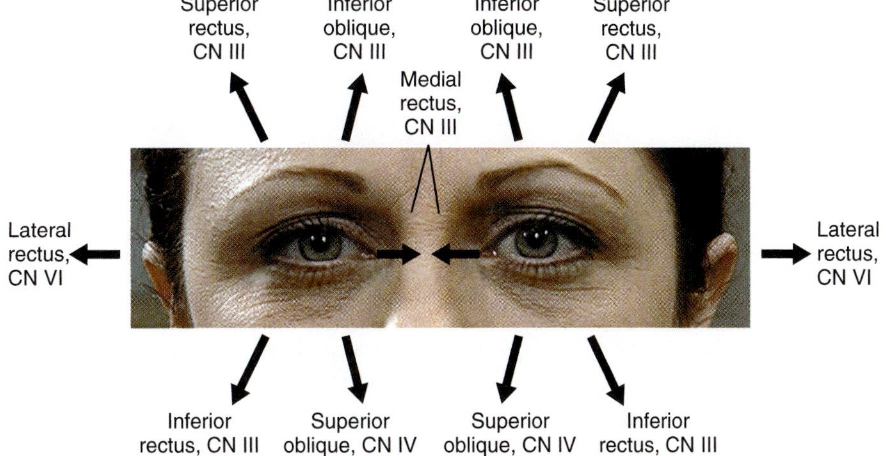

■ **Figure 1-26** The six cardinal fields of vision with their associated cranial nerves and extraocular muscles. *CN*, Cranial nerve. (From Seidel H, Ball J, Dains J, et al: Mosby's guide to physical examination, ed 6, St Louis, 2006, Mosby.)

TABLE 1-5 Cranial Nerves and Their Functions

Nerve #	Name	Function	Assessment
I	Olfactory	Sense of smell	Ask patient to close her eyes. Place spirits of ammonia or an alcohol wipe under her nose. The patient should be able to identify the odor.
II	Optic	Sense of sight	Evaluate visual acuity using a Snellen visual acuity chart or Rosenbaum card. Ask the patient to cover one eye and tell you how many fingers you're holding up. Then evaluate the opposite eye.
III	Oculomotor	Size, symmetry, and shape of pupils Eye movement	Test the pupil response to light for equality, reactivity, and roundness. Pupils should briskly constrict with light and dilate in darkness.
IV	Trochlear	Downward gaze	Hold the patient's chin to prevent movement. Ask the patient to follow a penlight or object in an "H" pattern to track the six visual fields.
V	Trigeminal	Cheek Jaw motion Chewing Facial sensation	Ask the patient to clench his teeth to determine the strength of the jaw and the ability to close the mouth without difficulty. The patient should feel a slight touch bilaterally.
VI	Abducens	Lateral eye movement	Same as for cranial nerve IV
VII	Facial	Strength of facial muscles Taste Saliva secretion	Assess for weakness or asymmetry by inspecting the face at rest and when speaking. Ask the patient to raise his eyebrows, frown, show his upper and lower teeth, smile, and puff out both cheeks.
VIII	Acoustic	Sense of hearing Balance	Occlude each ear independently to test for hearing and balance.
IX	Glossopharyngeal	Tongue and pharynx sensation Taste Muscles of swallowing	Ask the patient to say "ahhh," and observe the uvula and soft palate response. The soft palate should move up, and the uvula should remain midline.
X	Vagus	Sensation of throat and trachea Taste Muscles for voice production Heart rate	Same as cranial nerve IX
XI	Spinal accessory	Shoulder movement Ability to turn head	Ask the patient to raise and lower her shoulders against the resistance of your hand on her shoulder.
XII	Hypoglossal	Speech articulation Tongue movement	Ask the patient to stick out his tongue and move it side to side in several directions with symmetry.

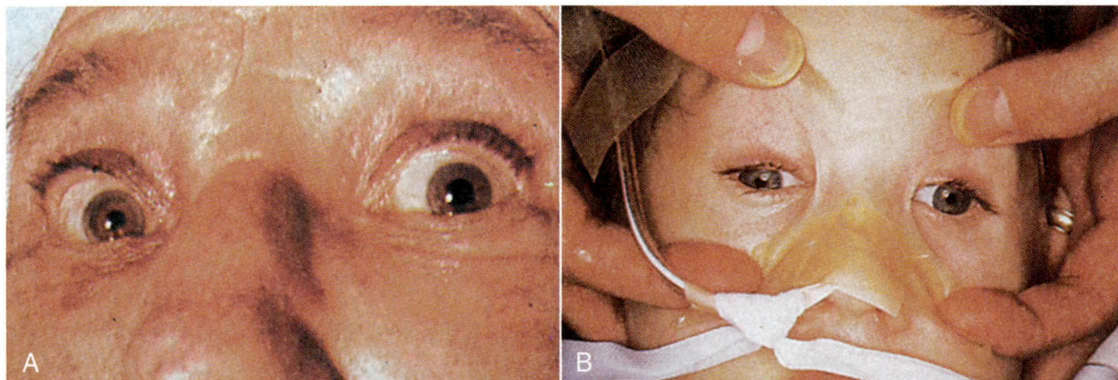

■ **Figure 1-27** **A**, Conjugate gaze. **B**, Disconjugate gaze. (From Sanders MJ: Mosby's paramedic textbook—revised reprint, ed 3, St Louis, 2007, Mosby.)

appear unequal in shape and size may also suggest glaucoma.

Reflexes

Reflexes are tested to evaluate symmetry and strength of response. Testing may include deep tendon reflexes (DTRs) and superficial reflexes, including superficial abdominal reflexes. Inappropriate responses may indicate damage to neuronal pathways at corresponding spinal segmental levels. All responses should be thoroughly documented.

Deep tendon reflexes are stretch reflexes, requiring the muscles being tested to be relaxed and the tendons gently

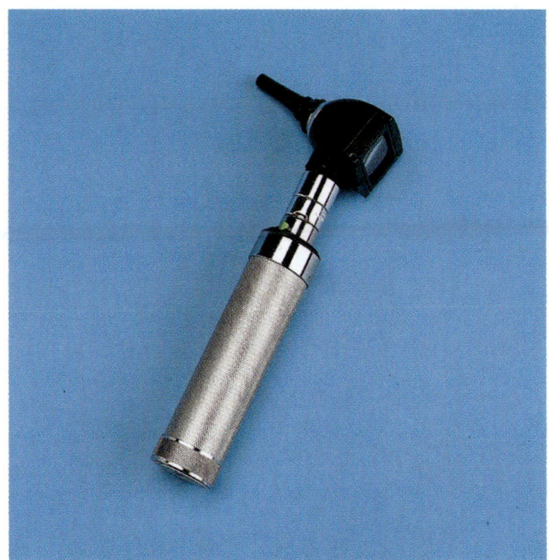

■ **Figure 1-28** Otoscope. (From Kidwell CS, Starkman S, Eckstein M, et al: Identifying stroke in the field: prospective validation of the Los Angeles Prehospital Stroke Screen (LAPSS), Stroke 31:71–76, 2000.)

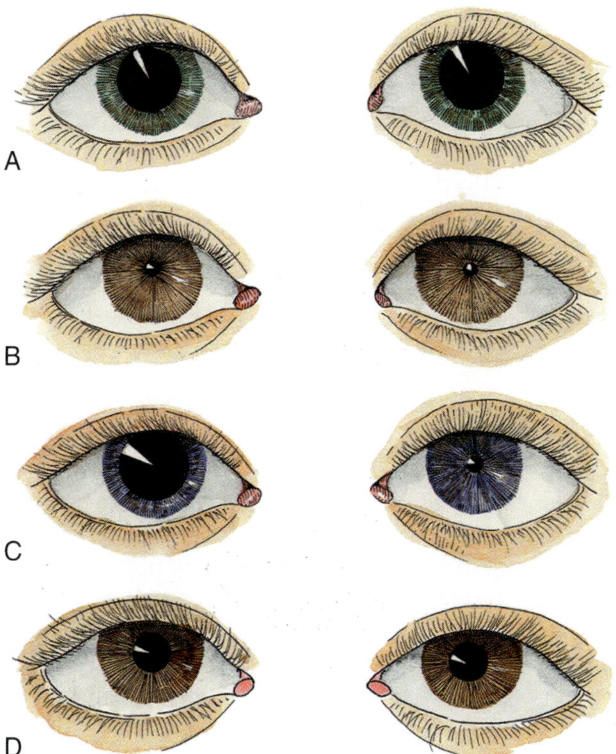

■ **Figure 1-29** A, Pupil dilation. B, Pupil constriction. C, Unequal pupils. D, Normal pupils. (From National Association of Emergency Medical Technicians: PHTLS: prehospital trauma life support, ed 6, St Louis, 2007, Mosby.)

stretched (Table 1-6). Using a reflex hammer and keeping the wrist relaxed, gently swing the hammer to tap the tendon. Support the joint or extremity being tested with your nondominant hand (Figure 1-30). Upper motor neuron lesions, such as in the brain or spinal cord, typically lead to hyperreflexia, whereas peripheral nerve lesions, such as with Guillain-Barré syndrome, cause hyporeflexia.

TABLE 1-6 Superficial and Deep Tendon Reflexes

Reflex	Spinal Level Evaluated
SUPERFICIAL	
Upper abdominal	T7, T8, and T9
Lower abdominal	T10 and T11
Cremasteric	T12, L1, and L2
Plantar	L4, L5, S1, and S2
DEEP TENDON	
Biceps	C5 and C6
Brachioradial	C5 and C6
Triceps	C6, C7, and C8
Patellar	L2, L3, and L4
Achilles	S1 and S2
SCORING DEEP TENDON REFLEXES	
Grade	**Deep Tendon Reflex Response**
0	No response
1+	Sluggish or diminished
2+	Active or expected response
3+	More brisk than expected, slightly hyperactive
4+	Brisk, hyperactive, with intermittent or transient clonus

From Sanders MJ: Mosby's paramedic textbook, ed 3, St Louis, 2009, Mosby.

Periodic reevaluation of the patient's response to questions about pain, discomfort, and difficulty breathing are important in gauging the effectiveness of interventions. The patient's physical exam should also be reevaluated, as appropriate, for diminished pain and discomfort, bleeding, and edema. Capillary refill time, distal pulses, and skin color, temperature, and moisture should also be reevaluated. Central nervous system function should be reassessed for improvement in GCS scores and motor, sensory, and pupil response.

Assessment Diagnostic Tools

Patient history, diagnostic tools, and physical exam can be targeted to a specific body system. Each body system presents a set of unique assessment options to rule in or rule out differential diagnoses. Using clinical reasoning, the provider can integrate new and unique information pertinent to the current patient with previous assessment and treatment knowledge discovered when responding to similar patients in the past and with evidence-based studies of the condition. Particularly in a hospital environment, providers will evaluate epidemiologic patterns, knowledge of the limitations of clinical findings, and an evidence-based understanding of the benefits and risks of various interventions. Interventions chosen take into account morbidity and mortality, short- and long-term effects, and projected quality of life for the patient.

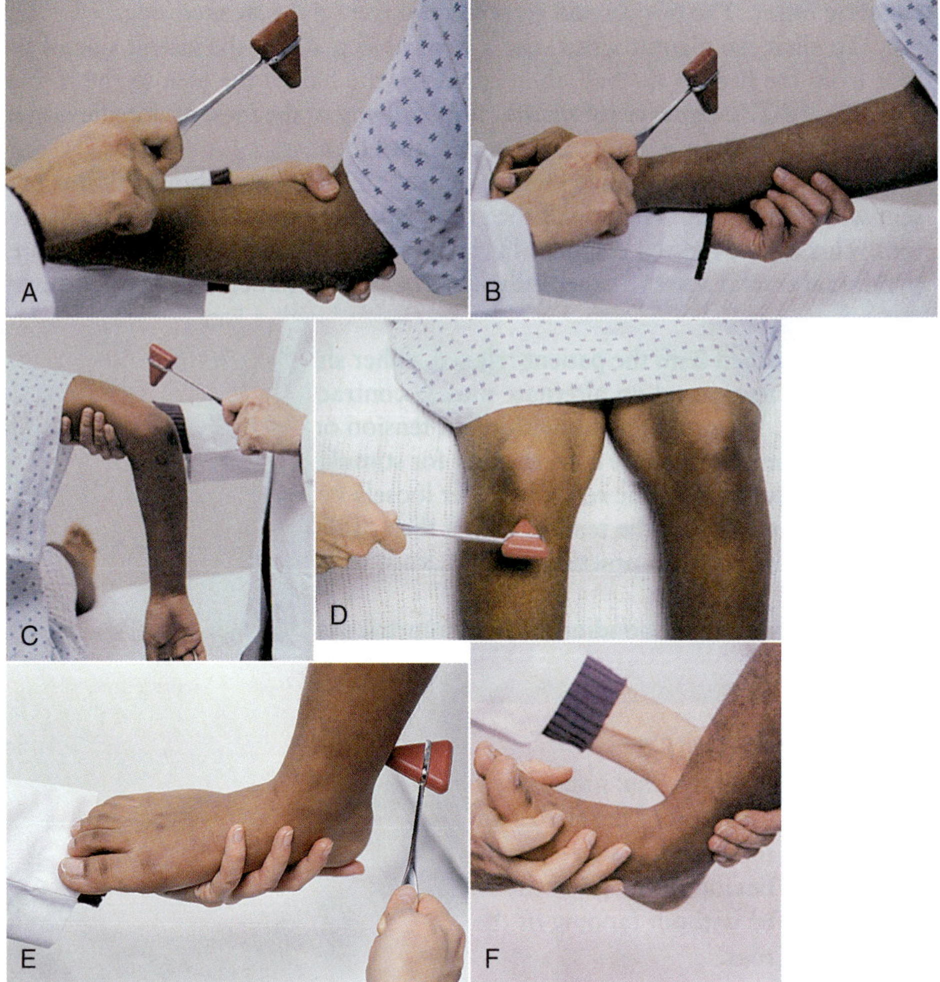

■ **Figure 1-30** Location of tendons for evaluation of deep tendon reflexes. **A**, Biceps. **B**, Brachioradial. **C**, Triceps. **D**, Patellar. **E**, Achilles. **F**, Evaluation of ankle clonus. (From Sanders MJ: Mosby's paramedic textbook—revised reprint, ed 3, St Louis, 2007, Mosby.)

Diagnostic Studies

Diagnostic tools can help identify a broad range of medical conditions. In-hospital technology may include computed tomography (CT), magnetic resonance imaging (MRI), cerebral angiography, ultrasonography, electroencephalography (EEG), and lumbar puncture, but prehospital diagnostic tools can also provide valuable information and prompt early, life-saving intervention.

Stroke Scales

Research indicates that using a stroke scale can help determine whether a patient has had a stroke. Although other assessment data and physical exam findings are needed to establish such a diagnosis, several consensus guidelines advocate using such a scale to make the rapid determination that a stroke is likely to have occurred. This early identification will prioritize the patient's treatment and transport. Many prehospital and in-hospital protocols also specify notification of a designated stroke team early in the assessment process (Box 1-10 and Figure 1-31).

Pulse Oximetry

This tool takes advantage of hemoglobin's propensity to absorb light, which results in an indirect measurement of oxygen saturation when a pulse oximetry probe is placed on a finger or toe (without nail polish) or earlobe. Oxygen saturation is an indication of how many hemoglobin-binding sites in the blood are occupied by (saturated with) oxygen molecules relative to the number available. This measurement is expressed as a percentage. Healthy people have an oxygen saturation of 97% to 99%. In a patient with a normal hemoglobin level, a saturation of 90% is minimally acceptable, but a saturation of 95% or better is preferable if it can be attained.

The tool is of minimal value in patients with poor perfusion attributable to autoimmune disease, endocrine emergencies, drug toxicity, or blood loss. In addition, pulse oximetry readings may be unreliable in patients with carbon monoxide poisoning, in smokers, and in diabetics with advanced peripheral vascular disease.

A patient whose oxygen saturation is 94% or lower may require supplemental oxygen delivered by a nasal cannula

■ **Los Angeles Prehospital Stroke Scale**

Criteria	Yes	Unknown	No
1 Age >45	☐	☐	☐
2 No history of seizures	☐	☐	☐
3 Symptome <24 hrs	☐	☐	☐
4 Not wheelchair-bound or bedridden at baseline	☐	☐	☐
5 Glucose 60-400	☐	☐	☐

Assess symmetry in facial movement, hand grip, or arm strength

	Normal	Right	Left
Facial smile/grimace	☐	☐ Droop	☐ Droop
Grip	☐	☐ Weak	☐ Weak
		☐ None	☐ None
Arm strength	☐	☐ Drifts down	☐ Drifts down
		☐ Falls rapidly	☐ Falls rapidly

	Yes	No
6 Based on exam, patient has only unilateral weakness	☐	☐

Items 1-6 all Yes or Unknown, then LAPSS criteria are met. If LAPSS criteria are met, then call the receiving hospital with a "cosde stroke"; if not, then return to the appropriate treatment protocol. (NOTE: The patient may still be experiencing a stroke even if the LAPSS criteria are not met.)

■ **Figure 1-31** Los Angeles Prehospital Stroke Scale. (From Aehlert BJ: Paramedic practice today: above and beyond, St Louis, 2009, Mosby.)

BOX 1-10 Cincinnati Prehospital Stroke Scale

Facial droop/weakness: Ask patient to "Show me your teeth" or "Smile for me."
- Normal: Both sides of face move equally well.
- Abnormal: One side of face does not move at all.

Motor weakness (arm drift): With eyes closed, ask patient to extend arms out in front 90 degrees (if sitting) or 45 degrees (if supine). Drift is scored if the arm falls before 10 seconds.
- Normal: Both arms move the same, or both arms do not move at all.
- Abnormal: One arm either does not move, or one arm drifts down compared with the other.

Aphasia (speech): Ask the patient to say "A rolling stone gathers no moss," You can't teach an old dog new tricks," "The sky is blue in Cincinnati," or a similar phrase.
- Normal: Phrase is repeated clearly and correctly.
- Abnormal: Patient uses inappropriate words, words are slurred, or the patient is unable to talk.

Reprinted from Kothari RU, Pancioli A, Liu T, et al: Cincinnati prehospital stroke scale: reproducibility and validity, Ann Emerg Med 33:373–378, 1999.

or nonrebreather mask (Figure 1-32). The percentage of supplemental oxygen administered will depend on assessment findings. Oxygen saturation findings are helpful to measure if assessed before and after application of supplemental oxygen.

Peak Flow Meter

Peak flow meters measure peak expiratory flow rate, or the rate at which a patient can breathe out. The rate is expressed in liters per minute (L/min). In patients with reactive airway disease, the rate diminishes because of increased resistance during exhalation. To participate in this test, the patient must be able to follow instructions to take deep breaths in and out (maximum inhalation and exhalation; see Figure 1-12, *A*).

End-Tidal CO_2 Monitoring

Capnography is used to monitor carbon dioxide levels in exhaled gases, or end-tidal carbon dioxide ($ETCO_2$). This

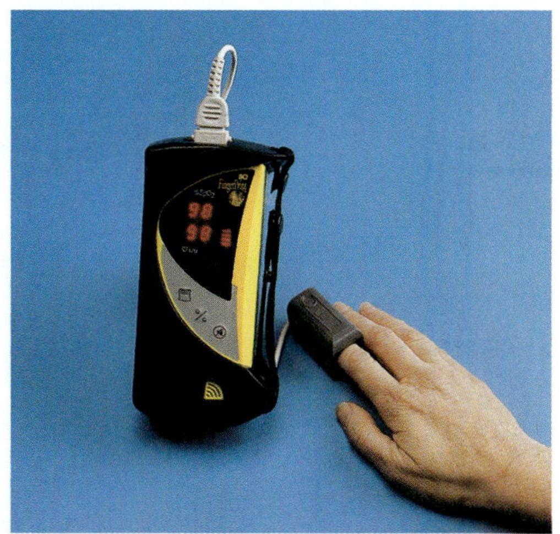

■ **Figure 1-32** Pulse oximeter. (From Sanders MJ: Mosby's paramedic textbook, revised ed 3, St Louis, 2007, MosbyJems.)

diagnostic assessment can give you a better understanding of the patient's ventilatory status. Capnography is projected as a waveform and a numerical value. The normal value of ETCO$_2$ in the blood is between 32 and 43 mm Hg.

Digital capnography can measure on a waveform tracing the exact amount of exhaled carbon dioxide. In addition, it can record air movement during inhalation and exhalation. This device allows continual monitoring of tracings. Abnormalities in inhalation or exhalation will alter the pattern of the waveforms.

Capnometry is the quantitative measurement of CO_2 without the waveform. A colorimetric capnometer provides semiquantitative information. This is a device with litmus paper that changes color in response to pH. The device can be placed between the airway and ventilating device. Exhaled air that contains no carbon dioxide will not change the paper color. Initially there is a dark purple color, and it turns to yellow/gold when there are near-normal levels of CO_2. If the litmus paper is exposed to stomach contents, it will also turn yellow/gold owing to acidity. The color should go from purple to yellow to purple with each ventilation to indicate the capnometer is accurately detecting CO_2.

Hypoventilation causes retention of CO_2, leading to respiratory acidosis (see Chapter 3). Increasing the percentage of supplemental oxygen, checking proper tracheal tube placement, and assisting ventilation with a bag-mask device is essential (Table 1-7).

Electrocardiography

An ECG records the electrical activity of the atrial and ventricular cells of the heart and represents this activity as specific waveforms and complexes. The ECG continuously detects and measures electrical flow on the patient's skin. Electrocardiographic testing is used to detect acute myocardial ischemia and to monitor a patient's heart rate, evaluate the effects of disease or injury on heart function, analyze pacemaker function, and assess response to medications. The ECG does not provide information about the heart's contractile (mechanical) function.

Whether using a 3-lead, 12-lead, 15-lead, or 18-lead ECG, reviewing various views of the frontal surface, horizontal axis, and left ventricle of the heart provides key information about ischemia and infarction. The standard 12-lead ECG visualizes the heart in the frontal and horizontal planes and views the surfaces of the left ventricle from 12 different angles. Having multiple views of the heart makes possible the recognition of bundle branch blocks, the identification of ST-segment changes such as ischemia, injury, or infarct, and the analysis of ECG changes associated with medications. Extended lead placement, as in the 15- and 18-lead devices, allows additional anterior and posterior views.

ECG monitoring is typically performed in patients who are having difficulty breathing or who have chest or abdominal discomfort or pain, particularly if the patient has both complaints. ST-segment elevation MI (STEMI) points toward an acute, evolving myocardial necrosis. Non-ST-segment elevation MI (NSTEMI) may show up on ECG as ST-segment depression and T-wave inversion. When reviewing 12-lead ECGs, several patterns may mimic ST elevation, including left bundle branch block (LBBB) and pericarditis. More detailed information is available in Appendix B.

Cardiac Enzymes

The most sensitive and specific enzymes to detect cardiac damage are the cardiac-specific troponins. This test is

TABLE 1-7 Capnography-Related Terms

Term	Description
Capnography	Continuous analysis and recording of CO_2 concentrations in respiratory gases Output displayed as a waveform Graphic display of the CO_2 concentration versus time during a respiratory cycle CO_2 concentration may also be plotted versus expiratory volume.
Capnometer	Device used to measure the concentration of CO_2 at the end of exhalation
Capnometry	A numeric reading of exhaled CO_2 concentrations without a continuous written record or waveform Output is a numerical value. Numeric display of CO_2 on a monitor
Capnograph	A device that provides a numeric reading of exhaled CO_2 concentrations and a waveform (tracing)
Exhaled CO_2 detector	A capnometer that provides a noninvasive estimate of alveolar ventilation, the concentration of exhaled CO_2 from the lungs, and arterial CO_2 content; also called an end-tidal CO_2 detector
Colorimetric ETCO$_2$ detector	A device that provides CO_2 readings by chemical reaction on pH-sensitive litmus paper housed in the detector The presence of CO_2 (evidenced by a color change on the colorimetric device) suggests tracheal placement.
Qualitative ETCO$_2$ monitor	A device that uses a light to indicate the presence of ETCO$_2$

ETCO$_2$, End-tidal carbon dioxide.
From Aehlert BJ: Paramedic practice today: above and beyond, St Louis, 2010, MosbyJems.

usually elevated within 4 to 6 hours of onset of the infarct, and elevation persists for 5 to 7 days. Besides signaling acute MI, these enzymes may also be elevated in the case of unstable angina, myocarditis, and congestive heart failure (CHF).

Damaged myocardial tissue cells also release the cardiac enzyme creatine kinase (CK); specifically, a subtype called *CK-MB* is released from heart muscle tissue. CK elevation is seen 4 to 8 hours after MI and returns to normal within 24 to 48 hours. Muscle damage, such as from bruising or rhabdomyolysis, renal failure, low thyroid hormones (triiodothyronine, thyroxine, thyroid-stimulating hormone [T_3, T_4, TSH]), and alcohol abuse can increase values unrelated to an MI.

Other hematologic studies frequently ordered include erythrocyte (red blood cell [RBC]) counts, leukocyte (white blood cell [WBC]) counts, hemoglobin, hematocrit, erythrocyte sedimentation rate (ESR), prothrombin time (PT), international normalized ratio (INR), and partial thromboplastin time (PTT). These values are important in patients suspected of having a thrombus or embolus.

Cardiac Stress Testing

Cardiac stress testing can demonstrate the presence of functional ischemia. Stress on the heart may be induced by exercise such as walking on a treadmill or pedaling on a bicycle while the patient is undergoing continuous cardiac monitoring in multiple leads. The ECG is then observed for signs of ischemia during exercise. Cardiac stress can also be induced by administration of vasodilating medications such as adenosine.

Stress testing can be combined with nuclear imaging before and after the cardiac stress portion. The imaging studies can then allow visualization of areas of the heart that show compromised blood flow during exertion. Such compromise is usually caused by stenosis in the coronary arteries.

Cardiac Catheterization

Cardiac catheterization may be warranted in patients with suspected cardiovascular abnormalities who have unstable angina, heart failure with a history that suggests coronary artery disease, or myocardial ischemia. Emergency cardiac catheterization is the treatment of choice for patients with acute STEMI.

Catheterization can be used to visualize either the right or left side of the heart as well as the coronary arteries. Stenosis, regurgitation, coronary artery occlusion, and ventricular ejection fractions can be identified. The information conveyed by a cardiac catheterization study can be critical in guiding clinical decision making.

Central Venous Pressure Monitoring

In patients with significant variances in fluid volume, central venous pressure (CVP) monitoring is performed. CVP measurements can be used to assess volume status and right heart function (Table 1-8). CVP catheters can have a single, dual, or triple lumen (Figure 1-33). The

TABLE 1-8 Central Venous Access Devices

Type of Catheter	Benefits	Maintenance Considerations
Peripherally inserted central catheter (PICC)	Used for therapy of short to moderate duration	Antecubital vein most common site (may limit movement of arm)
	Less costly	Risk of infection
		May become dislodged easily (most are not sutured into place)
Tunneled catheter:	Used for long-term therapy	Daily heparin flushes required
Hickman	Easy to use for self-administered infusions	Must be clamped or have clamp ready at all times
Broviac		Site must be kept dry
		Risk of infection
		Protrudes from body
		Susceptible to damage
		May be pulled out
		May alter patient body image
Implanted ports:	Used for long-term therapy	Must pierce skin to access port
Port-A-Cath	Reduced risk of infection	Pain associated with needle insertion (may use local anesthetic such as EMLA cream)
Infus-A-Port		
Mediport	Only slight bulge on chest; completely under skin	Special needle (Huber) required to access port
	Increased safety (under skin and minimal maintenance care)	Must prepare skin before injection
	Reduced cost for family	Catheter may dislodge from port, especially if child "plays" with site
	Regular physical activity (including swimming) not restricted	Generally not allowed to engage in vigorous contact sports
	Heparinized monthly and after each injection	Difficult for self-administered infusions

EMLA, Eutectic mixture of local anesthetics.
From DeNaras WC, Proctor BD, Lee CH: Income, poverty, and health insurance coverage in the United States: 2005, U.S. Census Bureau Current Population Reports, Washington, DC, 2006, U.S. Government Printing Office.

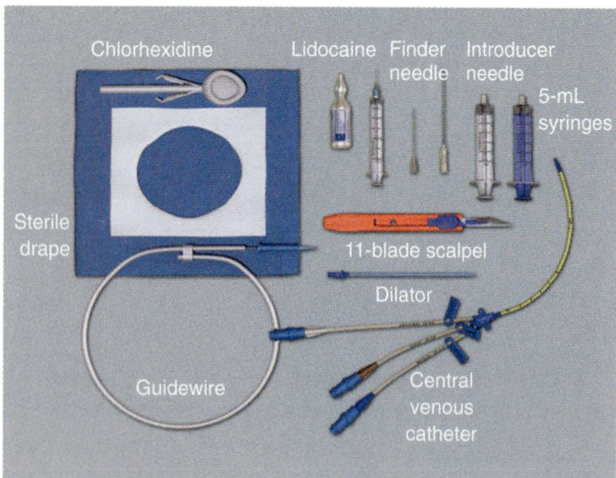

■ **Figure 1-33** Equipment used for central vein catheterization. (From Roberts JR, Hedges JR: Clinical procedures in emergency medicine, ed 5, Philadelphia, 2009, Saunders.)

subclavian and internal jugular veins are the vessels of choice for measuring right heart filling pressures. The CVP measurements are considered in combination with mean arterial pressure (MAP) and other clinical parameters to guide clinical reasoning and ensure hemodynamic stability. In the hypovolemic patient, CVP will fall before MAP and thus is an earlier harbinger of instability. CVP can be helpful in clinical decision making in patients with hypotension and uncertain intravascular volume status.

Laboratory Studies

Laboratory studies such as serum bilirubin, serum albumin, hemoglobin, hematocrit, blood urea nitrogen (BUN), and creatinine results are evaluated for blood loss, metabolic acidosis, renal or hepatic disease, dehydration, and malabsorption syndromes. Laboratory and radiographic tests are ordered to identify the presence of kidney stones, ulcers, and obstructions to the GI, GU, and reproductive systems.

Radiography

To assist in the neurologic exam, spine x-rays can help determine the size and shape of bony structures and can reveal degenerative processes, dislocations, and fractures (Figure 1-34).

A chest radiograph can assess the heart, aorta, and pulmonary vessels. It can also be used to confirm proper positioning of tubes and wires placed in the chest. Tracheal tubes, implanted defibrillators, and pacemaker devices can be viewed.

Bilateral alveolar infiltrates seen on a chest radiograph are a significant sign of acute respiratory distress syndrome (ARDS). Aspirated foreign bodies lodged in the airway passages may also be seen. Congestion with or without alveolar edema, as seen in CHF, and a focal infiltrate may represent pneumonia or a mass.

Noninvasive diagnostic tools such as single-plane radiographs are valuable in identifying chest abnormalities. Figure 1-35 shows the chest x-ray of a patient with heart failure. Chest x-ray can help detect cardiac conditions such as pulmonary congestion and pleural effusion from heart failure, an enlarged heart, aortic valve stenosis, and regurgitation.

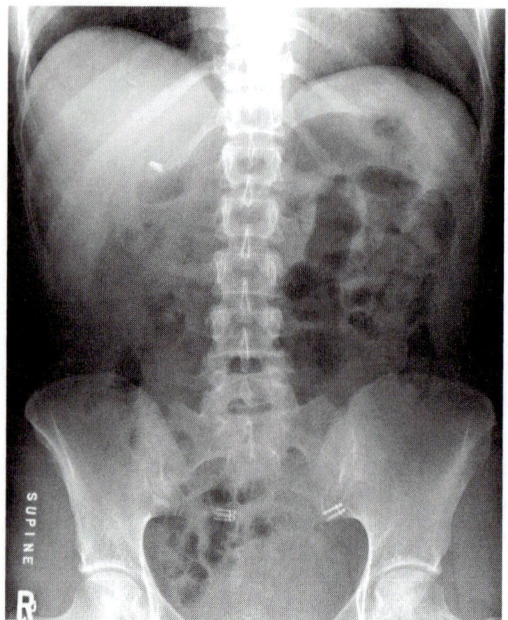

■ **Figure 1-34** Abdominal x-ray. (From McQuillen K: Radiographic image analysis, ed 2, St Louis, 2006, Saunders.)

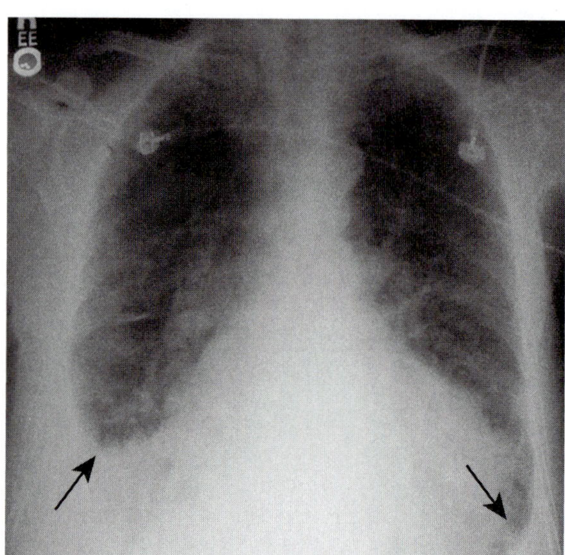

■ **Figure 1-35** Chest x-ray. (From Roberts JR, Hedges JR: Clinical procedures in emergency medicine, ed 5, Philadelphia, 2009, Saunders.)

SPECIAL POPULATIONS

Older Adult Patients

The American Geriatrics Society has estimated that more than a third of all EMS calls are in response to an older adult patient. Many older adults lead healthy, active lives, but others are plagued with chronic health problems. Assessment of the geriatric patient is more challenging than that of a younger adult for a variety of reasons. Let's consider a few of them.

Medications

Most older adults take three to five prescription medications, a situation referred to as *polypharmacy*. **Pharmacokinetics**—the absorption, distribution, metabolism, and excretion of medications—differs in older adults compared to younger patients. As a result, they tend to have adverse drug reactions more often, especially when they are also taking OTC medications or dietary supplements such as herbal preparations or nutritional drinks. The most common adverse reactions to medications are confusion, sedation, loss of balance, nausea, and electrolyte abnormalities.

Communication

Communication may be difficult if the patient has a hearing or speech-language impairment. However, most older adults are able to hear normally. If a patient does have hearing aids, make sure they're set at the proper volume.

Patience is vital when taking a history. Older adults often can't recall the names of medications or what conditions they've been prescribed for. In addition, they may process questions slowly and feel obligated to share information they believe is important before answering the question directly. Such extra information may prove helpful when trying to work through the differential diagnosis.

Breathing

The pulmonary system undergoes changes in the older adult. The kyphosis (curvature) of the thoracic spine that often occurs with advancing age can make expanding the lungs more difficult. The respiratory muscles weaken, causing respiratory fatigue and failure earlier than in younger adults. This decrement is perhaps attributable to lifelong exposure to environmental pollutants or to repeated lung infections over the years. In addition, the elasticity of the lungs and chest wall decrease with age, diminishing tidal volume. Because of these changes, the respiratory rate normally increases to compensate and maintain an adequate minute volume.

If a patient shows signs/symptoms of hypoxia, oxygen must be given in an effort to attain an oxygen saturation of 95% or greater. When transporting a patient who has shortness of breath, the patient may ask to sit upright. It's generally advisable to allow this, since patients are usually better able to determine for themselves which position makes breathing easier.

Cardiovascular System

Many changes occur in the cardiovascular system of an older adult patient. Large arteries become less elastic, creating more pressure in the arteriole system during systole. This raises systolic blood pressure, leading in turn to a widened pulse pressure (the difference between systolic and diastolic blood pressure). Peripheral vascular resistance (PVR) may increase, and diastolic blood pressure and MAP may rise, resulting in hypertension. Common cardiac problems among older adults include MI, heart failure, dysrhythmias, aneurysms, and hypertension.

When obtaining a history from the older adult patient complaining of chest pain or discomfort, try to ascertain his or her level of cardiovascular fitness. Older people who regularly engage in physical activity are able to maintain better cardiac function.

Assessment of the older adult for cognitive changes can be difficult without family members or friends to whom you can direct questions about the patient's history. If possible, determine the patient's baseline mental status, and then assess for any changes in behavior, thought processes, and mood (Figure 1-36). Ask family or friends

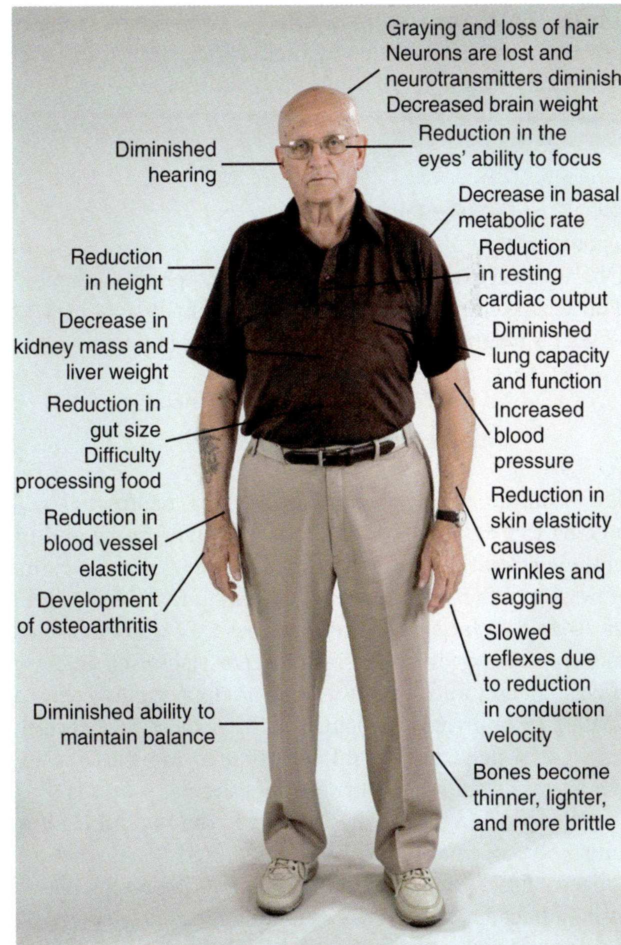

■ **Figure 1-36** The changes of aging. (From Aehlert BJ: Paramedic practice today: above and beyond, St Louis, 2009, Mosby.)

about any recent changes in the patient's hygiene and food preparation habits.

Physical Exam

In older adult patients, orthostatic hypotension attributable to diminished baroreceptor function can be a concern during the physical exam. Take care to have these patients move slowly to better accommodate blood volume changes.

Terminally Ill Patients

Hospice services include supportive social, emotional, and spiritual care for patients and their families at the end of life. Patients who are terminally ill, such as those with advanced cancer or acquired immunodeficiency syndrome (AIDS), often receive palliative care (comfort care). Medical needs vary depending on the disease but typically center on pain management.

The terminally ill patient may have medical and legal documents such as advance directives or do-not-resuscitate (DNR) orders. Some states have specific DNR paperwork, so healthcare providers should familiarize yourself with specific policies, procedures, and regulations in your part of the country. In many states, a provider's scope of practice governs whether a prehospital healthcare provider may honor legal DNR advance directives or living wills.

Bariatric Patients

Obesity is an excessive amount of weight relative to height. The CDC defines obesity in terms of body mass index (BMI), a height/weight ratio calculated as follows:

$$\text{BMI} = [\text{Weight (lb)} \div (\text{Height (inches)} \times \text{Height (inches)}] \times 703$$

For example, a person who is 5 feet 5 inches tall and weighs 135 lb has a BMI of 22.5, which falls in the middle of the normal range for a person of that height and weight. A person of the same height who weighs 180 lb has a BMI of 30 and is thus, by definition, obese. BMI is calculated more precisely for children and teens, factoring in their precise height and weight as well as their age and sex. A BMI of 39 or greater, or being 100 lb or more over recommended weight for height, constitutes morbid obesity, which carries more serious health risks.

Obesity is a chronic disease and is the second leading cause of preventable death in the United States (behind tobacco use). Obese (bariatric) patients are at increased risk of diabetes, hypertension, coronary heart disease, dyslipidemia, stroke, liver disease, gallbladder disease, sleep apnea, respiratory disorders, osteoarthritis, infertility in women, and certain types of cancer. Morbidly obese persons may develop pulmonary hypertension and right-sided heart failure, known as *cor pulmonale*. Early evidence, and perhaps common sense, suggests that obese patients are also more likely than their fit peers to suffer complications after contracting the H1N1 (swine flu) virus.

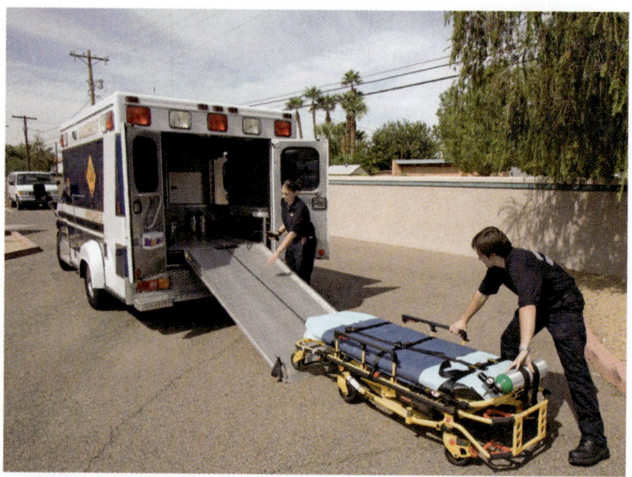

Figure 1-37 Some EMS services have specialized equipment and vehicles to care for bariatric patients. (From Aehlert BJ: Paramedic practice today: above and beyond, St Louis, 2009, Mosby.)

Moving the Bariatric Patient

EMS agencies must have policies for handling obese patients because of the additional risk they pose to providers and the extra demands they place on EMS staff and resources. Scene assessment is especially important, since the patient may first need to be extricated from his or her home or car, and extra staff may have to be called in to load and unload the obese patient into (ideally) a specially equipped bariatric ambulance (Figure 1-37). Be sure to ask the patient's weight—estimated, if the patient doesn't know it—and call for lift assistance if necessary.

Both provider and patient are at particularly high risk as the patient is being moved. Providers are subject to heavy-lifting injuries. Patients can be dropped or may roll off surfaces that were not designed to accommodate them, such as standard-sized backboards. High-capacity carrying sheets made of plastic with built-in side handles may be a good alternative to moving the patient on a stretcher.

Providing Specialized Medical Devices and Supplies

The agency should have on hand the proper equipment and supplies needed to care for obese patients, such as extra-large blood pressure cuffs, long-length needles for intramuscular injections or needle decompression, large cervical collars, extra-long straps and taping supplies, and large gowns, sheets, and blankets. Bariatric mannequins are now available for use in training EMS providers to care for bariatric patients, although they may be prohibitively expensive for most agencies.

Obstetric Patients

Emergent pregnancy-related problems include spontaneous abortion, ectopic pregnancy, premature labor, hemorrhage, blood clots, preeclampsia, infection, stroke, amniotic fluid embolism, diabetes, and heart disease. Begin by assessing the patient's skin color, temperature, and moisture. Maternal physiology changes as early as the first trimester. Heart rate quickens by 10 to 15 bpm. Respiratory rate also increases as the enlarging uterus pushes up on the diaphragm, causing breathing to become more rapid and shallow. Assess the patient's vital signs for evidence of dehydration and shock.

In early stages of pregnancy, usually the fifth to tenth weeks, abdominal pain, vaginal bleeding, and signs of shock can indicate ectopic pregnancy. These patients should be assessed for pregnancy-induced hypertension and gestational diabetes.

In later stages of pregnancy, patients who complain of tearing abdominal pain and vaginal bleeding with dark-colored blood may be experiencing an abruption, or separation of the placenta from the uterine wall. Painless vaginal bleeding in the last trimester can indicate a placenta previa, where the placenta is bleeding. Both conditions are life-threatening medical emergencies and require rapid transport.

Postpartum pathology may include hemorrhage, infection, and pulmonary embolism. Fever and severe abdominal pain are symptoms of endometritis (infection of the uterus), which can be very serious. A medical history related to the pregnancy must be obtained, including delivery by cesarean section.

SPECIAL CONSIDERATIONS

Air Transport

Depending on the proximity to the hospital and its specialization, some patients will be transported by air. Transfer from one facility to another, such as from a community hospital to a burn center, may also occur by air. Helicopters and fixed-wing aircraft (airplanes; Figure 1-38) have been used for patient transport by both civilian and military medical systems almost since the dawn of aviation. Patients who are critically ill and medically unstable may be considered for helicopter transport, especially when definitive care on the ground will be delayed. Box 1-11 gives examples of medical conditions that might be considered for air transport.

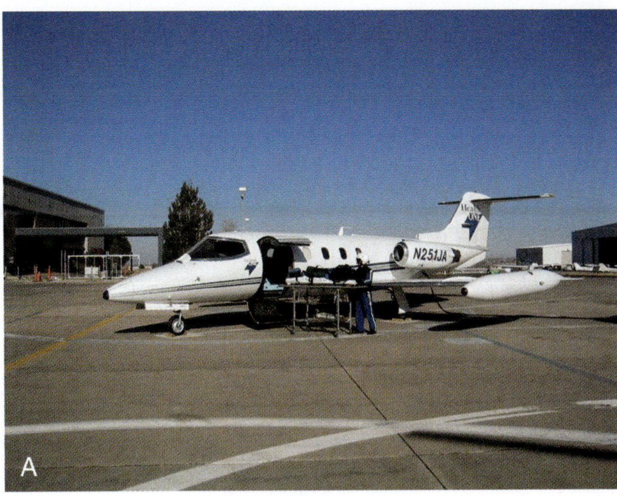

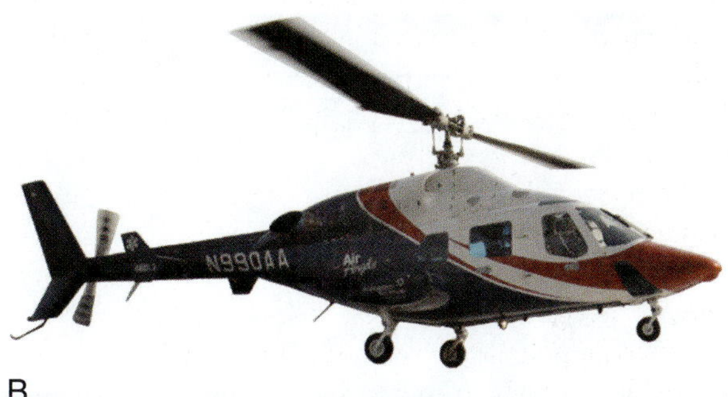

■ **Figure 1-38** **A**, Air medical fixed-wing aircraft. **B**, Air medical helicopter. (**A** from Lewis SM, Heitkemper MM, Dirksen SR: Medical-surgical nursing: assessment and management of clinical problems, ed 5, St Louis, 2000, Mosby. **B** courtesy Robert Vroman.)

BOX 1-11 Medical Conditions That May Necessitate Air Transport

- Bleeding or imminent rupture of a dissecting aortic aneurysm
- Intracranial bleeding
- Acute (time-dependent for treatment) ischemic stroke
- Severe hypothermia and hyperthermia
- Cardiac dysfunction requiring immediate intervention
- Status asthmaticus
- Status epilepticus

Each EMS provider should be familiar with the ground and air transport options in his or her geographic area. The decision to transport a patient by air has some advantages and some drawbacks (Box 1-12). Air transport allows the patient to be rescued in a remote area if necessary, transported quickly, and transferred rapidly to a specialty unit. In addition, specialized personnel or supplies (e.g., antivenin, blood products) can be delivered in minutes or hours rather than days. However, flying is often restricted in bad weather, and all aircraft have load restrictions that limit the number and weight of patients

BOX 1-12 Advantages and Disadvantages of Air Medical Transport

ADVANTAGES

- Rapid transportation
- Access to remote areas
- Access to specialty units such as neonatal intensive care units and burn centers
- Access to personnel with specialized skills
- Access to specialized equipment and supplies

DISADVANTAGES

- Weather and environmental restrictions to flight
- Limitations on patient weight
- Limitations on number of patients that can be transported
- Altitude limitations
- Airspeed limitations
- High cost
- Difficulties delivering patient care because of limited access and cabin size
- Limitations of the amounts of equipment and supplies that can be carried

From Aehlert BJ: Paramedic practice today: above and beyond, St Louis, 2009, Mosby.

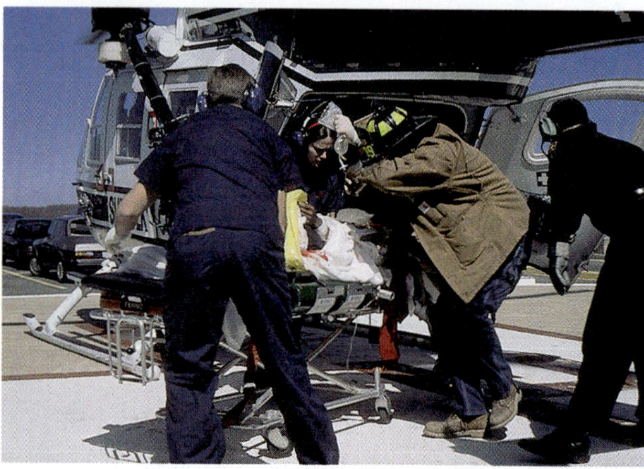

Figure 1-39 Helicopters can provide rapid transport to the hospital for critical patients. (From Applegate EJ: The anatomy and physiology learning system, Philadelphia, 1995, Saunders.)

who can be transported at once or at all. It's not just total passenger weight that counts, but the number of passengers, since the weight in an aircraft must be properly distributed. Each aircraft is different; one may be able to accommodate a tail-heavy load, whereas the same distribution pattern would be unsafe in another aircraft.

In addition, patients with certain conditions cannot easily tolerate high altitude, vibration, and rapid changes in barometric pressure. The altitude at which an aircraft flies depends on the type of aircraft, weather conditions, noise abatement procedures pilots must follow to reduce engine noise in certain areas, geography of the terrain below (for obvious reasons, aircraft fly higher over mountainous terrain and forested areas), altitude restrictions in heavily trafficked urban air corridors, and other factors.

Helicopter transport (Figure 1-39) requires observance of proper safety procedures, such as finding a landing zone of adequate size (at least 100 × 100 feet) and a location (downwind of the patient care area) that is relatively level, firm, and free of dangerous obstructions such as power lines, trees, poles, buildings, and rocks. Each EMS provider should be updated annually on local helicopter safety requirements and communications procedures.

Flight Physiology

The healthcare provider—in many instances, the paramedic—must select the most suitable mode of transportation for the patient, based on his or her condition, the specialty care offered at the receiving facility, and the safest, most efficient means available by which to move the patient. Likewise, in-hospital providers use similar criteria to determine whether to transfer a patient by air or ground.

If air medical transport is thought to be in the best clinical interest of the patient, you must prepare him or her for transport. Although the transport crew is responsible for the patient's safety during the flight, proper preflight preparation is the responsibility of the prehospital or in-hospital provider, who must be aware of factors that affect the patient during flight. For example, you should understand how factors such as vertigo (dizziness), changes in temperature and barometric pressure, gravity, and spatial disorientation might affect the patient (Figure 1-40 and Box 1-13).

Barometric Pressure

Patients with underlying pulmonary disease such as COPD, asthma, or pulmonary edema are at high risk of hypoxia when barometric pressure drops. Diminished barometric pressure during flight can reduce the PaO_2 in the alveoli, in turn reducing blood oxygen saturation. During flight, the patient may need supplemental oxygen or tracheal intubation to maintain adequate oxygen saturation.

Patients who have sinus infections may experience severe sinus pressure or pain during flight, or epistaxis (nosebleed) can occur during ascent as gases trapped in the sinus cavity expand. In such patients, nasal vasoconstrictors can be administered prophylactically before the flight.

Helicopters rarely fly above 1000 feet, so changes in barometric pressure are not clinically significant. However, with fixed-wing transport, this must be taken into consideration.

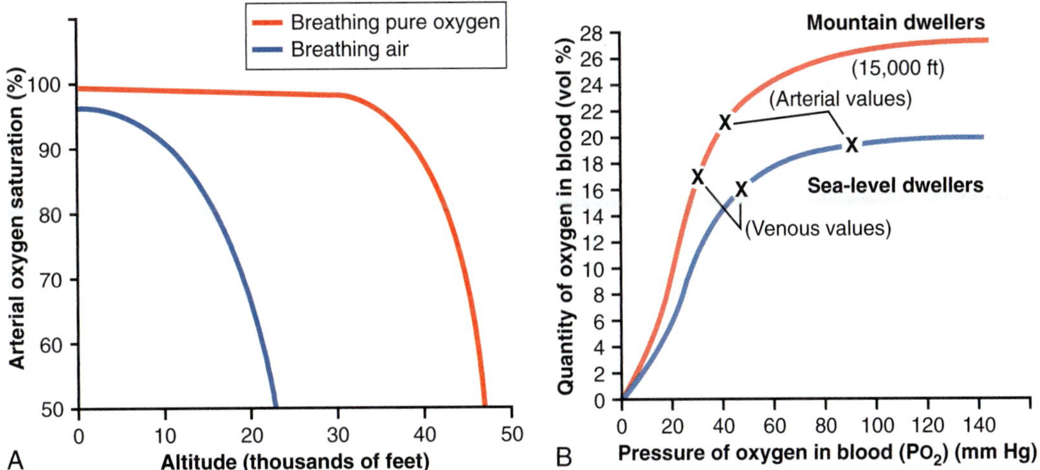

Figure 1-40 A, Effect of high altitude on arterial oxygen saturation when breathing air and when breathing pure oxygen. B, Oxygen-hemoglobin dissociation curves for blood of high-altitude residents *(red curve)* and sea-level residents *(blue curve)*, showing respective arterial and venous Po_2 levels and oxygen contents as recorded in their native surroundings. (Data from Oxygen-dissociation curves for bloods of high-altitude and sea-level residents. PAHO Scientific Publication No. 140, Life at high altitudes, 1966. In Guyton AC, Hall JE, editors: Textbook of medical physiology, ed 11, Philadelphia, 2006, Saunders.)

BOX 1-13 Landing Zone and Scene Operations

LANDING ZONE

- Ensure the landing zone is a minimum of 100 × 100 feet.
- Identify and mark any obstructions in the immediate area.
- Identify the landing zone by GPS coordinates or a major nearby intersection.
- Inform the flight crew of the landing surface and slope.
- Mark the corners of the landing zone with cones or other easily visible objects in the daytime. Place a fifth marker on the upwind side of the landing zone. Make sure markers are secured or heavy enough that they will not blow away.
- For night operations, mark the corners of the landing zone with ground strobes, secured flares, or vehicles with their lights on. Place a fifth lighted marker on the upwind side of the landing zone.

SCENE OPERATIONS

- Keep spectators at least 200 feet away.
- Ensure personal equipment is secured (e.g., no hats).
- Do not approach the helicopter until you are signaled by one of the crew members.
- Always approach from the front of the helicopter, never from the tail.
- Never bend over when approaching the helicopter. The rotors are 10 feet above the ground, and you are more likely to trip and fall if you are looking down.
- Do not hold anything above your head.
- Do not wear a hat.

GPS, Global positioning system.
From Aehlert B: Paramedic practice today: above and beyond, St Louis, 2009, Mosby.

Humidity

As altitude increases, the amount of moisture in the aircraft decreases as fresh air from the outside is drawn into the cabin. Therefore, supplemental oxygen should be administered with humidification to prevent dehydration of the patient's mucous membranes and nasal passages.

Temperature

The patient should be adequately protected from wind and cold to ensure that they remain normothermic. The transport team should be notified of the patient's hydration status and of any medications, such as sedatives, that have been administered. Alterations in cabin temperature with descent and ascent can disrupt a poorly hydrated and sedated patient's ability to maintain their core body temperature.

Other Considerations

Anxiety is an emotional factor to consider when a patient is being transported by air. If conscious, the patient should be briefed on the types of aircraft vibrations and sounds that might experienced during flight and on how long the flight is expected to take. Ill or injured patients can have physiologic signs and symptoms attributable to air turbulence or engine vibrations. The patient may have motion sickness or abdominal pain or trouble staying warm.

Patients with a history or risk of seizures should be visually protected from the flashing lights they might see during the aircraft's ascent and descent.

Safety

Take basic safety precautions when you are around fixed-wing or rotary aircraft. Navigate carefully around rotating helicopter and propeller blades. Always approach a helicopter from the front or side, in view of the pilot. Whether you are a prehospital or in-hospital provider, you must heed the flight crew's instructions when you are loading or unloading a patient.

Wilderness Conditions

EMS providers are often confronted with austere conditions that complicate the assessment process. Care delivery in such conditions is often called *wilderness medicine*. Loosely defined, wilderness medicine is medical management in situations in which care is limited by environmental considerations, prolonged extrication, or limited resource availability. You may encounter such situations in remote areas like national parks, or in cities or suburbs, such as when caring for a patient who is suffering from hypothermia or has been struck by lightning. Unfamiliar situations occurring in a familiar environment, such as an earthquake in your city, may call upon your wilderness medicine skills.

Wilderness EMS is a subset of EMS operations that requires specialized training. Personnel need training in technical rope rescue, prevention of hypothermia, and the safety precautions to follow when working in an unpredictable, unsafe outdoor environment that poses threats ranging from ravines to rattlesnakes. The National Association of Emergency Medical Technicians (NAEMT) has compiled a list of variables that affect wilderness EMS activities, shown in Box 1-14.

BOX 1-14 Variables in Wilderness EMS Activities

- Access to the scene
- Weather
- Daylight
- Terrain
- Special transport and handling times
- Access and transport times
- Available personnel
- Communications

From National Association of Emergency Medical Technicians [NAEMT]: PHTLS: prehospital trauma life support, ed 6, St Louis, 2007, Mosby.

The wilderness EMT's scope of practice may have to be expanded to include cervical spine clearance, administration of medications (e.g., steroids, antibiotics), and additional interventions such as shoulder reductions and sutures. According to the Academy of Wilderness Medicine, many programs in this specialty have been developed, and fellowship and residency programs are available within emergency medicine and paramedic programs. Programs that have been established in the field are offered by the U.S. National Park Service, the National Ski Patrol, the Mountain Rescue Association, the Divers Alert Network, and many other organizations.

SCENARIO SOLUTION

1 Auscultation of breath sounds will be difficult in a bariatric patient. If the patient needs an advanced airway, the vocal cords will likely be difficult to view. Moving the patient will be difficult and must be done with great care to preserve the patient's dignity and reduce the risk of injury to the patient and rescuers. Time on scene will be longer than normal.

2 You should consider heart failure (although right heart failure is more common in this group), pulmonary embolus or pneumonia (recent abdominal surgery and bed rest), asthma attack (history), sepsis related to wound infection, acidosis (related to drugs or metabolic causes), and anxiety or pain (unlikely because of the cardinal presentation).

3 Assessment should include complete vital sign assessment (including body temperature), auscultation of breath and heart sounds, observation for JVD and peripheral edema, wound assessment for signs of infection, pulse oximetry, electrocardiogram, blood glucose analysis, and waveform capnography.

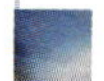

Putting It All Together

A systematic, thorough, efficient patient assessment is the backbone of effective management. The AMLS assessment pathway is built on the assumption that providers already have a broad understanding of human anatomy, physiology, pathophysiology, and epidemiology to complement the assessment and management processes. Beyond this foundation, your clinical reasoning, therapeutic communication, and clinical decision-making skills all affect your ability to integrate historical data, physical exam findings, and the results of diagnostic assessments to arrive at a working diagnosis. Implementation of appropriate treatment modalities hinges on the accuracy of this assessment information.

Since patients' cardinal presentations are often subtle, the dependability of your judgment is the key to timely, effective intervention. Most of the assessment information, especially in patients with emergent presentations, is obtained during history taking. Since patients tend to be poor historians, you must use your senses, and let your experience guide your decisions.

Initial observations begin with the dispatch information. Scene assessment gives you a preview of the patient's condition even before any direct interaction takes place. All scenes or situations, whether prehospital or in-hospital, should be evaluated for safety. Home environments should be assessed for medical devices, environmental issues, and indications of chronic disease processes. Once the area is deemed safe, you should begin to note the patient's affect and body position, breath sounds and respiratory pattern, coloring, odor, and other physical characteristics. Any life threats must be addressed immediately. Then you should proceed to the primary survey, which comprises an evaluation of the patient's LOC, airway, breathing, and circulation/perfusion status. This assessment, while finished in a matter of seconds, should be systematic and thorough to identify any emergent conditions for which urgent intervention is needed. Gather your first impression and determine how sick the patient is, whether he's likely to deteriorate, and if so, which body systems might be affected.

In the secondary survey, the provider applies clinical reasoning to the patient's cardinal presentation. Historical information is obtained by soliciting information about the present illness (OPQRST) and past medical history (SAMPLER) (see Rapid Recall boxes). Diagnostic information obtained from pulse oximetry devices, blood glucose meters, lab tests, radiographic imaging studies, 3-lead or 12-lead ECG monitoring, and $ETCO_2$ devices are analyzed to confirm or eliminate various diagnoses. Evaluation of pain or discomfort assessment is also performed during the secondary survey if the patient has such a complaint. In addition, vital signs and a physical exam help rule in or rule out differential diagnoses until you settle on a working diagnosis.

Associated symptoms are investigated to determine the acuity of the working diagnoses and to identify underlying conditions that need to be managed. A detailed head-to-toe physical exam is performed on patients with minimal LOCs if on-scene and transport time allow. A focused physical exam should be performed on patients with non-emergent presentations.

Communication, assessment, and management barriers can be encountered in patients with special challenges, such as bariatric patients, older adults, and obstetric patients. Transport decisions take into consideration the patient's condition but must also yield to exogenous factors such as weather, maximum aircraft load capacity, capabilities of the receiving hospital, and distance of the most appropriate facility.

All healthcare providers can apply the AMLS pathway to the care of every patient, especially those with medical emergencies. The AMLS pathway is a dynamic and ongoing assessment process in which conclusions are continually revised as more information about the patient's history and current status becomes available. The process promotes remarkable patient care from dispatch to delivery at the receiving facility.

SUMMARY

- The AMLS assessment pathway is a dependable framework allowing for early recognition and management of a variety of medical emergencies, with a goal of improved patient outcome.
- The patient's history, physical exam, risk factors, chief complaint, and cardinal presentation help suggest possible differential diagnoses.
- Therapeutic communication skills, keen clinical reasoning abilities, and expert clinical decision making are the foundation for the AMLS assessment.
- Patient assessment and management can be hindered by social, linguistic, behavioral, or psychological barriers.
- Effective clinical reasoning requires gathering and organizing relevant historical and diagnostic information, filtering out irrelevant or extraneous information, and reflecting on similar experiences to efficiently determine working diagnoses and management priorities.
- Clinical reasoning is a bridge between historical information and diagnostic test results, allowing the provider to draw inferences about underlying etiologies to formulate differential diagnoses.
- Barriers for efficient assessment and management of patient presentations involve the level of medical knowledge and experience and scope of practice of the healthcare provider.
- Clinical decision making is the ability to integrate diagnostic data and assessment findings with experience and evidence-based recommendations to improve patient outcomes.
- The primary survey consists of identifying and managing life-threatening medical emergencies related to the patient's level of consciousness, airway, breathing, circulatory and perfusion status.
- An emergent or critical patient is one who is hemodynamically unstable with decreased level of consciousness, signs and symptoms of shock, severe pain, and difficulty breathing.
- The provider's senses can contribute and enhance information obtained from observation of the scene and the cardinal presentation of the patient.

- The physical exam can be a focused exam related to the chief complaint or cardinal presentation, a rapid head-to-toe exam, or a comprehensive, thorough exam.
- All healthcare providers should be familiar with the benefits and risks in transportation options for patients.
- Wilderness medicine is medical management in situations where care is limited by environmental considerations, prolonged extrication, or limited resources.

BIBLIOGRAPHY

Aehlert B: Paramedic practice today: above and beyond, St. Louis, 2009, Mosby.

Centers for Disease Control and Prevention: Standard precautions. Modified October 12, 2007. www.cdc.gov/ncidod/dhqp/gl_isolation_standard.html. Accessed June 5, 2009.

Donohue D: Medical triage for WMD incidents, JEMS 33(5): 2008. www.jems.com/news_and_articles/articles/jems/3305/medical_triage_for_wmd_incidents.html. Accessed September 20, 2009.

Edgerly D: Assessing your assessment, Modified January 24, 2008. www.jems.com/news_and_articles/columns/Edgerly/Assessing_Your_Assessment.html. Accessed October 1, 2009.

Hamilton G, et al: Emergency medicine: an approach to clinical problem-solving, ed 2, Philadelphia, 2003, Saunders.

Iowa Critical Care Paramedic Standardized Curriculum, 2001.

Marx J, et al, editors: Rosen's emergency medicine: concepts and clinical practice, ed 5, St. Louis, 2002, Mosby.

Mock K: Effective clinician-patient communication, Physicians News Digest, February 2001.

Occupational Safety and Health Administration: General description and discussion of the levels of protection and protective gear. Standard 1910.120, App B. www.osha.gov/pls/oshaweb/owadisp.show_document?p_table=STANDARDS&p_id=9767. Accessed September 11, 2009.

Occupational Safety and Health Administration: Toxic and hazardous substances: bloodborne pathogens. Standard 1910.1030. www.osha.gov/pls/oshaweb/owadisp.show_document?p_table=STANDARDS&p_id=10051. Accessed June 5, 2009.

Pagana K, Pagana T: Mosby's diagnostic and laboratory test reference, St. Louis, 1997, Mosby.

Paramedic Association of Canada: National Occupational Competency Profile for Paramedic Practitioners, Ottawa, 2001, The Association.

Sanders M: Mosby's paramedic textbook, revised third edition. St. Louis, 2007, Mosby.

University of Maryland Baltimore County Critical Care Paramedic Curriculum.

Urden L: Priorities in critical care nursing, ed 2, St. Louis, 1996, Mosby.

U.S. Department of Transportation National Highway Traffic Safety Administration: EMT-Paramedic National Standard Curriculum, Washington, DC, 1998, The Department.

U.S. Department of Transportation National Highway Traffic Safety Administration: National EMS Education Standards, Draft 3.0, Washington, DC, 2008, The Department.

Chapter Review Questions

1. As you obtain historical information regarding your patient, you note that the patient's presentation and responses are very similar to several patient complaints you have treated in the past. Integrating this information from past experiences to this current experience is known as:
   a. Pattern recognition
   b. Active listening
   c. Clinical decision making
   d. Clinical reasoning

2. In which situation has the threat to your personal safety been reduced most significantly?
   a. An angry schizophrenic patient has been calmed using verbal diffusing techniques.
   b. A barking dog has been secured in a kennel in the yard.
   c. The perpetrator of a shooting has fled, and police are on the scene with you.
   d. Your partner has taken an angry family member into another room.

3. You evaluate the patient's environment to assess for:
   a. Safety concerns
   b. Room temperature
   c. Assistive devices
   d. All of the above

4. An unresponsive patient has a needle in his arm when you arrive. His pupils are pinpoint, and he is breathing four times per minute. You are preparing to administer naloxone. At this point, opioid overdose is your initial:
   a. Differential diagnosis
   b. Primary diagnosis
   c. Terminal diagnosis
   d. Working diagnosis

5. An 18-year-old male had a tonic-clonic seizure. Coworkers report no known seizure history. You can arouse him to voice. P 118, R 20, BP 102/68. The diagnostic test most likely to narrow your differential diagnosis would be:
   a. 12-Lead ECG
   b. Blood glucose analysis
   c. End-tidal CO_2 measurement
   d. Pulse oximetry

6. A 23-year-old female has an acute onset of left flank pain. You should investigate which of the following regarding her pain?
   a. Dysuria
   b. Fever with productive cough
   c. Increase in appetite
   d. Syncopal episodes

7. When you use an interpreter to question a 42-year-old female about her abdominal pain, what is the best way to ensure information has been conveyed accurately and completely?
   - **a.** Ask the interpreter to have the patient repeat back key information about your treatment plan to ensure understanding.
   - **b.** Have her husband interpret because it will save time, as he will know a significant amount of her history.
   - **c.** Let the patient write her answers, and have the interpreter restate them so you will have a record of her statements for your report.
   - **d.** Wait until you arrive at the hospital to find an interpreter to ensure an accurate interpretation of key findings.

8. After you ensure scene safety, your highest priority is to:
   - **a.** Form a working diagnosis
   - **b.** Form a differential diagnosis
   - **c.** Determine the root cause of the patient's problem
   - **d.** Rule out immediate life threats

9. Which of the following physical findings points most specifically to increased intracranial pressure?
   - **a.** BP 200/60 mm Hg
   - **b.** Both pupils are 5 mm and react sluggishly to light.
   - **c.** Glasgow Coma Scale score is 7.
   - **d.** Respiratory rate is 8 and irregular.

10. You are transferring a 65-year-old female with renal failure from the nursing home. She has a history of "abnormal lab values" and is drowsy and weak. You note the following lab values: serum calcium 10.0 mg/dL (0.55 mmol/L), pH 7.28, potassium 6.1 mEq/L. The patient goes into cardiac arrest after you load her into the ambulance. After epinephrine, you should first consider giving her:
    - **a.** Calcium chloride
    - **b.** Lactated Ringer's bolus
    - **c.** Magnesium sulfate
    - **d.** Sodium bicarbonate

CHAPTER

2 Altered Mental Status and Neurologic Changes

ASSESSING AND TREATING patients with neurologic problems can be some of the most challenging cases you will encounter. This is particularly true of the patient with altered mental status. The many causes of altered mental status and the frequent inability of patients to communicate effectively can present unique difficulties. This chapter will assist you by providing tools to complete a basic neurologic exam, formulate a differential diagnosis, and utilize history and assessment to process the differential and determine the most likely problems, with emphasis on life threats, appropriate intervention, and disposition.

Learning Objectives ***At the conclusion of this chapter, you will be able to:***

1. Recognize the signs and symptoms of altered mental status and abnormal neurologic function.
2. Perform a basic neurologic exam.
3. Apply the neurologic exam findings to help formulate a diagnosis.
4. Consider the appropriate differential diagnosis.
5. Gather pertinent historical data.
6. Provide physical and emotional supportive care on the scene and en route.
7. Recognize the signs that indicate a patient is or may soon become unstable.
8. Treat immediate life threats.
9. Consider special transport alternatives on the basis of the likely diagnosis.

Key Terms

altered mental status Any behavior that departs from what's normal for a given patient

Amyotrophic lateral sclerosis (ALS, Lou Gehrig's disease) The disease is characterized by degeneration of the upper and lower motor neurons, which causes voluntary muscles to weaken or atrophy.

ataxia An unsteady or altered gait due to brain dysfunction, often of the cerebellum, which controls coordination

cerebrospinal fluid (CSF) A transparent, slightly yellowish fluid that acts as a shock absorber for the brain

cerebrovascular accident (CVA) Another term for *stroke*

dysarthria Garbled speech (but of one's intended words) due to cranial nerve dysfunction (distinguish from expressive and receptive aphasia)

embolus A particle that travels in the circulatory system and obstructs blood flow when it becomes lodged in a smaller artery. A blood clot is the most common type of embolus, but fat (after long bone fracture) or air (diving) emboli can also occur.

expressive aphasia Inability to speak one's intended words due to dysfunction of the cerebral speech center (distinguish from dysarthria)

gait disturbance An altered gait pattern that may be caused by an injury to or pathology of the brain, spine, legs, feet, or inner ear

hemiparesis Unilateral weakness, usually occurring on the opposite side of the body from the stroke

hemiplegia Paralysis or severe weakness on one side of the body

hemorrhagic stroke A stroke that occurs when a diseased or damaged vessel ruptures

ischemic stroke A stroke that occurs when a thrombus or embolus obstructs a vessel, diminishing blood flow to part of the brain

Korsakoff syndrome Chronic and irreversible condition involving cognitive dysfunction, especially memory loss, due to prolonged thiamine deficiency

ophthalmoplegia Abnormal function of the eye muscles

proprioception Information that comes to the brain from the body to help determine where the body or a body part is located in space; spatial orientation

stroke Sometimes called a *brain attack* or *cerebrovascular accident* (CVA), a stroke is a brain injury that occurs when blood flow to a part of the brain is obstructed or interrupted, causing brain cells to die.

thrombus A blood clot or a cholesterol plaque that forms in an artery, occluding blood flow

weakness Any localized loss of neurologic function in part or all of an extremity or one side of the face

Wernicke encephalopathy A disorder often caused by deficiency of thiamine, or vitamin B_1, and characterized by a triad of symptoms: acute confusion, ataxia, and ophthalmoplegia

SCENARIO

AS YOU PULL UP to the well-kept bungalow you see an elderly couple seated in folding chairs on the front porch. Your patient is a 68-year-old female. Her husband explains that she has some regular memory problems, but today she's been complaining of a severe headache and says she is seeing some things "fuzzy." You notice a walker next to her, and her husband hands you a paper sack full of her medicines. He says he is not really sure what she takes them for. "Oh my," you think, "this is going to be a big puzzle to solve."

1 ***What specific assessments should you perform on this patient?***

2 ***What conditions are in your differential diagnosis?***

This chapter will help you evaluate, treat, and make transport decisions for patients with altered mental status. We hope to build on your current foundation to develop the clinical judgment necessary to form a differential diagnosis, treat immediate life threats, monitor the patient's status, and intervene if necessary. Here we'll review the causes of mental status changes and neurologic deficits and their associated signs and symptoms. We also suggest key findings and indicate which historical information is likely to prove most important in arriving at a working diagnosis that can be confirmed and definitively treated in the hospital setting. Any behavior that departs from what's normal for a given patient constitutes **altered mental status**. Behavior that's normal for one person might not be typical of another, so altered mental status manifests differently from one individual to the next. The signs of altered mental status range from mild confusion to significant cognitive deficit.

Altered mental status is a common sign of morbidity in the prehospital setting, and early recognition and treatment of its underlying cause can be life saving. The condition is often associated with comorbid conditions such as trauma and infection. Identification of these conditions is helpful in determining the patient's course of treatment.

Providing appropriate emergency care and formulating a differential diagnosis for any patient, whether he or she has an altered mental status or not, depends on having a solid understanding of the human body and on conducting a methodical, detail-oriented assessment. To carry out an adequate neurologic assessment of the patient with altered mental status, you can't rely on vital signs alone. Close observation of the patient's symptoms and behavior, a skillful physical examination, and additional diagnostic tests, such as blood glucose measurement and end-tidal carbon dioxide ($ETCO_2$) monitoring (capnography), give you a clearer picture of the cause of a patient's distress.

The Brain and Spinal Cord

The brain represents only 2% of body weight, yet it defines who we are. Billions of neurons allow us to interact with the world around us, regulate our thoughts and behavior, determine our intelligence and temperament, make it possible for us to perceive pleasure and pain, mold our personalities, and store a lifetime of memories. Thanks to advances made in neurologic research—including revolutionary functional and structural imaging modalities—we now know more about the brain than at any other time in human history.

The brain is not fully developed until after 20 years of life, and new evidence suggests that even an adult brain has some plasticity and can create new neurons in a process called *neurogenesis*.

Protective Anatomic Structures

The central nervous system (CNS), which consists of the brain and spinal cord, accounts for 98% of all neural tissues of the body. The brain itself is composed of nervous tissue (called white matter or gray matter, depending on its location and function) and occupies about 80% of the cranial vault, or skull. The average adult brain weighs about 1.5 kg (≈3 lb) and is cushioned inside the skull by the **cerebrospinal fluid** (CSF). The CSF is a transparent, slightly yellowish fluid that acts as a shock absorber for the brain. It's made up primarily of water but also contains proteins, salts, and glucose. The flow of CSF within the cranial vault is depicted in Figure 2-1.

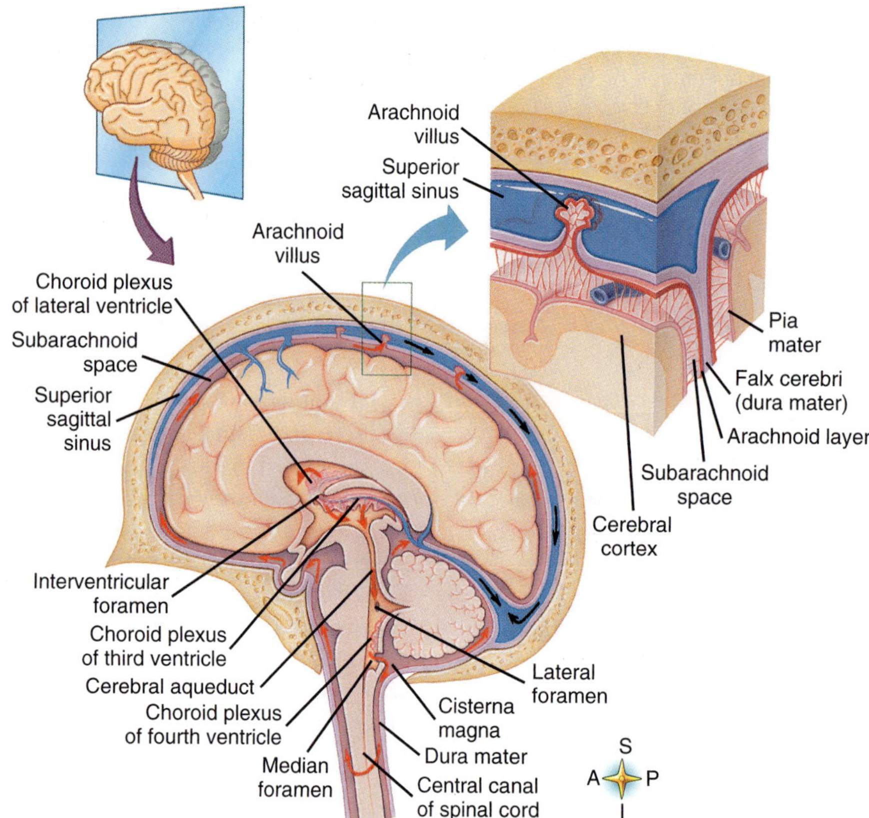

■ **Figure 2-1** Flow of cerebral spinal fluid. (From Patton K, Thibodeau G: Mosby's handbook of anatomy and physiology, St Louis, 2000, Mosby.)

Additional protection for the brain and spinal cord is provided by the three membrane layers called *meninges* (Figure 2-2). Each layer of the meninges is called a *meninx*, from a Greek word meaning "membrane" that can be traced back at least to Aristotle's texts on the human body.

The innermost meninx, which attaches directly to the brain's surface, is a delicate membrane called the *pia mater* (meaning "tender mother" or "soft mother"). The pia mater is highly vascular, containing the blood vessels that supply the surfaces of the brain and spinal cord. The middle layer of the meninges is a tangle of collagen and elastin fibers that takes its name from its appearance. The meshlike vascular network of this meninx resembles a cobweb, so it's known as the *arachnoid* (meaning "spider-like") *membrane*. CSF circulates in the space between the arachnoid and the pia mater (the subarachnoid space), protecting the brain against mechanical injury and providing an immunologic shield. The outermost meninx, which lines the cranial vault, contains arteries that supply the bones of the skull. It's called, appropriately, the *dura mater*—"tough mother." Composed of two fibrous layers, the dura mater is the most impregnable layer of the meninges.

Blood Supply

The brain, made up of billions of neurons, must be perfused by oxygenated blood. When blood flow is inadequate, the brain becomes hypoxic, and the person becomes agitated and restless. Too much carbon dioxide in the blood, and the person becomes stupefied or drowsy.

The brain uses oxygen and glucose greedily, consuming 20% of the body's total circulating blood supply. In the absence of a constant supply of fuel in the form of oxygenated blood and glucose, mental status will decline. Therefore, it's important to include blood glucose readings in every patient's baseline vital signs when a neurologic condition is suspected.

The capillaries that nourish the brain have a dual barrier that prevents certain particles (including extracellular ions and many proteins and toxins) from flowing into the brain while still allowing oxygen, water, and glucose to pass freely through the capillary membrane. This buffer is known as the *blood-brain barrier* (BBB). The BBB normally maintains the cellular environment of the brain, but head trauma and resulting cerebral edema may disrupt the BBB for several hours after a traumatic brain injury and lead to an influx of extracellular ions, proteins, and toxins, causing secondary brain injury.

Four major arteries supply blood to the brain: two internal carotid arteries and two posterior vertebral arteries. The two posterior vertebral arteries merge to become the basilar artery just inside the base of the skull. The basilar artery provides a blood supply to the brainstem and the cerebellum. These arteries bifurcate again at the circle of Willis, as shown in Figure 2-3.

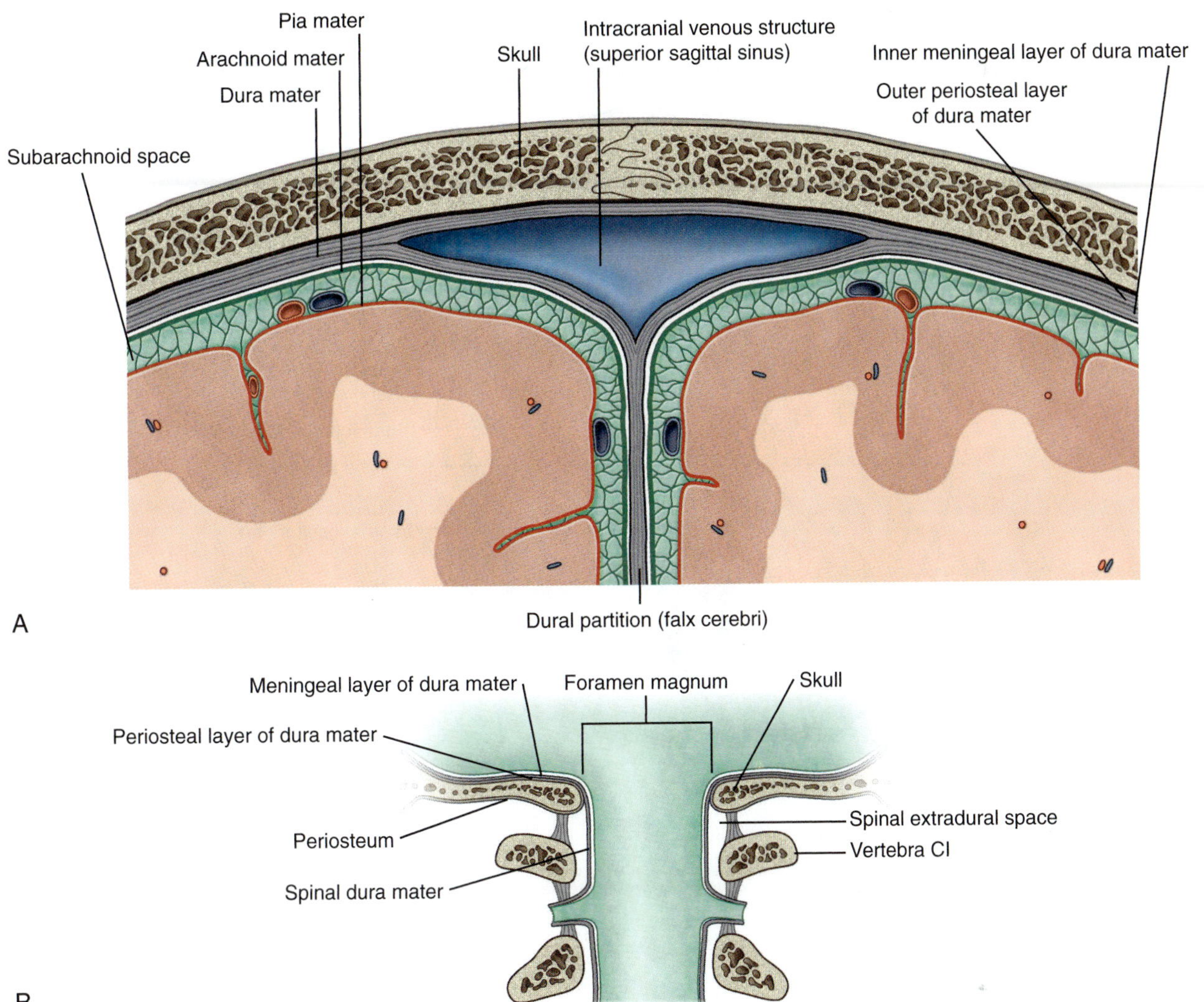

■ **Figure 2-2** The dura mater, arachnoid mater, and pia mater are the three layers of the meninges. **A,** Superior coronal view. **B,** Continuity with the spinal meninges. (From Drake R, Vogl W, Mitchell A: Gray's anatomy for students, New York, 2005, Churchill Livingstone.)

Cerebral blood flow is regulated by constriction and dilation of the cerebral vessels in response to various changes such as serum level of carbon dioxide (CO_2). In response to hypocarbia, alkalosis, and hypertension, the cerebral vessels constrict. Hypercarbia, on the other hand, causes vasodilation. It's important to check CO_2 measurements, because they may give you significant insight into the cause of a patient's deteriorating mental status.

Understanding cerebral vasoactivity is important in managing patients with altered mental status or suspected traumatic brain injury or stroke. The role of oxygen, free radicals, and neuroprotective antioxidants is discussed in greater detail later in the chapter.

Functional Regions

The brain is divided into five regions: the cerebrum (or cerebral cortex), the cerebellum, the diencephalon (meaning "double brain"), the limbic system, and the brainstem.

Cerebrum

The cerebral cortex, also called the *neural cortex* or *gray matter,* is the outermost layer of the cerebrum. This cortex is the highest-functioning part of the brain and comprises more than two-thirds of its mass. Because of its many convolutions, grooves, and ridges, the surface area of the cerebral cortex is actually 30 times larger than the space it occupies. Each ridge, or gyrus, and groove, or fissure, is associated with a specific highly selective cognitive function. Figure 2-4 depicts the cerebrum and the other major structures of the brain.

Right and Left Hemispheres The cerebrum is divided into left and right hemispheres. Structurally and functionally, they control opposite sides of the body. The hemispheres are interconnected by constantly communicating nerve fibers (in the corpus callosum) that transmit as many as 4 billion impulses per second.

The brain's structure is not identical from one individual to the next. In more than 90% of right-handed

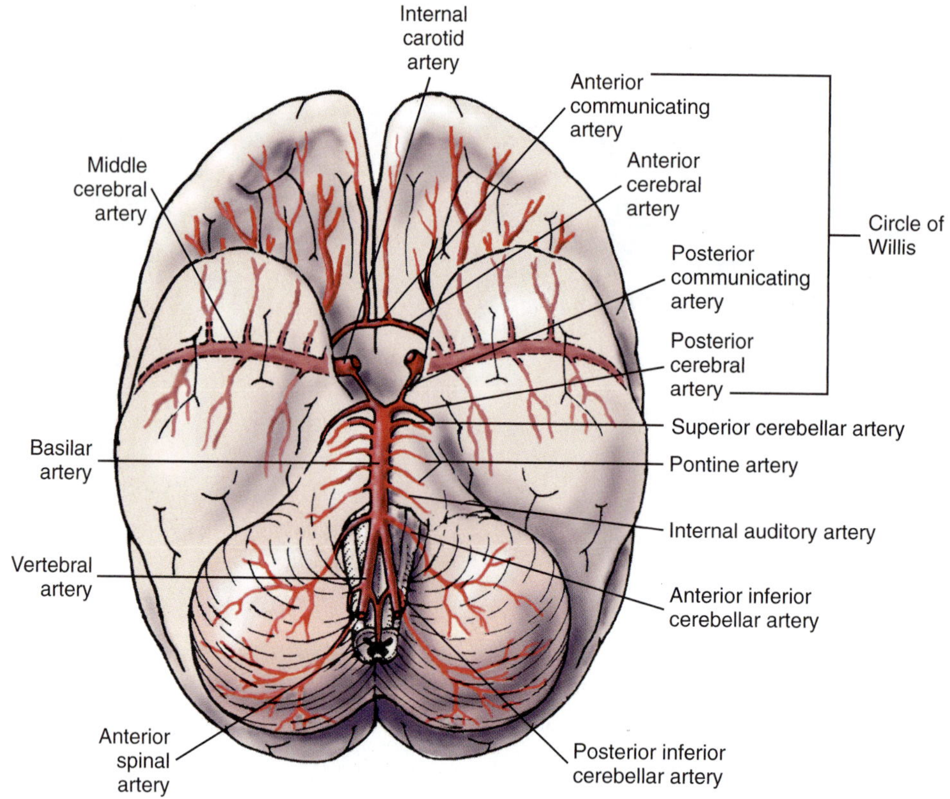

■ **Figure 2-3** Cerebral circulation and the circle of Willis at the base of the brain. (From Seidel H, Ball J, Dains J, et al: Mosby's guide to physical examination, ed 6, St Louis, 2006, Mosby.)

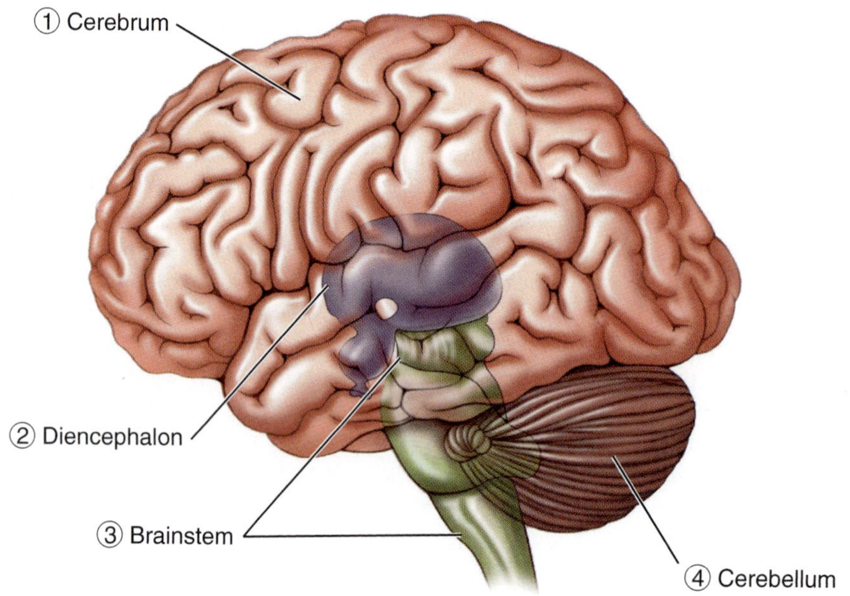

■ **Figure 2-4** The four primary areas of the brain are the brainstem, diencephalon, cerebrum, and cerebellum. (From Herlihy B: The human body in health and illness, ed 3, Philadelphia, 2007, Saunders.)

people and more than 70% of left-handed people, the interpretive speech center is located in the left hemisphere. The left hemisphere, often called the "logical brain," is also responsible for reading, writing, mathematical calculation, and sequential and analytic tasks. The right hemisphere, known as the "creative brain," interprets sensory information and processes spatial awareness. Interestingly, many musicians, dancers, and artists are left handed, and the right hemisphere of the cerebral cortex in such people appears to be more active than the left.

Lobes The cerebrum is further subdivided into lobes, each of which is named for the cranial bone that lies above it. For example, the frontal lobe lies beneath the frontal bone. The other lobes are the parietal, temporal, and occipital. Each lobe and its corresponding region of the cerebral cortex has a specific function. The frontal lobe controls motor function, determines personality and elaborates thought and speech, the parietal interprets bodily sensations, the temporal stores long-term memory and interprets sound, and the occipital is responsible for sight.

Cerebellum

The second-largest part of the brain, the cerebellum lies above the brainstem and posterior to the cerebrum (see Figure 2-4). The cerebellum coordinates movements, balance, and posture.

Diencephalon

Toward the center of the brain is the diencephalon (see Figure 2-4). The diencephalon includes the thalamus and the hypothalamus. The thalamus, composed of gray matter, connects sensory input between the spinal cord and the cerebral cortex and houses much of the reticular activating system, which is responsible for arousal (sleep/wake transitions). The tiny hypothalamus, not much bigger than a cherry pit, is responsible for maintaining homeostasis in the body. It links the sympathetic and parasympathetic nervous systems by way of the pituitary gland. The hormones of the hypothalamus stimulate or inhibit the release of hormones from the pituitary gland to regulate circadian rhythm (the body's innate sleep cycle), thirst and hunger, and other functions.

Limbic System

Surrounding the thalamus are the structures of the primitive brain, known collectively as the *limbic system* (Figure 2-5). The limbic system comprises two structures: the amygdala and the hippocampus. The system is connected to the prefrontal cortex of the frontal lobe.

The limbic system is referred to as the "primitive brain" because it controls basic survival instincts and many of the behavioral responses that constitute key features of our personalities, such as whether we have a positive or negative outlook. It's responsible for intense feelings—fear, frustration, anxiety, tension, anger, rage, sexual desire, appetite, the desire or ability to bond, and the storage of our emotional memories. The limbic system allows us to interpret events as they're happening and helps us predict the consequences of actions or events.

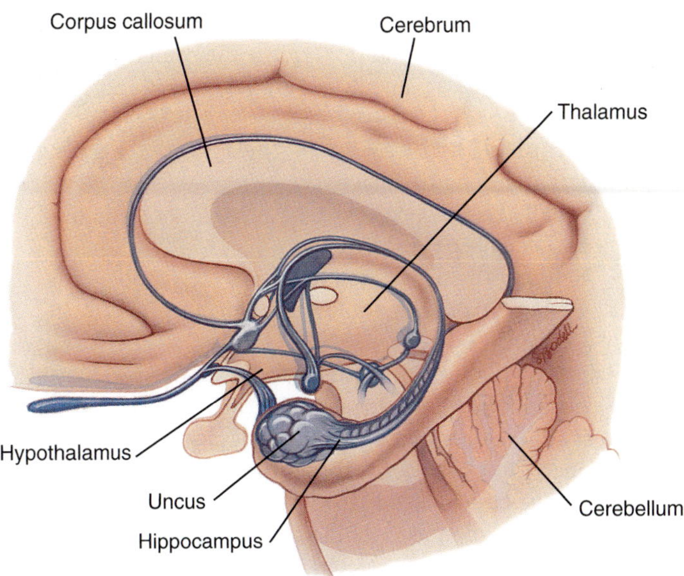

■ **Figure 2-5** The limbic system. (Modified from Thibodeau GA, Patton K: Anatomy and physiology, ed 5, St Louis, 2003, Mosby.)

Brainstem

Connecting the spinal cord to the brain is the brainstem, which includes the medulla and pons (see Figure 2-4). Some texts also classify the midbrain as part of the brainstem. The medulla controls basic physiologic functions such as breathing and heart rate. The pons (meaning "bridge") connects the cerebellum to the medulla and is responsible for facial expression.

Ventricles

The ventricles (meaning "little bellies") are cavity-like spaces filled with circulating CSF, which is constantly produced by the capillary network within the ventricles.

AMLS PATHWAY FOR PATIENTS WITH SUSPECTED NEUROLOGIC DYSFUNCTION

Evaluation of a patient with altered mental status requires a thorough and carefully performed initial assessment, and repeating your history and physical multiple times so that any new or worsening problems will not be overlooked. As described in Chapter 1, the AMLS approach consists of the following steps:

1. Initial observation, which involves noting the cardinal presentation and performing the primary survey, including assessment of airway, breathing, and circulation
2. Identifying and treating life threats and generating initial differential diagnosis
3. Detailed assessment (history, physical examination, and diagnostic testing)
4. Refining the differential diagnosis
5. Ongoing management and assessment

Patients with altered mental status may not be able to give a clear history or understand the caregiver. It's helpful to have other family members around if possible to collect additional information at the scene that could prove useful. If the patient is able to give some history, it should be obtained as soon as possible after the primary survey, since mental status can deteriorate within only a few minutes. If you're working with a partner, the history and physical exam can often be conducted simultaneously.

If the patient is becoming agitated or aggressive, take this behavior into account as part of your scene safety evaluation. If the scene becomes unsafe, call for appropriate backup or assistance. The area surrounding the patient may also provide clues to the cause of the altered mental status. Be alert to objects in the patient's environment (e.g., oxygen canisters, glucometers, drug paraphernalia, prescription drug bottles) that can help you formulate a differential diagnosis.

Initial Observation

For your own safety as well as that of the patient, make sure the scene is safe before you approach. If you're called to a scene at which the patient shows signs of altered mental status and you see a gun or knife, the patient may be violent, delirious, or confused, make sure the scene has been secured by law enforcement before you approach.

Arriving at a scene that has been secured, take in the surroundings. Your observations will help keep you safe and could suggest a diagnosis. Is the area clean and neat, or is it dirty and untidy? Is there any evidence that the patient is a victim of neglect or abuse? Who is the patient's caregiver if he or she does not live independently or is a minor? Check for anything out of place in the room. Is the phone on the floor, as if the patient had attempted to call 9-1-1 but dropped the receiver before doing so? This may tip you off to consider stroke as a potential diagnosis.

Send your partner to do a little investigation (ask permission of a family member if necessary) to check the cabinets and refrigerator to see whether there seems to be enough food. If not, or if the food on hand appears to be spoiled, the patient's condition could be attributable to malnutrition or electrolyte abnormalities. Look for insulin or oral hypoglycemic medications. Are there empty or nearly empty pill bottles lying scattered about? Are the prescription labels out of date? If so, an accidental or intentional overdose might be responsible for the patient's altered mental status.

Primary Survey

The primary survey includes an evaluation of the patient's airway, breathing, and circulation, as well as any necessary interventions suggested by your findings.

Airway

If the patient has a decreased level of consciousness (LOC), the airway may also be compromised. In most cases, a patient who is able to speak has a patent airway, but any neurologic condition that impairs mental status may quickly progress to a patient's being unable to maintain a functional airway. Once an individual becomes unconscious, the support of the oropharyngeal muscles is lost, and either the tongue or secretions can obstruct the airway. Keeping the airway open is of the utmost importance. It might become necessary to provide interventions such as suctioning, patient positioning, placement of an oral or nasopharyngeal airway, and initiation of advanced airway adjuncts such as intubation.

Breathing

Evaluation of the patient's respiratory rate, depth, and pattern may also indicate the underlying cause of altered mental status. Acidosis, stroke, metabolic disease, and other pathologic conditions cause changes in breathing patterns. Hypoventilation may indicate CNS depression, which might be attributable to drug overdose, stroke, or intracranial swelling. Provide oxygen and ventilatory support to maintain an oxygen saturation of at least 95% and $ETCO_2$ of 30 to 40 mm Hg. (Recall that $ETCO_2$ is about 5 mm Hg lower than serum $ETCO_2$.) Monitor the patient's response to oxygenation and ventilation. If possible, obtain a baseline oxygen saturation measurement (with the patient breathing ambient air) before you provide assistance, but in cases of respiratory distress, do not delay treatment just to obtain a baseline reading. Adequacy of ventilation (minute ventilation) is best assessed by measuring the partial pressure of carbon dioxide ($PaCO_2$). In the field and in other emergency settings, you can approximate $PaCO_2$ by measuring $ETCO_2$. If the $ETCO_2$ is markedly elevated, ventilatory assistance is needed. If the patient has been intubated, use capnography to monitor tube placement and assess the effectiveness of ventilation.

Circulation

Assessment of circulation can also help you pinpoint the cause of an altered mental status. Tachycardia (rapid heart rate) could be a sign of infection, temperature elevation, postictal (post seizure) state, or hypovolemia (low blood volume). Bradycardia may suggest cerebral herniation, hypothermia, or drug toxicity. An irregular pulse should lead you to consider cardiac dysrhythmia, which may be triggered by an electrolyte disturbance, acidosis, hypoxia, or ingestion of a toxic substance.

Forming a general impression of the patient requires you to establish the patient's LOC. The AVPU mnemonic is a fast, widely accepted method of accomplishing this task (see Rapid Recall box in Chapter 1). Recall that this mnemonic stands for *alert,* responsive to *verbal stimuli,* responsive to *painful stimuli,* and *unresponsive.*

Evaluate the temperature, color, and moisture of the patient's skin. Your findings may point toward environmental factors, infection, shock, organ dysfunction, or respiratory dysfunction.

Cardinal Presentations

This section will provide a brief overview of some of the most common cardinal presentations in patients with neurologic dysfunction. Many disease processes have similar presentations, or one finding may mask another. For example, delirium may lead to hypoglycemia, hypoglycemia may cause a seizure, and seizure may mask a stroke. In addition, although a patient's neurologic symptoms may seem pressing, sometimes they herald more worrisome medical conditions that should be considered in the differential diagnosis. Syncope (fainting), for instance, may be a harbinger of pulmonary embolism.

Altered Mental Status

Patients with altered mental status may show signs of confusion or exhibit changes in their typical behavior. In a patient with altered mental status, it's often difficult to sort out cause and effect. Hypoglycemia and electrolyte abnormalities (such as hyponatremia) can be responsible for disorientation, and depression, intoxication, and overdose can trigger unusual or disturbing behavior. Such behavioral alterations should be confirmed by a family member or someone else who knows the patient well.

A patient who has a significantly depressed mental status or is comatose cannot give a history, of course, and requires immediate resuscitation. Ominous mental decline of this sort can be attributable to hemorrhagic stroke, overdose, and other grave conditions.

Delirium

Delirium is an acute alteration in cognition characterized by impaired awareness, confusion, and disturbances of perception such as hallucinations or delusions. It is seen more often in women than men and is often caused by illness among the very young and those older than 60. These alterations can cause decrements in alertness, orientation, emotional or behavioral response, perception, language expression, judgment, and activity. Causes of delirium include intoxication, infection, trauma, seizure, endocrine disorders, organ failure, stroke, shock, infection, conversion disorder, intracranial bleeding, and tumor.

Dementia is sometimes confused with delirium but represents a chronic loss of brain function, particularly short-term memory function. It also affects thinking, language, judgment, and behavior. Unlike delirium, dementia is degenerative, occurring over time and usually irreversible.

In a patient with delirium, short-term memory becomes clouded, and the person becomes disoriented to time or place. Level of awareness may fluctuate over brief periods, and speech may be incoherent, tense, or rambling. The patient usually has no discernible focal neurologic deficit. Nevertheless, infection, intoxication, dehydration, cardiac dysrhythmia, thyroid problems, and medication issues (such as toxicity, undermedication, and skipping doses) may cause alterations in vital signs and physical exam findings.

The patient who demonstrates any level of delirium must be fully evaluated. Appearance, vital signs, hydration, and evidence of trauma should all be taken into account. A mini-mental status exam can be given to document the severity, nature, and progress of mental status changes. When you encounter an individual in an acute delirious state, remember that the patient is confused and is likely to have poor judgment. Your safety and that of the patient are the highest priorities. The patient may require physical or chemical restraints, using a benzodiazepine or antipsychotic agent.

Provide supplemental oxygen. Perform appropriate airway management measures to maintain an open airway and reduce the risk of aspiration if the patient is unconscious, has poor gag reflex, or you note snoring or noisy breathing. If you suspect a traumatic injury, take precautions to protect the cervical spine. Also be sure to test the patient's serum glucose level.

The patient will be evaluated in the emergency department (ED) with the aid of laboratory and radiologic studies. He may need a surgical, neurologic, or psychiatric evaluation.

You should also be aware of a syndrome called *agitated delirium,* in which the patient initially appears to be grossly psychotic and may exhibit strength out of proportion to your expectations. The patient may be extremely distraught, hyperstimulated, and uncontrollable. Attempts to restrain the agitated delirium patient may only worsen these findings. When restrained physically or with electrical devices (Taser devices), the patient's violent struggling may suddenly cease. The patient with agitated delirium may then have an irregular respiratory pattern followed shortly (typically within a few minutes to 1 hour) by death. Cardiac dysrhythmias have been noted in these patients, but asystole is the primary presenting rhythm. They may be hyperthermic and often have elevated circulating levels of epinephrine and metabolic acidosis. All patients who exhibit signs of agitated delirium must be medically evaluated and should not be restrained in a prone position, which is thought to exaggerate the acidosis by impeding ventilation. Monitor the patient and use continuous pulse oximetry. If active struggling stops abruptly, be immediately on the lookout for respiratory arrest, usually followed by cardiac arrest. Aggressive airway management and cardiac support may be life saving.

Syncope/Lightheadedness

Syncope, a transient loss of consciousness associated with decreased brain perfusion, has many possible causes. Lightheadedness, near-syncope, and syncope have the same differential diagnosis. It includes conditions such as aortic valve stenosis, hypertrophic cardiomyopathy, cardiac dysrhythmia, hypovolemia (dehydration, ectopic pregnancy rupture, aortic aneurysm rupture), CNS event (e.g., subarachnoid hemorrhage), pulmonary embolism, and vasovagal reflex (often due to situational or emotional triggers).

Dizziness/Vertigo

When patients complain of dizziness, it is essential to differentiate whether the patient is referring to a feeling of lightheadedness (or near-syncope) versus vertigo, a sense of spinning or abnormal sensation of movement. This section addresses the latter complaint.

Patients who complain of alterations in proprioception (spatial orientation of one's own body) and balance are usually able to give a history of such. You may not be able to assess intermittent alterations such as those secondary to transient ischemic attack (TIA). Many patients, however, including those with stroke, positional vertigo, overdose, vertebral artery dissection, and electrolyte abnormalities, may still be symptomatic as you complete your assessment.

Vertigo is more a symptom than a diagnosis. It originates in the CNS or vestibular organs. Central vertigo may be caused by hemorrhagic or ischemic insult (stroke), concussion, tumors, infection, migraine headache, multiple sclerosis, toxic ingestion or inhalation, Wernicke-Korsakoff syndrome, or lesion of the eighth cranial nerve nucleus in the brainstem. Peripheral vertigo is due to a disruption in the vestibular system or eighth cranial nerve.

The vertebrobasilar arterial system supplies the brainstem, cerebellum, and labyrinth of the ear. For this reason, occlusion of the vertebral or basilar arteries may cause stroke, TIAs, or cerebellar hemorrhage, all of which are associated with vertigo. Acoustic neuromas, tumors that originate on the eighth cranial nerve in the proximal internal auditory canal, can cause vertigo symptoms and compression and destruction of other cranial nerves.

A patient with vertigo has a feeling of imbalance or difficulty maintaining an upright posture. He may complain that he's feeling drunk or that the room is spinning around as if he's on a merry-go-round. He may have nausea or vomiting. The vertigo may have an abrupt onset, and the patient may also complain of tinnitus, a buzzing or ringing in the ears. It's important to question the patient about history of stroke, atrial fibrillation, and hypertension, since all of these can suggest stroke-related vertigo. A patient may have a decreased LOC, or the eyes may be moving quickly back and forth, a condition known as *nystagmus*. Nystagmus may be horizontal, vertical, or rotatory and may or may not diminish spontaneously. Nystagmus can result from a lesion in the cerebellum, brainstem, or vestibular organs.

Abrupt onset of vertigo associated with a change in position suggests benign positional vertigo. Recurrent transient symptoms usually indicate a TIA. Patients who have vertigo lasting longer than 48 hours, accompanied by a loss of balance and difficulty maintaining their posture, standing, and walking are often found to have cerebellar infarction. The patient who has other cranial nerve deficits needs to be evaluated for brainstem or cerebellar issues.

Vertigo may also be due to dysfunction of the vestibular system, usually the inner ear. This is commonly referred to as *peripheral vertigo*. Symptoms may be more acute, abrupt, severe, and of shorter duration than central vertigo and are often worsened or triggered by movement or change in position of the head. Patients may prefer to face one side or the other during transport and may not want to turn toward you to answer questions, because it exacerbates symptoms.

Seizure

You may be able to obtain a history from a patient who has had a seizure if his mental status has improved sufficiently, but usually in the immediate postictal period, you will have to rely on bystanders for information. The seizure may be generalized (involving loss of consciousness), such as a grand mal, associated with tonic-clonic movements, incontinence, and tongue biting, or it may be a focal seizure that affects only one part of the body.

During your scene survey, you may notice antiseizure medications or a MedicAlert bracelet. In addition to epilepsy, however, it's important to consider that the seizure may have been precipitated by other conditions such as head injury, stroke, meningitis, and toxins.

Headache

Headache can be an ambiguous, puzzling symptom. Provided there has been no loss of consciousness, as may happen with ischemic stroke or intracranial hemorrhage, the patient will probably be able to describe the symptoms to you. Pay special attention to the patient's description of the nature and location of the pain, since this information can be useful in pinpointing specific etiologies such as temporal arteritis and migraine.

Note any associated symptoms like vision changes—for example, ipsilateral vision changes (on the same side of the body as the headache) occur with temporal arteritis.

Patients with migraine may have photophobia (light sensitivity) and phonophobia (sound sensitivity), and they may perceive flashing lights. Patients who have experienced trauma and complain of headaches may have a subdural or epidural hematoma or a vertebral artery dissection. A severe headache that has a sudden onset, with or without vomiting, may indicate subarachnoid bleeding. A history of comorbidities (coexisting medical problems) such as hypertension and vascular abnormalities points to bleeding or aneurysm. A history of intravenous (IV) drug use or improper cleaning of implanted port sites before accessing may suggest epidural abscess. Finally, be alert for abnormal vital signs, including fever, which could indicate meningitis.

Ataxia/Gait Disturbance

Gait disturbance may be caused by an injury to or pathology of the brain, spine, legs, feet, or inner ear. **Ataxia** is an unsteady or altered gait due to brain dysfunction, often of the cerebellum, which controls coordination. The patient or a family member may report that the patient is unable to walk normally, and any of the following may be noted:

- Drags one foot
- Has trouble coordinating movements
- Feels pain in a particular area (such as a spasm in the foot) when walking
- Feels weak or unstable (off balance or about to fall) when walking

Associated symptoms such as incontinence or altered mentation (as occurs with normal-pressure hydrocephalus) or nausea, vomiting, and visual changes (as may occur with a posterior-circulation stroke) may also be present. Causes of ataxia are summarized in Table 2-1.

Focal Neurologic Deficit

Focal neurologic deficit refers to any localized loss of neurologic function, such as **weakness** or numbness in part or all of an extremity or one side of the face. Unless the patient has an associated neurologic insult that hinders speech, a condition known as **expressive aphasia**, he or she will probably be able to describe the onset of the deficit. Stroke is a particularly time-sensitive etiology of focal neurologic deficits. The history may reveal a preceding illness (e.g., Guillain-Barré syndrome) or chronic neurologic disorder (e.g., neuromuscular degenerative disease [Lou Gehrig's disease], multiple sclerosis, myasthenia gravis). Be sure to ask about bowel and bladder function, since incontinence typically accompanies the lower-extremity weakness of cauda equina syndrome. Note any change in the patient's ability to understand or follow instructions. Such deficit may indicate stroke, intoxication, electrolyte abnormality, or hepatic encephalopathy.

TABLE 2-1 Causes of Ataxia

Gait Disturbance	Description	Differential Diagnosis
Broad-based gait	Person walks with an abnormally wide distance between the feet, which increases stability Patient may hesitate, freeze, lurch, or be unable to walk in a straight line	Acute alcohol intoxication Cerebellar atrophy caused by chronic alcohol abuse Diabetic peripheral neuropathy Stroke Ingestion of antiseizure medications such as Dilantin Normal-pressure hydrocephalus Increased intracranial pressure
Propulsive (festinating) gait	Stooped, rigid posture, with the head and neck bent forward Shuffling gait Often accompanied by urinary incontinence	Advanced Parkinson's disease Carbon monoxide poisoning Chronic exposure to manganese (in those who handle pesticides and in welders and miners) Ingestion of certain medications such as antipsychotics
Spastic gait	Characterized by stiffness and foot dragging Caused by long-term unilateral muscle contraction	Stroke Liver failure Spinal cord trauma or tumor Brain abscess or tumor Head trauma
Scissors gait	Crouching posture, with legs flexed at the hips and knees Knees and thighs brush together in a scissors-like movement when patient walks Patient takes short, slow, deliberate steps Patient may walk on toes or on balls of feet	Stroke Liver failure Spinal cord compression Thoracic or lumbar tumor Multiple sclerosis Cerebral palsy
Steppage gait	Characterized by foot drop; foot hangs down causing toes to scuff the ground while walking	Guillain-Barré syndrome Lumbar disk herniation Peroneal nerve trauma

Life-Threatening Diagnoses

Hypoglycemia

A patient with hypoglycemia may seem depressed, sluggish, or dull witted. He may have focal weakness or seizure, or be completely unresponsive. When these signs are present, serum glucose should be checked; if low, a 50% dextrose solution should be administered IV according to protocol. If the patient is unconscious, or if there is any delay or difficulty in checking the blood glucose level, it's preferable to give the IV dextrose rather than withhold it until the level can be obtained. When IV access is not available, glucagon should be administered by IM injection.

Hypoventilation (CO_2 Narcosis)

A patient requires ventilatory assistance if unconscious or if respiratory effort is compromised, which may be due to a significant stroke, accidental or intentional medication overdose, or trauma or a medical event. When ventilation is impaired, $Paco_2$ climbs to dangerous levels, causing confusion, drowsiness, tremors, and convulsions. This condition is known as *CO_2 narcosis,* and it will lead to death if ventilatory assistance is not provided. Such assistance may be given with a bag-mask or advanced airway device or by intubating the patient. Initially the ventilation rate can be slightly higher than normal to bring down the $Paco_2$ level quickly, but the patient must be monitored carefully to prevent alkalosis.

Hypoxia

In the setting of altered mental status, hypoxia is usually associated with hypoventilation, and supplemental oxygen will be required, with or without assisted ventilation. Special attention should be paid to patients with certain toxicities (e.g., carbon monoxide or cyanide poisoning) and to those who have metabolic abnormalities associated with toxic ingestions (e.g., methemoglobinemia).

Hypoperfusion with Cerebral Ischemia

Many acute medical conditions, major trauma, and certain kinds of medications can cause hypoperfusion that leads to cerebral ischemia (lack of blood flow to the brain). The cause of the shock should be quickly discerned and targeted treatment implemented when possible. Chapter 4 offers an in-depth discussion of what to do in cases of shock.

Intracranial Hypertension

Elevated intracranial pressure (ICP) can significantly compromise perfusion to the brain, especially with significant acute elevations. This may be due to mass effect, such as from acute hemorrhage or malfunction of a ventriculoperitoneal shunt. Head trauma can lead to cerebral edema (swelling of the brain). If pressure becomes too high, herniation of the brain into the lower skull or through the foramen magnum may occur. This condition is often characterized by a unilateral blown pupil and a significant decrease in mental status or a coma, and has a high mortality.

Treating intracranial hypertension with hyperventilation must be done very cautiously. Hyperventilation decreases the amount of CO_2 dissolved in the blood, which induces vasoconstriction. Vasoconstriction decreases blood volume in the brain, thereby reducing ICP elevated by edema. However, vasoconstriction also decreases blood flow. The net effect on perfusion is difficult if not impossible to predict, so the patient's neurologic status must be monitored closely. In deciding whether to perform hyperventilation, follow local protocol and the preference of the receiving hospital. In life-threatening situations with herniation, mild to moderate hyperventilation may be indicated as a short-term measure. Adequate oxygenation and systemic perfusion must be maintained.

Detailed Assessment

After you have stabilized the patient by treating life threats discovered during the primary survey, you'll want to form a general impression of the patient's status and develop a list of possible differential diagnoses. Before you perform the secondary survey and the remaining physical examination, you should try to get an idea of how distressed the patient is, taking into account your general assessment findings as well as vital signs, the results of the serum glucose test, and pulse oximetry readings. Decide whether the patient must be immediately transported to the hospital or if you can take more time for evaluation on scene. Because patients with altered mental status tend to be unstable and may decompensate quickly, much of the rest of your evaluation and examination will probably be performed en route to the hospital. Remain alert for traumatic injuries and for any information that could prove diagnostically useful, such as unusual sights, sounds, and odors. Note the patient's positioning and any clues in visual appearance that may suggest causes of distress. You may wish to review Chapter 1 for detailed discussions of these topics.

History

When you treat a patient with altered mental status, gather information from witnesses or bystanders that might help describe the patient's baseline mental status and how it has changed recently. Ask about the degree of change, and inquire when the patient was last seen or known to be acting normal. Collect any other potential clues to the cause of the mental status change, such as information about the patient's medication regimen, blood pressure, and any recent trauma that might have been sustained.

The OPQRST and SAMPLER mnemonics (see the Rapid Recall boxes in Chapter 1) should be used to obtain the patient's complete history using a systematic approach. Talk to the patient directly when the neurologic status allows. Ask the patient what's wrong. They may give you valuable historical clues that will help generate your differential diagnosis. A teenage girl may tell you she has a fever and a stiff neck. An older man may admit he took the wrong medication by mistake. Conversely, if the patient has difficulty speaking, a stroke or other severe medical problem becomes a stronger possibility. You may want to review Chapter 1's discussion of therapeutic communication techniques for tips on how best to interview such patients.

Secondary Survey and Physical Examination

The secondary survey should be performed after the patient has been stabilized during the primary survey. The secondary survey is meant to help generate a more complete set of differential diagnoses that can then be ruled in or out with the aid of sound clinical reasoning. Document a history of the complaint and related issues, a timeline indicating when each of the patient's symptoms began, and a list of exacerbating factors.

During the physical examination, identify any injuries or other abnormalities in the patient's physical condition, and complete as much of a neurologic exam as possible. During your initial contact with the patient, you will have completed your evaluation of the patient's LOC, ability to speak, and general orientation, but other neurologic functions should be tested, including the presence or absence of cranial nerve function, motor function in the upper and lower extremities, and sensation and strength in those extremities. A more detailed discussion of how to perform the components of a complete neurologic exam can be found in Chapter 1. Document incontinence if present, and if the patient is able to walk, document whether the gait is normal.

Evaluate the patient's mental status more thoroughly. The easiest and most widely used means of evaluation is the AVPU mnemonic (see the Rapid Recall box in Chapter 1). The Glasgow Coma Scale is another tool used to evaluate LOC and mental status (see Table 1-3 in Chapter 1). You'll recall that this standardized neurologic test is scored on the basis of three responses: eye opening, motor response, and verbal response. It is often used to assess for brain injury in patients with head trauma.

Diagnostics

The arsenal of diagnostic tools in an ambulance or helicopter is limited, but the tools you do have, along with careful observation, may be all you need to formulate an accurate diagnosis. As noted earlier, vital signs including temperature when possible, serum glucose, and pulse oximetry measurements should be taken, recorded, and acted on as appropriate. If indicated, a 3- or 12-lead electrocardiogram (ECG) should be performed. Other lab tests may be carried out using an i-STAT device, a handheld blood analyzer available on some critical care transport vehicles and at some mass gathering events. In addition, some services may be equipped with portable ultrasound.

The mnemonics in the Rapid Recall boxes may assist you in formulating a differential diagnosis on the basis of history, physical exam, and laboratory findings.

RAPID RECALL

Causes of Decreased Level of Consciousness: AEIOU-TIPS

A Alcohol, anaphylaxis, acute myocardial infarction

E Epilepsy
Endocrine abnormality
Electrolyte imbalance

I Insulin

O Opiates

U Uremia

T Trauma

I Intracranial [tumor, hemorrhage, or hypertension]
Infection

P Poisoning

S Seizure

RAPID RECALL

Assessment of Acute Mental Status Changes: SMASHED

S Substrates—Substrates may include hyperglycemia, hypoglycemia, and thiamine
Sepsis

M Meningitis and other CNS infections
Mental illness

A Alcohol—Intoxicated or in withdrawal

S Seizure—Ictal (active) or postictal phase
Stimulants—Anticholinergic agents, hallucinogens, or cocaine

H Hyper—Hyperthyroidism, hyperthermia, hypercarbia
Hypo—Hypotension, hypothyroidism, hypoxia

E Electrolytes—Hypernatremia, hyponatremia, or hypercalcemia
Encephalopathy—Hepatic, uremic, hypertensive, or others

D Drugs—Any type

RAPID RECALL

Initial Assessment of Altered Mental Status: SNOT

Remember this mnemonic when performing initial assessment in the prehospital setting:

S Sugar
Stroke
Seizure

N Narcosis (CO_2, opiates)

O Oxygen

T Trauma
Toxins
Temperature

Be aware that this list is not a comprehensive survey of all possible causes of altered mental status.

Courtesy Vince Mosesso.

Management Strategies

Managing patients with suspected neurologic dysfunction should be undertaken similarly in all cases. As always, you should monitor airway, breathing, and circulation. A calm, supportive professional demeanor is of the utmost importance because the patient is usually frightened. A physiologic function he or she may have taken for granted is no longer working or not working properly. In addition, the patient may be confused and lash out physically or verbally. Use a composed, reassuring manner at all times.

Maintain the patient's oxygenation (95% oxygen saturation is the minimal level acceptable in stroke patients without supplemental oxygen, but oxygen at 2 to 6 liters per minute [LPM] by nasal cannula is almost always appropriate). Always check for hypoglycemia, which can mimic many neurologic disorders, and even if IV fluids are not needed, place an IV with a saline lock in case the patient decompensates.

If you have any suspicion that the patient may have suffered traumatic injury, you should assess for trauma during the history and physical exam.

After the steps outlined in the previous section have been completed and life threats have been ruled out, you and your team must decide which hospital can best treat the patient. You may select a stroke center, a trauma center, or a center that offers advanced specialized care. If the patient's condition is life threatening, of course, the closest facility is the most appropriate one. The medical staff there can stabilize the patient and transfer him or her for more definitive care if needed. If the decision is made not to transport the patient to the nearest hospital, the destination should be chosen on the basis of local point-of-entry protocols that specify which kind of facility is appropriate relative to each hospital's respective capabilities and the patient's medical needs. Online Medical Control can be a resource for additional guidance if needed.

SPECIFIC DIAGNOSES

Stroke

A **stroke**, sometimes called a *brain attack*, is a brain injury that occurs when blood flow to the brain is obstructed or interrupted, causing brain cells to die. According to the National Stroke Association, the term **cerebrovascular accident (CVA)** is being abandoned by the medical community because stroke is considered to be a preventable event, not an accident.

Strokes are classified as either ischemic or hemorrhagic, as shown in Figure 2-6. An **ischemic stroke** occurs when a thrombus or embolus obstructs a vessel, diminishing blood flow to the brain. A **thrombus** is a blood clot or a cholesterol plaque that forms in an artery, occluding blood flow. An **embolus** is a clot or plaque that forms elsewhere in the circulatory system, breaks off, and obstructs blood flow when it becomes lodged in a smaller artery. Rarely, an embolus may be composed of fat from a broken bone or an air bubble introduced during IV therapy, surgery, trauma, or severe decompression sickness. Ischemic stroke is much more common than **hemorrhagic stroke**, which occurs when a diseased or damaged vessel ruptures.

Pathophysiology

During an ischemic stroke, blood flow to a portion of the brain is disrupted, and ischemia of the brain occurs (see Figure 2-6, *B*). Ischemia is insufficient blood flow to an organ or tissue—in this case the brain—causing inadequate perfusion. Death of neurons and cerebral infarction (tissue death) follow. Blood flow may be restricted by an embolism or thrombus, or cerebral blood flow can be decreased by blood pressure relative to ICP or shock.

A blood clot, or embolus, may arise from the heart or its vessels and travel to the smaller vessels of the brain. The most common sites of thrombotic stroke are in the branches of the cerebral arteries, the circle of Willis, and the posterior circulation. When lack of perfusion to a portion of the brain causes infarction, an area of potentially reversible ischemia surrounds the region. Damage to the brain tissue, characterized by inflammation and microvessel compromise, causes larger and larger areas of stroke. The goal of treatment is to reverse or stop the ischemia in order to prevent further destruction and permit oxygenation of affected brain tissue.

Strokes in the middle cerebral artery typically produce **hemiparesis**, or unilateral weakness, on the opposite side

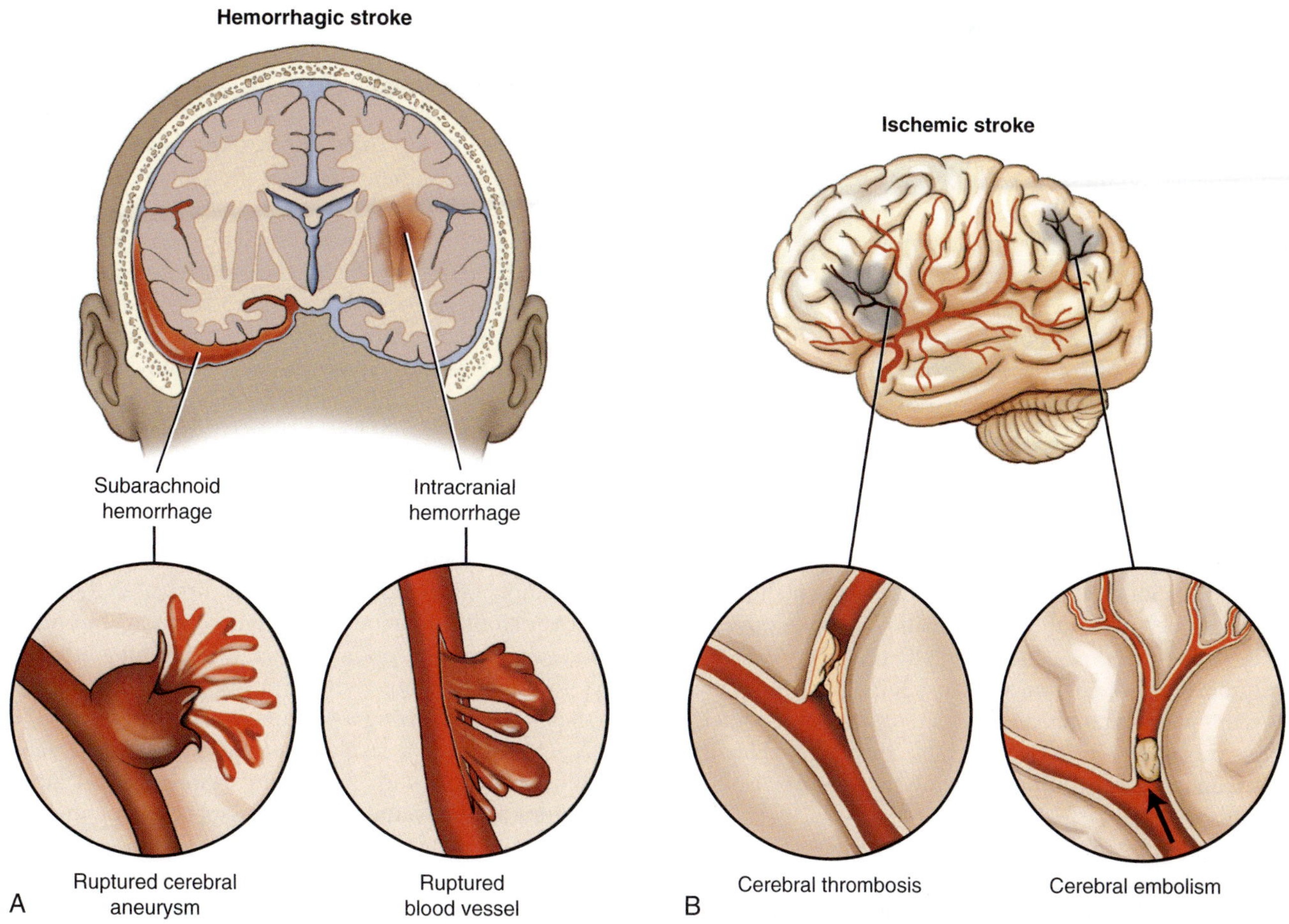

■ **Figure 2-6** Causes of stroke. **A**, Hemorrhagic stroke is the result of bleeding caused by an intracerebral hemorrhage or a subarachnoid hemorrhage, usually a result of a ruptured cerebral aneurysm. **B**, Ischemic stroke is the result of a blocked blood vessel caused by a cerebral thrombosis or cerebral embolism. (From LaFleur Brooks M: Exploring medical language: a student-directed approach, ed 7, St Louis, 2009, Mosby.)

of the body from the stroke (Figure 2-7). Patients often show a gaze preference toward the side of the lesion. If the ischemic lesion is in the dominant hemisphere, the patient may have receptive or expressive aphasia. A stroke in the nondominant hemisphere may cause neglect of or inattention to one side of the body. Usually, weakness is more pronounced in the arm and face than in the lower extremity. A stroke in the distribution of the anterior cerebral artery can cause altered mental status and impaired judgment, opposite-side weakness (greater in the leg than in the arm), and urinary incontinence.

Posterior cerebral artery occlusion impairs thought processes, clouds memory, and causes visual field deficits. Finally, vertebrobasilar artery occlusions may cause vertigo, syncope, ataxia, and cranial nerve dysfunction, including nystagmus, double vision, and difficulty swallowing.

Patients with atherosclerosis may have turbulent blood flow, which increases the risk of blood clot formation and platelet adherence within the arteries. In addition, patients who have blood disorders such as sickle cell anemia, protein C deficiency, and polycythemia (a hereditary disorder characterized by an abundance of circulating red

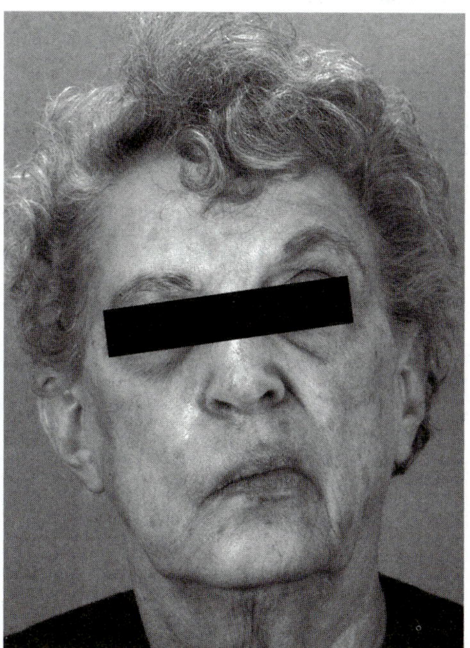

■ **Figure 2-7** A woman with right facial paralysis, often seen following a stroke. (From Cummings CW, Flint PW, Harker LA, et al: Otolaryngology: head and neck surgery, ed 4, St Louis, 2005, Mosby.)

blood cells) also have properties of the blood that increase the risk of stroke.

Presentation

Any patient who presents with an acute neurologic deficit should be evaluated for a stroke, whether the deficit is focal, such as a loss of strength or sensation in a particular body region, or diffuse, such as altered mental status.

A patient having a stroke usually experiences an abrupt onset of significant weakness on one side of the face, in one arm or leg, or on the entire one side of the body. A sudden decrease in or loss of consciousness altogether may also occur. A patient may lose vision in one or both eyes and have nausea or vomiting, a headache, or trouble speaking. This difficulty speaking may take the form of **dysarthria** or expressive or receptive aphasia.

Symptoms of stroke can occur alone, but patients usually have an array of symptoms. The presentation of a stroke can be either subtle or dramatic. A stroke can even occur while sleeping, and the patient doesn't feel any symptoms until he or she awakens. Sometimes the symptoms are incapacitating, and the patient cannot use a telephone or summon other help because of an altered mental status, aphasia, or **hemiplegia** (paralysis on one side of the body).

A very important point to differentiate here is the time the patient was last seen normal versus the time the patient was discovered with symptoms. If a patient is sitting with a family member and suddenly can't speak or has acute weakness on one side of the body (or other stroke symptoms), the time of discovery of symptoms and the time last seen normal are the same. If the patient went to bed the night before and was normal but woke up in the morning with stroke symptoms, then the time last seen normal was the night before. The same applies if a patient seemed normal when a family member left the house to go out but was showing symptoms of a stroke when the family member returned a few hours later. The time last seen normal is prior to the family member's leaving the house, not the time of arrival home (Box 2-1).

Differential Diagnosis

It is difficult to distinguish one kind of stroke from another in the field, but certain other causes of altered mental status can be quickly ruled out. A hypoglycemic episode, for instance, can mimic a stroke. For this reason, blood sugar should be checked in any patient who exhibits altered mental status or weakness. The symptoms of traumatic brain injury and spinal cord injury are also similar to those of a stroke. Migraine headaches or migraine equivalents, electrolyte abnormalities, CSF infections such as encephalitis and meningitis, demyelinating diseases of the nervous system like multiple sclerosis or Guillain-Barré syndrome, and psychiatric disorders also have stroke-like symptoms and should be ruled out as quickly and completely as possible, but this will have to be done at the hospital.

Other differential diagnoses to consider include acute intoxication with alcohol or other drugs, Bell's palsy, abscess or other infection, delirium, amnesia, carotid or vertebral artery dissection, intracranial bleeding attributable to trauma or hypertension, hemorrhagic stroke, and postictal state following a seizure.

A TIA mimics a stroke, but the symptoms resolve within 24 hours, with a majority resolving in 1 hour. According to the National Stroke Association, about 10% of these patients will suffer a stroke in 90 days and about half of them do so within 2 days (National Stroke Association, 2009). A TIA is a red flag that should not be ignored. However, a TIA precedes only 1 of every 8 strokes (National Stroke Association, 2009). For most people then, a stroke occurs without warning.

Key Findings

- Unilateral weakness
- Speech disturbance
- Lack of balance/vertigo
- Altered mental status

BOX 2-1 Onset of Symptoms: A Key Concept for Stroke Treatment

To treat stroke effectively, it's important to understand and differentiate between the time the patient was last seen acting normally and the time symptoms are discovered. For example, if a patient is sitting with his partner and suddenly can't speak or reports acute weakness on one side of the body (or other stroke symptoms), the time of discovery of symptoms and the time last seen normal are the same. If the patient seemed normal when he went to bed the night before but woke up in the morning with stroke symptoms, then the time last seen normal was the previous night. If the patient was normal when her husband left the house to run errands but was exhibiting stroke-like symptoms by the time he returned, the time the patient was last seen normal was before her husband left the house, not the time he arrived home.

If a patient has suffered a stroke in the past, it's important to know her baseline functioning and mental status. At the hospital, she will probably receive a CT scan and perhaps an MRI, and the physician will decide whether to administer a thrombolytic agent.

Management Strategies

The immediate priority in the prehospital setting is to consider stroke and transport the patient to a stroke center as quickly as possible if you believe the patient is having a stroke. A stroke scale will help you determine the severity of the stroke and indicate whether it warrants transport to a stroke center:

- The Cincinnati Stroke Scale compares facial droop and arm drift on each side of the body and takes into account slurred speech.
- The Los Angeles Stroke Scale measures smile or grimace, hand grip, and arm weakness on each side of the body and also factors in historical information about age, presence of a seizure disorder, duration of symptoms, glucose measurement, and ambulation at baseline.
- The National Institutes of Health Stroke Scale is a tool for more detailed evaluation of the neurologic and neuromotor deficits in stroke patients (Table 2-2). It also allows hospital providers to follow the patient's course.

Evaluate airway, breathing, and circulation and intervene as necessary. Check the patient's serum glucose. Provide supplemental oxygen if the patient's oxygen saturation dips below 94%. Patients treated with fibrinolytic agents within 3 hours of the last time definitely known to be normal (not time found with deficit) tend to have improved neurologic functioning and a lower mortality rate. Recent evidence suggests extending the time window for fibrinolytic treatment to 4½ hours for certain patients. Other interventions available at some centers to remove or dissolve clots include mechanical devices and directed intraarterial fibrinolytics, which can often be done beyond the 3- to 4½-hour window for intravenous therapy.

The most feared complication of administering thrombolytics is intracranial hemorrhage. The decision whether or not to administer an agent from this potent class of medications is a complex one and should be made by an experienced emergency physician or neurologist after discussing the risks and benefits with the patient and his or her family.

Patients should be kept in a comfortable supine position with slight head elevation if an ischemic stroke is suspected. Regulate blood pressure to maintain a mean arterial pressure (MAP) of at least 60 mm Hg, which will allow for cerebral blood flow. Do not lower blood pressure unless after multiple readings it exceeds 220/120 or the decision has been made to treat the patient with thrombolytics. (That decision will probably be made on arrival at the hospital.) Since hyperthermia accelerates ischemic brain injury, the patient's temperature should be lowered if it's higher than normal. Seizure-control medications and aspirin may be administered as directed by medical control.

Emergency Interventions

Patients who do not have a patent airway or who have signs of respiratory dysfunction require airway intervention. Blood glucose should be checked and corrected if necessary, according to protocol.

TABLE 2-2 National Institutes of Health Stroke Scale

Administer stroke scale items in the order listed. Record performance in each category after each subscale exam. Do not go back and change scores. Follow directions provided for each exam technique. Scores should reflect what the patient does, not what the clinician thinks the patient can do. The clinician should record answers while administering the exam and work quickly. Except where indicated, the patient should not be coached (i.e., repeated requests to patient to make a special effort).

Instructions	Scale Definition
1a. Level of Consciousness: The investigator must choose a response if a full evaluation is prevented by such obstacles as an endotracheal tube, language barrier, orotracheal trauma/bandages.	0 = **Alert;** keenly responsive 1 = **Not alert** but arousable by minor stimulation 2 = **Not alert;** requires repeated stimulation to attend 3 = **Responds** only with reflex motor or autonomic effects or totally unresponsive, flaccid, and areflexic
1b. LOC Questions: The patient is asked the month and his/her age. The answer must be correct—there is no partial credit for being close.	0 = **Answers** both questions correctly 1 = **Answers** one question correctly 2 = **Answers** neither question correctly
1c. LOC Commands: The patient is asked to open and close the eyes and then to grip and release the nonparetic hand. Substitute another one-step command if the hands cannot be used.	0 = **Performs** both tasks correctly 1 = **Performs** one task correctly 2 = **Performs** neither task correctly
2. Best Gaze: Only horizontal eye movements will be tested. Voluntary or reflexive (oculocephalic) eye movements will be scored, but caloric testing is not done.	0 = **Normal** 1 = **Partial gaze palsy;** gaze is abnormal in one or both eyes. 2 = **Forced deviation,** or total gaze paresis not overcome by the oculocephalic maneuver

Continued

TABLE 2-2 National Institutes of Health Stroke Scale—*Cont'd*

Instructions	Scale Definition
3. Visual: Visual fields (upper and lower quadrants) are tested by confrontation, using finger counting or visual threat, as appropriate.	0 = **No visual loss** 1 = **Partial hemianopia** 2 = **Complete hemianopia** 3 = **Bilateral hemianopia (blind)**
4. Facial Palsy: Ask—or use pantomime to encourage—the patient to show teeth or raise eyebrows and close eyes.	0 = **Normal** symmetrical movements 1 = **Minor paralysis** (asymmetry on smiling) 2 = **Partial paralysis** (total or near-total paralysis of lower face) 3 = **Complete paralysis** of one or both sides
5. Motor Arm: The limb is placed in the appropriate position: extend the arms (palms down) 90 degrees (if sitting) or 45 degrees (if supine). Drift is scored if the arm falls before 10 seconds. **5a.** Left arm **5b.** Right arm	0 = **No drift;** limb holds position for 10 seconds 1 = **Drift;** limb holds position but drifts down before full 10 seconds 2 = **Some effort against gravity;** limb cannot get to or maintain position, drifts down to bed, some effort against gravity 3 = **No effort against gravity;** limb falls 4 = **No movement** UN = **Amputation** or joint fusion
6. Motor Leg: The limb is placed in the appropriate position: hold the leg at 30 degrees (always tested supine). Drift is scored if the leg falls before 5 seconds. **6a.** Left leg **6b.** Right leg	0 = **No drift;** leg holds position for full 5 seconds 1 = **Drift;** leg falls by the end of the 5-second period but does not hit bed 2 = **Some effort against gravity;** leg falls to bed; by 5 seconds, has some effort against gravity 3 = **No effort against gravity;** leg falls to bed immediately 4 = **No movement** UN = **Amputation** or joint fusion
7. Limb Ataxia: The finger-nose-finger and heel-shin tests are performed on both sides with eyes open.	0 = **Absent** 1 = **Present in one limb** 2 = **Present in two limbs** UN = **Amputation** or joint fusion
8. Sensory: Sensation or grimace to pinprick when tested, or withdrawal from noxious stimulus in the obtunded or aphasic patient.	0 = **Normal;** no sensory loss 1 = **Mild to moderate sensory loss;** feels pinprick is less sharp or is dull on the affected side; or there is a loss of superficial pain with pinprick, but aware of being touched. 2 = **Severe to total sensory loss;** patient is not aware of being touched in the face, arm, and leg.
9. Best Language: Patient is asked to describe what is happening in the attached picture, to name the items on the attached naming sheet, and to read from the attached list of sentences. Comprehension is judged from responses here, as well as to all of the commands in the preceding general neurologic exam.	0 = **No aphasia;** normal 1 = **Mild to moderate aphasia;** some obvious loss of fluency or facility of comprehension, without significant limitation on ideas 2 = **Severe aphasia;** all communication is through fragmentary expression; great need for inference, questioning, and guessing by the listener. 3 = **Mute, global aphasia;** no usable speech or auditory comprehension
10. Dysarthria: An adequate sample of speech must be obtained by asking patient to read or repeat words from the attached list.	0 = **Normal** 1 = **Mild to moderate dysarthria;** patient slurs some words; can be understood with some difficulty. 2 = **Severe dysarthria;** patient's speech is so slurred as to be unintelligible; or is mute/anarthric. UN = **Intubated** or other physical barrier
11. Extinction and Inattention (formerly Neglect): Sufficient information to identify neglect may be obtained during prior testing. If the patient has a severe visual loss preventing visual double simultaneous stimulation, and the cutaneous stimuli are normal, the score is normal.	0 = **No abnormality** 1 = **Visual, tactile, auditory, spatial, or personal inattention** or extinction to bilateral simultaneous stimulation in one of the sensory modalities 2 = **Profound hemi-inattention or extinction to more than one modality;** does not recognize own hand or orients to only one side of space

Modified from National Institute of Neurological Disorders and Stroke at the National Institutes of Health: NIH stroke scale, 2003 (website). www.ninds.nih.gov. Accessed January 27, 2008.

Transport Decisions

Patients who are believed to be having a stroke should be brought to a stroke center with surgical capabilities in the event the stroke is found to be hemorrhagic and the patient requires emergency neurosurgery.

CEREBRAL VENOUS THROMBOSIS

Cerebral venous thrombosis is a blood clot that forms in the brain. The condition, once thought to be rare because it could be diagnosed only at autopsy, has been shown with advanced imaging techniques to be more common than previously believed. It affects women more often than men, and it tends to occur in early adulthood or middle age.

Pathophysiology

A patient with venous thrombosis will have stroke-like symptoms that are related to the area of the clot. A headache and a clinical picture resembling idiopathic intracranial hypertension may occur if the lateral sinus is thrombosed. Cranial nerve palsies can be seen with cavernous sinus thrombosis. Patients who have venous sinus thromboses may also present with cerebral hemorrhage.

Presentation

Thrombosis of the venous channels is relatively uncommon. Most clots in the brain occur in the arterial system. Headaches and cranial nerve palsies may be caused by venous system occlusion. A thunderclap headache usually indicates subarachnoid bleeding but may also be seen in sinus thrombosis. Nausea, vomiting, and a seizure or recurrent seizures are likely. The patient may have a focal neurologic deficit, depending on the area involved. Other symptoms may include hemiparesis, aphasia, ataxia (altered gait), dizziness, tinnitus (ringing in the ears), diplopia (double vision), and facial weakness.

Differential Diagnosis

The differential diagnosis for venous thrombosis includes acute stroke, head injury, idiopathic intracranial hypertension, nerve palsy, seizure, infection, and lupus.

Key Findings

- Headache
- Nausea/vomiting
- Visual changes
- Tinnitus

Management Strategies

Provide supportive care en route to the hospital. To prevent aspiration if the patient has altered mental status or hemiplegia, give nothing to eat or drink. Fluids may be given intravenously, and supplemental oxygen may be placed. Treat seizures according to protocol. Once at the hospital, the patient will usually be given a computed tomography (CT) scan or magnetic resonance imaging (MRI), and infectious processes will be ruled out. Laboratory studies, including lumbar puncture, may be done, and the patient may be placed on blood thinners to prevent further clotting.

Emergency Interventions

As with stroke, airway patency and adequate ventilation should be ensured.

Transport Decisions

The patient should be transported to a hospital that has neurologic consultative services. Since patients with blood clots in the venous sinuses are often given thrombolytic agents using a surgically placed microcatheter, interventional radiology or neurosurgery backup at the hospital is recommended.

CAROTID ARTERY DISSECTION

The internal carotid arteries, you'll recall, supply the brain with oxygenated blood. Carotid artery dissection, a key cause of ischemic stroke, begins with a tear in the innermost layer of the artery. Circulating blood enters the tear, quickly dissecting (separating) the innermost and middle layers. This mechanical process compresses the lumen (the hollow interior space) of the artery so that blood can no longer circulate through it, triggering an ischemic stroke.

Carotid artery dissection is an unusual cause of ischemic stroke (see Figure 2-6, *B*). This kind of stroke can occur in any age group but tends to appear most often in people younger than age 50. Carotid artery dissection represents about a quarter of all strokes that occur in teens and young adults, often striking while they are engaged in physical activity. Men and women are roughly equally affected.

Pathophysiology

The initial tear in the inner layer of the artery wall may be attributable to traumatic injury, connective tissue disease, hypertension, atherosclerosis, or some other pathologic process. In addition, the weakened outer layer of the diseased or damaged artery can begin to bulge, forming an aneurysm that may cause stenosis (narrowing) of the artery. In rare cases, the artery ruptures. A carotid aneurysm and a carotid dissection, however, are considered to be distinct pathologic processes.

The dissection of the internal carotid artery can occur inside or outside the skull. Extracranial dissection occurs most frequently because the skull tends to absorb the force of any traumatic impact. Sophisticated imaging studies are often required to make this diagnosis, since the signs and symptoms of the condition are ambiguous.

Presentation

Patients with carotid artery dissection may complain of unilateral headache, neck, or facial pain, and they may report a recent traumatic injury. You may note a Horner syndrome on the affected side, characterized by ptosis (drooping) of the eyelid, miosis (a constricted pupil), and facial anhidrosis (a lack of perspiration). The syndrome is usually the result of unilateral sympathetic nerve compression due to tumor, trauma, or vascular disorders.

The patient may present after physical activity or after an event that is normally innocuous, such as coughing or sneezing. Pain, usually in the head, back, or face, is often the initial symptom of a spontaneous, nontraumatic dissection. The headache is described as constant, severe, and unilateral. Transient vision loss may occur, and the patient may report a decreased sensation of taste. Physical findings may include hemiparesis, massive nosebleed, neck hematoma, cervical spine trauma, cervical bruit, or cranial nerve palsy.

Differential Diagnosis

The differential diagnosis for a carotid artery dissection includes neck trauma, other causes of stroke (either hemorrhagic or ischemic), subarachnoid hemorrhage, intoxication or toxicity, TIA, electrolyte abnormality, headache, cervical spine fracture, near-hanging injury, vertebral artery dissection, and retinal artery or vein occlusion.

Key Findings

- Unilateral pain in head or neck
- Vision changes
- Pupil constriction, especially unilaterally

Management Strategies

If trauma preceded the dissection, immobilize the patient's spine. Provide supportive care and monitor airway, breathing, and circulation. Once in the ED, blood pressure should be regulated, and the physician may choose anticoagulation or surgical/neuroradiologic intervention on the basis of MRI or angiographic findings.

Emergency Interventions

Airway patency and adequate ventilation should be maintained.

Transport Decisions

The patient should be transported to a hospital that has neurologic and vascular capabilities and is able to perform interventional radiologic procedures.

Intracerebral Hemorrhage

The term *intracerebral hemorrhage* is used interchangeably with *hemorrhagic stroke* (see Figure 2-6, *A*). In a hemorrhagic stroke, small arteries rupture and bleed directly into the tissues of the brain. Intracerebral hemorrhage accounts for 10% to 15% of all strokes and carries a higher likelihood of mortality than ischemic stroke. Mortality during the first month after this kind of stroke ranges from 40% to 80%. About half of all deaths, however, occur within 48 hours of presentation. Only 20% of patients with intracranial hemorrhage regain full functional independence.

Certain people are at higher risk of intracerebral hemorrhage: patients who receive excessively high doses of anticoagulants (for example, from iatrogenic or medication errors), those who have plaques in the cerebral arteries attributable to various other disease processes, and those who use cocaine or amphetamines.

Pathophysiology

The stage is set for intracranial hemorrhage when small intracerebral arteries—that is, arteries within the brain rather than on its surface—are damaged by disease processes such as hypertension and atherosclerosis. In patients who have had a previous stroke, the vascular tissue may be weaker and more friable and bleed more readily. Smoking may also weaken blood vessels. In fact, smokers with a systolic blood pressure greater than 150 mm Hg are nine times more likely to suffer a hemorrhagic stroke than nonsmokers.

Bleeding most often occurs in the thalamus, putamen, cerebellum, or brainstem. Brain tissue beyond the immediate area of the bleeding may be damaged by pressure produced by the mass effect of the hemorrhage itself. This mass effect increases ICP, which may cause symptoms such as nausea, vomiting, altered mental status, coma, respiratory depression, and/or death.

Presentation

A patient with intracerebral hemorrhage is likely to have an altered mental status. Frequent complaints include headache, nausea, and vomiting. The patient may have a seizure, with or without marked hypertension. However, in the prehospital setting, it is very difficult to distinguish between intracranial bleeding and an ischemic stroke. That determination will have to be made on arrival at the ED by obtaining a CT scan of the brain.

Differential Diagnosis

The differential of a hemorrhagic stroke includes ischemic stroke, migraine headache, tumor, and metabolic abnormalities. Vomiting may be gastrointestinal in origin, but it may also suggest increased ICP, as occurs with an intracerebral hemorrhage. A TIA may also mimic the presentation of intracranial bleed.

Key Findings

- Alteration in vital signs (hypertension, pulse and respiration changes)
- Altered LOC
- Stiff neck or headache
- Focal neurologic deficit (weakness, gaze preference)
- Difficulty with gait, fine motor control
- Nausea, vomiting
- Dizziness or vertigo
- Abnormal eye movements

Management Strategies

The most important thing to do when hemorrhagic stroke is suspected is transport the patient as quickly as possible. Recognize the signs and symptoms of stroke, and be able to take control of any difficulties that arise with airway, breathing, or circulation. Protocol may mandate that you use a stroke scale or ask specific questions about anticoagulation and bleeding problems. Obviously, treating life-threatening problems should take precedence over information gathering.

Many patients who have intracranial bleeding also have hypertension. In general, blood pressure will not be treated in the field unless otherwise ordered by protocol or by local Medical Control. However, you should minimize stimuli that could further increase ICP. Make phone notification as quickly as possible, and transport the patient to a stroke center, preferably one with neurosurgical backup. Monitor the patient, establish IV access, and check blood glucose, since hypoglycemia may mimic stroke symptoms, and hyperglycemia has been associated with poor outcomes in stroke patients.

Patients with intracranial bleeding may have ECG changes or seizures. Treat abnormal ECG findings and seizures according to institutional protocol. The receiving hospital will perform an immediate CT scan on the patient. Other possible imaging includes CT angiography, CT perfusion, and MRI (including MR angiography and venography). Patients who are on anticoagulants or hypocoagulable from other causes may be treated by a number of different modalities. Vitamin K, fresh frozen plasma, or recombinant factor VIIa may be administered in an attempt to limit bleeding. Blood pressure may be tightly controlled for the same reason. Emergent neurosurgical consultation may be necessary.

Emergency Interventions

Patients who do not have a patent airway or who have signs of respiratory dysfunction, including apnea, require intervention.

Transport Decisions

Patients believed to have had a hemorrhagic stroke should be brought to a stroke center that has neurosurgical capabilities.

Subarachnoid Hemorrhage

Subarachnoid hemorrhage is a kind of hemorrhagic stroke that occurs when arteries on the brain's surface bleed into the subarachnoid space, the area between the pia mater and the arachnoid. The blood often seeps into the ventricles, causing irritation. The volume of blood may also cause a mass shift. This kind of bleeding can be triggered by trauma such as a car accident, but it's more often a type of stroke that occurs when a cerebral aneurysm or arteriovenous malformation (AVM) ruptures (see Figure 2-6, *A*).

Pathophysiology

A cerebral aneurysm is an outpouching that develops in the weakened wall of a diseased or damaged vessel. An AVM is a genetic developmental defect of the vascular system in which certain arteries connect directly to veins rather than to a capillary bed, creating a tangle of vessels that can rupture. However, any part of the brain that has a tumor, thrombosis, or an abnormal blood vessel malformation may bleed. Uncontrolled hypertension and congenital aneurysms can be predisposing factors. Patients who have certain systemic diseases, such as Ehlers-Danlos syndrome, Marfan syndrome, aortic anomalies, or polycystic kidney disease, may also be at increased risk of subarachnoid hemorrhage. Patients with vessel-wall deficits due to age, hypertension, smoking, or atherosclerosis are also at risk.

Presentation

Subarachnoid hemorrhage should be suspected in any patient who describes a sudden, severe headache that came on like a thunderclap. Loss of consciousness may have occurred. About half of patients who present with subarachnoid bleeding have elevated blood pressure. Middle cerebral artery bleeding may cause seizures, motor deficits, nausea and vomiting, neck stiffness, back pain, photophobia, and visual changes.

About 30% to 50% of patients have prodromal headaches that stem from minor blood leakage into the subarachnoid space. The headache often has the

BOX 2-2 Grades of Hemorrhage

Grade	Description
Grade 1	Mild headache, with or without meningeal irritation
Grade 2	Severe headache and nonfocal examination, with or without pupillary change
Grade 3	Mild alteration in neurologic examination
Grade 4	Depressed level of consciousness or focal deficit
Grade 5	Comatose, with or without posturing

same characteristics as that of a larger subarachnoid hemorrhage, particularly a sudden onset and pain perceived as worse than usual. Seizures may occur very close to the acute onset of the bleed. Box 2-2 summarizes the five grades of hemorrhage.

Differential Diagnosis

The differential diagnosis of subarachnoid hemorrhage includes any pathologic occurrence that could lead to headache, nausea and vomiting, loss of consciousness, and altered mental status, including other causes of stroke, migraine headache, tumor, infection, medication use, overdose, and trauma.

Key Findings

- Sudden onset of severe headache
- Weakness (focal) or neglect
- Altered mental status
- Nausea/vomiting
- Vision changes/nystagmus
- Neck stiffness with associated headache

Management Strategies

At the hospital, a CT scan will be performed, and perhaps an MRI or cerebral angiogram will be done to locate the source of the bleeding. A patient with no obvious bleeding on initial imaging studies may receive a lumbar puncture to look for blood in the CSF or for changes consistent with blood being degraded in the CSF (xanthochromia), which is usually seen 12 hours after the onset of bleeding.

From a prehospital standpoint, support of airway, breathing, and circulation is of utmost importance. If at all possible, do not sedate the patient en route. Blood pressure control is usually not recommended in the field, but any stimuli that might increase ICP should be minimized.

Emergency Interventions

Obtain IV access and prepare to secure the airway if the patient exhibits an acute change in mental status or consciousness.

Transport Decisions

Appropriate triage and transport of the patient to a hospital that has CT scanning and neurosurgical support capabilities are critical.

Subdural Hematoma

A subdural hematoma is a collection of blood between the dura mater and arachnoid membrane. The hematoma may be acute, subacute, or chronic. The acute period is measured from the time of the injury to the third day. The subacute period lasts from day 3 to about 2 weeks after the injury, and the chronic phase begins 2 to 3 weeks after the injury. Subdural hemorrhage has a mortality rate of about 20% and usually occurs in patients older than age 60.

Pathophysiology

Subdural hemorrhage is usually caused by a tearing of the bridging veins that communicate between the cerebral cortex and the venous sinuses. This is usually precipitated by direct trauma or acute deceleration. The blood then clots in the subdural space. In the subacute phase of a subdural bleed, the clotted blood may liquefy and thin out. In the chronic phase, the blood has disintegrated, and serous fluid remains in the subdural space.

The phenomenon of coup-contrecoup injury can lead to subdural hematoma. The coup, or blow, causes trauma to the brain directly under the area of the skull that absorbs the direct force of impact. After the impact, the brain recoils within the closed container of the skull and is injured on its opposite side (contrecoup) when it rebounds against the cranium. This may cause bleeding or neurologic damage on both sides of the brain and generate separate but distinct findings on physical exam and imaging studies of the brain.

Presentation

After blunt head trauma, the patient may present with a subdural hematoma, often accompanied by loss of consciousness or amnesia for the event. The patient may either be asymptomatic or have personality changes, signs of increased ICP (headache, visual changes, nausea, or vomiting), hemiparesis, or hemiplegia. Patients with bleeding abnormalities, such as hemophiliacs and those on anticoagulant medications, may develop a subdural hematoma after only minor trauma, as can alcoholics and older adults.

Differential Diagnosis

The differential for subdural hematoma is the same as that for any other intracranial hemorrhage, infections such as meningitis, or ischemic stroke. Intracranial neoplasm may also have a similar presentation.

Key Findings

- Headache
- Loss of or alteration in LOC
- Focal or general weakness
- History or signs of trauma

Management Strategies

Evaluate the patient in the prehospital setting to assess for a change in mental status. Focal neurologic deficits can be a sign of subdural hematoma. If external trauma is evident, alert the physician to the possibility of associated injury. Because of the potential for a worsening mental status, watch carefully for any signs of increasing confusion or airway compromise, and rectify them immediately. If trauma is evident or suspected, use proper procedures to protect the cervical spine.

Emergency Interventions

Check the patient's serum glucose, and correct it if necessary as discussed earlier. If the patient has an altered LOC or airway compromise, take corrective action.

Transport Decisions

The patient should be transported to a trauma center or, if that's not possible, taken to a hospital where neurosurgical backup is available.

Special Considerations

The elderly may have a smaller brain volume as a result of the aging process and be at greater risk for tearing of the bridging veins between the skull and brain during any type of traumatic or deceleration injury leading to a subdural bleed.

Epidural Hematoma

An epidural hematoma is an accumulation of blood between the inner table of the skull and the dura mater, the outermost of the meninges. This condition is usually caused by trauma. The trauma is nearly always a skull fracture, usually in the area of the middle meningeal artery on the temporal aspect of the skull. Prompt surgical decompression is necessary for patients with significant neurologic dysfunction. The likelihood of recovery is directly related to the patient's preoperative neurologic condition.

Pathophysiology

About 80% of epidural hematomas are located in the temporoparietal region over the middle meningeal artery or its branches. The condition is usually precipitated by direct trauma to the head. Epidural hematomas in the frontal and occipital regions account for about 10% of epidural hematomas. Most of the time, the bleeding is arterial, but in a third of patients, it's the result of venous injury. Venous bleeding occurs almost exclusively with depressed skull fractures, and the resulting hematoma tends to be smaller and more benign.

The pressure associated with arterial epidural bleeding can result in a midline shift and herniation of the brain. Compression of the third cranial nerve can cause contralateral hemiparesis and ipsilateral pupil dilation. Although epidural hematomas usually attain their maximum size rapidly, in about 10% of patients, the size of the hematoma increases during the first 24 hours after injury.

Presentation

The patient may or may not lose consciousness after the trauma, or may lose consciousness and then awaken (the so-called lucid interval) for a period of time until again becoming obtunded or unresponsive. The patient may complain of severe headache and have vomiting or seizures. Increased ICP may cause Cushing's triad: systolic hypertension, bradycardia, and irregular respiratory pattern.

A pupil that is dilated, fixed, or slow to respond on the same side of the injury may indicate herniation due to increased ICP. The classic symptoms of an increasing herniation are coma, fixed and dilated pupil, and decerebrate posturing (see the heading *Pupils* under Physical Examination in Chapter 1 for a review).

Differential Diagnosis

The differential diagnosis of an epidural hematoma includes another type of intracranial hemorrhage, diffuse axonal injury, and concussion.

Key Findings

- Trauma
- Altered mental status
- Nausea/vomiting
- Dizziness/generalized weakness
- Altered LOC
- Unilateral dilated pupil

Management Strategies

In all patients with suspected epidural hematoma, start an IV, administer oxygen, and place the patient on a monitor.

Take precautions to protect the cervical spine as indicated. If the patient has a decrease in LOC, secure the airway and take steps to ensure hemodynamic stability.

Some studies of head-injured patients have associated increased mortality with prehospital intubation, and this has become a topic of intense debate within the EMS community. The best current recommendation is for advanced providers to maintain a high level of proficiency at advanced airway intervention through continued training and quality assurance procedures. Effective bag-mask ventilation is a skill that all providers must maintain, and it may be an option for difficult airways in lieu of endotracheal intubation.

In the ED, the patient will be evaluated according to trauma protocol, and a CT scan is usually performed. Further management includes neurosurgical consultation and control of ICP. Dilantin or another anticonvulsant may be given to reduce the incidence of early seizures but will not prevent development of a seizure disorder in the future.

Emergency Interventions

Because LOC may deteriorate, be prepared to manage the airway at any time.

Transport Decisions

Patients with suspected epidural hematoma should be brought to a trauma center with neurosurgical capability.

Special Considerations

The patient may feel fine and be acting appropriately and wish to refuse treatment. Special care must be taken to explain that this period may represent a so-called lucid interval that precedes the onset of symptoms. The patient may decompensate after refusal.

Cauda Equina Syndrome

Cauda equina syndrome is a disorder in which the nerve roots exiting from the end of the spinal cord in the lumbar region of the spine become compressed, causing lower-extremity pain, weakness or paralysis, bladder and bowel incontinence, and loss of sexual function. This syndrome is an emergent condition, and surgical intervention is necessary to prevent permanent loss of function.

Pathophysiology

Anatomically, the cauda equina resembles a horse's tail. It is formed by the nerve roots distal to the end of the spinal cord between T12 and L2. Cauda equina syndrome may be due to any compression of the nerve roots, including compression caused by trauma, disk herniation, tumors and other spinal cord lesions, and spinal stenosis (narrowing of the spinal canal). The nerve roots in the lumbar part of the spinal cord are susceptible to injury because they lack a well-developed covering, or epineurium, which may protect against stretch and compression injury.

Presentation

The patient affected by cauda equina syndrome may have low back pain, sciatica on either side or sometimes bilaterally, saddle sensory disturbances in the area of the perineum, and bowel or bladder dysfunction. Variable lower-extremity motor and sensory changes caused by compression of the nerve roots may also be present, and lower-extremity reflexes may be diminished or absent. Back pain is the most common complaint. If the patient doesn't voluntarily relate a history of urinary or bowel incontinence or numbness and tingling, be sure to ask.

Differential Diagnosis

The differential diagnosis includes back pain attributable to trauma and other causes, tumor, Guillain-Barré syndrome, spinal cord compression, metabolic abnormality, and other nerve disorders.

Key Findings

- Low back pain, often with radiation down legs
- Bowel or bladder incontinence or retention
- Recent manipulation of the spine (such as during a lumbar puncture or surgery)
- Trauma

Management Strategies

Prehospital care is mainly supportive. On arriving at the ED, various imaging studies (x-ray, CT, MRI, etc.) can be done and are most diagnostic. The patient may require neurosurgical intervention.

Emergency Interventions

Although prehospital intervention is not usually necessary, and cauda equina syndrome is not fatal, neurologic impairment may be permanent if not treated with emergency surgery.

Transport Decisions

A patient who is believed to have cauda equina syndrome should be transported to a hospital where orthopedic or neurosurgical spinal surgery can be performed.

Special Considerations

A patient suspected of having cauda equina syndrome may require spinal immobilization for transport in case there is an underlying traumatic cause that could be worsened with movement.

Tumor

A brain tumor, or intracranial neoplasm, is the inappropriate proliferation of cells into a mass that invades and compresses the surrounding healthy parenchymal tissue. Tumors are classified as either primary or metastatic and benign or malignant. *Primary* means the tumor originates in the brain. A metastatic tumor arises when cells migrate from a tumor elsewhere in the body, such as cutaneous melanoma or lung cancer, travel through the bloodstream, and begin to grow in the brain. Primary malignant lesions account for about half of all intracranial neoplasms and tend to be aggressive, invasive, and life threatening. Primary benign tumors tend to grow more slowly and are less aggressive, but they can still be life threatening if they arise in vital areas such as the brainstem.

Tumors are often classified by cell type, such as meningioma or glioma, but prehospital treatment is the same regardless of cell type.

Pathophysiology

Brain tumors may damage neural pathways by mass effect or infiltration of normal brain tissue. Tumors that arise near the third and fourth ventricles may obstruct the flow of CSF, causing hydrocephalus. Blood vessels that form to support the tumors may disrupt the BBB and cause edema or may rupture, leading to hemorrhage.

Presentation

The signs and symptoms of a brain tumor are nonspecific. The patient may have headache, altered mental status, nausea, vomiting, weakness, alterations in gait or even subtle behavioral changes. Focal seizure, visual changes, speech deficit, and sensory abnormalities are also possible. The patient may not notice symptoms, even as the tumor grows rather large, but often seeks treatment when an acute change in symptoms occurs. Such a change is often precipitated by an obstruction of CSF flow or hemorrhage.

Tumors in the frontal lobe may cause behavioral disinhibition, memory loss, decreased alertness, or a diminished sense of smell. Tumors in the temporal lobe may lead to emotional changes and behavioral disturbances. Pituitary tumors may cause visual changes, impotence, or changes in the menstrual cycle. Tumors in the occipital lobe may produce visual field deficits. Brainstem or cerebellar tumors can cause cranial nerve palsies, reduced coordination, nystagmus, and sensory deficits on either side of the body.

Differential Diagnosis

The differential diagnosis for brain tumor includes infection, stroke, and intracranial bleeding.

Key Findings

- Focal weakness
- Visual changes
- Dizziness/vertigo
- Nausea/vomiting

Management Strategies

Provide supportive care on the basis of the patient's symptoms. Edema, hydrocephalus, intracranial hemorrhage, pituitary infarction, infarction of the parenchyma (usually caused by compression of blood vessels), and seizures can cause the patient to deteriorate abruptly.

Emergency Interventions

Be prepared to intervene in the event the patient's LOC suddenly diminishes.

Transport Decisions

Patients with suspected brain tumor should be brought to a hospital that has oncology and neurosurgical backup.

Meningitis

Meningitis is an inflammation of the meninges, the membranes that surround the brain and spinal cord. By extension, the CSF will also show signs of infection and inflammation. Meningitis has many different infectious and noninfectious causes, but life-threatening acute meningitis is frequently a bacterial infection.

Pathophysiology

Bacterial meningitis usually occurs when bacteria migrate from the bloodstream to the CSF. If there is not an obvious source of infection, invasion of the CSF is usually presumed to have been caused by the bacteria that colonize the nasopharynx. In some cases, bacteria may spread from contiguous structures (e.g., sinuses, nasopharynx) that are infected or have been disrupted by trauma or surgical instrumentation.

Once in the CSF, the lack of antibodies and white blood cells allows bacteria to proliferate. The presence of bacterial components in the CSF makes the BBB more permeable and allows toxins to enter. As the bacteria multiply, inflammatory cells respond, changing the cell count, pH, lactate, protein, and glucose composition of the CSF. Intracranial pressure may rise as inflammation develops, causing occlusion of CSF outflow.

At a certain point, pressure in and around the brain reverses the flow of CSF. This development is associated with further deterioration of mental status. Ongoing damage to the brain triggers vasospasm, thrombosis, and septic shock, and the patient usually dies from diffuse ischemic injury.

Meningitis in neonates and infants is usually caused by group B *Streptococcus* or *Escherichia coli*. In children beyond the first year, *Streptococcus pneumoniae* and *Neisseria meningitidis* become increasingly common; these bacteria are the most common in adult meningitis as well. *Haemophilus influenzae* type B, once the most prevalent cause in children, is rarely seen since the advent of immunization for this organism, but there are some cases caused by different *Haemophilus* subtypes in children and adults. Other causative bacteria in adults include *Listeria monocytogenes* (particularly in the elderly), *Staphylococcus aureus*, various other streptococci, and gram-negative species. A different spectrum of bacteria are seen in meningitis after neurosurgical procedures; these include various staphylococci, streptococci, and gram-negative rods, including *Pseudomonas* and *Aeromonas*.

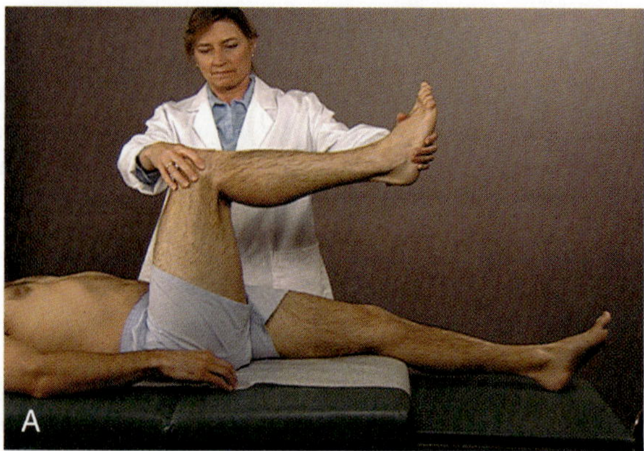

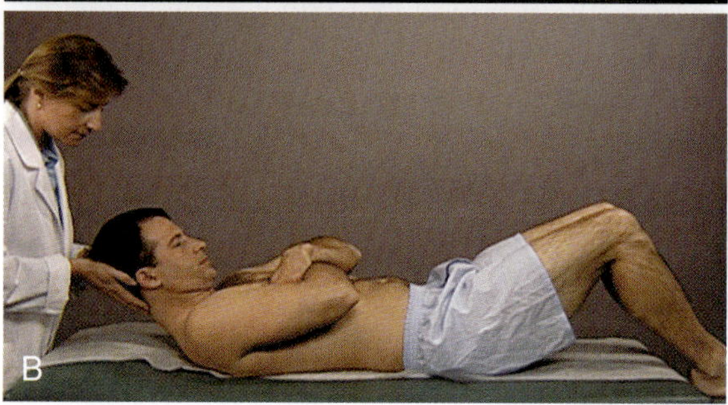

Figure 2-8 A, Kernig's sign. B, Brudzinski's sign. (From Seidel H, Ball J, Dains J, et al: Mosby's guide to physical examination, ed 6, St Louis, 2006, Mosby.)

Presentation

Patients with acute bacterial meningitis may decompensate quickly and require emergency care and antibiotics. The classic symptoms of meningitis include headache, nuchal rigidity, fever and chills, and photophobia. The infection can also cause seizures, altered mental status, confusion, coma, and death. The condition is usually precipitated by an upper respiratory illness.

Nearly a fourth of patients with bacterial meningitis present acutely within 24 hours of the onset of symptoms. Most patients with viral meningitis have symptoms that develop slowly over the course of a week. Patients who have a fever and headache should be examined for nuchal rigidity or discomfort with flexion of the neck, Kernig's sign (positive when the leg is flexed at the hip and knee, and subsequent extension of the knee is painful, leading to resistance and flexion of the torso), and Brudzinski's sign (involuntary flexing of the legs in response to flexing of the neck; Figure 2-8).

Altered mental status is often seen and can range from irritability or confusion to coma. In infants, the patient may present with a bulging fontanelle, decreased tone, and paradoxical irritability (calm when left alone, crying when held). Meningitis should be considered in older adults and in young children, especially those with diabetes, renal insufficiency, or cystic fibrosis. Patients with immune-system suppression, those who live in crowded conditions (e.g., military recruits, correctional facilities, college dorm residents), splenectomy patients, patients with alcoholism or other cirrhotic liver disease, patients receiving chemotherapy, patients who use IV drugs, and patients who have been exposed to others with meningitis are all at high risk of contracting this illness.

Differential Diagnosis

The differential diagnosis for meningitis includes brain abscess or tumor, encephalitis, delirium tremens, bleeding, and stroke.

Key Findings

- Fever
- Altered mental status, especially confusion or diminished LOC
- Neck stiffness/meningismus, a triad of nuchal rigidity, photophobia, and headache

Management Strategies

Be sure that the airway, breathing, and circulation have been stabilized, and begin IV fluids to treat the patient for shock or hypotension. Because patients with meningitis are at high risk for seizures, take seizure precautions, and administer treatment according to protocol. If the patient does have altered mental status, consider airway protection. If the patient is alert and may have an early stage of meningitis, monitor closely, administer oxygen, establish IV access, and transport rapidly to the ED.

While at the ED, the patient will be stabilized, and a head CT may be performed to rule out stroke and bleeding. Testing will usually include a lumbar puncture for evaluation of CSF. If bacterial meningitis is suspected, the patient will receive IV antibiotics. The patient may also receive steroids.

Emergency Interventions

A patient with meningitis may decompensate en route, so be prepared to control airway and breathing and treat seizures if they occur.

Transport Decisions

Patients with suspected meningitis can generally be treated in most EDs. If the patient is younger than 14 years of age, consider transport to a pediatric hospital if within reasonable distance.

Special Considerations

If you suspect the patient has meningitis, you should protect yourself, using droplet precautions including a mask, gown, and gloves to prevent airborne transmission of particles. Potential exposures of crew to patients should be reported immediately to a supervisor or the occupational health department. Prophylactic antibiotics are needed if there is a high likelihood a provider has been exposed to bacterial meningitis due to meningococcus (*N. meningitidis*); prophylaxis for meningitis due to other organisms is not indicated.

Because of the effect of the infection on the CNS, the patient may be confused, agitated, or violent. Remember that any patient with psychiatric symptoms may have an underlying medical problem.

Encephalitis

Encephalitis is a general inflammation of the brain that causes focal or diffuse brain dysfunction. This disorder has signs and symptoms similar to those of meningitis, including lethargy and headache. The key distinguishing feature is that encephalitis usually causes some alteration of brain function—disorientation, behavior change, motor or sensory deficits—whereas meningitis does not. However, keep in mind patients may have both conditions at once.

Pathophysiology

Encephalitis is most often a viral infection that damages brain parenchyma. A virus can enter the body by many different vectors. Some viruses are transmitted by humans, some are mosquito or tickborne, and some are transmitted by animal bites. A common culprit is herpes simplex virus type 1, known more commonly for causing cold sores. Patients with compromised immune systems are more likely to contract certain viruses, such as cytomegalovirus and varicella zoster. This latter virus, also known as *herpes zoster,* lies dormant in sensory nerve ganglia after initial infection (chickenpox) and is reactivated under circumstances that are still obscure, causing shingles. Rabies must be considered if there was potential exposure such as an animal bite or contact with a bat. Geography plays a role as well, with persons in North America at risk for St. Louis encephalitis and those in Asia for Japanese encephalitis.

Usually the virus replicates outside the CNS and enters through the bloodstream or a neural pathway. Once the virus has crossed over into the brain and entered the neural cells, the cells begin to malfunction. Hemorrhage, inflammation, and perivascular congestion all occur more frequently in the gray matter.

Postinfectious encephalitis is an immune-related disorder in which the body's immune response attacks brain tissue after a viral infection. This is difficult to distinguish clinically from acute viral infection at the time of initial presentation.

Presentation

The course of encephalitis varies widely among patients. The acuity and severity of presentation usually correlate with the prognosis. Generally the patient reports a history of a viral prodrome consistent with the common cold or flu. It might include fever, headache, nausea and vomiting, myalgia, or lethargy. The patient may also have behavioral or personality changes, decreased alertness or altered mental status, a stiff neck, photophobia, lethargy, generalized or focal seizures, confusion or amnesia, or flaccid paralysis. In the case of encephalitis associated with one of the viruses that causes chickenpox, measles, mumps, or Epstein-Barr, the patient may have a rash, lymphadenopathy, or glandular enlargement. Infant patients may have skin, eye, or mouth lesions, a rash, decreased alertness, increased irritability, seizures, poor feeding, and shock-like symptoms. Positive human immunodeficiency virus (HIV) status may predispose patients to encephalopathy secondary to toxoplasmosis infection.

Differential Diagnosis

The differential diagnosis for encephalitis includes most bacterial and viral illnesses that can affect the brain. Lupus, tickborne illnesses, seizures, cerebral hemorrhage, electrolyte abnormalities, intoxication, stroke, syphilis, trauma, and brain abscess may also appear in this fashion.

Key Findings

- Fever
- Altered mental status, such as confusion or diminished LOC

- Neck stiffness/meningismus
- Headache

Management Strategies

The mortality rate for encephalitis is up to 75%, and those fortunate enough to survive often have long-term motor or mental disabilities. In the case of rabies encephalitis, the mortality is thought to be 100%.

As with any patient who may have an infectious disease, the prehospital provider should practice strict blood and body-fluid isolation precautions and should wear a mask at all times. For additional safety, a mask should also be placed on the patient.

In the hospital, the patient will undergo a series of blood tests, radiologic and other imaging studies, and CSF studies, including viral serologies. A brain biopsy may be performed.

Emergency Interventions

Patients with encephalitis may decompensate quickly, so be ready to take control of the airway and provide resuscitative support of blood pressure. Patients who have a seizure or are in status epilepticus should be treated according to protocol. Antiviral medications will usually be given in the ED early in the course of treatment. Signs of hydrocephalus and increased ICP will usually be treated conservatively at first and then with more aggressive methods such as diuresis, mannitol, and steroids.

Transport Decisions

The patient should be transported to a facility that has intensive care, a neurologist, and neurosurgery backup (in case a brain biopsy has to be performed). If a hospital has an infectious disease specialist available, he or she may be of assistance. Pediatric patients should be transported to a pediatric facility with intensive care capabilities.

Special Considerations

If you suspect a patient has encephalitis, protect yourself by wearing a mask, gown, and gloves to prevent airborne transmission of particles.

Because of the effect of the infection on the CNS, the patient may be confused, agitated, or violent. Remember that any patient with psychiatric symptoms may have an underlying medical problem.

Abscess

A brain abscess is an infection that begins when an organism from a site beyond the CNS penetrates the BBB to enter the brain. Initially, inflammation occurs, turning into a collection of pus around which a well-vascularized capsule usually forms.

Pathophysiology

Certain bacteria (*Streptococcus, Pseudomonas, Bacteroides*) typically enter from the sinuses, mouth, middle ear, or mastoid through veins that drain directly into the brain from these sites. Other bacteria (*Staphylococcus, Streptococcus, Klebsiella, Escherichia, Pseudomonas*) usually spread by seeding of the blood from distant sites. Direct spread from penetrating trauma or surgical procedures may also be a source of bacterial infection (*Staphylococcus, Clostridium, Pseudomonas*) in the brain. About a fourth of abscesses have no clear source. Patients who have immune-system compromise, use IV drugs, have prosthetic valves, or are chronic steroid users, as well as near-drowning patients and patients who have extensive dental procedures, are at risk for brain abscesses caused by the spread of bacteria.

Presentation

A patient who has a brain abscess most often complains of a headache. A focal neurologic deficit consistent with the site of infection may be present. The triad of headache, fever, and focal neurologic deficit is seldom seen. Seizures, altered mental status, nausea or vomiting, and stiff neck may also indicate a brain abscess. A sudden worsening of the headache may indicate rupture of the abscess into the CSF.

Differential Diagnosis

Beyond the wide range of bacterial infections that must be considered, the differential diagnosis for a brain abscess includes headache, hypertension, intracranial bleeding, fungal infection, and tumor.

Key Findings

- Fever
- Altered mental status, such as confusion or diminished LOC
- Neck stiffness/meningismus
- Headache
- Nausea/vomiting
- Focal deficit consistent with the location of the abscess

Management Strategies

Brain abscesses are life threatening. With early recognition and intervention, however, morbidity and mortality have declined. Provide supportive care for the patient, monitor airway, breathing, and circulation, administer oxygen, and give IV fluids. If the patient has a seizure or decompensates, be prepared to provide lifesaving intervention.

At the hospital, laboratory and radiologic studies and perhaps a lumbar puncture or brain biopsy will be performed, and antibiotics will be administered.

Emergency Interventions

Although these patients are at risk of dying as a result of the mass effect of the abscess, its interference with brain function, and sepsis, this rarely happens acutely. Nevertheless, the abscess may rupture or cause bleeding in the brain, and the patient may quickly become sicker.

Transport Decisions

A patient suspected of having a brain abscess should be transported to an institution where neurosurgical services and a neurologic intensive care unit are available.

Special Considerations

Patients who are immunocompromised, either due to medication or underlying illness such as AIDS, are at particular risk of brain abscess.

Seizure

A seizure is an abnormal sudden burst of neuronal discharges in the brain that can cause loss of or alteration in consciousness, convulsions or tremors, incontinence, behavior changes, subjective changes in perception (taste, smell, fears), and other symptoms.

Seizures are a common nonspecific manifestation of neurologic injury and disease. They can be classified into generalized onset and partial onset. Partial-onset seizures are further categorized as either simple or partial complex seizures. In a generalized-onset seizure, electrical activity begins in both cerebral hemispheres simultaneously, whereas partial onset implies one specific focus in the brain.

Pathophysiology

Seizures are thought to occur when there is an imbalance between the excitatory and inhibitory forces within the brain, and the scales tip in favor of the excitatory forces. Researchers believe seizures are caused by decreased inhibition of the γ-aminobutyric acid (GABA) neurons, the inhibitory neurons in the brain. Benzodiazepines are used for treatment to increase the rate at which the GABA neurons fire, which slows down the seizure activity.

The pathophysiologic explanation of a seizure is that seizure activity represents an opening of ion channels in cell membranes, which changes the electrical potential of the cells. Various cellular receptors in the neurons mediate this depolarization of the ion channels.

Presentation

Generalized seizures tend to start out tonic (flexion or extension of the head, trunk, or extremities), then become clonic (rhythmic motor jerking of the extremities or neck, with or without a loss of consciousness), and then resolve with the patient becoming postictal (entering a period of sleep or confusion for an indeterminate period of time). Other forms of generalized seizure include tonic only, clonic only, diffuse myoclonic jerking, drop attacks, and absence seizure.

Partial-onset seizures begin in a focal area of the cerebral cortex. During simple partial seizures, the patient often remains conscious, and there may be uncontrolled jerking or movement of one body part. The patient may experience an aura (a perception of flashing lights, buzzing noises, or visual disturbances), which may precede a seizure or constitute a seizure in its own right.

Complex partial seizures are often preceded by an aura. The patient remains awake but has some alteration in consciousness and often does not recall the seizure event, which usually includes behavioral changes and automatisms (lip smacking, fumbling with the hands, mumbling, and chewing). These seizures are followed by a postictal period of variable length.

Differential Diagnosis

The differential diagnosis for seizure includes stroke, migraine, amnesia, hemorrhage, tumor, metabolic abnormality, sleep disorders, movement disorders, and psychiatric conditions.

Key Findings

- Altered mental status
- Focality of movement disorder
- Shaking or staring
- Postictal state described by family, friends, or caregivers

Management Strategies

The patient may activate EMS if they believe they are about to have a seizure. Seizures are often signaled by an aura, which may be a certain sound, smell, or taste and for some is a warning they are about to have a seizure. Protect the patient from injury by placing padding or removing hazards. Administer oxygen, since the patient's oxygen saturation is likely to drop during the seizure. Provide ventilatory assistance if respiratory rate or ventilatory effort is inadequate.

During the postictal state, supportive care is the best treatment. Postictal patients will probably be confused, upset, and perhaps aggressive or violent. Use deescalation techniques, and try to explain what happened. If possible, place IV access so the seizure can be treated with benzodiazepines according to local protocol. In the event of loss of consciousness or a compromised airway, be prepared to maintain the patient's airway.

Emergency Interventions

Oxygenation, ventilation, and protection from harm are the most important interventions in the prehospital scenario. Blood glucose testing should be performed on all patients with seizures or altered mental status, because hypoglycemia is a common cause. An ECG should also be performed, since syncope due to serious causes such as ventricular tachycardia can also be mistaken for an apparent seizure.

Patients actively seizing for more than 1 or 2 minutes should be treated with a benzodiazepine to stop the seizure. The fastest and most effective method of administration is IV, but when IV access is difficult, other routes may be used such as rectal, nasal, and intramuscular. Lorazepam (Ativan) and diazepam (Valium) are commonly used benzodiazepines for seizure control. If these do not stop the seizure, second-line agents include phenytoin (Dilantin) and phenobarbital. The last resort is general anesthesia. Patients who have repeated seizures and do not regain consciousness between seizures are said to be in status epilepticus, a neurologic emergency which may result in permanent brain injury and so must be treated aggressively.

Transport Decisions

The patient should be brought to a hospital that has neurologic backup. If the seizure is thought to have been precipitated by trauma, a hospital with surgical/trauma treatment abilities is preferable.

Special Considerations

Be cautious of attributing violent or confused behavior to a psychiatric condition, since patients may be confused, slow to respond, agitated, or violent during the postictal phase of a seizure.

Hypertensive Encephalopathy and Malignant Hypertension

Hypertensive emergencies are those that involve damage to the brain, kidney, or heart in the setting of severe hypertension. *Hypertensive encephalopathy* describes the neurologic symptoms associated with an extremely elevated blood pressure; malignant hypertension comprises retinal hemorrhage and papilledema. These symptoms are usually reversible when blood pressure is lowered.

Most patients with hypertensive encephalopathy already have a history of hypertension. For those who don't, your history taking may require specifically focused questions to identify the cause of the high blood pressure, including the use of drugs.

Pathophysiology

In healthy patients, cerebral autoregulation preserves steady-state cerebral blood flow through a range of mean arterial pressure, roughly from 50 to 150 mm Hg. In chronically hypertensive patients, the range of effective autoregulation is shifted to a higher range to allow protection at higher blood pressures. When blood pressure elevates dramatically, cerebral autoregulation is overcome, leading to increased pressure in the intracranial vessels, vascular damage, and compromise of the BBB. This leads to capillary fluid leak and resultant cerebral edema. In the eye, the increased ICP can cause retinal hemorrhages and lead to edema of the optic nerve, called *papilledema*.

Presentation

The patient may have a headache, confusion, visual disturbances, seizure, nausea, or vomiting. Be alert for other end-organ damage, such as aortic dissection, congestive heart failure, angina, palpitations, papilledema, or hematuria (blood in the urine).

Differential Diagnosis

A patient who has symptoms consistent with hypertensive encephalopathy may also have renal disease, pheochromocytoma, or preeclampsia or eclampsia (in pregnant patients). The patient may have ingested a specific food or medication that caused a blood pressure spike or may be in withdrawal from antihypertensive agents. Bleeding in the brain, trauma, and stroke should also be considered as part of the differential diagnosis.

Key Findings

- Hypertension
- Headache
- Nausea/vomiting
- Visual changes
- Altered mental status or focal neurologic deficits

Management Strategies

Give supplemental oxygen and start an IV. Specific intervention to lower blood pressure is generally warranted only if the systolic blood pressure (SBP) is above 220 or the diastolic blood pressure (DBP) is above 120. Medications commonly used for this purpose include labetalol and hydralazine as IV boluses, nitroprusside, nicardipine and nitroglycerin as IV drips, and clonidine by oral route. Remember to be cautious if antihypertensive medications are initiated, because lowering blood pressure rapidly can cause serious complications like ischemic stroke or myocardial infarction. Blood pressure should not be lowered by more than 25% acutely, with a DBP of 100 mm Hg a reasonable goal within 3 to 6 hours.

Emergency Interventions

Because patients who are acutely hypertensive may have a sudden intracranial hemorrhage and lose consciousness or become unable to protect their own airway, be prepared to take appropriate steps if the airway is lost.

Transport Decisions

The patient should be transported to a facility that has cardiology consultation and an intensive care unit.

Temporal Arteritis

Temporal arteritis, also known as *giant cell arteritis,* is an inflammation of the temporal arteries that causes throbbing or burning pain in the area of the temples, often accompanied by difficulty swallowing or chewing, visual disturbances, and other symptoms. Other arteries may be inflamed as well. The condition tends to affect adults age 50 and older, especially women in their 70s.

Pathophysiology

The exact pathophysiology of temporal arteritis is unknown. Some researchers speculate that it has an infectious cause, but this has never been proven. Another hypothesis implicates an autoimmune response that stimulates T-cell proliferation in the arterial walls.

Presentation

The patient usually complains of a headache and scalp tenderness in the area of the temporal artery. The headache has an acute onset but affects only one side of the head. In addition, the patient typically has jaw claudication and a swollen area in the temporal region, difficulty swallowing, hoarseness, and cough. Fever is also common. A headache usually precedes the onset of visual disturbances, which may be described as double vision, unilateral loss of one field of vision, or decreased visual acuity. Sometimes the patient reports hearing loss or vertigo. Other signs and symptoms include diaphoresis, anorexia (loss of appetite) with accompanying weight loss, muscle aches, fatigue, weakness, mouth sores, and bleeding gums.

Differential Diagnosis

The differential diagnosis for temporal arteritis includes other inflammatory rheumatic diseases, malignancies, migraine headache, and infection. Electrolyte changes and hypothyroidism may also mimic this disease.

Key Findings

- Headache (usually temporal)
- Visual changes (usually in one eye)
- Older adult

Management Strategies

Provide supportive care and monitor airway, breathing, and circulation. At the receiving facility, the patient may undergo a battery of tests, including blood tests, radiologic studies, and temporal artery biopsy. Patients who are believed to have temporal arteritis are usually also prescribed steroids to reduce vascular inflammation.

Transport Decisions

The patient should be transported to a hospital at which ophthalmologic follow-up is available.

Bell's Palsy

Bell's palsy is a unilateral facial paralysis that has an abrupt onset and uncertain cause. It is one of the most common cranial neuropathies, but it may frighten the patient by mimicking a stroke. Bell's palsy accounts for about half of cases of facial nerve palsy, with the other half associated with specific etiologies. Because of the significant facial abnormalities associated with this disorder, the patient may fear the facial deficits will be permanent.

Pathophysiology

The exact pathophysiology of Bell's palsy is unknown. Inflammation and swelling of the sheath of the seventh cranial nerve is typically present where it passes through the temporal bone. Some data suggest that Bell's palsy has an infectious origin, particularly herpes simplex, herpes zoster, and a variety of other viruses.

Presentation

A patient with Bell's palsy typically calls EMS or comes to the ED after having facial weakness that leads the person to believe they've had a stroke. Some patients have pain in the mastoid region or external ear, decreased tearing of the eye on the affected side, and an altered sense of taste.

On exam, weakness or paralysis of the entire face on the affected side may be present, and the eye may not close completely on that side. If you watch carefully, you may see that the eye on the affected side rolls upward and inward. Facial signs of a stroke differ in that only the lower half of the face will be weak, but the forehead and upper eyelid retain normal motor function. In some patients, this can be difficult to differentiate, so the patient should be treated as having had a stroke until proven otherwise.

Differential Diagnosis

Facial nerve palsy has a variety of potential causes other than Bell's palsy. These include Lyme disease, acute HIV infection, tumor, and otitis media. It is important to rule out a CNS (also called *upper motor neuron*) etiology such as stroke. This is a concern when there is sparing of the forehead muscles, as this part of the face has bilateral cerebral control.

Key Findings

- Unilateral weakness of entire side of face
- No arm or leg weakness
- Difficulty closing eyes

Management Strategies

The management of Bell's palsy in the prehospital setting primarily revolves around providing patient transport, supporting vital signs, and offering emotional support to the patient. Because of the impaired eyelid closure on the affected side, you should protect the affected eye with an eye shield or gauze taped lightly over the eye to keep it closed. Periodically placing a small amount of normal saline in the eye or on the gauze to keep it moist is also an acceptable option. In the ED, after ruling out other etiologies mentioned above, steroids and antiviral agents may be prescribed, with neurology follow-up for further testing and observation.

Transport Decisions

Bell's palsy is not life threatening and is usually self-limiting. For this reason, emergency transport is not necessarily indicated, but if there is any question whether the patient may be having an acute stroke, he or she should be brought urgently to the nearest stroke center.

Migraine

Migraine headaches are severe, recurrent headaches accompanied by incapacitating neurologic symptoms such as cognitive or visual disturbances, dizziness, nausea, and vomiting. The headache may be either unilateral or bilateral. Migraines often begin in childhood and become more frequent during adolescence. About 80% of patients develop their first migraine before age 30, and the headaches tend to become less frequent after age 50. Common migraine triggers are listed in Box 2-3.

BOX 2-3 Common Migraine Triggers

- Stress
- Illness
- Physical activity
- Changes in sleep pattern
- High altitude and other barometric pressure changes
- Skipping meals
- Use of certain medications (such as oral contraceptives)
- Ingestion of caffeine, alcohol, and certain foods
- Exposure to bright lights, loud noises, or unpleasant odors

Pathophysiology

The pathophysiology of migraine headaches is not completely understood. Recent research shows that neurotransmitters in the brain, such as serotonin and dopamine, stimulate an inflammatory cascade that causes vasodilation, which is responsible for the pain. Some of the symptoms associated with migraine headaches, such as nausea and vomiting, are also associated with dopamine receptor activation. Many dopamine antagonists have been clinically shown to be effective in treating migraines.

Presentation

Migraines usually last 4 to 72 hours, and the patient often prefers to be in a quiet, dark room and may initially attempt to treat the headache with over-the-counter medication. An aura consisting of dizziness, tinnitus, a perception of flashing lights, photophobia, phonophobia, or zigzagging lines in the visual field may signal or accompany the migraine. Some patients have myalgia, fever, jaw claudication, focal neurologic abnormalities, confusion, and irritability. Visual disturbances such as a lateral field deficit, balance problems, and syncope may also be reported.

Differential Diagnosis

The differential diagnosis for migraine headaches includes headaches of a different nature, infections (such as meningitis and sinusitis), temporal arteritis, and ischemic or hemorrhagic stroke or bleeding. In addition, increased ICP from a brain tumor, idiopathic intracranial hypertension, a leaking aneurysm, or opiate withdrawal may also cause headaches that resemble migraines.

Key Findings

- Headache
- Photophobia

- Nausea/vomiting
- Increased sensitivity to sound or smell
- Patient knowledge of the disorder

Management Strategies

Transport the patient to the hospital in a way that minimizes visual and auditory stimulation. Although patients may appear to be uncomfortable, they are usually stable. Opioid analgesia should be withheld until the patient can be fully evaluated by a physician. Treatment with antiemetics may help break the cycle and intensity of the migraine as well as treat the accompanying nausea.

Emergency Interventions

Patients with a history of migraine may mistake a stroke or other emergent condition for an especially bad migraine headache. Be alert for sudden changes in neurologic status should one of these other conditions be present.

Transport Decisions

Because the differential diagnosis includes stroke and intracranial hemorrhage, take care to transport the patient to a facility that can handle these medical problems. Supportive care is usually all that is necessary during transport.

Special Considerations

The patient may prefer to be transported without lights/sirens or with eyes closed or covered, because they may be highly sensitive to light and sound.

Idiopathic Intracranial Hypertension

Idiopathic intracranial hypertension used to be known as *pseudotumor cerebri*, or "false tumor," because its symptoms mimic those of a brain tumor. The condition is characterized by the poor uptake of CSF into the subarachnoid space. It predominantly affects obese women in their childbearing years. Papilledema, or the swelling of the optic nerve, is the most worrisome problem and is due to chronically elevated ICP. Papilledema leads to progressive optic nerve atrophy and blindness.

Pathophysiology

The cause of idiopathic intracranial hypertension, as its name suggests, remains elusive. Some studies have found a decreased outflow of CSF into the dural venous sinus. Others believe that increased blood flow impedes the brain's ability to drain CSF.

Presentation

Elevated ICP may lead the patient to seek medical attention for headaches that are nonspecific and tend to vary in type, location, and frequency. Pulsatile ringing in the ears and horizontal diplopia (double vision) are other symptoms. Uncommonly, the patient may have pain that radiates into the arms. Affected individuals may have orthostatic hypotension after bending over and standing up again, causing episodes of syncope. Papilledema may lead to intermittent dimming or blacking out of the vision in one or both eyes. The patient may have progressive loss of peripheral vision, usually starting in the nasal lower quadrant and then moving to the central visual field, followed by loss of color vision.

Differential Diagnosis

The differential diagnosis for idiopathic intracranial hypertension includes aseptic meningitis, Lyme disease, vascular tumors such as meningioma, arteriovenous malformation, stroke, hydrocephalus, intracranial abscess, intracranial bleeding, migraine headache, and lupus.

Key Findings

- Headache
- Vision disturbance and papilledema
- Younger, heavier female patients

Management Strategies

Little can be done for the patient in the prehospital arena. Visual acuity testing, direct ophthalmologic examination, lumbar puncture, and imaging studies may be required once the patient is hospitalized. Blood and CSF must be examined to rule out differential diagnoses.

Emergency Interventions

Prehospital care is typically supportive only. At the hospital, the patient may be placed on medication and may require drainage of CSF by lumbar puncture or surgical care, including placement or adjustment of an intracranial shunt.

Transport Decisions

The patient should be transported to an institution that offers ophthalmologic, neurologic, and neurosurgical specialty care.

Normal-Pressure Hydrocephalus

Normal-pressure hydrocephalus is characterized by excessive volume of CSF in the ventricles but normal CSF pressure when determined by lumbar puncture. The classic triad of symptoms includes urinary incontinence, abnormal gait, and cognitive disturbance, which are often reversible.

Pathophysiology

A patient with normal-pressure hydrocephalus has an increased volume of CSF in the ventricles. The excess CSF is believed to put pressure on the nerve fibers exiting the cerebral cortex, leading to the clinical findings. CSF accumulation is generally believed to be due to inadequate absorption across the arachnoid membrane into the dural sinuses.

Presentation

The patient with normal-pressure hydrocephalus typically presents with the triad of gait disturbance, urinary incontinence, and cognitive impairment. The patient tends to have a shuffling, widened gait and usually has difficulty taking the first step, much like a patient with Parkinson's disease. Urinary rather than bowel incontinence is experienced, and in the early stages, the patient may have urinary urgency and frequency. Cognitive impairment typically consists of apathy, psychomotor slowing, decreased attention span, and inability to concentrate.

Differential Diagnosis

The differential diagnosis for normal-pressure hydrocephalus includes Alzheimer's disease and other causes of dementia, stroke, Parkinson's disease, electrolyte abnormalities, toxicity, and idiopathic increased ICP.

Key Findings

- Altered gait
- Urinary incontinence
- Altered mental status

Management Strategies

On the scene and during transport, provide physical and emotional support to the patient. Once the diagnosis has been made by means of radiologic and laboratory studies in the inpatient setting, the patient may have CSF fluid removed and a shunt placed to allow continuous CSF shunting to decrease volume and pressure.

Emergency Interventions

Careful monitoring and documentation of vital signs, historical data, and physical exam findings will be useful to the ED team at the receiving facility. Emergency interventions are usually not necessary, but remain alert in case the patient has a seizure.

Transport Decisions

Transport the patient to a hospital that offers neurosurgical support.

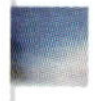

Neuromuscular Degenerative Disease

Neuromuscular degenerative disease is known in the United States as *Lou Gehrig's disease* or **amyotrophic lateral sclerosis** (ALS). This disease is characterized by degeneration of the upper and lower motor neurons, which causes voluntary muscles to weaken or atrophy. Patients usually die 3 to 5 years after diagnosis, which is commonly made between ages 40 and 60. More men than women are affected.

Pathophysiology

Neuromuscular degenerative disease has no single known cause. Scientists have recently identified a mutation in a gene that controls protein synthesis and synaptic function of motor neurons in some patients. However, this explanation accounts for only a small percentage of cases of neuromuscular degenerative disease. Glutamate toxicity, mitochondrial dysfunction, and autoimmunity may all play a role in ALS, but researchers are still trying to find out precisely how.

Presentation

Upper motor neuron findings in patients with neuromuscular degenerative disease include spasticity and hyperreflexia. Lower motor findings include weakness, ataxia, and fasciculations. Death is attributable to respiratory muscle weakness and aspiration pneumonia. Medical complications of immobility add to the morbidity and mortality of patients with this disorder.

The patient may seek acute medical care for limb weakness, difficulty speaking and swallowing, visual disturbances, and limb spasticity. Motor problems typically present from the periphery inward, starting with wrist drop, loss of finger dexterity, foot drop, and tongue fasciculations. Emotional lability may be present and may cause the patient to overreact to sad or humorous events or comments. The patient is aware of his lack of control over his emotions. Ocular, sensory, and autonomic dysfunction occur late in the disease, usually in patients who require ventilatory support. Weakness is often asymmetric and begins in the arms or legs. Difficulty chewing and swallowing occurs late in the illness.

Differential Diagnosis

The differential includes Guillain-Barré syndrome, multiple sclerosis, myasthenia gravis, spinal cord tumor, and stroke.

Key Findings

- Ascending and peripheral weakness moving upward and inward
- Mixed upper and lower motor neuron findings

Management Strategies

Prehospital care centers on transporting the patient and on supporting airway, breathing, circulation, and vital signs. Give oxygen and fluids for general weakness according to protocol.

At the hospital, the patient will undergo a battery of tests, including neurology consults and nerve conduction studies. Care is mainly symptomatic, and emotional support should be available to the patient and family. If the patient has a living will or DNR orders, he should be kept comfortable and not challenged. Complications such as pneumonia or other infections, deep vein thrombosis, or respiratory problems are common. These problems should be managed according to protocol.

Emergency Interventions

Patients with neuromuscular degenerative disease may decompensate from extreme weakness in the respiratory muscles, and corrective action must be taken (see Special Considerations heading).

Transport Decisions

The patient should be brought to the hospital, where he will be cared for by his neurologist, especially if this is a chronic condition. As with most patients who have altered mental status, the patient should be brought to a stroke center or a center that has neurologic and neurosurgical backup, since the diagnosis of neuromuscular degenerative disease is usually made during the course of a hospital stay.

Special Considerations

Because patients with neuromuscular degenerative disease may decompensate from extreme weakness of the respiratory muscles, if the decision is made to intubate, the provider, patient, and family should realize that it is unlikely the patient will ever be able to be weaned from the ventilator.

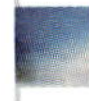

Wernicke Encephalopathy and Korsakoff Syndrome

Wernicke encephalopathy and Korsakoff syndrome are thought to be different stages of the same pathologic process, with the former progressing to the latter. Acute deficiency of thiamine, or vitamin B_1, can cause the disorder known as **Wernicke encephalopathy**, which is characterized by a triad of symptoms: acute confusion, ataxia, and **ophthalmoplegia** (abnormal function of the eye muscles). However, only a third of affected patients demonstrate all three features of the triad.

Korsakoff syndrome is the term given to the symptoms in the late stages of the disease, especially memory loss. The syndrome is often seen in alcoholics, but it can occur in any patient who has malnutrition, such as those on long-term hemodialysis and patients with acquired immunodeficiency syndrome (AIDS). The average age at diagnosis of the syndrome is about 50, but the syndrome can occur in younger patients who have metabolic disorders, receive parenteral nutrition, or have a diet deficient in thiamine or other vitamins.

Pathophysiology

Thiamine plays a key role in the metabolism of carbohydrates. It is a cofactor for essential enzymes in the Krebs cycle and the pentose phosphate pathway. If too little thiamine is available, these cellular systems fail, leading to inadequate usable energy and subsequent cell death. The systems most critically affected are those that have rapid turnover because of high metabolic needs, such as the brain. Energy production decreases, and neuronal damage occurs, causing cellular edema and further nervous system injury.

Presentation

A diagnosis of Wernicke encephalopathy should be considered for any patient who has evidence of alcohol abuse or malnutrition and acute symptoms of confusion, ocular dysfunction, and memory disturbance. The ocular problems most commonly seen are nystagmus, bilateral lateral rectus palsies, and disconjugate gaze. Blindness is not usually seen.

The encephalopathy may manifest as global confusion, apathy, agitation, or inattentiveness. Significant mental status changes, such as coma or low LOC, are rarely seen. About 80% of patients have some peripheral neuropathy. Hypotension, nausea, and temperature instability may also be caused by thiamine deficiency. Infants may have constipation, agitation, vomiting, diarrhea, anorexia, eye disorders, or altered mental status, including seizures and loss of consciousness.

Differential Diagnosis

The differential diagnosis includes alcohol or illicit drug intoxication, delirium, dementia, stroke, psychosis, closed head injury, encephalopathy secondary to liver failure, and postictal state.

Key Findings

- Malnutrition or chronic alcoholism
- Gait ataxia
- Abnormal eye movements, especially nystagmus
- Confusion

Management Strategies

At the hospital, the patient will undergo an array of laboratory and radiologic tests, such as blood tests, electrolyte measurement, lumbar puncture, arterial blood gas readings, and CT scan and MRI to evaluate differential diagnoses.

Focus on stabilizing the airway, ensuring oxygenation, and maintaining blood pressure and volume control. If the condition is suspected, empirical thiamine replacement should be initiated. This can be given orally but to assure absorption is often administered IV or intramuscularly (IM). The initial dose of thiamine is typically 100 mg, but over time as much as 500 mg may be needed to reverse the encephalopathy.

Some clinicians have expressed concern about giving patients dextrose before administering thiamine if they are in a thiamine-deficient state. The concern is that dextrose will exacerbate the encephalopathy by providing a substrate (dextrose) for the cellular pathway without the thiamine coenzyme. However, this effect is seen only in patients receiving long-term dextrose administration without concurrent thiamine administration. It is safe to give dextrose alone in the prehospital setting for hypoglycemic events, even if thiamine is not immediately available.

Emergency Interventions

Thiamine and glucose should be given to patients who have an altered mental status if there is a chance that Wernicke encephalopathy is being considered as a diagnosis.

Transport Decisions

No special transport decisions must be made. The patient may be brought to any hospital, but children should be brought to a pediatric specialty center if one is available.

Guillain-Barré Syndrome

Guillain-Barré syndrome refers to a group of acute immune-mediated polyneuropathies, demyelinating disorders that cause weakness, numbness, or paralysis throughout the body. The incidence of Guillain-Barré is 1 to 3 per 100,000 people in the United States. Although it can occur at any age, it's usually found in young adults and older adults. The condition affects men and women equally.

Pathophysiology

Guillain-Barré syndrome is believed to represent an autoimmune response to a recent infection or to many different types of medical problems. Researchers believe the body forms antibodies against the peripheral nerves, in particular the axons, which become demyelinated. Recovery is typically associated with a brief remyelination period. It has been shown that many patients with Guillain-Barré syndrome are seropositive for *Campylobacter jejuni*.

Presentation

The patient with Guillain-Barré often presents initially with lower-extremity muscle weakness, mainly in the thighs. The weakness usually appears a few weeks after a respiratory or gastrointestinal illness. Over the course of hours to days, the weakness may progress to involve the arms and chest muscles, facial muscles, and respiratory muscles. Approximately 12 days out, most patients will be at their worst and then will gradually begin to improve during the next few months.

Many patients with Guillain-Barré syndrome require mechanical ventilation during their illness to compensate for respiratory muscle weakness. In many cases, the patient cannot stand or walk even though she feels strong. Lack of deep tendon reflexes is a relatively strong indicator of Guillain-Barré. In addition, the patient usually has paresthesias that progress from the toes and fingertips upward, but not beyond the wrist or ankles. Pain may be present with the most minimal movements and is most impressive in the shoulder, back, buttocks, and thighs. The patient may experience a loss of ability to sense vibration, loss of proprioception and touch, and impressive autonomic dysfunction, including wide variation in vital signs, heart rate, and blood pressure. The patient may also have urinary retention, constipation, facial flushing, hypersalivation, anhidrosis, and tonic pupils.

Differential Diagnosis

The differential diagnosis of Guillain-Barré is the same as that of a spinal cord infection or injury. Electrolyte abnormalities such as hyper- and hypokalemia can cause weakness. Infections such as meningitis, encephalitis, and botulism, as well as tickborne infections, also mimic this disease. In the early stages of the disease, Guillain-Barré may also be mistaken for multiple sclerosis, myasthenia gravis, toxic ingestion of alcohol, heavy metals, or organophosphates, diabetes, and HIV neuropathy.

Key Findings

- Progressive, symmetric weakness of legs, arms, face, and trunk
- Areflexia
- Preceding illness

Management Strategies

In the prehospital setting, management of airway, breathing, and circulation, administration of oxygen, and assisted ventilation (if needed) are of primary importance. Other prehospital treatments include IV placement and cardiac monitoring devices. If the patient does have autonomic dysfunction, hypertension is best treated with short-acting agents; symptomatic bradycardia is best treated with atropine, and hypotension usually responds to IV fluids. Temporary cardiac pacing may be required if the patient has a second- or third-degree heart block.

Emergency Interventions

Because this is a rapidly progressing disease, it is important to recognize the likelihood that a patient will decompensate. Provide airway control and maintenance as necessary.

Transport Decisions

Transport should be to a tertiary care center when possible; rapid imaging and neurologic consultation are often required.

Acute Psychosis

The patient with acute psychosis has disturbances in thinking, behavior, and perception but not in orientation. He or she may have delusions, hallucinations, speech problems, flattened affect, withdrawal, and apathy.

Pathophysiology

Psychosis is primarily associated with abnormalities of brain chemistry and development. Genetics may play a role in the development of psychosis, but psychosocial stressors are thought to serve as exacerbating factors. It is believed that overactivity of the dopamine receptors in the brain, ones that are blocked by antipsychotic drugs, may cause the active hallucinations and delusions that characterize acute psychosis. Decreased activity in the prefrontal cortex of the brain related to serotonin transmission may be associated with symptoms such as flattened affect and social withdrawal.

Presentation

About 50% of patients have an acute onset of psychosis. The patient may have a period of relative mental health before the acute break occurs. That period is usually characterized by declining functioning at home, at work, and in public. Some patients with acute psychotic issues may seek medical care for medication reactions, such as hypotension, dry mouth, sedation, and difficulty with urination or sexual activity. Other patients may not have taken medications prescribed for psychosis for some period of time.

Differential Diagnosis

The differential diagnosis for acute psychosis includes delirium, depression, panic disorder, intoxication, brain tumor, and infection.

Key Findings

- Agitation and behavioral changes
- Abnormal thought content, often with delusions and/or hallucinations
- Labile mood

Management Strategies

Your safety and that of the patient are of utmost concern when treating a person with psychotic issues. The patient may require chemical or physical restraint. Monitor vital signs if possible, and provide emotional support. If the patient becomes medically unstable, initiate appropriate treatment per protocol.

Emergency Interventions

Because a medical issue may be responsible for the patient's alteration of mental status, blood glucose should be checked, a traumatic injury assessment should be performed, and vital signs, including pulse oximetry, should be carefully evaluated and treated if necessary. In addition, a careful history of the precipitating events should be taken to evaluate for poisoning, intoxication, and inappropriate or accidental medication ingestion.

Transport Decisions

Since medical abnormalities might have to be ruled out first in a patient demonstrating psychotic behavior, check blood glucose, and transport the patient to a facility that has both medical and psychiatric consultation services.

Special Considerations

Patients with psychoses may require chemical or physical restraint or police escort, depending on local protocol.

Acute Depression/Suicide Attempt

Suicide occurs when a person deliberately ends his own life. A suicide attempt occurs when a person tries to commit suicide but is unsuccessful at doing so. According to the National Institute of Mental Health, for every person who commits suicide, 12 to 25 attempts are made. Among teens, perhaps as many as 200 attempts are made for every suicide. A suicide attempt can take many forms, and emergency care must be administered on the basis of the self-inflicted harm the person has committed.

Although teen suicide pacts and other sensational suicides dominate the news on this topic, the rate of suicide among older adults is much higher than that among teens, primarily because they select more lethal means of ending their lives. According to the Institute on Aging, firearms, hanging, and poisoning (including toxic overdose), in that order, are the first, second, and third most common methods of suicide chosen among adults aged 65 and older. About 1 in 4 suicide attempts among this age group is successful. White men aged 80 and older have a higher risk of suicide than people in any other age, gender, or ethnic group.

The rate of suicide has increased steadily among adults aged 35 to 64, however, and is now about equal to the rate among older adults. Suicide remains the third leading cause of death among teens aged 15 to 19. Men are at much higher risk than women, and their attempts succeed much more often because they tend to choose more lethal means. The ethnic groups at highest risk are American Indians, Alaskan natives, and non-Hispanic whites.

According to the 2008 National Survey on Drug Use and Health, 1.1 million adults attempted suicide during the previous year. About two-thirds of them received medical care afterward. The goals of treatment are to stabilize the patient, identify any underlying medical conditions, evaluate mental health status, and provide appropriate referrals.

Pathophysiology

The pathophysiology of depression is multifactorial, but it is believed to involve changes in the neurotransmitters of the limbic system. Serotonin, norepinephrine, and dopamine have all been investigated as possible causes of depression. A family history of depression is frequently encountered, including among those who attempt suicide, but no definitive genetic link to depression has been found. Alcohol and other substance abuse is also a risk factor for depression. Emotional stressors such as physical or sexual abuse, suicide in the immediate family, family violence or divorce, incarceration, and prior suicide attempts may also accompany or precipitate depression or thoughts of suicide.

Presentation

Depression can manifest in many different ways. Some patients become withdrawn, others appear agitated. Eating behavior and sleeping patterns are affected. The patient may feel fatigued, hopeless, helpless, or worthless, and no longer take pleasure in activities that were once enjoyed. He may become forgetful, have changes in appetite or weight, and experience physical symptoms that have no obvious cause. The patient may have a slowing of normal functions, such as thinking and speech, and often has poor concentration. In severe cases of depression, the patient may come to the attention of medical providers when he or she attempts suicide.

Differential Diagnosis

The differential diagnosis for depression includes intoxication, anxiety, abuse or violence, electrolyte abnormality, headache, psychosis, infection, tumor, and other stressors.

Key Findings

- Flat or depressed affect
- History of depression/suicidal ideation
- Trauma (such as cutting or strangling oneself)
- Ingestion of a toxic substance

Management Strategies

Initiate supportive interventions, staying alert for a decreasing LOC, especially if the patient is suspected of having taken a drug overdose or has otherwise attempted to commit suicide. In these cases, management of airway, breathing, and circulation are the highest priorities. Render treatment consistent with the manner in which the patient has attempted suicide. For example, take spinal precautions if the person has attempted to hang himself, provide oxygenation for carbon monoxide poisoning, and use trauma packaging in patients with penetrating or blunt trauma. For potential poisonings, monitor cardiac rhythm, and watch for QRS widening.

Emergency Interventions

In a patient who makes a suicide attempt, take special care to evaluate for traumatic injury from causes such as jumping and hanging. Be on the lookout for stridor in hanging, deceleration injury in jumps, and electrolyte and rhythm abnormalities in ingestions.

Transport Decisions

The patient should be transported to a hospital with psychiatric facilities unless trauma or medical issues are present.

Special Considerations

Any suicide attempt should be taken seriously. The patient should not be left alone at any time. It is important to secure the back doors of the ambulance and to make sure the patient does not have easy access to potentially lethal objects in the back of the ambulance.

Putting It All Together

The patient with alterations in mental status or acute neurologic changes is often challenging for healthcare providers. When mental function is altered, it's difficult to obtain an accurate history and perform a reliable examination, so you must be especially observant and astute in looking for diagnostic clues and interpreting the information obtained. After assessing airway, breathing, and circulation for life threats, it is critically important to check every patient for those fundamental conditions that can be rapidly identified and managed. The SNOT mnemonic may help you do so. Once screening for these threats has been completed, guided by the patient's cardinal presentation, more detailed evaluation using the SAMPLE/OPQRST device for history should be carried out, the secondary survey should be conducted, and a differential diagnosis developed. This stepwise process allows prioritization of diagnostic testing and treatment interventions and, in the prehospital setting, determination of the most appropriate transport destination. Repeated reassessment until care is transferred is particularly important in patients with acute neurologic conditions and accompanying altered mental status.

SCENARIO SOLUTION

1. **After you ensure that she has a patent airway, is breathing adequately, and has adequate perfusion, you should obtain vital signs. Your head-to-toe assessment should include examination of her pupils, her vision (including peripheral vision), and her extraocular movements. Ask if she has photophobia. Note any redness, swelling, or tenderness in her temporal area. Evaluate the symmetry of her face. Auscultate her carotid arteries for bruits. Determine if she has any nuchal rigidity. Assess her periphery for presence of pulses, sensory function, and motor strength. Obtain additional history to determine whether she has sustained trauma. Evaluate her medications to obtain clues regarding her past medical history. Perform a stroke scale. Consider other diagnostic tests based on your findings.**

2. **Differential diagnosis for this patient could include stroke, intracranial hemorrhage, temporal arteritis, meningitis, and migraine headache.**

SUMMARY

- Reviewed the anatomy and physiology of the central nervous system
- Identified the components of the general impression and the elements of the primary survey for patients with a wide variety of neurologic emergencies
- Recognized the signs of altered mental status
- Applied the AMLS assessment pathway to rule in or out differential diagnoses based on a patient's cardinal presentation
- Identified the components of the secondary assessment using the mnemonics OPQRST and SAMPLER for pain assessment, physical examination, and key diagnostic findings
- Reviewed the importance of gathering pertinent patient historical data
- Applied the neurologic exam findings to help formulate a diagnosis after considering the differentials
- Reviewed the importance of providing physical and emotional supportive care on the scene and en route
- Based on patient condition, discussed the treatment options for immediate life threats
- Considered special transport alternatives on the basis of the likely diagnosis

BIBLIOGRAPHY

American Brain Tumor Association: A primer on brain tumors. Des Plaines, Ill., 2009, The Association. Modified January 2009. www.abta.org/index.cfm?contentid=170. Accessed September 26, 2009.

Hackam DG, et al: Most stroke patients do not get a warning: A population-based cohort study, Neurology 73:1074, 2009.

Institute on Aging: Suicide and the elderly. San Francisco, Calif. www.ioaging.org/services/counseling_healing/elderly_suicide.aspx. Accessed September 26, 2009.

National Institute of Mental Health: Suicide in the U.S.: Statistics and prevention. NIH Publication No. 06-4594. Modified July 27, 2009. www.nimh.nih.gov/health/publications/suicide-in-the-us-statistics-and-prevention/index.shtml. Accessed September 26, 2009.

National Stroke Association: National Stroke Association's complete guide to stroke, Centennial, Colo., 2003, The Association.

National Stroke Association: What is TIA? www.stroke.org/site/PageServer?pagename=TIA. Accessed September 29, 2009.

Pearce JMS: Meningitis, meninges, meninx, Eur Neurol 60:165, 2008. Published online July 16, 2008. http://content.karger.com/ProdukteDB/produkte.asp?Doi=145337. Accessed September 28, 2009.

Ruoff G, Urban G: Standards of care for headache diagnosis and treatment, Chicago, 2004, National Headache Foundation. www.guideline.gov/summary/summary.aspx?doc_id=6578&nbr=004138&string=migraine. Accessed September 26, 2009.

Substance Abuse and Mental Health Services Administration: 2008 National Survey on Drug Use and Health: Suicidal thoughts and behaviors among adults. Modified September 17, 2009. http://oas.samhsa.gov/2k9/165/Suicide.htm. Accessed September 26, 2009.

Chapter Review Questions

1. Which of the following describes a behavior that represents normal mental status? A person who:
   a. Asks you repeatedly what day of the week it is
   b. Does not respond when you call her name, but pushes your hand away when you perform a sternal rub
   c. Is drowsy and slow to respond to questions after awakening from a nap
   d. Is oriented to person, place, and time and has voices telling her she is evil

2. Which assessment evaluates at least one aspect of cranial nerve function?
   a. Blood glucose analysis
   b. Cincinnati Prehospital Stroke Scale
   c. Glasgow Coma Scale
   d. Mini-mental status examination

3. A 72-year-old male had a syncopal episode in church. He is now awake but confused. His wife said he has been complaining of a headache for about a week. He has early Alzheimer's disease. Home medicines include Lipitor and Exelon (rivastigmine). Which of the following questions may help narrow your differential diagnosis?
   a. Did he fall or hit his head recently?
   b. Does he have any allergies?
   c. Did he take his prescribed medication this morning?
   d. When was he diagnosed with Alzheimer's disease?

4. A 56-year-old female experiences a sudden onset of headache and blurred vision during yoga class. Her right eyelid is drooping, and the pupil on that side is small compared to the left pupil. You should take her to a hospital with:
   a. A STEMI center
   b. Ophthalmology surgical capability
   c. Psychiatric specialists
   d. Specialized neurologic and vascular capability

5. A 32-year-old complains of headache and dizziness. He vomited once and is walking with a staggering gait. His blood pressure is 148/72, pulse 92, respirations 20. He has a steady stare up toward his right ear. Which sign or symptom makes you consider intracerebral hemorrhage more strongly than migraine headache as a cause of his emergency?
   a. Abnormal gaze
   b. Blood pressure
   c. His age
   d. Dizziness and vomiting

6. Which is the most reliable indicator that ventilation should be assisted in a patient with altered mental status?
   a. Blood glucose is 600 mg/dL
   b. End-tidal CO_2 is 60 mm Hg
   c. Glasgow Coma Scale score is 10
   d. Oxygen saturation is 80%

7. A 24-year-old male complains of a sudden explosive headache. He asks you to lower the lights. He has vomited once. Which of these findings would increase your index of suspicion for subarachnoid hemorrhage?
   a. Bradycardia
   b. Hypertension
   c. Pupil dilation
   d. Stiff neck

8. Which of the following findings indicates the need to increase the rate of ventilation in an intubated patient you suspect to have an epidural hematoma?
   a. Flexion to painful stimulus
   b. Hypotension
   c. Positive Babinski sign
   d. Unilateral blown pupil

9. A 25-year-old helmeted female was thrown from a horse. She is complaining of weakness in her upper extremities. You ask her to close her eyes and identify whether you are moving her thumb up or down. She is unable to do so. This indicates she does not have normal:
   a. Fine motor movement
   b. Proprioception
   c. Sensation of touch
   d. Spinal accessory nerve function

10. A 44-year-old male is postictal after a witnessed grand mal seizure. He is arousable to light pain and is presently snoring. His vital signs are BP 142/86, P 120, R 20, SaO_2 98%. You should:
    a. Assist ventilation with a bag-mask
    b. Insert a nasopharyngeal airway
    c. Prepare to intubate his trachea
    d. Place in supine position

CHAPTER

3 Respiratory Disorders

IN THIS CHAPTER, you'll read about the anatomy and function of the respiratory system and learn about common diseases and conditions that generate respiratory complaints. More important, you'll be asked to apply your knowledge to patient assessment, determining whether pathology is present, identifying its cause from among several plausible diagnoses, and using cogent clinical reasoning to select the best treatment plan for your patient. In addition, you'll review several critical procedures for monitoring and treating patients with respiratory complaints.

Learning Objectives ***At the conclusion of this chapter, you will be able to:***

1. Explain the anatomy, physiology, and pathophysiology of diseases and conditions often accompanied by respiratory complaints, and describe their typical clinical presentations.
2. Describe how to obtain a thorough history from the patient with a respiratory complaint.
3. Carry out a comprehensive physical examination of a patient with a respiratory complaint.
4. Form an initial impression and generate a list of likely differential diagnoses on the basis of a patient's history, signs, and symptoms.
5. Order or recommend appropriate diagnostic tests, and apply the results to aid in diagnosis.
6. Perform critical procedures necessary to stabilize and treat patients with emergent respiratory conditions.
7. Follow accepted evidence-based practice guidelines for the overall management of each condition.
8. Provide an ongoing assessment of the patient, revising your clinical impression and treatment strategy on the basis of the patient's response to interventions.

Key Terms

abscess (peritonsillar) An abscess in which a superficial soft-tissue infection progresses to create pockets of purulence in the submucosal space adjacent to the tonsils. This abscess and its accompanying inflammation cause the uvula to deviate to the opposing side.

acute lung injury/acute respiratory distress syndrome (ALI/ARDS) A systemic disease that causes lung failure

aerobic metabolism The process in which glucose is converted into energy in the presence of oxygen

anaerobic metabolism A process in which when denied oxygen, cells can generate small amounts of energy but release excessive acids as byproducts, especially lactic and carbonic acids

angioedema A disorder characterized by a sudden swelling, usually of a head or neck structure such as the lip (especially the lower lip), earlobes, tongue, or uvula

apneustic center Located in the pons, this center regulates the depth of respiration.

atelectasis Alveolar collapse

chemoreceptors Chemical receptors that sense changes in the composition of blood and body fluids. The primary chemical changes registered by chemoreceptors are those involving levels of hydrogen (H^+), carbon dioxide (CO_2), and oxygen (O_2).

end-tidal carbon dioxide ($ETCO_2$) monitoring Analysis of exhaled gases for CO_2, this is a useful method of assessing a patient's ventilatory status.

gas exchange The process in which oxygen from the atmosphere is taken up by circulating blood cells and carbon dioxide from the bloodstream is released to the atmosphere

history of the present illness (HPI) The most important element of patient assessment. The primary elements of the HPI can be obtained by using the OPQRST and SAMPLER mnemonics.

Ludwig's angina A deep-space infection of the anterior neck just below the mandible. The name derives from the sensation of choking and suffocation reported by most patients with this condition.

noninvasive positive-pressure ventilation (NPPV) A procedure in which positive pressure is provided through the upper airway by some type of mask or other noninvasive interface

pneumotaxic center Located in the pons, this center generally controls the rate and pattern of respiration.

respiration The reciprocal passage of oxygen into the blood and carbon dioxide into the alveoli

respiratory failure A disorder in which the lungs become unable to perform their basic task of gas exchange, the transfer of oxygen from inhaled air into the blood and the transfer of carbon dioxide from the blood into exhaled air

thoracentesis A procedure to remove fluid or air from the pleural space

thoracic duct Located in the left upper thorax; the thoracic duct is the largest lymph vessel in the body. It returns to the venae cavae the excess fluid from the lower extremities and abdomen that is not collected by the veins.

thoracostomy A procedure in which a tube may be connected to a Heimlich valve, a one-way valve that lets air escape but not enter the pleural space

ultrasound Also called *sonography* or *diagnostic medical sonography,* this is an imaging method that uses high-frequency sound waves to produce precise images of structures within the body.

SCENARIO

YOUR 57-YEAR-OLD PATIENT complains of a "sore throat." As you greet him you note that he appears ill. His eyes are injected and he constantly dabs sputum from the corners of his mouth. With a muffled voice, he explains that his symptoms began today. He says he feels achy, has had chills, and is experiencing pain in his ear and lower teeth. His medical history includes type 2 diabetes and hypertension. Initial vital signs are BP 104/72, P 124/min, R 20, T 103°F (39.4°C). As your exam continues, the patient becomes more anxious and restless. You note a high-pitched noise as he breathes in.

1 *What differential diagnoses are you considering based on the information you have now?*

2 *What additional information will you need to narrow your differential diagnosis?*

3 *What are your initial treatment priorities as you continue your patient care?*

No longer shall I paint interiors with men reading and women knitting. I will paint living people who breathe and feel and suffer and love.

—Edvard Munch

From Byron to Billy Ray Cyrus, the fluttering, palpitating, achy-breaky heart has come to symbolize love. Likewise, breathing has become synonymous with expressiveness, with freedom—with life itself. Perhaps because we can hear, feel, and even see our respiration, the practical necessity of breathing is often elevated to a poetic ideal. In this chapter, we'll confine our discussion to the practical, leaving the poetic to the realm of music, art, and literature.

Anatomy of the Respiratory System

The pulmonary system is housed primarily within the chest, but it has far-reaching effects on every cell in the body. The system has two primary functions:

1. Ventilation: the movement of air in and out of the lungs. The process of ventilation is the first step in providing oxygen (O_2) to the cells and removing carbon dioxide (CO_2) and other waste products from the circulation. Delivery of clean, humidified air to the alveoli in sufficient quantities to maintain an appropriate level of oxygen in the blood is the function of the oropharynx, pharynx, trachea, bronchi, and bronchioles.
2. Respiration: the process of **gas exchange** in which oxygen from the atmosphere is taken up by circulating blood cells, and carbon dioxide from the bloodstream is released to the atmosphere.

The respiratory system can be divided into the upper and lower airways. The upper airways comprise all structures above the vocal cords, and the lower airways comprise the structures that fall below that anatomic point. Most of the respiratory system lies within the thorax, sharing space with the cardiovascular and gastrointestinal systems. The patient who complains of chest pain, cough, shortness of breath, or a choking sensation may have pathology arising from any of these three thoracic systems.

Upper Airway

The respiratory tract opens to the outside of the body through the nasal and oral cavities. From a respiratory standpoint, each route serves a different function. Air that passes through the mouth to the posterior pharynx does not become as moist as air that passes through the nasal cavity, but it still contributes to ventilation. Let's take a closer look first at the nasal cavity.

Nasal Cavity

The nasal cavity is composed of the following structures:

- The nares (nostrils)
- The nasal cavity, which contains the nasal turbinates (curved bony plates that extend from the lateral wall of the nasal cavity)
- The nasopharynx

The nasal cavity serves several important purposes. It humidifies and warms inhaled air, protecting the lower mucosa. The mucus-producing cells that line the nasopharynx capture large airborne particles, preventing lower respiratory tract infections. In addition, the nasopharynx functions as a resonating chamber, giving the voice its timbre and pitch.

Pharynx and Oral Cavity

While not dedicated to ventilation, the structures of the mouth—the lips, teeth, gums, tongue, and salivary glands—function in mastication and speech creation.

Inhaled air that passes through the oral cavity reaches the pharynx and then the hypopharynx, which is immediately behind the base of the tongue (Figure 3-1). This area also houses the tonsils, lymph tissue that helps fight infection. Directly below the hypopharynx is the

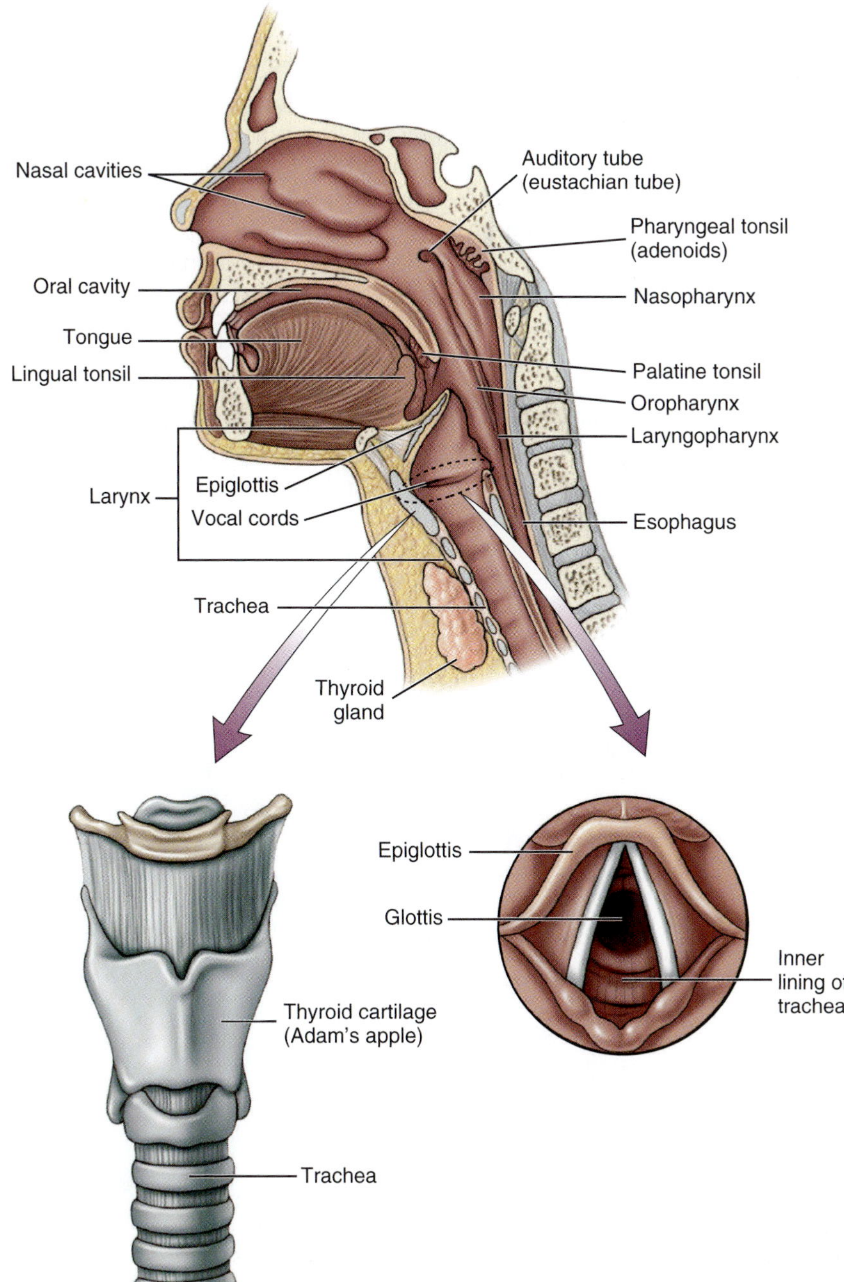

■ **Figure 3-1** Airway anatomy. Structures above glottis compose upper airway; below glottis, lower airway. Lower airway structures include trachea, bronchial tree, alveoli, and lungs. (Modified from Herlihy B: The human body in health and illness, ed 3, Philadelphia, 2007, Saunders.)

epiglottis, a cartilaginous flap that covers the trachea during swallowing. This flap, which normally remains open, protects the airway from aspiration by closing involuntarily during swallowing when a bolus of liquid or food passes over it. In unconscious patients, this reflex is often absent, putting them in grave danger of aspirating vomitus. Such aspiration can be life threatening because of the volume and acidity of stomach contents.

Below the epiglottis lie three glottic structures:

1. The thyroid cartilage, which surrounds everything
2. The arytenoid cartilages, which help support the vocal cords
3. The false vocal cords and true vocal cords, mobile structures that partially cover the glottis and move back and forth to create basic sounds that are tuned by the oropharynx and nasopharynx. The false vocal cords are made up of fibrous connective tissue and are attached to the true vocal cords. The true vocal cords are composed of fine ligamentous tissues. The space between the two true vocal cords, where air passes for ventilation to the lower respiratory tract, is referred to as the *glottis*.

Lower Respiratory Tract

When air enters the lower respiratory tract (Figure 3-2), it passes through the trachea and bronchi to the lungs, where it sweeps through the bronchioles and finally reaches the alveoli, the tiny sacs in which gas exchange takes place.

Trachea

After passing through the glottis, air next flows into the trachea. The trachea is a membranous tube supported by incomplete C-shaped cartilaginous rings. The first is the cricoid cartilage, the only ring with a circumferential cartilage framework. Below the cricoid are successive rings connected posteriorly by small muscles that help determine the diameter of the cartilage as they relax and contract. This structure keeps the trachea from collapsing with vigorous coughing or bronchial constriction.

The trachea is lined with a tissue called *columnar epithelium,* which produces mucus, a viscous substance that helps trap foreign particles. Microscopic hairs called *cilia* help move the mucus and trapped particles up the respiratory tract to be eventually expelled by coughing and expectoration.

Bronchi and Lungs

Proceeding down the trachea, the C-shaped cartilaginous rings continue to where the trachea divides into the left and right mainstem bronchi. The bronchi are the only source of ventilation for each lung. The right mainstem bronchus is straighter and larger in diameter than the left, making it more susceptible to aspiration and inadvertent intubation. These bronchi are also composed of C-shaped rings, connected in the back by a small muscle. The columnar epithelial lining extends into the bronchi, providing humidification and secreting mucus to protect the lower airway against harmful particulates.

The right and left lungs are the next structures in the path of airflow. The lungs are enveloped by a dual-layered membrane called the *pleura.* The visceral pleura adheres to the lungs, whereas the parietal pleura lines the inner surface of the chest wall and mediastinum. Between these two pleurae is an airtight space (potential space) containing a thin layer of lubricating fluid that allows the membranes to glide over each other when no disease is present.

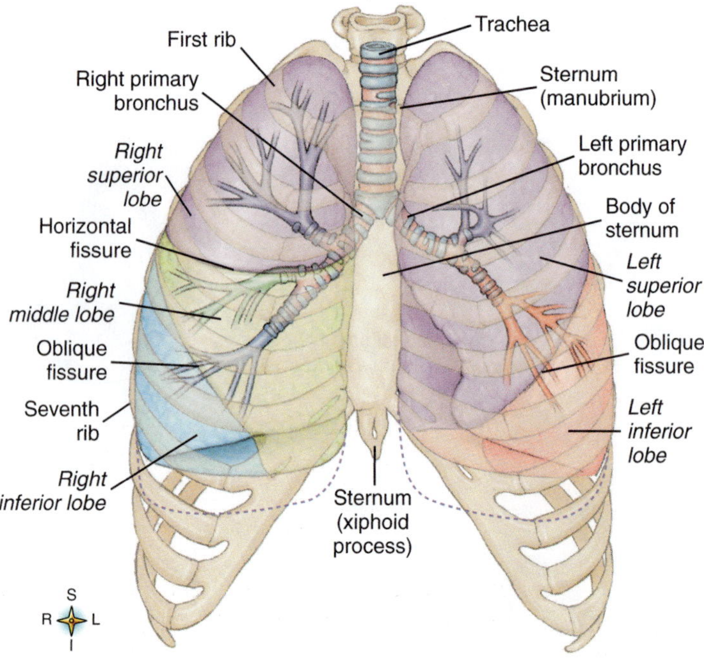

Figure 3-2 Lower airway structures. (From Thibodeau GA, Patton KT: Structure and function of the body, ed 12, St Louis, 2004, Mosby.)

Although they function similarly, the lungs differ somewhat in structure. The right lung has three main lobes: upper, middle, and lower. The left lung shares its side of the intrathoracic space with the heart, so it has only two lobes—the upper and lower.

Bronchioles and Alveoli

On entering the lungs, the mainstem bronchi split into successively smaller bronchioles: primary, secondary, and tertiary. These increasingly smaller tubes distribute inhaled air to all areas of the lung for effective ventilation. The linings of the tertiary and smaller bronchioles produce less and less mucus, which becomes progressively more difficult for the body to move up and out of the airway the farther down the bronchioles are in the respiratory tract. Note that although all of these structures have a role in conducting air to the lungs, they are not all involved in the act of respiration.

The bronchioles eventually terminate in alveoli, small sacs with walls only a single cell thick so as to allow gas exchange (respiration) to occur. Millions of alveoli exist in a healthy lung, forming grapelike clusters. Gas exchange takes place across the few layers of cells that separate the alveoli from the pulmonary capillaries. This reciprocal passage of oxygen into the blood and carbon dioxide into the alveoli is called **respiration.** As it leaves the alveoli, gas passes through the single layer of cells that makes up the alveolar wall, through a thin layer of interstitial tissue, and finally through the single layer of cells that makes up the capillary wall. Any increase in the thickness of this cell layer can profoundly jeopardize respiration.

Alveoli are held open and in position by connective tissue in the interstitial tissues that surround the alveoli. A chemical called *surfactant* coats the inner walls of the alveoli, helping keep open these tiny pouches. Surfactant is a chemical that acts much like soap, reducing surface tension and providing an interface between oil and water so the alveoli will not readily collapse on exhalation. Premature infants can have a deficiency of surfactant, which leads to serious respiratory problems. But whatever the patient's age, even normal amounts of surfactant and adequate connective-tissue support can't prevent alveolar collapse. **Atelectasis** occurs secondary to infection, trauma, or inflammation. Atelectasis is a major risk factor for pneumonia.

Musculoskeletal Support of Respiration

The bones, muscles, and connective tissues serve an integral function in ventilation. Without the support of these structures, effective ventilation would be impossible. Structural support ranges from the cartilaginous trachea to the bony vault of the thorax, which maintains the pressure necessary for ventilation.

The main muscle of ventilation is the diaphragm, a thick muscle that separates the thorax from the abdomen. The diaphragm is under both voluntary and involuntary control. The phrenic nerve, which signals the diaphragm to contract and relax, originates in the brainstem and exits from the cervical spine at C3, C4, and C5. These levels are important, particularly in trauma, since injury to the cervical spine at these levels may cause fatal apnea.

The thoracic cage is the truss that supports and shelters the structures within the thoracic cavity, including the lungs. Its architecture facilitates the intrathoracic pressure changes necessary for ventilation. The ribs, sternum, and thoracic spine form a protective framework (Figure 3-3). In addition to shielding the intrathoracic organs, the ribs help create the pressure necessary for inspiration and expiration.

The intercostal muscles are considered accessory muscles to respiration, meaning they're insufficient to serve as the primary muscle of ventilation but can assist the diaphragm in creating the pressure changes necessary for ventilation. There are other accessory muscles, including the abdominal and neck muscles. If you note that a patient is having to use accessory muscles to breathe, respiratory compromise or impending **respiratory failure** should be on your watch list.

Just behind the trachea lies the esophagus, which collapses easily with any negative pressure, since it's a muscular tube. The posterior muscular wall of the trachea lies next to the anterior esophagus. When swallowing large bites of food, the esophagus accommodates the bolus while the trachea retains its shape. Esophageal strictures and lesions may create a feeling of burning or fullness in the thorax because of this elasticity.

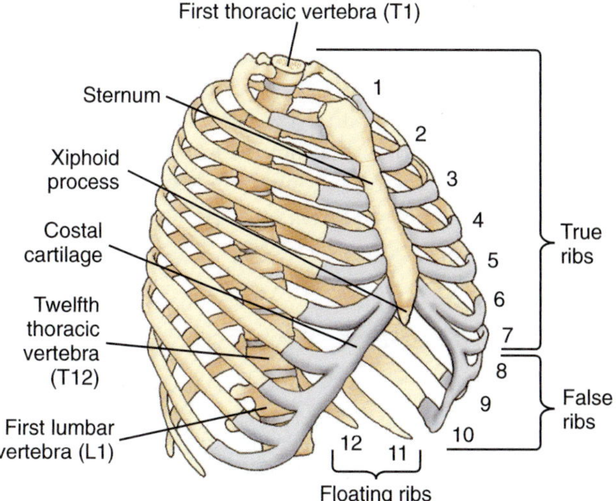

Figure 3-3 Thoracic cage. Ribs exist in pairs, 12 on either side of chest, and are numbered from the top rib, beginning with 1. Upper seven pairs join directly to sternum by a strip of cartilage and are called *true ribs*. Remaining five pairs are known as *false ribs* because they do not attach directly to sternum. Last two pairs of false ribs, called *floating ribs*, are attached only on posterior aspect. (From Leonard PC: Building a medical vocabulary: with Spanish translations, ed 7, St Louis, 2008, Saunders.)

Intrathoracic Relationship of Cardiac and Vascular Structures

The anatomic structures that support ventilation and respiration share the intrathoracic space with several other important structures, including the heart, venae cavae, aorta, pulmonary trunk, and thoracic duct. These vascular structures circulate oxygenated blood to tissues and return deoxygenated blood to the lungs for lymph exchange and removal of waste materials such as carbon dioxide.

The heart is the main pump of the circulatory system, and proper functioning is critical to distribution of blood throughout the body. Deoxygenated blood returns to the heart via the superior and inferior venae cavae. The superior vena cava returns the blood from the head, arms, and shoulders (that is, parts above the heart), and the inferior vena cava returns blood from the lower body (that is, parts below the heart). Deoxygenated blood passes from the venae cavae into the right atrium and is then pumped into the right ventricle, then into the pulmonary trunk. The pulmonary trunk branches into the right and left pulmonary arteries, which flow into the lungs. Oxygenated blood returns to the heart and left atrium through the pulmonary veins. This is the only place in the body where the arteries carry deoxygenated blood and the veins carry oxygenated blood.

From the left atrium, blood is pumped into the left ventricle, the most robust chamber of the heart. The left ventricle is strong enough to counter the force of aortic pressure in order to eject blood into the aorta. Blood is then distributed to the body by successively smaller arteries and arterioles.

The **thoracic duct**, located in the left upper thorax, is the largest lymph vessel in the body. The thoracic duct returns to the venae cavae any excess fluid from the lower extremities and abdomen that is not collected by the veins. The amount of lymph fluid returned is small compared with the blood volume that flows through the veins, but its evacuation is important, since the fluid would otherwise pool in the lower extremities.

Physiology of the Respiratory System

The respiratory system is governed by a complex set of physiologic processes, including activation of the immune response, regulation of respiration and ventilation, and support of acid-base balance. Let's take a brief look at each of these processes.

Activation of Immune Response

When air from the environment enters the respiratory tract, the potential for infection is always present, but the body is quite efficient in responding to this threat. The respiratory system has several strategies for preventing disease-causing organisms (pathogens) from entering from the upper respiratory tract and reaching the alveoli.

If a pathogen bypasses the skin (which acts as a primary barrier against injury and infection) and enters the body through the respiratory tract, the lining of epithelial cells in the trachea acts as a secondary barrier against infection. The epithelium is made up of mucus-secreting goblet cells. The sticky mucus intercepts would-be invaders. Other cells contain microscopic hairs (cilia) that help move the mucus to the upper respiratory tract, where it can be expectorated by coughing.

Mucus also contains an immune antibody called *immunoglobulin A (IgA)*. IgA is secreted into bodily fluids and binds to pathogenic organisms, allowing white blood cells to recognize and destroy them.

In the lower respiratory tract, white cells can physically enter the alveoli and bronchioles by squeezing between the cell borders. White cells attack pathogens and engulf any small particles not carried away in the mucus of the upper airway. These white cells are often expectorated in mucus and account for the yellow-green color of sputum in patients with certain kinds of respiratory infections.

Neuroregulation of Respiration and Ventilation

Three major mechanisms regulate ventilation:

1. The central nervous system (CNS)
2. The peripheral nervous system and the muscles of ventilation
3. Chemical and mechanical sensors in the body

Central Nervous System

The CNS governs ventilation from various locations within the brain and spinal cord. The medulla and pons, which make up the brainstem, are both involved in this central control. The medulla modulates the basic rhythm of ventilation and triggers a ventral group when a rapid respiratory rate is needed. The pons limits inhalation and triggers exhalation through the **pneumotaxic center**, which generally controls the rate and pattern of respiration. The **apneustic center**, also located in the pons, regulates the depth of respiration.

The cerebral cortex allows voluntary command of ventilation, overriding the automatic systems controlled by the medulla and pons. This is important when you want to laugh, cry, sing, or talk. CNS disorders can lead to respiratory compromise.

Peripheral Nervous System

The peripheral nervous system and the muscles of respiration must function in a coordinated fashion. During inspiration, contraction of the diaphragm forces it to move downward while contraction of the intercostal muscles causes the ribs to rise and expand. These actions increase intrathoracic volume, which in turn lowers pressure in the thorax. This reduction, or negative pressure, allows environmental air to rush into the lungs.

During expiration, the opposite occurs—the diaphragm and intercostal muscles relax, and positive pressure in the thorax forces air out of the lungs into the atmosphere.

Chemical and Mechanical Sensors

Sensors in the body are located centrally in the brain and cerebrospinal fluid, and peripherally in the aortic arch, kidneys, and lungs. Mechanical receptors, or mechanoreceptors, sense when irritating substances are present or when too much stretch in the muscles is occurring. When the stretch receptors are stimulated at the peak of inhalation, the muscles recoil so that overventilation does not damage the lungs. This reflex is also stimulated when coughing is triggered by a foreign object or particles in the airway.

Chemical receptors, or **chemoreceptors**, sense changes in the composition of blood and body fluids. The primary chemical changes registered by chemoreceptors are those involving levels of hydrogen (H^+), carbon dioxide (CO_2), and oxygen (O_2):

- H^+: the chemoreceptors sense when an increase in the hydrogen level in the fluid surrounding the cells of the medulla stimulates an increase in the rate of ventilation. The opposite occurs when H^+ levels fall. This change can be detected in the bloodstream by measuring pH. Normal pH in the human body is 7.35 to 7.45.
- CO_2: the CO_2 level in the blood will rise if respiration is too slow or shallow, causing CO_2 retention, or if the blood becomes too acidic. The excess CO_2 spills over into the cerebrospinal fluid, triggering an increase in H^+ and in turn precipitating an increase in the respiratory rate. This level can be measured in the blood by measuring the partial pressure of CO_2 ($Pa{CO_2}$). Normal $Pa{CO_2}$ is 35 to 45 mm Hg. CO_2 level is the principal regulator of respiration.
- O_2: when peripheral chemoreceptors sense an excessive drop in the oxygen level, the respiratory rate increases. Normal $Pa{O_2}$ is 80 to 100 mm Hg.

Normal ventilation is controlled by the hypercarbic (high CO_2 level) drive, whereby ventilation increases when CO_2 becomes even slightly elevated. Chemoreceptors undergo a change when chronic lung disease causes a perpetual elevation of the CO_2 level. The patient is said to convert to a hypoxic drive, whereby he or she is dependent on a low level of oxygen to stimulate a rise in ventilation rate or depth. This fact explains why patients with chronic lung disease should not be given long-term excessive amounts of oxygen.

Preservation of Acid-Base Balance

Respiration and ventilation are regulated by a complex interaction of nerves, sensors, and hormones. The level of carbon dioxide in the body is the primary modulator of respiration. CO_2 is the chief waste product of metabolism. Metabolism is the process of breaking down sugars (dextrose, or glucose) into energy for use by the cells of the body. A high CO_2 level damages the cellular machinery responsible for this metabolism. **Aerobic metabolism**, in which glucose is converted into energy in the presence of oxygen, is the basic process of life. This process is very efficient but relies on a steady supply of both oxygen and glucose, since the cell cannot stockpile either resource.

When denied oxygen, the cells resort to **anaerobic metabolism**, which allows the cells to generate small amounts of energy but releases excessive acids as byproducts, especially lactic and carbonic acids. This excess of acid must be removed by the circulation, or too much CO_2 will be produced and acidosis will result. Often, though, the same problem that impaired oxygen delivery also compromises the circulation, and acids build up, causing cellular injury or tissue death.

Blood Buffer System

The body neutralizes pH by means of three mechanisms: the blood, the respiratory system, and the kidneys. The blood is capable of buffering out some of the excess acid through the carbonic acid–bicarbonate system, which can be described by the carbonic acid–bicarbonate equation. This equation spells out the balancing function the blood performs in an almost immediate effort to maintain a normal pH. Excess CO_2 is combined with water to form carbonic acid ($H_2O + CO_2 = H_2CO_3$). This carbonic acid is only temporary, rapidly breaking down into hydrogen ions (acids) and HCO_3^- (H^+ and HCO_3^-). Note that the arrows in the equation point both ways, indicating that these key elements shift back and forth depending on the concentration level of each substrate:

$$CO_2 + H_2O \leftrightarrow H_2CO_3 \leftrightarrow HCO_3^- + H^+$$

Respiratory System

Besides the buffer system, which works continuously to neutralize pH, the respiratory system itself can make some adjustments in acid-base balance. When sensors detect an increase in the CO_2 level, the respiratory system speeds up respiration to “blow off” the excess CO_2 by means of exhalation. Conversely, when the CO_2 level is too low, the system slows down the rate of respiration.

Kidneys

The third system that helps maintain acid-base balance is the renal system. When acidosis persists for longer than 6 hours or so, the kidneys begin to retain HCO_3 and excrete H^+ ions, primarily in the form of ammonium (NH_4^+). This is a slow process, and it may take days for enough H^+ to be eliminated to achieve acid-base balance.

The kidneys can sense decreased oxygen levels in the blood. Sensors in the renal artery note hypoxia and then release erythropoietin, a hormone that stimulates the creation of red blood cells. When the sensors register chronic low levels of oxygen, more red blood cells are created. Patients who suffer from chronic bronchitis, for instance, often have an elevated number of red blood cells, a condition called *polycythemia*. This disorder increases the risk of forming blood clots. Erythropoietin has been chemically synthesized and is used as an injectable medication in patients who are receiving chemotherapy, in an effort to encourage the body to generate red blood cells.

Ventilation Volume

Analysis of the volume of air involved in ventilation can help us understand the pathology of many respiratory diseases and evaluate how well a patient is responding to treatment (Figure 3-4).

Tidal Volume

Tidal volume is the normal volume of air inspired per breath at rest. The precise volume can be affected by many variables, including lung disease, body size, physical fitness, and less obvious factors such as elevation above sea level. Normal tidal volume for an adult is about 500 mL. Minute volume is the tidal volume multiplied by the number of breaths per minute. This metric quantifies the amount of air inspired in 60 seconds.

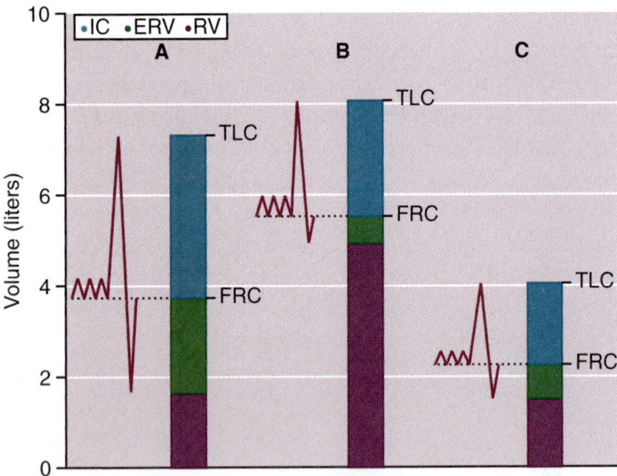

■ **Figure 3-4** Lung volumes. Leftmost tracing (**A**) shows typical breathing pattern in normal subject, including change in lung volumes associated with maximal inspiration (to total lung capacity [TLC]), followed by maximal expiration to residual volume (RV). Using techniques described in the text, lung volume measurements can allow accurate calculation of RV, TLC, and other components of lung volume, including functional residual capacity (FRC), inspiratory capacity (IC), and expiratory reserve volume (ERV). Also shown are typical lung volume profiles of a patient with severe asthma with hyperinflation and gas trapping (**B**) and a patient with restrictive lung disease causing severe reduction in lung volumes (**C**). (From Walsh D, et al: Palliative medicine, Philadelphia, 2009, Saunders.)

Residual Volume

Residual volume is the amount of air that remains in the lungs after maximum expiration. This air maintains partial inflation of the lungs.

Dead Space

Any area of tissue in which gas exchange cannot take place is known as *dead space*. The amount of dead space can increase when a disease process like atelectasis occurs (see Lower Airway Diseases later in the chapter).

Reserve Capacity

There are two kinds of reserve capacity: expiratory and inspiratory. Expiratory reserve capacity is the difference between a normal exhalation and an exhalation of the remaining air in the lungs. You can demonstrate this concept by forcing as much air out of the lungs as possible after a normal exhalation—this volume of air is the expiratory reserve capacity. Likewise, inhaling as deeply as possible after a normal inhalation allows you to take in an additional volume of air, the inspiratory reserve capacity. The inspiratory reserve capacity helps keep the alveoli inflated. It is often expelled in yawning.

Vital Capacity and Total Lung Capacity

Vital capacity is the total amount of air exchanged during a forced inhalation after a forced exhalation. Total lung capacity is calculated as vital capacity plus dead space. Although it depends on many factors, total lung capacity is the maximum capacity of the lungs, including any dead space.

Pulmonary Function Tests

Pulmonary function tests (PFTs) are breathing tests often ordered by pulmonologists for a patient with breathing difficulties in order to better characterize the nature and severity of the illness. PFTs often measure the capacities just discussed, as well as forced expiratory volume in one second (FEV_1) and other metrics.

Normal FEV_1 is calculated on the basis of the patient's height and weight and ranges from about 400 mL/sec to 600 mL/sec. FEV_1 is effort dependent, so patients who are unable or unwilling to put forth a genuine effort may skew the test to an artificially low value.

In the field or emergency department (ED), you may measure a peak expiratory flow rate, or peak flow, in patients with bronchospasm. This rate is a measure of airflow and is evaluated against an expected norm based on age, height, and sex or against the patient's known baseline.

SPECIAL CONSIDERATIONS

Advancing Age

Aging patients undergo multiple changes in the respiratory system, all of which ultimately impair the body's ability to oxygenate the blood. A wide range of physiologic changes can occur both within the respiratory tract and in the body structures that support ventilation. A summary of physiologic changes associated with advancing age is listed in Box 3-1.

Since these changes occur gradually, often over a period of years or even decades, the body has time to adapt to a significant decrease in function. If these same changes were to happen over a compressed period of days or weeks, the sudden loss of function could be fatal. A good example is the decrease in respiratory surface area that occurs as a person ages. The blood oxygen level (called the *partial pressure*) in a young adult normally averages 95 mm Hg. In the older adult, a value as low as 60 mm Hg is not uncommon. If the partial pressure of oxygen was noted to be 60 mm Hg in a young, seemingly healthy individual, you would be quite concerned.

The likelihood of pathologic changes in the respiratory system and supporting structures increases as a patient ages. Some intrapleural diseases impair the ability of the lungs to inspire and expire air. Others inhibit diffusion of oxygen into the blood and carbon dioxide out of the blood. In addition, tumors can occupy lung space, decreasing the area available for ventilation. Chronic smoking can ravage alveoli, narrow bronchi and choke them with mucus, and displace functioning alveoli with large blebs, or air pockets. Circulatory changes can result in delivery of less or thinner blood to the lung capillaries, impairing oxygenation. Decreased hemoglobin can reduce the oxygen-carrying capacity of red blood cells.

All these changes can combine to make it more difficult for an individual to perform normal activities of daily living. In the elderly, a relatively minor respiratory infection can pose a life threat. Pneumonia may cause an already marginally hypoxic elderly patient to become severely hypoxic, requiring respiratory support and mechanical ventilation.

Bariatric Considerations

Increased body mass can impede or complicate many functions of the respiratory system in the following ways:

- The larger body mass increases the need for energy for routine activities, with a consequent increase in the need for delivery of oxygen and removal of carbon dioxide and other waste products.
- The body's sheer physical mass limits the range of motion of the chest, reducing contraction of the diaphragm and subsequent expansion of the lungs.
- When lying supine, excessive weight in the anterior abdomen can shift to the upper abdomen, limiting expansion of the chest and perhaps decreasing tidal volume.

The lungs can expand somewhat in response to increased demand, but their size is limited by the abdomen and its contents. The chest can increase in diameter, a response often seen in patients who chronically abuse tobacco (an indicator of chronic bronchitis), but the size of the chest is also limited. The heart can become more efficient by pumping faster and harder, but these adjustments may have long-term cardiovascular side effects including heart failure.

Assessment

Dyspnea is both a sign and a symptom. An outward sign of dyspnea, for example, is the use of accessory muscles. The patient may complain of breathlessness or express an uncomfortable awareness that he is having breathing difficulties, using terms like "shortness of breath" or "chest tightness."

Dispatch and Situational Awareness

When responding to an emergency dispatch, the chief complaint of the patient with respiratory difficulties (sometimes expressed by bystanders when the patient is unable to speak) varies from the obvious shortness of

BOX 3-1 Age-Related Changes That Affect the Respiratory System

- Thinning of epithelial linings
- Decreased mucus production
- Flagging activity of respiratory cilia
- Reduced lung compliance due to calcification of cartilage in the trachea and bronchioles and calcification of interstitial tissues
- Decreasing respiratory surface area as the number of alveoli dwindles
- Reduced intrathoracic volume secondary to fractures, slumping, or bony changes
- Less vigorous immune response, including fewer immunoglobulins and leukocytes
- Weakened muscles of respiration, including diaphragm, intercostals, and accessory muscles

breath to weakness or altered mental status. The dispatcher may have obtained additional information from the caller, or your memory of having responded to this patient's residence before may clue you in to the fact that he or she has chronic disease.

Scene Survey

Evaluating the scene for hazards is a key step in the AMLS assessment pathway (see Chapter 1 for a review). Patients with respiratory distress rarely pose a threat to emergency responders, but caution must be exercised when dealing with any hypoxic patient who is restless. You must also consider the potential for violence by family members or bystanders who find it distressing to watch a patient, particularly a loved one, struggle to breathe. Extreme frustration combined with few coping resources is a recipe for aggression. Gaining a command of the scene with tact and empathy can lay the groundwork for good patient care.

A note of caution about settings in which drug overdoses may have occurred: in communities that have a high crime rate, police protection should usually be requested early in the dispatch process. Be alert for loud voices and other red flags that danger may be at hand.

The presence of medical devices in the patient's environment should prompt you to ask questions once you enter the home. Some chronic respiratory patients require airway and ventilatory support 24/7, from relatively simple oxygen tanks to sophisticated ventilators. When a complication arises, emergency services are implemented to help solve the acute problem.

Hazardous Materials

When patients show evidence of mucous membrane irritation and increased work of breathing, especially when there are isolated groups of victims, special attention to scene safety is warranted. Hazardous materials (hazmat) equipment and teams may have to be dispatched before you enter the scene.

Evaluation of any scene, whether a business or a private home, should be done using all your senses. You shouldn't be able to see particulates suspended in the air, and you shouldn't enter an area where the air is smoky, foggy, or dusty. If your patient is in such an area, respiratory complications are likely. Look for chemical placards within business settings. Obtain personal protection equipment and hazmat resources to gain safe entry to such scenes. Be sure to smell the air. Chemical odors may alert you to the presence of invisible chemicals in the air. The same protection and resources must be used if you detect this hazard. Within industrial scenes, unusual sounds should alert you to gas leaks or the potential for hazardous situations.

Standard Precautions

Any combination of respiratory complaints with a stated history of fever warrants barrier protection of your mucous membranes, especially while performing suctioning and airway procedures. Putting on a mask seems so simple, but it's a precaution that's easy to forget when you view a very sick patient from across the room.

Environmental Stressors

Social, psychological, and physiologic stressors assail the body's immune systems and create an environment conducive to respiratory disorders. Hypothermia, for instance, leads to respiratory compromise and failure. Heat and humidity combined with environmental pollution is also a hazard for chronic respiratory patients. Secondary smoke pollutes the air of everyone in the general vicinity but especially triggers reactive airway difficulties in those with asthma or chronic obstructive pulmonary disease (COPD).

Initial Assessment

Gaining knowledge of the anatomy, physiology, and pathophysiology that can affect breathing is the first step in being able to perform a thorough physical exam and obtain an appropriate history from the patient to determine the cause of the complaint. Chapter 1 outlined the process of forming that clinical impression, and a section devoted to assessment of the airway and treatment of airway compromise is included in Appendix D of this manual.

Observation

Your initial observation, no matter how you first encounter the patient, is important. In certain circumstances, the family will bundle up an ill patient having respiratory problems and go to the emergency department (ED), without calling for the aid of emergency services. Occasionally, emergency care is rendered in a clinic. Regardless of the setting, assess for overall consciousness and work of breathing, and do a quick check of perfusion status. You can do so while helping the patient out of the car or wheelchair or onto a gurney.

All healthcare providers must be aware of the safety and environmental clues that can be assessed when first encountering the patient.

Primary Airway Assessment and Management of Life Threats

Whether in an ED, a triage area, or the prehospital environment, you assess the patient's work of breathing and consciousness from across the room but assess the airway at the patient's side. Look for the work of breathing. Normal breathing should be peaceful and subtle while at rest. If you are able to note the patient's breathing from across the room, he or she is probably using accessory muscles to breathe, which indicates labored breathing and signals that the patient is probably unstable. The airway must be carefully evaluated.

Immediately open the airway with your gloved hands, using jaw thrust or head tilt and chin lift. Look for signs of upper airway obstruction, such as secretions or blood inside the mouth. Listen to the sounds of the airway. Are there unusual noises that indicate upper airway compromise, even with the head and jaw in proper position? Suction should always be readily available for your use in the primary exam.

If you need to provide ongoing manual airway management, an immediate plan for positioning or initiation of invasive techniques should be instituted. Preoxygenation/ventilation is always the first step in the plan while you map out a safe, effective means of managing the airway on the basis of your resources, the differential diagnosis, your location, and the patient's anatomy.

If the patient already has an artificial airway in place, evaluate its effectiveness and the patient's tolerance of the device. Confirm proper placement of the device before moving on to assess breathing.

Breathing Assessment

Assessment of breathing begins at your first encounter with the patient. Look, listen, and feel. Observe the patient's chest wall for symmetrical motion. Listen to lung sounds, and feel the chest for tenderness or fremitus. Tactile (or vocal) fremitus is a vibration palpable when a person speaks; pneumonia will cause vibration to be more prominent, whereas pneumothorax and pleural effusion leads to a decrease in fremitus. Listen to the patient speak. Is she hoarse or does she complain of dysphagia? How many words can she use in a sentence before taking a breath? The ability to use six- or seven-word sentences rather than two- to three-word sentences says a great deal about how the patient is breathing.

If the patient is not working hard to breathe and reaches out to shake your hand when you introduce yourself, most of the primary exam is complete, and you can rest assured the patient is relatively stable and safe from immediate life threats.

Distinguishing Respiratory Distress from Respiratory Failure When a patient reports dyspnea or has an observable increased work of breathing, you must pause and ask yourself a question: Is this patient in respiratory distress, or does he have signs of respiratory failure? If the patient improves with simple resuscitation maneuvers, then respiratory distress is the answer. If on the other hand the patient does not improve with basic interventions, or if any patient with respiratory distress has signs of fatigue or altered mental status, respiratory failure is imminent. Box 3-2 lists some of the indicators of impending respiratory failure. Immediate resuscitation measures should be implemented to support the patient's airway and ventilation.

After the primary or initial survey, you may have already initiated some basic resuscitation maneuvers if warranted by the patient's condition. You may have supplied oxygen or administered positive-pressure ventilation with a bag-mask device. Reevaluate how the patient is tolerating these interventions. Does he feel better? Have his vital signs improved? Is his chest rising symmetrically with bag-mask ventilation?

While gathering the patient's history, don't forget to use the OPQRST mnemonic (see the Rapid Recall box in Chapter 1). Even if the patient does not have pain, those who have had dyspnea before can give you many key pieces of information. For instance, an asthma patient might rate the severity of their discomfort of a current episode at an 8. It is important to determine how the patient compares this discomfort to previous episodes of discomfort. Identifying if they have ever been intubated when experiencing this type of discomfort can be a key indicator of the need for imminent airway management interventions and the likelihood of respiratory failure.

BOX 3-2 Indicators of Imminent Respiratory Failure

- Respiratory rate > 30 or < 6 breaths/min
- Oxygen saturation < 90%
- Use of multiple accessory muscle groups
- Inability to lie supine
- Tachycardia with a rate > 140 bpm
- Mental status changes
- Inability to clear oral secretions/mucus
- Cyanosis of nail beds or lips

Secondary Examination

Vital Signs

You should take baseline vital signs—temperature, pulse, respiration, blood pressure—and oxygen saturation, and repeat these periodically guided by the patient's acuity. Record your readings in the patient's chart, noting the time they were obtained.

Because of the shared cardiothoracic space, closely allied physiology, and marked influence on respiration, cardiopulmonary and neurologic function must be the focus of your assessment. In monitoring vital signs, it's especially important to keep a close eye on how respiration and perfusion are affecting the patient's mental status.

Respiration You've already sized up the patient's work of breathing: quiet (normal) or increased. You've also determined whether the patient is in respiratory distress (obvious from across the room) or has signs of impending respiratory failure (increased work of breathing with altered mental status).

BOX 3-3 Best Practices for Proper Auscultation

To perform auscultation properly, good habits must become hardwired into your assessment routine. Follow these simple rules each time you auscultate breath sounds:

- Use the diaphragm of the stethoscope.
- Place the diaphragm on the patient's skin if possible.
- To eliminate outside interference, do not allow the stethoscope tubing to touch anything during auscultation.
- To avoid abnormal airway noises, ask the patient to breathe with the mouth open and the head in a neutral position or slightly extended.
- Always move with purpose: superior to inferior, side to side, and site to site.
- If you hear something unusual, stop, move the stethoscope to a new site, and listen again for comparison.

Your attention then turns to the patient's respiratory rate. In the primary or initial assessment, you didn't have time to dwell on numbers—you were attending to vital functions and addressing life threats. During the secondary exam, however, you should pay particular attention to actually counting the patient's breaths per minute to determine the respiratory rate.

An extremely high or low respiratory rate may alert you that a secondary organ system is responsible for the respiratory distress. Take, for instance, a patient who is breathing without difficulty, using no accessory muscles, but at a fast rate. The patient is exhibiting quiet tachypnea. This subtle finding has ominous implications for shock. Quiet tachypnea occurs when the chemoreceptors sense a rise in acidity (metabolic acidosis), stimulating the respiratory system to breathe faster in an attempt to blow off excess CO_2. At the other end of the spectrum, a patient who is breathing slowly, with no accessory muscle use, is exhibiting quiet bradypnea, which can be caused by a CNS disturbance or by the action of depressant drugs.

Count the respiratory rate—it can tell you a lot. Put it together with the work of breathing, and you'll know even more.

Proximal and Distal Perfusion/Pulse Checks The radial pulse is the point most commonly assessed in a stable patient, but you can gather additional information by evaluating the pulse at alternative arterial sites like the carotid, femoral, and dorsalis pedis. Proximal pulses correspond to larger arteries. The body can shift circulation to these larger vessels during times of stress or hemorrhage. When this occurs, the peripheral pulses may be weak or absent while central circulation is preserved.

Like extremes of respiratory rate, extremes of heart rate can also help you form a differential diagnosis. In a patient with signs of respiratory compromise, for example, you would expect to see tachycardia. When the body's cells fail to receive enough oxygen, the heart beats faster in an effort to deliver more oxygen to the cells. A patient in respiratory distress who has a slow heart rate, then, is probably in trouble. Respiratory failure may be fast approaching. A bag-mask device should be readily available to resuscitate such patients, especially when their mental status is declining.

Lung Sounds

One of the key assessments of a patient with respiratory difficulty is auscultation of breath sounds. Evaluate all fields of respiration, both anterior and posterior. Auscultate each of the three lobes of the right lung and the two lobes of the left lung during both inspiration and expiration, paying close attention to ensure that breath sounds are equal bilaterally. Best practices for performing auscultation are outlined in Box 3-3.

Breath sounds can be categorized simply as normal or abnormal. You might hear normal sounds in one area and abnormal sounds in another. Abnormal sounds, sometimes called *adventitious breath sounds,* can be heard in any lung area. Sounds associated with particular respiratory disease processes are summarized in Table 3-1. You may also wish to review Box 1-6 in Chapter 1 for an additional list of abnormal breath sounds.

Wheezing The wheeze is the classic sound of airway obstruction or a reactive airway. Usually heard on expiration, wheezing can have a musical quality or a harsh discordant tone. The pitch varies with the size of the airway. Expiratory wheezes are heard in asthma, bronchitis, and chronic obstructive lung disease. Wheezes associated with other diseases, such as pneumonia and heart failure, signal a reactive airway. The area is inflamed, and bronchi are edematous.

Crackles (Rales) The auscultation of crackles (also known as *rales*) on inspiration is associated with accumulated fluid in the alveoli. The sound has a fine, high-pitched, shrill quality and sometimes clears with coughing. If the sound clears after a few deep breaths, the patient probably has atelectasis. Pneumonia, congestive heart failure (CHF), and pulmonary edema are the conditions most often associated with crackles.

Rhonchi The word *rhonchi* (the plural of rhonchus) derives from the Greek word *rhonkos,* meaning "snoring." Auscultation of rhonchi indicates accumulation of secretions in the larger airways. Rhonchi are often described as bubbly or slurpy sounds heard on expiration. The sounds are generated as air passes through secretions trapped in

TABLE 3-1 Breath Sounds Associated with Selected Conditions

Location	Sound	Phase	Disease Process
Upper airway	Stridor	Inspiration	Viral croup Epiglottitis Foreign-body aspiration
Lower airway	Rhonchi	Primarily expiration	Frank aspiration Bronchitis Cystic fibrosis
	Wheeze	Primarily expiration	Reactive airway disease Asthma Congestive heart failure Chronic bronchitis Emphysema Endobronchial obstruction
	Rales (crackles)	End inspiration	Pneumonia Exacerbation of congestive heart failure Pulmonary edema
	Diminished breath sounds	Either or both	Emphysema Atelectasis Tension pneumothorax Flail chest Neuromuscular disease Pleural effusion
Chest wall	Pleural rub	Either	Pleuritis Pleurisy Pleural effusion

the airways. Bronchiectasis, cystic fibrosis, and aspiration pneumonitis are often accompanied by rhonchi.

Pleural Friction Rub As noted earlier, fluid between the pleural layers reduces friction, helping the lungs expand and contract during normal respiration. When this fluid buffer is absent, a pleural friction rub can be auscultated. This sign is associated with chest wall pain caused by pneumonia, pleurisy, and lung contusion. The friction rub may be heard in an area adjacent to the site of pain.

Diminished Breath Sounds Diminished or distant breath sounds are heard in patients with the following respiratory difficulties:

- Disorders that lead to increased functional residual capacity—that is, an increase in the resting volume of gas in the lung
- Diminished air exchange
- Inappropriate presence of air or fluid

Auscultation of diminished breath sounds is a classic sign of emphysema. This disease process destroys the alveolar walls, creating greater surface area in the lungs. Gas flow becomes less turbulent, producing a softer sound. Other disorders associated with diminished breath sounds are atelectasis, pneumothorax, pleural effusion, and neuromuscular disorders that limit inspiratory volume.

Stridor Stridor is a sound produced by inflammation or a large obstruction in the upper airway. It is heard only on inspiration. Viral croup and epiglottitis are two respiratory disorders accompanied by stridor. In the critical care arena, **angioedema** and trauma are most commonly associated with stridor.

Mental Status

Normal mental status is a good rough indicator of adequate perfusion and oxygenation of the CNS. The CNS, and the brain in particular, is intolerant of prolonged interruption of its supply of blood, oxygen, or glucose. Mental status can deteriorate rapidly when any of these three components is deficient for as little as a few minutes. Dysfunction of the pulmonary system can lead to hypoxia and decline of mental status even in the presence of a functioning circulatory system.

Evaluation of mental status is an important part of patient examination. Assess the patient's orientation to person, place, and time (see Chapter 1). Assess clarity of speech, verbal coherence, and response time. Slurred speech, poor articulation, mumbling or rambling speech, and aphasia can all be attributable to hypoxia. The combination of new-onset altered mental status and respiratory distress is a hallmark of respiratory failure.

Jugular Venous Distention

Evaluating a patient for jugular venous distention is difficult, subjective, and sometimes unreliable. Place the patient supine with 30 to 45 degrees of head elevation. Measure the jugular appearance in centimeters from the base of the neck to the highest point of jugular vein distention. Remember, you're looking at the *internal* jugular vein, which lies beside and over the carotid, and assessing it in comparison to the clavicle. The internal jugular vein inserts just beneath the clavicle where it joins the sternum. You're not looking at the external jugular vein.

Elevated pressure indicates high right-sided heart pressure and possible heart failure. When a patient has an acute onset of dyspnea, jugular venous distention may indicate heart failure to the exclusion of COPD.

Heart Sounds

Careful auscultation of heart sounds can be important in forming a differential diagnosis, especially in an emergent situation. Ask the patient not to speak, and listen at three critical points: the right side of the sternum at the fourth intercostal space, the left side of the sternum at the fourth intercostal space, and the midclavicular line at the fifth intercostal space. The normal heart sounds are recorded as S_1S_2, where S_1 equates to the first heart sound, or the "lub," and S_2 is the second heart sound, the "dub." The sound of S_1 represents the closing of the atrioventricular valves (the tricuspid and mitral valves), and S_2 represents the closing of the semilunar valves (the aortic and pulmonary valves).

Occasionally, two additional heart sounds are heard—S_3 and S_4. An S_3 sound, often called the "S_3 gallop," is most often associated with increased pulmonary artery pressure. The three syllables of the word *Kentucky* are often said to represent the sound of the S_3 gallop: S_1 = *ken*, S_2 = *tuck*, and S_3 = *y*. The S_3 gallop is a cardinal sign of CHF.

An S_4 heart sound is also considered abnormal and suggests the presence of left ventricular hypertrophy and reduced left ventricular compliance. It may be heard in the older adult patient with hypertension and heart disease. The word *Tennessee* is often used to represent the fourth heart sound, with S_4 composing the first syllable (*tenn*). The sound of S_4 precedes S_1 and coincides with atrial contraction; S_3 may merge with S_4 to create a "summation gallop"—that is, the summation of S_3 and S_4.

History

The **history of the present illness (HPI)** is perhaps the most important element of patient assessment. As is often quoted in medical education, "95% of your diagnosis is made by asking the right questions." The primary elements of the HPI are easily remembered by using the OPQRST and SAMPLER mnemonics. (You may wish to review the Chapter 1 Rapid Recall boxes.) Using these memory aids, you can obtain a basic HPI.

Your history should include an exploration of risk factors to help you narrow your differential diagnosis. For example, the patient may have risk factors for the development of venous thrombosis and pulmonary embolus: use of oral contraceptives, obesity, smoking, and a sedentary lifestyle. Always ask a patient with a history of a complaint similar to the current one to compare today's symptoms with those experienced previously—same or different from last time? A patient with a history of heart failure and an acute onset of dyspnea may relate that the symptoms today are the same as the last time he developed pulmonary edema. *Ask the patient what he or she thinks is wrong.* Some patients are so familiar with their disorder, they can relate current symptoms to how they felt on previous occasions and what the cause turned out to be.

Also elicit information from the patient about aggravating or alleviating factors—what makes the symptoms worse, and what makes them better? A detailed HPI is decisive in developing an accurate differential diagnosis and formulating an effective treatment plan. Box 3-4 lists specific questions to ask when taking a pulmonary history. Box 3-5 outlines key findings you're likely to see in the patient with dyspnea.

BOX 3-4 Important Elements of a Pulmonary History

- Fever or chills
- Ankle edema
- Calf swelling or tenderness
- Back, chest, or abdominal pain
- Vomiting
- Orthopnea
- Cough
- Dyspnea on exertion
- History of bronchitis:
  - Asthma
  - COPD
- Blood in sputum:
  - Color of sputum
  - History of sputum production
- Prior respiratory admissions
- History of smoking or passive smoke exposure
- Prior intubations
- Home nebulizer use

Diagnostic Tools in Assessment

Chest X-Ray

The chest radiograph (Figure 3-5) is an invaluable evaluation tool for assessing patients with chest pain and dyspnea. A plain radiograph conveys a surprising amount of information about the lungs, heart, chest wall, bones, diaphragm, and soft tissues of the chest. A routine two-view chest radiograph is usually performed laterally and posteroanterior (PA), with the patient's chest against the film.

For more critically ill patients, a chest radiograph may be done at the bedside using a portable machine that yields only one view—the anteroposterior (AP) view. The two-view chest radiograph is better for diagnosing pulmonary disease, but an AP view is sufficient to identify most disorders. Since the unit is portable, an AP film tends to have some image degradation and is subject to more

BOX 3-5 Key Findings in the Patient with Dyspnea

DURATION

- Chronic or progressive dyspnea is usually related to cardiac disease, asthma, COPD, or neuromuscular disease (e.g., multiple sclerosis).
- An acute dyspneic spell may be due to exacerbation of asthma, infection, pulmonary embolus, intermittent cardiac dysfunction, a psychogenic cause, or inhalation of a toxic substance, allergen, or foreign body.

ONSET

- Sudden onset of dyspnea should raise suspicion of pulmonary embolism or spontaneous pneumothorax.
- Dyspnea that develops slowly (hours to days) points toward pneumonia, congestive heart failure, or malignancy.

PATIENT POSITION

- Orthopnea can be attributed to congestive heart failure, COPD, or a neuromuscular disorder.
- Paroxysmal nocturnal dyspnea is most common in those with left heart failure.
- Exertional dyspnea is associated with COPD, myocardial ischemia, and with the abdominal loading that occurs in obesity, ascites, and pregnancy.

variance in technique than a two-view chest x-ray. In addition, the AP portable chest unit can somewhat magnify the size of the heart.

Radiographic examination should include these basics:

- To detect pneumothorax, confirm full expansion of the lungs on both sides.
- Examine the borders of the lungs and margins of the diaphragm to look for fluid collection that suggests pleural effusion, hemothorax, or empyema.
- Explore the interior of each lung to identify pneumonia or any free air that suggests a pneumomediastinum.
- Evaluate the heart's size and position.
- Check both sides for air beneath the diaphragm that might indicate a perforated bowel.
- Confirm that the trachea is in the middle of the mediastinum and any endotracheal tubes are above the carina.

Ultrasound

Ultrasound examination, also called *sonography* or *diagnostic medical sonography,* is an imaging method that uses high-frequency sound waves to produce precise images of structures within your body. The images produced through ultrasound examination often provide information that's valuable in diagnosing and treating a variety of diseases and conditions.

Ultrasound imaging is a valuable tool in emergency settings and has been increasingly used to detect aneurysmal rupture and other life-threatening hemorrhages. Used in its early days primarily for evaluation of pregnancy, new-generation real-time ultrasound imaging is now used by some emergency care providers to detect ectopic pregnancy, pericardial tamponade, abdominal aneurysm, pleural effusion, pneumothorax, and intraabdominal hemorrhage. The equipment is relatively expensive, however, and reliable ultrasound evaluation requires training and significant expertise. Such drawbacks tend to limit the availability of this diagnostic tool.

Transcutaneous Respiratory Monitoring

Transcutaneous Oxygen Saturation Transcutaneous oxygen saturation monitoring, known variously as "pulse ox," "O_2 sat," and "sat monitoring," has become an easy, commonplace way to assess blood oxygenation. Transcutaneous oxygen saturation monitors are relatively inexpensive and can quickly approximate the level of oxygen in the blood without the need for an invasive procedure. The technology depends on hemoglobin's ability to absorb infrared light to varying degrees (Figure 3-6), depending on the number of hemoglobin-binding sites occupied by (i.e., saturated by) oxygen molecules. The monitor calculates the amount of light absorption and translates it into a percentage that represents the level of oxygen saturation. This percentage is displayed on the monitor.

At rest, most healthy individuals have an oxygen saturation of 95% to 100%. More accurate oxygen levels are assessed through invasive arterial blood gas (ABG) monitoring. The normal partial pressure of oxygen dissolved in arterial blood (PaO_2), expressed in millimeters of mercury (mm Hg), is 80 to 100. Generally, if oxygen saturation stays above 92%, the PaO_2 is above 60 mm Hg. As the oxygen level drops, the saturation monitor will show a declining reading. Because of the relationship between the partial pressure of oxygen and the saturation percentage, the latter is not very sensitive to changes in PO_2 above 90%. When oxygen saturation is 90%, PaO_2 is approximately 60 mm Hg. However, below 90%, the saturation will decrease markedly when decreases in the O_2 partial pressure occur. A minor dip in oxygen saturation at this level can translate to significant hypoxia. As the reading tumbles further, the oxygen level in the blood falls significantly. In some cases, readings below 90% can be used only to evaluate qualitative improvements in ventilation, not absolute improvements in oxygenation. For example, when intubating a severely hypoxic patient, if the patient initially shows 70% saturation, his PaO_2 may be in the 40s. After intubation, the oxygen saturation might improve to 80%, but the PaO_2 may actually have improved only marginally, to about 50 mm Hg.

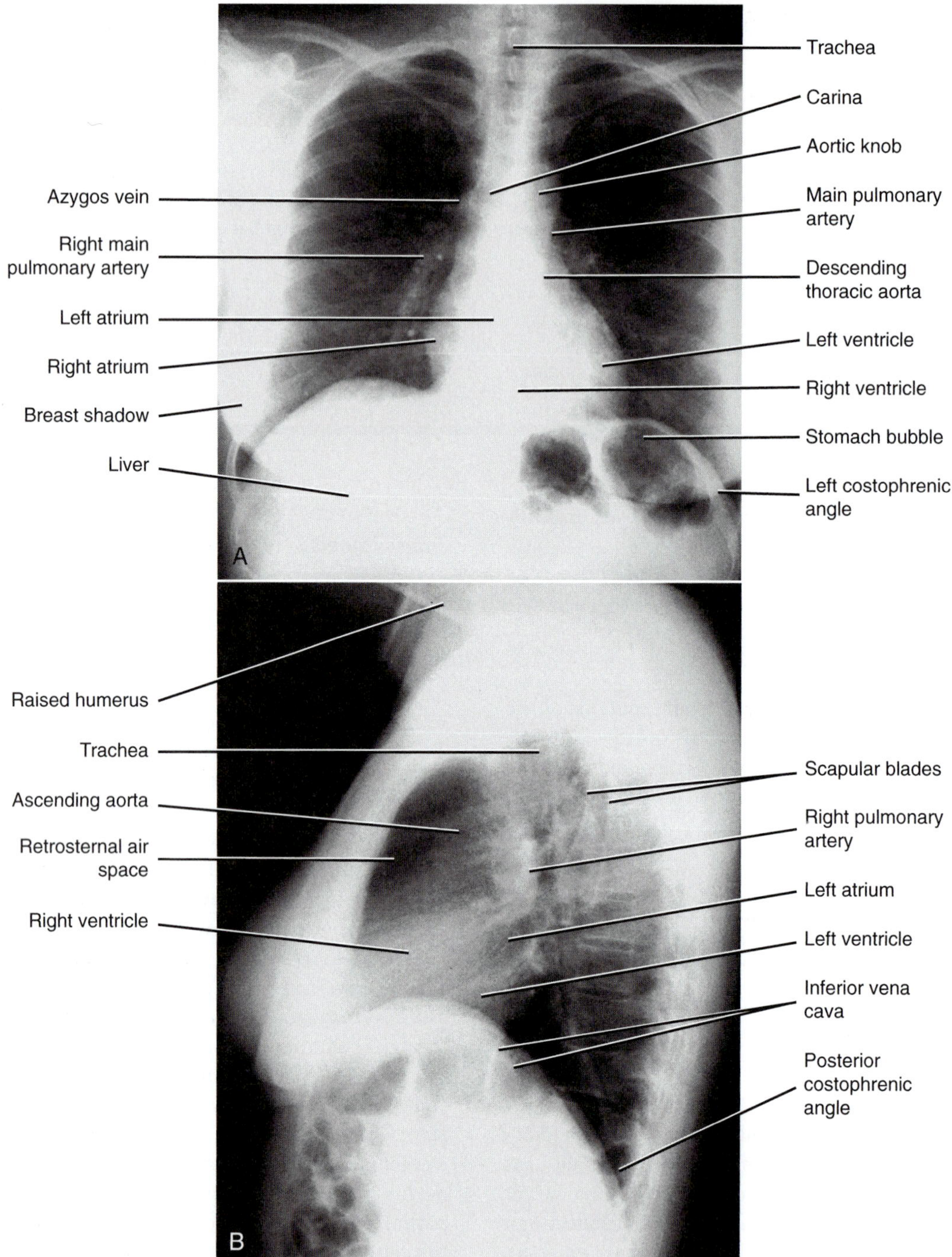

■ **Figure 3-5** Normal chest radiograph. (From Mettler FA: Essentials of radiology, ed 2, St Louis, 2004, Saunders.)

Other factors can compromise the reliability of oxygen saturation monitoring. Nail polish, paint, or stain on the fingers; cool extremities or a cold environment; shock; and poor sensor-to-skin contact can cause inaccurate readings. Carbon monoxide poisoning can cause falsely high readings; the saturation may be 100%, but the patient may nevertheless be severely hypoxic due to carbon monoxide binding.

Carbon Monoxide Sensors Relatively new in the healthcare industry, carbon monoxide oximeters have now become reliable indicators of the attachment of carbon monoxide molecules to hemoglobin. Hemoglobin likes carbon monoxide more than oxygen—it's said to have a much higher *affinity* for carbon monoxide than for oxygen when both are available for attachment. When a patient has been exposed to a toxic carbon monoxide inhalation, it's clinically useful to have a simple method of detecting the precise amount of carbon monoxide binding that has occurred. The highly accurate sensor attaches to the patient the same way a traditional oximeter device does, but it relies on different wavelengths of light on the

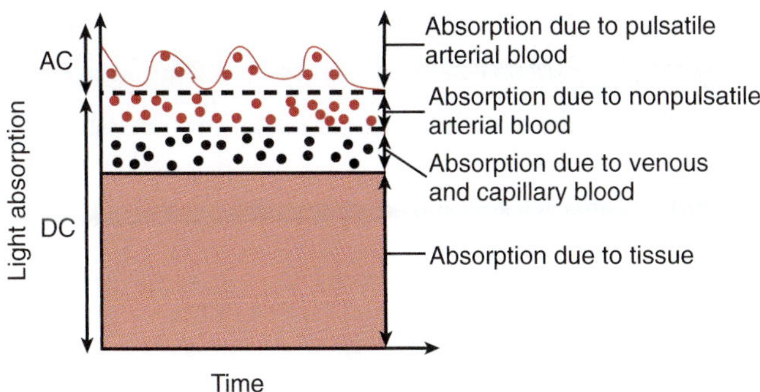

■ **Figure 3-6** Oxygen saturation monitoring. Light passing through blood is absorbed by arterial, capillary, and venous blood. Pulsatile (arterial, or AC) portion is measured and calculation performed to estimate blood oxygen level. (From Miller RD: Miller's anesthesia, ed 6, Philadelphia, 2004, Churchill Livingstone.)

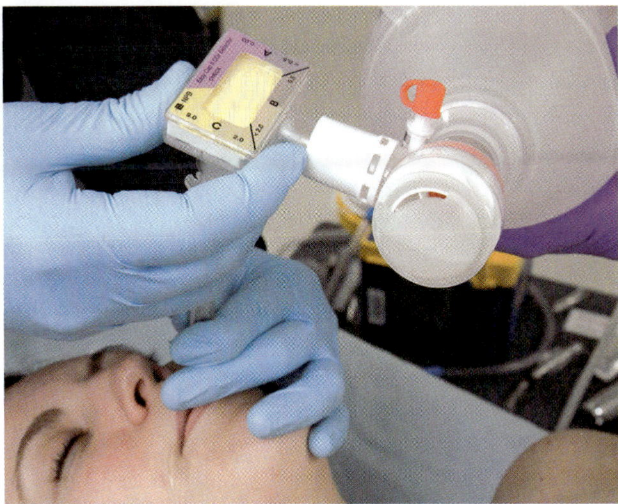

■ **Figure 3-7** Colorimetric end-tidal carbon dioxide ($ETCO_2$) detector connected to endotracheal tube. (From Aehlert B: Paramedic practice today: above and beyond, St Louis, 2009, Saunders.)

spectrum to detect carbon monoxide. Comparing the results of carbon monoxide oximetry and standard carboxyhemoglobin detection using ABG analysis, an invasive laboratory test, the oximetry method comes within 0.5% to 4.3% of the ABG result.

Conjunctival Saturation A relatively uncommon way of measuring peripheral oxygenation is through the conjunctiva, the membranous tissue that lines the inner eyelid and the sclera. The measurements obtained can be used to estimate arterial oxygen tension. In clinical studies carried out during anesthesia for pulmonary surgery, a close correlation was found between PO_2 and conjunctival oxygen tension ($PcjO_2$) readings. $PcjO_2$ is also thought to mirror the adequacy of peripheral perfusion. Though not currently used in emergency care, this technology may eventually become available as an alternative evaluation modality.

Transcutaneous Oxygen Sensors Transcutaneous monitoring of the actual blood oxygen level (PaO_2) by noninvasive means is termed *$tcPO_2$*. Special electrodes are applied to the skin surface and heated to 44°C to 45°C. The $tcPO_2$ has been used for monitoring oxygenation of neonates in respiratory distress since the early 1970s, but it has not been widely used in monitoring adult PO_2 levels. When the technology is applied to adults, the readings are significantly lower than actual PO_2 levels. Researchers attribute this discrepancy to the fact that $tcPO_2$ reflects oxygen tension as well as oxygen delivery and cardiac output. Should the equipment be available, $tcPO_2$ can be used to identify shock and hypoxia and help guide resuscitation efforts.

Monitoring Exhaled Carbon Dioxide

When using skin sensors to measure oxygen levels, an accurate reading depends on the patient's distal perfusion. Perfusion strongly influences the accuracy of CO_2 detection as well; CO_2 can't be detected if there is no perfusion. Analysis of exhaled gases for CO_2, known as **end-tidal carbon dioxide** ($ETCO_2$) monitoring (Figure 3-7), is a useful method of assessing a patient's ventilatory status.

Capnometry and Capnography Capnometry is a reliable method of confirming proper initial placement of an endotracheal tube, since the esophagus normally has a low level of CO_2 or none at all. It is also useful in detecting inadvertent extubation. Capnometry often employs a detector placed between the endotracheal tube and the ventilator or bag-mask device. One type of detector contains a paper indicator that is sensitive to pH changes. Exhaled CO_2 causes the paper to change color, serving as a visual indicator of the presence of CO_2. The degree of color change approximates the amount of CO_2 present, so this type of capnometry is referred to as *colorimetric CO_2 detection*. These devices provide only semiquantitative measurements. Colorimetric detectors have limited clinical use and a short shelf life. The pH-sensitive paper must remain in sealed packaging until needed, it must be used within 15 minutes of opening, and aspiration of gastric acid into the device will render it useless, as will administration of acidic drugs through the endotracheal tube.

As explained in Procedure 3-1, digital capnometry provides a true quantitative reading, with the patient's CO_2 level expressed numerically after each exhalation. Capnography takes carbon dioxide detection a step farther by making the measurement graphic and dynamic, mapping the CO_2 level throughout the respiratory cycle and over time, providing information about the rate of airflow and quality of respiration. The resulting waveform can be broken down into several phases that represent metabolism in the body:

- Phase I is the initial exhalation, consisting of dead space air that contains no significant amount of CO_2 and thus doesn't move the graph.

Procedure 3-1 Continuous End-Tidal Carbon Dioxide Monitoring Using Capnometry and Capnography

OVERVIEW

Measuring blood gases has been the gold standard for evaluating ventilatory status, but acquiring and evaluating blood samples quickly—especially in the field—is tricky. New technology and monitoring equipment enables us to easily assess the patient's spontaneous respiratory effort and the effectiveness of positive-pressure ventilation.

CO_2 is a waste product of oxygen and glucose metabolism. You might say that CO_2 is the product of good respiration. To evaluate a patient's ventilatory status, it's helpful to know his or her CO_2 level. Since CO_2 is released in air expelled through the lungs, CO_2 can neither dissipate nor be measured if the lungs are not being perfused. Both ventilation and blood flow to the lungs must be occurring if CO_2 is to be measured. Because the reading is taken near the end of exhalation, the term *end-tidal* is used.

Let's take a quick look at how CO_2 is produced during respiration. When venous blood is returned to the lungs, CO_2 in the venous circulation diffuses from the capillaries back into the alveoli. Normal $PvCO_2$ is 45 mm Hg, and normal $PaCO_2$ is 40 mm Hg. This pressure differential of 5 percentage points is enough to force CO_2 to diffuse out of the capillaries and into the alveoli where it is eliminated during expiration. As the blood passes through the capillaries, the pressure equalizes.

End-tidal CO_2 (sometimes abbreviated $ETCO_2$ or $PETCO_2$), the carbon dioxide concentration of expired air near the end of each breath, is normally 1 to 5 mm Hg less than $PaCO_2$. The patient's $ETCO_2$ reading, then, allows us to estimate $PaCO_2$—*if* the patient's respiratory status is normal. In patients with poor perfusion or respiratory impairment, the difference between $ETCO_2$ and $PaCO_2$ is >5 mm Hg. This gap is due to dead space ventilation, which means ventilation is occurring in areas of the lungs where there is little or no perfusion—therefore, no gas exchange.

Measuring CO_2 can help you identify V/Q abnormalities, monitor pulmonary blood flow, and correct tracheal tube placement. Two distinct means of measurement exist:

1. Capnometry: the measurement of CO_2 by means of a device called a *capnometer*. The capnometer projects a number which is the CO_2 measurement, but it doesn't represent the exhalation on a graph.
2. Capnography: the measurement of CO_2 by means of a device called a *capnograph*. This device takes a series of CO_2 measurements over time and plots them on a graph called a *waveform*. Because a waveform can reveal trends such as hypoventilation, capnography is more valuable than capnometry in clinical decision making.

Exhaled gas is measured by infrared analysis, usually with the aid of an exhalation port. The capnometer or capnograph captures a sample using one of two methods. In the aspiration (sidestream) method, the exhaled gas is transported through a small-bore tube to the monitor for analysis. In the nonaspiration (mainstream) method, the infrared device measures the gas sample directly at the ventilation circuit.

Sublingual Capnometry

Sublingual devices used to measure CO_2 not only assess the patient's ventilatory status but indicate the patient's overall perfusion status. Rackow and colleagues showed that sublingual capnometry may indicate the severity of circulatory failure. Other studies have likewise shown that sublingual capnometry can identify patients at risk of poor perfusion and multiple organ dysfunction syndrome (MODS).

Sublingual capnometry works by measuring blood flow within the gastrointestinal (GI) system. The GI system is sensitive to low-flow states and reflects the systemic CO_2 level with 90% accuracy. A gastric CO_2 reading is thus a good marker of systemic perfusion.

Instead of measuring exhaled gases, the sublingual device relies on a specialized sensor tip placed beneath the tongue. This gas-permeable sensor encapsulates a dye that can detect CO_2. When a fiberoptic light is beamed onto the tip, the capnometer calculates the amount of CO_2 present.

INDICATIONS FOR CAPNOMETRY AND CAPNOGRAPHY

- Baseline and continuous $ETCO_2$ monitoring and waveform analysis
- Continuous monitoring of endotracheal tube placement, airway patency, and ventilatory status
- Early detection of abnormal patterns of ventilation, perfusion, or CO_2 production
- Guidance in hyperventilation therapy
- Measurement of perfusion

EQUIPMENT

- Gloves, gown, mask, eye protection or face shield for compliance with Standard Precautions
- Gas measurement disposable device (mainstream attachment to tracheal tube or sidestream device for the nonintubated patient) as supplied by the manufacturer
- Manufacturer's cable that attaches to the gas measurement device at one end and to the monitoring system at the opposite end

PROCEDURE

1. Comply with Standard Precautions for infection control.
2. Follow your medical director's protocol for use of capnometry and capnography.
3. Assess for proper functioning of the capnograph or capnometer, including airway adapter, sensor, and display monitor; ensure all connections are secure.
4. Turn on the device, and allow it to calibrate. If monitoring is expected to be prolonged, ensure the batteries are adequately charged, or plug the unit into a grounded source.
5. Follow the manufacturer's recommendations for insertion of the airway adapter and sensor. Plug the cable into the monitor. In general, the closer the sensor is to the patient, the better. NOTE: This connection will add fairly significant weight to the end of your tracheal tube. Allow the sensor and connection to lie on patient's lower anterior neck or on the chest. Allowing the heavy connection to lie to the side of the mouth may precipitate extubation.
6. Set monitor alarms according to protocol and in compliance with the manufacturer's recommendations. (It's common to set the parameters ±5% of the standard.)

Procedure 3-1 Continuous End-Tidal Carbon Dioxide Monitoring Using Capnometry and Capnography—*Cont'd*

7. Be aware that a poor waveform probably means the $ETCO_2$ reading is false.

TIPS AND TROUBLESHOOTING

Interpretation of an Increasing CO_2 Level

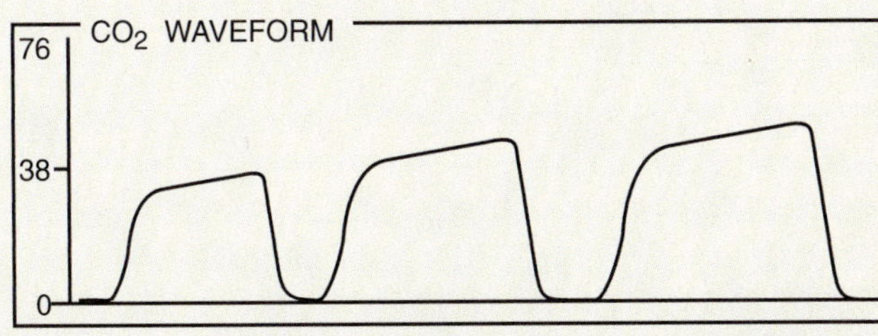

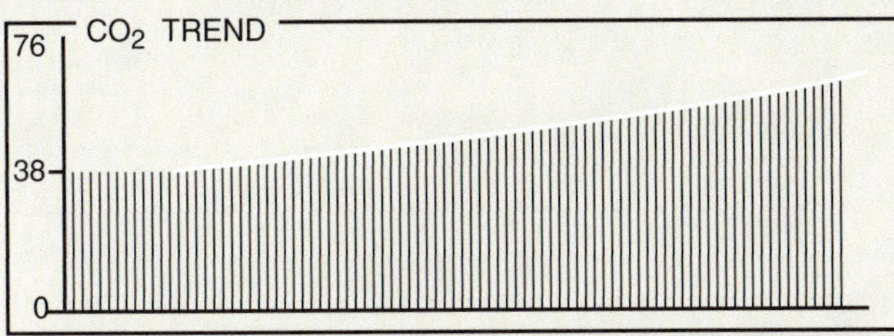

Gradually increasing $PETCO_2$. (Reprinted by permission of Nellcor Puritan Bennett Inc., Pleasanton, Calif.)

An increase of more than 10% from baseline measurements must be investigated. Common causes include:

- Hypermetabolic state
- Sepsis
- Fever
- Hypoventilation (inadequate minute ventilation)
- Partial airway obstruction
- Respiratory depressant drugs or neuromuscular blockade
- Metabolic alkalosis
- Ventilator malfunction

Interpretation of a Falling CO_2 Level

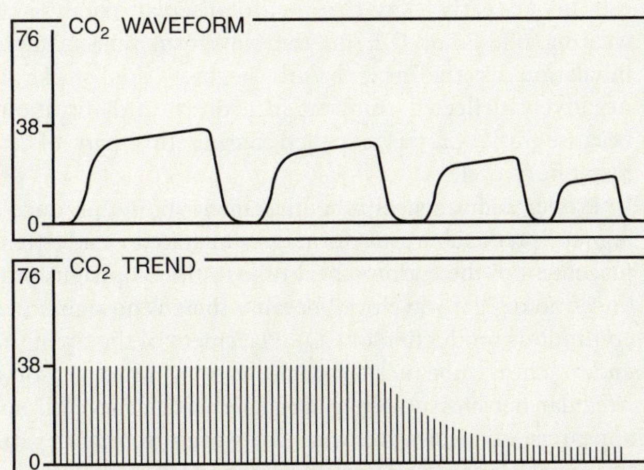

Exponential fall in $PETCO_2$. (Reprinted by permission of Nellcor Puritan Bennett Inc., Pleasanton, Calif.)

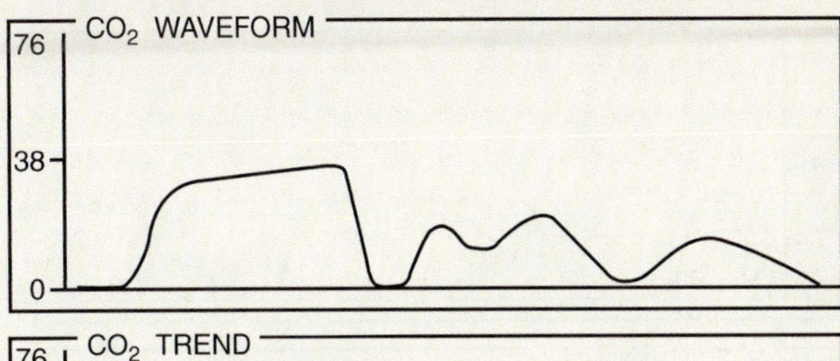

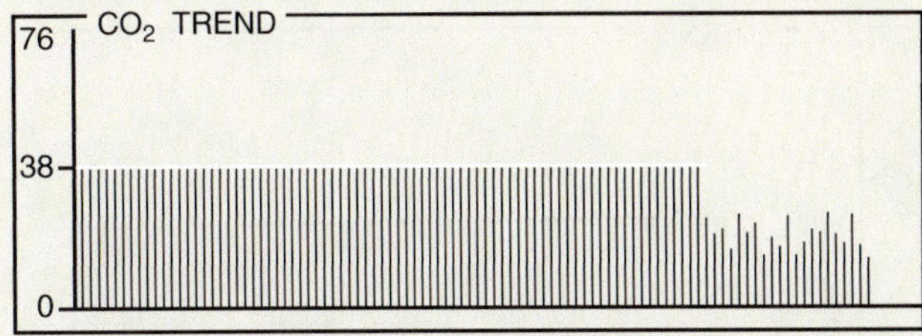

Sudden decrease in $PETCO_2$ values. (Reprinted by permission of Nellcor Puritan Bennett Inc., Pleasanton, Calif.)

A decrease of 10% or more from the baseline reading must be investigated. Such a decline reflects either a true decrease in blood PCO_2 or an increase in dead space ventilation. Common causes include:

- Diminished or absent perfusion (as in shock and cardiac arrest)
- High minute volume
- Hypothermia
- Metabolic acidosis
- Airway obstruction or leak

Interpretation of a Sustained Low CO_2 Level

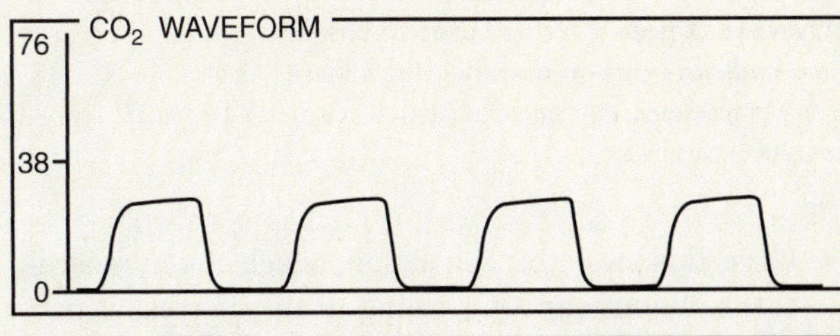

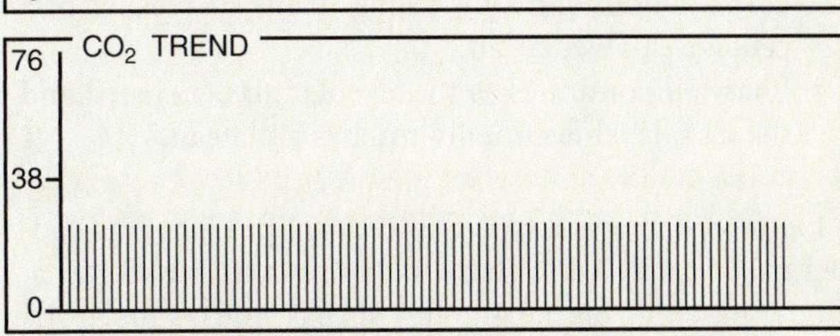

Decreased $PETCO_2$. (Reprinted by permission of Nellcor Puritan Bennett Inc., Pleasanton, Calif.)

Continued

Procedure 3-1 Continuous End-Tidal Carbon Dioxide Monitoring Using Capnometry and Capnography—*Cont'd*

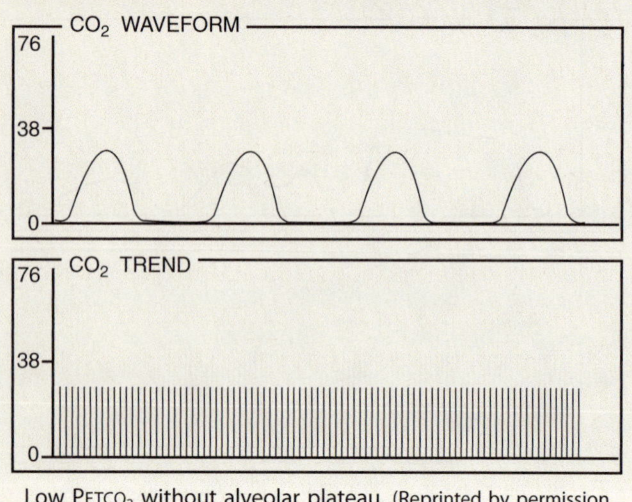

Low P_{ETCO_2} without alveolar plateau. (Reprinted by permission of Nellcor Puritan Bennett Inc., Pleasanton, Calif.)

Sustained low $ETCO_2$ levels indicate hyperventilation, large-volume dead space ventilation, or very poor circulation, as in:

- Cardiac arrest or severe shock
- Large pulmonary embolism
- Hyperventilation (excess rate or tidal volume)
- Poor expiration time on the ventilator

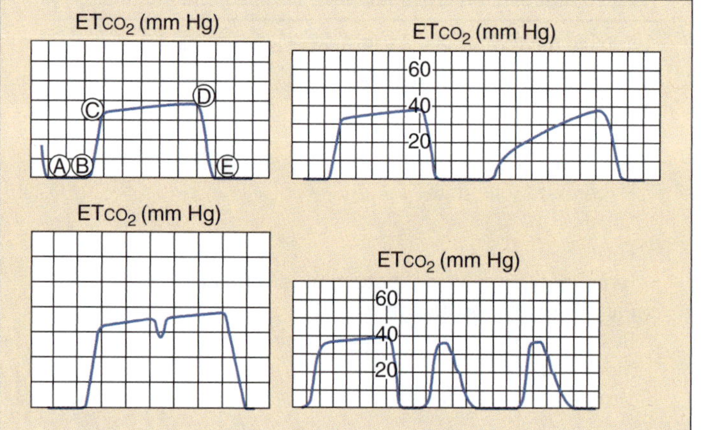

Figure 3-8 Four phases of normal capnogram. **A-B**, Carbon dioxide–free portion of respiratory cycle. **B-C**, Rapid upstroke of curve, representing transition from inspiration to expiration and mixing of dead space and alveolar gas. **C-D**, Alveolar plateau, representing alveolar gas rich in carbon dioxide and tending to slope gently upward with uneven emptying of alveoli. **D-E**, Respiratory downstroke, a nearly vertical drop to baseline. $ETCO_2$, End-tidal carbon dioxide. (From Marx J, et al: Rosen's emergency medicine: concepts and clinical practice, ed 6, St Louis, 2006, Mosby.)

- Phase II is the active exhalation, which contains escalating amounts of CO_2 owing to the increasing percentage of alveolar air.
- Phase III continues as the alveolar air is exhaled and the CO_2 level eventually reaches a plateau.

Figure 3-8 shows a typical waveform produced by capnography. Point A-B (phase I) shows the waveform at zero, or baseline, on the graph. This baseline occurs at the end of inspiration, just before exhalation. As exhalation begins, an upstroke appears on the waveform, represented by point B-C (phase II). This positive deflection occurs as the device immediately begins to detect CO_2. Point C-D (phase III) indicates a slowing of the velocity of the exhalation, with point D representing the peak of exhaled CO_2 at the end of exhalation. As the plateau of the wave is graphed, a negative deflection (dip), or cleft, may indicate the patient's spontaneous respiratory effort. This can be an early sign that neuromuscular paralysis is wearing off. Point D-E on the waveform reflects rapid inhalation as the next breath begins. This stroke is negatively deflected (moving in a downward direction) because little CO_2 is expelled during this part of the respiratory cycle.

Proper endotracheal tube placement should produce a regular, predictable waveform, as illustrated. Inadvertent placement of the endotracheal tube in the esophagus produces no regular waveform, because there is no significant continuous production of CO_2. Placement of the tip of the endotracheal tube near the glottis may produce some irregular but measurable readings; however, they will not appear as a typical waveform. Any waveform that departs the expected contours should prompt immediate reevaluation of intubation status.

Sidestream CO_2 Evaluation in the Nonintubated Patient Another valuable means of evaluating the patient's CO_2 level at the end of exhalation occurs in the nonintubated patient through sidestream capnography. A CO_2 sampling tube is placed within the patient's nose or mouth, and samples of the patient's exhalation are sent to a sensor in the machine itself. Monitoring of nonintubated patients can occur while simultaneously providing supplemental oxygen via mask or cannula. This technique provides breath-to-breath information and will detect problems such as apnea, respiratory depression, and hypoperfusion. Changes will be seen almost immediately, whereas it may take minutes for oxygen saturation to decrease. Sidestream $ETCO_2$ can be used to assess the severity of COPD or an asthma exacerbation and the effectiveness of interventions. With a mild exacerbation, the patient may initially hyperventilate, and $ETCO_2$ will decrease, but with a severe exacerbation, there will be retention of CO_2 that may signal respiratory failure.

Initial and Basic Management Techniques

Airway

Please refer to Appendix D for a discussion of airway assessment and management using rapid-sequence intubation.

VENTILATION AND OXYGENATION

Supplemental Oxygen

Supplemental oxygen is the easiest, quickest, and most efficient way to improve oxygenation in a breathing patient. Oxygen is usually delivered by nasal cannula, which can effectively provide 24% to 40% oxygen. Higher flow rates can cause patient discomfort, especially when given long term. Oxygen may be administered with humidification, reducing the drying effect of the inspired air.

Use of a face mask can increase the concentration of oxygen administered up to 60% when 15 L/min of oxygen is given. The Venturi (air entrainment) mask is a specialized face mask that gives the provider more precise control over the amount of inspired oxygen, from 28% to 40%. The Venturi mask and the standard face mask have one problem in common: placing a device over both the nose and mouth of a dyspneic patient will almost certainly increase the patient's anxiety and often results in the patient's removing the mask.

The nonrebreather face mask adds an oxygen reservoir to the standard face mask, increasing the inspired oxygen level to 100% at 15 L/min of oxygen flow. The nonrebreather mask often functions as a bridging device to another modality, since a patient who needs 100% oxygen typically requires some other type of ventilatory support such as bilevel positive airway pressure (BiPAP) or intubation. If aggressive care is successful, the patient can be weaned down to a lower fraction of inspired oxygen (FIO_2) instead of being intubated.

BOX 3-6 Criteria to Establish Ventilation

$PaO_2 < 55$ mm Hg
$PaCO_2 > 50$
pH < 7.32

Data from Amitai A, Skinert RH: Ventilator management (website). http://emedicine.medscape.com/article/810126-overview. Accessed June 5, 2009.

Positive-Pressure Ventilation

Patients with respiratory failure need positive-pressure ventilation (Box 3-6) to improve gas exchange, relieve respiratory distress, and allow for uncomplicated lung healing. You can provide this ventilatory support noninvasively through a bag-mask device, continuous positive airway pressure (CPAP), or BiPAP.

Bag-Mask Device

The bag-mask device has become a standard respiratory resuscitation tool for patients of all ages. Certain considerations are typical regardless of which manual resuscitator system you purchase and use. You must stock and select the correct size bag and masks for all patients. For instance, if you're caring for a 7-year-old child who weighs 40 kg, a 250-mL "premie" bag will not provide the necessary tidal volumes to the patient. Your resuscitation equipment should include at least a 450- to 500-mL and a 1-L bag. Many providers misinterpret the generic terms "pediatric" and "adult" as they apply to bag sizes. Within those two broad categories, there are many sizes of pediatric bags and at least two sizes of adult bags. Research your needs on the basis of the patients you will be transporting.

The manual resuscitator should have positive end-expiratory pressure (PEEP) valve capability, especially in the hospital and interfacility transport setting. If you need to administer temporary manual ventilation to a patient who just came off a bedside intensive care unit (ICU) ventilator equipped with PEEP, that parameter must be maintained. In addition, oxygenation is improved when a reservoir bag or tube is added, *and* you administer ventilation slowly with just enough tidal volume to raise the chest.

Another misconception about manual (self-inflating) bag-mask systems is that they all deliver 100% oxygen if you add 12 to 15 L of oxygen to the reservoir. *If* you administer ventilation slowly, with moderate tidal volume, you can approach 100% oxygen using those devices, but it is difficult to do so. A more realistic estimate is 65% to

80% oxygenation. Non–self-inflating devices or anesthesia bags do deliver 100% oxygen to the patient. Although not easy to use in practice, providers in many critical care areas prefer these bags because they give you a more sensitive feel for the patient's lung compliance while you're administering ventilation. The flow-control valve on an anesthesia bag gives it built-in PEEP capability.

Continuous Positive Airway Pressure

Continuous positive airway pressure (CPAP) is a ventilatory technique used to apply a modest amount of continuous pressure in the airway to keep smaller airways open, reduce the work of breathing, and improve alveolar oxygenation. CPAP devices can be beneficial for patients who are having moderate to severe respiratory difficulty, such as those with asthma, emphysema, and CHF. The technique reduces left ventricular preload and afterload in patients with CHF.

For the device to be effective, the patient must keep a seal between the mask and his or her face. Use of CPAP, including face mask considerations, is outlined in Procedure 3-2.

Procedure 3-2 Administering Continuous Positive Airway Pressure (CPAP)

OVERVIEW

Noninvasive positive-pressure ventilation is a temporary resuscitation measure in which continuous positive airway pressure (CPAP) is maintained throughout the respiratory cycle. This technique is used to decrease the work of breathing, improve oxygenation, and facilitate movement of fluids and oxygen across the alveolar-capillary membrane.

INDICATIONS

Respiratory failure in patients with:

- Chronic obstructive pulmonary disease (COPD)
- Asthma
- Congestive heart failure (CHF) with pulmonary edema

NOTE: Use only in patients who can follow commands and clear their own airway secretions.

CONTRAINDICATIONS

- Altered mental status (patient unable to follow commands or clear secretions)
- Copious secretions
- Maxillofacial trauma
- Congenital malformations of the lower face that preclude an adequate mask seal
- Pneumothorax or pneumomediastinum
- Acute myocardial infarction
- Hypotension
- Dysrhythmia
- Active vomiting

EQUIPMENT

- Gloves, gown, mask, eye protection or face shield for compliance with Standard Precautions
- CPAP device, including prefitted CPAP mask with straps
- Connecting tubing
- Oxygen source

PROCEDURE

1. Comply with Standard Precautions for infection control.
2. Evaluate the patient with respiratory complaints, and develop a treatment plan. Supply supplemental oxygen as you determine whether the patient would benefit from CPAP.
3. Monitor the patient using pulse oximetry and capnography or capnometry.
4. Once you determine CPAP is the appropriate treatment option, choose an interface (mask) in the correct size (see manufacturer's recommendations). Several types of interfaces are available, including a mask worn over the nose and a full face mask that covers the nose and mouth.
5. Explain the procedure to the patient.
6. After you select and place the mask, pay particular attention to how it fits over the patient's face. Facial hair and other variables can interfere with a tight seal.
7. Assemble and set the CPAP airway pressure at 5 cm H_2O with 95% to 100% oxygen (use 5 cm H_2O for asthma and COPD, 10 cm H_2O for CHF).
8. Ask the patient to hold the mask to his face as you guide the application. Doing so facilitates correct placement but gives the patient some control as you provide psychological support. Placement of a CPAP mask can make the patient feel claustrophobic and as if he's being smothered.
9. As the seal is made, adjust airway pressure as needed for the patient's comfort.
10. Once the patient is comfortable with the application, apply head straps to maintain a secure seal.
11. Monitor the patient every 5 minutes for improvement in respiratory function and for any signs of discomfort.

TIPS AND TROUBLESHOOTING

- If your patient doesn't improve in 5 minutes or signs of respiratory failure escalate, remove the CPAP and provide positive-pressure ventilation using a bag-mask device until advanced airway techniques can be initiated and invasive ventilatory management instituted.
- Increase airway pressure by 2 to 5 cm H_2O until signs of improvement are noted: less accessory muscle use, improved oxygenation, and less anxiety. Maximum airway pressure is usually considered to be 20 cm H_2O.
- If the patient resists placement of the mask, don't fight him; doing so will increase his work of breathing. Instead, use a calm voice to reassure and coach him as you move the mask into position and help him hold it there.
- If the patient vomits, he is at risk of aspiration. Administration of IV antiemetics may be of benefit.

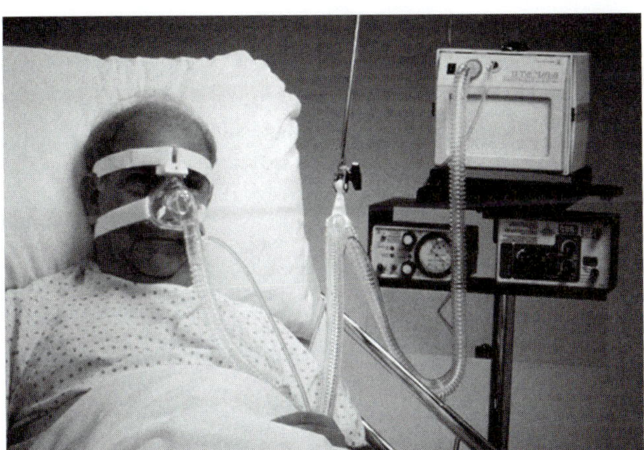

■ **Figure 3-9** Patient with bilevel positive airway pressure (BiPAP) mask applied. (From Marx J, et al: Rosen's emergency medicine: concepts and clinical practice, ed 5, St Louis, 2002, Mosby.)

Bilevel Positive Airway Pressure

BiPAP (Figure 3-9) is a modality being used more frequently in the emergency setting. This noninvasive technique can ease the work of breathing, improve ventilation, and greatly reduce the morbidity of intubation and possible subsequent ventilator dependence. BiPAP holds great promise for avoiding at least some intubations.

BiPAP is a form of CPAP, but it has two different levels of pressure support. One level is higher and supports inspiration (IPAP). The second, lower level assists expiration (EPAP) and helps keep the airway open. Ventilation is delivered through a mask that covers either the nose only or both the face and nose. The mask is often secured to the face with adjustable straps, allowing the patient to relax rather than worry about holding the mask in place.

Both CPAP and BiPAP are valuable noninvasive tools for supporting a patient's respiratory effort, but they are not without drawbacks. Some patients, especially those prone to claustrophobia, cannot tolerate having their nose and mouth covered. The continuous positive pressure can impede venous return and thus reduce blood pressure; it may also contribute to gastric distention and raise the risk of aspiration. Finally, increased positive airway pressure carries the risk of barotrauma, specifically pneumothorax or tension pneumothorax (see later discussion).

Invasive Positive-Pressure Ventilation

Emergent ventilatory management is always or almost always performed in response to a clinical presentation of respiratory distress and a declining level of consciousness. Since this treatment is temporary, the initial goal of invasive positive-pressure ventilation (PPV) is to ensure the airway is secure and protected and ventilation and oxygenation are adequate. The secondary goal then is to successfully wean the patient from the support without complications. The selection of ventilatory mode should take into consideration the patient's level of consciousness, pulmonary function, degree of respiratory distress, prior intubation history, coexisting medical conditions, and degree of hypoxia.

Invasive techniques for intubated patients include pressure- and volume-cycled ventilators. With the ultimate goal of successful extubation, you should select the mode that will allow the patient to exercise as much control as possible over his or her own breathing.

Pressure-Cycled Ventilation

In pressure-cycled ventilation, a breath is delivered until a preset airway pressure has been reached. This predetermined level is called the *peak inspiratory pressure (PIP)*, and the ventilator carefully maintains ventilation within this parameter. Higher pressure allows air to move from the ventilator until the PIP has been achieved and inspiration occurs. Passive exhalation follows inspiration, because the pressure is higher in the chest than in the ventilator.

Pressure-cycled ventilation is most beneficial in the ICU, where patients often have reduced compliance of the lungs or chest wall (as in acute respiratory distress syndrome [ARDS]) or increased lung pressure (as in asthma). In treating such patients, the ability to control peak pressure dictates the selection of pressure-cycled ventilation.

Volume-Cycled Ventilation

In volume-cycled ventilation, a preset tidal volume is programmed into the device. Inhalation is terminated when the limit has been reached. A major advantage of this type of ventilator is that it delivers the tidal volume regardless of changes in lung compliance. Assist/control and intermittent mandatory ventilation are types of volume-cycled ventilators.

Modes of Ventilatory Support

Four principal methods of ventilation are used to deliver volume-cycled and pressure-cycled ventilation:

1. Controlled mechanical ventilation (CMV): the ventilator delivers breaths at a preset interval, regardless of the patient's respiratory effort. This mode is appropriate only for apneic patients and for those who have been pharmacologically paralyzed.
2. Assist/control (A/C) ventilation: assists the patient once he summons his own breath, but if no respiratory effort is forthcoming by the patient, the ventilator provides a complete breath. This is a common ventilator setting during the early phase of ventilatory support.
3. Intermittent mandatory ventilation (IMV): combines CMV with the patient's spontaneous ventilation. The background CMV breathes for the patient regardless of his or her own respiratory effort. If the patient puts forth a respiratory effort, the ventilator does not support it with positive pressure. Instead, it supplies only warm, humidified oxygen. This mode is often used in the hospital to wean the patient from mechanical ventilation.

4. Synchronous intermittent mandatory ventilation (SIMV): supports the patient's spontaneous breaths with A/C ventilation. Synchronous delivery prevents stacking one breath on top of another and causing potentially serious complications.

Determine how the ventilator should respond to a patient's spontaneous respiration. Consider the patient's mental status, and take into account whether or not he or she will be aware of the ventilator's response. Attempting to breathe and receiving no response from the ventilator can make even the calmest patient extremely anxious. Conscious patients can be placed on SIMV, and totally awake patients who are being prepared for extubation may be placed on pressure-support ventilation.

A heavily sedated patient or one with severe brain injury, on the other hand, may put forth no respiratory effort. Such patients require near-total mechanical control and are candidates for A/C ventilation.

Mechanical Ventilator Settings

When initiating mechanical ventilation, you must select ventilatory mode, tidal volume, respiratory rate, and initial oxygenation concentration. Supplemental choices include pressure support or PEEP. The parameters can be altered to meet clinical requirements, such as an anxious patient with respiratory failure and COPD who prefers to breathe at a rate of 20 breaths/min but whose tidal volume is less than that predicted on the basis of body weight. Table 3-2 summarizes typical ventilator settings.

Minute Volume Minute volume is the amount of air inspired per minute. Minute volume combines tidal volume with rate to ensure that enough air is inspired to support adequate ventilation.

Tidal Volume Tidal volume (ventilation volume) and respiratory rate should approximate the patient's own normal rate. Most adults draw a tidal volume of between 5 and 10 milliliters per kilogram (mL/kg) of body weight. Typical settings for an adult who is not in distress are a volume of 6 to 8 mL/kg of body weight and a respiratory rate of 12 breaths/min. Several calculations used to determine tidal volume on the basis of weight are shown in Box 3-7.

Pressure Support Initially, choose the ventilatory mode on the basis of the patient's spontaneous respiratory effort and sedation level. Pressure-support ventilation is a mode used in patients who have retained a spontaneous respiratory drive. It allows the operator to set minimum parameters for breaths per minute, tidal volume, and minute volume. Pressure support can be used to hold a constant positive pressure in the airways, much like BiPAP.

Positive End-Expiratory Pressure Most ventilators accommodate PEEP, a small amount of positive pressure that remains even at the peak of expiration. This pressure opens alveoli clogged with mucus, vomitus, infiltrate (in patients with pneumonia), and edema (in patients with CHF), and it helps keep them open. PEEP can help patients who have alveolar collapse, as is seen in pneumonia and pulmonary edema, but larger tidal volumes and high-pressure support increase the risk of pneumothorax.

TABLE 3-2 Common Ventilator Settings

Setting	Description	Common Settings	Comments
Rate or frequency (*f*)	Number of breaths delivered per minute	6–20 per minute	
Tidal volume (VT)	Volume of gas delivered to the patient	6–8 mL/kg	
Oxygen (FIO_2)	Fraction of inspired oxygen delivered	21%–100%	Blender required if <100%
PEEP	Positive pressure delivered at the end of exhalation	5–20 cm H_2O	This mode improves oxygenation.
Pressure support (PS)	Pressure support to augment inspiratory effort	5–20 cm H_2O	
Inspiratory flow rate/time	Speed with which VT is delivered	40–80 L/min Time: 0.8–1.2 seconds	
Inspiration/expiration (I/E) ratio	Duration of inspiration to expiration	1:2	
Sensitivity	This determines the amount of effort the patient must generate to initiate a breath.	0.5–1.5 cm H_2O below baseline pressure	
High pressure limit	The maximum pressure with which the ventilator can deliver the tidal volume	10–20 cm H_2O above peak inspiratory pressure	The ventilator will stop the breath and release the rest to the atmosphere when the limit is reached.

Adapted from Urden L, et al: Thelan's critical care nursing, ed 5, St Louis, 2006, Elsevier.

BOX 3-7 Weight-Based Formulas for Calculating Tidal Volume

When choosing an appropriate tidal volume for your patient, you must consider what the patient's ideal weight is—not his or her actual weight. Many formulas have been devised to calculate ideal body weight. Most rely on the patient's height and sex.

DEVINE FORMULA

For women: 45.5 kg + 2.3 kg for every inch more than 5 feet of height

For men: 50 kg + 2.3 kg for every inch more than 5 feet of height

BROCA'S FORMULA

Women: 100 lb for the first 5 feet + 5 lb for every inch above that

Men: 110 lb for the first 5 feet + 5 lb for every inch above that

HAMWI FORMULA

Women: 45.5 kg for the first 5 feet, then 2.2 kg for every inch above that

Men: 48 kg for the first 5 feet, then 2.7 kg for every inch above that

GENERIC HEIGHT-WEIGHT FORMULA

Women: 105 lb + 5 × (Height in inches − 60)

Men: 105 lb + 6 × (Height in inches − 60)

Let's say your patient is a man who is 6 feet tall and weighs 225 lbs. If you convert his weight to kilograms, you might set his tidal volume at 800 mL if you calculate 8 mL/kg. Instead, you should calculate that his ideal body weight is 177 lb, or about 81 kg. Your setting, then, should be closer to 650 mL.

The fraction, or concentration, of oxygen in the inspired air (FIO_2) is also chosen as an initial ventilator setting. Choices range from 100% down to 21%. A severely dyspneic patient who has low PO_2 may benefit from an initial setting of 100% until his or her condition has stabilized. Few patients who require emergent or urgent intubation will tolerate 21% oxygen, which is the same as room air. Virtually all patients requiring aggressive airway management will need some oxygen supplementation, but the precise degree will vary from patient to patient. Settings typically fall between 40% and 80%.

Complications of Mechanical Ventilation

A number of serious risks are associated with invasive mechanical ventilation. Volutrauma (also known as *barotrauma*) is lung injury or alveolar rupture from overdistention of the alveoli. Pneumothorax and tension pneumothorax are the primary concerns in ventilator-induced barotrauma; pneumomediastinum and pneumoperitoneum are less frequent complications. Prolonged administration of high-concentration oxygen can damage cells by formation of free radicals and can lead to nitrogen washout and resultant atelectasis. Persistent high intrathoracic pressure can cause decreased cardiac return and low systolic blood pressure.

Another complication can occur while providing positive-pressure ventilation. You already know from earlier discussions that applying PEEP can help keep distal alveoli open and improve oxygenation. But using too much ventilation or administering ventilation to patients who have air-trapping diseases such as asthma or COPD may cause a complication called *auto-PEEP*. In this condition, too little time for exhalation leads to progressively increased air trapping. This phenomenon can compromise gas exchange and allow intrathoracic pressure to become so high that hemodynamic compromise occurs as a result of decreased cardiac output, placing a squeeze on the heart itself.

Special Circumstances

Closely monitoring the patient during intubation and subsequent mechanical ventilation is imperative, since adequate sedation to allow mechanical ventilation can preclude the patient's sharing symptoms of an evolving complication. Immediately investigate and address any unexplained tachycardia, bradycardia, hypotension, or hypertension. Use capnographic and oxygen saturation monitoring—including periodic measurement of ABGs—to direct your selection of ventilator settings. Reduce the FIO_2 as soon as possible, consistent with maintaining an adequate PO_2.

Patients with asthma or COPD may require a high inspiratory pressure and increased pressure support. These patients tend to retain air volume and have high airway pressure, putting them at markedly increased risk of barotrauma. The use of BiPAP in patients with COPD has been shown to reduce the need for intubation by 59%. Should intubation become necessary, adding PEEP may help reduce the air retention that puts these patients at higher risk.

Upper Respiratory Conditions

The upper respiratory tract is vulnerable to many conditions that can obstruct the airway and consequently impair ventilation. Infection is the most common cause of such conditions, but allergic reactions and foreign bodies can also obstruct airflow.

These patients may have no obvious outward signs of illness (e.g., swelling and positional breathing) but may have difficulty swallowing (dysphagia) to the point of drooling. Abnormal sounds may be generated when they breathe or speak. Some of these airway diseases can become life threatening, and you must have a safe and smart plan for airway management that includes proper positioning of the patient.

Mechanical Obstruction: Foreign Body

Aspiration of foreign objects can be a source of significant anxiety for patients and their caregivers. With a peak incidence among infants and toddlers, aspiration of foreign bodies is perhaps a predictable result of young children's tendency to mouth everything they handle. Older children and adults are not seized by this temptation so frequently; aspiration of a foreign object by an adult should prompt assessment for intoxication and mental impairment. In the United States in 2007, there were between 350 and 2000 deaths a year caused by foreign-body airway obstructions. Among children, food—especially popcorn, nuts, and carrots—is the most frequently aspirated item.

Sudden onset of coughing, dyspnea, and signs of choking are the hallmarks of aspiration of a foreign object. Depending on the size and position of the object and the diameter of the airway, the patient may have a total or partial obstruction. Partial obstruction of the lower airway may cause air trapping, with a sudden change in thoracic pressure leading to pneumothorax or pneumomediastinum. Sudden onset of wheezing, especially in an infant or child and particularly in one lung, should raise suspicion that a foreign object has been aspirated.

In some cases, aspirated foreign objects may remain trapped in the airway for several days, weeks, or even months (Figure 3-10). Chronic blockage of a bronchus can cause bronchial collapse and obstructive pneumonia. Even those in the esophagus can be responsible for airway compromise (Figure 3-11).

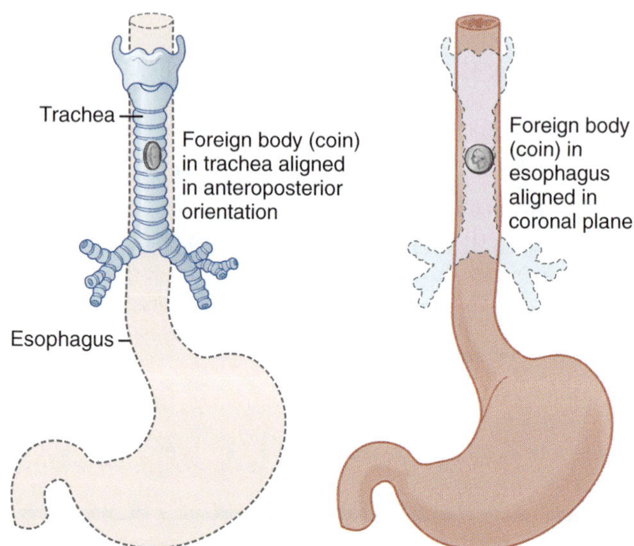

Figure 3-10 Orientation of foreign objects may depend on where object lodges. Coins lodged in trachea generally will orient anterior-posterior *(left)*, and in the esophagus will orient laterally *(right)*. (From Marx J, et al: Rosen's emergency medicine: concepts and clinical practice, ed 6, St Louis, 2006, Mosby.)

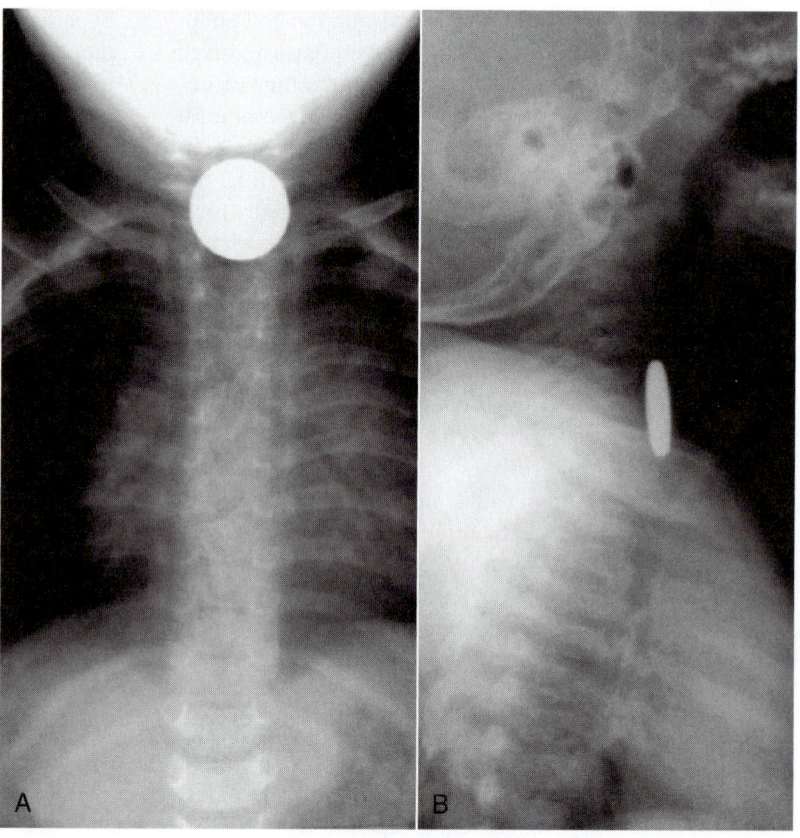

Figure 3-11 Coin lodged in esophagus.

Management of an aspirated foreign object should be dictated by the patient's ability to breathe or cough effectively. Supplemental oxygen may alleviate symptoms sufficiently to allow transport to the ED. Patients who exhibit severe stridor, low oxygen saturation, cyanosis, or signs of impending respiratory failure must receive immediate intervention. Management of such scenarios is challenging for even the most experienced provider—not just the physical act of removing a foreign object from an anxious, dyspneic patient, but calming the distressed parents or other family members.

For conscious patients with partial obstruction who cannot clear the obstruction on their own, abdominal thrusts may simulate a deep cough. If the patient loses consciousness, initiation of chest compressions has been found to be the best method of helping the patient clear the airway obstruction. Preoxygenate the patient if possible, and prepare an alternative rescue airway. Ready the equipment necessary for endotracheal intubation, and have forceps handy. Preparing the family with a brief, simple description of the procedure before you attempt removal can alleviate some anxiety. Using direct laryngoscopy may let you see well enough to grasp and remove the offending object. Suction should be nearby to prevent aspiration in case the patient vomits.

An object visualized below the glottis may be difficult to grasp and not easily removed. Blindly passing an endotracheal tube into the trachea in an effort to move the object to a less obstructive position has been known to be successful, but this is a maneuver that should only be attempted if you're a skilled, experienced provider faced with a complete obstruction.

After removal of a foreign object, intubation may still be indicated if the patient has a decreased level of consciousness, is intoxicated or bleeding, or requires oxygenation and respiratory support. Retain the object so it can be inspected at the receiving facility. The patient's post-transport condition or suspicion that portions of the aspirated object have been retained may warrant bronchoscopy. Bronchoscopy is performed under general anesthesia in the ICU or operating room.

Pharyngeal Infections

The term *pharyngeal infections* refers collectively to pharyngitis, tonsillitis, and peritonsillar abscess.

Pharyngitis and Tonsillitis

Pharyngitis and tonsillitis are both infections of the posterior pharynx. While sharing many of the same causes, *tonsillitis* specifically refers to infection of the tonsils, whereas *pharyngitis* refers to infection of the pharynx, which often includes some degree of tonsillitis.

The etiology of pharyngitis and tonsillitis is usually either viral or bacterial; about 40% to 60% of infections are viral, and 5% to 40% are bacterial. Most bacterial infections are caused by group A *Streptococcus*. A very small percentage of cases are due to trauma, cancer, allergy, or a toxic exposure.

Bacterial and viral infections cause inflammation of the local pharyngeal tissues. In addition, streptococcal infections release local toxins and proteins that may trigger additional inflammation. This inflammation and infection are usually self-limiting, but streptococcal infections have two important side effects. First, the bacterial surface carries antigens that are similar to proteins found normally in the heart. In the process of fighting off a streptococcal infection, the body can inadvertently attack the heart and heart valves, causing rheumatic fever. Second, the glomeruli in the kidneys can become damaged by the antibody-antigen combination, causing acute glomerulonephritis.

Symptoms of pharyngitis and tonsillitis may include:

- Sore throat
- Fever
- Chills
- Muscle aches (myalgia)
- Abdominal pain
- Rhinorrhea
- Headache
- Earache

Physical exam will reveal a red and swollen posterior pharynx, enlarged and tender anterior cervical lymph nodes, and sometimes a fine red rash that feels like sandpaper. Called scarlatina, this rough-feeling red rash begins on the torso and spreads to the entire body; this is caused by streptococcal infection. In addition, whitish exudates (pockets of pus) on the tonsils may be seen. These exudates are more common with streptococcal infection, although their presence does not confirm a bacterial infection. Viral infections are more often associated with the presence of other upper respiratory infection (URI) signs and symptoms such as cough and nasal congestion. A particular viral infection, mononucleosis, is associated with anterior and posterior cervical lymph node swelling and tenderness and should be identified because of potential complications such as splenic rupture.

Viral pharyngitis and tonsillitis are best treated symptomatically with fluids, antipyretic medications, and anti-inflammatory agents. Bacterial infections require antibiotics, usually penicillin or amoxicillin. Erythromycin is often used as an alternative in patients who are allergic to penicillin.

Peritonsillar Abscess

In peritonsillar **abscess**, a superficial soft-tissue infection progresses to create pockets of purulence in the submucosal space adjacent to the tonsils. This abscess and its accompanying inflammation cause the uvula to deviate to the opposing side (Figure 3-12).

Peritonsillar abscess is the most common infection of the peritonsillar region. The incidence of peritonsillar abscess in the United States is about 3 in 10,000 people

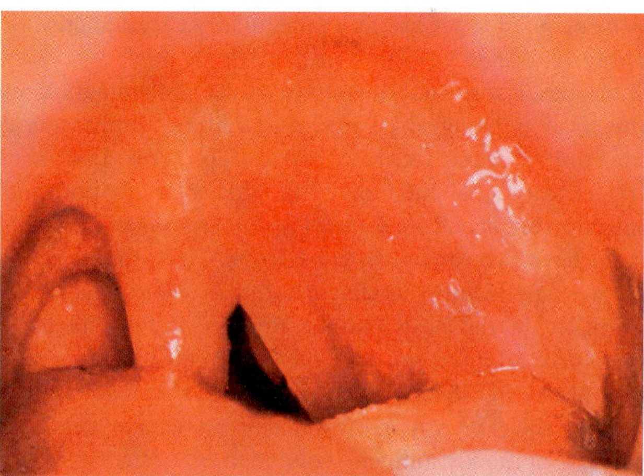

■ **Figure 3-12** Peritonsillar abscess. Note extensive swelling of left tonsil and deviation of uvula. (From Goldman L, Ausiello DAA: Cecil's textbook of medicine, ed 23, Philadelphia, 2008, Saunders.)

annually. *Streptococcus* is often isolated in cultures of peritonsillar abscess, along with other bacteria such as *Peptostreptococcus*. Symptoms of peritonsillar abscess may include:

- Sore throat (especially unilaterally)
- Dysphagia
- Fever
- Chills
- Muscle aches
- Neck and anterior throat pain
- Hoarseness

Signs of peritonsillar abscess include fever, tachycardia, dehydration, "hot potato" or thickened voice, cervical lymph nodes, difficulty swallowing, asymmetric bulging of the tonsils in the posterior pharynx, which often causes the uvula to deviate to the other side of the mouth, and exudates on the tonsils.

The differential diagnosis of peritonsillar abscess includes other serious illnesses such as retropharyngeal and prevertebral abscess, epiglottitis, bacterial tracheitis, mononucleosis, herpes pharyngitis, carotid artery aneurysm, and cancer. Treatment includes hydration with intravenous (IV) fluids and administration of antiinflammatory agents and antibiotics. If an abscess is present, surgical drainage is often indicated and can be performed in the operating room. Occasionally, needle drainage is performed in the ED.

Epiglottitis

Epiglottitis is a life-threatening infection that causes inflammation of the epiglottis and often the supraglottic region. This swelling can obstruct the trachea, inducing hypoxia or anoxia.

Once considered a disease of toddlers, the incidence of epiglottitis has changed dramatically since the United States began immunizing against *Haemophilus influenzae*.

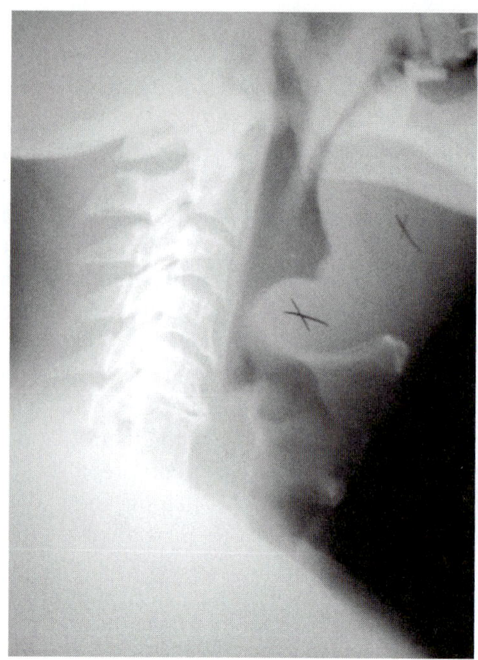

■ **Figure 3-13** Epiglottitis—marked by lower *X*. (From Marx J, et al: Rosen's emergency medicine: concepts and clinical practice, ed 6, St Louis, 2006, Mosby.)

Adults are more likely to present with this illness in the emergency setting; men develop epiglottitis about three times more often than women. The infection remains most common in children 2 to 4 years of age. Mortality is estimated at 7% in adults and 1% in children.

Signs and Symptoms

Epiglottitis often begins with a sore throat and progresses to pain on swallowing and a muffled voice. Physical exam may reveal a patient in moderate or severe distress assuming a tripod position, with fever, drooling, stridor, respiratory distress, notable pain when the larynx is palpated, tachycardia, and perhaps low oxygen saturation. The stridor may be of a softer, lower pitch than that caused by croup. The differential diagnosis should include bacterial tracheitis, retropharyngeal or prevertebral abscess, Ludwig's angina, and peritonsillar abscess.

Pathophysiology

Before a vaccine to *H. influenzae* type b (Hib) became available, epiglottitis occurred 2.6 times more often in children than in adults. *Streptococcus* spp. have now edged out *H. influenzae* as the pathogen most often responsible for causing epiglottitis.

Diagnosis

A diagnosis of epiglottitis should be suspected on the basis of clinical presentation and history, but it can be confirmed with plain-film lateral neck radiographs that reveal findings similar to those shown in Figure 3-13. Computed tomography (CT) imaging may be performed but is often unnecessary, since plain-film radiographs are usually sufficient. Fiberoptic laryngoscopy may provide direct information about the extent of airway edema and can assist in placement of an endotracheal tube.

Treatment

Emergency treatment should be limited to assisting oxygenation and ventilation. Humidified oxygen can be of some relief to the patient, but the severity of this condition cannot be overstated. Intubation should be undertaken in the field only if absolutely necessary. Manipulating the epiglottis with a laryngoscope blade while the tissue is inflamed may irritate the airway and make further intubation attempts extremely difficult. Endotracheal intubation in this setting is best achieved in the surgical suite with an ear, nose, and throat (ENT) surgeon nearby. Antibiotics are indicated, often amoxicillin/sulbactam (Unasyn) or clindamycin, as well as steroids, inhaled β-agonists, and nebulized epinephrine. If respiratory failure occurs with this condition, it is comforting to note that positive-pressure ventilation is usually successful, even without endotracheal intubation.

Infections of the Lower Face and Neck

Infections of the lower face and neck can range from mild to very serious. The neck contains deep spaces, has a plentiful blood supply, houses several structures connected to other body regions, and is in close proximity to vital structures such as the esophagus, trachea, lungs, arteries, veins, and soft tissues.

Signs and Symptoms

Patients with infections of the lower face and neck often have obvious symptoms, including swelling, pain, and redness. They may also exhibit an unusual wavelike motion when the infected portion of the face, neck, or jaw is palpated. This motion is called *fluctuance*. Without radiologic imaging, it is often impossible to rule out extension to deep neck spaces.

Pathophysiology

Widespread use of antibiotics has significantly decreased the frequency and severity of infections of the lower face and neck. In children, the most common cause of such infections is *Streptococcus*. In adults, dental caries most commonly initiate the portal for infection. Spread of infection from the teeth, face, or superficial neck to the deep neck tissues significantly increases the severity of disease. Spread to the lung cavity or mediastinum can cause mediastinitis or empyema, and spread to the carotid sheath can cause jugular vein thrombosis, bacterial endocarditis, pulmonary embolus, or stroke.

Treatment

Emergency management includes providing oxygenation and ventilation, paying particular attention to ensuring a patent airway. A patient with an airway obstructed by either cellulitis or abscess can present a tremendous challenge if you are an experienced emergency provider. Direct endotracheal visualization may be difficult or impossible. Alternative techniques include blind nasotracheal intubation, fiberoptic intubation, and transtracheal illumination. In some cases, you may need to create a surgical airway using needle cricothyrotomy or open cricothyrotomy. Before doing so in the field, consider using a supraglottic airway, such as the King airway, laryngeal mask airway, or Cobra airway. These airway techniques are described in Appendix D. Obtain and monitor vital signs, and initiate IV access. If the patient becomes hypotensive, initiate volume replacement, and consider the possibility of septic shock.

Ludwig's Angina

Named for the physician who first described it in the early 19th century, **Ludwig's angina** refers not to chest pain but to a deep-space infection of the anterior neck just below the mandible. Sensations of choking and suffocation are reported by most patients with this condition.

Signs and Symptoms

Because it often arises from dental decay and subsequent infection, Ludwig's angina is characterized by:

- Severe gingivitis and cellulitis, with firm swelling and rapidly spreading infection in the submandibular, sublingual, and submental spaces (Figure 3-14)
- Swelling of the sublingual area and tongue
- Drooling
- Airway obstruction
- Elevation and posterior displacement of the tongue as a result of edema

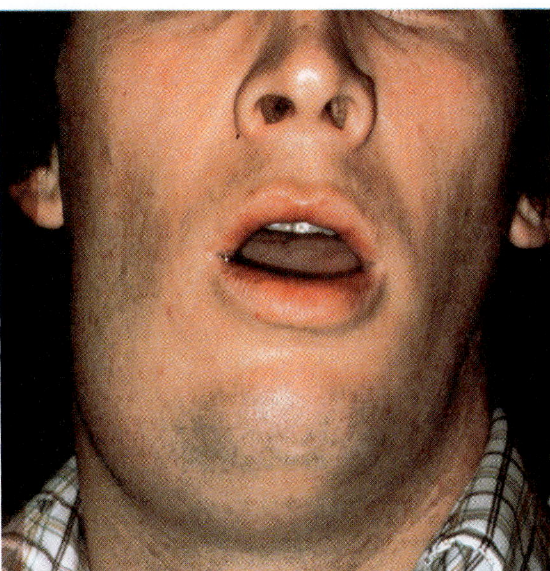

Figure 3-14 Ludwig's angina. Rapid progression may compromise airway in a few hours. (From Roberts JR, Hedges JR: Clinical procedures in emergency medicine, ed 5, Philadelphia, 2009, Saunders.)

Symptoms of Ludwig's angina include sore throat, dysphagia, fever, chills, dental pain, and dyspnea. The patient tends to look anxious and toxic, with poor dentition and a firm, red, pronounced swelling in the anterior throat area. The location of caries may suggest which primary spaces are affected. The patient's tongue may be elevated, portending a difficult intubation should a mechanical airway become necessary.

Pathophysiology

Swelling, redness, and warm tissue (induration) between the hyoid bone and the mandible may be the most notable sign on clinical exam. This inflammation is caused by bacteria in the oral cavity. *Streptococcus* spp. are often cultured, but such infections are rarely due to a single organism and may contain anaerobic organisms.

Submental (beneath the chin) infection often migrates from dental caries in the incisors. Sublingual infection can usually be attributed to infection in the anterior mandibular teeth and can manifest as tongue elevation caused by swelling. Submandibular infection, which usually originates in the molars, is characterized by swelling in the angle of the jaw.

Since fluoridation of public drinking water became widespread in the 1970s, the prevalence of dental caries has decreased in developed countries. However, dental caries remains the most common chronic disease in the world.

Differential Diagnosis

Your differential diagnosis should include retropharyngeal and prevertebral abscess, bacterial tracheitis, and epiglottitis. Patients who have recently had chemotherapy or organ transplant with immunosuppression are at increased risk of developing this infection, including abscess.

Treatment

A patient suspected of having Ludwig's angina should be considered to have a life-threatening illness, perhaps accompanied by a compromised airway. Maintaining a patent airway is of paramount importance. In a rapidly progressing infection, prophylactic intubation may be performed electively in the ED or operating room. Stridor, dysphagia with difficulty controlling secretions, and dyspnea may prompt intubation. In the prehospital environment, supplemental humidified oxygen can make the patient more comfortable. Electrocardiographic monitoring and IV placement should be initiated. Antibiotics are initiated in the ED, and an ENT surgeon may be consulted.

Bacterial Tracheitis

Sometimes difficult to differentiate from epiglottitis and retropharyngeal abscess, bacterial tracheitis is a rare infection of the subglottic trachea. Since *H. influenzae* vaccination became widespread, bacterial tracheitis may rival epiglottitis as the least common obstructive airway infection. One study showed that of 500 children hospitalized for croup over a 3-year period, 2% had bacterial tracheitis. While it may occur in any age group, tracheitis is more common in children because of their smaller airways and the narrow diameter of the subglottic tissues. Twice as many male patients as females contract the infection.

Signs and Symptoms

Bacterial tracheitis begins as an URI and progresses to become a life-threatening infection of the subglottic tracheal lining (Figure 3-15). Symptoms include productive cough, voice changes, high fever, chills, and dyspnea. Signs include rapid progression to a toxic state over as little as 8 to 10 hours, stridor, a brassy cough, and occasionally neck or upper chest pain. Unlike epiglottitis, drooling is uncommon, and the patient may be able to lie supine.

Pathophysiology

Tracheitis is caused by multiple organisms, such as *Staphylococcus aureus* (including community-associated

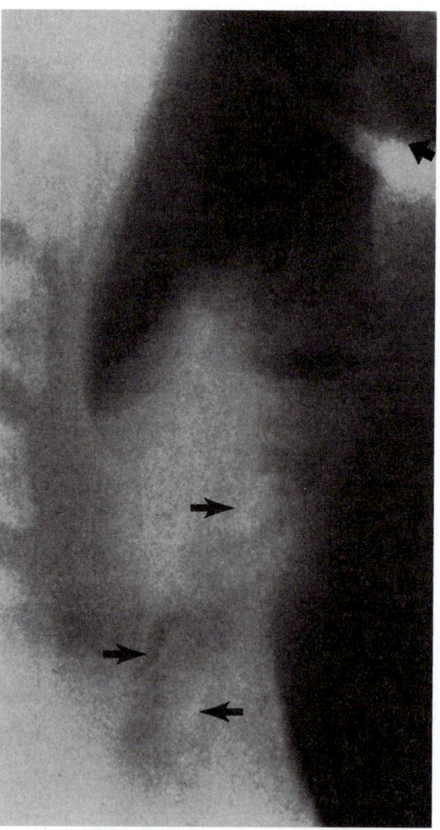

Figure 3-15 Neck x-ray showing bacterial tracheitis in lateral soft tissue. Note obscured airway due to sloughed tracheal linings *(lower two arrows)*. Epiglottis *(upper arrow)* is normal. (From Cummings CW, et al: Otolaryngology: head and neck surgery, ed 4, Philadelphia, 2005, Mosby.)

methicillin-resistant *S. aureus* [CA-MRSA] and healthcare-associated [HA]-MRSA), *Streptococcus* spp., *H. influenzae*, *Klebsiella* spp., and *Pseudomonas* spp.

Treatment

As with any airway infection, maintaining a patent airway is of primary importance. Provide supplemental oxygen, initiate electrocardiographic monitoring, and obtain IV access. Many patients with bacterial tracheitis will require intubation, but the procedure is best performed under controlled circumstances unless the patient is in acute respiratory failure. If intubation is absolutely necessary in the field, you should be ready to implement a backup airway if necessary. If intubation is successful, be alert for tracheal exudates and mucus clogging the tube, and provide appropriate suction. These patients may have features of sepsis, so initiate an appropriate fluid challenge.

Retropharyngeal and Prevertebral Abscess

Retropharyngeal and prevertebral abscesses are both infections that develop behind the esophagus and in front of the cervical vertebrae (Figure 3-16). As noted earlier, an abscess is a localized collection of pus in a tissue or other confined space in the body. A retropharyngeal abscess may originate in the sinuses, teeth, or middle ear. Up to 67% of these patients report having had a recent ENT infection. Retropharyngeal infections can be life threatening if they begin to cause airway obstruction. Infection that spreads to the mediastinum, called *mediastinitis*, is a grave complication that carries a startlingly high mortality rate of nearly 50%.

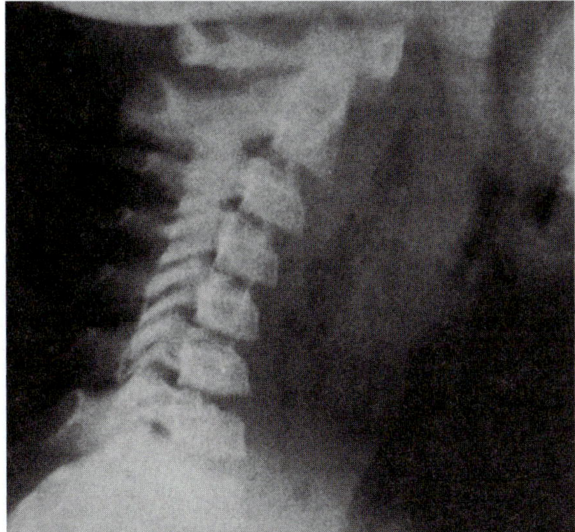

Figure 3-16 Retropharyngeal abscess. Note dark line in front of cervical spine, representing a gas-producing infection. (From Cummings CW, et al: Otolaryngology: head and neck surgery, ed 4, Philadelphia, 2005, Mosby.)

Signs and Symptoms

Early retropharyngeal abscess may be misdiagnosed as unspecified or streptococcal pharyngitis. If the patient's condition rapidly declines, you should consider more threatening illnesses such as epiglottitis, bacterial tracheitis, and meningitis. Signs of retropharyngeal abscess include:

- Pharyngitis
- Dysphagia
- Dyspnea
- Fever
- Chills
- Neck pain, stiffness, swelling, or erythema
- Drooling

The following are worrisome signs of possible airway compromise:

- Difficulty opening the mouth (trismus)
- Vocal changes
- Inspiratory stridor

Pathophysiology

Common causal organisms in retropharyngeal abscess are *Staphylococcus* spp., *Streptococcus* spp., and *H. influenzae*, although the infection can be attributed to other organisms, especially anaerobes from the mouth. Retropharyngeal lesions can be seen in adults as well as in children but usually affect those aged 3 to 4 or younger.

Treatment

Management includes ensuring a patent airway and providing supplemental oxygen. Be careful not to puncture the abscess during intubation, since aspiration of the purulent contents may be fatal. Initiate electrocardiographic monitoring, and obtain IV access. Initiate appropriate fluid replenishment if the patient is dehydrated from decreased oral intake.

Definitive care often involves intubation in the operating suite (or under other controlled circumstances), surgical drainage of the lesion, and antibiotics. With aggressive management of retropharyngeal abscess before it progresses to mediastinitis, many patients recover promptly and can be extubated immediately following or a few days after the procedure.

Angioedema

Angioedema is a sudden swelling, usually of a head or neck structure such as the lip (especially the lower lip), earlobes, tongue, or uvula, but it has been described in other tissues including the bowel. While not fully understood, angioedema is considered to be an allergic reaction and is treated as such. Sometimes the cause is idiopathic (of unknown cause). A few cases are hereditary, referred to as *hereditary angioedema*.

BOX 3-8 Selected Triggers of Angioedema

- ACE inhibitors (captopril, enalapril, and others)
- Radiologic dyes
- Aspirin
- NSAIDs (ibuprofen, naproxen, and others)
- Hymenoptera insect stings (wasps, yellow jackets, and others)
- Food allergies
- Animal hair or dander (shed skin cells)
- Sunlight exposure
- Stress

Up to 15% of the general population has episodic idiopathic angioedema. No racial predominance exists. Women are more likely to have angioedema than men, and the condition is most often seen in adults. Exposure to certain agents increases the risk of angioedema. Common triggers are listed in Box 3-8.

Signs and Symptoms

Signs of angioedema include clearly demarcated swelling with or without a rash and occasionally with dyspnea or anxiety. Stridor, wheezing on chest auscultation, or history of intubation should prompt careful observation for deterioration. Angioedema of the bowel may cause bowel obstruction with consequent nausea, vomiting, and abdominal pain.

Pathophysiology

In angioedema, some insult triggers leakage from the small-vessel circulation, prompting interstitial tissues to swell. Edema can originate in the epidermal and dermal tissues, in the subcutaneous tissues, or both. This inflammation is a response to the actions of circulating hormones and histamines, serotonin, and bradykinins.

Treatment

Although extensive angioedema may threaten the airway, many cases are self-limiting or require only minimal treatment. Carefully assess the patient for other life-threatening illnesses, such as cellulitis/abscess, retropharyngeal abscess, and Ludwig's angina. If the patient has hives, consider the possibility of anaphylaxis.

Allow the patient to assume a comfortable position. If there are no signs of respiratory failure, the patient will maintain his or her own airway with simple positioning.

Emergent intubation can be extremely difficult in severe cases of angioedema, since the swollen tissue may prevent adequate visualization of the vocal cords. In addition to normal intubation equipment, prepare rescue airway equipment before you attempt intubation. If time permits, intubation should be performed under controlled circumstances, where the services of the anesthesia service and an ENT surgeon or general surgeon are available. In nonemergent patients, it is prudent to initiate electrocardiographic monitoring, obtain IV access, and transport the patient to a nearby emergency facility.

LOWER AIRWAY DISEASES

Air-Trapping Diseases

Asthma and COPD are air-trapping diseases of the lower airway. These patients typically have an increased work of breathing, dyspnea, and a history of previous episodes. What distinguishes asthma from COPD? The reactive airway process in asthma, unlike in COPD, is largely reversible.

Asthma

Asthma is a common disease, prompting millions of ED visits a year and accounting for 20% to 30% of hospital admissions. Patients have a high relapse rate, with 10% to 20% returning within 2 weeks of treatment. Despite a declining mortality rate for asthma since 1996, about 4500 Americans die of the disease each year. In the United States, 6% to 10% of the population (about 25 million people) has asthma, and at least half of them are children. While mortality has declined, the prevalence continues to increase.

Children who have wheezing that begins before age 5 and persists into adulthood have a greater likelihood of compromised lung function. Children who begin to wheeze after age 5 have a lower incidence of pulmonary disease even if the wheezing persists into adulthood. As many as 80% to 90% of patients with asthma have their first symptoms before age 6. Some children present with nocturnal coughing as a symptom, without the typical wheezing.

Signs and Symptoms

Asthma patients are usually acutely aware of their symptoms, even if the symptoms are considered clinically mild. Early symptoms of asthma include some combination of the following:

- Wheezing
- Dyspnea
- Chest tightness
- Cough
- Signs of a recent URI, such as rhinorrhea, congestion, headache, pharyngitis, and myalgia

- Signs of exposure to allergens, such as rhinorrhea, pharyngitis, hoarseness, and cough
- Chest tightness, discomfort, or pain

The patient initially hyperventilates, causing a decrease in CO_2 levels (respiratory alkalosis). As the airways continue to narrow, it becomes more and more difficult to exhale completely, and air trapping results. The lungs become overinflated and stiff, increasing the work of breathing. Tachypnea, tachycardia, and pulsus paradoxus may occur, with accompanying agitation. Few retractions should be seen. Oxygen saturation should be near normal, even on room air.

Patients with moderate exacerbations may show increased tachycardia and tachypnea, with increased wheezing and decreased air movement. Oxygen saturation may dip, but it should be easily restored with supplemental oxygen. Retractions may be seen, and the degree and types will increase with the severity of the episode. Recruitment of more muscle sets (e.g., intercostals, subcostal) augurs a worsening condition.

Certain factors in a carefully taken patient history may help predict the severity of an asthma episode: respiratory illness, exposure to potential allergens, compliance with home inhaled medications, and the frequency of ED visits, hospital admissions, and steroid use.

Pathophysiology

Asthma is a chronic inflammation of the bronchi with contraction of the bronchial smooth muscle, resulting in narrowed bronchi and the associated wheezing. The airways become overly sensitive to inhaled allergens, viruses, and other environmental irritants—even strong odors can precipitate an episode. This oversensitivity is responsible for the reactive airway component of the disease.

Inflammation is at the center of asthma symptoms such as dyspnea, wheezing, and coughing. The body may respond to persistent bronchospasm with bronchial edema and tenacious mucous secretions that can cause bronchial plugging and atelectasis.

Allergens such as animal material and airborne ragweed and pollen particles are common precipitants of asthma episodes. Inhalation of smoke or cold dry air may also touch off a flare-up. Factors that indicate it is likely the patient is having a severe asthma exacerbation are listed in Box 3-9.

Differential Diagnosis

When gathering a history, new-onset wheezing is not enough to make an asthma diagnosis. Repeated bouts of this disease are usually necessary for a clinician to make a definitive diagnosis, since many other conditions are characterized by wheezing. Bacterial pneumonia, such as that caused by *Streptococcus* spp., can cause wheezing, as can atypical infections such as *Mycoplasma* and *Chlamydia*. Viral infections are also potential causes of wheezing, especially respiratory syncytial virus (RSV), a common infection among infants during the winter and early spring months.

What other diseases present with wheezing? The differential diagnosis should include both primary pulmonary and systemic disease. COPD often has at least some component of asthma, but it can also have features of bronchitis and emphysema. Consider upper airway obstruction, such as that caused by croup, epiglottitis, bacterial tracheitis, or retropharyngeal infection, especially if stridor is present. Congestive heart failure may present with new-onset wheezing, as can aspiration of a foreign object (see earlier discussion). Chest pain may prompt evaluation for cardiac ischemia, especially if the quality of the pain is different from that of previous asthma episodes.

In children, congenital heart disease should be considered in the differential diagnosis, as should aspiration of a foreign object, bronchiolitis, and gastroesophageal reflux disease (GERD). Fever is not a sign typically associated with asthma, and it should prompt evaluation for pneumonia or another infectious process.

Treatment

Therapy should be scaled to the severity of the exacerbation. First-line treatment for actively wheezing patients includes inhaled β-agonists such as albuterol and levalbuterol (Xopenex). β_2-Agonists used early and aggressively in the course of disease can reduce the likelihood of hospitalization. Albuterol 2.5 to 5 mg is given every 20 minutes for three doses, or it can be given continuously, followed by 2.5 to 10 mg every 1 to 4 hours as needed. The pediatric dose is 0.15 mg/kg (with a minimum dose of 2.5 mg) every 20 minutes, followed by 0.15 mg to 0.3 mg/kg every 1 to 4 hours as indicated by the patient's clinical condition, up to 10 mg.

BOX 3-9 Indicators of Severe Asthma Exacerbation

- Presenting oxygen saturation < 92%
- Tachypnea
- Recent ED visit or hospitalization
- Frequent hospitalizations
- Any history of intubation for asthma
- Peak flows < 50% to 60% of predicted values
- Accessory muscle use and retraction
- Duration of symptoms > 2 days
- History of frequent steroid use
- Currently taking theophylline

Parenteral β_2-agonists may be a useful supplement for severe asthma episodes. Terbutaline 0.25 mg, or 0.3 mg of 1:1000 epinephrine administered intramuscularly or subcutaneously, can assist inhaled β_2-agonists. Because of their tendency to cause hypertension and increase myocardial workload and oxygen demand, however, they should be used with caution, especially in patients who have coexisting ischemic disease. IV or intraosseous (IO) administration of terbutaline or epinephrine may also be indicated, but you should seek consultation first.

Ipratropium 0.5 mg is occasionally given and has the greatest effect on patients with coexisting COPD or a history of tobacco use. Ipratropium can be given every 20 minutes for three doses and then as indicated.

IV corticosteroids help tamp down the inflammatory response, thereby reducing the edema that narrows bronchial passageways. In adults, 40 to 125 mg methylprednisolone (Solu-Medrol) is given, or 2 mg/kg IV in pediatric patients. In adults, triamcinolone (Aristocort) 60 mg IM can be given. In children older than age 6, use 0.03 to 0.3 mg/kg IM. Remember that steroids may take hours to work. Emergency medical service (EMS) providers may initiate corticosteroid treatment rather than wait until the patient reaches the ED, so that the agents can begin to take effect as quickly as possible in the course of treatment.

Magnesium sulfate given intravenously has shown promise in controlling severe exacerbations of asthma. It's typically given as a 2-g dose over 30 to 60 minutes to help relax smooth bronchial muscles.

While not widely used, Heliox is another inhaled agent that has shown promise for severe exacerbations. Given either in an 80:20 or a 70:30 mixture, helium acts as a lighter-than-air carrier to help distribute oxygen and nebulized agents and decrease the work of breathing. Albuterol given with Heliox uses twice the normal dose of albuterol, at a flow rate of 8 to 10 L/min.

Despite aggressive pharmacologic therapy, some patients still face severe respiratory distress or respiratory failure.

Chronic Obstructive Pulmonary Disease

COPD is an airflow obstruction caused by chronic bronchitis or loss of alveolar surface area associated with emphysema. It is characterized by some degree of wheezing and airway edema, and even though the mechanism is slightly different from that of asthma, both are air-trapping diseases of the lungs. COPD is a chronic devastating disease ranked as the fourth-leading cause of death in the United States. About 14 million people have COPD. Of those, 12.5 million have chronic bronchitis, and 1.7 million have emphysema. The number of patients diagnosed with COPD has increased by 41.5% since 1982. The incidence of this disease in the United States is between 6.6% and 6.9% for mild and moderate COPD. It is more prevalent in men than women and in the caucasian than the black population. According to the National Health and Nutrition Examination Survey [NHANES], the rate of COPD climbs with age, especially in those who smoke.

The primary cause of COPD is cigarette smoking. Most patients with clinically significant COPD have smoked at least 1 pack a day for 20 years. An estimated 15% of all smokers develop clinically significant COPD. Many factors affect the rate at which COPD evolves, including the age at which the person began smoking, the number of packs per day, the existence of other illnesses, the person's level of physical fitness, and his or her current tobacco abuse. Second-hand smoke contributes to reduced pulmonary function, asthma exacerbations, and increased risk of upper respiratory tract infections. The only genetic risk factor known to cause COPD in nonsmokers is a deficiency of alpha$_1$-antitrypsin, a protein that inhibits neutrophil elastase, a lung enzyme.

Signs and Symptoms

Symptoms of acute exacerbation of COPD may include:

- Dyspnea
- Cough
- Intolerance of exertion
- Wheezing
- Productive cough
- Chest pain or discomfort
- Diaphoresis
- Orthopnea

You may note the following clinical signs of COPD:

- Wheezing
- Increased respiratory rate
- Decreased oxygen saturation
- Use of accessory muscles
- Elevated jugular pulse
- Peripheral edema
- Hyperinflated lungs
- Hyperresonance on percussion
- Coarse, scattered rhonchi

Critical episodes are indicated by:

- Saturation below 90%
- Tachypnea (about 30 breaths per minute)
- Peripheral or central cyanosis
- Mental status changes caused by hypercapnia

A patient with COPD can have single or multiple triggers of acute exacerbations. As noted, cigarette smoking is the primary cause of COPD, and continued tobacco abuse can be a seminal trigger of a critical episode. Exposure to environmental allergens can precipitate an episode or exacerbate an existing flare-up. Air pollution can contribute to a COPD exacerbation but by itself usually does not touch off a critical episode.

Pathophysiology

Chronic inflammation from exposure to inhaled particles injures the airways. The body tries to repair this injury by remodeling the airways, which causes scarring and narrowing. Changes in the alveolar walls and connective tissue permanently enlarge the alveoli. On the other side of those alveoli, the important connection to the capillary membrane is remodeled with a thickened vessel wall, which impedes gas exchange. Mucus-secreting glands and goblet cells multiply, increasing mucus production. Cilia are destroyed, limiting the elevation and clearing of this abundant mucus.

External changes in the body, such as a barrel-shaped chest, occur in response to the remodeled airways and chronic air trapping. Chronic shortness of breath and chronic cough are also manifestations of this remodeling. Because of chronic hypoxia, chemoreceptors fail to react to fluctuations in the blood's oxygen level. Unfortunately, these changes reflect a permanent adjustment of the body in response to chronic inhalation of irritants.

Lung function gradually declines, and body remodeling slackens. Sputum production increases, and the patient has retained secretions with a chronic cough. The classic air trapping is caused by the limited ability of the lungs to move air out of enlarged distal airways. The lungs become hyperinflated, and only limited gas exchange occurs, which leads to hypoxia and high CO_2 levels, a condition known as *hypercarbia* or *hypercapnia*. Chronic hypercarbia blunts the body's normal chemoreceptor sensitivity, and hypoxia becomes the primary mechanism for ventilation control. At this stage, the patient is vulnerable to infection and intolerant of exercise. Any condition that increases the work of breathing may quickly lead to respiratory failure.

Differential Diagnosis

The presentation of COPD should prompt you to consider other serious diseases, particularly since the chief complaint of dyspnea may be associated with chest pain. The differential diagnosis of COPD should include asthma, bronchitis, emphysema, pneumonia, pneumonitis, pulmonary fibrosis, respiratory failure, pneumothorax, and cardiac causes of dyspnea such as acute myocardial infarction, angina, CHF, pulmonary embolus, and pulmonary hypertension.

Management

Management of a COPD exacerbation hinges on maintaining oxygenation and ventilation. Emergency management includes supplemental oxygen delivered by either nasal cannula or Ventimask and sufficient to maintain saturation of at least 92%. If the patient remains hypoxic with low-flow oxygen, apply a nonrebreather mask with high-flow oxygen, and prepare for aggressive airway and ventilation management. Poor peak flow performance, saturation that falls into the 80s, and pale or cyanotic extremities also indicate a need for aggressive intervention. Endotracheal intubation, either rapid sequence or nasotracheal, may be indicated in severe cases. COPD patients may require extended periods of intubation, so nasotracheal intubation may have some advantages, since it requires less sedation and may allow for earlier extubation.

Never withhold oxygen from a hypoxic patient. It is a common misconception that giving oxygen to COPD patients with dyspnea will eliminate the drive to breathe. Although elevated oxygen levels may marginally decrease the drive to breathe, permissive hypoxia is a poor management plan.

Once you have secured the airway, administer β_2-agonists early and often. Even though these agents are not as effective in COPD as in asthma, they are a mainstay of treatment. Three nebulized doses can be administered 20 minutes apart for stabilization. In emergent cases, these doses can be administered back to back. Anticholinergic agents such as ipratropium bromide are beneficial, particularly in concert with β_2-agonists. Although they don't act as quickly as the β_2-agonists, the anticholinergics can provide an additional 20% to 40% bronchodilation when combined with β_2-agonists.

Systemic corticosteroids, usually in the form of injectable Solu-Medrol, are considered routine treatment in moderate to severe episodes. Although oral steroids, notably prednisone, are useful in mild exacerbations, they are not used in moderate to severe episodes.

Theophylline was often used before the advent of β_2-agonists. Since its maximum effectiveness is reached at near-toxic levels, however, it is now rarely used when alternatives are available. In severe cases of respiratory distress, you may consider giving theophylline, weighing its narrow therapeutic window against the likelihood of adverse effects and toxicity.

COPD patients in acute respiratory failure require positive-pressure ventilation in the form of **noninvasive positive-pressure ventilation** (NPPV) or endotracheal intubation with invasive ventilation through a ventilator. COPD patients may benefit from NPPV if they are hemodynamically stable, have a patent airway, have minimal secretions, and are alert and oriented. If tolerated, NPPV is usually better for short-term ventilatory support because it tends to have fewer side effects.

Conversely, the COPD patient who must be placed on invasive mechanical ventilation may be difficult to wean from that therapy and is vulnerable to ventilator-associated pneumonia. Mechanical ventilation is indicated when, despite aggressive therapy, the patient has mental status changes, acidosis, respiratory fatigue, and hypoxia. The patient may have discussed the use of long-term ventilatory support with his or her family. Be sure to ask the family whether the patient has an advance directive and what the patient's wishes are in regard to long-term mechanical ventilation.

Infection and Immune Response

Pneumonia and acute lung injury/acute respiratory distress syndrome (ALI/ARDS) are lower airway diseases that often have atypical presentations. Patients with pneumonia usually have the classic symptoms of cough and fever, but they may also have more subtle signs, such as abdominal pain, low-grade fever, and weakness with accompanying tachycardia. ALI/ARDS is a lung failure that occurs after a critical event, usually somewhere else in the body.

Pneumonia

Lung infection that causes fluid to collect in the alveoli is referred to as *pneumonia* (Figure 3-17). The resulting inflammation can cause dyspnea, fever, chills, chest pain, chest wall pain, and a productive cough. There are three broad types of pneumonia: community acquired, hospital acquired (nosocomial; begins 48 or more hours after hospital admission), and ventilator associated. The cause may be viral, bacterial, fungal, or chemical in nature (aspiration of gastric contents).

More than 3 million cases of pneumonia are diagnosed annually in the United States. Untreated pneumonia has a mortality rate approaching 30%. Even with appropriate and timely treatment, coexisting medical conditions (comorbidities) can drastically increase the likelihood of mortality. Advanced age increases susceptibility to pneumonia. In a 20-year study, overall mortality in pneumonia caused by *Staphylococcus pneumoniae* was 20%, but in patients older than age 80, mortality exceeded 37%.

Recovery may be complicated by comorbid conditions such as human immunodeficiency virus (HIV) infection, CHF, diabetes, leukemia, and pulmonary diseases like asthma, COPD, and bronchitis. Development of pneumonia in an already compromised patient can touch off a downward spiral of dyspnea, destruction of lung tissue by infection, further infection, more dyspnea, a worsening condition, and so on. Ravaged alveoli can be replaced by pus-filled saccules. This inflammatory material perpetuates the cycle, resulting in empyema or lung abscess, which can be difficult to treat without surgical intervention. Even in patients who recover, scarring from the infection can compromise respiratory gas exchange, reducing pulmonary reserve capacity and increasing susceptibility to another infection.

Signs and Symptoms

An acute onset of symptoms and a rapid progression are more suggestive of a bacterial than a viral cause. Clinical signs and symptoms of pneumonia may include any of the following:

- Fever
- Chills
- Cough
- Malaise
- Nausea and vomiting
- Diarrhea
- Myalgia
- Pleuritic chest pain
- Abdominal pain
- Anorexia
- Dyspnea
- Tachypnea
- Tachycardia
- Hypoxia
- Abnormal breath sounds, including rales, rhonchi, and even wheezing

Pathophysiology

Pathogens that can cause community-acquired pneumonia include *Streptococcus pneumoniae, Legionella* spp., *H. influenzae, S. aureus,* respiratory viruses, *Chlamydia,* and *Pseudomonas*. Hospital-acquired pneumonia can be caused by the same pathogens, along with *Klebsiella* and *Enterococcus* spp. The two pathogens most commonly associated with ventilator-assisted pneumonia are *S. aureus* and *Pseudomonas aeruginosa*. Pneumonia most commonly develops because of a defect in the host's immune system or an overwhelming burden of strong pathogens.

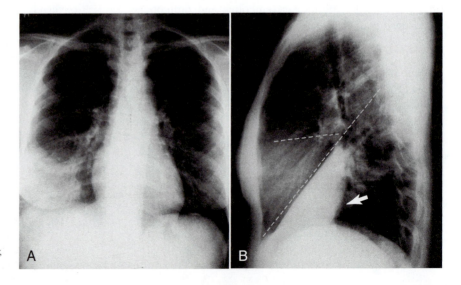

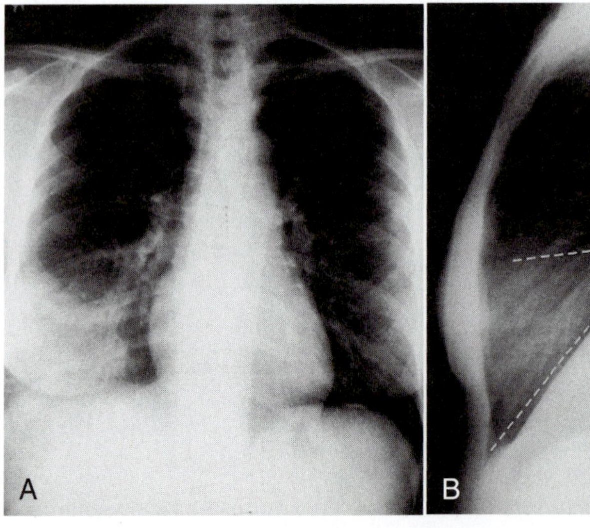

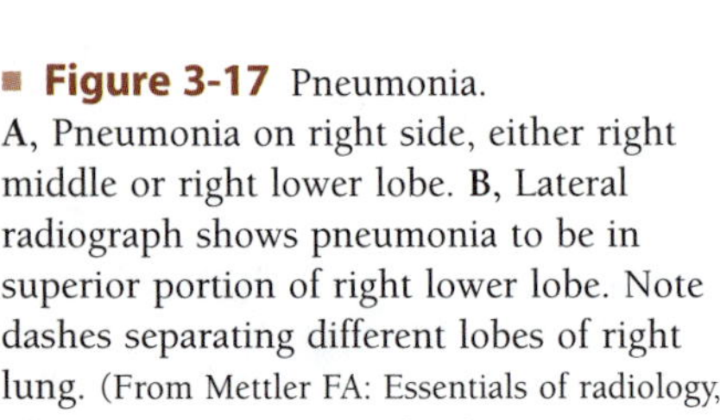

■ **Figure 3-17** Pneumonia. **A**, Pneumonia on right side, either right middle or right lower lobe. **B**, Lateral radiograph shows pneumonia to be in superior portion of right lower lobe. Note dashes separating different lobes of right lung. (From Mettler FA: Essentials of radiology, ed 2, St Louis, 2004, Saunders.)

Diagnosis

While auscultating the lungs over an area with decreased breath sounds, ask the patient to make an *e* sound and hold it. The tone transmitted may more closely resemble an *a* than an *e*. This phenomenon is known as *egophony*, derived from the Greek words for "goat" and "sound," since the pitch is said to mimic a goat's bleating. There may also be dullness to percussion over the affected lobe and increased tactile fremitus. Altered mental status and cyanosis are signs of severe illness.

Diagnosis can be made on the basis of clinical presentation, a careful HPI, and a thorough physical exam. Radiologic evaluation, including anteroposterior and lateral chest x-rays, shows fair to good sensitivity to infiltrate, although a negative study does not rule out pneumonia. CT is sensitive to pneumonia but exposes the patient to higher radiation than plain films.

The differential diagnosis of pneumonia should include asthma, bronchitis, COPD exacerbation, tracheal or supraglottic foreign objects, epiglottitis, empyema, pulmonary abscess, CHF, angina, and myocardial infarction.

Management

Supplemental oxygen is helpful for any patient with a clinically significant pneumonia. It should be provided by nasal cannula, with the goal of maintaining saturation above 92%. Consider more aggressive airway maneuvers for patients who require more intensive oxygenation. Use of a CPAP mask may alleviate the need for intubation in patients who are able to tolerate having the mask covering the face (see earlier discussion).

Blood cultures are often obtained, but antibiotics are administered empirically as soon as possible, before the results of such cultures become available. Studies have shown that administration of antibiotics within 6 hours of arriving in the ED decreases morbidity and mortality in patients with pneumonia. Hydration may also be effective, especially if the patient is bordering on septic shock. In such patients, vigorous fluid resuscitation and possibly vasopressor therapy may be needed. Fluid resuscitation in dehydrated patients may make the pneumonia visible on plain radiograph by making enough fluid available to cause an infiltrate. In such cases, a decrease in oxygenation may be seen as alveoli labor to carry out gas exchange under an increasing burden of collected fluid. Chest physical therapy and regular ambulation can loosen such infiltrates and collections of mucus.

Acute Lung Injury/Acute Respiratory Distress Syndrome

Acute lung injury/acute respiratory distress syndrome (ALI/ARDS), is a systemic disease that causes lung failure. Direct causes of ARDS include events and conditions that damage the epithelial cell layer, such as aspiration of gastric contents, near-drowning, toxic inhalation, pulmonary contusion, pneumonia, oxygen toxicity, and radiation therapy (Figure 3-18). The condition can be caused indirectly by a massive immune response in which chemical mediators are transported in the bloodstream. This creates a chain reaction where all organs, including the lungs, may be affected. This is called *multiple organ dysfunction syndrome (MODS)*. It occurs with massive transfusion, bypass surgery, severe pancreatitis, embolism, disseminated intravascular coagulation, and shock.

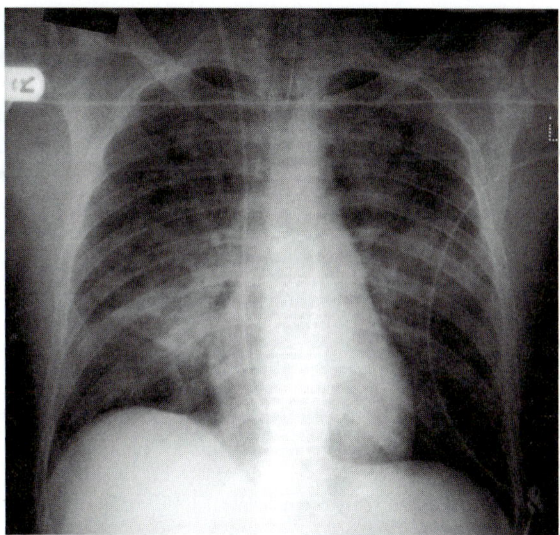

Figure 3-18 Acute respiratory distress syndrome (ARDS). Note increased diffuse lung opacity, suggesting diffuse infiltrates. (From Adam A, et al: Grainger & Allison's diagnostic radiology, ed 5, Philadelphia, 2008, Churchill Livingstone.)

When the lungs fail in ALI/ARDS, a noncardiogenic pulmonary edema develops, accompanied by respiratory distress, pulmonary edema, and respiratory failure. Ventilatory support may be required to treat the associated severe hypoxemia. Criteria for diagnosing ALI/ARDS are given in Box 3-10.

Signs and Symptoms

Development of progressive dyspnea and hypoxemia within hours to days after an acute traumatic or medical event characterizes ALI/ARDS; ARDS is most often seen in hospitalized patients, usually in the ICU. A typical patient has recently undergone major surgery, seems to recover and is in a non-ICU bed, and then develops phase 1 ALI/ARDS and must be readmitted to the ICU. Physical signs of ALI/ARDS include:

- Dyspnea
- Hypoxemia, sometimes accompanied by cyanosis of the mucous membranes
- Tachypnea
- Tachycardia
- Increasing demand for supplemental oxygen to maintain adequate saturation
- Fever and hypotension in patients with sepsis

BOX 3-10 American-European Consensus Conference Criteria for Diagnosing Acute Lung Injury/Acute Respiratory Distress Syndrome (ALI/ARDS)

Because ALI/ARDS is a relatively new disease and there is much confusion about its clinical nature, a consensus committee was established to outline the criteria that constitute a diagnosis of ALI/ARDS:

1. Acute in onset
2. Ratio of Pa_{O_2} to $F_{IO_2} \leq 300$ mm Hg (regardless of ventilation PEEP pressure)
3. Bilateral infiltrates on chest radiograph
4. Pulmonary artery occlusion pressure (PAOP) ≤ 18 mm Hg, or no clinical evidence of left atrial hypertension. This measurement comes from hemodynamic monitoring through a central venous pulmonary artery catheter, introduced in the ED or ICU.

- Rales/crackles (may or may not be heard on auscultation)

Pathophysiology

The onset of ALI/ARDS begins with a breakdown of the alveolar-capillary border that allows fluid to seep into the alveoli, decreasing gas exchange in the lungs. These pathologic changes may occur in response to a damaged capillary cell lining (as occurs in sepsis) or to a damaged alveolar cell lining (as occurs in pneumonia). In severe cases, high levels of oxygen are required to maintain adequate oxygenation.

The disease is generally said to have three phases:

1. Exudative phase. In the first 72 hours after the initial event, an acute phase develops during which immune system mediators injure the epithelial alveolar-capillary membrane. Fluid leaks, microemboli develop, and the pulmonary artery pressure rises, making it more difficult to perfuse blood around the heart and lungs. Alveolar edema sets in, the hyaline membrane and surfactant layer are disturbed, and alveolar collapse ensues.
2. Fibroproliferative phase. In the body's attempt to heal this fresh tissue injury, scarring develops in the alveolar-capillary membrane. Alveoli become distended and misshapen. The lungs become stiff, and pressure increases with prolonged hypoxemia.
3. Resolution phase. Over the next several weeks, gradual recovery occurs if the patient has survived the initial phases. The alveolar-capillary membrane and hyaline membrane heal. Fluids diffuse out of the alveoli and back into the tissues. Cellular debris is eliminated.

Treatment

Supporting oxygenation and assisting respiration are the cornerstones of ALI/ARDS treatment. No specific remedy exists other than aggressively managing the inciting medical or traumatic event. Intubation and mechanical ventilation, along with pressure support and suctioning as needed, are indicated.

Once the diagnosis of ALI/ARDS has been made and ventilatory support has been instituted, critical care staff must begin formulating a plan that emphasizes lung protective strategies. This plan may include use of high-frequency/low-tidal-volume ventilators, administration of pulmonary vessel–dilating drugs, and complete bypass of the lungs for oxygenation, a modality known as *extracorporeal membrane oxygenation (ECMO)*.

Diseases of the Pleura

In this group of lower airway pathologies, the patient may present with a sudden onset of pleuritic chest pain varying from a minor ailment to a severe, life-threatening event. Pleuritic chest pain is pain that increases with deep breath or cough. If air or excessive fluid is trapped between the pleural layers, the patient's difficulty breathing is likely to escalate.

PNEUMOTHORAX

Pneumothorax is best defined as gas in the pleural cavity. As discussed earlier, normally the pleural space is occupied by only a small amount of fluid which lubricates the pleura to minimize friction. Pneumothoraces can occur spontaneously or they can be induced by trauma, including barotrauma from positive-pressure ventilation. Other traumatic causes are beyond the scope of this book, so our discussion will be limited to primary and secondary spontaneous pneumothorax.

Primary Spontaneous Pneumothorax

Primary spontaneous pneumothorax (PSP) can occur without an obvious cause. Nearly all patients who develop PSP have bullae, or air pockets, that rupture to cause the pneumothorax (Figure 3-19).

PSP is much more prevalent among men, with an incidence of 7.4 cases per 100,000 per year, compared with just 1.2 cases per 100,000 per year among women. The peak incidence of PSP is in patients aged 20 to 30.

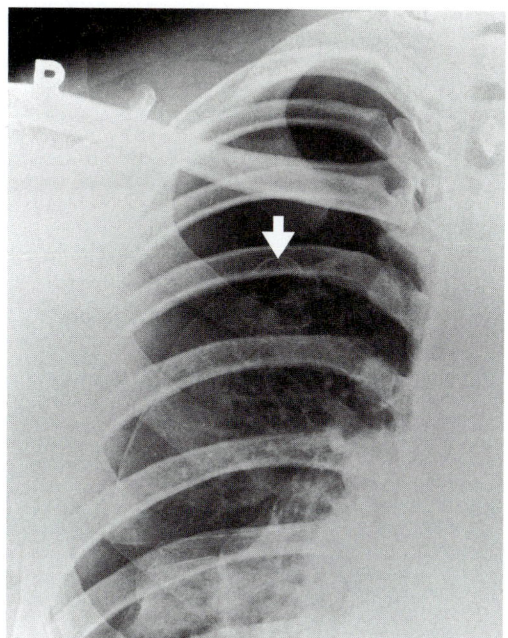

■ **Figure 3-19** Primary spontaneous pneumothorax, showing apex *(arrow)* of collapsed lung. (From Hansell DM, et al: Imaging of diseases of the chest, ed 4, Philadelphia, 2010, Mosby.)

The 5-year recurrence rate is 28% for PSP (versus 43% for SSP).

PSP is seen predominantly in patients without a prior diagnosis of lung disease. However, more than 90% of those who develop PSP are smokers; an increased rate of smoking equates to an increased rate of PSP. The condition is also more common in tall, thin young men. Developing evidence suggests that certain genetic factors may predispose patients to spontaneous pneumothorax. Use of inhaled or injected cocaine is also a known risk factor for spontaneous pneumothorax.

Secondary Spontaneous Pneumothorax

Secondary spontaneous pneumothorax (SSP) can be caused by a variety of lung diseases but occurs primarily in patients with COPD and is most often due to tobacco abuse. Pulmonary fibrosis, sarcoidosis, tuberculosis, and infection with *Pneumocystis jirovecii* (almost exclusively in patients with acquired immunodeficiency syndrome [AIDS]) are other reported causative factors. SSP occurs more frequently in patients aged 60 to 65, and COPD patients with SSP are 3.5 times more likely to die of the condition than SSP patients without COPD as a cofactor.

Signs and Symptoms

The cardinal signs of a spontaneous pneumothorax (both PSP and SSP) are chest pain and dyspnea. The chest pain is often described as sudden, sharp, or stabbing and made worse by breathing or other chest wall motion. Decreased lung reserve capacity, as in COPD, may make dyspnea more pronounced in patients with SSP. Additional symptoms of pneumothorax may include diaphoresis, anxiety, back pain, cough, and malaise.

Look for the following clinical signs of PSP and SSP:

- Tachypnea
- Tachycardia
- Pulsus paradoxus
- Decreased breath sounds
- Hyperresonance on percussion
- Hypoxia and altered mental status (in some patients)

The presence of breath sounds on the affected side cannot rule out a pneumothorax. Hypoxia, cyanosis, and increased jugular venous distention should prompt you to consider tension pneumothorax.

Diagnosis

Other pneumothoraces may occur as a result of volume or barotrauma from high intrathoracic pressure during positive-pressure ventilation. If you're administering positive-pressure ventilation and your patient exhibits acute status changes, barotrauma with pneumothorax must be immediately ruled out. In fact, in the intubated patient, a rapidly declining condition usually warrants a quick assessment of the most common causes of acute deterioration in the intubated patient, using the DOPE mnemonic shown in the Rapid Recall box.

RAPID RECALL

DOPE: Assessing Causes of Acute Deterioration in the Intubated Patient

When evaluating for acute deterioration in the intubated patient, begin by taking the patient off of the ventilator and performing ventilation with a bag-mask device while assessing DOPE:

D Displaced tube. Has the tube been accidentally displaced? Auscultate for bilateral breath sounds and absence of epigastric sounds. Use capnography/capnometry.

O Obstructed tube. Does the patient have thick secretions that have plugged the distal tube? Perform sterile suctioning. Is the patient biting on the tube to obstruct it? Insert a bite block.

P Pneumothorax. Has pneumothorax occurred during positive-pressure ventilation? Listen for breath sounds. Sense lung compliance while ventilating. Is it hard to squeeze the bag because of high intrathoracic pressure? If a tension pneumothorax is present, perform needle decompression until a chest tube can be inserted.

E Equipment failure. Has the ventilator run out of oxygen to drive the ventilatory pressure? Check the oxygen tank and ventilator for correct function.

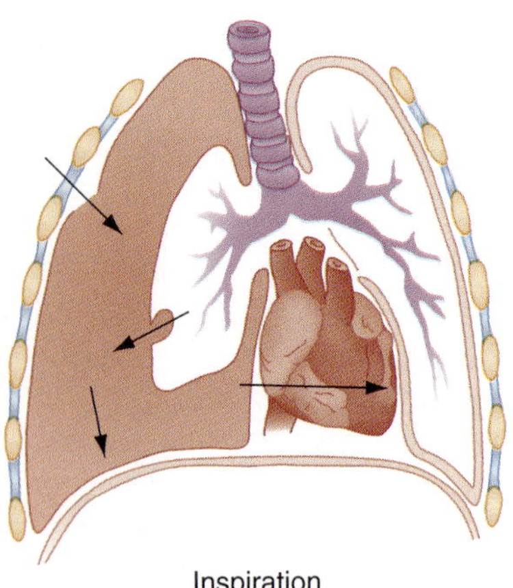

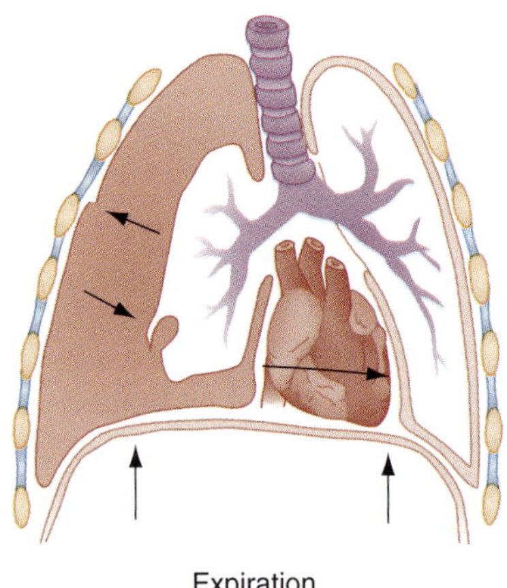

■ **Figure 3-20** Development of a tension pneumothorax. (From Marx J, et al: Rosen's emergency medicine: concepts and clinical practice, ed 6, St Louis, 2006, Mosby.)

Although diagnosis can be made on the basis of clinical exam findings, a chest radiograph can confirm the degree of pneumothorax. Performing a chest radiograph while the patient is exhaling will allow the practitioner to see the severity of the pneumothorax, although a regular chest radiograph is also acceptable. CT can also demonstrate a pneumothorax and can be especially useful when the pneumothorax is small and the patient has a comorbidity. Bedside ultrasound is also helpful in diagnosing pneumothorax. When the patient is in severe respiratory distress, diagnosis of a tension pneumothorax must be clinical, not radiographic.

The differential diagnosis of PSP and SSP includes tension pneumothorax, pleurisy, pulmonary embolism, pneumonia, myocardial infarction, angina, pericarditis, esophageal spasm, and cholecystitis.

A distinction should be made when differentiating pneumothorax from tension pneumothorax (Figure 3-20). Accumulation of air in the pleural space on the affected side eventually forces the mediastinum to shift against the "good" lung and the vena cava (Figure 3-21). These changes cause worsening dyspnea, increased work of breathing, and a drop in cardiac output, leading to obstructive shock. The patient with unilateral diminished breath sounds who is clinically deteriorating and slipping into shock should be diagnosed with tension pneumothorax. Immediate lifesaving chest decompression must occur. Tension pneumothorax is best diagnosed by clinical exam. Waiting for radiologic confirmation can prove a fatal delay.

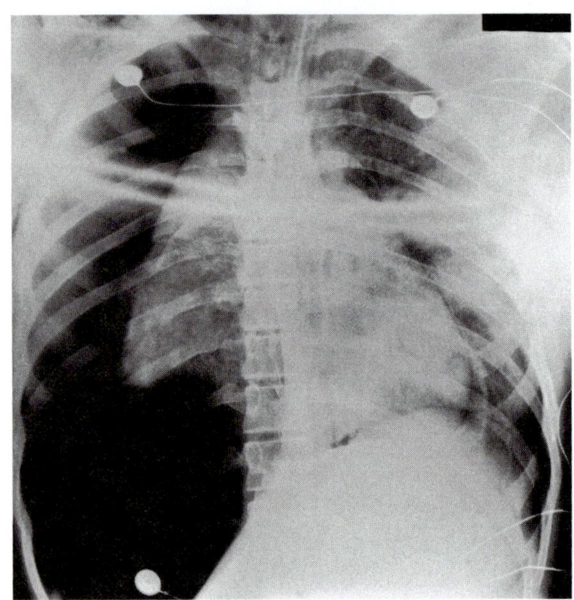

■ **Figure 3-21** Tension pneumothorax. Note deviation of mediastinal contents to patient's left side. (From Hansell DM, et al: Imaging of diseases of the chest, ed 4, Philadelphia, 2010, Mosby.)

Treatment

The goal of treating pneumothoraces is to restore an air-free pleural space. The treatment you select should be guided by the patient's medical history, comorbid conditions and clinical status, the likelihood of resolution, and follow-up avenues.

The least invasive management strategy is simple observation; this approach is ideal for stable patients with no comorbid conditions who have good oxygenation and reserve capacity and a small pneumothorax. These patients may be observed in the ED for a period of 6 hours. If a repeat chest radiograph shows no increase in the size of the pneumothorax, they can be discharged in 24 to 96 hours, provided they receive close follow-up.

Simple aspiration may be performed on certain patients whose condition is unlikely to resolve without intervention. Candidates include symptomatic but stable patients and those who have a small pneumothorax but comorbid conditions such as COPD. To perform this procedure, a needle is introduced into the chest under local anesthesia, and air is aspirated to induce reexpansion of the lung. The patient is then observed, usually as an inpatient. Needle aspiration is the treatment of choice if possible for patients with AIDS, since placement of a chest tube in such patients often leads to a protracted hospital stay. The steps for performing needle **thoracentesis** are summarized in Procedure 3-3.

Procedure 3-3 Performing Needle Thoracostomy (Thoracentesis)

OVERVIEW

Most patients with a tension pneumothorax can't wait for the completion of a tube thoracostomy procedure. The air accumulating between the pleura must be removed more rapidly with the insertion of a long IV or spinal needle. This procedure should be performed when ongoing examination of the patient reveals hypotension or respiratory failure associated with increasing work of breathing and dyspnea with unilateral breath sounds.

INDICATIONS

- Tension pneumothorax

CONTRAINDICATIONS

- Simple pneumothorax (clinical distinction from tension pneumothorax)

EQUIPMENT

- Gloves, gown, mask, eye protection or face shield for compliance with Standard Precautions
- Needle decompression kit containing the following:
  - A 14- or 16-gauge hollow catheter-over-needle device (the needle must be at least 2 inches [5 cm] in length)
  - A skin cleansing agent
  - A 5- to 10-mL syringe with 2 mL of saline drawn up
  - One-way (flutter/Heimlich) valve (optional)

NOTE: These kits should be ready and available at all times. They should be positioned in jump kits, transport, or on easily accessible emergency trays or packets within easy reach of the crew.

PROCEDURE

1. Comply with Standard Precautions for infection control.
2. Identify the second intercostal space in the midclavicular anatomic line on the side with no breath sounds. This can be done using one of two methods:
   - Find the angle of Louis on the sternum, and move your fingers laterally. This is the second rib.
   - Palpate the clavicle on the affected side, and consider that the first rib is curved under it. Count down one more rib to the second and then the third rib.
3. Take the time to confirm that you are performing the procedure on the correct side.
4. Cleanse the skin lying above the third rib at the midclavicular line on the affected side.
5. Remove the protective covering from a 2-inch needle.
6. Use your nondominant hand to identify the top of the third rib at the midclavicular line on the affected side while you use your dominant hand to insert the needle at the top of the third rib at a 90-degree angle.
7. Skin drag will be quickly reduced as the needle tip enters the thoracic cage. Remove the hollow needle and discard appropriately.
8. Confirm that air is being released:
   - The saline that partially fills the attached syringe should bubble. This technique can be quite helpful when your environment does not allow you to hear subtle sounds.
   - Feel for a rush of air from the open end of the catheter.
9. Reassess the patient for the following critical clinical signs of improvement:
   - The work of breathing has eased.
   - The complaint of dyspnea has diminished.
   - Evidence of obstructive shock has been eliminated.
10. The catheter may be kept within the insertion site until a tube thoracostomy is performed. It serves as a reminder that the patient has had a needle decompression performed on that side. If circumstances dictate, remove the catheter and apply a simple dressing to the site. Report the completion of the procedure during handoff to the hospital healthcare staff.
11. A one-way (flutter/Heimlich) valve may be attached, but its placement is optional, since a 14- or 16-gauge catheter does not have a large enough opening to allow air to enter the thoracic cavity once pressure has nearly equalized.
12. Prepare the patient for chest tube insertion (tube thoracostomy) by the clinician.

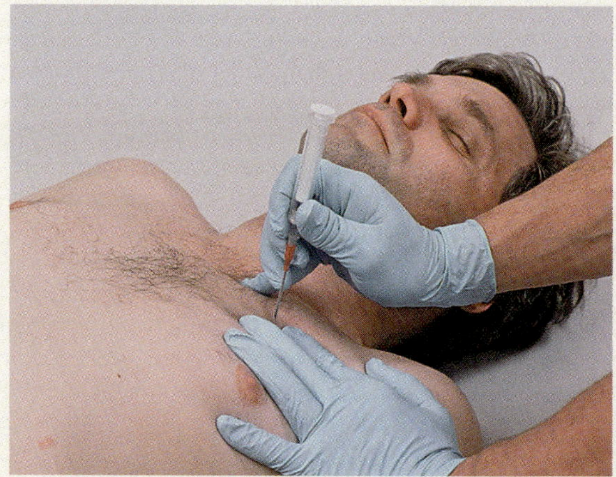

(From PHTLS: Prehospital Trauma Life Support, ed 6, St Louis, 2007, MosbyJems.)

TIPS AND TROUBLESHOOTING

- An alternative site for needle thoracentesis is the midaxillary line. In an emergency, quick access to the air in the top of the thorax is preferred. (Picture what happens when a partly full water bottle is tipped on its side. Where does the air go? To the top, of course.)
- A standard 1¼-inch IV needle is not long enough to access the pleural space in most older children and adults. Make sure you're using a needle that is at least 2 inches long.
- If no air is obtained, report having performed the procedure to the staff at the receiving facility. A tube thoracostomy should still be performed, since the patient will have incurred a pneumothorax when your needle was inserted.

Patients who are significantly symptomatic often warrant tube **thoracostomy.** If time permits, local anesthesia and conscious sedation are provided. The tube may be connected to a Heimlich valve, a one-way valve that lets air escape but not enter the pleural space. Alternatively, the tube may be connected to continuous wall suction. Patients in whom a Heimlich apparatus has been placed may be eligible for discharge sooner than those who require continuous suction. Surgical intervention may be necessary in severe or prolonged cases, or in cases in which tube thoracostomy does not rectify the pneumothorax. Procedure 3-4 outlines how to perform a thoracostomy. Procedure 3-5 describes maintenance of a closed chest-tube drainage system.

EMS responders and members of the resuscitation team should have a working knowledge of chest tube insertion. Even if you never perform the procedure yourself, knowing how the procedure is accomplished will help you assist and anticipate the needs of the clinician who does so.

Pleurisy

Inflammation of either the visceral or parietal pleura, often referred to as *pleurisy*, is a common and worrisome

Text to be continued on page 135

Procedure 3-4 Performing Tube Thoracostomy (Chest Tube Insertion)

OVERVIEW

For normal respiration to occur, the alveoli—the delicate air sacs in the lungs—must exert pressure against the surrounding tissue when fully inflated. The recoil that occurs when air is released during expiration forces the sacs to deflate. For the alveoli to maintain the necessary pressure, the thoracic cavity itself must remain at a negative pressure relative to the atmosphere, creating a slight vacuum. Disease or trauma can release this negative pressure, making it difficult or impossible for the lung to expand. In trauma, an accumulation of air (pneumothorax), blood (hemothorax), or fluid (pleural effusion) can cause the affected lung to collapse. Insertion of a chest tube allows air or fluid to be drained, negative pressure to be reestablished, and the lung to be reinflated.

The chest tube is a sterile, flexible catheter connected to an underwater seal drainage system. The catheter has nonthrombogenic properties to keep dangerous blood clots from forming in the tube and entering the pulmonary circulation. Each tube has a radiopaque line that aids in confirming its location on chest x-ray.

Selecting an Appropriate Catheter

Catheters are about 20 inches long, ranging from sizes 12 French to 40 French. The diagnosis dictates the size of the catheter; a larger diameter is needed to drain blood and fluid than to release air:

- Pneumothorax or tension pneumothorax: size 12F to 26F catheter
- Hemothorax: 36F to 40F catheter
- Pleural effusion: 26F to 36F catheter

Determining the Proper Insertion Site

- Drainage of air: distal tip of tube placed near lung apex (second intracostal space)
- Drainage of fluid: distal tip should rest near the base of the lung (fifth to sixth intracostal space)
- Postoperative cardiac: mediastinum

INDICATIONS

Drainage of air or fluid from the thoracic or mediastinal space in patients with the following conditions:

- Pneumothorax
- Tension pneumothorax
- Hemothorax
- Pleural effusion:
  - Postoperative
  - Empyema (accumulation of pus in the pleural space in patients with pneumonia or other lung infections)
  - Hydrothorax (accumulation of serum in the pleural cavity in patients with cancer, heart disease, and other conditions)

A chest tube may also be placed as a preventive measure in unstable patients during transport.

RELATIVE CONTRAINDICATIONS

There are no absolute contraindications to the insertion of a chest tube. Multiple adhesions, large blebs, and coagulopathies put patients at risk of pain, bleeding, infection, thrombus, and air embolus, but the need to reestablish negative pressure within the thorax usually outweighs the risks of placement.

EQUIPMENT

- Gloves, gown, mask, eye protection or face shield for compliance with Standard Precautions
- Sterile towels or drapes
- Skin cleansing agent(s)
- Small procedure instruments:
  - Three large Kelly clamps
  - Scalpel with #11 blade
  - 4 × 4 gauze sponges
  - Needle holder
- Local anesthetic
- Syringe
- 18-gauge and 25-gauge needles
- Sterile chest tube (NOTE: Open onto sterile field. Place large Kelly clamp over proximal end.)
- Pleural drainage system (NOTE: Assistant should set up system according to manufacturer's recommendations and prepare collection tubing for chest tube attachment.)
- Connecting tubing and Y connector for suctioning
- Tape (dovetailed), Parham bands, or plastic straps to secure each connection
- Dressings (4 × 4s, split dressings, self-sealing wide tape, and petroleum gauze)

Procedure 3-4 Performing Tube Thoracostomy (Chest Tube Insertion)—*Cont'd*

PROCEDURE

1. Comply with Standard Precautions for infection control. In particular, don a sterile gown and gloves, and wear a mask.
2. Position patient supine with arm abducted and extended to at least a 90-degree angle if possible on the affected side.
3. Surgically prepare and drape the insertion site. This should never be inferior to the nipple line.
4. Inject local anesthetic into subcutaneous tissue, muscle, and periosteum.
   - Use a 25-gauge needle to inject local anesthetic subcutaneously, creating a wheal at the insertion site.
   - Continue administering local anesthesia by advancing a 1½-inch needle, using aspiration as the needle is inserted into deeper tissue. Inject local anesthetic into deeper tissue, and continue as the needle is withdrawn.
5. Make a 3- to 4-cm transverse incision into the subcutaneous tissue directly over the inferior edge of the rib just below the insertion site.

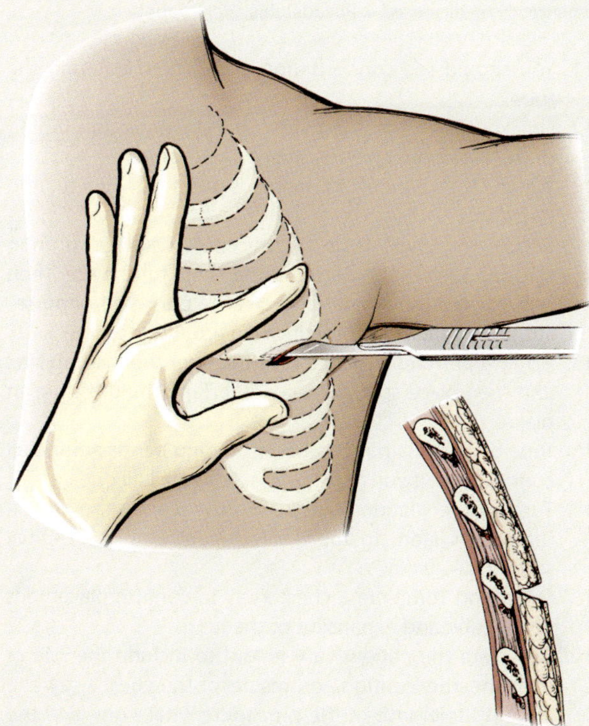

Transverse skin incision is made directly over inferior aspect of anesthetized rib down to the subcutaneous tissue. (From Dumire SM, Paris PM: Atlas of emergency procedures, Philadelphia, 1994, Saunders.)

6. Insert a closed Kelly clamp into the incision, tips directed upward, and then open the clamp. Repeat this motion with the clamp as you bluntly dissect the tissue. The goal is to create a pathway toward the superior portion of the rib and into the thorax. NOTE: The chest tube must enter the thorax over the superior margin of the ribs to avoid injuring the neurovascular bundle that lies beneath each rib.

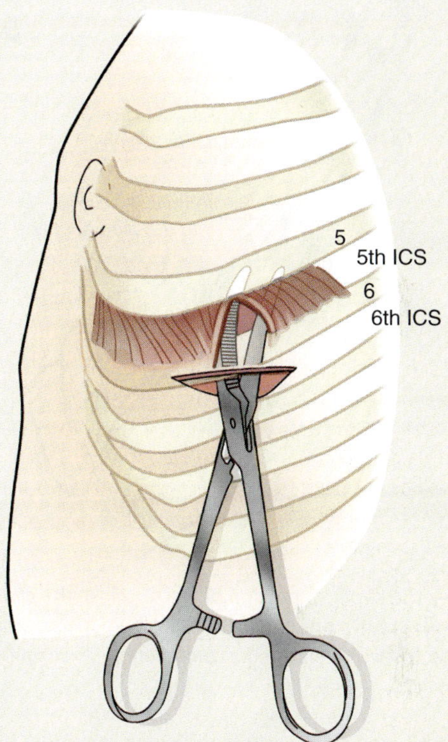

Blunt dissection is accomplished by forcing a closed clamp through the incision and using an opening-and-spreading maneuver to create a tunnel to the pleura. *ICS,* Intercostal space. (From Aehlert B: Paramedic practice today: above and beyond, St Louis, 2010, MosbyJems.)

Continued

Procedure 3-4 Performing Tube Thoracostomy (Chest Tube Insertion)—*Cont'd*

7. When blunt dissection has achieved a pathway to the thorax, stop and close the Kelly clamp again. Place the first finger of your dominant hand over the upper edge (tips) of clamp. Direct firm pressure there until the clamp enters the pleural space. Open the Kelly and create an entrance pathway in which to insert your finger and then the chest tube.

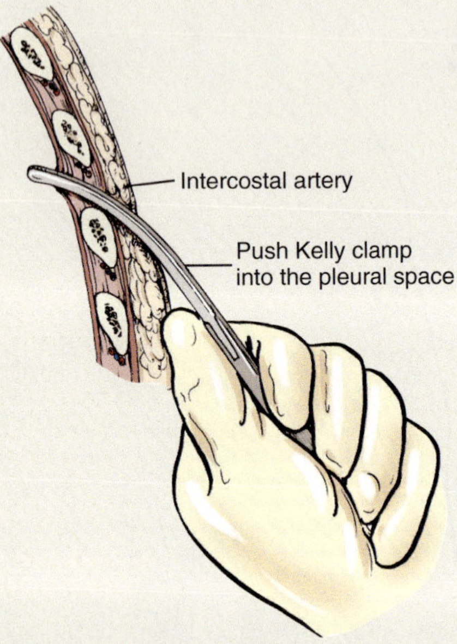

Just over the superior portion of the rib, close the clamp, and push with steady pressure into the pleura. (From Dumire SM, Paris PM: Atlas of emergency procedures, Philadelphia, 1994, Saunders.)

8. Remove the clamp as you slide your forefinger over and into the newly created pathway. Dilate the pleural hole with your finger, and then sweep a curved finger around inside the hole to release any adhesions. Keep your finger in the pleural opening.
9. Pick up the second Kelly clamp, which was previously placed on the proximal chest tube. Direct this clamp into the pleural opening, placing the tips of the clamp (and the chest tube) under your finger.
10. As the proximal tip enters the chest, remove the clamp and your finger. Direct the tip of the chest tube to the desired area of the thorax with a rotating motion. Once the last drainage hole enters the thorax, you may stop inserting the tube.

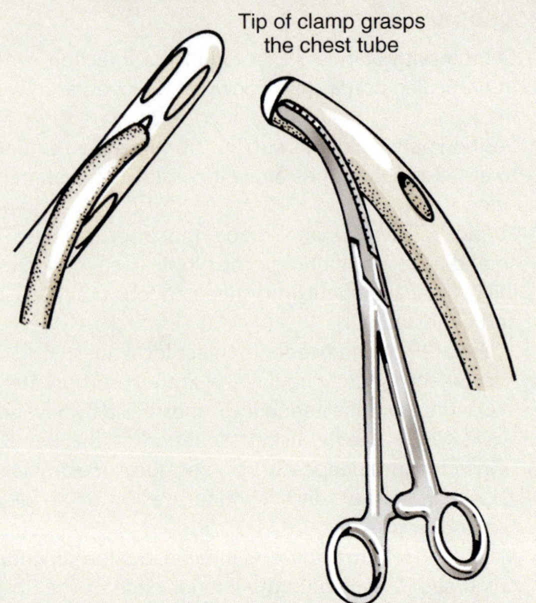

Tube is grasped with curved clamp, with tube tip protruding from jaws. (From Roberts JR, Hedges JR: Clinical procedures in emergency medicine, ed 4, Philadelphia, 2004, Saunders.)

11. You should see condensation, air, or fluid entering the tube.
12. Quickly attach the chest tube to the connecting tubing of the assembled pleural drainage system.
13. Watch the pleural drainage system for fluctuation (tidaling).
14. Secure the chest tube to the chest wall by suturing through the skin and around the chest tube twice. Then pull up the suture material to create a puckered, or purse-string, appearance of the incision around the tube.
15. Apply a petroleum gauze dressing over the incision site, and then place split 4 × 4s over it. Tape the dressings in place.
16. Tape or place Parham bands or binding bands around all connections. If you're using tape, dovetail all ends.
17. Turn on the suction source. Turn the dial on the pleural drainage system to the desired level. The usual initial setting is −20 cm.
18. Order and complete a chest x-ray to confirm placement of the tube and expansion of the lung.
19. Complete the patient care record to include the size of the tube, the location and results of the chest x-ray, the patient's tolerance of the procedure, vital signs, and the initial fluid output in the pleural drainage system.

Procedure 3-4 Performing Tube Thoracostomy (Chest Tube Insertion)—*Cont'd*

TIPS AND TROUBLESHOOTING

- To avoid kinking or clamping of the chest tube system, drape the tubing along the length of the patient. Avoid positioning the patient on top of the tubing.
- Monitor the pleural drainage system output at least every 2 hours. A thoracic surgeon will need to be notified if bloody pleural drainage is initially more than 1200 to 1500 mL or if the output is more than 200 mL per hour for several hours. Mark the time on the face of the collection chamber every 2 hours at the level of the drainage.
- Monitor the chest tube, incision site, and pleural drainage system (also see Procedure 3-5):
  - The chest tube should have condensation (fog) within it.
  - The skin around the incision site should not have air beneath it (subcutaneous emphysema).
  - The tubing should be clear of clots and kinks.
- Continuous bubbling (with suction off) indicates an air leak. Follow local protocol for maintenance of the pleural drainage system and for troubleshooting an air leak.

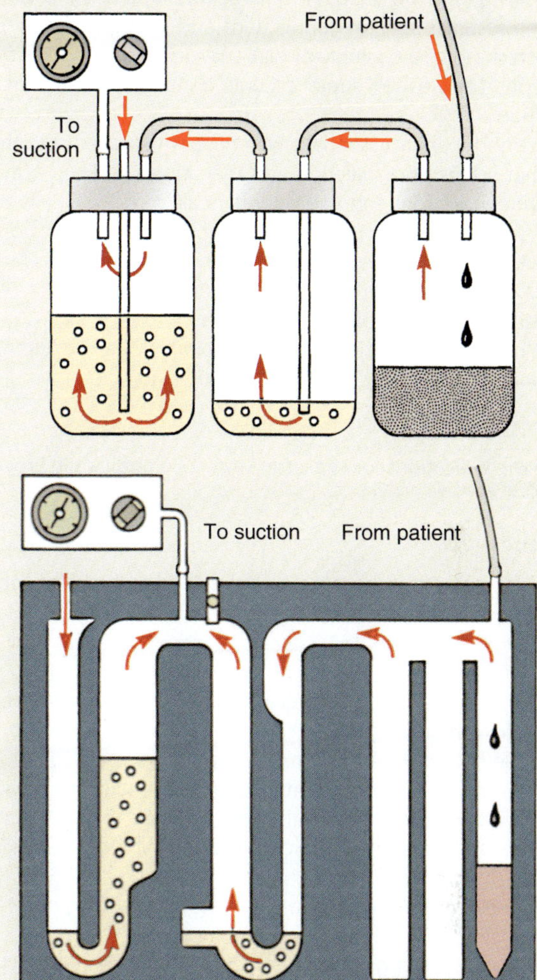

Disposable system correlates with three-bottle system. (From Luce JM, Tyler ML, Pierson DJ: Intensive respiratory care, Philadelphia, 1984, Saunders.)

Procedure 3-5 Maintaining a Closed Chest Drainage System

OVERVIEW

As explained in Procedure 3-4, a tube may be placed in the mediastinum or pleural space to drain air, infectious matter, blood, or other fluid in a closed sterile setting. A chest tube may be placed emergently when trauma disturbs the negative pressure of the thoracic cavity in which the lungs are suspended, or a tube may be placed in the operating room for certain surgical procedures.

A system that allows accumulated air or fluid to be released or drained from the thorax must have some special features to reestablish or maintain appropriate vacuum pressure within the chest:

- The system must take advantage of gravity to allow negative pressure within the thorax.
- It must have a one-way valve or mechanism to prevent backflow into the chest.
- It must be maintained below the patient's chest, with no kinks in the tubing, so the pressure within the drainage system is higher than that within the chest.

Continued

Procedure 3-5 Maintaining a Closed Chest Drainage System—*Cont'd*

- To enhance the drainage of large amounts of air or fluid, the system's suction connections and gauges must allow attachment to portable or wall suction.

Special features of some pleural drainage systems may include:

- A dry-dry drain, essentially waterless, with a one-way valve that opens on exhalation and then closes to keep atmospheric air from entering during inhalation
- A self-sealing port to allow access to the device for laboratory analysis of chest drainage or to withdraw excess fluid when the chamber becomes too full
- Autotransfusion collection chambers
- A manometer portion to observe for and measure fluctuations in inspiratory and expiratory tidaling

INDICATIONS

See the indications for chest tube insertion outlined in Procedure 3-4.

EQUIPMENT

- Gloves, gown, mask, eye protection or face shield for compliance with Standard Precautions

PROCEDURE

1. Comply with Standard Precautions for infection control.
2. Follow the manufacturer's recommendations for setup of a pleural drainage system.
3. Depending on the patient setting, either hang the device from the lower edge of the cart or swing the unit stand into position and secure it to the floor. *Maintain the device lower than the patient.*
4. If you're not using suction, leave the short tubing open to the air.
5. If you are using suction, fill the suction chamber with sterile water (usually provided) to the marked level on the unit. Connect the short tubing to the suction connecting tubing and to the suction source.
6. If the suction chamber becomes overfilled, access the corresponding grommet with a syringe and needle to withdraw excess fluids. If it is underfilled, instill sterile saline through the grommet.
7. Dial the pleural drainage system unit to the prescribed amount. Suction pressure is usually set initially at −20 cm. Setting suction pressure higher than −40 cm is not recommended.
8. Turn the wall suction on, and observe the pleural drainage unit indicator window in the suction section. Turn the wall suction up until the indicator shows the appropriate level, consistent with the manufacturer's recommendation. NOTE: You should observe constant gentle bubbling within the chamber.
9. Uncoil longer tubing from the drainage unit, and arrange it adjacent to the sterile field you established for the tube thoracostomy procedure. Keep the cap on the end of the tubing to maintain sterility until it's connected to an appropriately inserted chest tube.

TIPS AND TROUBLESHOOTING

- Clamping the patient's chest tube with tools or instruments is contraindicated. All connections of tubing coming from the patient (chest tube to connector, connector to pleural drainage system tubing) are to be secured with tape or strapping devices:
  - If you're using tape, fold the end of the tape over on itself to make it easier to remove later. Use strong tape.
  - If you're using plastic straps, follow the manufacturer's recommendations for securing them.
- Follow your local protocol for routine assessment of the patient's ventilation and perfusion status, but at a minimum, evaluate initially, every 2 hours thereafter, and any time the patient's condition changes suddenly. The exam should include assessment of the chest tube insertion site and subcutaneous tissue for possible air leaks.
- When you perform your initial patient assessment, you should evaluate the pleural drainage system to confirm proper functioning and rule out air leaks before transport.
- Once the chest tube has been inserted, the initial output should be marked with the date and time, written directly on the face of the pleural drainage unit. With continuous output, hourly or other routine notations can help the healthcare staff identify trends despite shift and staff changes.
- In addition to initial and hourly or routine measurements, documentation should include the color of drainage and a record of any fluctuation or tidaling. NOTE: Initial output of more than 1200 mL or an hourly collection of 200 mL for more than 2 hours indicates the need for surgical consultation. The facility's autotransfusion policies should be followed.
- You can obtain a sample from the pleural drainage system by aspirating a specimen from the indicated self-sealing site with a syringe and 20-gauge needle.

Maintaining the Patency of Tubing

- Keep the tubing free of kinks, looped at or below the level of the patient, and free of thick secretions or clots that may create an obstruction.
- If clots or other debris have created an obstruction, milking the tube may be indicated. You can accomplish this by gently squeezing the tubing between your fingers and moving the debris along toward the drainage unit. Do not strip the length of the tubing.
- Observe for fluid fluctuations in the chamber. If no fluctuations (tidaling) occur, the tubing may be kinked or the patient's lung may have reexpanded.

Assessing for Air Leaks

- Be aware that some systems feature an air-leak assessment chamber. Check the manufacturer's documentation for details.
- *With the suction off,* you should suspect an air leak when the unit bubbles continuously.

Procedure 3-5 Maintaining a Closed Chest Drainage System—*Cont'd*

- To find the leak, begin at the patient's chest wall (at the insertion site) and intermittently occlude the tubing with your fingers. Hold it for a few seconds, and proceed toward the drainage unit if the bubbling continues. If the bubbling stops as you are occluding the tubing, the air leak is between the manual occlusion and the drainage unit. Replace the tubing or drainage unit.
- If the bubbling stops at the insertion site, the air leak is within the patient. Make sure all chest tube eyelets are within the site and dressing. Apply another dressing, and notify the physician. If this is a mediastinal tube, there should never be bubbling in the chamber. An air leak indicates incorrect placement of the chest tube within the pleural cavity.

condition for patients. The condition is characterized by a sudden onset of sharp chest pain.

Signs and Symptoms

The cardinal symptom of pleurisy is chest pain exacerbated by taking a deep breath. Expiration mostly or totally relieves the pain. The patient may have a history of a recent cold or cough. Physical findings may include a pleural friction rub, but few other physical findings are typically present.

Pathophysiology

The cause of the inflammation in pleurisy is unclear. Researchers speculate that viral infection or focal trauma is involved, but little evidence of the true etiology exists.

Differential Diagnosis

Pleurisy is a diagnosis of exclusion. You must first consider pulmonary embolus, pneumonia, pneumothorax, and other possible causes of the chest pain. Consider other diagnoses if the patient has fever, chills, rash, constant chest pain, a productive cough, pedal edema, dyspnea on exertion, nausea and vomiting, or abdominal pain. Pleurisy is treated with antiinflammatory agents in scheduled dosing. Care must be taken to reduce gastrointestinal side effects, and as always, nonsteroidal antiinflammatory drugs (NSAIDs) should be used with caution in those with renal insufficiency.

Pleural Effusion

Pleural inflammation (pleurisy) and pleural effusion often go hand in hand, since the presence of a pleural effusion—an excessive accumulation of fluid between the pleural layers—is suggestive of pleural inflammation. Like pleurisy, pleural effusion can cause dyspnea as well as chest pain. About 1 million people in the United States are diagnosed with pleural effusion each year; most cases are associated with CHF, malignancy, infection, or pulmonary embolus.

Pleural effusions are classified as either transudates or exudates. (The terms can also be used to refer to the accumulated pleural fluid itself.) Transudative effusions occur when increased pressure or a lack of protein causes fluid to seep out of blood vessels and into the pleural space, whereas in exudative effusions, the leakage can be traced to pleural inflammation (Figure 3-22).

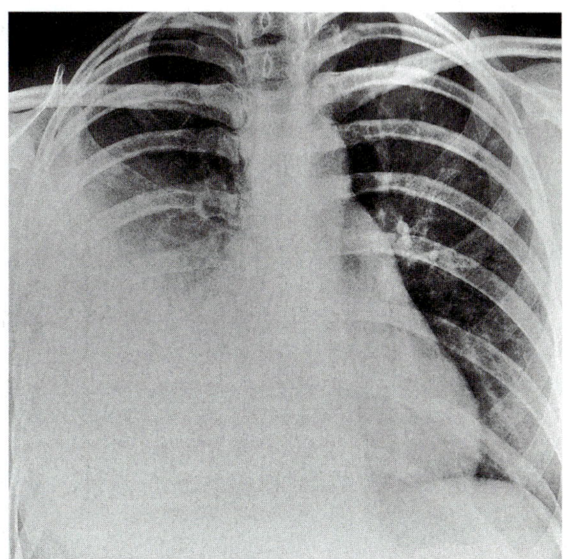

Figure 3-22 Right-sided pleural effusion. Note consistent appearance of effusion and lack of aeration below top of effusion. This effusion was caused by tuberculosis. (From Hansell DM, et al: Imaging of diseases of the chest, ed 4, Philadelphia, 2010, Mosby.)

A chronic pleural effusion is characterized by a slowly accumulating collection of fluid. This kind of slowly evolving effusion, as might occur in a patient with cancer, is better tolerated than the kind of rapidly developing effusion that can accompany heart failure. The acute effusion leaves the patient with less pulmonary reserve, and the patient can decompensate more rapidly when faced with additional challenges.

Signs and Symptoms

The most common symptom of patients with effusion is dyspnea. Chest pain (particularly pleuritic), cough, dyspnea on exertion, or orthopnea may also be present. The absence of a pleuritic component of chest pain does not rule out effusion. Certain etiologies of effusion may carry additional symptoms (e.g., pneumonia causing fever and productive cough), and systemic effects such as hypotension and hypoxia may suggest sepsis.

Physical findings of effusion include decreased breath sounds, egophony, shifting dullness and decreased breath sounds when supine versus upright, and dullness to percussion. Physical findings may be absent in patients with less than 300 to 400 mL of effusion. Effusions exceeding 1000 mL may cause deviation of the mediastinum toward the affected side. It's possible for several liters of fluid to collect.

Pathophysiology

Transudate effusions form when fluid is either forced out of blood vessels or fails to be resorbed back into them. As a result, the transudate tends to be thinner because it contains less protein, fewer white cells, and is less likely to be the result of infection and inflammation. Transudate effusions are seen in CHF, low-protein states (e.g., malnutrition, alcoholism, liver disease/dysfunction), atelectasis, and renal failure.

Exudate effusions form as a result of inflammation or infection, and thus contain many more components of serum, including protein, white blood cells, clotting factors, and antibodies. An exudate effusion can be precipitated or worsened by poor lymphatic drainage, cancer, pulmonary embolism, sarcoidosis, Dressler's syndrome, trauma, esophageal injury, radiation injury, and pancreatitis.

Diagnosis

Effusions can be confirmed on chest radiograph, which can help guide treatment. Lateral decubitus films can help image smaller effusions but may be unnecessary with larger effusions. Approximately 200 mL of fluid is required to produce a layer of fluid throughout the lung when the patient is placed in the decubitus position. Supine films can help determine whether the fluid is loculated (within a cavity), which may suggest empyema.

Pneumonia, pulmonary abscess, empyema, pulmonary embolism, and hemothorax can have symptoms and physical findings similar to pleural effusion. Of these, hemothorax often has a traumatic etiology, whereas the other causes are medical. Consider malignancy in patients who present with new pulmonary effusion. Consider tuberculosis in patients known to have been exposed to the infection and in those who have a newly converted purified protein derivative (PPD) test.

CHF should also be part of the differential diagnosis, as well as myocardial infarction and ischemia with accompanying heart failure. Collection of fluid in the pericardial space or in both the pericardial and pleural spaces after a recent myocardial infarction should prompt you to consider Dressler's syndrome.

Treatment

Fluid from significant effusions can be extracted by needle thoracentesis for both diagnostic purposes and symptomatic relief (see Procedure 3-3). Chemical and microscopic examination of the aspirated fluid can determine its etiology and distinguish between a transudate and an exudate. In rare cases, tube thoracostomy or surgery may be required to relieve very large effusions or to treat the cause of the effusion, as in the case of certain aggressive cancers. Imaging with CT may be performed in patients who have a new-onset effusion; this study can help diagnose lung cancer and tuberculosis that may be associated with the effusion.

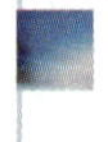

Respiratory Complaints Originating from Nonrespiratory Causes

Heart Disease

The clinical presentation of a patient with dyspnea who is working hard to breathe, is weak, and even has a cough and fever can often be misleading. The disease responsible for the patient's signs and symptoms may not originate in the respiratory system at all but elsewhere. Because the respiratory system shares its thoracic space with the cardiovascular system, heart disease can mimic respiratory disorders.

Cardiomyopathy, CHF, inflammatory heart conditions, valvular diseases, ischemic heart disease, and myocardial infarction can all be characterized by respiratory complaints. You should perform your exam and gather the HPI with that in mind.

VASCULAR DISEASE

Pulmonary Embolus

Pulmonary embolus (*pl.*, emboli) is the sudden blockage of an artery in the lung with a blood clot, an air bubble, a fatty plaque, or even a group of tumor cells. Deep venous thrombosis (DVT), a blood clot that has traveled to the lung from a deep vein in the leg, is one of the most common causes of pulmonary embolism.

Because this vascular event tends to generate only vague, nonspecific symptoms, it's one of the most challenging diagnoses to make in the ED. Patients at risk of pulmonary embolism include those who have recently had surgery or major trauma and those with indwelling catheters. Symptoms suggesting pulmonary embolism include:

- Chest pain
- Chest wall tenderness
- Dyspnea
- Tachycardia
- Syncope
- Hemoptysis (blood-tinged sputum)
- New-onset wheezing
- New cardiac arrhythmia
- Thoracic pain

The classic triad of chest pain, hemoptysis, and dyspnea is seen in fewer than 20% of patients. Early symptoms of pulmonary embolism may be minimal, but massive pulmonary embolism evolves quickly and may rapidly become symptomatic.

On physical exam, massive pulmonary embolism can cause hypotension secondary to cor pulmonale. More subtle pulmonary embolism can evolve into atelectasis that appears much like pneumonia over the course of a few days. New wheezing may be noted and can be deceptive, especially in COPD and asthma patients. Chest radiograph is typically normal, and the classic triad of S wave in lead I, Q wave in lead III, and ST-segment changes in lead III cannot be used to rule in or out pulmonary embolism. Tachycardia is often seen but is a nonspecific finding.

Pulmonary Artery Hypertension

Pulmonary hypertension is a rare chronic disease characterized by elevated pulmonary artery pressure. The high pressure in the pulmonary artery makes it difficult for the heart to pump enough blood to the lungs, eventually affecting both the heart and the lungs.

Affecting only 1 to 3 people per million in the U.S. population, the disease can have a genetic component. Side effects from drugs such as cocaine, methamphetamine, and fenfluramine/phentermine/dexfenfluramine (known as *fen/phen* and withdrawn from the market in 1997 because of safety concerns) have also been implicated. The disease is most common among women of childbearing age and women in their 50s and 60s. Severe chronic lung disease is another cause.

Signs and symptoms of pulmonary hypertension include:

- Dyspnea (cardinal symptom)
- Weakness
- Fatigue
- Syncope
- Increased second heart sound (S_2)
- Tricuspid murmur
- Jugular venous pulsations
- Pitting edema

Lung sounds are often normal. Echocardiography and blood tests can be performed to help confirm the diagnosis. Management is generally dictated by the patient's symptoms. Administering oxygen to dilate pulmonary vessels is an important part of treatment. A pulmonary vessel dilator or an antiinflammatory agent may be prescribed, along with medications that hinder the growth of endothelial layers that can narrow the pulmonary artery.

Central Nervous System Dysfunction

A wide range of CNS diseases can impair respiratory tract function, as shown in Box 3-11. CNS disorders can be divided into three categories:

- Acute: illnesses lasting less than 1 week
- Subacute: diseases and disorders lasting between 1 week and 2 months
- Chronic: conditions lasting 2 months or longer

Acute

Acute CNS dysfunction has a wide array of medical and traumatic causes. We will focus on acute medical illnesses of the CNS that impair respiratory function. The primary concern in such illnesses is maintaining a patent airway. An occluded airway may lead to rapid deterioration and cerebral anoxia. Stroke, seizure, CNS infection, and other acute neuromuscular disorders may cause a decreased level of consciousness and place the patient at great risk for poor airway and ventilation control.

BOX 3-11 CNS Conditions That Can Impair Respiration

Acute	Subacute	Chronic
Intoxication	Guillain-Barré syndrome	HIV/AIDS
Overdose	Encephalopathy	Neuromuscular degenerative disease (ALS)
Stroke/TIA	Meningitis	Dementia
Tick paralysis	Delirium	Myasthenia gravis paralysis
Myasthenia gravis paralysis	Myasthenia gravis paralysis	
Guillain-Barré syndrome		
Meningitis		
Encephalopathy		
Delirium		
Psychiatric illness		
Seizure		
Epidural abscess		

ALS, Amyotrophic lateral sclerosis; *HIV/AIDS*, human immunodeficiency virus/acquired immunodeficiency syndrome; *TIA*, transient ischemic attack.

BOX 3-12 Abnormal Breathing Patterns

Pattern	Description
Kussmaul's respiration	Hypertachypneic, hyperpneic respiration that points to metabolic acidosis, particularly diabetic ketoacidosis.
Cheyne-Stokes respiration	Apnea alternating with tachypnea in a crescendo-decrescendo sequence, suggesting injury to the respiratory centers in the brainstem.
Biot's respiration	Characterized by groups of quick, shallow inspirations followed by regular or irregular periods of apnea. This rhythm, which may be caused by opioid overdose, indicates injury to the medulla oblongata in the brainstem.
Apneustic respiration	Deep, gasping breaths with a pause at full inspiration, followed by an incomplete release that suggests injury to or infection of the pons or upper medulla section of the midbrain. It may also be caused by ketamine sedation.
Ataxic respiration	Characterized by a disorganized pattern and depth of respiration that often progresses to apnea. Damage to the medulla oblongata is responsible for this chaotic pattern.

General changes in respiration such as hyperpnea, tachypnea, or both often accompany CNS dysfunction. Abnormal respiratory patterns, summarized in Box 3-12 and Figure 3-23, sometimes suggest the etiology of the disturbance. A look back at Table 1-4 in Chapter 1 will also provide a useful review of irregular breathing patterns.

Subacute

Subacute CNS dysfunction can be responsible for prolonged respiratory compromise, including respiratory failure, atelectasis, pneumonia, lobar collapse, or infiltrate. An extended period of immobility can impair the ability to expel mucus, increase the risk of mucous plugging of bronchi, and raise the risk of pneumonia as the alveoli lose their ability to expand. Persistent immobility can increase the threat of deep venous thrombosis and pulmonary embolus.

Chronic

Chronic CNS dysfunction carries many of the same unwelcome risks as subacute CNS dysfunction, such as an increased chance of DVT and pulmonary embolism. Prolonged respiratory compromise may necessitate a tracheostomy to maintain a secure airway. Inspired air thereby skirts the defenses of the upper airway, increasing the risk that a lower airway infection might gain a toehold.

Furthermore, long-term care of CNS dysfunction is associated with exposure to hospitals and healthcare facilities, where serious infection with *Pseudomonas* spp., HA-MRSA, and vancomycin-resistant *Enterococcus* (VRE) is more likely.

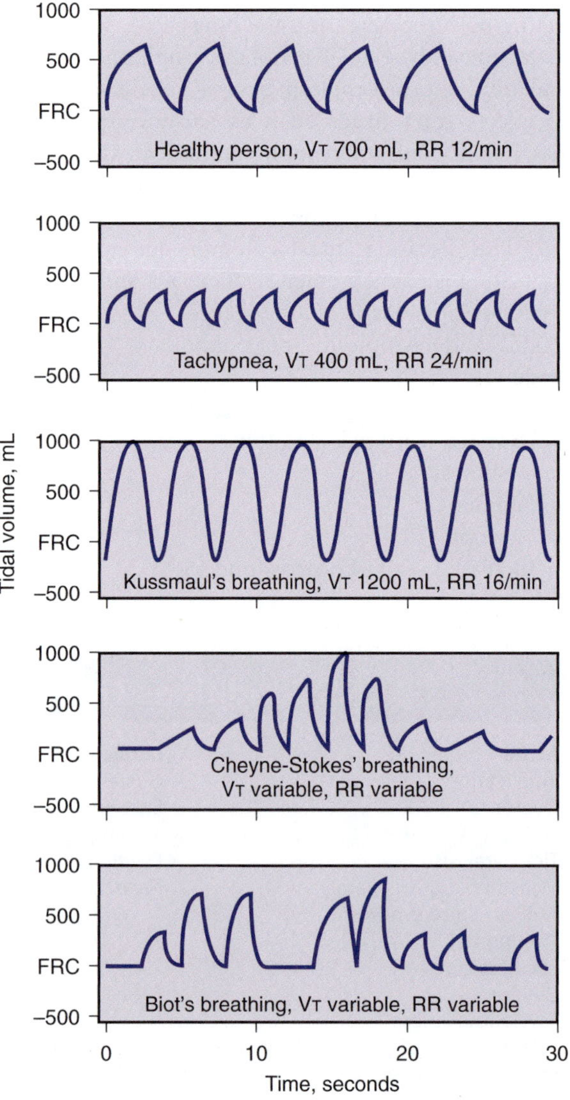

Figure 3-23 Abnormal respiratory patterns. (From Mason RJ, et al: Murray & Nadel's textbook of respiratory medicine, ed 4, Philadelphia, 2005, Saunders.)

Generalized Neurologic Disorders

Neuromuscular diseases such as myasthenia gravis and neuromuscular degenerative disease, often called *amyotrophic lateral sclerosis (ALS)*, or *Lou Gehrig's disease*, are chronic diseases that rarely cause death but can nevertheless have profound effects on the respiratory tract. Respiratory muscle weakness or ineffective nervous system control can cause hypoventilation, resulting in atelectasis. Subsequent pneumonia can be life threatening in patients who are already debilitated by disease. Acute respiratory failure can be superimposed on pneumonia or, conversely, pneumonia may precipitate respiratory failure.

A few chronic neuromuscular diseases bear mention individually. Guillain-Barré syndrome is an ascending paralysis believed to represent an overzealous immune system response to a viral infection. Patients with this disease may report having had a recent URI and may develop an ascending paralysis over a period of a few days. Respiratory compromise may be seen if the disorder progresses to involve the chest muscles and muscles of breathing. You may wish to review Guillain-Barré syndrome in Chapter 2 for additional information.

Neuromuscular degenerative disease (ALS/Lou Gehrig's disease) is a chronic muscle-wasting disease that affects extremity muscles, some skeletal muscles, and respiratory muscles. Respiratory muscle paralysis can be partial or complete and may make the patient permanently dependent on a ventilator. Chapter 2 offers an in-depth discussion of this neurologic disorder.

A few final tips and cautions are in order:

- Do not use depolarizing neuromuscular blocking agents (i.e., succinylcholine) for medication-assisted intubation in patients with chronic neuromuscular diseases.
- Since many nontraumatic respiratory complaints of CNS origin are infectious, follow Standard Precautions.
- Consider suctioning for any patient who is producing sputum. Suctioning may induce coughing, offering the bonus of helping to clear plugs of mucus.
- Provide supplemental oxygen and initiate endotracheal intubation with any necessary sedation if you have any concern about the patient's ability to protect the airway.

Remember, all situations—acute, subacute, and chronic CNS dysfunction—should prompt meticulous attention to airway maintenance.

Endocrine Dysfunction

Metabolic Encephalopathy

Metabolic encephalopathy is a brain pathology caused by diseases like liver or kidney failure, HIV, hypertensive crisis, Lyme disease, and dementia. The toxic effect of these diseases causes disordered brain function and can lead to respiratory dysfunction, distress, and failure.

Medication Side Effects

Many medications have pulmonary side effects. Among them is one of the most common and most commonly abused categories of drugs—narcotics. As the name suggests, narcotics induce sleep as well as respiratory depression. Both illicit and prescription narcotics are prone to abuse. In a well patient, small to moderate doses of narcotics induce pain relief and mild sedation. In larger doses, narcotics induce respiratory depression and eventually respiratory arrest, to which almost all fatal narcotics overdoses can be attributed. Both naloxone (Narcan) and naltrexone (ReVia) are effective in reversing opioid toxicity, although naloxone is more frequently given emergently because it's available in IV form. Naloxone is administered to an adult as 0.4 to 2 mg IV push, and its effects are both naloxone-dose and opioid-dose dependent. Alcohol has a synergistic effect with opioids, and acute intoxication with both substances increases the risk of respiratory depression.

Benzodiazepines such as diazepam (Valium), lorazepam (Ativan), alprazolam (Xanax), and midazolam (Versed) may also cause respiratory depression or, in significant quantities, respiratory failure. Among the most commonly prescribed medications, agents in this class of drugs also have significant potential for abuse. Nevertheless, benzodiazepines have a relatively low toxicity, with less than 1% resulting in death. Like opioids, benzodiazepines have synergistic effects with alcohol, and combined ingestions increase the likelihood of an adverse outcome. Hypoventilation, respiratory depression, and respiratory failure can accompany major toxicity. Flumazenil (Romazicon) can be administered as a reversal agent, given intravenously in a 0.1- to 0.2-mg dose, up to a total of 1 mg. If the patient has not responded after 5 minutes or a total dose of 5 mg, consider other causes.

Use caution with any reversal agent in the setting of chronic use or abuse. Naloxone use may precipitate opioid withdrawal, which is rarely life threatening but almost always unwelcome. Benzodiazepine withdrawal may precipitate seizures in severe cases. Treatment with flumazenil may make treating withdrawal seizures problematic. Both medications have variable duration, so monitor the patient carefully if airway compromise is suspected.

Panic Attack/Hyperventilation Syndrome

Panic disorder is a distressing phenomenon for patients. What makes it especially worrisome is that the diagnosis must be made by ruling out other more serious disorders. Asthma, arrhythmia, pneumonia, COPD, pneumothorax, pulmonary embolism, and pericarditis are all conditions that may mimic panic disorder. Be sure to consider hormonal disorders such as thyroid storm, pheochromocytoma, and hypoglycemia as well. Panic disorder is estimated to have a 1% to 5% prevalence in the U.S. population, and it's about twice as prevalent in women as in men. It may be present with other psychiatric illness, such as personality disorder, schizophrenia, or agoraphobia.

Frequent symptoms of panic disorder include:

- Sudden onset of fear or anxiety
- Palpitations
- Shaking
- Dyspnea
- A smothering sensation
- Chest pain or discomfort
- Dizziness
- Light-headedness
- Chills or hot flashes
- A dread of dying

A personal or family history of similar episodes may be elicited. Abuse of drugs, especially methamphetamine, cocaine, PCP, ecstasy, and LSD can exacerbate symptoms and the frequency of their occurrence. Over-the-counter (OTC) medications such as caffeine, stimulants, and weight-loss products can also exacerbate the disorder.

Physical exam may show only tachycardia and anxiety. The patient may hyperventilate, but perhaps not dramatically. Evaluation is directed at excluding life-threatening illness. Treatment is symptomatic only. Old-fashioned treatment included breathing into a paper bag to limit the amount of carbon dioxide removed from the body, but this remedy is no longer recommended because of the potential to retain excessive CO_2. Supplemental oxygen should not be necessary, but a dip in oxygen saturation suggests you should investigate other diagnoses.

Neoplasms

Lung cancer is the most common cause of cancer-related death in the United States and the world. An estimated 1.5 million cases of lung cancer were diagnosed globally in 2007, making lung cancer the most common malignancy in the world. The highest 5-year survival rate (14%) has been reported in the United States, but the disease remains highly lethal.

Lung cancer too often progresses to an advanced stage silent and undiagnosed, significantly increasing mortality. Most patients who develop lung cancer have a history of tobacco abuse or are current tobacco abusers. They often have pulmonary compromise (COPD), and the resultant lung damage may limit their cancer treatment options.

Like all cancers, lung cancer arises from a defect in the control mechanism that limits cell division, allowing cells to multiply unchecked. Tobacco use is the leading cause of lung cancer, but genetic differences seem to make some people more susceptible than others. A small number of lung cancers appear to be related to passive smoke exposure. An even smaller number of lung cancers develop in patients who have never smoked and have not had significant exposure to second-hand smoke; such cancers have a strong genetic component.

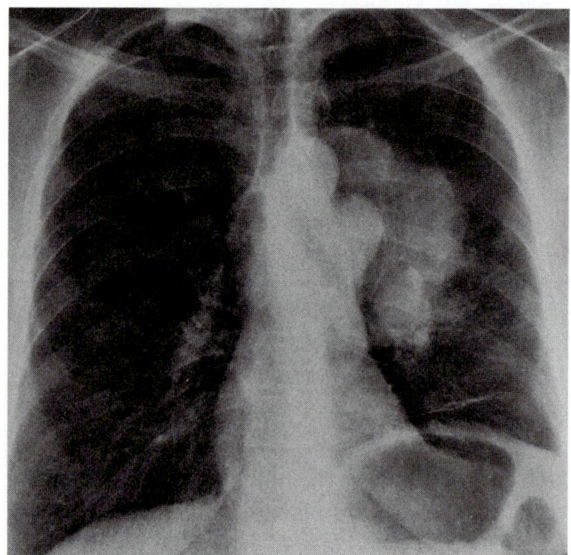

Figure 3-24 Lung cancer in a 50-year-old smoker. Note large mass in middle of left lung. (From Haaga JR: CT and MRI of the whole body, ed 5, Philadelphia, 2009, Mosby.)

Clinical symptoms mirror the extent of disease and spread of metastasis but may include:

- Cough
- Dyspnea
- Dyspnea on exertion
- Wheezing
- Hemoptysis
- Chest wall pain from pleural irritation or pleural effusion (decreased breath sounds may not be noted until a significant pleural effusion develops)

Regional spread of the cancer can compress structures or destroy tissue, generating a broad range of symptoms. For example, superior vena cava obstruction can cause extensive central thrombus and emboli formation, paralysis of the recurrent laryngeal nerve can cause hoarseness, pressure on the esophagus can cause swallowing difficulties, and so on. The cancer may cause markedly elevated calcium, which may be responsible for muscle pain, renal problems, kidney stones, and mental status changes.

A chest radiograph will often demonstrate the malignancy (Figure 3-24) as well as any associated effusion. Treatment involves administering supplemental oxygen, assisting respiration, ensuring a patent airway, and providing appropriate suctioning. Pneumothoraces are extremely rare with lung cancer, but consider this condition if the patient has had a recent lung biopsy. Pleural effusions, if present, are rarely drained emergently (see earlier discussion).

Barotrauma

Barotrauma emergencies can arise from extremes of altitude or water depth. Divers have long feared "the bends," the colloquial name for decompression sickness. Blast injures may also be responsible for some cases of barotrauma. Decompression sickness, sinus or middle ear injury, and arterial gas emboli are the major metabolic consequences of pressure extremes.

Diving barotrauma is explained by the laws of physics that govern the behavior of gases under pressure. Pressure changes affect the volume in air-filled spaces—in the case of the mostly fluid-filled human body, these spaces are the lungs, bowel, sinuses, and middle ear. According to Boyle's law, these spaces compress on descent and expand on ascent because as pressure increases, the gas volume is reduced; conversely, as pressure eases, gas volume increases.

In addition, the solubility of a gas in liquid is governed by the amount of pressure exerted on that gas, so a gas will become decreasingly dissolved in the liquid (i.e., blood) as the body ascends. The body can tolerate this if the amount of gas separating from the blood is small enough to be exhaled. If the ascent is rapid, large amounts of gas are liberated, and life-threatening gas bubbles can block the circulation—the phenomenon known as *decompression sickness.*

The location and size of the gas bubbles will determine their clinical effects. Bubbles trapped in the muscles or joints cause pain in corresponding areas. In fact, the source of the nickname "the bends" is that this condition leaves the afflicted person doubled over for long periods of time. Gas bubbles in the spinal cord can cause paralysis, paresthesia, and anesthesia. Gas bubbles in the arterial circulation can cause limb ischemia, in the pulmonary arteries can cause pulmonary gas embolism, and in the cerebral arteries can cause stroke.

The average risk of severe decompression sickness is slightly more than 2 cases per 10,000 dives. Asthma, pulmonary blebs, and patent foramen ovale increase the risk and severity of symptoms. Decompression sickness generally arises within 24 hours of the first symptoms, which may begin with sinus and ear pressure, pressure in the back, and joint pain and aches that worsen with motion. More severe decompression sickness may be characterized by dyspnea, chest pain, altered mental status, or shock. The most severe illness is seen with arterial gas embolism. Gas emboli often occur a few minutes after surfacing. Acute-onset dyspnea and severe chest pain are common in people with acute gas emboli, and the condition can be fatal.

Physical exam should center on detecting emergent symptoms, including gas emboli. Pay particular attention to performing a complete cardiovascular exam, looking for decreased breath sounds, muffled heart sounds, and heart murmurs. Jugular venous distention or petechiae on the head or neck can indicate more severe decompression sickness. Palpate the skin to detect crepitus, and palpate all pulses.

Emergency care includes careful attention to maintaining the airway with supplemental oxygen. IV hydration should be given to maintain systolic blood pressure. Placement of a urinary catheter can help in monitoring renal function. Tube thoracostomy is indicated if pneumothorax occurs. Consider hyperbaric therapy in patients having neurologic symptoms, unstable blood pressure, respiratory compromise, or altered mental status.

Nitrogen narcosis, a change in mental status while scuba diving, is a slightly different clinical entity. Its effect is similar to alcohol or benzodiazepine intoxication. The condition may occur at shallow depths, but it typically doesn't set in unless the diver has gone below 30 meters. The effect is explained by the increased solubility of nitrogen under higher pressure, with consequent impairment of cognition, motor function, and sensory perception. Nitrogen narcosis also impairs judgment and coordination, potentially causing serious errors that can jeopardize underwater safety. Fortunately, the condition is reversible and resolves over several minutes once the diver has ascended.

Toxic Inhalations

The respiratory tract can serve as the portal of entry for airborne toxins that cause local irritation of the airways and occasionally have systemic effects on the body. Chronic inhalation of these toxins can occur inadvertently while working a day-to-day job (occupational exposure), or the exposure can be dramatic and obvious, as in an industrial incident. Asking the right questions during the history taking can help you correctly identify the toxic agent. Questions should cover time of day, location and circumstances, presence of combustion or odors, and number and condition of other victims. Identifying the specific inhalant is generally unnecessary, however, since therapy is determined on the basis of the patient's signs and symptoms.

This section will review general strategies to use in assessing and caring for patients who have inhaled simple asphyxiants and pulmonary irritants. Chapter 9 includes specific information on treatment for various types of inhaled toxins, including carbon monoxide and cyanide.

Simple Asphyxiants

The inhalation of simple asphyxiants is usually associated with workplace exposure, such as environments using liquefied gas or in confined spaces. These toxins generally cause hypoxia by displacing oxygen. When oxygen content drops to less than 21%, the autonomic nervous system automatically creates tachycardia and usually quiet tachypnea. The sensation of dyspnea is not an early finding, nor is increased work of breathing. Oxygen deprivation in the brain leads to ataxia, dizziness, uncoordinated movements in the body, and mental confusion. If the victim is removed from this deoxygenated environment, the symptoms usually resolve. By the time EMS arrives or the patient reaches the ED, most have dramatically improved. If the patient does not improve, complications of the ischemic event may be present. Seizures, coma, cardiac arrest, and a poor outcome can be predicted.

Diagnosis and Management The first and most important element in assessing and caring for the patient is safety for all—bystanders, coworkers, EMS colleagues, and the public at large. The diagnosis is based on the history of the event and the resulting rapid resolution of the signs and symptoms when the patient is removed from the exposure. Scene investigation by trained personnel will evaluate and correct the initial problem to prevent its recurrence. Treatment begins and usually ends with removing the victim from the deoxygenated environment. Supportive care and administration of oxygen are helpful adjuncts. Standard resuscitation protocols should be used if the patient has neurologic injury or cardiopulmonary arrest. Those with mild symptoms are usually observed and discharged. Those with major ischemic symptoms are supported in the hospital ICU.

Pulmonary Irritants

Gases that cause pulmonary irritation produce a common syndrome when inhaled. Some of these gases are found in the home (usually in smaller quantities). When stored for industrial use, these gases can pose a serious hazard if they cannot be properly contained. In 1984, for example, the release of methyl isocyanate in Bhopal, India, caused 2000 deaths and 250,000 injuries.

Irritant gases are grouped according to water solubility, since the primary target when inhaled is the mucous membrane of the airways. Dissolved in that tissue, most toxic gases produce an acid or alkali as a byproduct. When a person is exposed, the eyes and airways become immediately irritated, as evidenced by tearing, nasal burning, and cough. The irritation and odor will prompt the victim to exit this atmosphere very quickly if it's possible to do so, thus limiting the toxic exposure. If circumstances are such that escape is impossible, prolonged exposure causes laryngeal edema, laryngospasm, bronchospasm, and ALI.

Some gases don't dissolve easily in water but can still have devastating effects on the respiratory system. Irritation of the mucous membranes occurs less quickly, and the toxic gas may even have a neutral or pleasant odor. Phosgene, which has an odor similar to hay, is one such gas. The exposed person will have none of the immediate symptoms of irritation described earlier, and as a result will remain in the environment, and the gas will be able to reach the alveoli. Deep pulmonary tissues can be injured, causing an initial presentation of mild ALI symptoms (e.g., tachypnea) but rapidly progressing to respiratory failure within 24 hours.

Diagnosis and Management Initial and ongoing assessment for laryngeal edema is the key to an effective management plan for the victim of pulmonary irritant inhalation. Even if normal tissues are found on direct laryngoscopic exam, the patient may subsequently develop rapid swelling and airway compromise. Continuous monitoring, repeated chest auscultation, and listening to the patient's voice and complaints are important for several hours after exposure. Findings of dyspnea, cough, hypoxia, or other abnormal findings during your assessment should prompt a chest x-ray and blood gas analysis. Many of these patients will progress to ALI, so your assessment and management plan should include close monitoring for potential respiratory failure.

If the patient has hoarseness and stridor, secure the airways with endotracheal intubation. If wheezing is present, administer β-adrenergic agonists. Use of ipratropium and steroids is not recommended. Identification of ALI requires aggressive airway support and ventilation by intensive care specialists experienced in the care of high-risk patients.

Impression and Differential Diagnosis: Systemic Review

You should perform certain diagnostics, ask particular questions, and select assessments on the basis of the patient's chief complaint, such as dyspnea, weakness, fever, altered mental status, syncope, or chest pain. The following tables will help you formulate a set of differential diagnoses associated with common complaints. Differential diagnosis of dyspnea by body system is summarized in Table 3-3. Differential diagnosis by sign or symptom is outlined in Table 3-4.

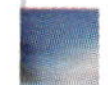

Special Tests and Devices

Arterial Blood Gases and Venous Blood Gases

ABGs and venous blood gases (VBGs) are used to evaluate both the oxygenation and the acid-base balance of the blood. ABGs are obtained by needle perforation and aspiration of arterial blood into a syringe. The blood is then analyzed rapidly and used to direct clinical management of a patient in respiratory distress. A sample ABG result is listed in Box 3-13.

BOX 3-13 Sample Arterial Blood Gases Laboratory Result

pH	7.38
Po_2	86
Pco_2	42
Hco_3	24
Sao_2	98%
Fio_2	24%
BE	−1
Na^{++}	138
K^+	3.5

TABLE 3-3 Differential Diagnosis of Dyspnea by Body System

Critical	Emergent	Nonemergent
PULMONARY DIAGNOSES		
Airway obstruction	Spontaneous pneumothorax	Pleural effusion
Pulmonary embolus	Asthma	Neoplasm
Noncardiogenic edema	Cor pulmonale	Pneumonia
Anaphylaxis	Aspiration pneumonia	COPD
CARDIAC		
Pulmonary edema	Pericarditis	Congenital heart disease
Myocardial infarction		Valvular heart disease
Cardiac tamponade		Cardiomyopathy
ABDOMINAL		
Abdominal dissection	Ischemic bowel	Ascites
Bowel perforation	Pancreatitis	Ileus
Perforated diverticula	Cholecystitis	Obesity
Gangrenous gallbladder	Bowel obstruction	
Perforated esophagus	Herniated diaphragm	
PSYCHOGENIC		
Wernicke encephalopathy	Catatonia	Hyperventilation
		Panic disorder
METABOLIC		
Diabetic ketoacidosis	Hyperglycemia	
Thyroid storm	Hyperthyroidism	
INFECTIOUS		
Sepsis	Pneumonia, viral	Influenza
Pneumonia	Pneumonia, bacterial	Bronchitis
Epiglottitis	Pneumonia, fungal	Human immunodeficiency virus (HIV) infection
Bacterial tracheitis	Pneumonitis	Tuberculosis
Retropharyngeal abscess	Aspiration pneumonitis	
Foreign object aspiration	Lung abscess	
Meningitis	Empyema	
HEMATOLOGIC		
Severe anemia	Anemia	Chronic anemia
Hemorrhage, gastrointestinal	Leukemia	
	Lymphoma	
NEUROMUSCULAR		
Intracerebral hemorrhage	Encephalopathies	Neuromuscular degenerative disease (amyotrophic lateral sclerosis [ALS])
Cerebrovascular accident	Alcohol intoxication	Myasthenia gravis
Transient ischemic attack	Basilar artery syndrome	Multiple sclerosis

The pH is a reflection of the acidic or alkalemic condition of the blood. Normal pH in the human body ranges between 7.35 and 7.45. A decreased pH level, such as 7.20, represents acidosis caused by a body malfunction. An elevated pH level, such as 7.55, represents alkalosis.

Acidosis and alkalosis can be further divided into respiratory and metabolic components. Acidosis of a respiratory nature—that is, respiratory failure—can evolve rapidly. Metabolic conditions can also cause acidosis; diabetic acidosis is a primary example, although shock is the most common cause of metabolic acidosis.

Measuring the Po_2 is essential in evaluating the presence and degree of hypoxia. Normal values for patients who are able to breathe room air range from 80 to 100 mm Hg. Values exceeding 500 can be seen in patients receiving pure oxygen. Hypoxia ranging from 50 to 70 mm Hg is not uncommon in patients with longstanding lung disease such as COPD. Patients with acutely decreased levels (between 50 and 70 mm Hg) may have a more severe clinical presentation because of the tolerance that occurs with chronic hypoxia. The HCO_3, or bicarbonate level, reflects the body's acid-base status from a

TABLE 3-4 Differential Diagnosis of Dyspnea by Sign or Symptom

Critical	Emergent	Nonemergent
WEAKNESS		
Sepsis	Electrolyte abnormality	Dehydration
Intracerebral hemorrhage	Pneumonia	Heat exhaustion
Myocardial infarction	Basilar artery syndrome	
Pulmonary embolus		
Pneumothorax		
Drug overdose		
FEVER		
Sepsis	Pneumonia	Bronchitis
Heat stroke	Empyema	Urinary tract infection
Epiglottitis		
Bacterial tracheitis		
Retropharyngeal abscess		
SYNCOPE		
Sepsis	Congestive heart failure	Dehydration
Pulmonary embolus	Myocarditis	Vertigo
Myocardial infarction		Vasovagal stimulation
Myocardial ischemia		
Cardiac arrhythmia		
CHEST PAIN		
Acute myocardial infarction	Pericarditis	Bronchitis
NSTEMI	Myocarditis	Chest wall pain
Pericardial tamponade	Pericardial effusion	Costochondritis
Aortic dissection	Pneumonia	Hiccough
Status asthmaticus	Dressler's syndrome	Tietze's syndrome
Arrhythmia	Cholecystitis	
	Hepatitis	
	Superior vena cava embolus	
ALTERED MENTAL STATUS		
Hypoglycemia	Drug intoxication	Alcohol intoxication
	Acute coronary syndrome	
Stroke/TIA	Hypercalcemia	
Sepsis	Hyperkalemia	
Respiratory failure	Hyponatremia	
Aortic dissection	Pneumonia	
Intracerebral hemorrhage		
Status epilepticus		

NSTEMI, Non–ST-segment elevation myocardial infarction; *TIA,* transient ischemic attack.

metabolic perspective. A low HCO_3 indicates a metabolic acidosis, and a high HCO_3 level indicates a metabolic alkalosis. The base excess (BE) or base deficit can also be used to evaluate the presence of a metabolic or respiratory condition. Normally ranging from −3 to +3, a negative value indicates metabolic acidosis. A positive value indicates metabolic alkalosis.

Arterial Blood Gas Interpretation

Blood gas analysis can be confusing to healthcare providers. It's important that you have a basic understanding of these findings and their application. This becomes particularly important when providing proper mechanical ventilation to your patient. You can't just turn on a ventilator and hope it works. You must guide the settings on the basis of precise clinical findings, some of which include blood gases (Table 3-5).

TABLE 3-5 Key Blood Gas Results

		Abnormal Findings	
Parameter	**Normal Range**	**Acid**	**Alkali**
pH	7.35–7.45	↓	↑
Pco_2	35-45	↑	↓
Base excess	−2 to +2	↓	↑
Bicarbonate	22-26	↓	↑

Note that an acid or base change in the Pco_2 is proportionately opposite of the pH and reflects a respiratory abnormality or adjustment. Also keep in mind that the BE

TABLE 3-6 Blood Gas Abnormalities

Abnormality	pH	P_{CO_2}	HCO_3
Uncompensated metabolic acidosis	Low	Normal	Low
Uncompensated respiratory acidosis	Low	High	Normal
Compensated metabolic acidosis	Low normal	Low	Low
Compensated respiratory acidosis	Low normal	High	High
Mixed metabolic and respiratory acidosis	Low	High	Low
Uncompensated metabolic alkalosis	High	Normal	High
Uncompensated respiratory alkalosis	High	Low	Normal
Compensated metabolic alkalosis	High normal	Low	High
Compensated respiratory alkalosis	High normal	Low	Low
Mixed metabolic and respiratory alkalosis	High	Low	high

and HCO_3 levels generally move in the same direction as the pH when a metabolic reason exists for the abnormality or body adjustment.

When you review the blood gas results from the lab, a shortcut way to guide you toward the correct interpretation is to place an arrow next to the result. Is the result from the patient higher than normal? If so, use an arrow pointing up. Is the result lower than the normal range? If so, use a down arrow.

Let's suppose your patient's blood gas results read as follows:

pH: 7.20
P_{CO_2}: 78
BE: −2
HCO_3: 22

You note that the pH is down, the P_{CO_2} is up, and the BE and HCO_3 levels are normal. These findings, taken together, indicate acidosis—respiratory acidosis. All laboratory results must be correlated with the patient's clinical condition. In this case, you know that the way to correct the acidosis is to increase the patient's minute volume. If you were providing mechanical ventilation to the patient, you could correct the minute volume by increasing the rate (frequency), the tidal volume, or both. Blood gas abnormalities are summarized in Table 3-6.

The body continually tries to recalibrate its balance, or homeostasis. The mechanisms by which the body adjusts for acid or alkali abnormalities come first and most rapidly through the buffer system, second and more slowly through the respiratory system, and third—days later—through the renal system.

An example of successful compensation is a patient who is in early hemorrhagic shock, with the following blood gas results:

pH: 7.36
P_{CO_2}: 25
BE: −8
HCO_3: 15

Clinically this patient is demonstrating tachypnea (an early sign of shock) and is blowing off CO_2 to minimize the availability of carbonic acid. In fact, the respiratory system has done so well that the patient's pH remains normal. This is termed *complete compensation*. Alternatively you could say the metabolic acidosis is fully compensated.

Using Blood Gas Results to Manage Ventilation

Adjusting positive-pressure ventilation on the basis of blood gas results is standard practice in the critical care arena. One way to do this is from a practical standpoint:

1. P_{CO_2} is largely a function of rate (*f*) and tidal volume (V_T).
   - For increased P_{CO_2}: increase $f \times 2$ to 5 or $V_T \times 50$ to 100 mL
   - For decreased P_{CO_2}: decrease $f \times 2$ to 5 or $V_T \times$ 50 to 100 mL
2. For acute changes in Sp_{O_2}, changes in F_{IO_2} and PEEP should occur. Changes in PEEP must be undertaken with caution, especially where PEEP levels are greater than 7 to 10 cm H_2O.
   - For increases in Sp_{O_2} greater than 95%: decrease F_{IO_2} in increments of 5% to maintain Sp_{O_2} above 92%

Venous Blood Gas Analysis

Some EDs are beginning to rely on VBG values in certain clinical circumstances. This practice has obvious clinical advantages: it reduces the number of high-risk arterial punctures required to obtain laboratory samples, it provides enough data for physicians to determine the presence of some metabolic disorders, and it eliminates a painful experience for the patient. VBG values, except P_{O_2}, serve as predictors of arterial values.

One disadvantage to VBG testing is the necessity of drawing ABGs in the event that clinical correlation cannot be made with venous values. Another is the obvious gap in reliable P_{O_2}. Pulse oximetry may be used as an adjunct to VBG sampling. Table 3-7 demonstrates the differences in normal venous and arterial blood gas values.

TABLE 3-7 Comparison of Arterial and Venous Blood Gas Values in Healthy Volunteers

	Arterial	Venous
pH	7.38–7.42	7.35–7.38
P_{CO_2}	38–42 mm Hg	44–48 mm Hg
P_{O_2}	90–100 mm Hg	40 mm Hg
H_{CO_3}	24 mEq/L	22-26 mEq/L

From Sherman SC, Schindlbeck M: When is venous blood gas analysis enough?, Emerg Med 38:44–48, 2006.

Putting It All Together

Disorders that result in respiratory compromise are common to all ages of patients and are seen by all levels of healthcare providers. Respiratory complaints can result in significant ventilation, perfusion, and diffusion compromise. A thorough patient history, physical exam, and evaluation of diagnostic findings will aid your early recognition of the underlying etiologies of respiratory distress and respiratory failure.

As a healthcare provider, your understanding of the anatomy, physiology, and pathophysiology of the respiratory system and the diseases that contribute to inadequate ventilation, perfusion, and diffusion can be critical in evaluating your patient's level of distress and initiating proper care.

Ineffective work of breathing may be due to a variety of dysfunctional processes. Be familiar with the differences and similarities of reactive airway diseases, bacterial versus viral infections, and the causes of airway occlusion—accidental, traumatic, and idiopathic. Maintain your skill levels at peak performance, and be ready to initiate prompt basic life support (BLS) and advanced life support (ALS) airway adjunct interventions. The expertise you bring to the work of responding to and attending patients with respiratory disorders can save lives.

SCENARIO SOLUTION

1 Differential diagnoses may include: pharyngitis, tonsillitis, peritonsillar abscess, epiglottitis, Ludwig's angina, bacterial tracheitis, retropharyngeal abscess, and prevertebral abscess.

2 To narrow your differential diagnosis, you will need to complete the history of past and present illness. Perform a physical examination of his mouth and throat. Do not insert anything into the mouth to examine the throat. This could worsen airway swelling. Assess his oxygen saturation. Palpate his submental area and his neck. This examination should not delay transport or transfer to an area where advanced airway management is possible.

3 The patient has signs of impending airway obstruction. Airway management in these patients is best provided by anesthesia or ENT physicians when immediately available. Administer humidified oxygen. Prepare to suction his oropharynx (provide him with an emesis basin to spit secretions if he prefers). Establish vascular access, and deliver IV fluids. Prepare to intubate. Select several tube sizes. Prepare equipment for cricothyrotomy if the airway cannot be secured by oral endotracheal intubation. Consider medication for fever, antibiotics, and pain once the airway is managed.

SUMMARY

- Upper and lower airways conduct air (ventilation) to the alveoli, the site of gas exchange (respiration).
- Sensors tell the respiratory system when and how to adjust the respiratory cycle to meet the body's needs for oxygen and carbon dioxide (CO_2) and maintain its acid-base balance.
- The interdependence of respiratory anatomy on other thoracic structures helps it provide oxygen to all tissues and eliminate CO_2.
- Diseases of the cardiovascular system, which shares intrathoracic space with the respiratory system, should be included in the differential diagnosis when the patient complains of respiratory distress or failure, weakness, airway compromise, chest pain, altered mental status, cough, or fever.
- Specific disease processes that may compromise the upper airway include infections, altered mental status, aspiration, allergic reactions, and cancer.
- Specific disease processes characterized by lower airway dysfunction include respiratory system infection, cancer, organ failure, air-trapping diseases; heart diseases that cause ischemia, infection, cardiac failure, or pressure-gradient changes; and CNS effects from chronic neuromuscular disorders, drugs, and environmental exposures.
- Your assessment of the patient with respiratory complaints should include a standard emergency approach, with special techniques to help identify signs and symptoms of various conditions. Special monitoring and diagnostic clues can help you rule in or out differential diagnoses.
- Patient management includes airway and ventilatory support, with ongoing assessment that reassures the patient he or she is improving as you carry out your treatment plan on the basis of your field impressions.

BIBLIOGRAPHY

Acerra JR: Pharyngitis. http://emedicine.medscape.com/article/764304-overview. Accessed May 12, 2009.

Aceves SS, Wasserman SI: Evaluating and treating asthma, Emergency Med 37:20–29, 2005.

Amitai A, Sinert RH: Ventilator management. http://emedicine.medscape.com/article/810126-overview. Accessed June 5, 2009.

Asmussen J, et al: Conjunctival oxygen tension measurements for assessment of tissue oxygen tension during pulmonary surgery, Eur Surg Res 26:372–379, 1994.

Balentine J, Lombardi DP: Aortic stenosis. http://emedicine.medscape.com/article/757200-overview. Accessed June 12, 2009.

Bascom R, Benninghoff MG: Pneumothorax. http://emedicine.medscape.com/article/424547-overview. Accessed May 22, 2009.

Blackstock UA, Sinert R: Dilated cardiomyopathy. http://emedicine.medscape.com/article/757668-overview. Accessed May 23, 2009.

Brenner B: Asthma. http://emedicine.medscape.com/article/806890-overview. Accessed May 13, 2009.

Bowman JG: Epiglottitis, adult. http://emedicine.medscape.com/article/763612-overview. Accessed May 11, 2009.

Centers for Disease Control and Prevention: 2007–2008 National health and nutrition examination survey. http://www.cdc.gov/nchs/nhanes.htm. Accessed August 4, 2010.

Dodds NR, Sinert R: Angioedema. http://emedicine.medscape.com/article/756261-overview. Accessed May 12, 2009.

Fink S, Abraham E, Ehrlich H: Postoperative monitoring of conjunctival oxygen tension and temperature, Int J Clin Monit Comput 5:37–43, 1988.

Grossman S, Brown DFM: Congestive heart failure and pulmonary edema. http://emedicine.medscape.com/article/757999-overview. Accessed May 23, 2009.

Harman EM: Acute respiratory distress syndrome. http://emedicine.medscape.com/article/165139-overview. Accessed May 29, 2009.

Howes DS, Booker EA: Myocarditis. http://emedicine.medscape.com/article/759212-overview. Accessed May 24, 2009.

Huq S, Maghfoor I, Perry M: Lung cancer, non–small cell. http://emedicine.medscape.com/article/279960-overview. Accessed May 27, 2009.

Jenkins W, Verdile VP, Paris PM: The syringe aspiration technique to verify endotracheal tube position, Am J Emerg Med 12(4):413–416, 1994.

Kaplan J, Eidenberg M: Barotrauma. http://emedicine.medscape.com/article/768618-overview. Accessed May 28, 2009.

Khan JH: Retropharyngeal abscess. http://emedicine.medscape.com/article/764421-overview. Accessed May 13, 2009.

Lazoff M: Encephalitis. http://emedicine.medscape.com/article/791896-overview. Accessed May 29, 2009.

Maloney M, Meakin GH: Acute stridor in children. http://www.medscape.com/viewarticle/566588. Accessed May 13, 2009.

Mantooth R: Toxicity, benzodiazepine. http://emedicine.medscape.com/article/813255-overview. Accessed May 27, 2009.

Marx J, et al: Rosen's emergency medicine: concepts & clinical practice, ed 5, St Louis, 2002, Mosby.

Mehta N: Peritonsillar abscess. http://emedicine.medscape.com/article/764188-overview. Accessed May 12, 2009.

Murray AD: Deep neck infections. http://emedicine.medscape.com/article/837048-overview. Accessed May 13, 2009.

National EMS Education Standards (NEMSES), Draft 3.0, Education Standards Document, 2008, NHTSA.

National Occupational Competency Profile for Paramedic Practitioners, 2001, Paramedic Association of Canada.

Oudiz RJ: Primary pulmonary hypertension. http://emedicine.medscape.com/article/301450-overview. Accessed May 26, 2009.

Pappas DE, Hendley JO: Retropharyngeal abscess, lateral pharyngeal abscess and peritonsillar abscess. In Kleigman RM, et al, editors: Nelson textbook of pediatrics, ed 18, Philadelphia, 2007, Saunders.

Paul M, Dueck M, Kampe S, et al: Intracranial placement of a nasotracheal tube after transnasal trans-sphenoidal surgery, Br J Anaesth 91:601–604, 2003.

Peng LF, Kazzi AA: Dental infections. http://emedicine.medscape.com/article/763538-overview. Accessed May 13, 2009.

Petrache I, Sigua NL: Pleurodynia. http://emedicine.medscape.com/article/300049-overview. Accessed May 23, 2009.

Plewa MC: Panic disorders. http://emedicine.medscape.com/article/806402-overview. Accessed May 27, 2009.

Rackow E, et al: Sublingual capnometry and indexes of tissue perfusion in patients with circulatory failure, Chest 120:1633–1638, 2001.

Rajan S, Emery KC: Bacterial tracheitis. http://emedicine.medscape.com/article/961647-overview. Accessed May 13, 2009.

Rubins J: Pleural effusion. http://emedicine.medscape.com/article/299959-overview. Accessed May 23, 2009.

Sharma S: Chronic obstructive pulmonary disease. http://emedicine.medscape.com/article/297664-overview. Accessed May 15, 2009.

Shores C: Infections and disorders of the neck and upper airway. In Tintinalli J, editor: Emergency medicine: a comprehensive study guide, New York, 2004, McGraw-Hill Professional Publishing, pp 1494–1501.

Stephen JM: Pneumonia, bacterial. http://emedicine.medscape.com/article/807707-overview. Accessed May 20, 2009.

Stephens E: Toxicity, opioids. http://emedicine.medscape.com/article/815784-overview. Accessed May 26, 2009.

Sutherland SF: Pulmonary embolism. http://emedicine.medscape.com/article/759765-overview. Accessed May 25, 2009.

Tanigawa K, Takeda T, Goto E, et al: The efficacy of esophageal detector devices in verifying tracheal tube placement: a randomized cross-over study of out-of-hospital cardiac arrest patients, Anesth Analg 92:375–378, 2001.

Tatevossian RG, et al: Transcutaneous oxygen and CO_2 as early warning of tissue hypoxia and hemodynamic shock in critically ill emergency patients, Crit Care Med 28(7):2248–2253, 2000.

Urden L, Stacy K, Lough M: Thelan's critical care nursing: diagnosis and management, ed 5, St Louis, 2006, Elsevier.

Zevitz ME: Hypertrophic cardiomyopathy. http://emedicine.medscape.com/article/152913-overview. Accessed May 25, 2009.

Chapter Review Questions

1. Which of the following is most likely to impair ventilation?
   a. Anaphylaxis
   b. Carbon monoxide poisoning
   c. Congestive heart failure
   d. Pneumonia

2. Which sign or symptom indicates impending respiratory failure in a patient who is having an asthma attack?
   a. End-tidal CO_2 32 mm Hg
   b. Increased respiratory rate
   c. S_3 heart sounds
   d. Sleepiness

3. A 65-year-old female has progressive onset of dyspnea over several days. Her temperature is 102.2°F (39°C). Her prescription medicines include Accupril, spironolactone, Lanoxin, ipratropium, and salbutamol. Which of the following would be included in your differential diagnosis?
   a. Pneumonia
   b. Pulmonary edema
   c. Spontaneous pneumothorax
   d. Status asthmaticus

4. Which diagnostic test will quickly detect poor ventilation?
   a. Capnography
   b. Carbon monoxide sensors
   c. Chest x-ray
   d. Transcutaneous oxygen saturation

5. A patient presents with fever, sore throat, and swollen lower jaw. Which should be included in your differential diagnosis?
   a. Foreign-body airway obstruction
   b. Laryngotracheobronchitis
   c. Ludwig's angina
   d. Tonsillitis

6. A 62-year-old male has a sudden onset of dyspnea after a bout of coughing. Lung sounds are diminished on the right side. Which element of his past medical history would help confirm the diagnosis of spontaneous pneumothorax?
   a. Heroin abuse
   b. Pneumonia within 5 years
   c. Tobacco smoker
   d. Treatment with warfarin

7. Which sign or symptom may develop as a result of pulmonary embolism, COPD, or pulmonary hypertension?
   a. Bradycardia
   b. Jugular venous distention
   c. Rhonchi
   d. Right heart strain or right axis deviation

8. You have administered albuterol and parenteral epinephrine to a 21-year-old female who is having an asthma attack. Her PCO_2 is now 55 mm Hg. What additional treatment is indicated?
   a. Apply oxygen, and allow the patient's body to reverse the bronchospasm and hypercarbia.
   b. Coach the patient to slow her respiratory rate.
   c. No immediate treatment is indicated except to monitor the patient.
   d. Place the patient on a continuous positive airway pressure mask.

9. A 24-year-old male was diagnosed with Guillain-Barré syndrome 1 week ago. Which complication should you anticipate?
   a. Hypertension
   b. Metabolic alkalosis
   c. Pneumonia
   d. Spontaneous pneumothorax

10. The risk of barotrauma for the asthmatic patient who is receiving mechanical ventilation increases if you decrease the:
    a. Expiratory time
    b. Positive end-expiratory pressure
    c. Respiratory rate
    d. Tidal volume

CHAPTER

4 Shock

THIS CHAPTER EXPLORES the devastating phenomenon of shock. We'll begin by reviewing the anatomy and physiology of tissue perfusion and describing the pathophysiology of hypoperfusion. Then we'll compare the types of shock and describe how to recognize and treat shock at each stage. Finally, we'll discuss the important place of shock within the AMLS assessment pathway and offer concrete tools for diagnosing shock and arresting its ominous cascade of organ system dysfunction.

Learning Objectives

At the conclusion of this chapter, you will be able to:

1. Describe the anatomy and physiology of body systems as they relate to shock.
2. Describe the pathophysiology of each shock state.
3. Identify the key features of each type of shock.
4. Assess the patient for life-threatening findings during the primary and secondary surveys and ongoing assessment.
5. Describe laboratory and diagnostic tests used to verify diagnoses associated with shock.
6. Compare and describe hypovolemic, distributive, cardiogenic, and obstructive shock.
7. Apply appropriate treatment modalities for the management, monitoring, and continuing care of the patient in shock.
8. Describe the pathway used to address problems found during assessment of the shock patient.
9. Formulate a differential diagnosis, demonstrate sound clinical reasoning skills, and apply advanced clinical decision making in caring for the patient in shock who has an emergent cardiovascular, respiratory, or hematologic condition.
10. List effective ways of discovering a patient's allergies, current medications, incident and past medical history, and last oral intake, and correlate them to each of the types of shock.

Key Terms

acidosis An abnormal increase in the hydrogen ion concentration in the blood, resulting from an accumulation of an acid or the loss of a base, indicated by a blood pH below the normal range

afterload The force resisting shortening after the muscle is stimulated to contract. In the intact heart, it is the pressure against which the ventricle ejects blood, as measured by the stress acting on the ventricular wall following the onset of contraction. Afterload is determined largely by peripheral vascular resistance and the physical characteristics and volume of blood in the arterial system. It is often estimated by determining systolic arterial pressure.

cardiac cycle A complete cardiac movement or heartbeat. The period from the beginning of one heartbeat to the beginning of the next; diastolic and systolic movement, with the interval in between.

cardiac output (CO) The effective volume of blood expelled by either ventricle of the heart per unit of time (usually volume per minute); it is equal to the stroke volume multiplied by the heart rate (SV × HR = CO)

disseminated intravascular coagulation (DIC) A pathologic form of coagulation that is diffuse or systemic rather than localized. The process causes the clotting cascade to be activated, resulting in several clotting factors being consumed to such an extent that generalized bleeding or clotting may occur. Also known as *diffuse intravascular coagulation*.

hypovolemia Abnormally decreased volume of circulating blood in the body; the most common cause is hemorrhage.

intravascular volume The amount of circulating blood in the vessels

mean arterial pressure (MAP) The average pressure within an artery over a complete cycle of one heartbeat; expressed as: MAP = Diastolic pressure + (1/3 × Pulse pressure)

perfusion The act of pouring over or through, especially the passage of a fluid through the vessels of a specific organ

preload The mechanical state of the heart at the end of diastole; the magnitude of the maximal (end-diastolic) ventricular volume or the end-diastolic pressure stretching the ventricles. In isolated cardiac muscle, the force stretching the resting muscle to a given length prior to contraction; in the intact heart, the stress on the ventricular wall at the end of diastole, determined largely by the venous return, total blood volume and its distribution, and atrial activity.

pulse pressure The difference between the systolic and diastolic blood pressures

shock A condition of profound hemodynamic and metabolic disturbance characterized by failure of the circulatory system to maintain adequate perfusion of vital organs. It may result from inadequate blood volume, cardiac function, or vasomotor tone.

stroke volume The amount of blood ejected by the left ventricle at each heartbeat. Amount varies with age, sex, and exercise. Also called *systolic discharge*.

SCENARIO

YOUR PATIENT IS a 78-year-old male whose chief complaint is difficulty breathing. When you examine him, you note severe dyspnea with accessory muscle use and cyanosis. His skin is warm. The nursing home reports that he has had a cough for several days, but he suddenly became worse about 20 minutes ago. His medical history includes emphysema, prostate cancer, and according to nursing home staff, "a little kidney failure." He has an indwelling urinary catheter. His breath sounds are diminished over the left lung, and his vital signs are BP 88/66 mm Hg, P 128/min, R 28 and labored. You are unable to obtain a saturation reading.

1 ***What differential diagnoses are you considering based on the information you have now?***

2 ***What additional information will you need to narrow your differential diagnosis?***

3 ***What are your initial treatment priorities as you continue your patient care?***

Celebrated 19th century trauma surgeon Samuel Gross described shock as "a manifestation of the rude unhinging of the machinery of life." R. Adams Cowley, the U.S. Army physician who promulgated the concept of the "golden hour," called shock "a momentary pause in the act of dying." As the organizer of the first statewide emergency medical services (EMS) system in Maryland and the founder of one of the first shock trauma centers in the nation, however, Dr. Cowley wasn't content to accept death as the inevitable consequence of shock. He and others, including William Harvey, Walter Cannon, George James Guthrie, William Bayliss, and George Crile, helped pioneer many of the treatments we'll discuss in the following sections. First, though, we must define *shock*, albeit in less poetic words than those of Drs. Gross and Cowley.

Anatomy and Physiology of Shock

Shock is a progressive state of cellular hypoperfusion in which insufficient oxygen is available to meet tissue demands. Either oxygen intake, absorption, or delivery fails, or the cells are unable to take up and use the oxygen to carry out cellular functions. Shock is a complicated, often catastrophic clinical phenomenon that can be difficult to identify until it has become irreversible. As a healthcare provider, you must understand the pathophysiology, assessment, and management of this condition, since each year in the United States, more than 1 million people arrive at emergency departments (EDs) in varying states of shock.

The initial signs of shock can be subtle and their progression insidious. Even with aggressive early treatment, the mortality rate for all types of shock can be quite high and poses a real threat to our patients. The rapid recognition of the physiologic state of shock is an essential skill for every healthcare provider. It begins with an understanding of the anatomy, physiology, and pathophysiology of tissue perfusion.

The word **perfusion** derives from the Latin verb *perfundere,* meaning "to pour over." In the body, then, the blood supplies oxygen to cells as it spills over them by way of the circulatory system. The three main determinants of cellular perfusion are cardiac output (discussed in the next section), intravascular volume, and vascular capacitance. **Intravascular volume** is the amount of circulating blood in the vessels. Vascular capacitance is the size of the vascular space and is a function of volume and pressure (to be precise, it's calculated by dividing the change in volume by the change in pressure).

Shock begins at the cellular level. The cellular changes that occur during shock impact every system of the body, including the gastrointestinal (GI), endocrine, and neurologic systems. The symptoms of shock are consistent with the degree of metabolic impairment, but they're generally similar regardless of etiology. In other words, the compensatory mechanisms of the body tend to respond in the same way to enhance organ and tissue perfusion no matter what type of shock is presenting.

Heart

The heart is a cone-shaped muscular organ situated in the mediastinum, posterior to the inferior aspect of the sternum. It lies at an oblique angle, with two-thirds of its mass to the left of the body's midline and one-third to the right. The heart comprises four chambers: the left and right atria, which are located at the base of the heart, and the left and right ventricles, which make up the apex.

The left and right atria are smaller than the larger, more muscular ventricles. Deoxygenated blood enters the heart through the right atrium and then flows through the tricuspid valve into the right ventricle. From the right ventricle, the blood travels through the pulmonary valve into the pulmonary artery. Once the blood has been oxygenated in the lungs, it proceeds through the pulmonary vein to the left atrium. (The four pulmonary veins, two for each lung, are the only veins in the body that carry oxygenated blood.) The mitral (bicuspid) valve allows blood to pass from the left atrium to the left ventricle, where it is then pumped to the aorta through the aortic valve.

A complete heartbeat is called a **cardiac cycle**. Systole (contraction) and diastole (relaxation) in all four chambers, atria and ventricles, are the components of the cardiac cycle. The contraction of the heart occurs in stages. The atria squeeze first, followed quickly by the much stronger ventricles as the atria begin to relax.

Cardiac Output

For blood to "pour" through the body, it must be pumped. The heart is magnificently designed for this purpose. In a healthy person, the heart is remarkably efficient at moving oxygenated blood through the body, ensuring adequate perfusion. **Cardiac output (CO)** is the amount of blood ejected by the ventricles per unit of time, usually expressed as liters per minute (L/min). For this reason, CO is also known as *minute volume*. The CO of a healthy adult varies from 3 to 8 L/min, with 5 L/min being about average.

CO is determined by **stroke volume**—the volume of blood ejected with each contraction of the heart—and heart rate. The equation is as follows:

$$\text{CO} = \text{Stroke volume} \times \text{Heart rate}$$

The stroke volume of a healthy adult is typically about 70 mL—about as much liquid as would fit inside an egg—but the amount is variable because of individual physiologic differences. The primary mechanical variable that affects stroke volume is explained by Starling's law, also known as the *Frank-Starling mechanism*. Starling's law describes the ability of cardiac muscle fibers to stretch and contract to regulate the strength of the heart's contraction. According to this law, the more the heart is stretched, the stronger it contracts, but only up to a point. Once the heart muscle has stretched beyond its optimal elasticity, the contraction will become weaker and less effective. Figure 4-1 shows an overview of stroke volume and Starling's law.

Neural and endocrine mechanisms also influence stroke volume through neurotransmitters. Sympathetic nerve fibers in the cardiac nerves release norepinephrine, and the adrenal medulla releases epinephrine. These two adrenergic agents boost the strength of the contraction.

Inadequate CO is one cause of hypoperfusion. To generate adequate CO, the heart must be able to contract with sufficient vigor, and the heart rate must be within an effective range. Four primary factors determine stroke volume and CO:

1. **Preload:** the stretch of the myocardial tissue by the blood in the ventricles just before the start of a contraction. You can grasp the concept of preload by comparing it with the tension created when a bowstring is drawn back. If there's not enough tension on the string, the arrow will drop to the ground near the archer's feet. A strong pull, on the other hand, will propel the arrow toward its target. In the heart, the pull or stretch on the muscle is from the volume of blood returning to the heart and accumulating in the ventricle prior to a contraction. Starling's law holds that the greater the stretch—up to a point—the stronger the cardiac contraction and output.
2. **Afterload:** the force the ejected blood meets as it exits the ventricle. You may think about afterload as the pressure it takes to push through a swinging door. If someone or something is pushing against the other side of the door, it takes more pressure to open it. In the systemic circulation, afterload is represented by aortic systolic pressure and systemic vascular resistance.
3. Contractility: the force of cardiac contraction for a given level of preload. Positive inotropic stimulation, such as that provided by administration of epinephrine or dopamine, heightens the force and velocity of contraction. This stronger contraction will in turn increase the stroke volume for a given level of preload, but more oxygen will be required to support it.
4. Synchrony: to pump effectively, cardiac contractions must be synchronized, with the atria contracting before the ventricles and the left ventricle depolarizing just slightly before the right ventricle. Loss of atrioventricular synchrony, such as occurs during atrial fibrillation, decreases ventricular preload. Conduction disorders such as bundle branch block disturb coordination among the ventricular muscle fibers, which reduces the efficiency of contraction.

DECREASED BLOOD PRESSURE

↓ Peripheral resistance (dilation)
• Nitric oxide ↑
• Prostacyclin ↑
• Kinins ↑
• Atrial natriuretic peptide (ANP) ↑
• Neural factors (β-adrenergic) ↓

↓ Cardiac output
• Blood volume ↓ (ANP) ↑
• Heart rate ↓
• Contractility ↓

Blood pressure

↑ Cardiac output
• Heart rate ↑
• Contraction ↑
• Blood volume ↑ (aldosterone)

↑ Peripheral resistance (constriction)
• Angiotensin II ↑
• Catecholamines ↑
• Thromboxane ↑
• Endothelin ↑
• Neural factors (α-adrenergic) ↑

INCREASED BLOOD PRESSURE

A

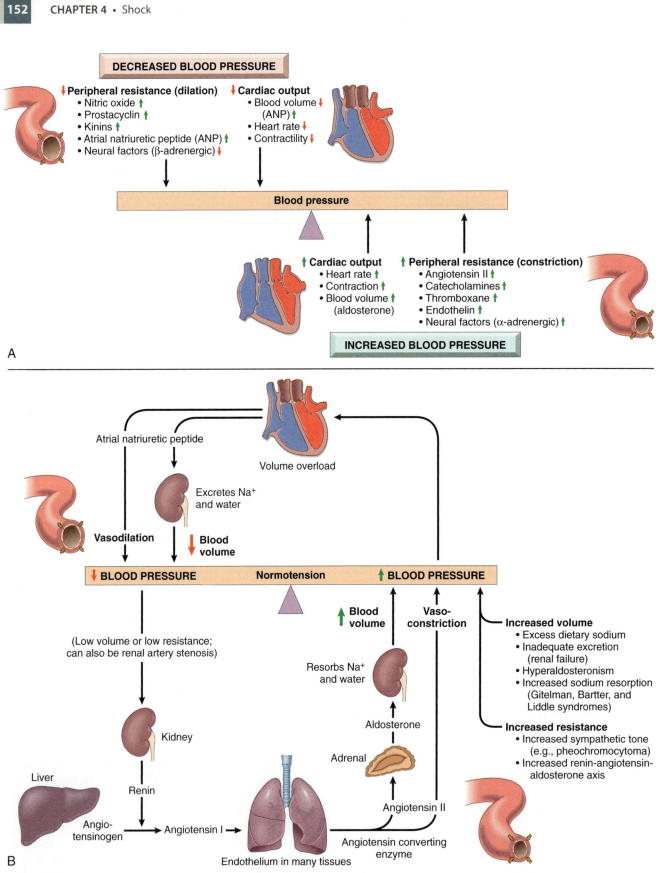

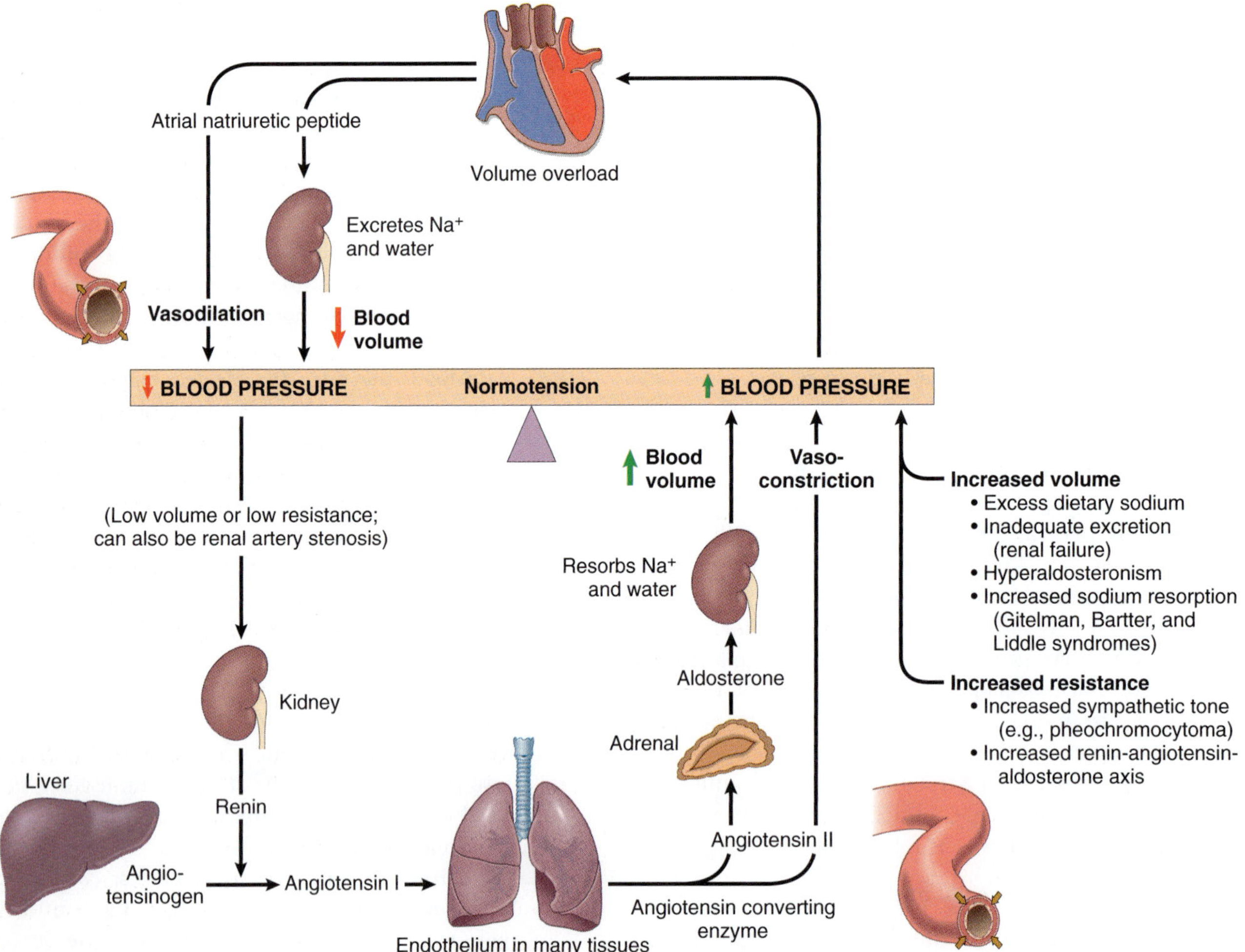

■ **Figure 4-1** Blood pressure regulation. **A**, Critical roles played by cardiac output and peripheral resistance in modulating blood pressure. **B**, Interplay of renin-angiotensin-aldosterone and atrial natriuretic peptide in maintaining blood pressure homeostasis. (From Kumar V, et al: Robbins and Cotran pathologic basis of disease, ed 8, Philadelphia, 2009, Saunders.)

Vascular System

The vascular system is similar to the plumbing in a house. It's a conduit for moving blood through the body. The arteries and arterioles, which make up the arterial vascular system, carry oxygenated, nutrient-rich blood. The veins and venules, which make up the venous system, return deoxygenated blood to the heart and transport waste products to be eliminated from the body. The capillaries communicate between the blood and tissues by acting as the site of transfer of oxygen and other nutrients to the tissues and removal of wastes from the tissues. The precapillary sphincters dilate to allow blood to flow into the capillaries when a fresh supply is needed.

In fact, all parts of the vascular system can contract (vasoconstrict) and dilate (vasodilate) in response to various stimuli. The arteries and arterioles constrict and dilate more vigorously than the veins and venules do because their vessel walls are stronger. The increased force of the blood in the arteries relative to the veins keeps the blood flowing quickly. Since the residual pressure is lower in the venous system, valves are necessary to prevent the backflow of blood.

Blood Pressure

Blood pressure is the pressure the blood exerts against the walls of the arteries. For perfusion to be effective, the heart must continue to force fluid into the system, and the arterial vessels must maintain their tone. We call this resistance of blood flow through the circulatory system *peripheral vascular resistance,* and it's determined by the degree of vasoconstriction of distal arteries and arterioles. Vasoconstriction exerts compressive force on the blood, which increases pressure within the vascular space. When peripheral resistance increases, arterial blood pressure rises, promoting blood flow through capillary beds and effectively perfusing the tissues.

As vessels shrink in diameter, friction—and thus resistance—increases. Friction is created as blood, a viscous fluid, courses along the vessel walls and through the vessels. Red blood cells (RBCs) are responsible for much of the blood's viscosity, but protein molecules contribute too. As the composition of blood changes, it becomes more or less viscous. For example, the percentage of the fluid component of blood, called *plasma,* may increase or decrease. If it drops, as evidenced by an increased hematocrit level, the blood becomes more viscous.

As the volume of blood ejected from the heart increases, so does the arterial blood pressure. Thus arterial blood pressure is an indirect indicator of tissue perfusion. The amount of pressure exerted against the arterial wall, stated in millimeters of mercury (mm Hg), determines the measured pressure. Blood pressure is expressed as the systolic pressure over the diastolic pressure. The systolic blood pressure represents the ventricular volume ejection and the response of the arterial system to that ejection, and it is thus the higher number. The diastolic pressure represents the residual pressure in the arterial system after the ventricles relax.

Mean arterial pressure (MAP) is the mean systolic and diastolic pressure required to perfuse the myocardium and brain. It is generally thought to be 70, with normal considered to be 80 to 100 mm Hg. Patients may have higher or lower MAPs in response to their medical conditions. Patients with chronic hypertension may require a pressure higher than the average to maintain adequate perfusion. The formula used to calculate the MAP is as follows:

$$\text{MAP} = \text{Diastolic pressure} + (1/3 \times \text{Pulse pressure})$$

Pulse pressure is the difference between the systolic and diastolic pressures. The pulse pressure is normally about 40 mm Hg. Changes in cardiac output or vascular resistance are responsible for changes in pulse pressure. The body's response to hypovolemic shock is an example of the effect of each on pulse pressure. A decrease in cardiac output and an increase in peripheral vascular resistance presents as a narrowing pulse pressure. As volume is lost, a decrease in blood returning to the heart causes a decrease in cardiac output. The body responds by activating the sympathetic nervous system, which secretes epinephrine. This causes an increase in heart rate, an increase in contractility, and vasoconstriction. The result is an increase in diastolic blood pressure in the presence of a lower systolic blood pressure, causing a narrowing pulse pressure. The changes may be subtle and easily missed. For example, the blood pressure may change from 118/68 to 108/82. This represents a decrease in pulse pressure of nearly 50% (50 to 26). When looking at the blood pressure alone, the decline in pulse pressure may not be noticed, but when the pulse pressure is calculated, a significant decrease is noted. A decline of greater than 50% indicates a 50% downturn in stroke volume. Pulse pressure is a helpful indicator of shock, especially when the measurement is taken repeatedly so that an emerging pattern can be identified. Like any other sign or symptom, it should be a part of the whole assessment and be used to direct you to collect other findings to confirm the patient's status.

Blood

Blood has two main functions: transportation of oxygen and nutrients to the body's cells and removal of waste from the body. Hemoglobin, an iron-containing protein in RBCs, carries oxygen to the tissues. Carbon dioxide (CO_2), one of the primary waste products of metabolism, is dissolved in the plasma and must be eliminated quickly, since a buildup of CO_2 contributes to a state of **acidosis**.

Other components of the blood include:

- White blood cells (WBCs): help defend the body against infection by bacteria, fungi, and other pathogens
- Platelets: initiate the process of clotting

- Proteins: perform various functions involving blood clotting, immunity, wound healing, and transport
- Hormones: control organ system function, regulate growth and development, and perform other vital functions
- Nutrients: fuel cells so that they can function properly (Glucose, for example, is a nutrient carried by the blood to cells throughout the body.)
- Plasma: carries the solid components in blood; a fluid composed of about 92% water and 7% protein

An equilibrium must be maintained between the interstitial (extracellular) fluid, which occupies the spaces between the cells, and the intracellular fluid, which remains inside the cells. Plasma proteins are critical in the regulation of fluid equilibrium. The plasma proteins albumin and globulin are large and cannot easily pass out of the vessels. Their presence within the vessels creates an osmotic pressure that draws fluid back into the vasculature.

Nervous System

The autonomic nervous system controls involuntary actions of the body, such as the respiratory drive. The two branches of the autonomic nervous system are the sympathetic nervous system and the parasympathetic nervous system. The sympathetic nervous system helps maintain normal bodily functions and allows the body to respond to threats that demand an instant reaction—the so-called fight-or-flight response. During such events, the sympathetic nervous system plays a direct role in tissue perfusion by temporarily redirecting blood away from nonessential functions, such as digestion, and toward the heart and brain. The parasympathetic nervous system maintains bodily functions when no such danger looms. Table 4-1 summarizes the functions of the sympathetic and parasympathetic nervous systems.

Pathophysiology of Shock

Shock is a complicated and subtle process that involves every body system. When the cardiovascular system is unable to maintain adequate tissue perfusion, shock ensues, causing widespread impairment of cellular metabolism in the tissues of the body. The mitochondria are the first cellular component affected by shock. Most of the oxygen in the body is consumed by mitochondria, which produce 95% of the aerobic energy used by every body system. When the oxygen has been depleted in the mitochondria, they begin to convert fats, carbohydrates, and ketones into lactate, thereby creating an acidotic environment. An elevated lactate level in the blood, then, is a red flag for shock.

Metabolic Acidosis

During normal cell metabolism of glucose, oxygen is consumed. This process is called *aerobic metabolism*. When insufficient oxygen is present, glucose is metabolized through an alternative pathway that does not require oxygen. This process is termed *anaerobic metabolism*. The anaerobic pathway is much less efficient, yielding less energy (in the form of adenosine triphosphate [ATP]) per molecule of glucose and generating many more waste products, primarily lactic acid.

When the body tissues no longer have ample oxygen, and cells begin producing lactic acid as a byproduct of anaerobic metabolism, metabolic acidosis sets in. If shock persists, this alternative pathway will not be able to generate enough ATP, the primary means of energy storage. Because ATP helps maintain the integrity of cell walls, a deficiency of ATP will allow sodium and water to enter cells, causing cellular edema. Breakdown of the cell wall also permits potassium and lactic acid to seep out of the cell and into the serum. As a result, lactic acidosis and hyperkalemia (high blood potassium) develop. The edema forming within the cells and mitochondria eventually damages the cell. As interstitial edema develops, intravascular volume decreases, resulting in a decreased flow to surrounding cells. This causes a choking off of fluid flowing into adjacent capillaries and leads to additional ischemia. Ischemic cells create lactate, free radicals, and inflammatory factors that increase damage to the cells. These toxins are flushed back into the circulatory system when perfusion is restored, contributing to damage to other organs as well. If the damage is severe, no amount of reoxygenation and perfusion can repair the damage, and

TABLE 4-1 Functions of the Sympathetic and Parasympathetic Nervous Systems

	Sympathetic	Parasympathetic
Cardiac muscle	↑ Rate and strength	↓ Rate and strength
Coronary blood vessels	Constriction (alpha receptors) Dilation (beta receptors)	Dilation
Bronchioles	Relaxation (beta)	Constriction
Digestive tract	↓ Peristalsis	↑ Peristalsis
Urinary bladder	Relaxation	Contraction
Skin	Sweat	No effect
Adrenal medulla	↑ Epinephrine secretion	No effect

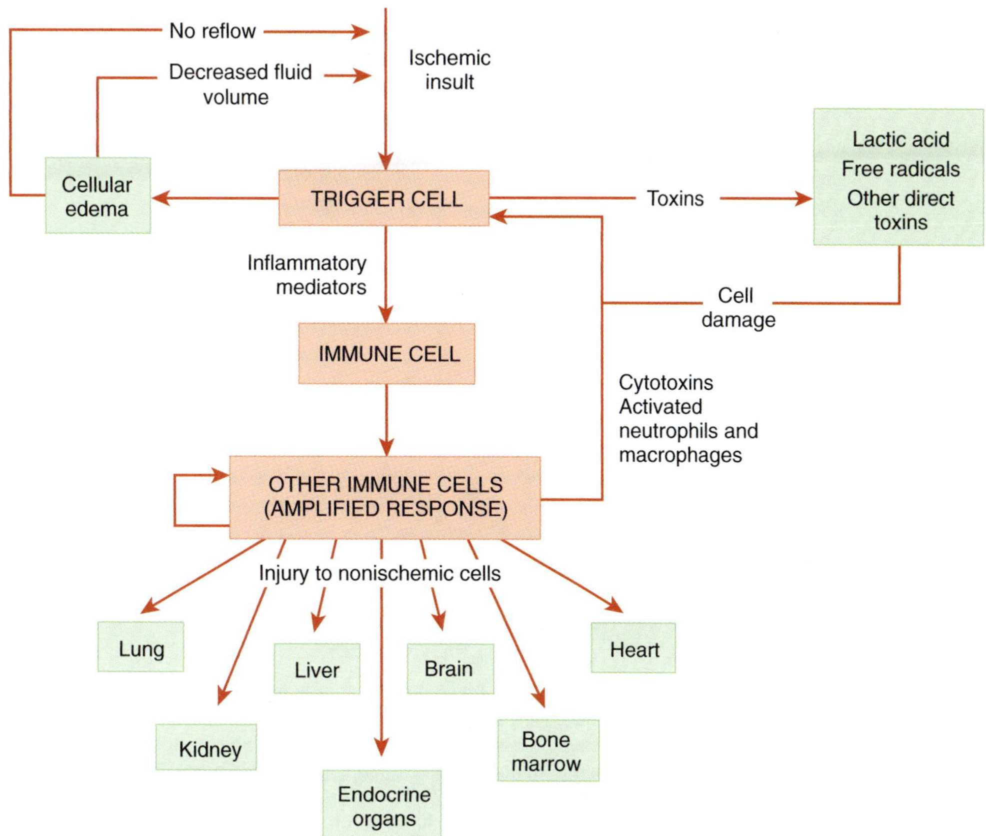

Figure 4-2 The "shock cascade." Ischemia of any given region of the body will trigger an inflammatory response that will have an impact on nonischemic organs even after adequate systemic perfusion has been restored. (Reprinted with permission from Dutton RP: Shock and trauma anesthesia. In Grande CM, Smith CE, editors: Anesthesiology clinics of North America: trauma, Philadelphia, 1999, Saunders.)

cellular death occurs. As seen in Figure 4-2, the shock cascade for the inflammatory response is associated with hypoperfusion.

Three events can compromise cellular oxygen use: activation of the clotting cascade, lysosomal enzyme release, and a drop in circulatory volume. Each of these events triggers a cycle that progressively impairs the body's ability to maintain adequate oxygenation. As each state advances, a greater response is activated. The clotting cascade (Figure 4-3) may be responsible for tubular necrosis and disseminated intravascular coagulation. Lysosomal enzyme release injures the affected cell and neighboring cells, contributing to additional damage and problems such as systemic immune response (SIRS) and acute respiratory distress syndrome (ARDS) or acute lung injury (ALI). The response to a drop in circulatory volume is discussed below in compensatory mechanisms.

Compensatory Mechanisms

A number of compensatory mechanisms can be activated to help maintain adequate oxygenation: increased minute ventilation, increased cardiac output (increased heart rate and/or contractility), and vasoconstriction. Increased minute ventilation raises arterial oxygen content. The body boosts CO by elevating heart rate, increasing cardiac contractility, or both. Constriction of vessels improves perfusion pressure in the tissues. In the aortic arch and carotid arteries, sympathetic nerve fibers called *baroreceptors* constantly monitor arterial blood pressure. When pressure is adequate or high, baroreceptor firing leads to sympathetic inhibition and parasympathetic activation. When pressure falls, baroreceptor firing subsides, allowing greater sympathetic nervous system activation and less parasympathetic activity. The physiologic result is vasoconstriction and an increase in heart rate and cardiac contractility.

Compensatory mechanisms are effective only up to a point. Once that critical threshold has been reached, hypoxia develops, and shock overtakes the body. Ultimately, insufficient oxygen is available to meet oxygen demands throughout the body. If left untreated, multiple organ dysfunction and death are inevitable. The stages of shock are summarized in Table 4-2.

Adrenal Response

The adrenal glands, located on top of the kidneys, release epinephrine and norepinephrine in response to declining cardiac output. These hormones stimulate alpha and beta receptors in the heart and blood vessels. Alpha 1 triggers vasoconstriction, and beta 1 stimulates heart rate and cardiac contractility (Table 4-3). Receptor distribution

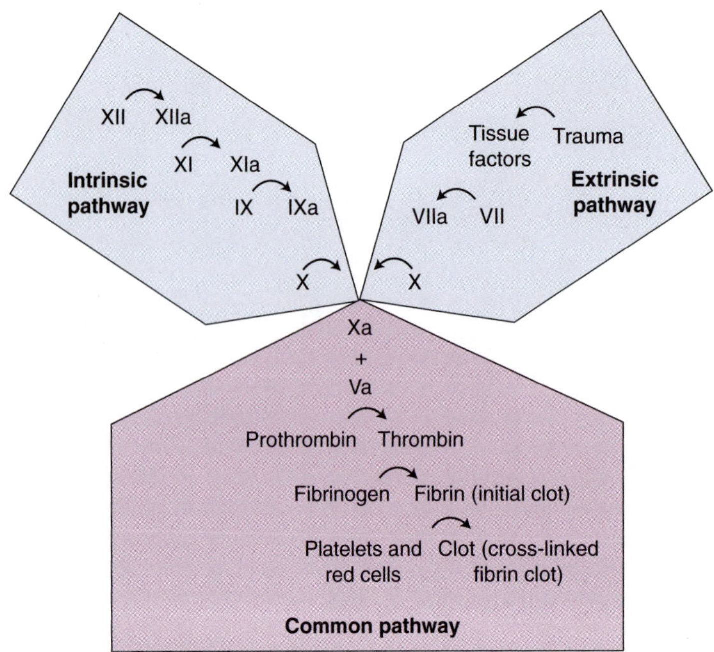

When a blood vessel is injured, the body responds through two pathways - the **intrinsic and extrinsic**. The **Extrinsic pathway** begins when tissue factor (TF) is released from injured tissue outside the blood vessel. The tissue factor activates Factor VII which activates Factor X. The **Intrinsic pathway** begins when clotting factors within the blood vessel are activated in a domino-type effect, leading to activation of Factor X. Once Factor X is activated, the **Common pathway** is set in motion. Activated Factors Xa and Va combine to convert prothrombin to thrombin. Then thrombin converts fibrinogen to fibrin to form an initial clot. The fibrin fibers become cross-linked and red blood cells and platelets become enmeshed to form a more stable clot.

■ **Figure 4-3** Coagulation cascade.

TABLE 4-2 Stages of Shock

Stage	Vital Signs	Signs and Symptoms	Pathophysiology
Compensated	Normal blood pressure Normal to slightly ↑ heart rate Tachypnea Delayed capillary refill	Cool hands and feet Pale mucous membranes Restlessness, anxiety Oliguria	Vasoconstriction maintains blood flow to essential organs, but tissue ischemia occurs in less essential areas.
Decompensated	Blood pressure decreasing Tachycardic >120 bpm Tachypneic >30–40 bpm	Waxen, cool, clammy skin Pale or cyanotic mucous membranes Profound weakness Metabolic (lactic) acidosis Anxiety Absent or ↓ peripheral pulses	Blood pressure decreases as vascular tone decreases. Dysfunction to all organs is imminent. Anaerobic metabolism ensues, causing lactic acidosis.
Irreversible	Profound hypotension	Lactate > 8 mEq/L	Metabolic acidosis causes postcapillary sphincters to open and release stagnant and coagulated blood. Excessive potassium and acid causes dysrhythmias. Cellular damage is irreversible.

usually leads to greater constriction in noncritical tissues such as fat, skin, and tissues of the digestive tract. Vasoconstriction also occurs within the kidneys.

Pituitary Response

The anterior pituitary gland releases antidiuretic hormone (ADH) in response to shock. ADH, which is synthesized in the hypothalamus, is released during early shock when symptoms are difficult to detect. As it circulates to the distal renal tubules and the collecting ducts in the kidneys, ADH causes fluid to be reabsorbed. Intravascular volume is maintained, and urine output decreases. ADH is also called *vasopressin* (from *vaso-*, meaning "vessel," and the Latin verb *pressor,* meaning "to press"). ADH stimulates smooth muscle contraction in the digestive tract and blood vessels.

TABLE 4-3 Alpha-Beta Response to Shock

	Location	Action
Alpha 1	Arterioles in skin, viscera, mucous membranes Veins Bladder sphincters	Constriction, increased peripheral vascular resistance
Alpha 2	Digestive system	Decreased secretions, peristalsis
Beta 1	Heart, kidneys	Increased heart rate, force of contraction, oxygen consumption Release of renin
Beta 2	Arterioles of the heart, lungs, and skeletal muscles Bronchioles	Dilation with increased organ perfusion Dilation

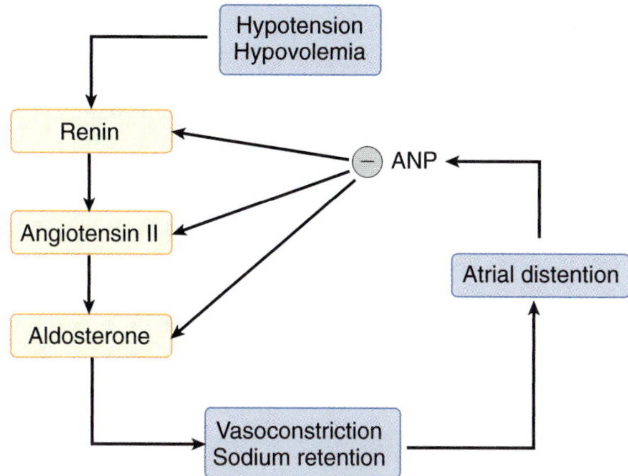

■ **Figure 4-4** Interactions between atrial natriuretic peptide (ANP) and the renin-angiotensin-aldosterone system. Hypotension or hypovolemia triggers release of renin from afferent arteriole, causing formation of angiotensin II, which stimulates release of aldosterone from adrenal cortex. Angiotensin II and aldosterone cause vasoconstriction and sodium retention, ultimately resulting in reexpansion of intravascular volume; this causes atrial distention, which triggers release of ANP. ANP inhibits release of renin, renin's action on angiotensinogen to form angiotensin II, angiotensin-induced vasoconstriction, stimulation of aldosterone secretion by angiotensin II, and actions of aldosterone on collecting duct. Actions of ANP promote vasodilation and sodium excretion. Therapeutic administration of fluids to distend atrium and release ANP is an important intervention to curtail renal vasoconstriction and sodium retention. (From Miller RD, Eriksson L, Fleisher L, et al: Miller's anesthesia, ed 7, Philadelphia, 2009, Churchill Livingstone.)

Renin-Angiotensin System Activation

The kidneys are vital to maintaining blood pressure. When blood flow to the kidneys is restricted, the renin-angiotensin system is activated (Figure 4-4). Renin is an enzyme released from the juxtaglomerular cells in the kidneys. It converts angiotensinogen to angiotensin I, which is in turn converted to angiotensin II in the lungs by angiotensin-converting enzymes (ACE). Angiotensin II is a potent but short-lived vasoconstrictor. During shock, it triggers constriction of the vessels farthest from the heart, creating resistance that increases the heart's afterload. Shunting from the less essential organs is enhanced, which increases preload. This selective perfusion occurs during the ischemic phase of shock. While perfusion of essential organs—the brain, heart, lungs, and liver—is enhanced, organs that are less essential become ischemic.

Aldosterone Angiotensin I and II are proteins that stimulate the production and secretion of aldosterone from the adrenal cortex, which causes the kidneys to reabsorb sodium from the renal tubules. The sodium carries water back into the vasculature instead of excreting it in the urine, thereby increasing vascular volume and driving up blood pressure. The release of aldosterone signals the kidneys to halt the release of renin and restore perfusion to the kidneys. Aldosterone secretion also creates the sensation of thirst, one of the early signs of shock.

Types of Shock

If you consider each type of shock relative to its respective portion of the cardiovascular system, you'll be better able to identify the condition, anticipate problems, and take the appropriate corrective action. In the following sections, we'll outline the types of shock and describe the differences among them. Keep these variations in mind as you explore the AMLS pathway for a patient with signs of shock.

Shock can be categorized into four types: hypovolemic, distributive, cardiogenic, and obstructive, depending on which portion of the cardiovascular system fails (Table 4-4). Failure can occur in any of the three major components of the cardiovascular system: the pump (the heart), the pipes (the blood vessels), or the fluid within them (the blood).

Hypovolemic Shock

It's easy to remember the cause of inadequate tissue perfusion in hypovolemic shock by taking a closer look at the

TABLE 4-4 Types of Shock

Category	Cardinal Signs	Causes	Management
HYPOVOLEMIC SHOCK			
	Cool, clammy skin Pale, cyanotic skin Decreased BP Altered LOC Decreased capillary refill	Hemorrhage: trauma, GI bleeding, ruptured aortic aneurysm, pregnancy-related bleeding Severe dehydration: gastroenteritis, diabetic ketoacidosis, adrenal crisis	Administer oxygen. Stop the bleeding. Give IV fluid bolus. Splint fractures. Perform surgery.
DISTRIBUTIVE SHOCK			
Septic	Hyperthermia or hypothermia Decreased BP Altered LOC	Infection	Administer oxygen. Give IV fluid bolus. Administer antibiotics.
Anaphylactic	Pruritus, erythema, urticaria, angioedema Increased HR Decreased BP Anxious Respiratory distress, wheezing	Antibody-antigen release	Give epinephrine 1:1000, 0.3–0.5 mg subcutaneously or intramuscularly for mild reaction. Epinephrine 1:10,000, 0.3–0.5 mg IV for severe reaction over 3–10 min, and repeat every 15 min as needed. Intravenous fluid bolus Diphenhydramine, 1–2 mg/kg IV (max 50 mg) Consider corticosteroids. Consider vasopressors.
Neurogenic	Warm, dry, pink skin Decreased BP Alert Normal capillary refill time		Administer oxygen. Give IV fluid bolus. Consider dopamine.
Toxins	Based on specific agent (See Chapter 9 for a discussion of toxic agents.)	(See Chapter 9.)	Based on specific agent (See Chapter 9.)
CARDIOGENIC SHOCK			
	Cool, clammy skin Pale, cyanotic skin Tachypnea Tachycardia or other abnormal rhythm Decreased BP Altered LOC Decreased capillary refill time	Pump failure: AMI, cardiomyopathy, myocarditis, ruptured chordae tendineae, papillary muscle dysfunction, toxins, myocardial contusion, acute aortic insufficiency, ruptured ventricular septum Dysrhythmia	Administer oxygen. Give IV fluid bolus. Rate correction (medication or pacing/cardioversion) Inotropes Vasopressors Intraaortic balloon pump
OBSTRUCTIVE SHOCK			
	Decreased blood pressure Difficulty breathing, tachycardia, tachypnea JVD, unilateral decreased breath sounds, muffled heart tones	Acute pericardial tamponade, massive pulmonary embolus, tension pneumothorax	Administer oxygen. Perform needle decompression for tension pneumothorax. Consider surgery.

AMI, Acute myocardial infarction; *BP*, blood pressure; *GI*, gastrointestinal; *HR*, heart rate; *IV*, intravenous; *LOC*, level of consciousness.

term **hypovolemia** itself. The prefix *hypo-* means "below" or "low," *vol-* refers to volume, and the combining form *-emia* means "in or pertaining to the blood."

A reduction in the amount of circulating fluid leads to a diminished CO, which prevents adequate oxygenation to the tissues and cells. The classic signs and symptoms of hypovolemic shock are tachycardia, hypotension, and increased respiratory rate, but signs will vary depending on how much fluid has been lost. Bleeding, vomiting, diarrhea, and many other conditions can lower the volume of circulating fluid (Figure 4-5).

Hemorrhagic Shock

Hemorrhagic shock is the most common cause of hypovolemic shock. Significant blood loss can occur without obvious bleeding. Internal or external hemorrhage can accompany traumatic injuries or medical problems such as ruptured or dissected aortic aneurysm, ruptured spleen, ectopic pregnancy, GI bleeding, or other causes of significant blood loss. The bleeding may be obvious, as in a patient vomiting blood, or insidious, as in a patient with a small GI bleed that has been presenting over time. In hemorrhagic shock, oxygen-carrying capacity diminishes as RBCs are depleted.

Hemorrhagic hypovolemic shock is best treated by stopping the bleeding. If the bleeding is obvious, direct pressure should be applied. If direct pressure to an extremity is ineffective, a tourniquet should be used. In the past, concern about tissue and nerve destruction discouraged tourniquet application. Although such damage is a legitimate risk, survival of the whole person outweighs survival of an extremity. Elevation of an extremity has not been shown to diminish bleeding, so it is considered unnecessary. Application of pressure to specific pressure points is no longer recommended.

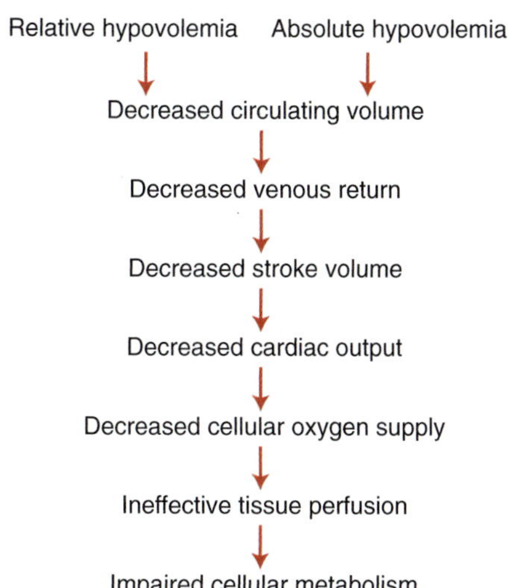

■ **Figure 4-5** Pathophysiology of hypovolemic shock. (Redrawn from Urden LD: Thelan's critical care nursing: diagnosis and management, ed 5, St Louis, 2006, Mosby.)

Other Causes of Hypovolemic Shock

Loss of fluids other than blood can also cause hypovolemic shock. For example, extreme interstitial fluid loss may follow vomiting, diarrhea, and massive diuresis in patients with diabetes mellitus or diabetes insipidus. Excessive plasma loss in patients with untreated burn injuries may cause delayed hypovolemic shock.

The severity of shock depends on the percentage and rate of fluid loss. Insidious fluid loss gives the body time to compensate. In a healthy adult, a 10% to 15% blood loss is well tolerated. Children and older adults are more sensitive to even a small amount of blood loss, but compensatory mechanisms or medications may delay outward signs. Table 4-5 summarizes the stages of hypovolemic shock.

Distributive Shock

Distributive shock is also due to an inadequate volume of blood to fill the vascular space, but the problem doesn't stem from blood or fluid *loss*, but from a precipitous *increase* in vascular capacity as blood vessels dilate and the capillaries leak fluid. This fluid leaks into extravascular and interstitial spaces, which is called the "third space." Such vasodilation can occur in sepsis, anaphylaxis, neurogenic shock, toxic shock syndrome, and toxin exposure. Too much vascular space translates into too little peripheral vascular resistance and a decrease in preload, which in turn reduces CO and sets the stage for shock.

Septic Shock

Septic shock is the result of a massive systemic inflammatory response to infection by gram-negative or gram-positive aerobes, anaerobes, fungi, or viruses. Gram-negative organisms appear to be the primary cause of sepsis, especially in hospitalized patients.

Several changes in health care have contributed to a recent rise in the incidence of sepsis. More patients are remaining at home with medical devices prone to causing

TABLE 4-5 Classes of Hypovolemic Shock

	% Blood Loss	Stage of Shock	Mental Status	Blood Pressure	Heart Rate	Respiratory Rate	Skin
Class I	<15%	Compensated	Slightly anxious	Normal	Normal	Normal	Pink, normal
Class II	15%–30%	Compensated (early)	Mildly anxious	Low normal	Mild tachycardia	Mild tachypnea	Pale, cool skin, >2 sec capillary refill
Class III	30%–45%	Decompensated (late)	Altered, lethargic	Hypotension	Severe tachycardia	Moderate tachypnea	Pale, mild cyanosis, cool, >3 sec capillary refill
Class IV	>45%	Irreversible	Extremely lethargic, unresponsive	Severe hypotension	Severe tachycardia to bradycardia	Severe tachypnea to agonal	Pale, central and peripheral cyanosis, cold, >5 sec capillary refill

From Aehlert B: Paramedic practice today: above and beyond, St Louis, 2009, Saunders.

infection, such as indwelling catheters. Many of these patients also have compromised immune systems, putting them at even greater risk for sepsis. In addition, infection by antibiotic-resistant gram-positive organisms such as *Staphylococcus aureus* and *Streptococcus pneumoniae* is increasing in incidence. Factors that predispose a patient to septicemia are summarized in Box 4-1.

The basis of septic shock and systemic inflammatory response syndrome (SIRS) is a complex process of inflammatory response and multisystem organ failure (Figure 4-6). Two or more of the following criteria must be met for a diagnosis of SIRS:

- Temperature > 38°C (100°F) or < 36°C (97°F)
- Heart rate > 90 beats per minute (bpm)
- Respiratory rate > 20 breaths/min or $PaCO_2$ < 32 mm Hg
- White blood cell count > 12,000/mm³, < 4000/mm³, or > 10% band neutrophilia

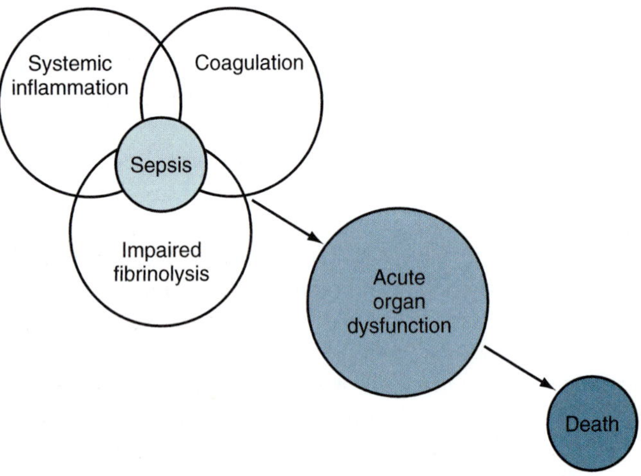

■ **Figure 4-6** Pathophysiologic consequences of sepsis syndrome result from an imbalance between proinflammatory and antiinflammatory mediators, activation of the coagulation cascade, and inhibition of fibrinolysis. The syndrome can progress to acute multiorgan dysfunction and death. (From Long S, Pickering L, Prober C: Principles and practice of pediatric infectious diseases, ed 3, Philadelphia, 2008, Churchill Livingstone.)

Sepsis syndrome is a precursor to septic shock. In a patient who has SIRS compounded by organ dysfunction or hypotension, sepsis can be said to have progressed to septic shock when the hypotension continues despite adequate fluid resuscitation. Sepsis may present in the hyperdynamic phase or the hypodynamic phases, described later.

Treatment Care of the patient in septic shock can be complicated. Relative hypovolemia develops in sepsis because the vasculature dilates. Actual hypovolemia may develop secondary to massive GI fluid loss or if third-spacing of fluid from capillary leakage occurs. Figure 4-7 reviews the management of septic shock.

Heart function is depressed in sepsis even in the early hyperdynamic phase. This phase, formerly known as "warm shock," is characterized by decreased systemic vascular resistance and occasionally by elevated CO. As inflammatory mediators circulate, the heart bears the brunt of the impact. Inflammation and altered metabolism can cause heart muscle injury. The heart rate may increase, and a fever may be present. The patient's skin will still be warm.

In the hypodynamic phase, formerly "cold shock," hypotension becomes evident, and an altered level of consciousness (LOC) develops. In this phase, the patient's skin will feel cool and clammy.

Prehospital treatment of septic shock must be aggressive. You should ensure adequate oxygenation and rapid fluid infusion. Pay close attention to airway management. Simple oxygen therapy may be adequate, but some patients require advanced airway support measures such as intubation. Establish vascular access (intravenous [IV] or intraosseous [IO]), and administer isotonic fluid in 500- to 1000-mL increments in adults (20 mL/kg in children), and reassess the patient after each bolus. The goal of fluid resuscitation is to restore perfusion, as indicated by a decreased heart rate, revived blood pressure, and diminished respiratory distress. If the patient's blood pressure doesn't improve, repeat the fluid challenge up to 2000 mL. Perform fluid resuscitation cautiously, since fluid overload is possible, particularly in older adults and children. If

BOX 4-1 Selected Predisposing Factors for Sepsis

INADEQUATE IMMUNE RESPONSE

- Patients with diabetes mellitus, liver disease, or HIV/AIDS
- Neonates
- Older adults
- Pregnant women
- Persons with alcoholism

PRIMARY INFECTIONS

- Pneumonia
- Urinary tract infection
- Cholecystitis
- Peritonitis
- Abscess

IATROGENIC SOURCES

- Indwelling vascular catheter
- Foley catheter
- Major abdominal or pelvic surgery

HIV/AIDS, Human immunodeficiency virus/acquired immunodeficiency syndrome.

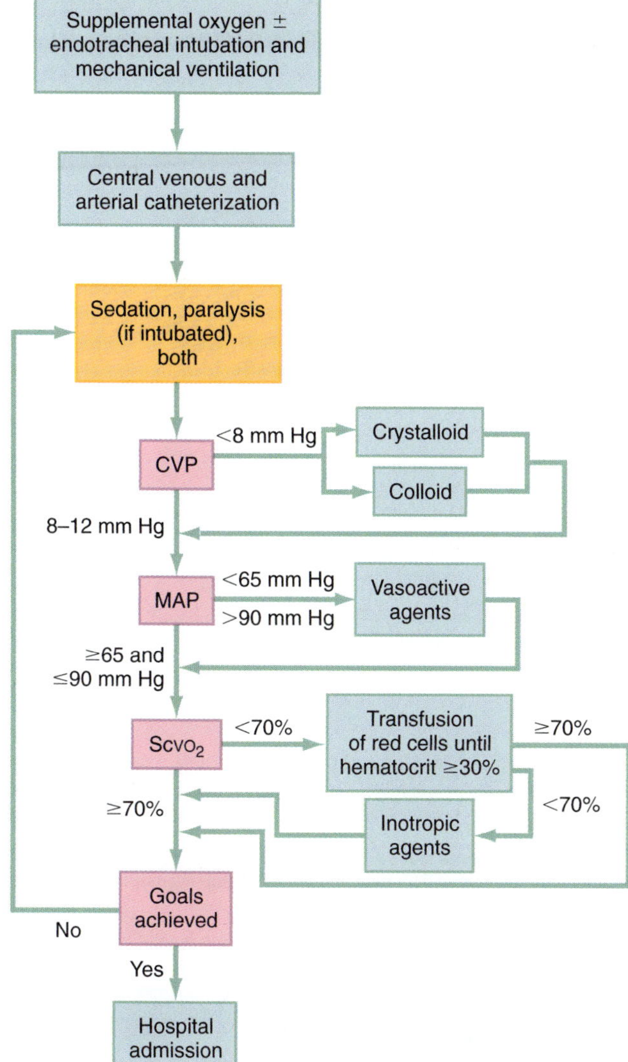

■ **Figure 4-7** Management of septic patients. Protocol outlines specific hemodynamic and physiologic parameters the clinician should seek to achieve within the first 6 hours of care. It focuses on resuscitation and should be used in conjunction with standard clinical care for patients with suspected infection (e.g., appropriate diagnostic studies to determine the focus of infection and appropriate antimicrobial agents to treat it). *CVP,* Central venous pressure; *MAP,* mean arterial pressure; *Scv*O_2, central venous oxygen saturation. (Redrawn from Rivers E, et al: Early goal-directed therapy in the treatment of severe sepsis and septic shock. N Engl J Med 345:1368, 2001.)

resuscitation is ineffective, a vasopressor and/or inotrope infusion titrated to effect may be beneficial. This may include epinephrine, phenylephrine, or dopamine.

During transport, relay the possibility of sepsis or SIRS to the receiving facility so the protocol to address these patients can be initiated as soon as possible. Once the patient arrives at the hospital, appropriate cultures should be collected *before* antibiotics are infused, so long as there is no significant delay. The cultures typically include two sets of blood cultures and a urine culture. In certain instances, ED personnel will collect a wound culture or a culture of a medical device (e.g., Foley catheter or central line). Typically, two broad-spectrum antibiotics will be initiated, and a more targeted antibiotic will be used when the results of the cultures become available.

Recombinant human activated protein C (rhAPC) has been approved for use in sepsis along with antibiotics. Activated C protein inhibits thrombin production, which is important because stimulation of the coagulation cascade is believed to promote the inflammatory process in patients with sepsis. (See Figure 4-7 to review management of septic patients.)

Anaphylactic Shock

For patients with known hypersensitivities, anaphylaxis is a frightening possibility. Signs and symptoms such as hypotension, tachycardia, difficulty breathing, wheezing, rales, rhonchi, anxiety, urticaria, and pruritus can begin within minutes or up to 1 hour after exposure to the antigen. Once the symptoms have resolved, they can return 1 to 12 hours later, at which time they may be either milder or more severe. Yet despite the sudden onset and dramatic nature of an anaphylactic reaction, the condition precipitates only 400 to 800 deaths per year in the United States. Figure 4-8 illustrates the management of anaphylaxis.

An antibody-antigen hypersensitivity response is the primary cause of anaphylactic shock. Not all hypersensitivity reactions evolve into shock. Most allergic reactions produce only mild symptoms such as pruritus and urticaria. Not all people have repeated anaphylactic reactions to additional exposures, but of the 40% to 60% who do, the most common trigger is the sting of an insect belonging to the *Hymenoptera* order—wasps, bees, and ants. Almost any substance can provoke a reaction in a sensitive individual, but some other common triggers of anaphylaxis are eggs, milk, shellfish, and peanuts (Box 4-2). Box 4-3 discusses latex allergy, a trigger that has become increasingly common among patients and healthcare workers since 1987, when the Centers for Disease Control (now the Centers for Disease Control and Prevention, but still abbreviated *CDC*) issued recommendations for Universal Precautions to prevent the transmission of bloodborne pathogens.

During anaphylaxis, biochemical mediators such as histamine, eosinophils, chemotactic factor of anaphylaxis, heparin, and leukotrienes are released. Vasodilation, increased capillary permeability (including pulmonary capillary permeability), bronchoconstriction, excessive mucus secretion, coronary vasoconstriction, inflammation, and cutaneous reactions ensue. The cutaneous reaction may be observed as flushed, warm skin resulting from vasodilation and urticaria.

As with other causes of distributive shock, peripheral vasodilation in anaphylaxis causes a relative hypovolemia. Fluid volume would be sufficient except that the vessels have dilated, so more space must be filled to maintain adequate perfusion. The sudden loss of volume and

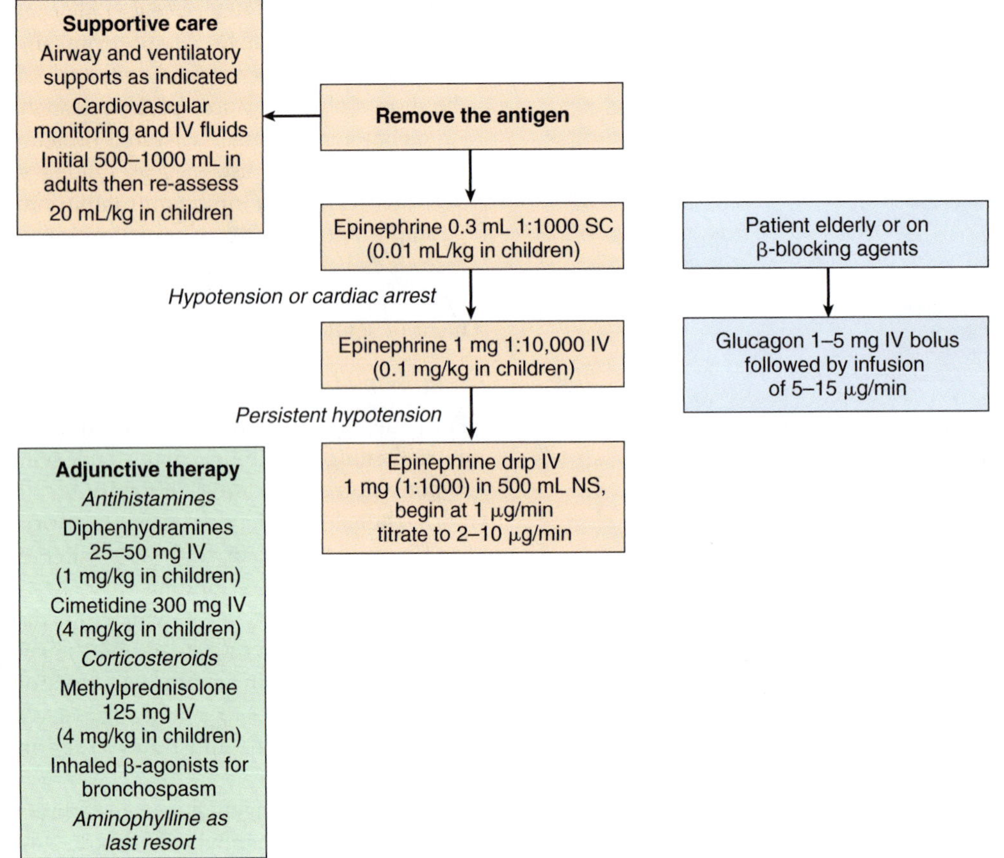
Supportive care
Airway and ventilatory supports as indicated
Cardiovascular monitoring and IV fluids
Initial 500–1000 mL in adults then re-assess
20 mL/kg in children
Remove the antigen
Epinephrine 0.3 mL 1:1000 SC (0.01 mL/kg in children)
Hypotension or cardiac arrest
Epinephrine 1 mg 1:10,000 IV (0.1 mg/kg in children)
Persistent hypotension
Epinephrine drip IV 1 mg (1:1000) in 500 mL NS, begin at 1 μg/min titrate to 2–10 μg/min
Patient elderly or on β-blocking agents
Glucagon 1–5 mg IV bolus followed by infusion of 5–15 μg/min
Adjunctive therapy
Antihistamines
Diphenhydramines 25–50 mg IV (1 mg/kg in children)
Cimetidine 300 mg IV (4 mg/kg in children)
Corticosteroids
Methylprednisolone 125 mg IV (4 mg/kg in children)
Inhaled β-agonists for bronchospasm
Aminophylline as last resort

■ **Figure 4-8** Management of anaphylaxis. (From Shannon M, Borron S, Burns M: Haddad and Winchester's clinical management of poisoning and drug overdose, ed 4, Philadelphia, 2007, Saunders.)

BOX 4-2 Some Triggers of Anaphylactic Shock

FOODS

- Eggs
- Milk
- Fish and shellfish
- Nuts and seeds
- Legumes and cereals
- Citrus fruits
- Chocolate
- Strawberries
- Tomatoes
- Avocados
- Bananas

FOOD ADDITIVES

- Food coloring
- Preservatives

DIAGNOSTIC AGENTS

- Iodine contrast material

BIOLOGICAL AGENTS

- Blood and blood components
- Gamma globulin
- Vaccines and antitoxins

ENVIRONMENTAL

- Pollen, mold, spores
- Animal hair
- Latex

DRUGS

- Antibiotics
- Aspirin
- Narcotics

ANIMAL VENOM

- Bees, wasps
- Snakes
- Jellyfish

From Urden LD, Stacy KM, Lough ME: Critical care nursing: diagnosis and management, ed 6, St Louis, 2010, Mosby.

BOX 4-3 Latex Allergy

Latex allergy is a response to a protein found in natural tropical rubber, from which latex products are manufactured. This allergy is an important concern for medical providers, since latex is found in so many medical products—gloves, IV catheters, endotracheal tubes, anesthesia equipment, tourniquets, and adhesive tape, to name a few. The latex protein itself or additives used during the manufacturing process can initiate a hypersensitivity response. Exposure can occur when latex comes into contact with the skin, mucous membranes, or internal tissues (including intravascular tissues) or when the patient inhales airborne latex components.

The patient's reaction can range from simple skin irritation (contact dermatitis) to anaphylaxis, a dangerous systemic response. Several patient populations are at increased risk for latex allergy:

- Patients with neural tube defects, such as spina bifida
- Those who have congenital urologic disorders
- Those who have had cumulative exposure to latex, including patients who have undergone multiple surgeries and workers in health care, rubber manufacturing, and glove manufacturing

Remember, simply inhaling invisible latex proteins can cause a life-threatening anaphylactic reaction in extremely sensitive individuals. Asking about latex allergy while taking the patient history is important so that nonlatex substitutes can be used if necessary. Sensitive patients must learn which common medical and nonmedical products may contain latex—rubber bands, pacifiers, and even children's toys, such as dolls.

BOX 4-4 Common Agents Used to Treat Anaphylaxis

EPINEPHRINE

- **Class:** catecholamine, sympathomimetic, adrenergic, inotrope
- **Action:** binds with alpha and beta receptors, thereby increasing blood pressure, heart rate, and bronchodilation
- **Dosage:**
  - 1:1000: 0.3–0.5 mg for mild reaction. Repeat every 5–15 minutes as needed.
  - 1:10,000: 0.3–0.5 mg over 3–10 minutes for severe reactions. Repeat every 15 minutes as needed.
- **Route:**
  1:1000: subcutaneous or intramuscular
  1:10,000: intravenous
- **Adverse effects:** palpitations, tachycardia, hypertension, anxiety, nausea, vomiting

DIPHENHYDRAMINE

- **Class:** antihistamine, anticholinergic, histamine-1 (H_1) receptor antagonist
- **Action:** binds and blocks H_1 receptors. Provides symptomatic relief but does not reverse anaphylaxis.
- **Dosage:** 1–2 mg/kg (maximum 50 mg) IV every 4 to 8 hours
- **Route:** oral, IV, IM
- **Adverse effects:** hypotension, palpitations, drowsiness, anxiety, chest tightness

resistance causes CO to drop. Cardiovascular collapse and/or airway obstruction are typically the direct cause of death.

Because shock can quickly overwhelm such patients, prompt intervention is critical. As the ABCs—airway, breathing, circulation—are initiated, it's important to ascertain the following:

- Does the patient have a history of previous allergic reactions?
- Has the patient been exposed to an offending agent? If so, when?
- Is there a complaint of urticaria, rash, throat swelling, or shortness of breath? Laryngeal edema can have a rapid onset, so intervention must be swift.
- When did the symptoms begin? The more rapid the onset, the more likely it is the reaction will be severe.
- How long have the symptoms lasted? Symptoms typically resolve within 4 to 6 hours.

Treatment The treatment of anaphylactic shock requires removing the allergen and reversing the effects of the biochemicals that have been released. It may be necessary to support vital functions by providing oxygen, initiating intubation or mechanical ventilation, and administering IV fluids. Drugs, especially epinephrine, should be administered without delay. Corticosteroids can stabilize the capillary membranes and reduce angioedema and bronchospasm, but because they don't take effect quickly, their use is limited to preventing or ameliorating the late-phase component of anaphylaxis, not to treating an initial attack. The two most common drugs used to treat anaphylaxis, epinephrine and diphenhydramine, are summarized in Box 4-4.

Neurogenic Shock

Neurogenic shock is a rare form of distributive shock. When signal transmission in the sympathetic nervous system is interrupted, the body can't mount an appropriate fight-or-flight response. Spinal cord injury, usually at the sixth thoracic vertebra (T6) or higher, often leads to neurogenic shock. Vessels can no longer constrict and instead begin to dilate. For this reason, neurogenic shock is sometimes called *vasogenic shock*. The dilated vessels make the patient's skin warm and pink. Blood pressure slackens, peripheral vascular resistance falls flat, and the circulatory system below the level of injury fails to return enough venous blood to the heart. The heart rate slows—in fact, bradycardia is highly characteristic of neurogenic shock—because of the lack of sympathetic stimulation. Arterial pressure flags, and tissue ischemia sets in at values below 50 to 60 mm Hg.

Treatment If the patient with neurogenic shock is also a trauma patient, the cervical spine must be stabilized. Ensure that the airway is patent, and offer support as necessary. Maintain oxygenation by providing supplemental oxygen or assisting respiration as indicated. Establish vascular access, and initiate fluid resuscitation. If the patient does not respond to fluid resuscitation, consider vasopressor agents such as phenylephrine, norepinephrine, or dopamine. Atropine may be indicated as well if the patient is bradycardic and symptomatic. Be sure to keep the patient warm, and monitor him for increased intracranial pressure and other neurologic dysfunction; associated head injury may be present. Transport the patient as quickly as possible to definitive care.

Vasodilation may also occur as a result of exposure to a toxin, poison, or medication overdose. In these cases, provide supportive care as you address the exposure. See Chapter 9 for details of AMLS management of exposure to toxins.

Cardiogenic Shock

Cardiogenic shock is caused by a problem with the rate or strength of heart contractions. Either the right or left ventricle may be the site of the pathology, which might be a rhythm disturbance, a cardiac structural disorder such as ruptured chordae tendineae, or the action of certain toxins. The most common cause is myocardial infarction with greater than a 40% loss of heart muscle. This is usually due to a massive infarction of the anterior wall of the heart, but it can be caused by many smaller infarctions throughout the heart. Risk factors for cardiogenic shock include advancing age, female sex, congestive heart failure, previous myocardial infarction, and diabetes.

In patients with cardiogenic shock, blood is no longer effectively pumped because of a diminished stroke volume or a heart rate that is too slow or too fast. The blood overloads the pulmonary vasculature, causing pulmonary edema and impaired gas exchange.

The signs and symptoms of cardiogenic shock are diverse. The respiratory rate is increased, and crackles caused by pulmonary edema can be heard on auscultation. Because of the ineffective myocardium, diminished stroke volume, and dwindling CO, the heart rate may be >100 bpm, heart sounds are diminished, and the pulse is weak and thready. Dysrhythmias may be present. The patient's skin will be cool, moist, and pale. The patient may have an altered LOC. Systolic blood pressure will be low, and the patient may complain of chest pain and shortness of breath.

Cardiogenic shock requires early identification of the cause and initiation of decisive supportive care. An electrocardiogram (ECG) assists in diagnosing ischemia or infarction and arrhythmia. A chest radiograph can be performed to detect pulmonary edema and pleural effusion. Cardiac markers like creatine kinase MB (CKMB) and troponin should be sent for laboratory analysis. In addition to those labs, a test for the presence of elevated levels of a hormone called *B-natriuretic peptide (BNP)* in the serum may indicate heart failure. In certain patients, BNP is released in response to the stretch of the atria and ventricles. The vasodilation that occurs causes natriuresis (release of excessive sodium into the urine) and a reduction in blood volume. When BNP is elevated beyond the normal level of 100 pg/mL (<100 ng/L SI units), it's typically a sign that the patient's difficulty breathing is related to congestive heart failure. If the BNP level is normal, the difficulty in breathing is probably pulmonary, not cardiac.

Treatment Your initial treatment of a patient in cardiogenic shock must focus on stabilization. Managing the airway is always of paramount importance. Correct hypoxia as rapidly as possible, and obtain vascular access. If an acute myocardial infarction has occurred, administer aspirin and heparin unless a contraindication exists. Use nitroglycerin and morphine only if the patient has an adequate blood pressure. Although beta-blockers may be used in myocardial infarction, they are inappropriate in cardiogenic shock until the patient has been stabilized.

If hypotension is present, consider initiating small isotonic fluid challenges, about 250 mL each, before progressing to a dopamine infusion. Fluid must be administered cautiously, especially if high central venous pressure or pulmonary edema is present. Initiate dopamine, and titrate to effect. To limit the spike in heart rate dopamine often causes, administer the lowest effective dose. If tachycardia is present with hypotension, use a norepinephrine or phenylephrine infusion. Use dobutamine and/or milrinone if the patient's systolic blood pressure is 80 to 100 mm Hg. Emergency treatment of cardiogenic shock centers on maintaining the heart's pumping ability without significantly affecting the heart rate. Manage cardiogenic shock with signs of pulmonary congestion by placing the patient in a semi-Fowler's position with the feet dependent unless this causes more severe hypotension. Maintain oxygen saturation at above 95%. Use of continuous positive airway pressure (CPAP) or bilevel positive airway pressure (BiPAP) may assist in relieving pulmonary congestion at the alveolar level but is relatively contraindicated in hypotension. Follow local protocols to guide this decision.

An intraaortic balloon pump may be required to support the heart and promote revascularization of the coronary arteries.

Obstructive Shock

Obstructive shock occurs when blood flow in the great vessels or heart is occluded. Common causes are acute pericardial tamponade, massive pulmonary embolus, and tension pneumothorax. Each of these conditions is discussed in detail in Chapters 3 and 5.

Common signs and symptoms of patients in obstructive shock are shortness of breath, anxiety, tachypnea, and tachycardia. Breath sounds may be diminished if a pulmonary cause is involved. In later stages, the patient becomes hypotensive, and a declining level of consciousness and cyanosis become apparent.

Reversal of obstructive shock requires support of vital functions and removal of the obstruction, so your treatment of the patient will depend on the specific cause of the obstruction. Your initial management should focus on increasing vascular volume with fluid resuscitation and vasopressors as needed to maintain perfusion until a definitive diagnosis and treatment plan can be established.

Cardiac Tamponade

Cardiac tamponade is seen when fluid or blood accumulates in the pericardial sac surrounding the heart, diminishing the heart's ability to function. Trauma, ventricular rupture, and infection are possible causes of cardiac tamponade. The speed of fluid accumulation (blood or effusion) in the pericardium creates either a rapid deterioration with smaller amounts or a slow and chronic presentation with much larger amounts of fluid in the sac. It may help to remember Beck's triad, the classic indicator of cardiac tamponade: jugular venous distention, hypotension, and muffled heart sounds. But this is a late sign, present in only 10% to 40% of patients, and it's difficult to differentiate clinically.

Treatment A tamponade emergency may be treated by pericardiocentesis and inotropic medications but depends on the rate of fluid accumulation and cause.

Pulmonary Embolus

A pulmonary embolus is a life-threatening condition that occurs when a thrombus (a blood clot, cholesterol plaque, or air bubble) travels through the vasculature and lodges in the pulmonary artery. If a large component of the pulmonary vasculature is occluded, reduced blood flow back to the heart decreases cardiac output, resulting in hypoperfusion. A complete discussion of pulmonary embolus can be found in Chapter 5.

Treatment Pulmonary embolus interventions focus on oxygenation and ventilation. Be prepared to support the vasculature with fluids. The primary therapy is systemic anticoagulation with heparin or fractionated heparin medications such as enoxaparin (Lovenox). Thrombolytics may be considered for severe cases with shock.

Tension Pneumothorax

The most treatable cause of obstructive shock is tension pneumothorax. A tension pneumothorax develops when air becomes trapped outside the lung between the visceral and parietal pleura and applies pressure to the contents of the chest cavity. This pressure causes the mediastinum to shift to the unaffected side and interferes with respiration. Pressure and a subsequent torque of the venae cavae diminishes venous return to the heart, in turn leading to inadequate CO.

Although trauma is a common cause of a pneumothorax, the condition can develop spontaneously or as a result of positive-pressure ventilation. Patients with COPD have weakened areas of the lungs and are thus vulnerable to the effects of excessive pressure. Pneumothorax can also be caused by overzealous ventilation in an otherwise healthy patient; patients being ventilated with positive pressure are at increased risk for a tension pneumothorax.

Treatment Needle or tube thoracostomy must be performed on patients with this life-threatening emergency.

Primary Survey

The AMLS assessment pathway for shock is grounded in the conviction that your efficiency in recognizing, evaluating, and managing a patient in shock correlates directly with the likelihood your patient will survive. Initial assessment goals, then, should center on recognizing the presence or potential for hypoperfusion. Obtaining a thorough medical history and physical exam will help you identify shock early in its course. Prompt diagnostic assessment and accurate interpretation of the results will assist you in pinpointing the type of shock you may be dealing with.

Initial Observation

Scene safety is critical in approaching any patient. Chapter 1 includes an in-depth discussion of general scene survey and scene safety considerations. For the patient suspected of being in shock, you must further determine the following:

- Do I see any signs of a life threat as I approach my patient?
- Does the patient's skin show me signs of shock? Pale, gray-appearing, faded.
- Do the surroundings suggest the possibility of shock (vomitus, blood, infectious disease)?

The initial appearance of a prostrate patient who is pale and lethargic should warrant a quick movement to the patient's side to rule out threats to the patient's life, including shock.

Level of Consciousness

Any patient who has an altered LOC or seems anxious, combative, or confused should be evaluated for hypoxia and signs of shock. Assessing the patient using the AVPU mnemonic and the Glasgow Coma Scale can help you determine whether the patient has altered mentation. A look back at Tables 1-2 and 1-3 and the Chapter 1 discussions on these topics will provide a review.

Airway, Breathing, and Circulation

Each patient's treatment evolves as new diagnostic information is discovered. In the patient whose condition is critical, your immediate focus should be on airway, breathing, and circulation until definitive care is reached. If you see or suspect trauma, immediately stabilize the cervical spine in a neutral, in-line position before initiating assessment or treatment.

Once you've completed the initial assessment, you have to decide whether the patient is critically ill, emergent, or stable. Unexplained signs and symptoms of shock indicate possible internal bleeding and warrant immediate transport. Support oxygenation and ventilation, place the patient in a supine position, maintain normothermia, monitor cardiac status, and conduct pulse oximetry and capnography. Be aware that in patients with hemorrhagic shock, pulse oximetry may be unreliable because of the loss of hemoglobin, and the hemoglobin that is present may be fully saturated with oxygen, giving a misleadingly high reading. In such patients, initiate vascular access and provide fluid therapy and/or vasopressors en route to improve perfusion and volume expansion.

Airway

If the patient is unable to maintain a patent airway, you should provide basic airway management until definitive care is achieved, whether that be on scene or en route to the receiving facility. The key is to focus on the patient's needs and meet them in a timely manner. Appendix D and the discussions of establishing and managing the airway in Chapters 1 and 3 offer more details.

Breathing

Once you've secured the patient's airway, you should direct your attention to improving oxygenation. Remember, the oxygen level may drop significantly before symptoms of hypoxia become apparent. A surge in the rate and depth of respiration, often the earliest sign of shock, can be confused with anxiety. Prevention and prompt treatment of early acidosis can greatly improve patient outcome. If the ventilatory rate is slow, shock has reached an advanced state.

Circulation

Circulatory status can be rapidly assessed. Begin by looking for obvious bleeding as you approach the patient. Bloody vomitus or stool should raise suspicion of internal bleeding. Bright red blood in the stool indicates active bleeding from the lower GI tract. Dark red or maroon stool, called *melena,* is due to upper GI bleeding. Dark or black blood in the stool may indicate either old bleeding or the presence of digested blood.

If the patient is unable to speak, ask bystanders what they have witnessed. Then assess the patient's pulses by asking the following questions:

- Are the radial, carotid, and femoral pulses strong, or are they weak and thready?
- Is the rate too fast or too slow?
- Is the rate regular or irregular?

According to the National Association of Emergency Medical Technicians Pre-Hospital Trauma Life Support Committee, the emphasis during the assessment should be on the quality of the pulse (thready versus bounding), rather than on blood pressure. Evaluating pulse quality will give you more information in less time. A weak, thready pulse is an indicator of hypoperfusion. A bounding, strong pulse suggests adequate perfusion. While assessing pulse, note the color and temperature of the skin—peripheral vasoconstriction is common in shock.

Establish appropriate vascular access, and draw blood for laboratory analysis if you can do so without delaying appropriate care. Because metabolism ramps up during shock, glucose can become perilously low without warning. A bedside glucose test should be done if the patient's mental status is altered. Administering fluid boluses is controversial, since overhydration can dilute the blood and elevate blood pressure to a level that will destroy the blood's ability to compensate and clot in hemorrhagic shock. An initial bolus of 1000 to 2000 L of isotonic fluid should be given if the patient shows no signs of fluid overload (e.g., crackles or rales on lung auscultation). The purpose of fluid resuscitation should be to enhance perfusion to maintain MAP at 60 to 70 or systolic pressure at 80 to 90 mm Hg.

In the hospital setting, urine output should be maintained at a minimum of 0.5 to 1 mL/kg/h in adults (1 to 2 mL/kg/h in children) who do not have kidney disease. Urine output is an important metric, since it indicates renal perfusion. If the patient is at risk for fluid overload, a more modest bolus of 250 to 500 mL, followed by a reassessment, is appropriate. On the other hand, for patients with septic and neurogenic shock and patients with severe non–blood volume loss, such as hyperosmolar hyperglycemic nonketotic syndrome (HHNS), a large volume (5 to 6 L) of crystalloid fluid is often required for initial resuscitation.

Exposure/Environment

You must expose an adequate area of the patient's body to assess properly for further illness or injury. Exposure also allows you to search for clues to the patient's condition, such as surgical wounds or drains, insulin pumps, and other medical devices. You might wish to review this topic in Chapter 1 for tips on protecting the patient's modesty and preventing temperature and other environmental stresses related to body exposure.

Take care to keep the patient warm, since shock causes diminished peripheral perfusion. Shunting of blood to the essential organs, together with the switch to anaerobic metabolism, make it difficult for the patient to retain body heat. Consider administering warmed IV fluids to help maintain the patient's temperature. Any IV fluid that is cooler than normal body temperature will have to be warmed by the patient's body, putting additional demands on an already strained metabolism.

Secondary Survey

The secondary survey consists of determining what type of shock the patient is in, taking a detailed history, and performing diagnostic studies. Vital signs (blood pressure, heart rate, respiratory rate, and temperature) are essential to determining the patient's stability and pinpointing the type of shock. Most types of shock are characterized by hypotension, tachycardia, tachypnea, and cool skin, but there are several exceptions. Because the blood vessels are dilated in distributive shock, the patient will have hypotension and tachycardia, but his skin may be warm. In cardiogenic shock, the patient's heart rate may be bradycardic or tachycardic, depending on the underlying cause. In neurogenic shock, the patient is often both bradycardic and vasodilated. A look back at Types of Shock in this chapter will help you review.

Obtaining a thorough history, including an account of the present illness and a comprehensive past medical history, is essential to determining the type and stage of shock. The AMLS assessment pathway relies on the SAMPLER and OPQRST mnemonics to obtain historical information (see the Rapid Recall boxes in Chapter 1). This historical data, in combination with physical exam findings, will help you modify the diagnosis and select appropriate interventions. Box 4-5 lists hypoperfusion considerations in the patient history, and Table 4-6 details medications affecting shock.

BOX 4-5 Hypoperfusion

HISTORY OF VOLUME LOSS?

- Vomiting
- Diarrhea
- Excessive sweating
- Excessive urination
- Blood loss—internal or external (hemorrhagic)

OBSTRUCTIVE

Tension Pneumothorax

- Breath sounds—decreased on one side
- Jugular venous distension (JVD)
- Increasing respiratory distress

Pulmonary Emboli

- Risk factors
- Sudden onset
- Hypoxia
- Chest pain

Cardiac Tamponade

- Risk factors
- Muffled heart tones
- JVD

DISTRIBUTIVE

Neurogenic

- Cord injury
- Recent trauma
- Flushed skin

Anaphylaxis

- History of exposure to allergen
- Breath sounds—wheezing
- Hives

Sepsis

- History of infection (pneumonia)
- On antibiotics
- Fever (possible)
- Wounds, Foley catheter, drains, IVs, etc.
- Depressed immune system

OTHER

- Toxic exposure
- Drug overdose

CARDIOGENIC

- Cardiac history
- Acute myocardial infarction (AMI)
- 12-lead ECG changes
- Breath sounds—crackles in lungs
- JVD
- Peripheral edema

TABLE 4-6 Medications Affecting Shock

Medication	Effect	Shock
Steroids	May mask signs of infection; decreases potential for early recognition	Sepsis
Beta-blockers	Blocks an increase in heart rate, decreasing ability to compensate	All types
Anticoagulant/antiplatelet	Increases potential for bleeding	Hemorrhagic
Calcium channel blockers	Inhibit vasoconstriction, decreasing ability to compensate	All types
Hypoglycemic agents	May impair blood glucose regulation	All types
Herbal preparations	May contribute to bleeding	Hemorrhagic
	May increase workload on the heart	Cardiogenic specifically, but all types may be affected
Diuretics	Long-term diuretic therapy may cause hypokalemia.	All types

Assessment Tools

Assessment tools used to evaluate patients with signs of shock include monitoring (pulse oximetry, cardiac rhythm, possibly hemodynamic), electrocardiography, and radiographic and laboratory testing. Sometimes end-tidal carbon dioxide ($ETCO_2$) testing is available as an adjunct to monitor acidosis and respiratory status. In the hospital, laboratory studies, computed tomography (CT), ultrasonography, and x-ray studies are essential. Table 4-7 outlines laboratory studies typically used to evaluate patients in shock. Let's take a closer look at some of these tools.

Pulse Oximeter

A pulse oximeter is one of the simplest assessment tools to use. All it requires is placing a sensor on the patient's finger or skin, but despite its apparent straightforwardness, pulse oximetry presents many possibilities for error. A pulse oximeter measures the percentage of gas saturation in hemoglobin, but it can't differentiate between saturation with oxygen and saturation with carbon monoxide unless a specific spectrum analysis by a device made for carbon monoxide detection is used.

If the pulse oximetry monitor doesn't display a waveform, you should question the accuracy of the reading. Above all, patient care should never be delayed or withheld based on a pulse oximetry reading when other signs and symptoms indicate poor tissue perfusion.

Electrocardiogram

An ECG is helpful in assessing heart rhythm, ischemia, injury, and certain electrolyte abnormalities. Leads must be properly placed, the findings interpreted or transmitted, and the results used to guide transport of the patient to an appropriate healthcare institution. A multilead, diagnostic ECG should be completed in the secondary exam but early enough to help determine the patient's destination for definitive care (e.g., cardiac catheterization and intervention lab).

Radiographs

X-rays have limited usefulness in shock but can be used in the ED to quickly assess associated conditions such as fractures and chest abnormalities.

Computed Tomography

CT is a common radiologic imaging technique that can be rapidly performed in the ED. It offers a noninvasive, accurate diagnostic method of gathering more precise information about a range of internal reasons for signs and symptoms of shock: aortic aneurysms, GI obstructions, pulmonary emboli, hemorrhages, tumors, and cysts, to name a few.

Ultrasonography

An ultrasound is a noninvasive imaging study that can be performed at the bedside. High-frequency sound waves are emitted to penetrate the heart or abdominal organs, and the reflected sound waves allow internal structures to be visualized.

Ultrasonography can be useful for rapid assessment of the chest and/or abdomen when bleeding or other critical threats are suspected. It can be used to visualize the heart, lungs, and key abdominal areas when the patient shows signs of shock. Performing ultrasonography and accurately interpreting the findings requires a high degree of skill, however, and the test is not available in all emergency resuscitation areas.

Complications of Shock

Acute Renal Failure

During shock, blood is initially shunted from the least vital organs to the brain and heart. Because blood flow to the kidneys is reduced, acute renal failure is a common sequela. If circulation is impaired for too long, cellular dysfunction can be permanent. More specifically, if the

TABLE 4-7 Laboratory Tests for Patients in Shock

	Normal Values	Abnormal Values	Indications for Test
Glucose	70–110 mg/dL (3.8–6.1 mmol/L)	↑ Indicates hyperglycemia, diabetic ketoacidosis, steroid use, stress ↓ Indicates hypoglycemia, decreased reserves	All types of shock
Hemoglobin/ hematocrit	Hb, male: 14–18 g/dL (8.7–11.2 mmol/L) Hb, female: 12–16 g/dL (7.4–9.9 mmol/L) Hct, male: 42%–52% (0.42–0.52 SI) Hct, female: 37%–47% (0.37–0.47 SI)	↓ Indicates severe blood loss ↑ Indicates plasma loss, dehydration	All types of shock
Gastric/stool hemoglobin	Negative	+ Indicates GI bleeding	Suspected GI bleeding
Lactic acid	Venous: 5–20 mg/dL (0.6–2.2 mmol/L)	↑ Indicates tissue hypoperfusion and acidosis, prolonged use of tourniquet	All types of shock
Complete blood cell count	Total WBC count 5000–10,000/mm^3 (5–10 × 10^9/L)	↑ Excessive WBC count indicates sepsis.	More important in septic shock
Acid-base balance	pH 7.35–7.45	↑ pH indicates alkalosis ↓ pH indicates acidosis and impaired perfusion	All types of shock
	HCO_3 21–28 mEq/L	↓ Bicarbonate indicates it is being lost or used up rapidly. Diarrhea, intestinal fistula, or in response to increased acid such as renal failure, DKA, salicylate overdose ↑ Bicarbonate indicates excessive intake of bicarbonate or antacids, lactate administration, or loss of acid in conditions such as vomiting, gastric suctioning, low potassium, diuretics.	
Arterial blood gases	PCO_2 35–45 mm Hg PO_2 80–100 mm Hg	↑ PCO_2 indicates CO_2 retention, hypoventilation, pneumonia, pulmonary infections, pulmonary emboli, CHF, condition that impairs respiratory effort. ↓ PCO_2 indicates decrease in CO_2, hyperventilation, anxiety, fear, pain, CNS lesions, pregnancy, conditions that increase respiratory ventilation. ↓ O_2 indicates hypoxia.	All types of shock
Serum electrolytes	Na 136–145 mEq/L (136–145 mmol/L) K 3.5–5 mEq/L (3.5–5 mmol/L)	↑ Na may be present with osmotic diuresis. ↑ K is common in acidosis, vomiting, diarrhea, and DKA. ↑ K may cause abnormal ECG; peaked T waves may be present.	All types of shock
Renal function	BUN 10–20 mg/dL (3.6–7.1 mmol/L) Creatinine 0.5–1.2 mg/dl (44–97 mmol/L)	↑ BUN indicates severe dehydration, shock, sepsis ↑ Serum creatinine indicates >4 mg/dL (0.2 mmol/L) Indicates impaired renal function	All types of shock
Blood/urine cultures	Negative	+ Indicates infection	Septic shock

BUN, Blood urea nitrogen; *CHF,* congestive heart failure; *CNS,* central nervous system; *CO_2,* carbon dioxide; *DKA,* diabetic ketoacidosis; *ECG,* electrocardiogram; *GI,* gastrointestinal; *Hb,* hemoglobin; *Hct,* hematocrit; *K,* potassium; *Na,* sodium; *PCO_2,* partial pressure of carbon dioxide; *PO_2,* partial pressure of oxygen (oxygen saturation); *WBC,* white blood cell.
From Pagana KD, Pagana TJ: Mosby's diagnostic and laboratory test reference, ed 9, St Louis, 2009, Mosby.

renal tubules receive insufficient quantities of oxygen for more than perhaps 45 to 60 minutes—depending on the individual—irreversible damage is done. This phenomenon is known as *acute tubular necrosis*. Once kidney failure occurs, the body can no longer remove electrolytes, acids, or excess fluid from the bloodstream, so dialysis will be required either temporarily or indefinitely.

Acute Respiratory Distress Syndrome or Acute Lung Injury

During shock, capillary permeability allows proteins, fluid, and blood cells to exit the capillaries and collect in the alveoli, thereby impairing ventilation and adequate oxygenation. Inflammation and diffuse alveolar injury

BOX 4-6 Causes of Disseminated Intravascular Coagulation

ACUTE CAUSES

- Abruptio placentae or eclampsia in pregnant women
- Massive transfusions
- Obstructive jaundice
- Acute liver failure
- Aortic balloon pump
- Burns
- Trauma

CHRONIC CAUSES

- Cardiovascular disease
- Autoimmune disease
- Hematologic disorder
- Inflammatory disorder
- HIV/AIDS

HIV/AIDS, Human immunodeficiency virus/acquired immunodeficiency syndrome.
From McCance KL, Huether SE: Pathophysiology: the biologic basis for disease in adults and children, ed 6, St Louis, 2010, Mosby.

cause widespread edema in the lungs. Other mediators released by neutrophils cause pulmonary vasoconstriction. This constellation of events is known as *acute respiratory distress syndrome (ARDS)* or *acute lung injury (ALI)*. It can have many causes other than shock, including pneumonia, aspiration, pancreatitis, and drug overdose. Despite advances in treatment, the syndrome continues to carry a high mortality rate. If the patient does survive, he or she may require mechanical ventilation for an extended period. An in-depth discussion of ARDS/ALI is offered in Chapter 3.

Coagulopathies

Late shock can trigger an overstimulation of the clotting cascade in which clotting and bleeding begin to occur simultaneously. This condition is known as **disseminated intravascular coagulation (DIC).** In this pathologic clotting presentation, RBCs and other debris occlude the vessels, and they become ischemic distal to the blockage. Platelets bind where the blood is pooling, further promoting viscosity. Clotting factors that are normally present are rapidly exhausted. The widespread clots advance ischemia. In the pathologic bleeding presentation of DIC, hemorrhage begins as the coagulation components are broken down and the fibrinolytic system is activated. This complex condition can be acute or chronic.

Manifestations include rapid development of hemorrhage (e.g., oozing from venipuncture sites and bruising), shock that is more severe than is consistent with the apparent amount of blood loss, and a positive D-dimer lab test. Microvascular clotting may present with signs of ischemia in distal tissues. In isolation, standard laboratory coagulation tests, such as prothrombin time and partial thromboplastin time (PT/PTT), are unreliable. A low platelet count, prolonged thrombin time, and a low fibrinogen level in addition to a prolonged PT/PTT paint a more convincing diagnostic picture.

Treatment depends on the cause of DIC and will vary among patients. Management goals, though, are generally to reduce bleeding, discourage excess coagulation, and improve perfusion by eliminating the underlying etiology and restoring homeostasis. Causes of DIC are listed in Box 4-6.

Hepatic Dysfunction

Liver failure, as evidenced by persistently elevated liver enzymes, glucose abnormalities (hyper- or hypoglycemia), unremitting lactic acidosis, and jaundice may occur if shock is left untreated. The liver is essential in any shock state because of its ability to regulate glucose (which the body converts to energy) and manufacture clotting factors (which are important in healing from injury). But the liver can become ischemic as blood is shunted to more essential organs. Elevated hepatic transaminase levels and a serum bilirubin of >2 mg/dL (18 μmol/L [SI units]) indicate dysfunction. Liver failure is typically a late development that may be prevented with efficient early care.

Multiple Organ Dysfunction Syndrome

An uncontrolled inflammatory response can set in motion a progressive sequential dysfunction of interdependent organ systems. This calamitous condition, first recognized in the 1970s, is known as *multiple organ dysfunction syndrome (MODS)*. It typically occurs in response to injury or severe illness and carries a grim prognosis. In fact, it's the leading cause of death in intensive care units, with a mortality rate as high as 54% if only two organ systems have failed. Mortality is 100% if five organ systems have collapsed.

Sepsis and septic shock are the most common causes of MODS, but it can be brought on by any pathologic process that initiates a massive systemic inflammatory response. It's often precipitated by severe trauma, major surgery, acute pancreatitis, acute renal failure, ARDS, and the presence of necrotic tissue (e.g., eschar in a patient with burns). Older adults, those with preexisting medical disease, and those with extensive tissue damage are at the

BOX 4-7 Stages of Multiple Organ Dysfunction Syndrome

Multiple organ dysfunction syndrome (MODS) can be divided into primary and secondary stages. Primary MODS is evident immediately after a discrete insult such as chest trauma or overwhelming infection. Diminished perfusion is local and generalized, making it difficult to detect. A low-grade fever, tachypnea, dyspnea, acute respiratory distress syndrome (ARDS), altered mental status, and hypermetabolism may be present. Cardiovascular signs include tachycardia, increased systemic vascular resistance, and increased cardiac output (CO). Gastrointestinal indicators include abdominal distention, ascites, paralytic ileus, upper and lower gastrointestinal bleeding, diarrhea, ischemic colitis, and decreased bowel sounds. Jaundice, right upper quadrant pain, and elevated serum ammonia and liver enzyme levels indicate hepatic involvement.

A latent period occurs after the initial insult. Then, as macrophages and neutrophils are activated in response to the initial organ dysfunction, organs unaffected by the original insult begin to collapse. This systemic response constitutes secondary MODS. As the vascular endothelium becomes dysfunctional, coagulation and fibrin cascades are touched off, causing disseminated intravascular coagulation and thrombocytopenia. This systemic response leads to uncontrolled hypermetabolism, increased capillary permeability, and vasodilation. CO drops, and tissue perfusion becomes progressively more impaired as the imbalance between oxygen supply and demand widens. Ultimately, tissue hypoxia, myocardial dysfunction, and metabolic failure result in widespread total organ dysfunction.

greatest risk for MODS. The two broad stages of MODS are described in Box 4-7.

AMLS Management Summary

When assessing a patient, always consider the possibility of trauma, and protect the cervical spine if you suspect the patient may have been injured. Proper positioning depends on initial complaints and symptoms. If a patient is unable to tolerate the supine position because of respiratory distress or intolerable pain—or for any other reason—place the head as low as can be tolerated to ease the heart's workload and enhance perfusion.

Historically, hypotensive patients were transported in Trendelenburg position (head lower than the heart), but this older practice is not supported by contemporary research. In fact, such a position can negatively affect ventilatory status because the contents of the abdominal cavity apply pressure to the diaphragm.

To ensure adequate perfusion, optimal oxygenation must be maintained. Many patients become hypoxic before the symptoms of shock are overt. All critically ill or injured patients should receive oxygen through a nonrebreather mask. If the respiratory rate is inadequate, you may need to deliver 100% oxygen through a bag-valve device. If these measures are ineffective, consider using advanced airway techniques such as intubation.

Begin maintaining the patient's circulatory status by stopping any obvious bleeding. Although hemorrhagic hypovolemic shock is one of the most common types of shock, it's not the only cause of hypoperfusion. Most perfusion problems have complex causes that aren't simple to reverse, so your treatment may be limited to symptomatic care until the underlying etiology can be addressed at the receiving facility. Initiate vascular access, but don't let it delay transporting a gravely ill patient to definitive care.

Fluid Resuscitation

Initiate isotonic crystalloid fluid in patients with hypovolemic shock, but be mindful that it may be insufficient because it doesn't carry oxygen, hemoglobin, clotting factors, or any other essential blood components. Also remember that isotonic crystalloid fluid works as a temporary volume expander, but if too much is administered, the existing blood volume will become more dilute, compounding the edema that's already present.

Colloids, whole blood, packed RBCs, fresh frozen plasma, platelets, Dextran, and albumin are other volume expanders. Blood products replace blood volume while offering the additional advantage of oxygen-carrying capacity, but the presence of antibodies in human blood presents some risk. Ideally, type compatibility between the patient and the donor will have been established, diminishing the risk of an infusion reaction. In an emergent situation, uncrossmatched type O-negative blood can be given.

Dextran is a synthetic volume expander. It stays in the vessels longer than isotonic fluid, but it has no oxygen-carrying capability. Albumin is a human blood product that does not require typing or crossmatching, but it too has no oxygen-carrying capacity.

Temperature Regulation

The body expends a great deal of energy maintaining normothermia. Vasoconstriction shunts blood away from peripheral tissues, and the body will expend valuable energy trying to stay warm. To help the patient conserve metabolic reserves, try to keep him warm. The ambulance or the room should be kept very warm, and the patient should be covered with a blanket when practical. This can be difficult during assessment and physical examination, but it should be a high priority.

TABLE 4-8 Blood Products

Product	Clinical Application
Packed red blood cells (RBCs)	Low hemoglobin (usually <7.0)
Platelets	Prevent bleeding Thrombocytopenia
Fresh frozen plasma (FFP)	Coagulation deficiencies in liver failure, warfarin overdose, disseminated intravascular coagulation, or massive transfusion
Cryoprecipitate (cold FFP with fibrinogen, Factor VIII, and von Willebrand factor)	For bleeding disorder, massive transfusion
Massive transfusion	Aggressively bleeding patients where >10 units of blood given over 24 hours; coagulation factors and platelets added. Patient at risk for hypothermia, hypocalcemia.

BOX 4-8 Vasoconstrictors and Inotropes

VASOCONSTRICTORS

- Epinephrine
- Norepinephrine
- Dopamine
- Phenylephrine
- Vasopressin

INOTROPES

- Dopamine
- Dobutamine
- Epinephrine
- Isoproterenol
- Norepinephrine

Vasopressors in Hypoperfusion

Vasopressors are an efficient adjunct in patients with certain types of hypoperfusion. In cardiogenic shock, the heart isn't functioning effectively, and inotropic agents can improve CO by bolstering cardiac contractility and raising blood pressure. Distributive shock, especially neurogenic shock, is characterized by hypotension and bradycardia. Although volume replacement can be helpful, vasopressors may be required to arouse the responsiveness of the veins, and atropine may be needed to spur the heart rate. Box 4-8 lists vasoconstrictors and inotropes.

Administration of Blood Products

When the patient is considered anemic, in shock, or has a serious bleeding disorder, administration of blood products is indicated. As already noted, the overriding goal of a blood product transfusion is to increase the blood's oxygen-carrying capacity. Selection of the different blood products available will depend on the patient's underlying condition.

If blood products were stored as whole blood, the shelf life would be very brief, and the platelets within would deactivate quickly. The preferred process is to separate the blood components out and provide specific products with longer shelf life. For blood transfusions, packed red blood cells (PRBCs) are generally used. These packed cells have 80% of the plasma removed and a preservative added. Table 4-8 describes available blood products and their clinical applications.

Transfusion Reactions

There are generally two complications of blood product administration: infection and immune reactions. Improved methods of screening donors and blood products have decreased problems with the spread of infections. There remains a small risk, especially for cytomegalovirus (CMV), which is a common virus that is rarely serious in the general population. Some pathogens can infect blood even during cold storage.

Hemolytic Reactions When the recipient's antibodies recognize and react to transfused blood as an antigen, the donor RBCs are destroyed or hemolyzed. This hemolytic reaction can be quick and aggressive or slower, depending on the immune response.

Errors in the blood administration process can create fatal hemolytic reactions. When this occurs, most transfused cells are destroyed in an overwhelming immune response. When an immune response occurs, the coagulation cascade is also engaged, potentially creating bleeding disorders like DIC. With DIC and anaphylactic response, symptoms may include back pain, IV site pain, headache, chills and fever, hypotension, dyspnea, tachycardia, bronchospasm, pulmonary edema, coagulopathic bleeding, and renal failure.

At the first sign of transfusion reaction, the blood products must be stopped and appropriate lab analysis completed. Immediate supportive treatment is instituted and the blood bank notified. Every institution that credentials personnel to administer blood products has strict policies and procedures that guide the provider in these cases.

Febrile Transfusion Reactions During the transfusion or shortly thereafter, fever may develop that is usually responsive to antipyretics. Those patients prone to febrile reactions may be given diphenhydramine and acetaminophen as the transfusion is begun.

Allergic Transfusion Reaction An onset of hives and/or rash is usually self-limiting during transfusion of blood products, but some will progress to bronchospasm and anaphylaxis. Treatment may include antihistamines.

Transfusion-Related Acute Lung Injury Transfusion-related acute lung injury (TRALI) is a rare but complex immune response during or after transfusion, with subsequent development of noncardiogenic pulmonary edema, or ARDS/ALI, described earlier in this chapter and at length in Chapter 3.

Hypervolemia

For those patients with limited cardiovascular reserve (elderly, infants), transfusion of blood products can increase circulating volume and create problems for the patient's cardiovascular system with symptoms of dyspnea, hypoxia, and pulmonary edema.

Bleeding Disorders

In the earlier discussion of the cardiovascular system, blood was described in overview. Although the following disorders do not commonly cause shock, blood dyscrasias are an important subject within any medical emergencies topic. Disorders of platelets and hemophilia are presented next.

Thrombocytopenia

Platelets are irregularly shaped, colorless blood components that have sticky surfaces that, when joined with other agents (calcium, vitamin K, fibrinogen), form fibrin. Fibrin is a weblike mesh that traps more blood cells, creating a clot. When a bleeding disorder occurs in the body, platelet dysfunction is usually at fault.

Bleeding disorders cause problems when platelet numbers are decreased (decreased production or destruction) or platelets become dysfunctional. The disease is generally known as *thrombocytopenia*. Other disorders of bleeding can occur when part of the clotting cascade is disrupted because of a lack of specific clotting factors. Let's first briefly review platelet disorders.

Decreased Platelets

When platelets are not produced in adequate numbers or are destroyed, small bleeding episodes may occur. These usually present with petechiae (especially in the legs) and purpura. Petechiae are small (1 to 2 mm) red-purple, point-sized dots in the skin; they are not raised (nonpalpable). Petechiae indicate capillary leakage into the skin. Purpura are larger areas of capillary leakage that appear first as red, then purple, non-raised blotches and occur in clumps. When you press a purpuric area with your finger, it does not blanch (turn paler).

Conditions that cause a decreased platelet count may progress, if severe enough, to create bleeding emergencies. If you encounter a patient whose presenting signs and symptoms include bleeding (gums, nose, GI) for no obvious reason and petechiae and purpura, check the patient's medications and family history for bleeding episodes, and make sure blood is analyzed for platelet levels. Table 4-9 lists some conditions and drugs that may lead to thrombocytopenia.

Idiopathic Thrombocytopenic Purpura Idiopathic thrombocytopenic purpura (ITP) was so named because its cause was unknown, but it is now thought to be an autoimmune disorder. ITP rapidly destroys platelets and creates the characteristic thrombocytopenic bleeding disorder presentation already described. On closer examination of this patient, bone marrow will be normal, but antiplatelet antibodies may be detected. When the disorder begins, the bone marrow and immune system will attempt to keep up platelet production to keep bleeding under control. Steroid therapy is the common management technique for ITP.

TABLE 4-9 Causes of Thrombocytopenia

CAUSES OF DECREASED PRODUCTION OF PLATELETS	
Aplastic anemia	
Bone marrow disease (leukemia)	
Hereditary syndromes:	
Alport syndrome	
Bernard-Soulier syndrome (large platelets)	
Decreased production of thrombopoietin related to liver failure	
Viral/bacterial infection (sepsis)	
Medication induced:	
Glycoprotein inhibitors	Quinidine
Heparin	Sulfonamide antibiotics
Interferons, chemotherapy	Vancomycin
Measles/mumps/rubella vaccine	Valproic acid
CAUSES OF INCREASED DESTRUCTION OF PLATELETS	
Hemolytic-uremic syndrome (HUS)	
Disseminated intravascular coagulation (DIC)	
Systemic lupus erythematosus (SLE)	
Posttransfusion purpura	
Thrombotic/idiopathic thrombocytopenic purpura	
Viral infections (human immunodeficiency virus, mumps, chickenpox)	

Poor-Quality Platelets

When platelets become dysfunctional, bleeding times are prolonged, and signs of bleeding may become aggressive. Liver, spleen, and kidney disease may cause this type of thrombocytopenia. When chronic liver failure occurs, portal hypertension develops, where the pressure in the abdominal cavity is high. This can cause a backup of pressures into the spleen. Congestive hypersplenism and a pooling of blood in the spleen, called *splenic sequestration,* may occur. Treatment includes transfusion of platelets and (occasionally) splenectomy.

Hemophilia

The cascade of interlocking steps called *coagulation* involves both a cellular (platelets) and a protein (coagulation factor) component. This chain reaction begins as soon as a blood vessel is injured. Hemophilia is a bleeding disorder that occurs when there is a deficiency of one of the coagulation factors in the cascade. There are three main types of hemophilia:

1. Factor VIII (hemophilia A)—most common in the United States
2. Factor IX (hemophilia B), also called *Christmas disease*
3. von Willebrand disease

Hemophilia A and B present very similarly in the clinical setting. Affected patients usually have a bleeding disorder history in the family or, if new in onset, early and severe bleeding is experienced with minor trauma, especially in the joints and muscles. There is a common pattern to the bleeding in the patient's history as well. Bleeding into the joints is very common and leads to subsequent joint damage. Bleeding into the muscle body can cause compartment syndrome, and bleeding into the mouth can progress rapidly to airway compromise. Central nervous system bleeding may present as a new-onset headache with localized neurologic signs.

Treatment of hemophilia A and B entails factor replacement in those patients with known disease. Patients should carry at least one dose with them at all times, and as an EMS responder, you should remember to ask about this medication if your history taking uncovers a diagnosed bleeding disorder. Pain control is also a treatment goal but the provider should try to avoid intramuscular injection of analgesics.

von Willebrand Disease

A congenital inherited bleeding disorder, von Willebrand disease is characterized by missing or deficient von Willebrand factor, which like other clotting factors helps platelets stick or clump together. These patients have similar presentations to patients with hemophilia A and may have abnormal menstrual bleeding, bleeding of the gums, epistaxis, bruising, and petechiae. Treatment includes use of the synthetic hormone desmopressin (1-deamino-8-D-arginine-vasopressin [DDAVP]).

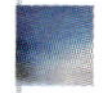

Special Considerations

The Older Adult Patient

Older adults are living longer and staying more active into their later years. Paradoxically, living longer gives a person more opportunities to become severely ill or injured.

The use of medications to control chronic disease states can complicate both the body's ability to save itself and our ability to recognize disorders such as shock. Platelet-inhibiting drugs can cause bleeding even when therapeutic levels are present; for example, a patient may develop a GI bleed. Excessive bleeding may result if too much is taken or if trauma occurs. Because platelet-inhibiting drugs affect the body's ability to stop bleeding, it is important to identify these or any drugs that may prolong bleeding and understand their potential to contribute to shock. Recognizing the need to control bleeding and possibly reverse the effects of certain drugs with antagonists or blood products is part of early intervention. Ask older patients whether they take any of the common drugs that inhibit platelet activity, including acetylsalicylic acid (aspirin) and clopidogrel (Plavix). Many older adults are also on anticoagulation therapy with warfarin (Coumadin.)

Some antihypertensive and vasoactive drugs limit the ability of the heart to increase its rate in response to a shock state. Beta-blockers and calcium channel blockers are two examples of medications that may keep the patient's heart rate low despite normal compensation mechanisms that would create tachycardia.

Other factors can complicate the early diagnosis of shock in an older adult patient. As a person ages, pulmonary and cardiac reserves diminish. The alveoli stiffen, and tidal volume becomes shallower. Resting CO declines, as does the basal metabolic rate. Shock-related compensatory mechanisms are more sluggish and less effective. The amount of adipose tissue decreases, muscle mass begins to atrophy, and it becomes more difficult to maintain body heat.

The Pregnant Patient

In caring for a pregnant patient, you must be cognizant that the survival of two patients depends on maintaining adequate perfusion. Pregnancy normally lasts about 40 weeks, and a woman's body undergoes tremendous changes during that time. The maternal heart rate accelerates by 10 to 15 bpm to compensate for the additional perfusion demands of the fetus. Blood volume expands by almost 1.5 times, and CO surges by 30%.

As the fetus grows, it places additional pressure on the internal organs, diaphragm, and vena cava. Because of the increased CO and intravascular volume, signs of hypoperfusion in a pregnant patient may be delayed. Vascular changes attributable to pregnancy can mask early signs of shock.

During the second half of pregnancy, position the patient left-lateral recumbent to avoid hypotension caused by pressure on the vena cava. Maintain adequate oxygenation, and initiate IV fluid therapy.

Putting It All Together

Early, accurate identification of the patient's stage and type of shock is essential in managing this condition. Seasoned clinical reasoning skills, a thorough assessment, and judicious interpretation of diagnostic findings are necessary to provide effective treatment for the patient in shock.

SCENARIO SOLUTION

1 **Differential diagnoses may include sepsis related to pneumonia or urinary tract infection, tension pneumothorax, pulmonary embolism, or pericardial tamponade.**

2 **To narrow your differential diagnosis, you'll need to complete the history of past and present illness. Perform a physical exam that includes assessment for jugular venous distention, tracheal deviation, muffled heart sounds, pulsus paradoxus, capnography, and body temperature.**

3 **The patient has signs of shock and hypoxia. Take immediate measures to secure his airway and administer oxygen. If tension pneumothorax is suspected, decompress the chest. Establish vascular access, and administer IV fluids. Monitor ECG and obtain a 12-lead ECG. Transport to the closest appropriate healthcare facility. During transport, it is important to relay to the facility if sepsis or SIRS is suspected, since some facilities are beginning sepsis intervention based on EMS findings.**

SUMMARY

- Understanding inadequate tissue perfusion requires a thorough knowledge of the anatomy, physiology, and pathophysiology of shock.
- Shock is a progressive state of cellular hypoperfusion in which too little oxygen is available to meet tissue demands in multiple organ systems.
- The three primary stages of shock are compensatory, decompensated, and irreversible.
- The three main determinants of cellular perfusion are CO, intravascular volume, and vascular capacitance.
- CO is determined by stroke volume and heart rate.
- The four primary determinants of stroke volume are preload, afterload, contractility, and synchrony.
- Mean arterial blood pressure is an indirect and often inaccurate indicator of tissue perfusion.
- Blood transports oxygen to and wastes from the body's cells. Hemoglobin, an iron-containing protein in RBCs, carries oxygen to the tissues.
- Underlying chronic medical illnesses, age, obesity, and immunosuppression adversely affect compensatory mechanisms of shock.
- Compensatory mechanisms include increasing minute ventilation, increasing CO, and vasoconstriction.
- The types of shock are hypovolemic, obstructive, distributive, and cardiogenic.
- When the body no longer has ample oxygen, and cells begin producing lactic acid as a byproduct of anaerobic metabolism, metabolic acidosis sets in.
- During the ischemic phase of shock, perfusion of the brain, heart, lungs, and liver is enhanced, while less essential organs become ischemic.
- Altered LOC, anxiousness, combativeness, and confusion may be early signs of shock.
- Most types of shock are characterized by hypotension, tachycardia, tachypnea, and cool skin. In distributive shock, however, the skin may be warm. Bradycardia can accompany cardiogenic or neurogenic shock.
- Assessment tools used to evaluate patients suspected of being in shock include pulse oximetry, electrocardiography, serum glucose testing, and end-tidal carbon dioxide testing. In the hospital, laboratory studies, CT, ultrasonography, and x-ray studies are used.
- Complications of shock include acute renal failure, ARDS, coagulopathies, hepatic dysfunction, and MODS.
- Initial treatment of shock consists of supportive measures, fluid resuscitation, temperature regulation, and administration of vasopressors. Specific interventions are based on the underlying cause.

BIBLIOGRAPHY

Aehlert B: Paramedic practice today: above and beyond, St Louis, 2010, Mosby/JEMS.

American College of Surgeons: ATLS student course manual, 8e, Chicago, 2008, American College of Surgeons.

Berne RM, et al: Berne & Levy physiology, ed 6, St Louis, 2008, Mosby.

Cairns CB: Rude unhinging of the machinery of life: metabolic approaches to hemorrhagic shock. Curr Opin Crit Care 7(6):437–443, 2001.

Centers for Disease Control and Prevention: Universal precautions for prevention of transmission of HIV and other blood-borne infections. Modified February 5, 1999. www.cdc.gov/ncidod/dhqp/bp_universal_precautions.html. Accessed October 16, 2009.

Copstead-Kirkhorn LE, Banasik JL: Pathophysiology, Philadelphia, 2010, Saunders.

Darovic GO: Handbook of hemodynamic monitoring, ed 2, Philadelphia, 2004, Saunders.

Gaugler MH: A unifying system: does the vascular endothelium have a role to play in multi-organ failure following radiation exposure? Br J Radiol 78:100–105, 2005.

Hamilton GC: Emergency medicine: an approach to clinical problem-solving, ed 2, Philadelphia, 2003, Saunders.

Hudak CM, Gallo BM, Morton PG: Critical care nursing: a holistic approach, ed 7, Philadelphia, 1998, Lippincott.

Kragh JF Jr, et al: Survival with emergency tourniquet use to stop bleeding in major limb trauma, Ann Surg 249:1–7, 2009.

McCance KL, Huether SE: Pathophysiology: the biologic basis for disease in adults & children, ed 5, St Louis, 2006, Mosby.

Miller RD, et al: Miller's anesthesia, ed 7, Philadelphia, 2009, Churchill Livingstone.

National Association of Emergency Medical Technicians (U.S.), Pre-Hospital Trauma Life Support Committee & Trauma, American College of Surgeons: PHTLS prehospital trauma life support, St Louis, 2007, Mosby/JEMS.

Pagana KP: Mosby's diagnostic and laboratory test reference, ed 9, St Louis, 2008, Mosby.

Patton KT, Thibodeau GA: Anatomy & physiology, ed 7, St Louis, 2010, Mosby.

Rosen P, et al: Rosen's emergency medicine: concepts and clinical practice, ed 6, St Louis, 2006, Mosby.

Solomon EP: Introduction to human anatomy and physiology, ed 3, Philadelphia, 2009, Saunders.

Swan KG Jr, et al: Tourniquets revisited, J Trauma 66:672–679, 2009.

Tintinalli JE, Kellen GD, Stapczynski S, et al: Tintinalli's emergency medicine: a comprehensive study guide, ed 6, The American College of Emergency Physicians, New York, 2003, McGraw-Hill.

University of Maryland Shock Trauma Center: R Adams Cowley Shock Trauma Center: Tribute to R Adams Cowley, MD. www.umm.edu/shocktrauma/history.htm. Accessed October 11, 2009.

Urden LD, Stacy KM, Lough ME: Thelan's critical care nursing: diagnosis and management, ed 5, St Louis, 2006, Mosby.

Chapter Review Questions

1. A 25-year-old woman was involved in a motor vehicle collision. Her initial vital signs were BP 122/80 mm Hg, P 128 bpm, R 20 breaths/min. Which of the following findings on repeat assessment would indicate that she is developing shock?
- **a.** End-tidal CO_2 35 mm Hg
- **b.** Heart rate 118 bpm
- **c.** Mean arterial pressure 86 mm Hg
- **d.** Pulse pressure 32 mm Hg

2. Which gland is responsible for some of the vasoconstriction in shock?
- **a.** Thymus
- **b.** Pancreas
- **c.** Pituitary
- **d.** Thyroid

3. The primary mechanism for septic shock is:
- **a.** Acute loss of intravascular volume
- **b.** Direct myocardial depression from endotoxins
- **c.** Suppression of normal compensatory mechanisms
- **b.** Widespread inflammatory response

4. A 24-year-old male was injured in a shallow diving incident. Which assessment finding would you anticipate if he is developing neurogenic shock?
- **a.** Blood pressure 102/88 mm Hg
- **b.** Heart rate 58 bpm
- **c.** Oxygen saturation 90%
- **d.** Pale, cool extremities

5. Which intervention for a patient in shock prevents an increase in myocardial oxygen demand?
- **a.** Administer oxygen by facemask.
- **b.** Maintain normal body temperature.
- **c.** Place the patient in Trendelenburg position.
- **d.** Start a vasopressor infusion.

6. Which diagnostic test most accurately assesses the presence and magnitude of anaerobic metabolism?
- **a.** Capnography
- **b.** Hemoglobin
- **c.** Lactic acid
- **d.** Serum potassium

7. Which patient is at highest risk for nontraumatic obstructive shock?
- **a.** 6-month-old with pneumonia
- **b.** 22-year-old who is 38 weeks pregnant
- **c.** 45-year-old female with right upper quadrant pain
- **d.** 67-year-old who has black tarry stools

8. A 19-year-old female is flushed, itchy, and wheezing after eating crab legs. Her vital signs are BP 90/64 mm Hg, P 128 bpm, R 24 breaths/min. Which intervention is indicated first?
- **a.** Albuterol updraft
- **b.** Diphenhydramine intravenous
- **c.** Epinephrine intramuscular
- **d.** Normal saline bolus

9. A 62-year-old male is vomiting coffee-ground emesis. Which of his home medicines may make it more difficult to control his bleeding?
   a. Acetaminophen
   b. Furosemide
   c. Hydrochlorothiazide
   d. Plavix

10. Shock related to tension pneumothorax is most directly secondary to:
   a. Decreased preload
   b. Hypovolemia
   c. Hypoxemia
   d. Pressure on the heart

CHAPTER

5 Chest Discomfort

THE COMPLAINT OF CHEST DISCOMFORT is a common reason for adults to seek medical attention each year. Chest pain is not only the most common presenting medical complaint, it can also be a symptom of a life-threatening medical emergency. In this chapter, we'll help you to quickly assess the causes, from life-threatening to nonemergent, by categorizing this common symptom into the three possible systems affected: cardiovascular, pulmonary, and gastrointestinal. We'll provide further descriptions to help you make an accurate field diagnosis, develop a treatment plan, and monitor the patient in order to adapt treatment as necessary.

Learning Objectives

At the completion of this chapter, you will be able to:

1. Apply your knowledge of anatomy, physiology, and pathophysiology to patients presenting with chest discomfort.
2. Use history collection and physical exam skills to direct the assessment for patients with chest discomfort.
3. Apply your knowledge of disease processes and the information obtained from the patient presentation, history, and physical to form a list of diagnoses based on the degree of life threat (life threatening, critical, emergent, and nonemergent diagnoses).
4. Manage patients with chest discomfort by making clinical decisions, performing diagnostic tests, and using the results to modify care as indicated. Decision making includes routing the patient to the correct resources and following accepted practice guidelines.
5. Provide an ongoing assessment of the chest discomfort patient to confirm or rule out potential diagnoses and adapt treatment and management based on patient response and findings.

Key Terms

acute coronary syndrome (ACS) An umbrella term that covers any group of clinical symptoms consistent with acute myocardial ischemia (chest pain due to insufficient blood supply to the heart muscle that results from coronary artery disease). ACS covers clinical conditions ranging from unstable angina to ST-segment elevation myocardial infarction (STEMI) and non–ST-segment elevation myocardial infarction (NSTEMI).

acute myocardial infarction (AMI) Commonly known as a "heart attack," AMI occurs when the blood supply to part of the heart is interrupted, causing heart cells to die. This is most commonly due to blockage of a coronary artery following the rupture of plaque within the wall of an artery. The resulting ischemia and decreased supply of oxygen, if left untreated, can cause damage and/or death of heart muscle tissue.

cardiac tamponade Also known as *pericardial tamponade,* this is an emergency condition in which fluid accumulates in the pericardium (the sac that surrounds the heart). If the amount of fluid increases slowly (such as in hypothyroidism), the pericardial sac can expand to contain a liter or more of fluid prior to tamponade occurring. If the fluid increases rapidly (as may occur after trauma or myocardial rupture), as little as 100 mL can cause tamponade.

ischemia A restriction in oxygen and nutrient delivery to muscle caused by physical obstruction to blood flow, increased demand by the tissues, or hypoxia, which leads to damage or dysfunction of tissue.

non–ST-segment elevation myocardial infarction (NSTEMI) A type of MI caused by a blocked blood supply that causes nontransmural infarction in an area of the heart. There is no ST-segment elevation on electrocardiogram (ECG) recordings, but other clinical signs of MI are present.

pericarditis A condition in which the tissue surrounding the heart (pericardium) becomes inflamed. This can be caused by several factors but is often related to a viral infection. If cardiac dysfunction or signs of congestive heart failure (CHF) are present, this suggests a more serious myocarditis or involvement of the heart muscle.

pleura A thin membrane that surrounds and protects the lungs (visceral pleura) and lines the chest cavity (parietal pleura)

pulmonary embolism The sudden blockage of a pulmonary artery by a blood clot, often from a deep vein in the legs or pelvis, that embolizes and travels to the lung artery where it becomes lodged. This can cause tachycardia, hypoxia, and hypotension.

pulsus paradoxus An exaggeration of the normal inspiratory decrease in systolic blood pressure. It's defined by an inspiratory fall of systolic blood pressure of greater than 10 mm Hg.

stable angina Symptoms of chest pain, shortness of breath, or other equivalent symptom that occurs predictably with exertion, then resolves with rest. This suggests the presence of a fixed coronary lesion that prevents adequate perfusion with increased demand.

ST-segment elevation myocardial infarction (STEMI) A type of MI caused by a blocked blood supply that causes transmural infarction in an area of the heart. These attacks carry a substantial risk of death and disability and call for a quick response by a STEMI system geared for reperfusion therapy.

tension pneumothorax A life-threatening condition that results from progressive worsening of a simple pneumothorax, the accumulation of air under pressure in the pleural space. This can lead to progressive restriction of venous return, which leads to decreased preload, then systemic hypotension.

unstable angina (UA) Angina of increased frequency, severity, or occurring with less intensive exertion than the baseline. This suggests the narrowing of a static lesion, causing further limitation of coronary blood flow with increased demand.

SCENARIO

A 37-YEAR-OLD FEMALE complains of dyspnea and chest pain. She has been feeling ill for about a week and vomited twice today. Her skin is flushed, and her heart rate is increased. She reports smoking two packs of cigarettes a day. Her only home medicines are birth control pills and insulin.

1. ***What differential diagnoses are you considering based on the information you have now?***
2. ***What additional information will you need to narrow your differential diagnosis?***
3. ***What are your initial treatment priorities as you continue your patient care?***

We have Dr. Werner Forssmann to thank for performing the first heart catheterization in 1929. Had the rest of the medical world listened to his critics—suggesting his methods were appropriate for a circus but not for a respected hospital—cardiac catheterization and the many procedures that have since evolved may have suffered serious setbacks. What was it that made his colleagues deem his ideas a "circus"?

Initially Dr. Forssmann experimented with cardiac catheterization on a cadaver. He found he could pass a catheter through a vein in the elbow and advance it all the way into the right ventricle. The success of his experiments motivated him to take the next obvious step: he'd need to complete the procedure on a living person. That person was himself. He had a colleague puncture his right brachial vein, and then Dr. Forssmann advanced the catheter. Success on the first attempt led to a second attempt a week later. This time, Dr. Forssmann cannulated his own vein and advanced the catheter 65 cm—its full length. To confirm its placement, he walked to the radiology department, which meant climbing the stairs from the operating room below. A nurse held a mirror in front of the x-ray machine to help him see that the catheter was indeed in the right atrium. Unable to advance the catheter any farther because he had introduced it to its full length, he did at least get a corroborating picture of what he had achieved. But the medical community wanted little to do with Forssmann and his revolutionary ideas; they felt he was too crazy to be given a clinical position. But in 1956, Werner Forssmann, Andre F. Cournand, and Dickenson W. Richard, Jr, shared the Nobel Prize in Physiology or Medicine for their work in cardiac studies.

Yes, caring for patients with chest discomfort can sometimes seem like a circus. The sheer number of associated life threats and the difficulty differentiating them can turn us into a crazy traveling show as emergency care providers. But thanks to Dr. Forssmann, we have a great prop in our kit for managing this presenting complaint. This chapter will work to help you sort out the circus.

Anatomy and Physiology

Several organs and structures within the chest can cause discomfort or pain if affected by disease or injury, including the chest wall, which contains the ribs, vertebrae, muscles, the pleurae and lungs; the heart and great vessels; the esophagus; and the diaphragm (Figure 5-1).

The Heart

We'll begin our discussion with one of the most important organs, the heart. The heart is a four-chambered, electrically driven, muscular pump located beneath the sternum, slightly offset to the left of midline, and roughly the size of a man's fist. It beats from birth to death and is the body's most exercised muscle, requiring a healthy blood supply of its own. Diseases of the heart are the leading cause of death in both men and women, and it's estimated that 13 million Americans suffer from heart disease. The heart and its connection to the great vessels are surrounded by a tough fibrous membrane known as the *pericardial sac* or *pericardium*. A small amount of pericardial fluid is normally in the pericardium and acts as a lubricant to allow normal heart movement within the chest.

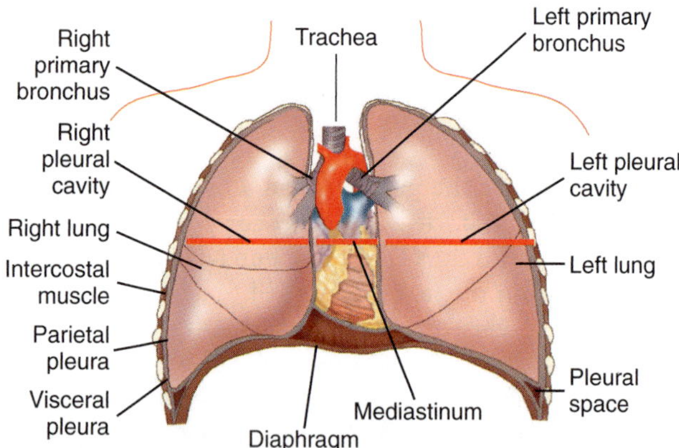

■ **Figure 5-1** Thoracic cavity, including ribs, intercostal muscles, diaphragm, mediastinum, lungs, heart, great vessels, bronchi, trachea, and esophagus. (From PHTLS: Prehospital trauma life support, ed 6, St Louis, 2007, MosbyJems.)

The Great Vessels

The great vessels include the aorta, superior and inferior venae cavae, pulmonary arteries, and pulmonary veins (Figure 5-2). The section of the aorta that runs through the chest is called the *thoracic aorta* and, as the aorta moves down through the abdomen, it's called the *abdominal aorta*. Serious, life-threatening illness occurs when the aorta becomes diseased and the layers begin to separate.

The Lungs and Pleurae

Chapter 3 has already covered respiratory disorders in depth, but let's briefly review the anatomy and physiology. The lungs are the large organs made of spongy lobes of elastic tissue that stretch and constrict as you inhale and exhale. The trachea and bronchi are made of smooth muscle and cartilage, allowing the airways to constrict and expand. The lungs and airways bring in fresh, oxygen-enriched air and get rid of carbon dioxide, which is a product of metabolism. When you inhale, the diaphragm and intercostal muscles contract and expand the chest. This expansion lowers the pressure in the chest below that of the outside air pressure. Air then flows in through the airways from an area of high pressure to low pressure and inflates the lungs. When you exhale, the diaphragm and intercostal muscles relax, and the weight of the chest wall along with the elasticity of the diaphragm forces the air out.

The lungs are also surrounded by the chest wall, which is lined with **pleura** (Figure 5-3). The visceral pleurae

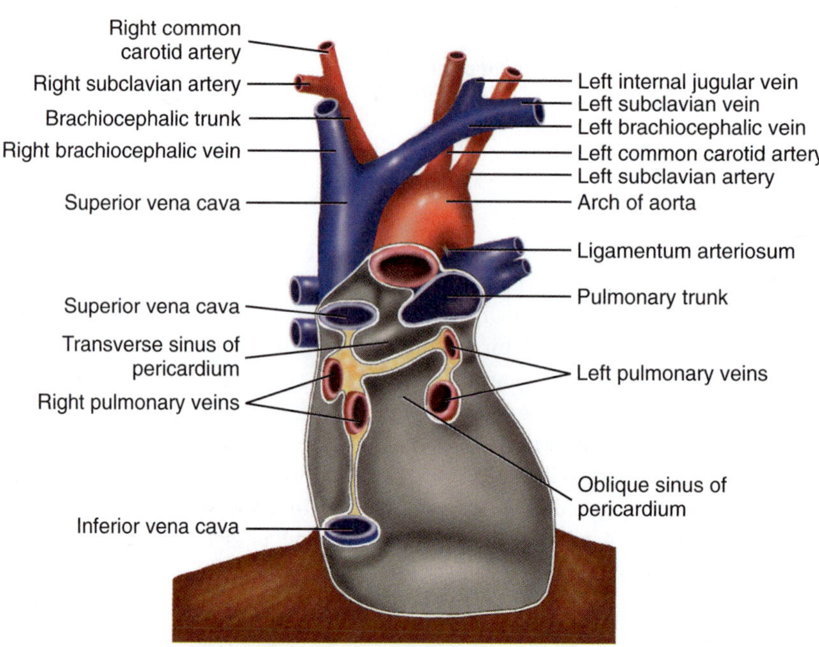

■ **Figure 5-2** Pericardial reflections near the origins of the great vessels, shown after removal of the heart. Note that portions of the caval vessels are within the pericardial space. (From Johnson D: The pericardium. In Standring S, et al, editors: Gray's anatomy, St Louis, 2005, Mosby.)

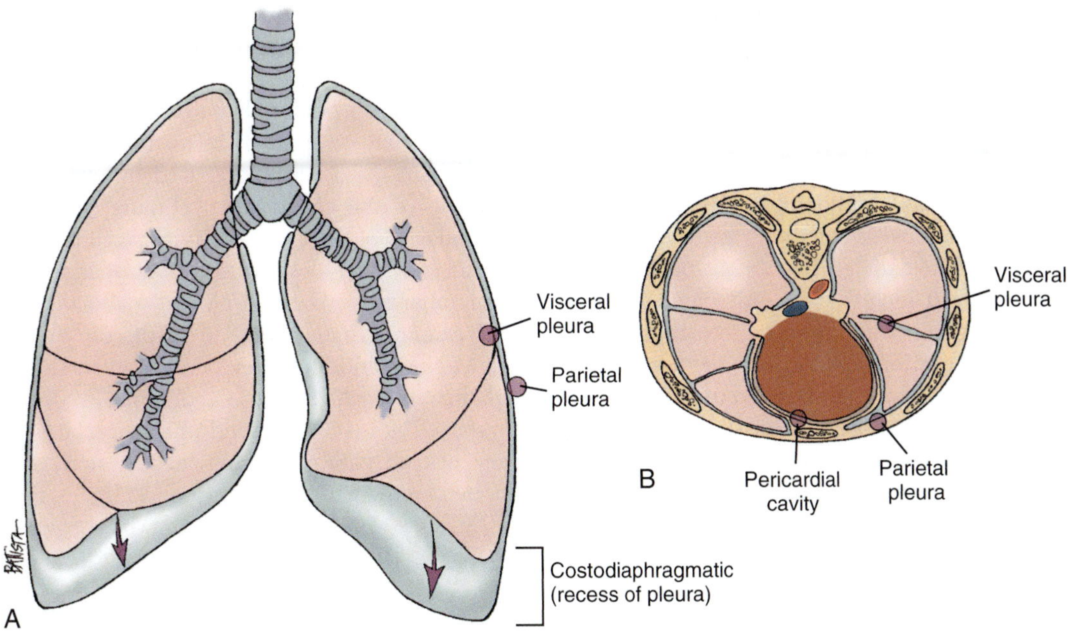

■ **Figure 5-3** A, Anterior view of visceral pleura and parietal pleura of the lungs. B, Cross-section of visceral pleura and parietal pleura of the lungs. (From Shade B, Collins T, Wertz E, et al: Mosby's EMT-intermediate textbook for the 1999 national standard curriculum, ed 3, St Louis, 2007, Mosby.)

surround the lungs, and the parietal pleurae line the chest wall. A small amount of visceral fluid acts as a lubricant to allow normal lung movement within the chest, and a small amount of parietal fluid causes the visceral and parietal pleurae to adhere together. This adherence keeps the lungs expanded and stretches the spongy tissue when the chest cavity expands during inhalation. (To illustrate how fluid can act as an adhesive, take two glass slides. If you place them together, you can easily separate them, but if you place just one small drop of water between them, it's very difficult to pull them apart.)

Oxygenation occurs in the alveoli, the terminal sacs of the lungs (Figure 5-4). The alveoli are covered by single-cell capillaries, where the exchange of gases (oxygen and carbon dioxide) takes place. Anything that causes disruption of diffusion between the alveoli and capillaries can interfere with oxygenation, leading to hypoxia. An example of this is a patient with pulmonary edema. In pulmonary edema, fluid accumulates in the interstitial space and alveoli, decreasing the ability for oxygen to cross from the alveoli to the capillaries and contributing to hypoxia.

The Esophagus

When food is swallowed, it passes from the pharynx into the esophagus, initiating rhythmic contractions (peristalsis) of the esophageal wall. This propels the food toward the stomach. Any alteration in these processes can lead to chest discomfort. Esophageal reflux often causes chest discomfort and may be confused with the discomfort caused by a cardiac event. In gastroesophageal reflux, or GERD, the contents of the stomach flow back up the

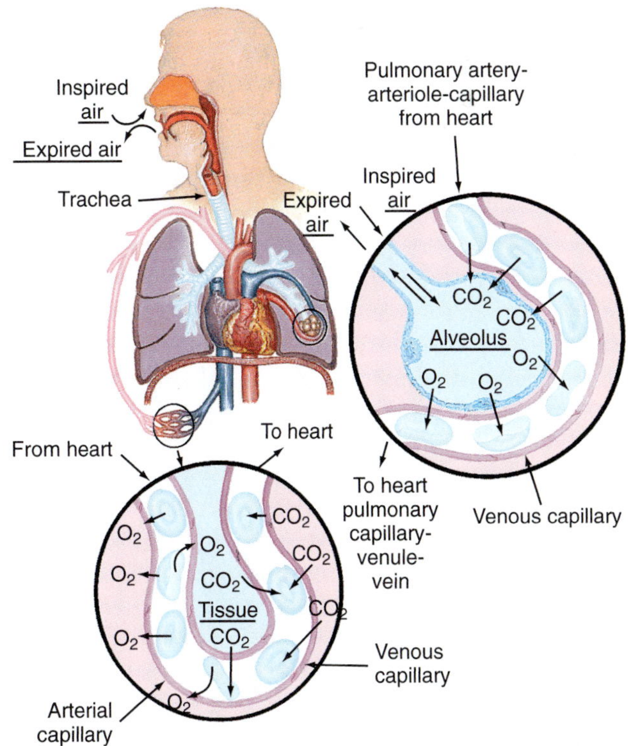

■ **Figure 5-4** Structures of the pulmonary system. Circles denote the alveoli. (Modified from Wilson SF, Thompson JM: Mosby's clinical nursing series: respiratory disorders, St Louis, 1990, Mosby.)

esophagus, causing a burning sensation or local discomfort.

The Sensation of Chest Pain

The scientific and clinical definition of *pain* is an unpleasant sensory and emotional experience associated with actual or potential tissue damage. For the purpose of this chapter, *chest discomfort* includes not only pain, but any feeling of discomfort to include burning, crushing, stabbing, or squeezing sensations. Chest pain or discomfort, then, is the direct result of the stimulation of nerve fibers from potentially damaged tissues within the chest. This potential damage may be caused by mechanical obstruction, inflammation, infection, or ischemia. For example, with an acute myocardial infarction (AMI), ischemic tissues send the brain sensory information that is interpreted as chest pain or discomfort.

All complaints of chest discomfort should be taken seriously until potential life threats can be ruled out. At times, it may be difficult to distinguish chest discomfort from pain or discomfort caused by organs or structures outside of the chest cavity (Figure 5-5). Although the boundaries of the chest cavity are well defined, organs or structures lying close to those boundaries may be served by similar nerve roots. A patient with gallbladder disease, for example, may complain of discomfort in the upper right chest and shoulder because even though the gallbladder is located in the abdominal cavity, pain can be "referred" to the chest and shoulder. The converse may also be true; pathophysiology inside the chest can be interpreted by the patient as symptoms outside the chest, such as in the abdomen, neck, and back. AMI commonly

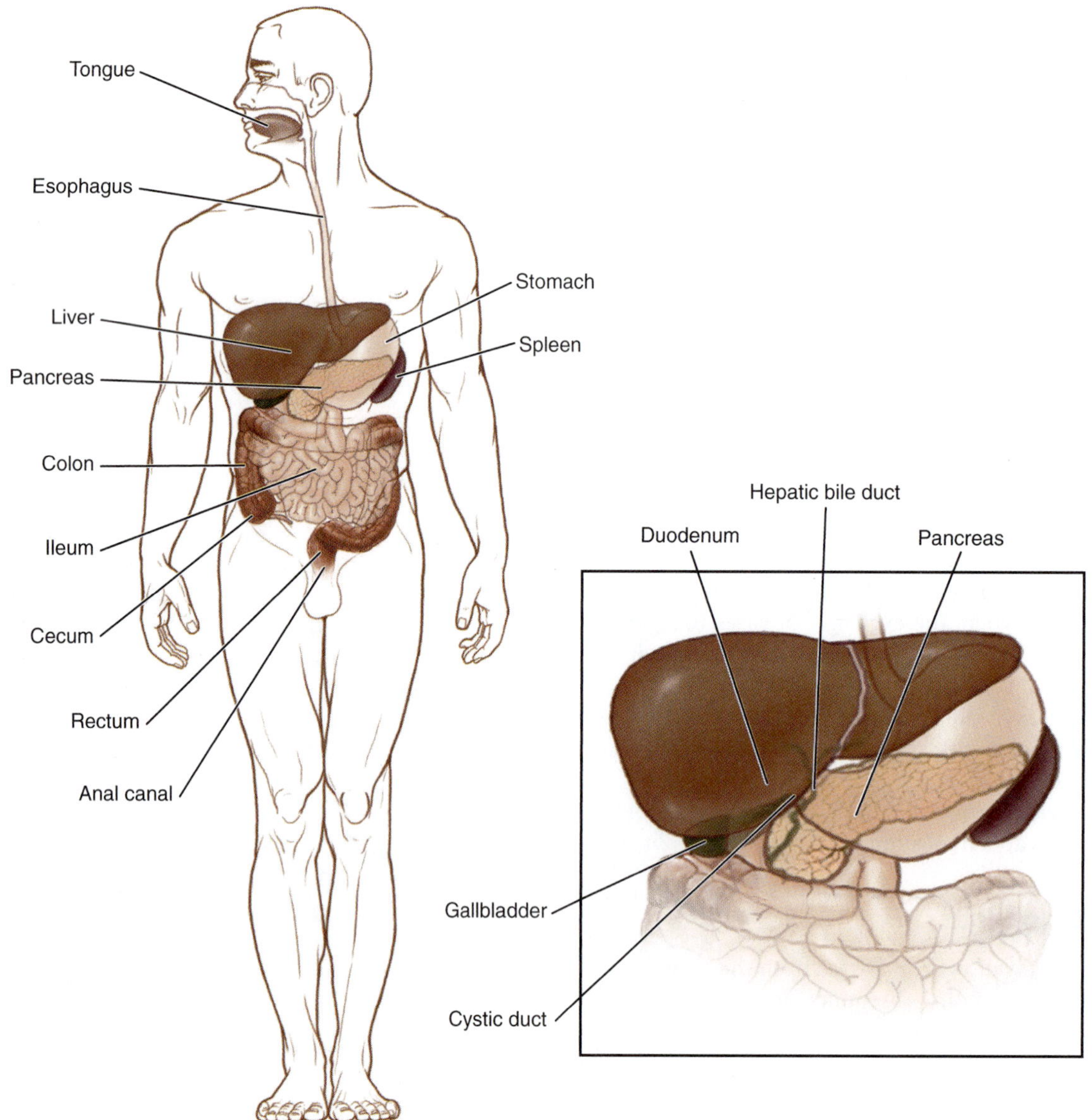

■ **Figure 5-5** Location of the spleen, liver, and gallbladder. (From Aehlert B: Paramedic practice today: above and beyond, St Louis, 2009, Mosby.)

presents with feelings of epigastric pain, nausea, and vomiting.

What may help us distinguish the location of the discomfort is to have an understanding of the types of pain: somatic and visceral. Patients will often describe the pain or discomfort in terms of how it feels to them: sharp, burning, tearing, or squeezing. These are actually descriptions of different types of pain. Somatic pain is well localized and described as sharp in nature. Visceral pain, on the other hand, originates in the viscera covering the organs within the chest and abdomen and is often described as heaviness, pressure, aching, or burning that is not easy to pinpoint. Visceral pain may also radiate to other areas of the body.

Assessment

Initial Process and Critical Diagnoses

When evaluating the patient with a complaint of chest pain, your knowledge of anatomy, physiology, and pathophysiology will help guide you toward the common causes of chest discomfort. Box 5-1 lists some of these. The most serious and common life threat is an AMI. (However, less than half of all patients suffering an AMI call 9-1-1.) Considering the wide range of possible causes, providers must have a high index of suspicion when dealing with potential intrathoracic pathophysiology.

When first assessing the patient, the top priority is looking for those life-threatening causes of chest discomfort. Early recognition of the patient with a critical medical or surgical cause should be your initial focus. Should your primary assessment reveal these life-threatening signs, triage decisions have to be made in both the prehospital and in-hospital setting, with a goal of quickly moving the patient toward definitive intervention.

Initial Observations

Is this situation or patient safe for my approach?

Look for clues in the environment that may give you insight and direct you toward certain diagnoses. What risk factors, medications, medical equipment, and sights or smells support the cause of the complaint? If the patient was brought to you, how did they arrive?

Do you have all the necessary resources to manage this patient right now? What resources do you need to request to help you manage this patient appropriately? If you're functioning within a basic life support (BLS) system of emergency medical services (EMS), should you request the additional resources of an advanced life support (ALS) or critical care team? If you're functioning within a small hospital without interventional catheterization lab resources, should you initiate an ALS or critical care transport as soon as possible?

From Across the Room

What can you discern from across the room? Is the patient awake? What position is he/she in? Is there increased work of breathing? Is there an appearance of shock or poor perfusion?

Your first impression of the patient may tell you whether they're sick or not. Are they in a tripod position indicating trouble breathing, or lying flat with minimal response to your presence? Simply put, are they going to die right now? Conduct a rapid primary survey assessing the patient's level of consciousness (LOC), airway, breathing, and circulation.

If multiple healthcare providers are available, essential monitoring equipment, diagnostics, and some early treatment can be initiated while you look for symptoms of those critical diagnoses.

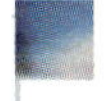

Initial Life-Threatening Diagnoses and Interventions

Life-threatening conditions associated with chest discomfort that requires immediate treatment include tension pneumothorax, pulmonary embolism, esophageal rupture, aortic dissection, cardiac tamponade, arrhythmia, and acute coronary syndromes (including congestive heart failure [CHF]/acute pulmonary edema [APE]). Some of these conditions are seen in the primary survey as chest discomfort with respiratory distress, chest discomfort with altered vital signs, or a combination of those three cardinal

BOX 5-1 Critical Differential Diagnosis of Chest Pain

Cardiovascular Causes	Pulmonary Causes	Gastrointestinal Causes
Acute MI	Pulmonary embolism	Esophageal rupture
ACS	Tension pneumothorax	
CHF, APE		
Aortic dissection		
Cardiac tamponade		
Arrhythmia		

ACS, Acute coronary syndrome; *APE,* acute pulmonary edema; *CHF,* congestive heart failure; *MI,* myocardial infarction.
Adapted from Marx JA, Hockenberger RS, Walls RM: Rosen's emergency medicine: concepts and clinical practice, ed 6, St Louis, 2006, Mosby.

signs and symptoms. Each has its own unique treatment that we'll discuss in this section.

Chest Discomfort with Respiratory Distress

In the patient with a patent airway, performing a quick primary exam of breathing is next. You and your team should apply appropriate supplemental oxygen to the patient as you assess for breath sounds. In the patient with increased work of breathing, unilateral absence or decreased breath sounds suggests a pneumothorax. If shock is also present, a tension pneumothorax has to be immediately recognized and treated.

Tension Pneumothorax

Tension pneumothorax is a life-threatening condition that results from a progressive deterioration and worsening of a simple pneumothorax (the accumulation of air under pressure in the pleural space). If allowed to continue, a tension pneumothorax can cause a mediastinal shift, putting pressure on the heart and great vessels and disrupting blood flow. Increased intrathoracic pressure will impede venous return, decreasing preload, leading to a drop in systemic blood pressure.

Assessment of a tension pneumothorax will reveal chest discomfort, severe respiratory distress, decreased or absent breath sounds on the affected side, and obstructive shock. Jugular venous distention (JVD) and tracheal deviation can be seen as well but are sometimes difficult to find and are late signs. Treatment is aimed at relieving the pressure inside the chest by decompressing the affected side. For most cases, that would mean a needle decompression, accomplished by placing a large-bore (12- to 14-gauge), long (2- to 3-inch) needle (for adolescents and adults) in the second intercostal space in the midclavicular line. An alternative location for needle thoracostomy is the fourth or fifth intercostal space in the midaxillary line. Some experts recommend this location because there is less risk for injury to the great vessels in the chest. This will provide a temporizing measure until a chest tube can be placed. See Chapter 3 for more information on pneumothoraces and treatment.

Pulmonary Embolism

Pulmonary embolism (PE) falls into the general category of venous thromboembolism (VTE), which includes both the deep venous thrombosis (DVT) and pulmonary embolism. A thrombus can form when the fine balance between clot development and clot breakdown is affected. Many factors can create an imbalance toward clot formation, such as malignancy, immobility, and medications such as oral contraceptive pills. In this condition, a vessel injury or sluggish blood flow in large vessels cause a fibrin formation or clot, and when this clot forms in a deep vein, a DVT is present.

The initial symptoms of DVT may be quite subtle and be limited to pain or discomfort only, without outward signs of inflammation. At times, local inflammation is obvious, and you can act quickly to help prevent the movement of this clot into the central circulation.

Pulmonary embolism occurs when a clot that has formed in those deeper veins (even weeks earlier) is dislodged and travels through the venous system (embolism), through the heart, and lodges in the pulmonary arteries. Rosen et al. estimate that as many as 50% of PEs go undiagnosed in the emergency department (ED). If the clot only occupies about 30% of the low-flow pulmonary vessel, and the patient is otherwise healthy, there will be few symptoms. For patients with long-standing disease like chronic obstructive pulmonary disease (COPD), symptoms of chest pain and dyspnea may be present.

If the clot occupies a large portion of the vessel, and blood flow to that portion of the lung is compromised, an infarction will occur, and symptoms will be evident. There may be sharp, very localized pain that increases with a deep breath or cough (pleuritic) and leads to subsequent "splinting" of the patient's breathing.

Ninety percent of all patients with PE (noninfarcting and infarcting) will have dyspnea, sometimes intermittently. This occurs when there is air going in and out, but blood flow to certain areas of the lung is redirected so the air is not being used. This is called a *ventilation-perfusion (V/Q) mismatch* or *dead space ventilation*. If there is hypoxia and no physiologic explanation, PE must be considered.

About half of all patients with PE will have tachycardia. This can be driven by a response to hypoxia or to hypotension from poor left ventricular filling. Computed tomography (CT), echocardiogram, or electrocardiogram (ECG—classically S_1,Q_3,T_3) may show a strain pattern due to increased pulmonary artery pressures. About 10% of PE patients present with hypotension, which suggests a poor prognosis. The patient will be hemodynamically unstable if one of the main branches of the pulmonary artery is occluded with a saddle embolus, and cardiac arrest will usually present in pulseless electrical activity (PEA).

Elements of patient history that suggest PE include an acute onset of shortness of breath, lightheadedness or syncope, chest pain, dry cough, or unexplained tachycardia (Box 5-2). Pulmonary infarction presents similarly to pneumonia, but high fever is usually only found in pneumonia. An acute onset of chest pain and hemoptysis in the same day suggest the possibility of a PE. There may be unilateral swelling of the leg and risk factors for DVT. Patients with PE will normally have clear lungs on exam.

Diagnostics in Pulmonary Embolism

1. A 12-lead ECG should be completed as soon as feasible. In patients with chest pain or shortness of breath, this is critical to evaluate for alternative diagnoses. The most common ECG finding in PE is sinus tachycardia.

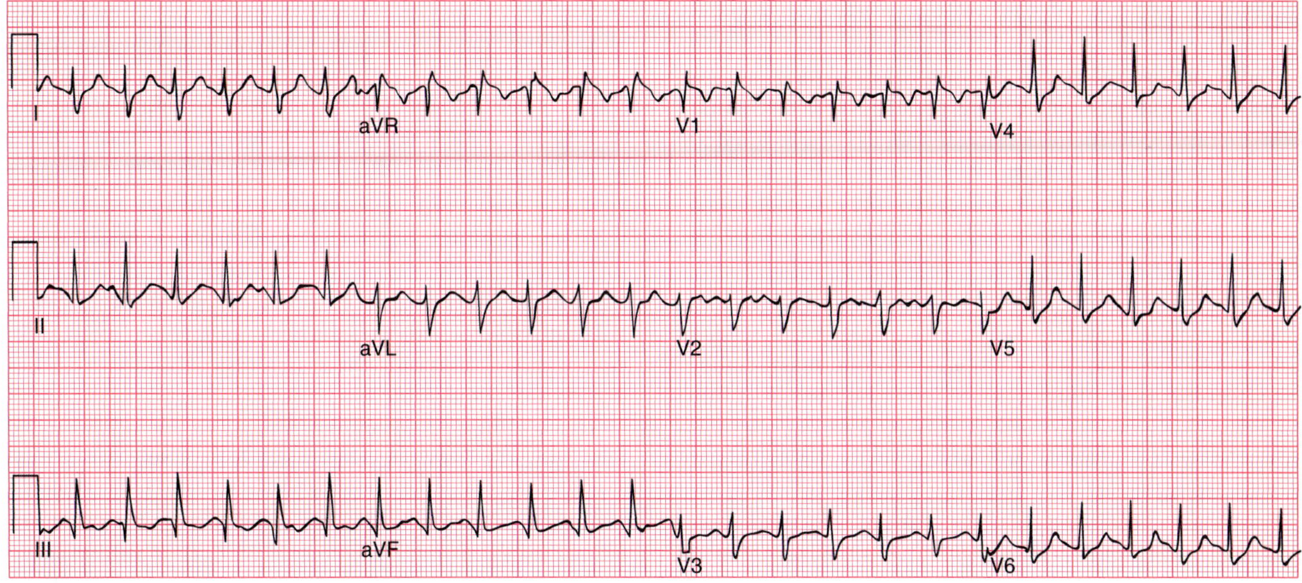

■ **Figure 5-6** 12-Lead electrocardiogram with S_1,Q_3,T_3. (From Marx JA, Hockberger RS, Walls RM: Rosen's emergency medicine: concepts and clinical practice, ed 6, St Louis, 2006, Mosby.)

BOX 5-2 Most Common Signs and Symptoms of Pulmonary Embolism

Tachypnea (96%)
Shortness of breath (82%)
Chest pain (49%)
Cough (20%)
Hemoptysis (7%)

Adapted from Goldhaber SZ, et al: Acute pulmonary embolism: clinical outcomes in the International Cooperative Pulmonary Embolism Registry, Lancet 353:1386–1389, 1999.

Other findings suggestive for PE, which are seen in the minority of cases, are related to pulmonary hypertension and RV strain. These include an S wave in lead I, a Q wave in lead III, and a T wave inversion in lead III (S_1,Q_3,T_3; Figure 5-6).

A constellation of symptoms along with ECG findings is called the *McGinn-White sign*. This sign includes:

- A Q wave and late inversion of the T wave in lead III
- Low ST intervals and T waves in lead II
- Inverted T waves in chest leads V_2 and V_3, the electrocardiographic evidence of right ventricular dilatation due to massive pulmonary embolism
- Clinical signs of acute cor pulmonale

2. Chest radiograph, although unable to show a PE in the hospital setting, is necessary to evaluate for other diagnoses that cause chest pain or shortness of breath. Findings on chest x-ray that are specific but not sensitive for PE include Hampton's hump (wedge-shaped, pleural-based triangular opacity which represents pulmonary infarction) and Westermark's sign (clearing of normal radiologic shadow of pulmonary tissue distal to a PE).
3. Other imaging of value in diagnosing PE includes echocardiography, computed tomography angiography (CTA), and V/Q scans. An ultrasound of the heart that shows right ventricular strain is common in the case of a large PE. CTA may be used in some hospitals and is fast and about 90% sensitive. Ventilation/perfusion scans may also be employed where the patient inhales radionuclide while an injectable form is used to compare V/Q mismatch.
4. Laboratory testing, like the standard chest radiograph in the hospital setting, is usually done to try to differentiate the many causes of chest pain and/or dyspnea. There really is no one definitive blood test sensitive enough to diagnose PE. Clotting function tests are usually within normal limits; D-dimer is reasonably sensitive but nonspecific so not diagnostic if positive. While helpful in low-risk patients, D-dimer can't be relied upon for patients who are clinically at high risk for DVT or PE. Blood gases can be done, but PE often fails to produce obvious abnormalities of pulmonary gas exchange.

Management of Pulmonary Embolism In the prehospital setting, the patient with acute chest pain, dyspnea, and/or alteration in vital signs should have oxygen, vascular access, electronic monitoring, and 12-lead ECG acquisition. Beginning standard therapy for acute coronary syndromes with aspirin is appropriate if the diagnosis is unclear. If the patient has been identified as having respiratory failure, airway control and ventilatory assistance is also required. Stabilization of vital signs may include crystalloids and use of vasopressor infusion to combat obstructive shock.

Once the patient enters the in-hospital setting, appropriate diagnostic tests should be performed. Anticoagulation therapy may include unfractionated or fractionated heparin, which will reduce the possibility of new clot formation. Placement of a filter in the inferior vena cava will help trap any traveling emboli from moving superiorly. Persistent hypotension and tachycardia usually indicate a more difficult course of treatment and poor outcome.

For a hemodynamically significant pulmonary embolism, thrombolytic therapy is a treatment option. In some patients, it can achieve quicker results than anticoagulation therapy, but it must be balanced with the increased risk for bleeding.

Surgical embolectomy requires a cardiothoracic surgeon and placing the patient on cardiopulmonary bypass. Catheter thrombectomy can be conducted in the interventional radiology suite of high-resource hospitals.

Esophageal Rupture

Chest pain with dyspnea may indicate esophageal rupture. When the esophagus is torn, gastric contents enter into the mediastinum, where an inflammatory infectious process ensues. The most common causes of esophageal perforation include iatrogenic injury from endoscopy or instrumentation, foreign bodies from poorly chewed food or sharp objects, caustic burns, blunt or penetrating trauma, spontaneous rupture (Boerhaave's syndrome from forceful vomiting), or postoperative complications.

Early clinical signs of esophageal rupture are vague. The patient may complain of pleuritic pain in the anterior chest and may be worse with swallowing when the head and neck are flexed. Dyspnea and fever often accompany the chest pain as the infectious process worsens.

As air and gastrointestinal (GI) contents enter the mediastinum, subcutaneous air will gather around the patient's chest and neck. Pneumomediastinum and pneumopericardium may be apparent on the chest x-ray. Auscultation of heart sounds may pick up the so-called Hamman's crunch, where a crunching sound is heard during systole. As the inflammatory process begins because of mediastinal contamination, sepsis, fever, and distributive shock will ensue. If the diagnosis of this ailment is delayed for more than 24 hours, the patient may deteriorate rapidly.

Management of this life-threatening disease begins with your recognizing its signs and symptoms, including it in your differential diagnosis, and conducting a good history and physical exam. This patient will present with symptoms as described and have one of the common causes in their recent history. Routine treatment includes oxygen, vascular access, application of monitors, and obtaining a 12-lead ECG, chest x-ray, and laboratory specimens. Quickly initiating antibiotics, volume replacement, and airway maintenance are other important elements of treatment. A surgery consult should be obtained as soon as possible.

Acute Pulmonary Edema/Congestive Heart Failure

Another life-threatening event that may be found in the primary survey is APE from heart failure. This patient typically has a combination of chest pain and increased work of breathing. In your primary assessment of breathing, you may note crackles or rales in the lung fields, often starting in the bases and moving progressively upward with increased severity. A quick assessment of circulation can help you pinpoint the problem, especially if cardiogenic shock is also present.

Heart failure is a complication of nearly all forms of heart disease, both structural and functional; the ventricles are unable to fill or eject blood in adequate amounts to meet the body's needs. Coronary artery disease is the most common underlying cause of CHF. Cardinal signs and symptoms are dyspnea, fatigue, exercise intolerance, and fluid retention that can lead to pulmonary and peripheral edema. Poor ventricular pumping function leads to an overall decrease in cardiac output (CO), and as more blood is left in the ventricle, pressure builds in the left or right heart circulatory pathways. If the left ventricle fails, the pressure in the pulmonary veins increases, and blood backs up into the lungs leading to pulmonary edema with poor gas exchange. In the chronic CHF patient, compensatory mechanisms work to redistribute blood to critical organs and adapt the body to diseased heart function. If the right side of the heart is also involved, blood backs up into the venae cavae, causing congestion of the venous system, which may present as pedal edema, JVD, or sacral edema.

Acute Pulmonary Edema with Shock This patient may be in the midst of suffering an MI and have signs of shock with pulmonary edema due to acute systolic dysfunction when you arrive on scene. From across the room, you might note the patient is sitting upright (due to orthopnea), working hard to breathe, and may be complaining of chest tightness or discomfort. They'll have signs of poor perfusion (weak distal pulses, cool skin, delayed capillary refill, poor urinary output, and acidosis). Systemic and pulmonary congestion will also be present—tachypnea, labored breathing, bilateral crackles (possibly with wheezing ["cardiac asthma"]), pale or cyanotic skin, hypoxemia, and sometimes frothy, blood-tinged sputum.

Diagnostics in the Patient with Acute Pulmonary Edema/ Congestive Heart Failure In the prehospital setting, standard protocols for acute coronary syndromes (see STEMI, NSTEMI later in the chapter) should be followed if they appear to be the cause of the CHF and APE. Overall care should focus on lowering the pressure. Oxygen, vascular access, and monitors should be applied, and a 12-lead ECG should be acquired to evaluate for evidence of AMI.

In the in-hospital setting, patients require aggressive treatment while a history, physical exam, chest x-ray, and laboratory assessment are completed. If not already performed, a 12-lead ECG should also be done. Arterial and/or venous blood sampling will help evaluate the patient's ability to oxygenate and ventilate. Besides a routine laboratory analysis, brain natriuretic peptide (BNP) elevation can be useful to help diagnose CHF in unclear cases. These peptides are released when there is stretch in the ventricular muscle. Cardiac enzymes should also be ordered to help evaluate for myocardial injury.

In the intensive care setting, left- and right-sided hemodynamic monitoring can help evaluate the various pressures throughout the heart, along with treatment effectiveness.

Management of Heart Failure Management of heart failure is geared toward improving gas exchange and CO. If the actual blood pressure is adequate (systolic blood pressure > 100 mm Hg), help the patient get into a comfortable position. Many times this can be done with the patient sitting with legs dependent. Supplemental oxygen should be provided as tolerated. Oxygen saturations above 90% are desired, so you should evaluate the patient for possible ventilatory assistance. If there are signs of respiratory failure along with altered mental status, intubation and invasive pulmonary ventilation will be necessary. If the patient is alert enough, noninvasive positive pressure ventilation (NIPPV) can be therapeutic in two ways: (1) decreasing venous return and preload, thereby reducing pulmonary edema, and (2) improving gas exchange. The use of positive end-expiratory pressure (PEEP), NIPPV, continuous positive airway pressure (CPAP), and bilevel positive airway pressure (BiPAP) are explained in Chapter 3.

Along with positive pressure ventilation, if the systolic blood pressure is above 100 mmHg, nitroglycerin has emerged as the primary treatment of pulmonary edema. This drug acts to decrease preload through peripheral vasodilation. Caution must be exercised when employing these strategies simultaneously; systemic blood pressure can drop quickly. Patients with subacute CHF who also feel volume overloaded may be given furosemide to initiate diuresis. Furosemide should also be used with caution in the prehospital setting, because many patients with "crackles" on exam are later found to have pneumonia. Diuresis in this group of patients can be detrimental. In addition, many of those who do have CHF are not total-body-fluid overloaded; the fluid is just not distributed correctly. Diuresis can be detrimental in these patients because many have poor renal function to begin with.

Angiotensin-converting enzyme (ACE) inhibitors are also currently used in the acute treatment of CHF. Nesiritide may be of value. In the intensive care setting, aquapheresis may help remove fluid overload without major derangements in electrolytes. Morphine has historically been used to treat acute CHF but has become controversial owing to studies that show increased mortality with its use in this group of patients, possibly as a result of depression of respiratory drive and hypotension.

If your patient's chest pain is complicated by low blood pressure, cardiogenic shock, and dyspnea, vasoactive medications to improve the blood pressure will also be necessary. Dopamine and/or dobutamine may be given to help increase blood pressure and inotropy/chronotropy.

Some APE patients may be found to have abnormal heart sounds indicating mitral regurgitation due to a ruptured papillary muscle or chorda. These patients are in immediate need of a cardiothoracic surgeon.

In conjunction with the medical management discussed, an intraaortic balloon pump will help reduce afterload and may improve overall perfusion. Procedure 5-1 details management of this very specialized device.

Chest Discomfort with Alteration in Vital Signs

Cardiac Arrhythmia

As the primary survey is being conducted, monitors should be applied by your team to obtain continuous vital signs and evaluate for arrhythmia or acute myocardial injury. Noting an arrhythmia early may help diagnose and speed treatment of a major cause of chest pain. An arrhythmia may cause chest discomfort and can be life threatening if CO is too low.

If the heart rate becomes too slow, CO will decrease. Depending on the effectiveness of the body's compensatory mechanisms, blood pressure may also drop, causing a decrease in coronary artery perfusion. If the heart rate is too fast, CO may decrease as the chambers of the heart are not allowed adequate time to fill. This decreases CO, dropping blood pressure and impairing cardiac function. If the coronary arteries are diseased, the increased workload on the heart may precipitate angina. The cardiogenic shock caused in either case may lead to APE, causing shortness of breath. Treatment is aimed at rate control, which will lead to improved pump function. Improving pump function will increase CO and raise blood pressure.

For treatment of bradycardia and tachycardia, follow current ACLS guidelines and/or your protocols. This patient may also be in the midst of suffering from an acute coronary syndrome. A 12-lead ECG and laboratory samples should be acquired early as the oxygen is applied and vascular access is obtained. If bradycardia is causing the patient to become clinically unstable (chest pain, dyspnea, APE, shock), measures should be implemented to increase the heart rate. This usually involves the use of medications such as atropine, and/or vasoactive agents (epinephrine, dopamine), and/or application of a transcutaneous pacemaker. Care should be taken not to increase

Text to be continued on page 192

Procedure 5-1 Intraaortic Balloon Pump (IABP) Management

OVERVIEW

This short-term therapy improves myocardial oxygenation by reducing afterload, thus reducing the workload of the heart, through counterpulsation.

INDICATIONS

- Patients with heart failure

CONTRAINDICATIONS

- Aortic insufficiency or aneurysms
- Severe blood clotting disorders

PROCEDURE

Preprocedure Preparation and Maintenance of the System

1. The practitioner will place a sterile intraaortic balloon pump (IABP) catheter in the femoral artery and position it in the descending thoracic aorta, just distal to left subclavian. Arterial pressure hemodynamic monitoring is usually also in place in the radial artery to assist in the proper assessment and timing of this device.
2. The patient's affected leg must remain extended; a full-leg knee immobilizer is effective to prevent flexion.
3. Follow the manufacturer's recommendations for:
   - ECG leads: maintain a prominent R wave for timing of the device.
   - Console maintenance: timing procedures and alarms
   - Helium source: inflates the IABP balloon. Make sure there is enough gas in the canister for the length of the trip.
   - Flushing of the device to prevent thrombus formation
   - Identify with marked tape which electrode goes to monitor and which goes to console.
4. Follow your institution's policies on heparinized flush solution.
5. Standard wound care and dressing procedures per your policies
6. Follow your protocols and policies for frequency of cardiovascular assessment. Assessment of the patient includes:
   - Level of consciousness (cerebral perfusion)
   - Vital signs and pulmonary artery pressure (IABP therapy effectiveness)
   - Arterial catheter and IABP waveforms (timing effectiveness)
   - Cardiac output, cardiac index, systemic vascular resistance (effectiveness of IABP therapy)
   - Distal perfusion: skin parameters (should be warm and dry) and urinary output (should be > 0.5 mL/kg/h)
   - Heart and lung sounds: to auscultate these sounds adequately, you may need to turn the IABP to standby and restart when completed.
   - Check all central and distal pulses to ensure that the catheter has not migrated and is not occluding any vessel. The catheter should be measured and marked for location at the femoral site.
7. Turn and position patient at least every 2 hours if able.
8. Monitor anticoagulation therapy via laboratory studies and clinical evidence of bleeding or clot formation. Check dressings frequently for bleeding.

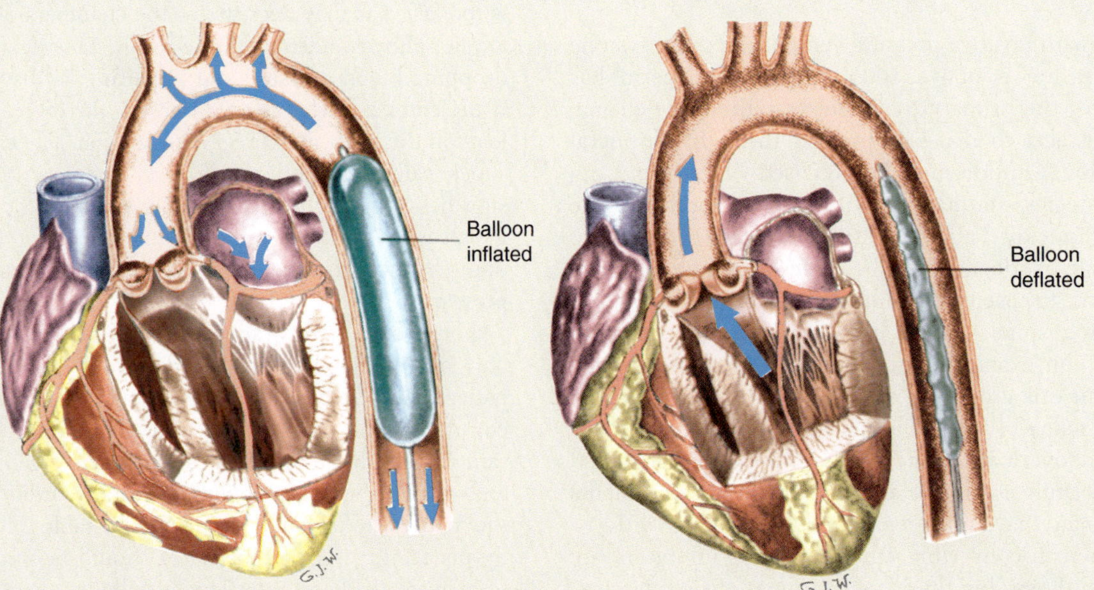

Mechanisms of action of the intraaortic balloon pump. A, Diastolic balloon inflation augments coronary blood flow. B, Systolic balloon deflation decreases afterload. (From Urden L: Thelan's critical care nursing, ed 5, St Louis, 2006, Mosby.)

Procedure 5-1 Intraaortic Balloon Pump (IABP) Management—*Cont'd*

Timing the Balloon Pump

1. ECG and arterial pressure waveform are monitored to verify proper timing of the device. Timing the inflation (during diastole) and deflation (during systole) effectively decreases workload of the heart and improves oxygenation.

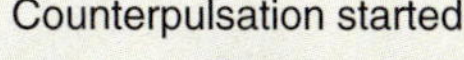

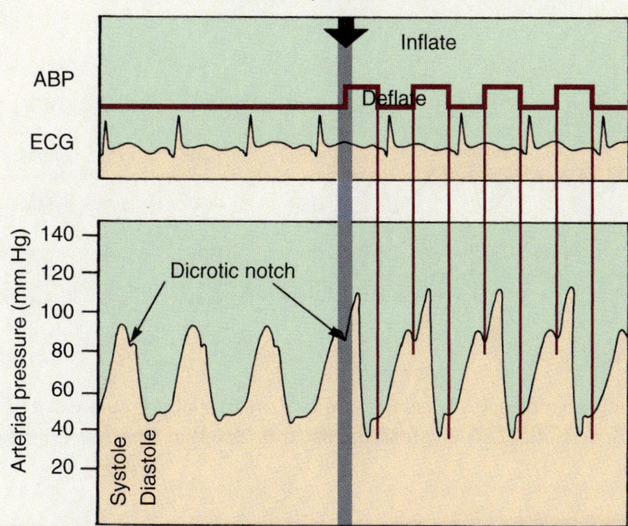

Timing and effect of balloon counterpulsations. Timing is adjusted by synchronizing balloon inflation with the dicrotic notch on the arterial waveform, resulting in an elevated diastolic pressure. Inflation is maintained throughout diastole to augment coronary perfusion. Deflation occurs just before the next systole, resulting in a reduced systolic pressure and decreased afterload. (From Guzzetta CE, Dossey BM: Cardiovascular nursing: holistic practice, St Louis, 1992, Mosby.)

2. A prominent R wave on the ECG and a properly maintained arterial waveform signals the IABP console when to time inflation and deflation of the balloon.
3. To start, set the IABP to 1:2 or 50% (every other beat augmented).

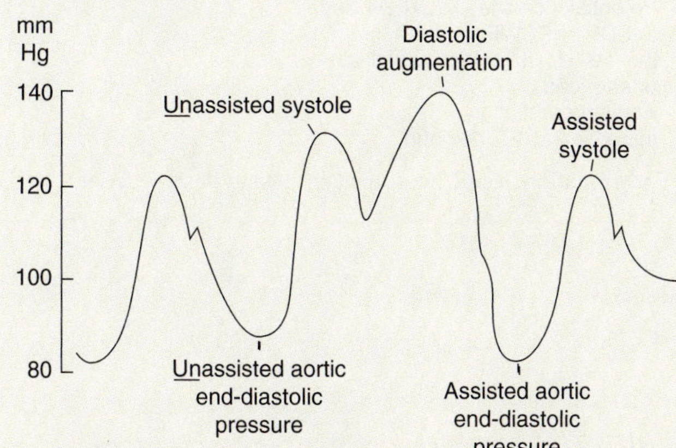

1:2 intraaortic balloon pump frequency. (From Datascope Corp., Montvale, New Jersey.)

4. Inflation:
   - Dicrotic notch identified in the arterial waveform (aortic valve closure)
   - Balloon inflation should occur after aortic valve closure. Adjust inflation on the console until the dicrotic notch disappears and a sharp V wave appears.

1:1 IABP Frequency

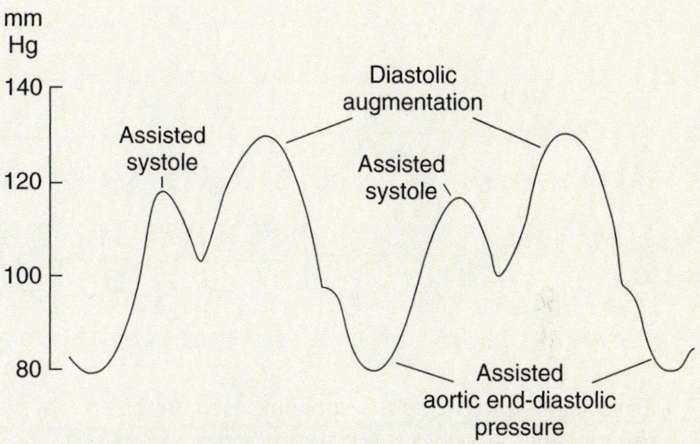

Correct intraaortic balloon pump timing (1:1). (From Datascope Corp., Montvale, New Jersey.)

5. Compare the augmented pressure with the unassisted systolic pressure. This pressure should be the same or slightly higher.
   - If augmented pressure is less: balloon too low, patient hypovolemic or tachycardic, or balloon volume is too low.
6. Adjust the console as needed to time the inflation of the balloon.
7. There are considerations for location of the arterial line:
   - Radial: time inflation 40–50 ms before notch.
   - Femoral: time inflation 120 ms before notch.
8. Deflation:
   - With IABP on 1:2 frequency (as above) identify unassisted end-diastolic pressure and assisted and unassisted systolic pressures.
   - Balloon should deflate so that end-diastolic pressure is as low as possible (<patient's unassisted diastolic pressure) while maintaining optimal diastolic augmentation and NOT interfering with the next systole.
9. Now that you have the timing set, turn the console augmentation to 1:1 (100%).

Balloon Pressure Waveform

1. Check the IABP console for balloon pressure waveform as helium is shuttled in and out of the catheter.

Continued

Procedure 5-1 Intraaortic Balloon Pump (IABP) Management—*Cont'd*

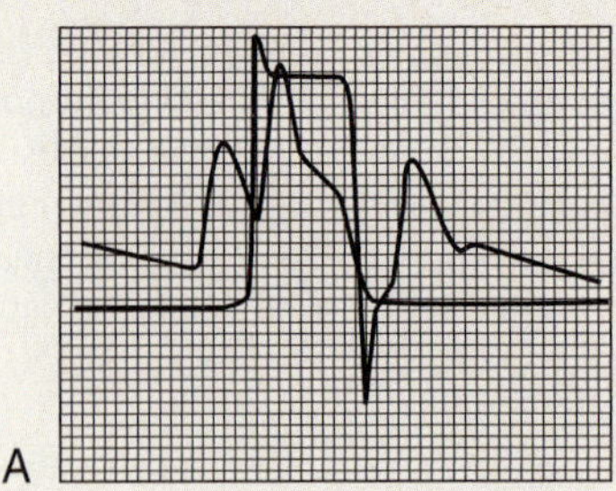

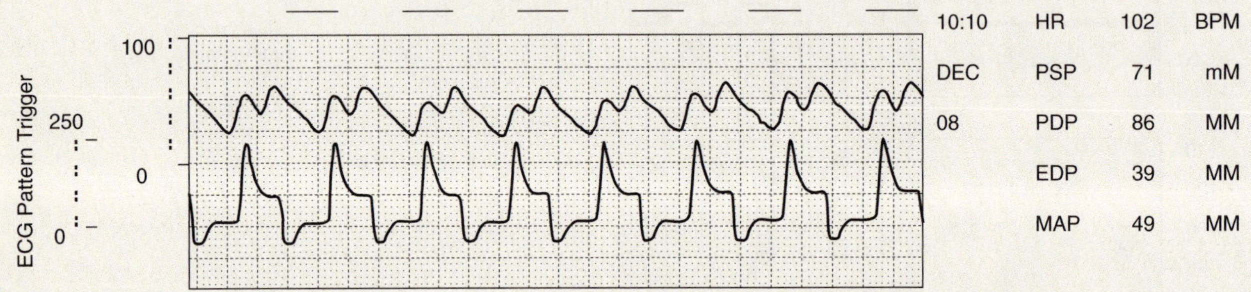

A, Balloon pressure waveform superimposed on the arterial pressure waveform. B, Actual recording of an arterial pressure waveform *(top)* and balloon gas waveform *(bottom)* from a balloon-pumped patient. (From Arrow International, Cleveland, Ohio.)

2. Refer to the manufacturer's guidelines on inflation errors reflected in the balloon pressure waveform.

Timing the Device with Dysrhythmias Present

1. Atrial fibrillation: set device to shuttle on most R waves, or (if available) use the atrial fibrillation mode on the console.
2. Tachycardia: set the frequency to 1:2 (50%).
3. Asystole: change the trigger to the arterial pressure. If compressions do not provide an adequate trigger, set device to internal trigger at 60–80/min, 1:2 frequency, and decrease augmentation to 50%.
4. Ventricular tachycardia or ventricular fibrillation: cardiovert or defibrillate as necessary, as the console is electrically isolated.

TROUBLESHOOTING THE IABP

Timing Errors

Early Inflation

Timing Errors

Early Inflation

Inflation of the IAB prior to aortic valve closure

Waveform Characteristics:
- Inflation of IAB prior to dicrotic notch
- Diastolic augmentation encroaches onto systole (may be unable to distinguish)

Physiologic Effects:
- Potential premature closure of aortic valve
- Potential increased in LVEDV and LVEDP or PCWP
- Increased left ventricular wall stress or afterload
- Aortic regurgitation
- Increased MVO_2 demand

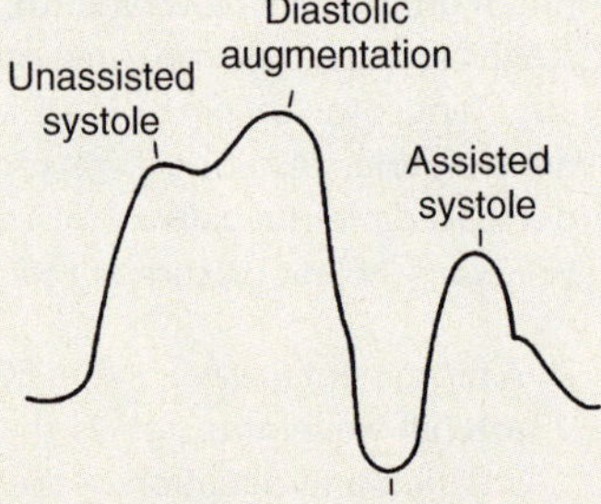

Early inflation. (From Datascope Corp., Montvale, New Jersey.)

Procedure 5-1 Intraaortic Balloon Pump (IABP) Management—*Cont'd*

Late Inflation

Timing Errors
Late Inflation

Inflation of the IAB markedly after closure of the aortic valve

Waveform Characteristics:
- Inflation of the IAB after the dicrotic notch
- Absence of sharp V
- Suboptimal diastolic augmentation

Physiologic Effects:
- Suboptimal coronary artery perfusion

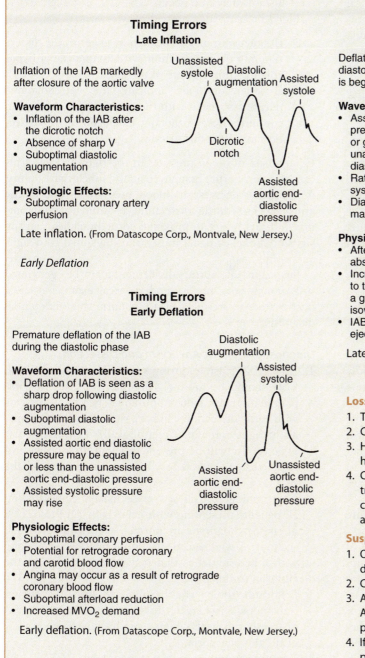

Late inflation. (From Datascope Corp., Montvale, New Jersey.)

Early Deflation

Timing Errors
Early Deflation

Premature deflation of the IAB during the diastolic phase

Waveform Characteristics:
- Deflation of IAB is seen as a sharp drop following diastolic augmentation
- Suboptimal diastolic augmentation
- Assisted aortic end diastolic pressure may be equal to or less than the unassisted aortic end-diastolic pressure
- Assisted systolic pressure may rise

Physiologic Effects:
- Suboptimal coronary perfusion
- Potential for retrograde coronary and carotid blood flow
- Angina may occur as a result of retrograde coronary blood flow
- Suboptimal afterload reduction
- Increased MVO_2 demand

Early deflation. (From Datascope Corp., Montvale, New Jersey.)

Late Deflation

Timing Errors
Late Deflation

Deflation of the IAB late in diastolic phase as aortic valve is beginning to open

Waveform Characteristics:
- Assisted aortic end-diastolic pressure may be equal to or greater than the unassisted aortic end-diastolic pressure
- Rate of rise of assisted systole is prolonged
- Diastolic augmentation may appear widened

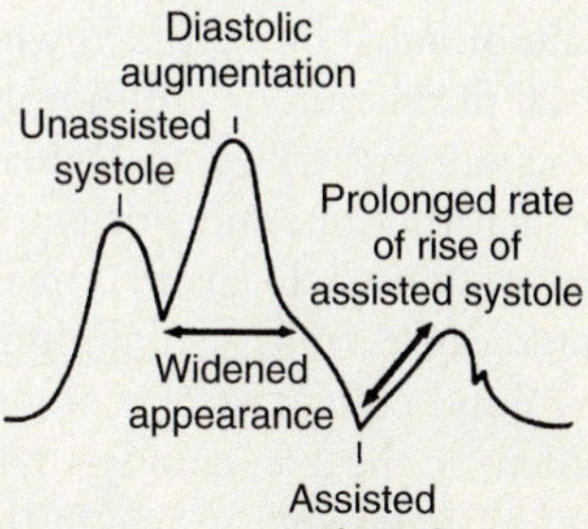

Physiologic Effects:
- Afterload reduction is essentially absent
- Increased MVO_2 consumption due to the left ventricle ejecting against a greater resistance and a prolonged isovolumetric contraction phase
- IAB may impede left ventricular ejection and increase the afterload

Late deflation. (From Datascope Corp., Montvale, New Jersey.)

Loss of Vacuum/IABP Failure

1. Tighten all connections in the tubing.
2. Check the device power source that drives the helium.
3. Hand inflate and deflate the balloon every 5 minutes with half the total balloon volume to prevent clot formation.
4. Change the IABP console if possible. If this happens during transport, call ahead to receiving hospital for an IABP console to be available on the helipad or the ED door upon arrival.

Suspected Balloon Perforation

1. Observe for loss of augmentation (alarms set to sound if a diastolic drop of 10 mm).
2. Check catheter; if blood present, balloon is perforated.
3. Assess for normal balloon pressure waveform on console. Absent waveform if balloon won't retain helium. Pressure plateau will decrease if the balloon is leaking.
4. If leak detected by machine, it will shut itself off. If not, place console on standby, and be prepared to remove the catheter within 15–30 minutes.
5. Clamp the IABP catheter to prevent arterial blood backup.
6. Disconnect the IABP catheter from the console. You may want to discontinue anticoagulation therapy.
7. Notify the licensed practitioner. Prepare for insertion of a new IABP catheter.

the rate excessively, however. Challenging the heart by causing too high a heart rate while it is suffering from **ischemia** could cause myocardial injury.

For the patient with chest pain who is having tachycardia (≥150) but normal blood pressure (>100 systolic), treatment is based on the source of the pacemaker (supraventricular versus ventricular) and the type of arrhythmia present. If the rhythm is tachycardic and very irregular, poor valve function and stagnant blood flow may be present, creating an increased risk of clot formation. Caution must be exercised when encountering new-onset atrial fibrillation or multifocal atrial tachycardia. Medications are prescribed to regulate the heart rate, restore a normal rhythm, and prevent blood clot formation. Such medications help avoid a major change in rhythm that could cause a release of multiple clots into the circulation, with subsequent stroke or other related complications. When applicable, antidysrhythmic agents may also be administered appropriate to the potential pacemaker site. If the tachycardic patient also has signs of alterations in mentation and evidence of cardiogenic shock, synchronized cardioversion may be necessary to immediately change the life-threatening rhythm.

Aortic Aneurysm and Dissection

The aorta is suspended from a fixed ligament near the bifurcations or branches of the left subclavian artery. It has three layers: intima, media, and adventitia. The middle or media layer is made up of smooth muscle and some elastic tissue. Normal aging causes this layer to lose its elasticity and the intimal layer to weaken. If chronic hypertension is present, the deterioration is intensified. Some patients have congenital changes in their aorta that also decrease wall strength and hasten the degeneration of the aortic wall. Marfan and Ehlers-Danlos syndromes create such changes.

If the aortic intima layer finally tears, high-pressure blood flow enters the medial layer. The amount of dissection depends on where this tear occurs, the degree of disease in the media layer, and blood pressure. This injury may move up or down the aorta and may extend back into the coronary arteries (usually right), pericardial sac, or pleural cavity. Control of blood pressure is a major factor in controlling the extension of this hematoma. Another management tactic depends on where the dissection is occurring—in the ascending or descending aorta. Ascending aortic dissections are much more lethal.

Chest pain is the most common complaint, and the patient may describe it as excruciating, sharp, tearing, or ripping. If the patient indicates that the pain is located in the anterior chest, the ascending aorta may be involved. Neck and jaw pain may be associated with injury to the aortic arch, and pain near the scapula may indicate dissection in the descending aorta. Auscultation of heart sounds may yield aortic regurgitation. CHF and APE may quickly develop. It is essential to look for the development of pericardial tamponade.

This tearing type pain is usually associated with nausea, vomiting, a feeling of lightheadedness, anxiety, and diaphoresis. Syncopal episodes are not very common but may be the only presentation in some patients. A change in mental status may also occur.

Blood pressure may present in two ways:

1. Hypotension may indicate movement of the dissection into the pericardium, with tamponade or hypovolemia from rupture of the aorta.
2. Hypertension may indicate the catecholamine release associated with the event or, if hypertension continues despite therapy, extension of the dissection into the renal arteries.

Comparison of blood pressure in the right and left arms can indicate aortic branch (usually subclavian) injury. A significant decrease in blood pressure in one of the arms suggests aortic dissection. Neurologic symptoms may indicate injury to proximal aortic branches, causing signs of stroke, or distal injury, causing spinal cord signs and symptoms.

Suspicion of aortic dissection may be generated just though your history and physical exam, but diagnostic studies are needed to confirm the differential diagnosis.

Diagnostics in Aortic Aneurysm and Dissection

1. As soon as feasible during your evaluation, a 12-lead ECG should be routinely done for any patient complaining of chest pain. Approximately 15% of patients with aortic dissection will have signs of ischemia, especially right coronary (inferior wall). Left ventricular hypertrophy will be present in about 26% because of hypertension, and 31% will have no changes on the ECG.
2. Chest radiograph: chest x-ray is usually completed on all patients presenting with chest pain. Of these, 12% of chest radiographs are normal, even with aortic dissections. A widened mediastinum may be seen, along with other subtleties that may or may not point the clinician to this disease.
3. Echocardiography can be obtained from two views: transthoracic (where aortic regurgitation may be seen) or transesophageal, which actually allows a good view of the thoracic aorta.
4. Computed tomography angiography (CTA): the primary diagnostic test chosen to find aortic dissection, which can be missed if intravenous (IV) contrast is not used with CT.
5. Magnetic resonance imaging (MRI) is very good at capturing the true image of an aortic dissection. However, it does require nonferrous equipment around the patient, and because of the prolonged time required for obtaining images, it is not helpful when the patient is unstable.
6. Angiography is another radiologic test for diagnosing and evaluating this condition.

Management of Aortic Dissection In general, use of your chest pain protocol is safe, even when this disease process is lurking within the chest cavity. Oxygen, vascular access, and application of monitors are routine. The use of antiplatelet therapy like aspirin in the aortic dissection that requires surgery is problematic but not contraindicated. Transporting the patient to a hospital with emergency cardiac capabilities is of high priority. Suspecting an aortic dissection and passing those signs and symptoms on to the in-hospital team may facilitate more rapid identification.

The most critical presentation of aortic dissection is the patient who presents with hypotension due to aortic rupture and/or pericardial tamponade. This patient needs to be resuscitated with IV crystalloids while moving toward the operating room. Pericardiocentesis may afford the patient more time with slight improvements in CO until the definitive repair can be done in surgery.

In the patient who presents with hypertension, beta-blocker administration (especially an infusion of esmolol) to decrease rate and strength of contractions is the most common management choice and may be combined with nitroprusside to decrease afterload and preload. Use of morphine may also decrease the workload of the heart while providing analgesia.

Pericardial Tamponade

You've now reviewed some of the most life-threatening conditions responsible for complaints of chest pain or discomfort. The focus has been on the very practical image of that patient who presents with chest pain and increased work of breathing and/or chest pain and altered vital signs. One rare event that may present with chest pain, cough, or dyspnea is pericardial tamponade (cardiac tamponade).

Cardiac tamponade occurs when fluid accumulates inside the layered pericardial sac surrounding the heart itself. This causes compression forces around the heart, restricting its movement and causing subsequent obstructive shock. Although you may think of cardiac tamponade as a traumatic injury, many medical causes for this condition also exist. The fluid that accumulates can come from cancerous lesions and exudate, pus, gas, blood, or a combination of factors. The most common causes, as described by Merce et al., were malignant diseases in 30% to 60% of cases, uremia in 10% to 15% of cases, idiopathic pericarditis in 5% to 15%, infectious diseases in 5% to 10%, anticoagulation in 5% to 10%, connective tissue diseases in 2% to 6%, and Dressler or postpericardiotomy syndrome in 1% to 2%. Tamponade can occur as a result of any type of pericarditis.

Rapidly accumulating fluid in a confining space usually brings on signs and symptoms very quickly with a minimal amount of fluid. The body space doesn't have time to compensate or adapt to the change in the environment. Slower accumulating fluid in a body space allows for adaptation, with slower onset of signs and symptoms with a much larger amount of fluid within the space.

There are generally three factors for the presentation of cardiac tamponade: how quickly the fluid accumulated, the amount of fluid, and the heart's health. When symptoms develop, the increased pericardial pressure has squeezed the heart and kept it from filling adequately, decreasing CO.

The signs and symptoms reflecting this squeeze are usually described as a series of three (triad), as described by Beck in 1935. These are: hypotension (low CO), distended neck veins (high right heart pressures), and muffled heart tones (fluid outside the heart). In a more subtle way (with slow accumulation), the patient may present with chest pain, cough, and dyspnea. While rare presentations, evaluation may note JVD and muffled heart sounds.

Other classic signs and symptoms that may be indicative of cardiac tamponade include:

1. **Pulsus paradoxus**, or paradoxical pulse. Normally the systolic blood pressure decreases slightly with each inhalation. When the heart is being squeezed in tamponade, this is exaggerated. Pulsus paradoxus is found when the pulse decreases in size or is non-palpable during inhalation. Kussmaul's sign, an increase in JVD during inspiration, may also be present.
   - Kussmaul's sign is also a paradox: listening to the heart sounds during inspiration, the pulse weakens or may not be palpable with certain heartbeats, while S_1 is heard with all heartbeats.
2. Dysphoria. Restless body movements will be observed with unusual facial expressions, restlessness, or a sense of impending death. Ikematsu reported that this unusual finding is present in as many as 26% of all patients with pericardial tamponade.

Diagnostics in Cardiac Tamponade

1. Chest x-ray will show a large heart if the fluid accumulated is 200 to 250 mL.
2. ECG will show low amplitude (decreased voltage).
   - Another diagnostic sign involving the ECG is called *electrical alternans*. This is a highly specific marker of chronic pericardial tamponade, rare in acute accumulation of pericardial fluid. The morphology and amplitude of the P, QRS, and ST-T waves in all leads will alternate in every other beat because of "swinging heart phenomenon." The normal heart swings back and forth with each contraction but returns to normal position before the next contraction. In pericardial tamponade, the heart is too heavy to swing back to a normal position in time, and the continuous ECG "sees" the heart out of position for one contraction (Figure 5-7).
3. Echocardiography shows pericardial effusion with RV collapse.
4. Hemodynamic monitoring will show that the right and left ventricular pressures are equal.

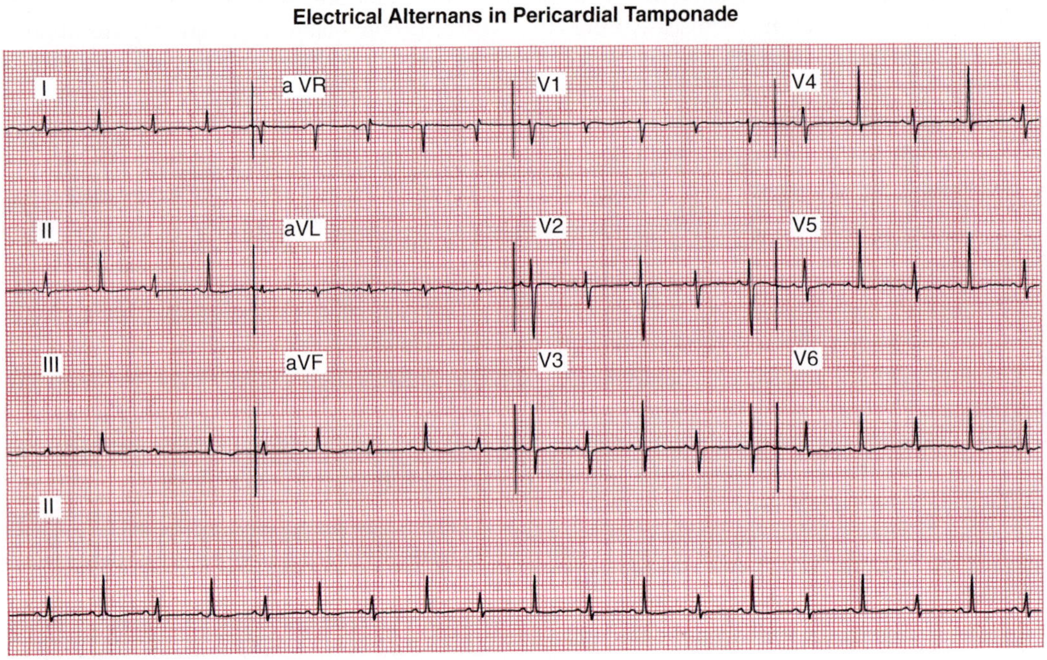

Electrical Alternans in Pericardial Tamponade

■ **Figure 5-7** Cardiac tamponade. Electrical alternans may develop in patients with pericardial effusion and cardiac tamponade. Notice the beat-to-beat alternation in the P-QRS-T axis; this is caused by the periodic swinging motion of the heart in a large pericardial effusion. Relatively low QRS voltage and sinus tachycardia are also present. (From Goldberger A: Clinical electrocardiography: a simplified approach, ed 7, St Louis, 2006, Mosby.)

Management of Cardiac Tamponade The patient with cardiac tamponade will be presenting to you with a complaint of chest pain and dyspnea, possibly with a cough. A high index of suspicion must guide you toward this diagnosis while reviewing the patient's risk factors for development of a medical cardiac tamponade. The application of oxygen, gaining vascular access, and applying monitors is routine. A 12-lead ECG is also necessary. Following standard chest pain protocols in the prehospital setting is warranted, but signs of shock may prevent administration of morphine and nitrates.

If hypotension is present, fluid resuscitation with crystalloids for the obstructive shock state may initially help fill the right heart and improve CO. This buys the clinician time until an ultrasound-guided pericardiocentesis can be performed.

Figure 5-8 shows pericardiocentesis being used to remove blood from the pericardial sac, and Procedure 5-2 details how pericardiocentesis is performed. Enough fluid should be removed to improve the patient clinically. If tamponade recurs, the procedure may be repeated, and a catheter may be left in with a 3-way stopcock. Surgical consultation is warranted if further drainage is required.

Acute Coronary Syndrome

Acute coronary syndrome (ACS) is a group of conditions that involve decreased blood flow to the heart muscle. This group of conditions often share the common underlying pathology of atherosclerosis. Atherosclerosis comes from the Greek words *athero* (meaning "gruel" or "paste")

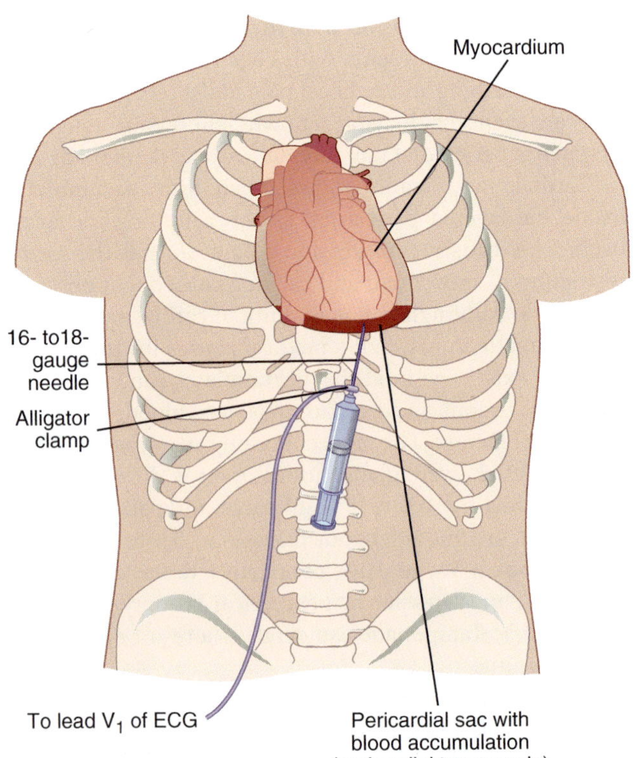

■ **Figure 5-8** Pericardiocentesis to remove blood from the pericardial sac during tamponade. *ECG,* Electrocardiogram. (From Black JM, Hokanson Hawks J: Medical-surgical nursing, ed 8, Philadelphia, 2009, Saunders.)

Procedure 5-2 Pericardiocentesis

OVERVIEW

Pericardial tamponade can occur through both medical and traumatic disease processes. The accumulation of serosanguineous fluid is called pericardial effusion. Whether blood or effusion, the rapid accumulation of fluid within the space creates a high-pressure environment outside of the heart, resulting in obstructive shock. A slower rate of accumulating effusion allows for the heart to accommodate and remodel into a hypertrophic state with distention of the heart. As much as 1 to 2 liters of fluid can accumulate before hemodynamic compromise occurs when slow effusion gathers in the sac. Pericardiocentesis is geared toward the emergent, life-saving removal of as little as 15 to 50 mL of blood following traumatic pericardial tamponade.

INDICATIONS

- Emergency: pericardial tamponade with obstructive shock
- Elective: removal of fluid for laboratory specimen analysis (effusion)

CONTRAINDICATIONS

- In the emergency setting, there are really no contraindications to this procedure when tamponade exists.

PREPARATION/EQUIPMENT

The critical care team must have protocols in place, and the professional credentialing agency must have approved of this procedure as being within the staff member's scope of practice. The employer should routinely reeducate and recredential each employee on this procedure in a skills lab.

- Small procedure tray with sterile instruments (4 × 4 gauze sponges, alligator clip and cable, two 3-way stopcocks)
- Sterile drapes or towels
- Skin cleansing agent
- 5-, 10-, 20-mL syringes
- 16- or 18-gauge, 3-inch cardiac needle or catheter-over-needle device
- 12-Lead ECG machine at bedside and prepared for procedure
- If available, bedside ultrasound machine and transducer gel

PROCEDURE

1. Identify the xiphochondral junction on the left side. This is the angle where the lowest rib meets the sternum at the lateral border and the xiphoid medially. Prep the site with skin cleanser.
2. Assemble a 16- to 18-gauge, 6-inch or longer over-the-needle catheter, and attach a 20- to 35-mL empty syringe with a 3-way stopcock. To guide the needle, either attach an alligator clamp on an electrode to the needle and watch for ECG changes (see diagram), or use the ultrasound device. Some providers use both devices to guide insertion.
3. The needle is inserted 1 to 2 cm inferior to the left side of the angle described in step 1. The direction of the needle is advanced toward the tip of the left scapula at a 45-degree angle.
4. If the needle is advanced too far, an injury called *current of injury* is seen on the ECG. Extreme ST wave changes or widened/enlarged QRS may be seen. This means the needle should be withdrawn until the ECG returns to the preprocedure baseline.
5. *Unclotted blood is aspirated into the syringe from the pericardial sac. Withdraw as much as possible. As little as 15 to 20 mL may relieve symptoms. If a current-of-injury pattern reappears, it means the epicardial layer may be touching the needle tip now that you have removed the blood. Withdraw the needle slightly, and continue to withdraw blood. If the injury pattern continues on the ECG, discontinue the procedure.
6. Once the blood is removed, the catheter may be left in place as the inner needle is withdrawn. The catheter along with the 3-way stopcock may then be secured into place so that any further bleeding into the space can be drained.
7. The patient's obstructive shock signs should subside.

*Unclotted blood would be aspirated from the pericardial sac, since cardiac motion removes fibrin from the blood.

and *sclerosis* (meaning "hardness"). The "gruel" or "paste" in this case is made up of calcium, lipids, and fats, and is called *plaque*. As plaque clings to the walls of coronary arteries, it narrows the lumen, reducing the amount of blood (carrying nutrients and oxygen) reaching the heart muscle (Figure 5-9). The plaque may harden or remain soft.

When atherosclerosis occurs within the coronary arteries, it is referred to as *coronary artery disease (CAD)*. Patients with CAD are at increased risk for ACS. The two most common ACS disorders are angina pectoris and AMI. AMI can be further divided into **ST-segment elevation myocardial infarction** (STEMI) and **non–ST-segment elevation myocardial infarction** (NSTEMI).

Angina Angina pectoris literally means "chest pain" and is caused by an inadequate blood supply from a narrowed coronary artery filled with plaque. **Stable angina** pain usually comes on with exercise or stress and lasts 3 to 5 minutes, sometimes up to 15 minutes. Angina pain is relieved by rest and/or nitroglycerin. Less common causes of angina may include coronary artery spasm, arterial inflammation resulting from an infection, and extrinsic causes not related to the coronary artery like hypoxia, hypotension, tachycardias, and anemia. Most patients who develop anginal pain from these extrinsic causes have a past medical history of CAD or angina. Another form of ACS may result from cocaine or methamphetamine; these drugs increase myocardial oxygen demand and may cause coronary artery spasm or dissection. In and of itself, angina is a sign of serious heart disease and may lead to an AMI if it becomes unstable. **Unstable angina** occurs at rest, is more severe than normal episodes of angina, and may also be caused by coronary artery spasms. If left untreated, unstable angina can lead to an AMI.

Acute Myocardial Infarction **Acute myocardial infarction (AMI)** is caused by a clot or thrombus that forms in a narrowed coronary artery where the plaque has ruptured, causing platelets to aggregate and a clot to form. If the coronary artery becomes completely obstructed, the ischemic cells in the heart muscle will begin to die. This can cause permanent damage to the heart muscle and is often referred to as a "heart attack."

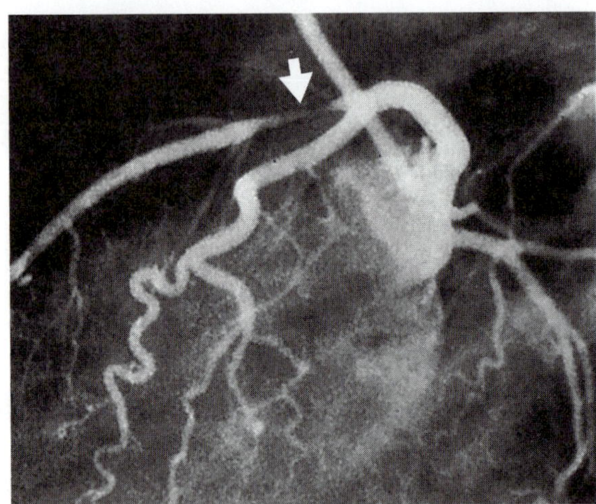

Figure 5-9 Coronary angiography shows stenosis *(arrow)* of left anterior descending coronary artery. (From Braunwald E: Heart disease: a textbook of cardiovascular medicine, ed 4, Philadelphia, 1992, Saunders.)

As already noted, AMI is divided into two types: STEMI and NSTEMI. Either diagnosis requires acquisition and interpretation of a 12-lead ECG to differentiate between them. Differentiation is key in providing treatment geared for the specific types of AMI. An AMI involving ST-segment elevation (Figure 5-10) or non–ST-segment elevation may lead to an irregular heart rhythm, a lethal heart rhythm like ventricular fibrillation, or CHF. CHF may lead to the development of APE or cardiogenic shock and death. Left ventricular infarction of 40% or more usually results in left heart failure, cardiogenic shock, and carries a high mortality rate. Right ventricular infarction or ischemia occurs in up to 50% of patients who present with an inferior wall AMI and usually results in right heart failure and hypotension. These conditions can be exacerbated if nitrates or morphine are administered for the complaint of chest pain.

Certain risk factors place the patient at a greater risk for developing an ACS. The more risk factors, the greater the chance of developing ACS. Some risk factors can't be modified, but others can.

Those risk factors we can't modify include age, sex, and heredity. The older you get, the more likely your chance of CAD is. Men have CAD at an earlier age and are more likely to die from their ACS. However, heart disease remains the leading cause of death in women, particularly post menopause. Estrogen in younger women is felt to perhaps have a cardioprotective effect, but after menopause, the incidence of ACS in men and women is similar. A family history of CAD increases your risk of developing ACS and may be directly linked to lifestyle. If your parents

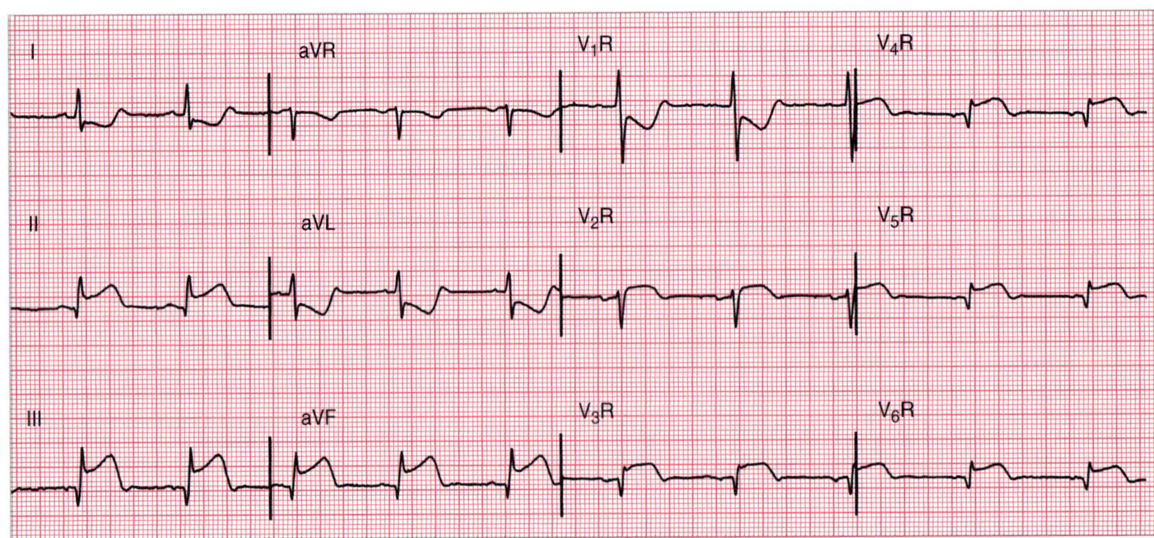

Figure 5-10 Acute right ventricular infarction with acute inferior wall infarction. Note the ST elevation in the right precordial leads, as well as in leads II, III, and aVF, with reciprocal change in I and aVL. ST elevation in lead III, greater than in lead II, and right precordial ST elevation are consistent with proximal to middle occlusion of the right coronary artery. The combination of ST elevation in conventional lead V_1 (lead V_2R here) and ST depression in lead V_2 (lead V_1R here) has also been reported with acute right ventricular ischemia or infarction. (From Libby P, et al: Braunwald's heart disease: a textbook of cardiovascular medicine, ed 8, Philadelphia, 2008, Saunders.)

led a lifestyle of high risk for CAD, chances are you will as well.

Those risk factors we can modify include hypertension, smoking, high cholesterol, diabetes, obesity, stress, and lack of physical activity. Hypertension is defined by the American Heart Association (AHA) as a blood pressure greater than 140/90, is easily diagnosed, and can usually be successfully managed with diet, exercise, and medications. Hypertension causes the heart to work harder than it should and, over time, causes it to enlarge and weaken. Smoking increases your risk of developing ACS. Smoking is the single most preventable cause of death in the United States. Smokers' risk of heart attack is more than twice that of nonsmokers. Smokers who have ACS are more likely to die. The nicotine and carbon monoxide in tobacco smoke reduces the amount of oxygen in the blood and damages blood vessel walls, causing plaque to build up. Tobacco smoke may trigger blood clots to form as well. Smoking promotes heart disease by reducing HDL ("good") cholesterol. Quitting smoking reduces your risk of having ACS even if you have smoked for years. High cholesterol is another easily diagnosed problem that can be managed with diet, exercise, and medications. A heart-healthy diet high in fruits and vegetables and low in fats and carbohydrates reduces LDL ("bad") cholesterol. Diabetes greatly increases the risk of heart disease. In fact, most people with diabetes die from some form of cardiovascular disease. One reason for this is that diabetes is usually linked with low HDL ("good") cholesterol and high LDL ("bad") cholesterol levels. It also affects the blood vessels themselves, accelerating atherosclerosis. Many people with diabetes also have high blood pressure, increasing their risk even more. Obesity, stress, and lack of exercise accelerate the atherosclerotic process, increasing the chances of having ACS.

Healthcare providers get frequent calls for the most common symptom associated with ACS, chest discomfort. Effective treatment for ACS is time sensitive, so it becomes important to quickly recognize its presence and provide essential treatment within the first hours of onset. Early intervention can reduce the likelihood of sudden cardiac death and/or myocardial damage. Quick recognition and diagnosis of an ACS starts with readily recognizing the signs and symptoms and obtaining a thorough history and physical exam.

Signs and Symptoms of Acute Coronary Syndrome The classic signs and symptoms of ACS may include a sudden onset of chest pain or pressure located in the center of the chest beneath the sternum. This pain or pressure may feel like it is radiating to the neck or jaw and down the left arm. It is described as constant, usually lasting longer than 15 minutes. The patient may also complain of shortness of breath, like the chest is in a vise or an elephant is sitting on the chest, making it difficult for them to breathe. They may also have the associated signs and symptoms of diaphoresis; pale, mottled, cool skin; and weakness or lightheadedness. They may complain of feeling nauseated, may vomit, and may have a feeling of impending doom. The presence of rales and rhonchi, with or without JVD, may be present with large AMI, indicating the presence of CHF.

These classic signs and symptoms of ACS may all be present, or only a few may be present. The elderly, diabetics, and postmenopausal women over 55 may present with no pain or discomfort, but instead present as though they are having a sudden onset of weakness. Women may also present with shortness of breath with or without chest discomfort. Nausea, vomiting, and back or jaw pain are also more common complaints in women. Failure to recognize the weakness as ACS in the elderly, diabetic, or postmenopausal woman may lead to the development of serious and life-threatening consequences.

You can organize your approach to the patient with chest discomfort using a SAMPLER history and the OPQRST mnemonic (see the Rapid Recall boxes in Chapter 1 for a review). Let's start with the OPQRST evaluation:

O—Onset: What was the patient doing when the chest discomfort started? Remember, you don't have to be working hard for an AMI to occur. In fact, most happen at rest. If the discomfort began suddenly with activity or during a stressful situation, assess further to determine a past medical history of angina. Gradual onset may suggest pericarditis. An onset a day after heavy lifting or forceful coughing may suggest a chest wall muscle involvement (diagnosis of exclusion only).

P—Provocation: What makes the discomfort better or worse? The pain from an AMI is usually constant and is worsened by exertion, but not normally worsened with a deep breath or with palpation on the area where the pain is being felt. It is not made better by a particular position or by splinting the chest with a pillow. If the discomfort is relieved by rest and/or nitroglycerin, then the ACS may be angina. If not, then the pain or discomfort could be the result of unstable angina or an AMI. If the pain increases with palpation or inspiration, pneumonia, pneumothorax, pericarditis, or pulmonary embolism may be the reason for the pain or discomfort. At that time, further assessment for those signs and symptoms should occur.

Q—Quality: Have the patient describe the discomfort in his or her own words. Mistakes like asking them if the pain is sharp or dull can limit their response to sharp or dull, which may not accurately describe how they feel. Heart-related pain is often accompanied by a sensation of pressure or squeezing, as it is visceral in nature. It can be described as indigestion. A tearing pain is associated with dissection of an aneurysm.

R—Radiation: Does the discomfort radiate? Typically the discomfort of an ACS will radiate to the neck or jaw or down the arms. However, it may also radiate to the back, into the abdomen, or down the legs. It could radiate anywhere. Discomfort felt in the shoulder may be referred and associated with gallbladder disease or spleen involvement. The discomfort of an aortic dissection classically radiates straight through to the back and may settle in the flank. Further assessment of those types of discomfort are warranted.

S—Severity: Ask the patient to rate the pain on a 1-to-10 scale, with 1 being the least amount of discomfort and 10 being the worst pain ever felt. Giving the discomfort a number informs you where on the scale the patient's experience of the chest discomfort is right now. If the treatment you provide is effective, that number should go down. If the number goes up, it should signal to you that your patient is not responding to treatment and probably getting worse. You may find gender differences in reporting: men typically rate their discomfort a higher number than women. At times the treatment for chest discomfort in men is taken more seriously because of how they describe its intensity. Women may have little or no complaints of discomfort, but instead complain of a sudden onset of weakness with the associated signs and symptoms of AMI like nausea, dizziness, malaise, and anxiety.

T—Time: How long have they had this discomfort? If a clot is the cause, the patient may need a fibrinolytic or "clot buster" to dissolve a clot in the coronary artery. This decision will depend on how close the patient is to a definitive therapy or chest pain center capable of cardiac catheterization, The window of opportunity in which administration of a fibrinolytic will be beneficial is narrow.

Healthcare providers should know the capabilities of the surrounding facilities to which they may be transporting the patient. Cardiac centers or STEMI centers are designated as the place a patient with an ACS should be quickly transferred to for specialty care. The evolving standard of care is to bypass hospitals not capable of 24-hour emergent percutaneous intervention (PCI) capabilities for patients with STEMI.

After completion of the OPQRST, you should have a good idea whether your patient is experiencing an ACS and whether the cause is angina, unstable angina, or AMI. For example, a patient states that he was shoveling heavy snow and suddenly developed chest discomfort. The pain is substernal, constant, radiates to the neck, jaw, and down the arms. He is having difficulty breathing because he feels pressure like an elephant is sitting on his chest. When asked to rate his pain, he describes it as above a 10. The pain has lasted for about an hour and has not been relieved by rest or his nitroglycerin. Chances are, he's having an AMI. We may not have completed a 12-lead ECG or have the ability to look at cardiac markers, but we can with some certainty develop the field impression of an AMI.

Importantly, the absence of a classic presentation should not falsely reassure you. For instance, the presence of tenderness to palpation of the chest, a pleuritic component, or presence of a cough does NOT rule out a cardiac etiology to the pain. These patients should be taken seriously and evaluated for possible ACS depending on age and risk factors. Alternative diagnoses such as GERD and musculoskeletal pain are diagnoses of exclusion.

Now, let's add a SAMPLER history to the findings of your OPQRST:

S—Signs and symptoms: Look for associated signs and symptoms, such as a sudden onset of weakness; dizziness; pale, cool, clammy skin; or the feeling of impending doom. Ventricular assistive devices can cause skin breakdown at the cannulation site, disturbances in sleep/wake cycles, alterations in mentation and behavior and depression due to the lifestyle changes that occur with end-stage heart failure. Pertinent negatives such as discomfort not being relieved by rest or nitroglycerin would be important to note and suggest unstable angina or AMI.

A—Allergies: Learning of allergies to any medications is important because this patient may be given aspirin along with other medications for their AMI.

M—Medications: All medications—prescription, herbal, and over-the-counter (OTC)—are important to note. They may indicate a past medical history of CAD or a previous heart condition. Medications like nitroglycerin, aspirin, cholesterol-lowering medications, high blood pressure medications like ACE inhibitors, beta-blockers, calcium channel blockers, and oral hypoglycemics would all be pertinent for the possibility of CAD. If the patient has taken any medications in the last 24 to 36 hours for erectile dysfunction (such as Viagra, Cialis, or Levitra), nitrates should be avoided; they may drastically lower blood pressure.

P—Pertinent past medical history: Does the patient have heart disease? Is there a family history of heart disease? Has the patient had an AMI? Have they ever had a coronary artery bypass graft (CABG) or a percutaneous transluminal coronary angioplasty (PTCA) with a stent to open a coronary vessel? Is there evidence of risk factors? These are all pertinent medical history questions you should attempt to answer.

You should also make note of a surgically implanted left ventricular assistive device (LVAD; Figure 5-11). This implanted mechanical device is used in patients with end-stage heart failure and those waiting for heart transplantation. Patients may also have devices that are right ventricular assistive devices (RVAD) and biventricular assistive devices (BiVAD). Such devices are a "bridge" to transplantation or aids for those who have had heart

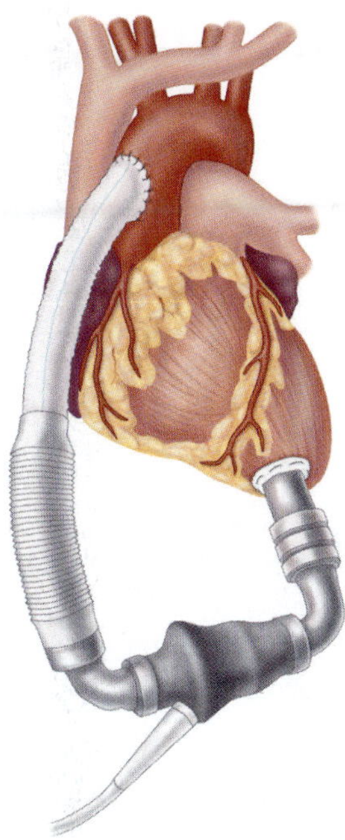

■ **Figure 5-11** Left ventricular assistive device (LVAD). A HeartMate II is a small continuous flow pump. The inflow cannula is connected to the cardiac apex, and the outflow graft is connected to the ascending aorta. (From Cleveland Clinic: Current clinical medicine 2009, ed 1, Philadelphia, 2008, Saunders.)

surgery and experience severe heart failure. Trials of these devices as permanent alternatives to transplantation are taking place.

L—Last oral intake: This may indicate the presence of a full stomach and an increased risk of vomiting should the patient become nauseated.

E—Events: What events led up to the call for 9-1-1? Was the patient engaged in physical activity, a high stress situation, or did they wake up from a sleep with the discomfort? Has there been any use of cocaine or methamphetamines? Has there been a long period of inactivity like an international flight or cross-country road trip (suggesting PE)?

R—Risk factors: Risk factors for the development of the disease as have been described as modifiable and nonmodifiable. If the patient has had previous episodes, have them compare this event with past presentations.

Your continued physical assessment would include a baseline set of vitals and continuous reassessment of those areas of the body associated with the chief complaints. The baseline vitals and application of monitors should be routine.

Diagnostics in Acute Coronary Syndrome Pulse oximetry should be monitored for the presence of hypoxia as defined by the complaint of shortness of breath, increased work of breathing, tachypnea, and oxygen saturations of less than 95%. Administering oxygen in ACS is a high priority and is one of the few interventions that is known to improve outcome. This should not be delayed to get a pulse oximeter reading. Since what you see on a pulse oximeter is not real time, applying oxygen will not have an instantaneous effect on the number you see on the oximeter. Delaying oxygen administration in a hypoxic patient in need of oxygen is strongly discouraged.

12-Lead ECG A heart monitor with 12-lead ECG capabilities should be placed on all patients with suspected ACS prior to giving medications for suspected ischemia (e.g., nitroglycerin, morphine). A 12-lead ECG should be immediately acquired on all patients with ischemic chest discomfort. If STEMI is present, a STEMI alert should be called and the patient transported following local or internal guidelines. Medications may be administered en route to shorten on-scene times. Extended on-scene times do little more than increase the time to definitive therapy and reperfusion.

Being trained in the interpretation of acute changes on a 12-lead ECG and notifying the receiving facility in advance of arrival can reduce door-to-drug times for patients who are candidates for fibrinolysis. Further classifying patients with ACS into one of three group subtypes based on 12-lead ECG findings will guide you in treatment options as well as predict the seriousness of the event and potential complications.

Patients with STEMI or new left bundle branch block (LBBB) are at the greatest risk of developing the serious complications associated with ACS and should be assessed for reperfusion candidacy. Patients with ST-segment depression, indicating ischemia rather than infarct, include the high-risk set of patients with unstable angina who do not qualify for definite early reperfusion. Finally, those with normal 12-lead ECGs but a history suspicious for ACS may be having an NSTEMI or may develop evidence of STEMI. These patients require serial ECGs and repeated assessment and should be treated with aggressive early medical therapy.

Knowing the location where the ischemia or injury is occurring in the heart and the expected complications associated with standard treatments will enhance your ability to provide the most appropriate treatments. As an example, you should suspect right ventricular infarction in patients with inferior wall infarction evidenced by elevated ST segments in leads II, III, and aVF. In patients with inferior wall infarction, the provider should obtain a right-sided ECG by placing the V leads on the left side of the chest to the right side of the chest. ST-segment elevation greater than 1 mm in lead V_4R is suggestive of right ventricular infarction. Patients with acute right ventricular infarction are dependent on maintaining right ventricular filling pressure to maintain CO. Any medication that decreases preload—nitrates, diuretics, or other vasodilators (morphine, ACE inhibitors)—should be avoided because they may cause severe hypotension. This hypotension should be treated with an IV fluid bolus, assuming you have an IV established before giving nitroglycerin. Basic EMTs administering nitroglycerin, not knowing the

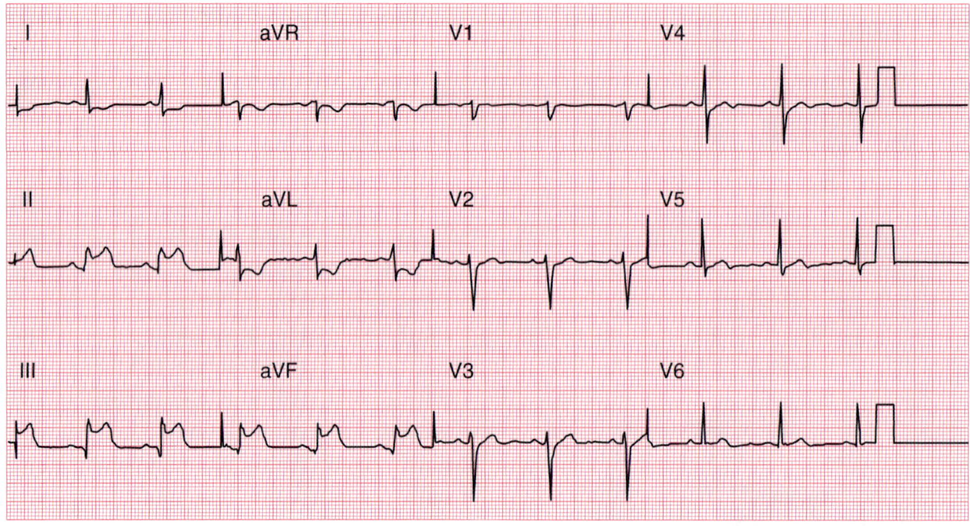

■ **Figure 5-12** (From Aehlert B: ECG made easy, ed 3, St Louis, 2006, Mosby.)

right ventricle is involved, may cause this sudden drop in blood pressure, which reinforces the need for an Advanced Life Support tier with 12-lead ECG capability when possible (Figure 5-12).

Early during the assessment of the patient with suspected ACS, a physical exam should be performed, focusing on the area of the body associated with the chief complaints. Lung sounds should be assessed for the presence of rales or rhonchi. Wet lungs may be the result of left heart failure and APE, indicating cardiogenic shock. The presence of a cough with frothy pink sputum may also be evidence of APE.

If the patient has a cough, do they normally have a cough? If so, why? Do they have a past medical history of COPD? If they normally cough, is it productive? Is what they are coughing up typical in amount and color? A patient with COPD or pneumonia may have a productive cough, so noting if this is different may help you determine whether or not what you are hearing is a new process to the patient. Jugular vein distention and pedal edema may be present if right heart failure has occurred secondary to left heart failure. Examining the chest for previous scars indicating the presence of a pacemaker or past heart surgery would be important findings as well and would support your diagnosis of ACS. Having completed your assessment, the diagnosis of ACS can be made and treatment specific to the type of ACS instituted.

Management of Acute Coronary Syndrome As a prehospital provider, you should be able to provide the following care for suspected ACS. Until risk stratification occurs with 12-lead ECG interpretation, your initial management of ACS is the same as for prehospital care. The common mnemonic *MONA* is often used to remember the interventions needed once the field impression of ACS has been determined. *MONA* stands for *morphine, oxygen, nitroglycerin,* and *aspirin*. It doesn't suggest a particular order of administering treatment or a particular importance of one over the other. Oxygen and aspirin are the only prehospital medications known to improve survival from ACS. Nitroglycerin is generally accepted to be a beneficial treatment for ACS, provided there is no RV involvement as described earlier. The use of morphine has been called into question by recent studies. Check with your medical director, and review regional protocols for the medications preferred in your area. The following protocol is typical:

- Aspirin 162 to 325 mg (2 to 4 baby aspirin), nonenterically coated, should be chewed and/or swallowed at the earliest sign of ACS. Make sure the patient is not allergic to ASA, has no history of recent bleeding ulcers, and is not having an asthma attack. Patients with asthma may develop a condition known as *aspirin-induced asthma* (AIA). When given aspirin, they may develop an asthma attack that occurs gradually but is more intense and difficult to break. Early administration of aspirin in ACS has been associated with decreased mortality rates in several clinical trials, so it should be given as soon as possible if no contraindications are present. The AHA is advocating that dispatchers give prearrival instructions to take aspirin if at all possible. Aspirin suppositories (300 mg) are safe and can be considered for patients with severe nausea, vomiting, or disorders of the upper GI tract.
- Oxygen, initially at 4 LPM via nasal cannula, would be appropriate; administering oxygen increases the supply of oxygen to the ischemic tissue. If there are signs of hypoxia, oxygen should be administered at 10 to 15 LPM via nonrebreather mask. If shortness of breath is severe or in the presence of APE secondary to left heart failure, oxygen should be administered with NIPPV/NPPV (CPAP or BiPAP), or at least using a bag-mask to provide positive pressure.
- Nitroglycerin may be administered sublingually as a 0.4-mg tablet or metered dose spray. It may be

repeated every 3 to 5 minutes three times as long as systolic blood pressure remains above 90 mm Hg. Administering nitroglycerin more than three times may be appropriate with medical direction as long as the blood pressure remains above 90 mm Hg. Nitroglycerin decreases the pain of ischemia by decreasing preload and cardiac oxygen consumption, and it dilates coronary arteries, increasing cardiac collateral flow. Nitroglycerin should be given in patients with ACS, ST-segment elevation or depression, and for the consequences associated with AMI, to include left ventricular failure (APE or CHF). Use with extreme caution in right ventricular infarct, because these patients require adequate preload. Nitroglycerin should not be given to patients with hypotension, extreme bradycardias, or tachycardias. Do not administer nitroglycerin to patients who have taken a phosphodiesterase inhibitor (Viagra, Cialis, Levitra) for erectile dysfunction within the last 24 to 36 hours. Nitroglycerin may lower the BP in a patient whose vascular system is already dilated. Watch for headache, a drop in BP, syncope, and tachycardia when nitroglycerin is given. The patient should sit or lie down during administration. An infusion of nitroglycerin may be started for more finite control of pain and blood pressure at 10 mcg/min. Titrate to relieve the pain by increasing the dose by 10 mcg every 3 to 5 minutes. Keep a close eye on the blood pressure; if not closely monitored, nitroglycerin infusion can lead to a dangerous drop in blood pressure.

Advanced EMS providers with knowledge of rhythms and 12-lead ECG interpretation may:

- Establish an IV of normal saline as a route for medications and fluid. If hypotension occurs following administration of nitroglycerin, fluid boluses should be infused quickly to increase right ventricular filling pressures. Some protocols call for 1 to 2 L in 500-mL boluses, checking blood pressure and lung sounds after each bolus. Fluids should be avoided in the presence of APE secondary to left heart failure, and medications like dopamine should be infused to improve the pumping function of the heart.
- Consider morphine, 2 to 8 mg IV, titrated for discomfort not relieved by nitroglycerin in STEMI patients. Morphine may be given once at 1 to 5 mg in an NSTEMI patient whose discomfort is not relieved by oxygen and nitroglycerin. Be alert for a drop in blood pressure, especially in patients with volume depletion or if right ventricular infarction is apparent. Respiratory depression may occur, so Narcan should be available. If the patient is allergic to morphine, other analgesics may be an option. Fentanyl is an option as a short-acting opioid with less effect on blood pressure than morphine. Check with your medical director and the scope of practice within your state for use of these drugs.

Determining the presence of acute changes indicating ischemia or injury on the 12-lead ECG may further support the need for the following:

- Heparin bolus, when used as adjunctive therapy with fibrin-specific lytics in STEMI: current recommendations call for a bolus dose of 60 Units/kg followed by infusion at a rate of 12 Units/kg/h. While most ground services will not be infusing heparin drips, some are giving a bolus in STEMI confirmed by history and 12-lead ECG. Local protocol, physician medical director involvement, and scope of practice within your state will determine if such treatment is appropriate for your service.
- IV beta-blocker administration is reported to reduce the size of the infarct and mortality in patients who do not receive fibrinolytic therapy. They may also reduce the incidence of ventricular ectopy and fibrillation. IV beta-blockers decrease postinfarction ischemia and nonfatal AMI in patients who do receive fibrinolytic agents. IV beta-blockers may also be beneficial for NSTEMI ACS.

Recent studies suggest that beta-blockers may increase the incidence of cardiogenic shock in the first 48 hours, so some clinicians are now recommending beta-blockers be reserved for patients who are hypertensive and/or tachycardic, rather than administering them routinely to all patients with ACS. Contraindications to beta-blockers are moderate to severe left ventricular failure and pulmonary edema, bradycardia, hypotension, signs of poor peripheral perfusion, second-degree or third-degree heart block, and asthma. Metoprolol, atenolol, propranolol, esmolol, and labetalol are acceptable, and paramedics should follow their local protocol. Vital signs should be taken between doses to ensure heart rate and blood pressure remain adequate. Sometimes once discomfort is relieved, the catecholamine release stops. If IV beta-blockers are on board, the patient then becomes hypotensive, and the condition may worsen. Be prepared to treat this with an IVF bolus. Local protocol, physician medical director involvement, and scope of practice within your state will determine if such treatment is appropriate for your service.

Out-of-hospital administration of fibrinolytics to patients with STEMI who have no contraindications is reasonable for patients with symptom duration up to 6 hours. Services offering out-of-hospital fibrinolytics require a strict adherence to protocols, 12-lead ECG acquisition and interpretation, experience in ACLS, the ability to communicate with the receiving institution, and a medical director with experience in management of STEMI. A continuous quality improvement (CQI) process to evaluate all calls where fibrinolytics are used is required. Most EMS services have short enough transport times that they focus on early diagnosis with 12-lead ECG, completing a fibrinolytic checklist, administering first line medications, and advance notification of the receiving facility for

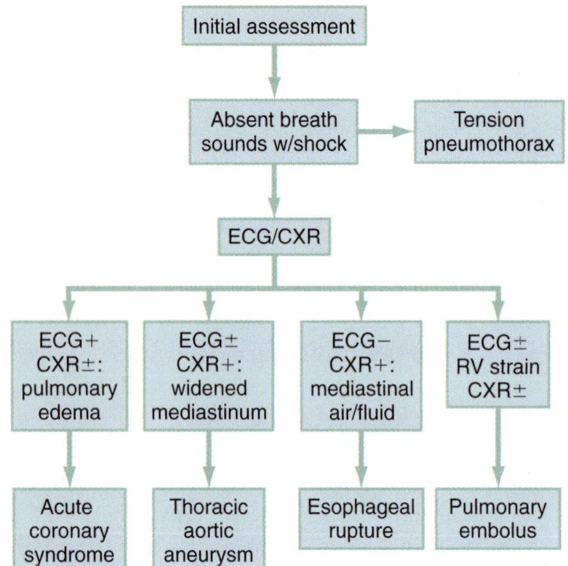

■ **Figure 5-13** In-hospital critical diagnoses in chest pain. (From Marx JA, Hockberger RS, Walls RM, et al: Rosen's emergency medicine: concepts and clinical practice, ed 7, 2010, Mosby.)

Cath Lab activation. Selecting the proper fibrinolytic requires a thorough understanding of their properties and complications. Not being able to obtain a chest x-ray to determine the presence of a widened mediastinum indicating an aneurysm is another reason for not considering prehospital fibrinolytics.

All complaints of chest discomfort or those patients presenting atypically with the associated signs and symptoms of an ACS should be assessed first for the presence of an ACS. After initial evaluation, if ACS appears less likely, other differential diagnoses must be investigated (Figure 5-13).

Pivotal Findings in the Patient with Chest Pain

The history, physical exam, and 12-lead ECG will identify 80% to 90% of the diagnoses with the presentation of chest pain. So far, you've identified those life-threatening causes of chest pain that are initially suggested in the primary survey when the patient is complaining of pain with obvious shortness of breath and/or signs of shock.

For those patients who are more stable, or for those conditions that cause fewer cardinal signs and symptoms, a more detailed history with secondary exam will aid you. When obtaining history, there are some key findings that may help narrow down the diagnostic list:

1. Character of the pain: crushing or pressure-like versus tearing should lead you to think ACS versus thoracic aortic aneurysm. Those with sharp pain can be suffering from a PE, pneumothorax, or a musculoskeletal cause. The complaint of burning or indigestion may lead you to think of GI complaints.
2. Activity with pain: pain with exertion is usually indicative of ACS. If at rest, MI is suggested. A sudden onset of pain usually points to aortic dissection, pulmonary embolism, or pneumothorax. Pain after meals may indicate GI problems.
3. The 1-to-10 pain scale: now universal. You should get this information from your patient early in the course of assessment and management. Onset and peak of pain should also be noted, along with an ongoing assessment related to management.
4. Pain location: localized pain in a small area is usually somatic (the patient can point to it with one finger, and there's no radiation). Visceral pain, on the other hand, is more difficult to localize (the patient circles the chest with their hand and talks about referral of pain). Peripheral chest wall pain is usually not cardiac in nature.
5. Radiation of pain: radiation into the back may guide you toward aortic dissection or GI causes. Pain located near the scapular area of the back and radiating into the neck suggests aortic dissection as well. Inferior MI may present as thoracic back pain. Any radiation of pain to jaw, arms, or neck usually points toward cardiac ischemia.
6. Duration of pain: very short-lived (measured in seconds) pain is rarely cardiac in nature. Pain that begins suddenly and is described as being worst at the onset is many times aortic dissection. Pain that may begin with exertion but goes away with rest may be cardiac ischemia. Pain that is constant and lasts for days is less commonly life threatening. On the other hand, pain that is intermittent and fluctuates is more likely serious.
7. Aggravation/alleviation: pain that worsens with exertion and improves with rest is usually coronary ischemia. Pain related to meals is associated with GI problems. Pain that worsens with deep breath or cough is generally tied to pulmonary, pericardial, or musculoskeletal problems.
8. Associated symptoms with chest pain:
   - Diaphoresis: serious or visceral causes
   - Hemoptysis: pulmonary embolism
   - Syncope or syncopal feeling: cardiovascular cause or pulmonary embolism
   - Dyspnea: cardiovascular or pulmonary causes
   - Nausea and vomiting: cardiovascular or GI causes

Non–Life-Threatening (Emergent) Causes of Chest Pain

Once you have reviewed the causes and the clinical signs and symptoms of life-threatening causes of chest pain, your focus on the secondary exam, history, diagnostic tests, and ongoing assessment may lead you to find the other causes for the patient's complaint. Some emergent diagnoses include unstable angina, coronary spasm, Prinzmetal's angina, cocaine-induced chest pain, infection (myocarditis, pericarditis), simple pneumothorax (see Chapter 3), and GI causes such as esophageal tear, cholecystitis, and pancreatitis (see Chapter 7).

Unstable Angina

Prolonged chest discomfort (lasting more than 15 minutes) that continues at rest or chest discomfort that awakens the patient at night (nocturnal) are features of unstable angina. The patient may describe the pain as increasing in duration and intensity over the last few days and is at risk for more serious complications such as plaque rupture. The patient is considered to be having an NSTEMI; they do not release cardiac biomarkers (cardiac enzymes).

This patient will present with the complaint of chest pain (with history as described) but on ECG, they may demonstrate ischemia or transient ischemic changes. Careful observation and consultation with cardiology is warranted.

Coronary Spasm or Prinzmetal's Angina

Coronary spasm is also known as *variant angina.* While the patient is at rest, a coronary artery will spasm and create a myocardial ischemic episode even without atherosclerotic plaque disease present. This chest pain may be relieved with rest or nitrates. ECG changes are noted, with ST-segment elevation that looks just like an AMI.

Because this condition is difficult at times to differentiate from STEMI and AMI, typical categorization, triage, and management should occur.

Cocaine-Induced Chest Pain

Cocaine or "crack" can be taken into the body in various forms, and the dangerous consequences to the heart are well documented. Cardiac toxicity occurs because of the direct effect on the heart with an increase in heart rate and myocardial contractility (beta effect). Additionally, there is a decrease in coronary artery blood flow, and a high risk for spasm exists (alpha effect). The bottom line is, when your heart is challenged by an increase in myocardial oxygen demand from the beta effects of cocaine, the heart is unable to meet the demand because of the alpha effects.

First-line treatment for cocaine-induced arrhythmias and hypertensive episodes is usually benzodiazepines, which temper the effects of cocaine on the CNS and cardiovascular system. Most patients having chest pain after use of cocaine will suffer transiently without change in ECG. Rarely, ACS and AMI occur, usually in those with other risk factors like cigarette smoking. Benzodiazepines should be added to the standard ACS management protocols. Because of the risk associated with cocaine, use of fibrinolytics is considered high risk. Beta-blockers are contraindicated, as the resultant unopposed alpha effect can precipitate dangerous hypertensive states. Keep in mind also that chronic cocaine/crack use accelerates atherosclerotic disease, so patients at younger ages than normal may be at risk for ACS.

Chest Pain Due to Infections

Pericarditis

Pericarditis is an inflammation of the pericardium or pericardial sac. It may be acute with a 48-hour duration or chronic, lasting longer and returning frequently. It is usually caused by a virus but may be caused by rheumatic heart disease, TB, leukemia, acquired immunodeficiency syndrome (AIDS), or cancer. Often the cause is unknown. The discomfort of pericarditis differs from ACS. It is often described as a dull ache that increases in intensity gradually over several days. The patient may find it difficult to lie flat and may lean forward or be propped up on pillows to make breathing easier (nocturnal dyspnea) while sleeping. Pain may increase on inspiration. Lungs will be clear, with no JVD or pedal edema early. Additional symptoms may include fever, weakness, fatigue, malaise, and pericardial friction rub. If a pericardial effusion is developing as a result of the pericarditis, you might hear the friction rub or pulsus paradoxus. A chest x-ray may show an enlarged cardiac silhouette due to pericardial effusion, and the 12-lead ECG will demonstrate global ST-segment elevation in almost every lead (Figure 5-14). Lab studies may show an elevated erythrocyte sedimentation rate (ESR), a test that indirectly measures inflammation in the body, and an elevated white blood cell count (WBC), which may indicate the presence of an infection.

Management is aimed at relieving discomfort with analgesics and nonsteroidal antiinflammatory drugs (NSAIDs). Corticosteroids and antimicrobials may be prescribed as well, but they are not initially given in the prehospital or ED setting until the definitive cause is known. The pericarditis patient requires continued monitoring, as more serious cases may develop pericardial tamponade.

Myocarditis

Inflammation of the myocardial layer of the heart is considered to be a form of dilated cardiomyopathy. Often undiagnosed clinically, this inflammation is usually caused by a virus (coxsackie B enterovirus, adenovirus) in the summer months. The 1/3 rule applies to the prognosis of this disease: 1/3 recover without consequences, 1/3 have chronic cardiac dysfunction, and 1/3 go on to have chronic heart failure with need for heart transplant, or they die.

The patient may present with an influenza-like illness (ILI) including fever, fatigue, myalgia, vomiting, and diarrhea. Then signs of myocarditis ensue: fever, tachycardia, tachypnea, with 12% complaining of chest pain. The ECG may show low voltage with a prolonged QT interval, AV

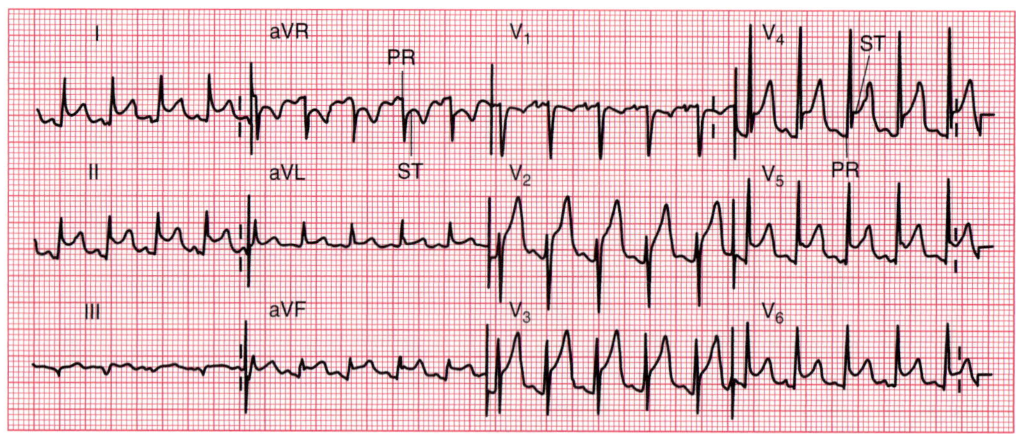

■ **Figure 5-14** A 12-lead electrocardiogram from a patient with acute pericarditis. Note the diffuse ST-T wave changes and PR elevation in lead aVR and PR-segment depression in leads II and aVF and in the precordial leads. (From Goldman L, Ausiello D: Cecil textbook of medicine, ed 23, Philadelphia, 2007, Saunders.)

block, or AMI patterns. Cardiac enzymes are usually elevated, along with the ESR.

Myocarditis can present just like AMI with CHF but the patient is usually young (<35 years) and may not have risk factors for heart disease. When sent to the Cath Lab, no coronary obstruction is noted. Management is supportive, and severe cases place the patient on the list for heart transplant.

Simple Pneumothorax

Another cause of chest discomfort might be a simple pneumothorax. A pneumothorax occurs as the result of a bleb rupturing on the lung, causing air to leave the lung and collect in the space between the visceral and parietal pleurae. With each ensuing breath, more air is trapped in that space, causing the affected lung to collapse. A simple pneumothorax may occur spontaneously in patients with connective tissue diseases like Marfan syndrome or in tall, slim males. They can occur as the result of barotraumas or other injury to the chest. Diseases like COPD, cystic fibrosis, and cancers may also cause a pneumothorax. Acute lung infections, like pneumonia, or chronic lung infections, like tuberculosis, may also cause a pneumothorax. The greatest threat of a pneumothorax is the development of a tension pneumothorax, which may require immediate intervention.

In addition to histories associated with the causes listed, the patient may actually feel a sudden tearing as the lung separates from the chest wall. This is often followed with sudden shortness of breath and a sharp pain that increases when a breath is taken. Dry cough with lung sounds diminished on the affected side occur if the pneumothorax is significant in size. Low oxygen saturations may accompany the simple pneumothorax. Treatment is aimed at maintaining near-normal oxygen saturations by administering oxygen by nasal cannula or mask. Assisting ventilations is usually not required and may worsen the situation, increasing the likelihood of a tension pneumothorax. Some smaller simple pneumothoraces may seal on their own and require only conservative monitoring. Significant pneumothoraces may require insertion of a chest tube to resolve the problem.

Intraabdominal Causes of Chest Discomfort

Cholecystitis

Because of the close proximity to the thorax, GI problems may also cause chest discomfort. Problems like cholecystitis, pancreatitis, and an esophageal tear can be emergent conditions needing immediate attention on the part of the healthcare provider.

Cholecystitis is inflammation of the gallbladder often caused by bile duct obstruction that leads to infection and inflammation of the walls of the gallbladder. The pain associated with cholecystitis is usually localized to the right upper quadrant, but it may radiate to the shoulders. The pain is sharp and colicky and often follows ingestion of a greasy meal. Because it may come on suddenly, it is often referred to as an "attack." Fever may or may not be present, depending on whether the attack is acute (no fever) or chronic (fever). Nausea and vomiting are commonly associated signs and symptoms. Lab studies may show elevated liver function tests and WBC count.

Treatment requires removal of the gallbladder, with supportive measures until that can occur. Relief of nausea and pain is a priority, as is ensuring the patient remains hydrated. Broad-spectrum antibiotics may be infused prior to going to surgery.

Pancreatitis

Pancreatitis is an acute inflammation of the pancreas and is often caused by gallstones or excessive alcohol use. Some common medications may also cause pancreatitis and include certain AIDS drugs, diuretics like furosemide and hydrochlorothiazide, some chemotherapy medications like L-asparaginase, and azathioprine. Estrogen replacement therapy may also cause pancreatitis because of its effect of raising blood triglyceride levels. Early complications of pancreatitis include shock from third-spacing, leading to dehydration, hypocalcemia, and hyperglycemia. Frequently, respiratory compromise also occurs with pancreatitis in the form of atelectasis from shallow breathing due to pain. Some degree of pleural effusion or pneumonitis may occur if pancreatic enzymes directly damage the lungs or from third-spacing.

Pancreatitis may be present with lower-left-quadrant abdominal pain, serum amylase or lipase more than three times normal, and positive CT scan.

Treatment of pancreatitis will depend on the severity of the disease. General principles include relieving pain with opiates, nausea control, and hydrating the patient. A nasogastric tube for feedings may help avoid pancreatic stimulation. If the patient shows signs of infection, an IV antibiotic may be started as well.

Esophageal Tear

A Mallory-Weiss tear in the esophagus usually follows forceful vomiting. The tear is usually about 1 to 4 cm in length at either the junction of the esophagus and stomach or in the stomach itself. Some GI bleeding will occur, but it is usually not severe.

Other GI causes of chest pain include esophageal spasm, esophageal reflux, peptic ulcer, and biliary colic. These disorders are described in Chapter 7.

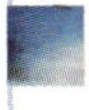

Nonemergent Causes of Chest Pain

Several causes of chest discomfort are neither emergencies nor life threats and merit a review by system. Most can be differentiated by the cause and description of the pain. Treatment is supportive, and finding the cause of the pain requires testing not routinely done in an ambulance. Diagnostic testing is often done as a follow-up to discharge from an ED, once serious life threats have been ruled out.

Neurologic Causes of Chest Pain

There could be neurologic causes of chest discomfort to include thoracic outlet syndrome, herpes zoster, and postherpetic neuralgia.

Thoracic Outlet Syndrome

Thoracic outlet syndrome (TOS) involves a compression of the brachial plexus (nerves that pass into the arms from the neck) and/or the subclavian vein or artery by muscle groups in the chest, back, or neck. When compressed, these nerves will cause chest discomfort that differs from ACS in that it is often associated with changes in position.

The two groups of people most likely to develop TOS are those with neck injuries from motor vehicle collisions and those who use computers in nonergonomic postures for extended periods of time. Young athletes (such as swimmers, volleyball players, and baseball pitchers) and musicians may also develop thoracic outlet syndrome, but significantly less frequently.

C8 and T1 nerve roots are usually affected, producing pain and tingling in the ulnar nerve distribution area (lower arm) or the C5, C6, and C7 nerve roots with pain that refers to the neck, ear, upper chest and upper back, and the outer arm.

One physical exam test that may lead you toward this diagnosis is called the *elevated arm stress test* or *EAST exam*. Direct the patient to raise the arms to 90 degrees while seated, with elbows flexed 90 degrees. With shoulders back, the patient is asked to open and close both fists slowly for about 3 minutes while they describe their symptoms. A negative test produces no complaints except perhaps fatigue. A positive test for thoracic outlet syndrome produces complaints of heaviness of the involved arm, gradual numbness of that hand, and progressive aching through the arm and top of shoulder. It is not unusual to see the patient drop the hand because of increasing pain. The involved arm and hand may have circulatory changes as well.

Often, stretching, practicing proper posture, and treatments such as physiotherapy, massage therapy, and chiropractic care will resolve the pain of TOS. Cortisone and Botox injections will lessen the symptoms during a course of treatment. The recovery process, however, is long term, and a few days of poor posture can often lead to setbacks. About 10% to 15% of patients undergo surgical decompression if 6 to 12 months of therapy fails to relieve the pain.

Herpes Zoster

Varicella-zoster virus is the primary agent of both chickenpox and herpes zoster, otherwise known as *shingles* (see Chapter 8 and Figure 8-10 for further information on this condition). Herpes zoster results from the varicella-zoster virus (VZV), left dormant in the body following a case of the chickenpox and later reactivated in a single sensory ganglion that follows a distinct dermatome. Herpes zoster can cause chest discomfort before, during, or after the signature rash develops. Patients who are immunocompromised from human immunodeficiency virus (HIV) or on chemotherapy are at a greater risk for herpes zoster outbreaks.

Unlike the pain of a heart attack, herpes zoster pain is described as a burning pain that typically precedes a rash by several days. The pain can persist for several months after the rash disappears, as in the case of postherpetic neuralgia. The pain and rash most commonly occur on the torso but can appear on the face, eyes, or other parts of the body. At first, the rash appears similar to hives, but unlike hives, it is has a tendency to follow dermatomes on one side of the body, appearing in a beltlike pattern and not crossing the midline. Later, the rash forms small fluid-filled blisters. The patient may develop a fever and general malaise. The painful blisters eventually become cloudy or darkened as they fill with blood, crust over within 7 to 10 days, and usually then fall off. Diagnosis is easy if the rash is present: herpes zoster is the only rash that follows a dermatome and is limited to one side of the body. If no rash is present, as in the case of postherpetic neuralgia, blood tests may be needed for definitive diagnosis. Direct contact with the rash can spread the virus to a person who has never had chickenpox. Until the rash has developed crusts, a person is considered contagious. A person is not infectious before blisters appear or during postherpetic neuralgia (pain after the rash is gone). The pain may persist well after resolution of the rash and can be severe enough to require medications for relief.

Herpes zoster is usually treated with oral antivirals, which are most effective when started within 72 hours after the onset of the rash. The addition of an orally administered corticosteroid can provide modest benefits in reducing the pain of herpes zoster and the incidence of postherpetic neuralgia. Patients with postherpetic neuralgia may require narcotics for adequate pain control.

Other Pulmonary Causes of Chest Pain

The many respiratory causes of chest discomfort include pneumonitis, pleurisy, lung tumor, and pneumomediastinum, to name a few. You may wish to have a look back at Chapter 3 for an in-depth review of these and other respiratory conditions responsible chest discomfort.

Pneumonitis

Pneumonitis refers to any inflammation of lung tissue and may be caused by a variety of conditions to include pneumonia, bronchitis, and aspiration. Productive cough and difficulty breathing are the most common symptoms of pneumonitis. Fever may occur with infection, and the cough may burn. Fatigue and malaise may also accompany pneumonitis. Treatment is generally supportive and is aimed at finding the cause. Treatment may be the avoidance of the trigger or may include medications like IV antibiotics. If the patient is complaining of shortness of breath, oxygen to maintain saturations above 94% would be appropriate. An IV should be established and a heart monitor applied. Place the patient in the position of greatest comfort. Obtain a CBC, chemistry panel, and chest x-ray to confirm or rule out pneumonia.

Pleurisy

Pleurisy is the term most used to refer to painful respiration and should alert you to conduct a thorough assessment to find the cause of the pain. Pleuritic pain usually increases with respiration and is the result of inflammation of the parietal and visceral pleurae lining the chest wall and lungs, a pathologic process described earlier in this chapter and dealt with in detail in Chapter 3. As the patient breathes, the inflamed pleurae rub against each other, causing a sharp pain that increases with inspiration. Fever and cough may be present and can be difficult to distinguish from pneumonia. A possible distinguishing sign may include the rough, scratchy sound heard with a stethoscope when the pleurae rub against each other, known as a *pleural friction rub*. It often sounds like leather stretching when the patient inhales deeply.

A chest x-ray may show air or fluid in the pleural space. It also may show what's causing the pleurisy (e.g., pneumonia, a fractured rib, a lung tumor). If significant fluid is present, it may have to be removed with thoracentesis in the inpatient setting. Collected fluid will be tested to determine its origin; fluid may accumulate from lung tissue disease or cancers.

Acetaminophen or NSAIDs may be used for pain, and a codeine-based cough syrup to suppress the cough may also be given. Treatment is generally supportive and aimed at finding the cause. As discussed earlier, life-threatening causes of heart-related chest pain have been ruled out by this point.

Other Heart-Related Causes of Chest Discomfort

Other causes of chest discomfort may include such structural changes in the heart like valvular heart disease, aortic stenosis, mitral valve prolapse, and hypertrophic cardiomyopathy. All may cause chest discomfort very similar to that of an ACS.

Aortic Stenosis

As we age, the protein collagen of the heart's valve leaflets are damaged, and calcium is deposited. Turbulence from blood flowing across the valve increases scarring, thickening, and stenosis or narrowing of the valve. Why this aging process progresses to cause significant aortic stenosis in some patients but not in others is unknown. The progressive disease causing aortic calcification and stenosis has nothing to do with healthy lifestyle choices, unlike the calcium that can deposit in the coronary artery to cause heart attack.

Rheumatic fever is a condition resulting from untreated infection by group A streptococcal bacteria. Damage to valve leaflets from rheumatic fever causes increased turbulence across the valve and similar damage. The narrowing from rheumatic fever occurs from the fusion of the edges of the valve leaflets. Rheumatic aortic stenosis usually occurs with some degree of aortic regurgitation. Under normal circumstances, the aortic valve closes to prevent blood in the aorta from flowing back into the left ventricle. In aortic regurgitation, the diseased valve allows leakage of blood back into the left ventricle as the ventricular muscles relax after pumping. These patients also have some degree of rheumatic damage to the mitral valve. Rheumatic heart disease is uncommon in the United States, except in people who have immigrated from underdeveloped countries.

Chest pain may be the first symptom in patients with aortic stenosis. Chest pain in patients with aortic stenosis resembles the chest pain experienced by patients with angina. In both of these conditions, pain is described as pressure below the breast bone brought on by exertion and relieved by rest. In patients with coronary artery disease, chest pain is due to inadequate blood supply to the heart muscles because of narrowed coronary arteries. In patients with aortic stenosis, chest pain occurs without any underlying narrowing of the coronary arteries. The thickened heart muscle must pump against high pressure to push blood through the narrowed aortic valve. This increases heart muscle oxygen demand in excess of the supply delivered in the blood, causing angina.

Syncope related to aortic stenosis is usually caused by exertion or excitement. Any time a patient's blood pressure drops suddenly, the heart is unable to increase output to compensate for the drop in blood pressure. Therefore, blood flow to the brain is decreased, causing syncope. Syncope can also occur when CO is decreased by an irregular heartbeat. Without effective treatment, the average life expectancy is less than 3 years after the onset of chest pain or syncope symptoms from aortic stenosis.

Shortness of breath from left heart failure is the most ominous sign and is caused by increased capillary permeability in the lungs due to the increased pressure required to fill the left ventricle. Initially, shortness of breath occurs only during activity but as the disease progresses, shortness of breath occurs at rest. Patients can find it difficult to lie flat without becoming short of breath. Strenuous activities should be avoided and may trigger syncope or angina, causing the patient to seek medical attention.

Care is similar to the care of the patient for angina and is usually relieved by rest and oxygen. Use extreme caution with medications such as nitroglycerin, which decrease preload. Lack of sufficient preload in these patients may lead to a significant drop in systolic blood pressure and worsening of their condition.

A thorough history and the presence of murmur are key to identification. Since valve infection is a serious complication of aortic stenosis, these patients are given antibiotics prior to any procedure in which bacteria may be introduced into the bloodstream. This includes routine dental work and minor surgery. When symptoms of chest pain, syncope, or shortness of breath appear, the prognosis for patients with aortic stenosis without valve replacement surgery is poor.

Mitral Valve Prolapse

Mitral valve prolapse is the most common heart valve abnormality (Figure 5-15), affecting 5% to 10% of the world population. A normal mitral valve consists of two thin leaflets located between the left atrium and the left ventricle of the heart. Mitral valve leaflets, shaped like parachutes, are attached to the inner wall of the left ventricle by a series of strings called *chordae*. When the ventricles contract, the mitral valve leaflets close snugly and prevent the backflow of blood from the left ventricle into the left atrium. When the ventricles relax, the valves open to allow oxygenated blood from the lungs to fill the left ventricle. In patients with mitral valve prolapse, the mitral valve leaflets and chordae degenerate, becoming thick and enlarged. When the ventricles contract, the leaflets prolapse (flop backward) into the left atrium, sometimes allowing leakage or regurgitation of blood through the valve opening.

Severe mitral regurgitation can lead to CHF and abnormal heart rhythms. Most patients are unaware of the prolapsing of the mitral valve, but others may experience a number of symptoms like palpitations, chest pain, anxiety, and fatigue. Sharp chest pain may be reported by the patient and would not respond to nitroglycerin. Auscultation of heart sounds with a stethoscope might reveal a clicking sound that reflects the tightening of the abnormal valve leaflets against the pressure load of the left ventricle. If there is associated regurgitation of blood through the abnormal valve opening, a whooshing sound can be heard immediately following the clicking sound.

Cardiomyopathy

Cardiomyopathy is the end product when heart muscle myocytes are injured by various causes, and the heart remodels itself to accommodate with hypertrophy or thickening of the muscle. There are genetic and immune causes of this debilitating disease process. The common look of the remodeled heart is one of dilation and failing muscle.

The diagnosis is one of exclusion, but a common presentation is a patient with chest pain, weakness, and dyspnea. Left-sided heart failure may be the first presentation, along with exertional chest pain. The ECG may be nonspecific, with intraventricular conduction delay or LBBB. Chest x-ray will usually show a large heart, and BNP may be mildly elevated if the patient is asymptomatic, very elevated if symptomatic (Figure 5-16).

Management is supportive and similar to that of CHF and APE. ACE inhibitors are the treatment of choice, along with other techniques to decrease the heart's

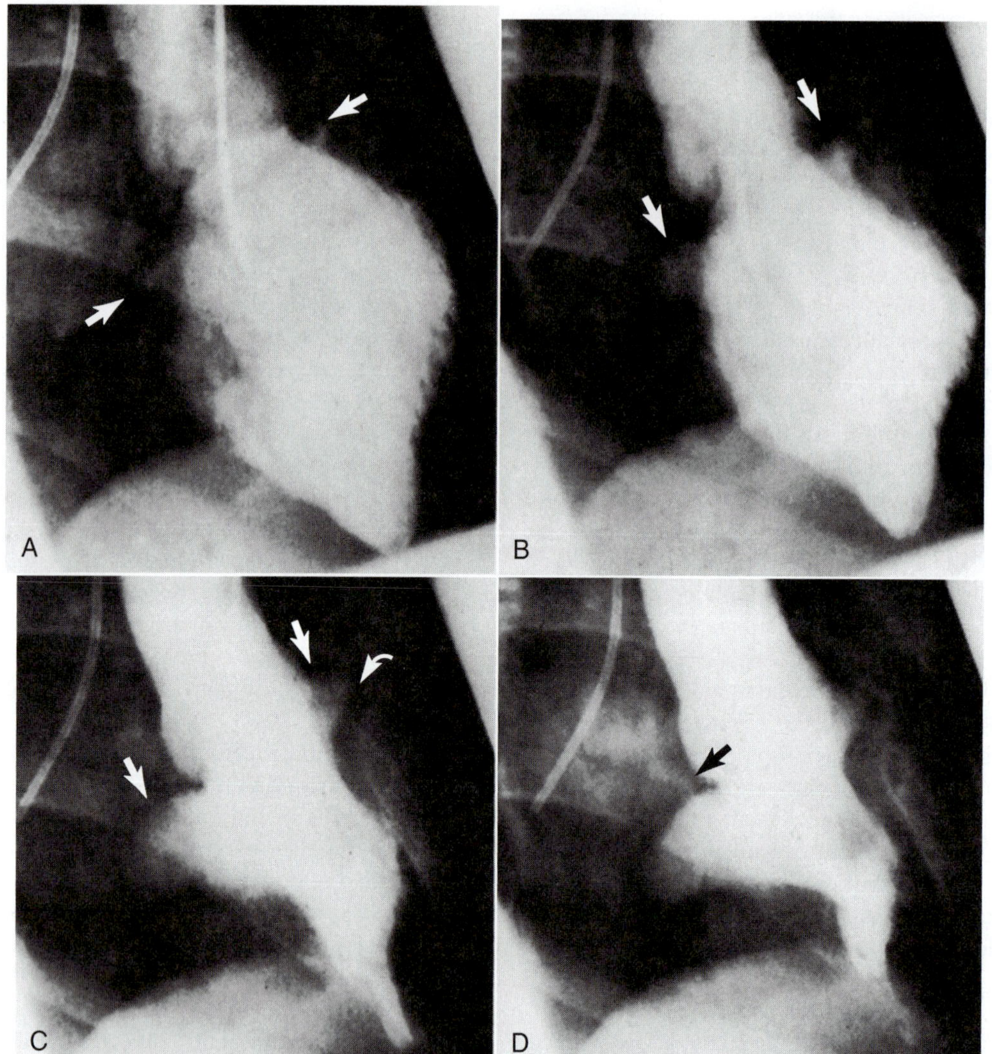

■ **Figure 5-15** Nonrheumatic mitral regurgitation due to mitral valve prolapse. Left ventriculography (right anterior oblique [ROA] projection). **A**, Diastole. Arrows indicate the recess under the mitral valve, which persists in diastole. **B**, Early systole. Prolapse of the mitral valve *(arrows)* is just appearing. **C**, Midsystole. Mitral valve prolapse *(arrows)* has reached its fullest extent. **D**, Late systole. After maximum prolapse, reflux into the left atrium *(arrowhead)* begins. (From Adam A, Allison D: Grainger and Allison's diagnostic radiology, ed 5, 2008, Philadelphia, Churchill Livingstone.)

afterload. This disease is the leading indication for heart transplantation. As discussed earlier, ventricular assistive devices can be used as bridge therapy to transplantation or as sustained therapy in and of themselves.

Musculoskeletal Causes of Chest Pain

As described in the assessment section, the thoracic cage is made up of musculoskeletal structures and can be a somatic cause for chest pain. Muscle strain, costochondritis, and nonspecific chest wall pain are usually well defined by the patient and sharp or aching in nature. You must rule out all other causes for the patient's chest pain before deciding on this as a diagnosis. As with most inflammation, use of NSAIDs, heat or cold therapy, and rest are the most common tactics for management.

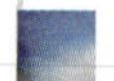

Special Considerations

■ Transporting Patients

Choosing the appropriate method of transport for a patient with ACS should be directed at the needs of the patient. First you must decide whether the patient is critically ill and determine which modes of transportation the patient can tolerate and which facility is best suited for the patient. A chest pain center should be a consideration for patients with ACS. Altitude changes and the stress of flight can increase myocardial demand, so the patient should be closely monitored and supported. Decreasing the

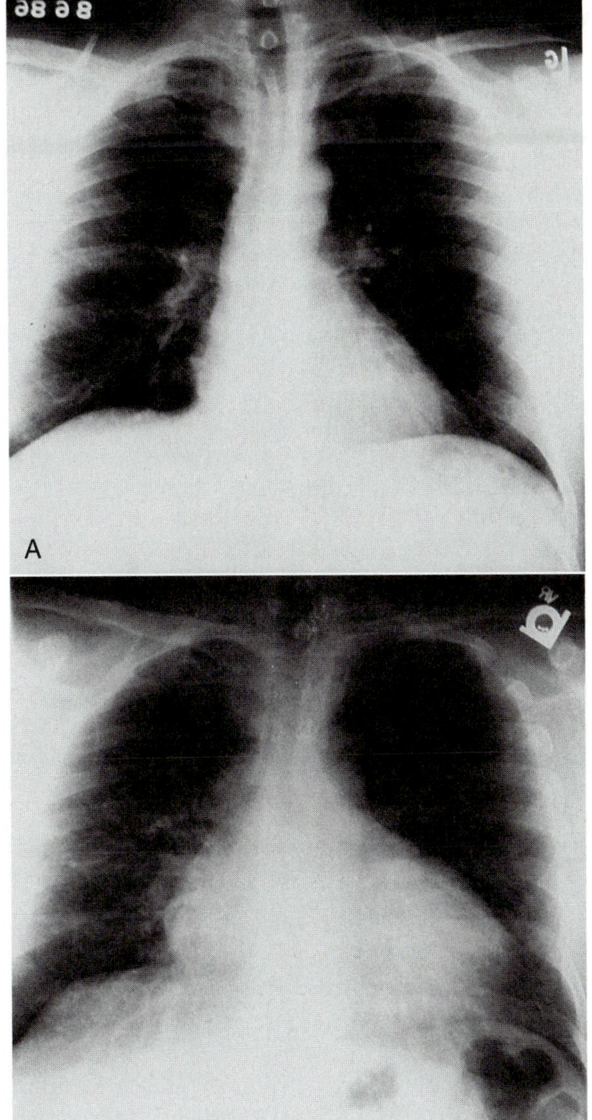

■ **Figure 5-16** Cardiomyopathy. In this case, cardiomyopathy is due to cancer chemotherapy with doxorubicin. An initial chest x-ray (A) demonstrates a normal-sized heart. After several therapeutic courses of doxorubicin (B), marked enlargement in the cardiac silhouette is due to multichamber dilatation. (From Mettler F: Essentials of radiology, ed 2, Philadelphia, 2005, Saunders.)

transport time to the appropriate facility can serve as a benefit to air transport.

Patients with support devices may need additional space and teams for transport. This should be prepared for prior to transport to eliminate delays.

Older Adult Patients

The older patient may present with ACS, but the symptoms may not be apparent. Weakness or a silent MI (no signs and symptoms) are common, so a high index of suspicion must be maintained. Since the elderly may be on medications (e.g., beta-blockers) that decrease their ability to compensate for hemodynamic compromise, you must be prepared to address these issues. Many older patients have multiple medical issues that can make diagnosis and management challenging because of the "muddy picture" presented.

Obese Patients

Owing to the decrease in mobility in the obese, blood clots in the legs may contribute to pulmonary emboli. The complaint of chest pain may be altered because of nerve distribution in the tissues due to torso mass. The increase in myocardial workload make these patients high risk for ACS. In addition, diabetes is more common and may contribute to cardiovascular issues as well. Electrolyte imbalance may follow bariatric surgery and result in dysrhythmias as the cause of chest discomfort in these patients.

Pregnant Patients

A pulmonary embolism should be high on your list of rule outs when assessing a pregnant patient; this may be due to the state of hypercoagulation and potential for developing blood clots. Pregnancy also places increased demands on the cardiovascular system and may exacerbate a previous diagnosed or undiagnosed condition. GERD is also common during pregnancy and may contribute to chest discomfort. Transport to a facility that cares for high-risk obstetric patients should be considered.

Putting It All Together

Caring for a patient with chest discomfort begins with your initial observation. When ordering your priorities, your immediate goal is to determine whether the patient is sick or not (see Chapter 1). Your first impression should tell you whether you have time to continue your assessment or if you should intercede immediately. Evaluate the patient for critical or emergent diagnoses first. Since the life-threatening diagnoses require immediate separation for management, begin your assessment to differentiate between these first. Include breath sounds to rule out a tension pneumothorax and APE/CHF, move to the ACS rule outs (consider a 12-lead ECG as patient condition allows, but do not delay aspirin, oxygen, or nitroglycerin), check blood pressures and pulses in both upper extremities, and compare them to the lower extremities as you consider an aortic aneurysm. Often the clue to an esophageal rupture, pulmonary embolism, or other life threat is in the history, so focus your history questions to rule these out as time allows.

At the receiving facility, add chest x-rays, lab work, and CTs as time allows. To confirm or rule out conditions that make up your differential diagnosis, use tools such as

SAMPLER, OPQRST, physical examination findings, and lab results. If your patient is unstable or deteriorates, support the ABCs as you work through the AMLS process. Immediate life threats take precedence over all else. Once these are ruled out, progress to the other causes of chest pain, but realize initial complaints of chest discomfort may be very vague; constant reassessment is essential so that that a life threat is not missed.

SCENARIO SOLUTION

1 **Differential diagnoses may include myocarditis, pneumonia, pulmonary embolism, acute coronary syndrome, cholecystitis, or pericarditis.**

2 **To narrow your differential diagnosis you will need to complete the history of past and present illness. Obtain a more thorough history of her present illness. Perform a physical examination that includes vital sign assessment and evaluation of heart and breath sounds, jugular vein assessment, ECG monitoring and 12-lead ECG, Sao_2, capnography, and blood glucose analysis.**

3 **The patient has signs that may indicate acute coronary syndrome, infection, or heart failure. Administer oxygen. Establish vascular access. Monitor ECG, and obtain a 12-lead ECG. Further treatment will depend on the rest of your assessment findings. If you suspect acute coronary syndrome, treat with aspirin, nitroglycerin, and morphine. If the patient has signs of congestive heart failure without shock, treat with continuous positive airway pressure and nitroglycerin. If the patient's examination points to cholecystitis, treat for pain. If she has diabetic ketoacidosis, administer a large volume of IV fluids. Transport to the closest appropriate healthcare facility.**

SUMMARY

- Your standard assessment practice for the patient with chest pain should include looking for life-threatening causes and managing them appropriately—even within the primary survey. In the patient with a patent airway, assessing for breath sounds and looking for shock are key.
- Life-threatening causes of chest pain usually include those diseases that produce both chest pain and increased work of breathing, or chest pain and alteration in vital signs (or a combination thereof).
- Standard protocols for chest pain include use of oxygen, vascular access, application of monitors, acquisition of ECG, chest x-ray, and laboratory studies. Healthcare providers need to triage the patient for additional resources (Cath Lab, Heart Center) and move the patient toward those specialties early in the process.
- Non–life-threatening causes of chest pain can arise from several body systems including cardiovascular, respiratory, gastrointestinal, immunologic, structural cardiac, neurologic, and musculoskeletal.

BIBLIOGRAPHY

Adam A, Dixon AK, Grainger RG, et al: Grainger and Allison's diagnostic radiology, ed 5, 2008, Churchill Livingstone.

Aehlert B: Paramedic practice today: above and beyond, St Louis, 2009, Mosby.

American Heart Association: ACLS for experienced providers, Dallas, TX, 2003, American Heart Association.

American Heart Association: 2005 AHA guidelines for CPR and ECC, Dallas, TX, 2005, American Heart Association.

American Heart Association. Atherosclerosis. http://www.americanheart.org/presenter.jhtml?identifier=4440. Accessed February 4, 2010.

Black JM, Hokanson Hawks J: Medical-surgical nursing, ed 8, Philadelphia, 2009, Saunders.

Braunwald E: Heart disease: a textbook of cardiovascular medicine, ed 4, Philadelphia, 1992, WB Saunders.

Dorland: Dorland's illustrated medical dictionary, Philadelphia, 2007, Saunders.

Field J: Advanced cardiac life support provider manual, Dallas, TX, 2006, American Heart Association.

Field J, Hazinski M, Gilmore D: Handbook of ECC for healthcare providers, Dallas, TX, 2008, American Heart Association.

Frownfelter D, Dean E: Cardiovascular and pulmonary physical therapy, ed 4, St Louis, 2006, Mosby.
Goldman L, Ausiello D: Cecil medicine, ed 23, Philadelphia, 2007, Saunders.
Johnson D, editor: The pericardium. In Standring S, et al, editors: Gray's anatomy, St Louis, 2005, Mosby.
Marx JA, Hockberger RS, Walls RM, et al: Rosen's emergency medicine: concepts and clinical practice, ed 6, St Louis, 2006, Mosby.
PHTLS: Prehospital trauma life support, ed 7, St Louis, 2010, MosbyJems.
Urden L, Stacy K, Lough M: Critical care nursing: diagnosis and management, ed 6, St Louis, 2010, Mosby.
U.S. Department of Health and Human Services: How is a heart attack treated? National Institutes of Health. http://www.nhlbi.nih.gov/health/dci/Diseases/HeartAttack/HeartAttack_Treatments.html. Accessed August 10, 2010.
U.S. Department of Transportation National Highway Traffic Safety Administration: EMT-paramedic national standard curriculum, Washington, DC, 1998, The Department.
U.S. Department of Transportation National Highway Traffic Safety Administration: National EMS education standards, Draft 3.0, Washington, DC, 2008, The Department. http://www.ems.gov/pdf/811077a.pdf. Accessed August 10, 2010.
Wilson SF, Thompson JM: Mosby's clinical nursing series: respiratory disorders, St Louis, 1990, Mosby.

Chapter Review Questions

1. The most common sign or symptom found in patients with pulmonary embolism is:
a. Coughing up blood
b. Crackles in the affected lung
c. Increased respiratory rate
d. Pleural friction rub

2. A 52-year-old male with a history of alcoholism complains of pleuritic chest pain. He states the pain increases when he swallows. He appears very ill and has subcutaneous emphysema around his neck. You suspect:
a. Boerhaave's syndrome
b. Cholecystitis
c. Esophageal varices
d. Pleurisy

3. A 73-year-old male awakens suddenly at 0200 complaining of dyspnea. You find him in the tripod position. Crackles are audible around his scapulae. He has a history of hypertension. You suspect his symptoms are related to:
a. Fluid overload
b. Increased cardiac output
c. Left heart failure
d. Reactive airway disease

4. A 70-year-old male suspected to have a dissecting aortic aneurysm has a blood pressure of 170/102 mm Hg. This sign may indicate:
a. Cardiac tamponade is developing.
b. Rupture of the aorta is imminent.
c. The aorta is not dissecting.
d. The renal arteries are involved.

5. Which of the following patients is at highest risk for pericardial tamponade?
a. 55-year-old with end-stage lung cancer
b. 62-year-old dialysis patient
c. 45-year-old with influenza
d. 72-year-old who takes warfarin

6. If you administer nitroglycerin to a patient with ST-elevation in leads II, III and aVF, you should be prepared to:
a. Administer a bolus of normal saline if the blood pressure drops.
b. Change to morphine, as nitroglycerin is rarely successful.
c. Start a dopamine drip if the patient becomes hypotensive.
d. Treat the patient for congestive heart failure.

7. A 45-year-old male with a history of hypertension complains of chest "pressure," about a 5 on a scale of 1 to 10, for 20 minutes. He just "wants to be checked out." Vital signs and 12-lead ECG are normal. You have already administered oxygen and aspirin. You should next:
a. Administer nitroglycerin 0.4 mg sublingual.
b. Advise him that his ECG is normal and no further care is needed.
c. Monitor and transport to the hospital for further evaluation.
d. Perform a right-sided electrocardiogram.

8. An 82-year-old female complains of chest heaviness. She has sinus tachycardia. Her vital signs are BP 108/72 (equal in both arms), P 98, R 20. Her breath sounds are clear in all fields. Aside from myocardial infarction, what should you suspect her chest pain could be related to?
a. Aortic dissection
b. Congestive heart failure
c. Esophageal rupture
d. Pulmonary embolism

9. A 40-year-old male has chest pain reported as an "elephant sitting on my chest." He confides that he snorted cocaine 5 minutes before his pain began. You should first administer:
a. A fibrinolytic drug
b. Lorazepam, 2 mg IV
c. Metoprolol, 5 mg IV
d. Naloxone, 2 mg IV

10. A 65-year-old female complains of chest pain that feels like "aching" in her chest. It has become progressively worse over several days. Her temperature is 38.3°C (101°F). Which finding will help narrow your differential diagnosis to pericarditis?
a. Pleural friction rub is audible.
b. Pulsus alternans is present.
c. S_3 gallop is auscultated.
d. ST-segment elevation in every lead

CHAPTER

6 Endocrine, Metabolic, and Environmental Disorders

THE PURPOSE OF THIS CHAPTER is to give you a fundamental understanding of endocrine, metabolic, and selected environmental disorders. You'll learn to integrate your knowledge of anatomy, physiology, and pathophysiology with the information gleaned from a focused and comprehensive Advanced Medical Life Support (AMLS) assessment in order to formulate differential diagnoses for life-threatening, critical/emergent, and nonemergent conditions. You'll also learn how to implement and adapt management strategies for a variety of endocrine, metabolic, and environmental disorders in prehospital and hospital settings.

Learning Objectives ***At the conclusion of this chapter, you will be able to:***

1. Describe the anatomy, physiology, and pathophysiology of common endocrine, metabolic, and environmental emergencies.
2. Outline primary, secondary, and ongoing assessment strategies for the patient with an endocrine, metabolic, or environmental disorder.
3. Describe the pathophysiologic processes responsible for electrolyte and acid-base derangements, explain their causes, and discuss common modalities used to treat them.
4. Formulate provisional diagnoses on the basis of assessment findings for a variety of endocrine, metabolic, and environmental disorders.
5. List the causes, diagnostic techniques, and treatment strategies for diseases of glucose metabolism and thyroid, parathyroid, and adrenal disorders.
6. Use clinical reasoning skills to formulate a differential diagnosis on the basis of a systematic, thorough secondary survey of a patient with a metabolic, endocrine, or environmental illness.
7. Implement effective treatment plans consistent with your assessment findings, and determine whether to continue the treatment on the basis of your ongoing assessment.
8. Compare and contrast normal and abnormal electrocardiogram (ECG) findings in the patient with an electrolyte derangement.
9. List and be able to recognize the signs and symptoms of acid-base imbalances, electrolyte derangements, and endocrine disorders.
10. Integrate your knowledge of approach, assessment, treatment, and transport to make sound decisions for a patient with a metabolic or endocrine disorder, and give your rationale for those decisions.
11. Identify the cardinal presentations of a broad range of endocrine, metabolic, and environmental disorders.
12. Describe the cardinal presentations and treatment strategies for patients with selected environmental emergencies.

Key Terms

Addison's disease An endocrine disease caused by a deficiency of corticosteroid hormones produced by the adrenal cortex. The disease is characterized by nausea, vomiting, abdominal pain, and tanning of the skin.

adrenal crisis An endocrine emergency caused by a deficiency of corticosteroid hormones produced by the adrenal cortex. The disease is characterized by nausea, vomiting, abdominal pain, hypotension, hyperkalemia, and hyponatremia.

diabetic ketoacidosis (DKA) An acute endocrine emergency caused by a lack of insulin. The condition is characterized by an elevated blood glucose level, ketone production, metabolic acidosis, dehydration, nausea, vomiting, abdominal pain, and tachypnea.

heatstroke A syndrome in which the body loses its ability to regulate temperature, resulting in altered mental status, an elevated core body temperature, and multiorgan failure.

hyperosmolar hyperglycemic nonketotic syndrome (HHNS) An endocrine emergency characterized by a high plasma glucose concentration, absent ketone production, and increased serum osmolality (>315 mOsm/kg). The syndrome causes severe dehydration, nausea, vomiting, abdominal pain, and tachypnea.

hypoglycemia A plasma glucose concentration of less than 70 mg/dL. This condition is often associated with signs and symptoms such as sweating, cold skin, tachycardia, and altered mental status.

hypothermia Core body temperature below 35°C (95°F). At lower temperatures, hypothermia may induce cardiac arrhythmia and precipitate a decline in mental status.

myxedema Severe hypothyroidism associated with cold intolerance, weight gain, weakness, and declining mental status.

thyroid storm An endocrine emergency characterized by hyperfunction of the thyroid gland. This disorder is associated with fever, tachycardia, nervousness, altered mental status, and hemodynamic instability.

thyrotoxicosis A condition of elevated thyroid hormone levels, which often leads to signs and symptoms of tachycardia, tremor, weight loss, and high-output heart failure.

SCENARIO

YOU'RE CARING FOR a 58-year-old female who is complaining of severe fatigue and weakness. She has a history of type 2 diabetes, polymyalgia rheumatica, hypertension, and heart failure. Her medicines include metformin, prednisone, lisinopril, furosemide, and digoxin. Her vital signs are BP 88/52, P 58 bpm, R 20/min.

1. ***What differential diagnoses are you considering based on the information you have now?***
2. ***What additional information will you need to narrow your differential diagnosis?***
3. ***What are your initial treatment priorities as you continue your patient care?***

Tongue in cheek, former astronaut and U.S. Senator John Glenn once stated "The good Lord only gave men so many hormones, and if others want to waste theirs growing hair, that's up to them." Hormones released by endocrine system glands affect far more than our visible physical characteristics (and penchants for being hurled through space at 17,000 miles an hour). Hormones stimulate growth and development throughout the body, regulate the flow of water in and out of cells, help muscles contract, control blood pressure and appetite, modulate the sleep cycle, and much more. The body carries out these metabolic processes with remarkable efficiency, yet occasionally something goes awry. The acid-base balance may tip too far in one direction. Body cells become resistant to insulin. Or perhaps too much sodium or potassium builds up in the blood. That's when the emergency medical services (EMS) provider might be asked to step in.

In this chapter, we'll take a look at endocrine, metabolic, and selected environmental emergencies whose successful management often depends on timely intervention, confidence, and sharp clinical acumen and skills.

ENDOCRINE SYSTEM AND RELATED DISORDERS

Anatomy and Physiology

The endocrine system is composed of seven main glands: the pituitary, thyroid, parathyroid, adrenal, pancreas, and the reproductive organs (ovaries in women and testes in men) (Figures 6-1 and 6-2). These glands modulate the function of specific organs by secreting special proteins called *hormones*. Once released into the bloodstream, hormones regulate homeostasis, reproduction, growth, development, and metabolism by transmitting messages directly to receptors located on their respective target organs.

The functions of the endocrine glands are so interdependent that it's impossible to describe one gland without discussing another. Take the thyroid gland, for instance. The thyroid is located in the anterior part of the neck at

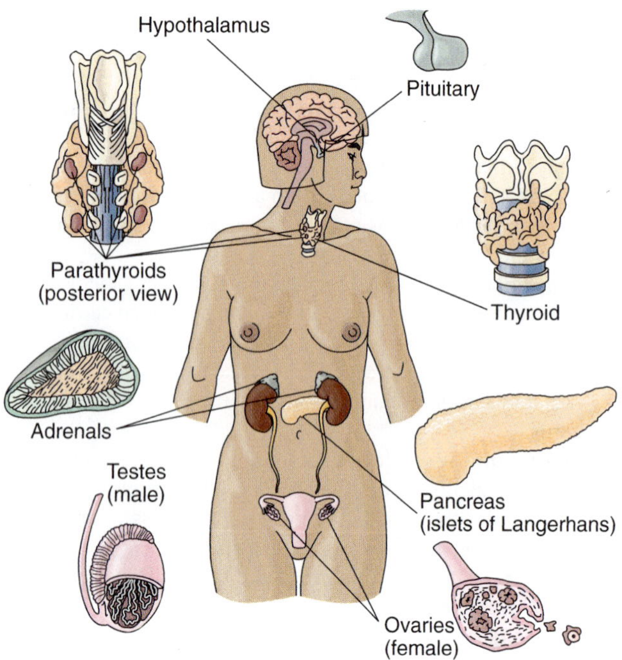

■ **Figure 6-1** The endocrine system communicates with every cell of the body through hormones made in the endocrine glands. (From Ignatavicius D, Workman ML: Medical-surgical nursing: patient-centered collaborative care, ed 6, Philadelphia, 2010, Saunders.)

the level between the fifth cervical and first thoracic vertebrae. It's located beneath the rigid cartilage palpable in the anterior neck. Hormones secreted by the thyroid affect many tissues and organs in the human body, including the heart, musculoskeletal and nervous systems, and adipose tissue. Thyroid hormones are regulated through a feedback process that involves the hypothalamus and the pituitary gland. Thyrotropin-releasing hormone (TRH), secreted by the hypothalamus, binds to a specific receptor for thyroid-stimulating hormone (TSH, or thyrotropin) in the thyroid gland, activating a biochemical cascade. This process stimulates the secretion of T_4 (thyroxine) and T_3 (triiodothyronine) by follicular cells in the thyroid gland. This free (circulating) T_3 and T_4 in turn inhibits TSH secretion by the pituitary gland by regulating synthesis of TRH in the hypothalamus. TSH secretion can be also inhibited by factors such as stress, glucocorticoids, and warmth.

Parafollicular cells, which constitute a minority of thyroid gland cells, are responsible for secreting calcitonin hormone, which controls calcium metabolism. Calcitonin regulation depends on serum level, rather than on a feedback process.

PARATHYROID GLAND AND RELATED DISORDERS

The parathyroid glands lie posterior to the thyroid gland and comprise three types of cells, each of which has a particular function. Chief cells are responsible for producing parathyroid hormone (PTH), which stimulates the production of active vitamin D in the kidneys, encourages the reabsorption of calcium by the renal tubules, and inhibits phosphate reabsorption in the kidneys. PTH also liberates calcium from bone to increase calcium levels.

Calcium receptors in the parathyroid gland detect changes in extracellular calcium concentration and in response inhibit calcitonin secretion. A low calcium concentration (Figure 6-3) stimulates PTH secretion, whereas an increase in calcium inhibits the production and liberation of PTH through a negative-feedback process.

Hypoparathyroidism

Hypoparathyroidism is a rare condition characterized by low serum levels of PTH or resistance to its action. Congenital, autoimmune, and acquired diseases are among its many causes. Regardless of etiology, the hallmark of the condition is hypocalcemia (see later discussion).

Signs and Symptoms

Patients suffering from acute hypoparathyroidism complain of muscle spasm, paresthesia, and tetany (Figure 6-4). The patient may even have seizures. These signs and symptoms are due to hypocalcemia.

Pathophysiology

The most common cause of acquired hypoparathyroidism is iatrogenic damage or inadvertent removal of the glands during thyroidectomy. Damage (during neck dissection, for example) can be transitory or permanent.

Diagnosis

In the prehospital setting, no laboratory studies are immediately available to confirm hypoparathyroidism, so you must have a high index of suspicion on the basis of history and physical examination findings. Recent anterior neck surgery is a risk factor for iatrogenic hypoparathyroidism.

You should be familiar with Trousseau's sign and Chvostek's sign, both of which will help you detect muscular irritability caused by hypocalcemia. To obtain a positive Trousseau's sign, place a blood pressure cuff around the arm, inflate it 30 mm Hg above systolic blood pressure, and hold it in place for 3 minutes. This will induce spasm of the muscles of the hand and forearm (Figure 6-5). The wrist and metacarpophalangeal joints flex, the distal and proximal interphalangeal joints extend, and the fingers adduct. You can elicit a positive Chvostek's sign by tapping the facial nerve against the mandibular bone just anterior to the ear, which produces an abnormal ipsilateral spasm of the facial muscles. This sign, however, is not as sensitive as Trousseau's sign.

Another tool available is the electrocardiogram (ECG). In patients with hypocalcemia, the QT interval is prolonged (Figure 6-6).

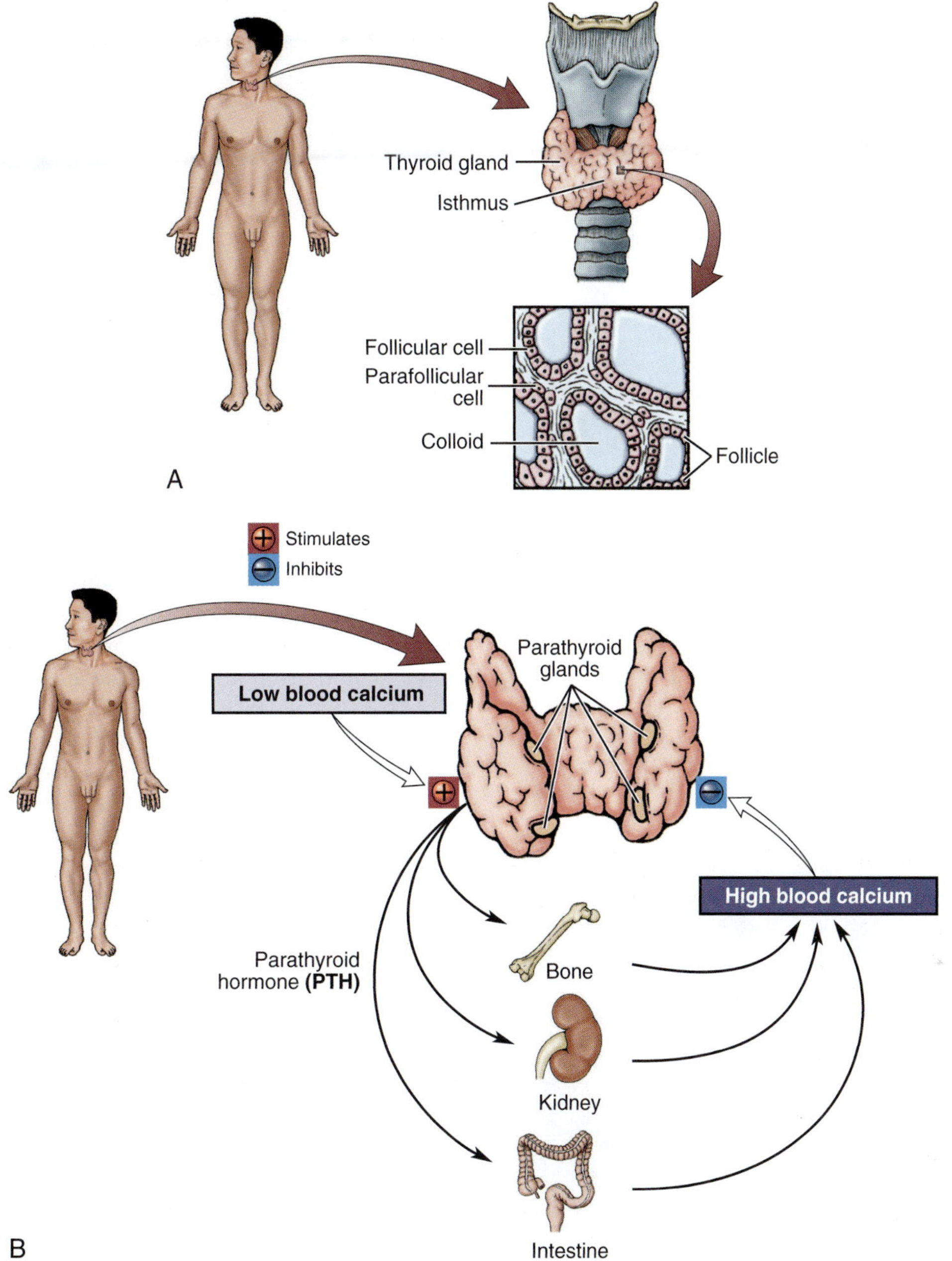

■ **Figure 6-2** A, Thyroid gland. B, Parathyroid glands and three target organs of parathyroid hormone (PTH). (From Herlihy B: The human body in health and illness, ed 3, Philadelphia, 2007, Saunders.)

Management

As in any emergent condition, you must assess and stabilize the patient's airway, breathing/ventilation, and hemodynamic status. Obtain intravenous (IV) access, and provide supportive treatment. If the patient is having seizures, administer benzodiazepines. When you have a strong clinical suspicion or laboratory analysis confirms hypocalcemia, give the patient IV calcium. In emergent situations, administer calcium chloride or calcium gluconate 0.5 to 1 g IV bolus. In nonemergent situations, administer 100 to 300 mg calcium diluted in 150 mL 5% dextrose in water (D_5W) solution over 10 minutes.

THYROID GLAND

The thyroid gland lies in the anterior part of the neck below the larynx (voice box). Its two lobes straddle the midline, joined by a narrow isthmus. Histologically, it's composed of secretory cells, follicular cells, and C cells (parafollicular cells).

Hyperthyroidism

Hyperactivity of the thyroid gland, or hyperthyroidism, is a common ailment that results in a hypermetabolic state called **thyrotoxicosis**. **Thyroid storm** is a rare

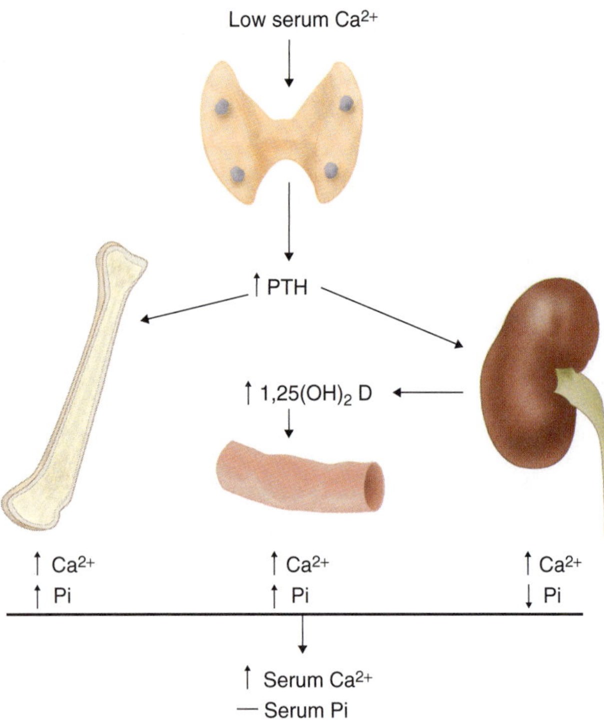

■ **Figure 6-3** Homeostatic response to a fall in serum calcium (Ca^{2+}). (From Goldman L, Ausiello D: Cecil textbook of medicine, ed 23, Philadelphia, 2007, Saunders.)

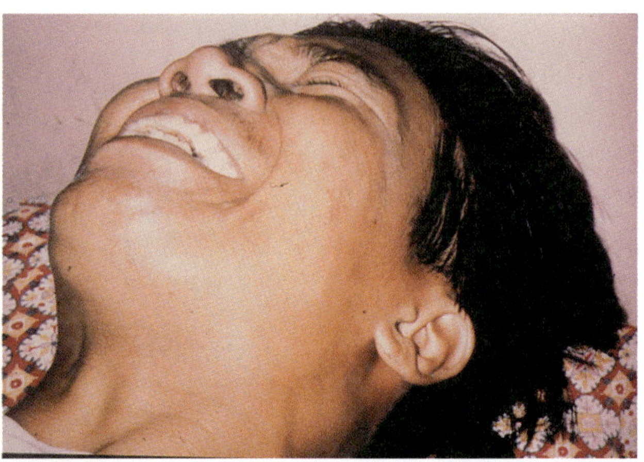

■ **Figure 6-4** Facial spasm and risus sardonicus in a patient with tetanus. (From Cohen J, Powderly W: Infectious diseases, ed 2, St Louis, 2004, Mosby.)

complication of hyperthyroidism that occurs in only 1% to 2% of patients, but it's a life-threatening condition characterized by hemodynamic instability, altered mental status, gastrointestinal (GI) dysfunction, and fever.

Signs and Symptoms

The characteristic clinical presentation of a patient with hyperthyroidism includes apprehension, agitation, edginess, heart palpitations, and weight loss of as much as 40 pounds over a few months. The heat intolerance caused by this hypermetabolic state is a frequent symptom.

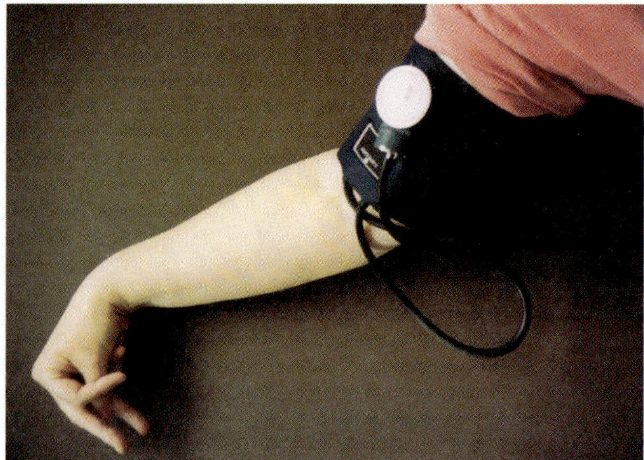

■ **Figure 6-5** Trousseau's sign. (From Ignatavicius DD, Workman ML: Medical-surgical nursing: patient-centered collaborative care, ed 6, Philadelphia, 2010, Saunders.)

A complete physical exam will reveal signs and symptoms of thyrotoxicosis, including the exophthalmos that is characteristic of the condition (Figure 6-7). Other signs and symptoms of hyperthyroidism are summarized in Box 6-1.

Apathetic thyrotoxicosis is a rare form of thyrotoxicosis seen only in older adults. In this condition, the characteristic symptoms of hyperthyroidism are absent. The patient is lethargic, has an apathetic affect, develops a goiter, and experiences weight loss.

Pathophysiology

Graves' disease, also known as *diffuse toxic goiter,* is the most common form of hyperthyroidism. An autoimmune disorder in which antibodies that mimic the role of TSH produce an increase in secretion of thyroid hormones, this condition most often strikes women of middle age, but it can occur at any age and can affect men as well. Other causes of hyperthyroidism include autoimmune destruction of the gland, acute intoxication with exogenous thyroid hormones, and (less commonly) as a result of amiodarone or iodinated IV contrast in susceptible individuals.

Thyroid storm occurs when the body is stressed by a diabetic emergency, an adverse drug reaction, or some serious challenge. You should suspect thyroid storm if the patient experienced cardiac decompensation after taking amiodarone, an antiarrhythmic agent rich in iodine. Other triggers of thyroid storm are summarized in Box 6-2.

Diagnosis

In the prehospital setting, no laboratory studies are immediately available to confirm hyperthyroidism or thyroid storm, so you must have a high index of suspicion on the basis of history and physical examination findings. You can begin to stabilize the patient and initiate early treatment on the strength of clinical judgment alone.

In the hospital, the most rapid and useful test for hyperthyroidism is TSH serum level; if it is low and the patient

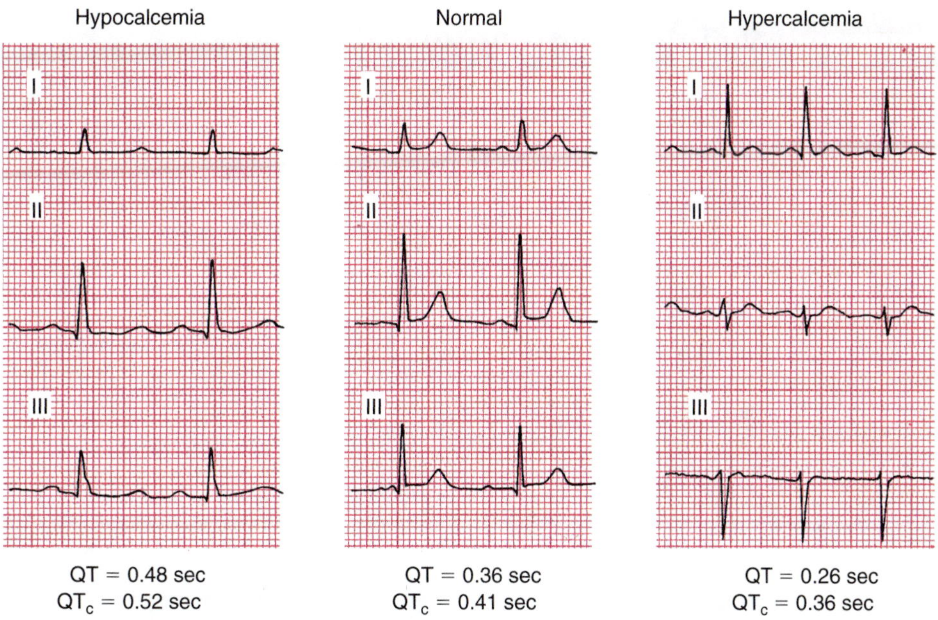

■ **Figure 6-6** Hypocalcemia prolongs QT interval by stretching out ST segment. Hypercalcemia decreases QT interval by shortening ST segment so that T wave seems to take off directly from end of QRS complex. (From Goldberger A: Clinical electrocardiography: a simplified approach, ed 7, St Louis, 2006, Mosby.)

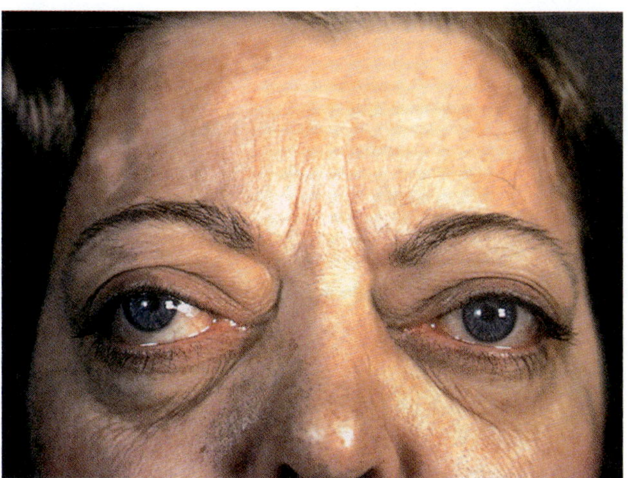

■ **Figure 6-7** Person with hyperthyroidism. Wide-eyed, staring gaze caused by overactivity of sympathetic nervous system is one feature of this disorder. In Graves' disease, one of the most important causes of hyperthyroidism, accumulation of loose connective tissue behind the eyeballs also adds to protuberant appearance of the eyes. (From Kumar V: Robbins and Cotran pathologic basis of disease, professional edition, ed 8, Philadelphia, 2009, Saunders.)

has clinical signs and symptoms of hyperthyroidism, the test is essentially diagnostic. To confirm this presumptive diagnosis, the levels of the actual thyroid hormones, usually T_4 and T_3, may be obtained. Imaging studies and biopsy can help determine the specific cause of the disorder.

As part of the differential diagnosis, consider stroke, diabetic emergencies, congestive heart failure (CHF), toxic ingestion (particularly ingestion of a sympathomimetic agent), and sepsis.

Management

To provide optimal patient care, you have to be able to differentiate among the various hypermetabolic states induced by thyroid disorders. These include subacute (chronic) hyperthyroidism, acute severe hyperthyroidism, and its most feared complication, thyroid storm. When dealing with chronic hyperthyroidism, the patient requires supportive care and early management of symptoms. If severe hyperthyroidism or thyroid storm is detected, it's imperative to stabilize the patient. As in any acute emergency, assess airway patency. Sometimes the patient shows evidence of altered mental status or is in a coma, in which case you must maintain the airway using a bag-mask device, oronasal airway device, or endotracheal intubation if necessary.

Maintain adequate ventilation to keep oxygen saturation at 95% or better. If saturation dips below this level, administer supplemental oxygen through a nonrebreather mask, especially if the patient has heart failure.

The patient with thyroid storm often has moderate to severe dehydration because of excessive diarrhea and sweating. For aggressive hydration, establish two peripheral IV lines early in the course of treatment. Continuously reassess your patient and be alert for adverse affects to overhydration such as pulmonary edema.

A patient with hyperthyroidism is prone to arrhythmias such as sinus tachycardia, atrial fibrillation, atrial flutter, and premature ventricular contractions. For this reason, you should begin continuous cardiac monitoring as soon as you suspect this diagnosis.

BOX 6-1 Signs and Symptoms of Thyrotoxicosis

COMMON SYMPTOMS

- Palpitations
- Shaking
- Weight loss
- Anxiety

LESS COMMON SYMPTOMS

- Shortness of breath
- Disorientation
- Abdominal pain
- Edema
- Diarrhea
- Chest pain

COMMON SIGNS

- Enlarged thyroid gland (palpable goiter)
- High-output cardiac failure
- Fever
- Increased sweating
- Thyrotoxic gaze
- Tachycardia
- Drug interactions

LESS COMMON SIGNS

- Altered mental status
- Shock
- Jaundice
- Weakness

BOX 6-2 Triggers of Thyroid Storm

MEDICAL TRIGGERS

- Infectious disease
- Cardiac ischemia
- Serious burns
- Thromboembolism
- Major surgery
- Trauma

ENDOCRINE TRIGGERS

- Hypoglycemia
- Diabetic ketoacidosis
- Nonketotic hyperosmolar state

PHARMACOLOGIC TRIGGERS

- Iodine therapy
- Amiodarone ingestion
- Administration of contrast medium
- Drug interactions

Patients with thyroid storm may have fever associated with the pathophysiologic process itself or with an infection. Always assess body temperature, and treat hyperpyrexia with acetaminophen. *Do not* use aspirin, since it's associated with decreased protein binding of thyroid hormones and correspondingly increased levels of unbound T_3 and T_4, which will exacerbate symptoms.

The goals of pharmacologic treatment in the prehospital setting are to block the peripheral adrenergic hyperactivity the thyroid hormones elicit (tachycardia, fever, anxiety, and tremors) and to inhibit the conversion of T_4 to T_3 in peripheral tissues. Both objectives can be achieved by administering beta-blockers. The drug of choice is propranolol, given 1 mg IV every 10 minutes up to a total of 10 mg IV or until symptoms have resolved. Propranolol is contraindicated in patients with bronchial asthma, chronic obstructive pulmonary disease (COPD), atrioventricular blocks, hypersensitivity, and severe heart failure. A patient with thyroid storm and concomitant heart failure most likely has a high-output cardiac failure. This is not considered a contraindication to the use of propranolol unless he or she also has significant cardiomyopathy with systolic dysfunction. Adjunctive corticosteroid therapy, either hydrocortisone, 100 mg IV, or dexamethasone, 10 mg IV, may be given to slow the conversion of T_4 to T_3.

Hypothyroidism

Hypothyroidism is an endocrine dysfunction characterized by decreased or absent secretion of thyroid hormones. Its incidence in the United States is 4.6% to 5.8%, but half of those with the condition are asymptomatic. Hypothyroidism is most common among white adult women between the ages of 40 and 50. It is highly associated with autoimmune conditions.

Signs and Symptoms

Hypothyroidism has a deleterious effect on many body systems, including the integumentary, metabolic, nervous, and cardiovascular systems. The skin of a patient with this condition is cool, dry, and yellow. The patient typically has thinning of the eyebrows, coarse hair and skin, marked intolerance to cold temperatures, and neurologic changes

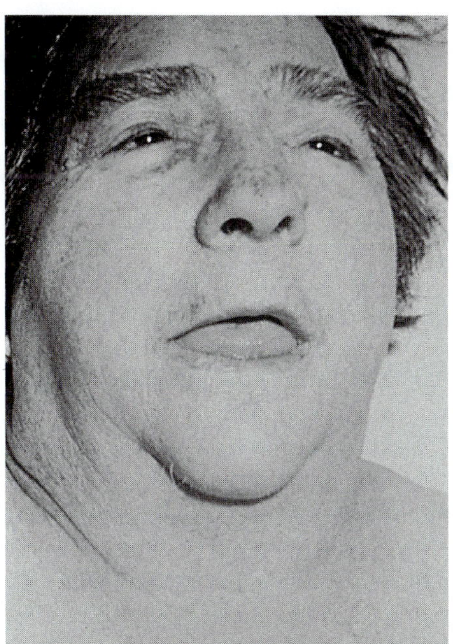

■ **Figure 6-8** Myxedema facies. Note dull, puffy skin; coarse, sparse hair; periorbital edema; prominent tongue. (Courtesy Paul W. Ladenson, MD. The Johns Hopkins University and Hospital, Baltimore.)

BOX 6-3 Precipitants of Myxedema Coma

- Lung infection
- Cold exposure
- Heart failure
- Stroke
- Gastrointestinal bleeding
- Trauma
- Stress
- Hypoxia
- Electrolytic disturbances
- Low serum glucose

such as altered mental status, ataxia, and prolonged deep tendon reflexes. When hypothyroidism becomes chronic and extreme, it may evolve into a life-threatening condition called **myxedema** coma (Figure 6-8), characterized by hypotension, bradycardia, hypoglycemia, and low serum sodium (hyponatremia). Precipitants of myxedema coma are listed in Box 6-3.

Pathophysiology

Defective thyroid hormone secretion is classified as either primary or secondary hypothyroidism. The causes of each are summarized in Box 6-4. Primary hypothyroidism involves direct thyroid injury caused by an autoimmune disorder or an adverse drug reaction. Patients who have had surgical thyroidectomy or radioablation therapy for a hyperthyroid state may have resultant hypothyroidism. In secondary hypothyroidism, damage to the hypothalamus or pituitary gland results in decreased stimulation of the thyroid gland (specifically, a decline in the production and release of TSH). Many complications result from clinical hypothyroidism, as shown in Box 6-5.

BOX 6-4 Etiologic Factors in Hypothyroidism

PRIMARY

- Autoimmune hypothyroidism
- Hereditary hypothyroidism
- Radiation therapy
- Iodine deficiency
- Use of lithium
- Use of antithyroid medications
- Idiopathic

SECONDARY

- Sarcoid infiltration
- Pituitary mass

BOX 6-5 Complications in Myxedema Coma and Hypothyroidism

- Hypoxia
- Hypothermia
- Hypoglycemia
- Sepsis
- Narcosis

Diagnosis

In the prehospital setting, no laboratory studies are immediately available to confirm hypothyroidism or myxedema coma. History and physical examination findings will suggest the diagnosis. Stabilization and early treatment must be initiated solely on the basis of clinical judgment.

In the hospital, TSH levels will be greater than 10 μU/mL or (10 mU/L). In addition, a free thyroxine (FT_4) study may be ordered to evaluate abnormal protein levels that may in turn affect the level of T_4. A T_4 level below 0.8 ng/dL (10 pmol/L) indicates that the thyroid gland is not producing adequate levels of the hormone. Ultrasound imaging can be performed to reveal the size, shape, and position of the thyroid gland and to identify cysts or tumors that may contribute to thyroid dysfunction.

Management

You should be able to differentiate among the various hypometabolic states induced by thyroid disorders: hypothyroidism, severe hypothyroidism, and its most alarming complication, myxedema coma. Patients with hypothyroidism require supportive care and early management of symptoms. You must have a high index of suspicion for this disorder. If severe hypothyroidism or myxedema coma is detected in the prehospital environment, it's imperative to stabilize the patient and transport him or her immediately to a facility with adequate resources to provide definitive treatment.

As in any acute emergency, begin by evaluating airway patency. Sometimes the patient shows evidence of altered mental status or is in a coma, which will preclude his keeping a patent airway. In such a patient, you must maintain the airway using a bag-mask device, oronasal airway device, or endotracheal intubation if necessary.

Maintain adequate ventilation to keep oxygen saturation at 95% or better. If saturation dips below that level, administer supplemental oxygen through a nonrebreather mask, especially if the patient has heart failure.

Initiate a peripheral IV line early during prehospital management to support conservative hydration. It's important to assess cardiovascular function, however, since the patient may have CHF.

If the patient has altered mental status, determine the serum glucose level. If the value is less than 60 mg/dL (3.3 mmol/L), administer 25 g 50% dextrose in water ($D_{50}W$) solution IV.

The hypothyroid patient is prone to developing heart arrhythmias, especially bradycardia, so begin continuous cardiac monitoring as soon as possible. Be aware, however, that standard treatment for bradycardia may be ineffective until thyroid hormone has been replaced.

A patient suffering from myxedema coma may be hypothermic as a result of the pathophysiologic process itself or because of an infection. Always assess body temperature, and treat hypothermia with blankets and other warming techniques. Rapidly transport the patient to a well-equipped hospital facility for definitive treatment, which may include L-triiodothyronine, 0.25 mcg IV; hydrocortisone, 100 mg IV every 8 hours; and subsequent daily oral replacement therapy if the condition proves irreversible.

ADRENAL GLAND AND RELATED DISORDERS

At the apex of each kidney is a triangular adrenal gland about 1.5 inches tall and 3 inches long. These two glands lie retroperitoneal and lateral to the inferior vena cava and abdominal aorta. Their venous and arterial blood supply is derived from upper and lower branches of the inferior vena cava and aorta, respectively (Figure 6-9). The cortex, or surface, of each adrenal gland secretes glucocorticoids such as cortisol, mineralocorticoids such as aldosterone, and supplemental sex hormones. The medulla, or body, produces epinephrine and norepinephrine.

The hypothalamus secretes corticotropin-releasing factor (CRF), stimulating the pituitary to produce adrenocorticotropin hormone (ACTH) and melanocyte-stimulating hormone (MSH). The adrenal gland reacts to ACTH by producing cortisol and aldosterone. Once a sufficient amount of cortisol has been produced by the adrenal glands, the hypothalamus automatically inhibits the production of ACTH and MSH.

Chronic Adrenal Insufficiency

Adrenal insufficiency, the failure of the adrenal cortex to produce a sufficient amount of cortisol, is classified as

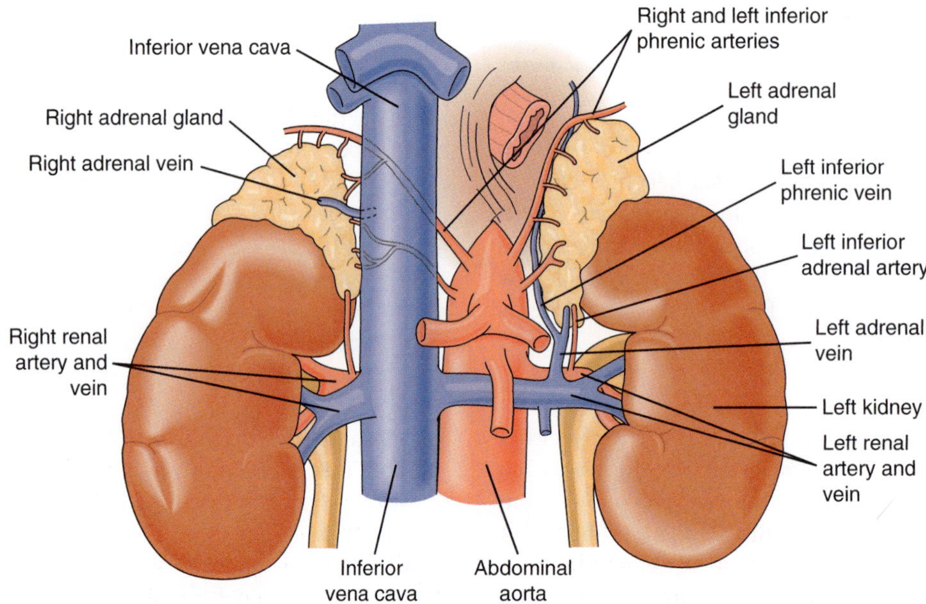

Figure 6-9 Anatomy of the adrenal glands. (From Townsend C, et al: Sabiston textbook of surgery, ed 18, Philadelphia, 2008, Saunders.)

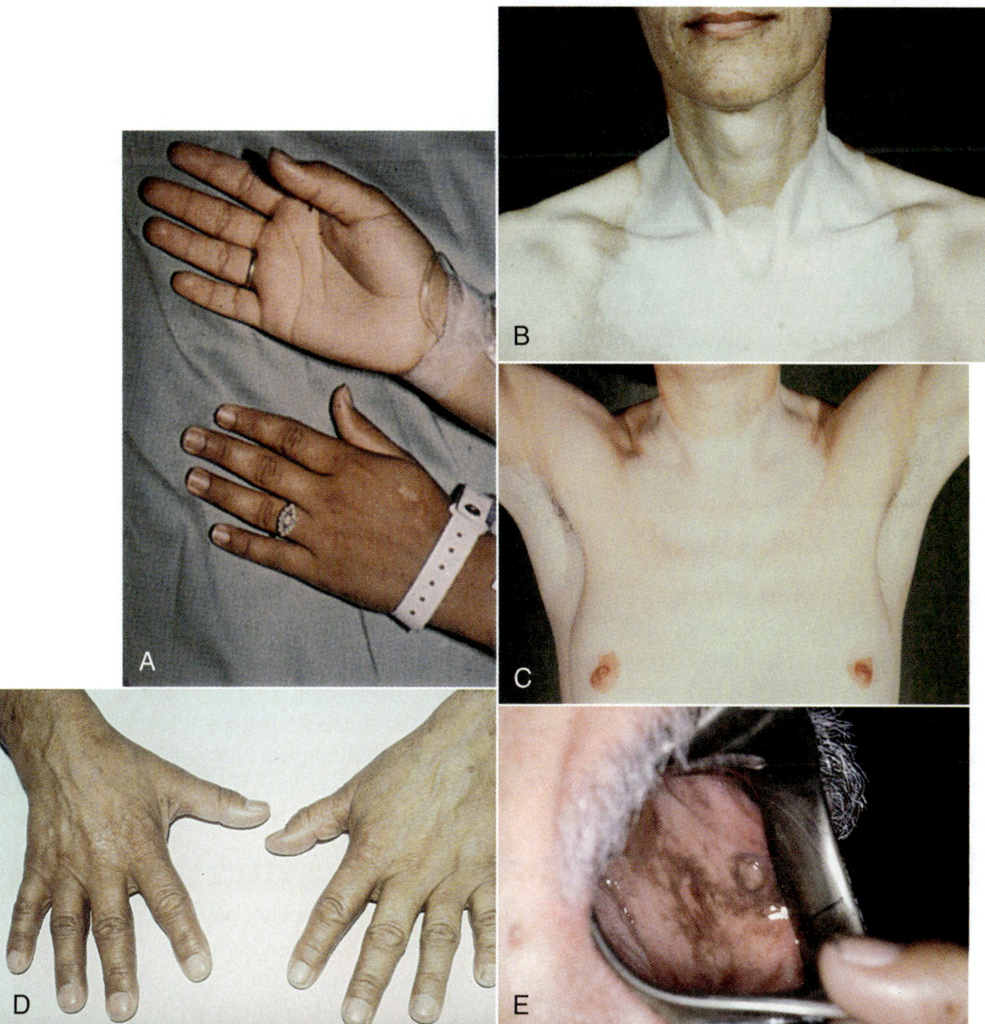

■ **Figure 6-10** Pigmentation in Addison's disease. **A**, Hands of an 18-year-old woman with Addison's disease. Pigmentation in a patient with Addison's disease before (**B**) and after (**C**) treatment with hydrocortisone and fludrocortisone. Note additional presence of vitiligo. **D**, Similar changes also seen in a 60-year-old man with tuberculous Addison's disease, before and after corticosteroid therapy. **E**, Buccal pigmentation in same patient. (From Kronenberg HM, Melmed S, Polonsky K, et al: Williams textbook of endocrinology, ed 11, Philadelphia, 2008, Saunders. **B** and **C** courtesy Professor C.R.W. Edwards.)

primary, secondary, or tertiary, depending on whether the cortex is damaged directly or indirectly. Primary adrenal insufficiency, known as **Addison's disease**, is a metabolic and endocrine ailment caused by a direct insult to or malfunction of the adrenal cortex. It is a chronic disease with a protracted onset. Almost any condition that directly harms the adrenal cortex can cause primary adrenal insufficiency, including autoimmune disorders, adrenal hemorrhage, and infectious diseases such as acquired immunodeficiency syndrome (AIDS), tuberculosis, and meningococcemia.

Signs and Symptoms

The clinical presentation of a patient with Addison's disease is consistent with the endocrine and electrolyte disorders brought on by the disease. The patient will have chronic fatigue and weakness, loss of appetite and consequent weight loss, and hyperpigmentation of the skin and mucous membranes (Figure 6-10). The hyperpigmentation is a result of uninhibited MSH secretion in conjunction with pituitary production of ACTH, which as a side effect stimulates melanocytes in the skin to produce melanin. The patient will have electrolyte disturbances associated with hyponatremia, hyperkalemia, and hypotension and might also have GI disturbances such as abdominal pain, nausea, vomiting, and diarrhea.

Pathophysiology

As noted previously (see Anatomy and Physiology), the adrenal cortex produces the corticosteroid hormones aldosterone and cortisol. Aldosterone is responsible for keeping serum levels of sodium and potassium in balance. When the body suffers any stress—trauma, infection, cardiac ischemia, or a severe illness, to name a few—the adrenal glands may become unable to produce sufficient amounts of corticosteroid hormones to supply the body's demands, triggering an acute exacerbation of Addison's disease.

Secondary adrenal insufficiency is so called because although the cortex itself is intact, it fails to receive a signal to produce cortisol because the pituitary gland fails to release ACTH—thus the adrenal insufficiency is one step removed. Tertiary (third-level) adrenal insufficiency, in which the pituitary's failure to release ACTH stems from a disorder of the hypothalamus, is even less direct. In contrast to primary adrenal insufficiency, the latter two types are not associated with hyperpigmentation of the skin, since they involve low rather than high levels of MSH.

Diagnosis

Diagnostic tools for chronic adrenal insufficiency are not available in the prehospital setting. It's important that you ask the patient for any old diagnostic laboratory reports that might be readily available. Past abnormal electrolyte findings that correlate with the patient's current clinical presentation, such as metabolic acidosis, hyponatremia, hyperkalemia, and hypoglycemia, should raise a red flag. Definitive diagnosis of this condition is made by measuring the patient's baseline serum cortisol level and then conducting stimulation testing, in which synthetic ACTH (called *cosyntropin*) is administered. If the cortisol level fails to rise shortly afterward, the patient can be diagnosed as having primary adrenal insufficiency.

Management

The prehospital management of an acute exacerbation of Addison's disease, known as an *addisonian crisis,* is limited to supportive care. If the patient has tachycardia and hypotension, administer a fluid bolus of normal saline solution, 20 mL/kg. Continual reevaluation of the patient's hemodynamic state, early administration of hydrocortisone (100 to 300 mg IV, or as dictated by local EMS protocol and Medical Control orders), and rapid transport to the emergency department (ED) are paramount in treating this condition. Provide correction of hypoglycemia, as well as symptomatic medical treatment of nausea and vomiting.

In the hospital, diagnostic testing will be carried out to identify electrolyte abnormalities such as hyponatremia and hyperkalemia. Elevated hematocrit levels are common. Management includes correction of electrolyte abnormalities, restoration of metabolic balance (e.g., by replacing glucocorticoids), and volume replacement for hypovolemia.

Acute Adrenal Insufficiency

Acute adrenal insufficiency is a condition in which the body's need for glucocorticoids and mineralocorticoids exceeds the delivery of these hormones by the adrenal glands. The most common cause is abrupt discontinuation of pharmacologic therapy after prolonged use by a patient with chronic adrenal insufficiency. It can also occur when such a patient fails to receive an adjusted dosage during times of stress, such as during illness or after major surgery or trauma.

Signs and Symptoms

The clinical picture of acute adrenal insufficiency will include nausea, vomiting, dehydration, abdominal pain, and weakness. When adrenal insufficiency is accompanied by hypotension, the condition is called **adrenal crisis** and constitutes a true life-threatening emergency.

Pathophysiology

Like chronic adrenal insufficiency, acute insufficiency is classified as primary, secondary, or tertiary, depending on the dysfunctional endocrine gland. *Primary adrenal insufficiency* refers to dysfunction of the adrenals, *secondary adrenal insufficiency* refers to pituitary dysfunction, and *tertiary insufficiency* is linked to hypothalamic dysfunction.

Diagnosis

The diagnosis of this condition in the prehospital setting can be challenging. Not only is the definitive confirmatory laboratory test available in the field, but the presentation of acute adrenal insufficiency can easily be confused with more common conditions such as GI pathology. As the EMS provider, you have to use your available tools to find indirect evidence for adrenal pathology. Assess for hypoglycemia with a glucometer, and look for evidence of hyperkalemia on the ECG. Assess for signs and symptoms of other abnormalities such as anemia, hyponatremia, and metabolic acidosis.

Historical clues, such as tan skin on a patient who denies sun exposure, may indicate chronic adrenal insufficiency. Ask the patient about recent medication changes that may have precipitated the symptoms.

Vital signs can also provide key clues. For example, hypotension that's poorly responsive to administration of IV fluids is seen in adrenal crisis. Confirmation of the disorder can be performed in the ED, using the cosyntropin stimulation test (see Chronic Adrenal Insufficiency).

Management

As with any life-threatening emergency, first evaluate the patient's ability to maintain airway, breathing, and circulation. For hypotension, immediate resuscitation with normal saline is warranted. Administer dextrose if hypoglycemia is present. Address a deficit of glucocorticoids with hydrocortisone, 100 to 300 mg IV, which must be ordered under medical direction in some systems. If a cosyntropin stimulation test is to be performed at a later time, dexamethasone, 4 mg IV, is preferable to hydrocortisone; it can prevent a false-positive test. Rapidly transport the patient to the ED for definitive treatment.

Hyperadrenalism (Cushing's Syndrome)

Cushing's syndrome is the clinical condition caused by long-standing exposure to excessive circulating serum levels of glucocorticoids, particularly cortisol, as a result of overproduction in the adrenal cortex. It's more common in women, especially those aged 20 to 50. Cushing's syndrome can be brought on by an adrenal gland or pituitary tumor or by chronic corticosteroid use.

Signs and Symptoms

Patients with Cushing's syndrome have a distinct appearance characterized by obesity, a moon face (Figure 6-11), and other cardinal features. Box 6-6 outlines signs and symptoms that tend to accompany this disorder.

Diagnosis

Definitive diagnostic testing for Cushing's syndrome is not available in the prehospital setting. Ask the patient for any old diagnostic laboratory reports that might be readily available as a part of recent discharge paperwork. Past abnormal electrolyte findings that correlate with the patient's current clinical presentation, such as metabolic alkalosis, hypernatremia, hypokalemia, and hyperglycemia, should raise a red flag.

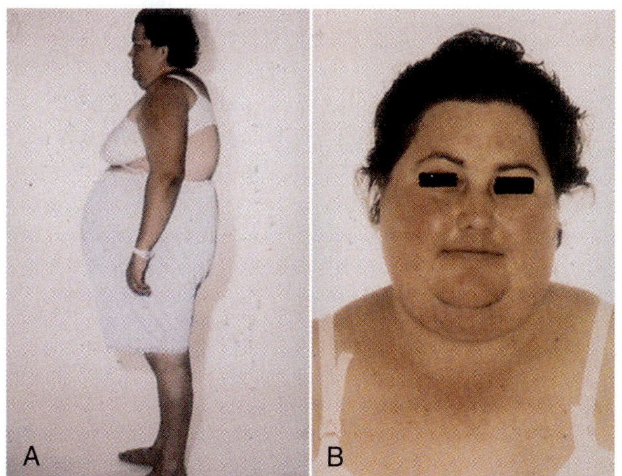

Figure 6-11 Patient with Cushing's syndrome, demonstrating (A) central obesity and (B) "moon facies." (From Kronenberg HM, Melmed S, Polonsky K, et al: Williams textbook of endocrinology, ed 11, Philadelphia, 2008, Saunders.)

Management

Patients with Cushing's syndrome often have chronic or subacute symptoms. Management is guided by the clinical presentation. Affected patients may have fluid retention or, because of the osmotic diuresis brought on by hyperglycemia, may be dehydrated. Thus fluid replacement should be dictated by volume status. Hypertension doesn't require specific therapy unless it has caused end-organ dysfunction or symptoms (e.g., CHF, cardiac ischemia, encephalopathy, acute renal failure). If such a condition is present, administer antihypertensive treatment. Monitor vital signs, mental status, and cardiac rhythm closely.

METABOLISM AND RELATED DISORDERS

Metabolic emergencies represent true diagnostic and management challenges for basic life support (BLS) providers because so few diagnostic tools are available in the prehospital setting. You often have to settle for generating a provisional diagnosis and initial treatment plan on the basis of historical information, physical examination findings, and clinical judgment. This is difficult when a patient has no known medical history or is unable to provide one. Advanced providers can benefit from key information gained through capnometry and (less often) point-of-care laboratory testing. Many metabolic conditions are associated with nonspecific symptoms, perhaps causing a delay in treatment. The following sections discuss the fundamental clinical facts to consider in order to arrive promptly at a diagnosis so you can begin appropriate management of metabolic emergencies.

Anatomy and Physiology

Glucose Metabolism and Control

Glucose is a vital fuel for key metabolic processes in organs, especially those controlled by the central nervous system (CNS). The interdependence of the CNS on glucose metabolism explains why, for example, acute episodes of

BOX 6-6 Signs and Symptoms of Cushing's Syndrome

- Chronic weakness
- Increased body and facial hair
- Plethoric (full, puffy) face
- Fatty "buffalo hump" at the back of the neck
- Central body obesity
- Purple striae on the abdomen, buttocks, breasts, or arms
- Atrophied proximal muscles
- Thin, fragile skin
- Amenorrhea
- Gonadal dysfunction, such as decreased fertility or diminished sex drive
- Diabetes mellitus
- Hypertension

hypoglycemia are manifested as mental status changes, and persistent episodes of hypoglycemia can lead to irreversible brain damage.

Cellular survival depends on preserving a balanced serum glucose concentration. Under normal circumstances, the body is able to maintain serum glucose in the relatively tight range of 70 to 150 mg/dL (3.9 to 8.3 mmol/L) before and after meals. This control essentially derives from three metabolic processes:

1. Gluconeogenesis: the formation of new glucose from precursors including pyruvate, glycerol, lactate, and amino acids
2. Glycogenolysis: glucose produced as glycogen breakdown occurs in the liver
3. GI absorption: direct intestinal absorption of glucose through the intestine

Hormones and neurohumoral factors interact with regulatory mediators, including insulin, epinephrine, norepinephrine, and glucagon, to maintain a normal serum glucose concentration. When the level of glucose in the blood is insufficient, glucagon is released from alpha cells in the pancreas to increase glucose production through gluconeogenesis. Glucagon release can also be triggered by exercise, trauma, and infection. These mechanisms increase glucose levels within minutes but do so only transiently. Epinephrine and norepinephrine increase glucose levels even more rapidly by enabling gluconeogenesis and hepatic glycogenolysis. Insulin, which is secreted by the pancreatic islet cells, is essential for efficient cellular glucose utilization and also drives glucose into the cells.

Diabetes Mellitus

Diabetes is the most common endocrine disorder, and hypoglycemia—a frequent complication of diabetes—is the most common endocrine emergency. Diabetes mellitus is characterized by defective insulin production or utilization, a high level of blood glucose, and unbalanced lipid and carbohydrate metabolism. Untreated diabetes results in hyperglycemia. A random plasma glucose level > 200 mg/dL (>11.1 mmol/L) or a fasting serum glucose > 140 mg/dL (>7.7 mmol/L) meets the threshold for a diagnosis of diabetes.

Hypoglycemia among people with diabetes is the result of inadvertent overdosage of insulin or (less commonly) oral hypoglycemic agents. Because glucose must be maintained within a narrow range, diabetes is a difficult disease to control, and diabetic emergencies account for between 3% and 4% of EMS calls, most of which are for hypoglycemia and 10% to 12% of which are for acute and chronic medical problems associated with hyperglycemia.

Because glucose fuels every cell in the body, patients with diabetes mellitus are prone to developing serious acute metabolic problems and chronic medical illnesses, especially if the blood glucose level is not well controlled.

BOX 6-7 Classification and Etiology of Diabetes Mellitus

TYPE 1

- Idiopathic; appears to have an immunologic basis

TYPE 2

- Dysfunction of pancreatic beta cells
- Defects of insulin action
- Infectious
- Medication induced

GESTATIONAL

- Impaired glucose tolerance

Besides hypoglycemia, ketoacidosis and hyperosmolar coma can occur. Chronically poor glucose control tends to cause microvascular problems in multiple organs and systems, including the heart, kidneys, eyes, and neurologic system.

Classification

Classification of diabetes mellitus is summarized in Box 6-7. You're likely to encounter patients with three presentations:

- Type 1 diabetes mellitus: characterized by pancreatic beta cell destruction, which renders the body incapable of producing the insulin necessary to carry out cell metabolism. This type of diabetes is typically diagnosed during childhood or adolescence and accounts for 5% to 10% of all cases of diabetes mellitus. Patients with type 1 diabetes usually require daily insulin administration to stay alive.
- Type 2 diabetes mellitus: accounts for 90% to 95% of all diabetes diagnoses. Rather than a defect of insulin manufacture, this type of diabetes is characterized by cellular insulin resistance and a gradual failure of pancreatic insulin production. Type 2 diabetes is most common among older adults and is associated with physical inactivity and obesity. Women with type 2 diabetes often have a history of gestational diabetes. It's common for patients with type 2 diabetes to remain asymptomatic for years before they begin to show signs and symptoms. Unfortunately, there has been a significant rise in the number of pediatric patients who are being diagnosed with type 2 diabetes. Increasing rates of childhood obesity and decreasing levels of physical exercise appear to be contributing factors.
- Gestational diabetes: a form of glucose intolerance that can occur among pregnant women. It typically has the same clinical presentation as type 2 diabetes. Patients usually have hyperglycemia but no acidosis.

Measurement of Glucose

Using a glucometer to quantify serum glucose at the patient's side has become a standard of care in modern EMS practice. In the past, dextrose was given empirically to all patients with altered mental status without first quantifying serum glucose. Later, researchers found that few patients benefited from such an approach. A glucometer gives rapid bedside glucose results, and its use in the prehospital setting has been found to be safe and accurate. Ideally, you should measure glucose using capillary blood samples, not venous blood obtained during placement of an IV line, since the latter can produce inaccurate readings. Store glucose strips in temperature-controlled, airtight compartments in the ambulance to ensure their accuracy and reliability.

DISORDERS OF GLUCOSE METABOLISM

Hypoglycemia

As already discussed, glucose is the principal fuel for metabolism in the body and its organs, especially the brain. **Hypoglycemia** is defined as a blood glucose level < 70 mg/dL (3.9 mmol/L). Keep in mind that individual responses to blood glucose levels vary, and those discussed here represent averages. Generally, as the plasma glucose level falls below 70 mg/dL (3.9 mmol/L), the following sequence of events occurs in quick succession:

1. First, the body decreases insulin secretion in an effort to arrest the blood glucose decline.
2. Next, there is an increase in the secretion of counterregulatory hormones, primarily epinephrine and norepinephrine.
3. Finally, signs and symptoms, including impaired cognition, become apparent. Once the level falls below 50 mg/dL (2.8 mmol/L), significant mental status changes occur.

Untreated hypoglycemia is associated with significant morbidity and mortality. To decrease these risks, you should be able recognize the signs and symptoms and be prepared to initiate treatment quickly and effectively.

Signs and Symptoms

Clinical manifestations of hypoglycemia usually evolve rapidly. The patient will seek treatment for a myriad of signs and symptoms directly related to the release of endogenous stress hormones, including diaphoresis, altered level of consciousness (LOC), tremors, and pale, cold, clammy skin. If hypoglycemia is not treated, the patient may develop life-threatening generalized seizures. It's important to check serum glucose in every patient who is having an active seizure, to rule out hypoglycemia as the cause.

However, the rate at which signs and symptoms appear and the patient's medical history, age, sex, and overall health contribute to the clinical presentation. For instance, an older adult with a complex medical history may have signs of severe hypoglycemia at a glucose level above 50 mg/dL (>2.8 mmol/L). On the contrary, a young adult may have signs of severe hypoglycemia at a level well below 50 mg/dL (<2.8 mmol/L).

Most clinical manifestations of hypoglycemia are generated by secretion of counterregulatory hormones (e.g., epinephrine) which are secreted in response to a low glucose concentration. Signs and symptoms may include:

- Sweating
- Tremors
- Nervousness
- Tachycardia
- Altered LOC or behavior
- Seizures
- Coma

You must consider that the patient may be taking a medication, such as a beta-blocker, whose effects initially mimic signs of hypoglycemia. Such patients can rapidly lose consciousness or begin having a seizure in the absence of any prodrome of hypoglycemia.

Pathophysiology

Diabetic management emphasizes tight plasma glucose control to prevent long-term complications such as renal failure and heart disease. Hypoglycemia is common among diabetic patients with a tight glucose control regimen, although it may occur in nondiabetic patients as well. Patients with diabetes are treated with a number of medications to help them maintain this careful control. Sometimes they're prescribed a combination of subcutaneously administered insulin and oral hypoglycemic agents, a therapeutic strategy that makes them susceptible to hypoglycemic episodes. Triggers of all types of hypoglycemia are listed in Box 6-8.

Hypoglycemia in Nondiabetic Patients Hypoglycemia in patients who have no history of diabetes is called *fasting* or *postprandial hypoglycemia*. Fasting hypoglycemia is usually the result of an imbalance between glucose utilization and production. Postprandial hypoglycemia is characterized by alimentary hyperinsulinism and is commonly seen in patients who have undergone gastric surgery.

A number of conditions may elicit fasting hypoglycemia. Among the most common are severe liver disease, pancreatic tumors (such as insulinomas), enzyme defects, drug overdoses (for example, insulin, sulfonylureas), and severe infection. The clinical characteristics are similar to those of diabetic hypoglycemia.

Management of hypoglycemia in nondiabetic patients is similar to management of the condition in patients with diabetes. However, hypoglycemia in nondiabetic patients may recur, especially in patients with drug overdose. Such patients may require more than one dose of dextrose or even a continuous infusion.

BOX 6-8 Triggers of Hypoglycemia

- Decreased food intake
- Exogenous insulin administration (factitious hypoglycemia)
- Medications:
  - Oral hypoglycemic agents
  - Beta-blockers
  - Antimalarial drugs
- Alcohol abuse
- Aggressive treatment of hyperglycemia:
  - Diabetic ketoacidosis
  - Nonketotic hyperosmolar state
  - Uncontrolled blood sugar
  - Administration of excessive doses of therapeutic insulin
- Malnutrition
- Medication adjustments
- Insulin pump failure
- Sepsis
- Volume depletion
- Kidney disease
- Liver disease
- Pancreatic tumors
- Endocrinopathy:
  - Thyroid disease:
    - Hypothyroidism
    - Hyperthyroidism
  - Adrenal disease:
    - Addison's disease

BOX 6-9 Key Treatment Considerations for Patients with Hypoglycemia

- Check for hypoglycemia in every patient with altered mental status.
- Administer oral glucose to patients awake enough to take fluids by mouth without risk of aspiration.
- Administer intravenous (IV) glucose (50 mL of a 50% dextrose [D_{50}] solution) to patients with depressed alertness.
- If giving glucagon, administer 1-2 mg intramuscularly (IM) or subcutaneously (SQ) in adult patients. You may repeat this dose every 20 minutes. (In children, administer 0.025-0.1 mg/kg IM or SQ. You may repeat this dose every 20 minutes.) Be aware that glucagon will not work in patients with depleted glycogen stores, such as those with alcoholism or malnutrition.
- Overdoses of oral hypoglycemic agents will cause profound, persistent, and severe hypoglycemia. Patients may need a continuous infusion with a 10% dextrose solution.
  - In infants and children younger than age 8, do not administer 50% dextrose in water ($D_{50}W$) solution. Use 25% ($D_{25}W$) or 10% ($D_{10}W$) dextrose in water solution instead.
  - In children, give 0.5-1 g/kg glucose IV in a $D_{25}W$ solution (2-4 mL/kg)
  - In neonates, give 0.5-1 g/kg glucose IV in a $D_{10}W$ solution (1-2 mL/kg)

Diagnosis

Severe hypoglycemia can be indicated by a comprehensive history and physical exam and confirmed with a serum glucose test. As part of the initial evaluation, obtain a complete set of vital signs. Use glucose strips that have been stored properly, since storage at improper temperatures may affect readings. Remember that the equipment has to be properly calibrated to give an accurate reading.

Management

To prevent further complications, such as seizures or permanent brain damage, begin providing glucose immediately. The simplest option is to give oral glucose in the form of a small snack or a sugar-containing beverage. This option should always be considered in awake and alert patients who are able to swallow. For patients who have altered mentation or cannot swallow, administration of $D_{50}W$ has been the standard, but such a high concentration of glucose can have serious complications if extravasation or infiltration occurs. Recently, EMS has begun to embrace the use of $D_{10}W$. Studies have found no difference in the amount of time necessary for a hypoglycemic patient to regain consciousness when the two solutions are compared. When patients are given $D_{10}W$, they receive a considerably lower amount of glucose while achieving the same therapeutic response and are less likely to have a high glucose level after treatment.

If quick IV access proves difficult, intramuscular (IM) glucagon can be an effective alternative. It may not work, however, in patients with chronic illness who have depleted glycogen stores (e.g., alcoholics and others with chronic liver disease). Recovery time with glucagon is significantly longer than with IV dextrose, and glucagon may cause side effects such as nausea and vomiting. If it is used, the standard dose is 1 to 2 mg IM. Key treatment considerations for patients with hypoglycemia are listed in Box 6-9.

An important distinction must be made between patients who have become hypoglycemic from taking oral agents and those who use insulin. Oral agents usually do not cause hypoglycemia, even if oral intake of food has been decreased. If they do, you should suspect the presence of a serious underlying condition (e.g., renal failure), and the patient should be transported to the ED for further evaluation and possible admission.

Diabetic Ketoacidosis

Diabetic ketoacidosis (DKA) is characterized by a plasma glucose concentration >350 mg/dL (>19.4 mmol/L), ketone production, a serum bicarbonate level < 15 mEq/L, and metabolic acidosis. The mortality rate for DKA ranges from 9% to 14%. DKA is an acute endocrine emergency in which insulin deficiency and an excessive glucagon level combine to create a hyperglycemic, acidotic, volume-depleted state. The condition is often associated with electrolyte imbalances.

Signs and Symptoms

Patients with DKA are dehydrated and will appear ill. They usually report polydipsia, polyphagia, and polyuria. Patients with severe DKA will exhibit altered mental status during the initial examination. Tachycardia, rapid and shallow breathing, and orthostatic changes are likely to be present. Expect:

- Nausea and vomiting
- Abdominal pain (especially common in children)
- Tachypnea
- Fruity breath odor
- Fatigue and weakness
- Increased diuresis
- Altered LOC
- Orthostatic hypotension
- Cardiac dysrhythmia
- Seizures
- Hemodynamic shock in severe cases

Pathophysiology

DKA may be elicited by certain metabolic stressors such as infection, myocardial infarction, trauma, and sometimes pregnancy. The common trigger among these conditions is the interruption of the insulin regimen of a person with diabetes. Lack of insulin prevents glucose from entering cells, and consequently, the cells become starved of glucose for cellular metabolism and turn to other sources of energy such as fat. As a result, glucose begins to accumulate in the bloodstream. This overflow of glucose is forced into the renal tubules, drawing water, sodium, potassium, magnesium, and other ions into the urine, creating significant diuresis. The renal tubules then release large amounts of glucose into the urine.

This diuresis, combined with vomiting, produces volume depletion and consequent shock. These osmotic changes are largely responsible for the declining mental status of a patient with DKA. The clinical hallmark of DKA is metabolic acidosis (see later discussion). Physiologically, the body attempts to compensate and eliminate acids by breathing faster (a pattern known as *Kussmaul's respiration*) and trying to use more bicarbonate. All this will have a direct impact on the body's electrolyte balance, especially potassium. Acidosis encourages the shift of potassium into the bloodstream in exchange for hydrogen (H^+), thereby increasing total body potassium loss, perhaps generating neurologic and cardiovascular complications.

Differential Diagnosis

Several conditions bear a clinical resemblance to DKA. It's difficult for you to distinguish among them in the field, however, without definitive diagnostic tests. Sepsis, for example, is an emergency that may mimic DKA. You should suspect sepsis if the patient has a fever, since patients with DKA rarely have an elevated body temperature. Prolonged fasting—for instance, in a third-trimester pregnant patient or nursing mother who is not eating properly—can also resemble DKA.

Other conditions can be mistaken for DKA as well. People who abuse alcohol may have a fruity breath odor, a rapid respiratory rate, and a recent history of having stopped drinking. Rapid breathing should raise your suspicion that the body is trying to compensate for an acidotic state. However, a significant percentage of such patients will have misleading glucose values that are normal or even low. This condition is known as *alcoholic ketoacidosis* (detailed later).

Make sure to perform a 12-lead ECG if you suspect DKA. The information it provides could change your management strategy (e.g., if the ECG reveals a myocardial infarction). In addition, electrolyte abnormalities often accompany diabetic emergencies, and a 12-lead ECG could reveal worrisome anomalies, the gravest of which is hyperkalemia.

As you can see, the differential diagnosis of DKA is tricky. To minimize confusion, tackle every case in an organized way and, most important, begin initial treatment without delay, since management for all these conditions is the same.

Management

Patients with severe DKA look critically ill and require immediate treatment. A patient with an altered LOC may be actively vomiting, putting him or her at risk of aspiration. In such cases, consider early intubation to protect the airway. Remember that DKA patients breathe rapidly to compensate for their metabolic acidosis. Therefore, if you intubate such a patient, maintain hyperventilation to prevent deterioration of acid-base status. Initiate aggressive fluid resuscitation using 0.9% normal saline administered through two peripheral lines. Patients with DKA usually require 3 to 6 L of fluid during initial resuscitation. Monitor them closely, since they can decompensate rapidly. Patients with a history of heart failure can easily go into fluid overload, so be cautious when administering IV fluids. Consider underlying causes of DKA, such as myocardial infarction, and treat them appropriately.

DKA cannot be reversed without insulin therapy, but insulin is not generally administered in the prehospital setting. However, on occasion, you may have to care for a patient who is already receiving an insulin infusion. Your EMS service should have a protocol in place to guide management of such patients during transport. You must be able to recognize potential and common side effects of continuous insulin therapy. High-dose insulin is associated with iatrogenic hypoglycemia and hypokalemia, for example. This is caused by a shift of glucose and potassium into the cells after insulin administration. Although patients in DKA initially appear to be hyperkalemic, this is only due to a shift caused by the acidosis. They are typically total body deficient in potassium. Abnormal potassium levels can result in life-threatening cardiac arrhythmias, so it would be prudent to confirm the patient's most recent potassium level before transport. Complications of DKA are listed in Box 6-10, and important treatment considerations are summarized in Box 6-11.

Hyperosmolar Hyperglycemic Nonketotic Syndrome

Hyperosmolar hyperglycemic nonketotic syndrome (HHNS) is a serious diabetic emergency, carrying a mortality rate of 10% to 50%. You may not be able to differentiate DKA from HHNS in the field, but there's a chance you can deduce it from the patient's history. HHNS is more common in patients with type 2 diabetes mellitus and is triggered by the same stressors that cause DKA. The condition is characterized by:

- Elevated plasma glucose concentration, often greater than 600 mg/dL (>33.3 mmol/L)

BOX 6-10 Complications of Treatment for Diabetic Ketoacidosis

The treatment of diabetic ketoacidosis is difficult and complex, requiring the participation of a multidisciplinary group of medical professionals. Even then, patients are not immune from developing complications. Five major complications increase morbidity and mortality in DKA:

1. Hypokalemia: can occur as a result of inadequate potassium replacement during treatment, since aggressive insulin treatment shifts potassium into the cells.
2. Hypoglycemia: can be attributed to aggressive treatment and failure to closely observe glucose. It's vitally important to begin administering a 5% dextrose in water (D_5W) solution when glucose falls below 300 mg/dL.
3. Fluid overload: aggressive fluid resuscitation in patients with congestive heart failure can cause fluid overload.
4. Alkalosis: overly aggressive treatment with bicarbonate causes alkalosis, which can further complicate electrolyte imbalances, specifically by increasing potassium requirements as potassium is displaced into body cells.
5. Cerebral edema: the most feared complication of DKA treatment. It occurs as a result of rapid osmolar shifts. Cerebral edema generally appears 6-10 hours after the initiation of therapy and carries a mortality rate of 90%. You should suspect this complication in a patient who becomes comatose after acidosis is reversed during treatment of DKA.

BOX 6-11 Key Treatment Considerations for Patients with Diabetic Ketoacidosis or HHNS

- If the patient is intubated, maintain hyperventilation to prevent worsening of acidosis.
- Provide fluid rehydration. You may need to rapidly administer 1 to 2 liters of normal saline. Monitor glucose regularly, since fluid resuscitation will decrease glucose levels.
- Evaluate ECG for signs of hyperkalemia (peaked T waves, widened QRS, loss of P waves, bradycardia, or sign wave morphology), and treat accordingly.
- In pediatric patients, administer fluid resuscitation of 20 mL/kg.

For extended Critical Care Transports, consider:

- Change the IV solution to D_5 in 0.45% normal saline when glucose falls below 300 mg/dL (<16.6 mmol/L).
- Correct electrolytes when indicated, using the following guidelines:
  - Potassium. If potassium is low, first ensure that the patient's renal function is adequate, and then add 20-40 mEq/L potassium chloride for each liter of fluid administered.
  - Magnesium. If magnesium is low, correct the level with 1 to 2 grams magnesium sulfate in the first 2 liters of fluid administered.
  - In the case of acidosis, correct acidosis if the pH falls below 7 by adding 44 to 88 mEq/L of sodium bicarbonate to the first liter of IV fluid administered.
  - Be aware of the potential complications of insulin infusions, such as hypokalemia and hypoglycemia.
- Remember, constant monitoring is essential. Treat underlying causes if possible, and transport the patient to a hospital with ICU capabilities.

- Absent ketone production
- Increased serum osmolality, usually > 315 mOsm/kg

HHNS is associated with significant dehydration and a decline in mental status. Occasionally it progresses to full coma. In contrast to DKA, acidosis and ketosis are usually absent.

Signs and Symptoms

Patients with HHNS are usually acutely ill, with marked volume depletion, nausea, vomiting, abdominal pain, tachypnea, and tachycardia. It's common for these patients to have a 25% fluid deficit. In addition, they may have focal neurologic deficits and seizures or signs of stroke. Signs and symptoms of HHNS include:

- Fever
- Dehydration
- Vomiting and abdominal pain
- Hypotension
- Tachycardia
- Rapid breathing
- Thirst, polyuria or oliguria, polydipsia
- Focal seizures
- Altered LOC
- Focal neurologic deficits

Pathophysiology

The pathophysiology of HHNS is complex but similar to that of DKA. The condition doesn't usually develop suddenly but evolves over a period of several days. The time frame varies, depending on the patient's overall health. HHNS usually occurs in older adults and in patients debilitated by a primary condition. As in DKA, the hallmark is decreased insulin action, which triggers a volley of counterregulatory mechanisms that increase serum glucose. Once insulin function decreases, gluconeogenesis, glycogenolysis, and decreased glucose uptake in the periphery begin to dominate. Hyperglycemia then pulls fluid into the extracellular space, triggering osmotic diuresis, which in turn causes hypotension and volume deficit. Patients are initially able to maintain intravascular volume with constant fluid intake, but the diuresis eventually overtakes the system. Keep in mind that other conditions such as sepsis may be causing further volume depletion. Common causes of HHNS include:

- Trauma
- Drugs
- Myocardial infarction
- Cushing's syndrome
- Sepsis
- Cerebrovascular accident (stroke)
- Dialysis
- CNS insult (e.g., subdural hematoma)
- Hemorrhage
- Pregnancy

Differential Diagnosis

Many conditions have signs and symptoms similar to those of DKA (see earlier discussion) and HHNS. In most cases, your initial intervention will be similar for all of these possible illnesses, but be alert for time-sensitive conditions that can cause DKA and HHNS, such as myocardial infarction and sepsis.

To differentiate HHNS from DKA, remember that the former is usually accompanied by a more profound decrease in mental status. Signs and symptoms of HHNS can be confusing, since they may be similar to those of hypoglycemia. If blood glucose cannot be rapidly evaluated, hypoglycemia must be assumed until proved otherwise. The administration of dextrose could minimally worsen glucose levels in HHNS, but it can be life saving in a patient with hypoglycemia.

Management

The initial management of a patient with HHNS is the same as that of a patient with DKA. Take immediate steps to stabilize airway, breathing, and circulation. The patient may have significant volume depletion, so begin IV fluid resuscitation immediately. The initial fluid of choice is 0.9% normal saline. Early boluses may be necessary to stabilize the patient hemodynamically. Use caution, however, when the patient has comorbidities such as CHF. Remember that fluid administration alone will correct much of the hyperglycemia. DKA management controversies apply to HHNS as well. For instance, rapid correction of serum osmolality can predispose patients—especially children—to the development of cerebral edema. (You may wish to review the summary of treatment considerations for HHNS in Box 6-11.)

ACID-BASE DISORDERS

Acid-Base Homeostasis

Healthy cellular function is directly related to a precise acid-base balance in the body. Essential organs that play a key role in maintaining this balance are the kidneys and lungs, which interact with serum buffers to maintain a narrow acid-base balance. This balance is expressed as a pH measurement, which must remain between 7.35 and 7.45. A pH below 7.35 constitutes acidosis. In contrast, a pH level above 7.45 constitutes alkalosis. These pH derangements are classified according to their primary etiology, either metabolic or respiratory. The body usually initiates a compensatory reaction to try to correct the underlying abnormality. In some cases, three different overlapping processes are at work. This situation may involve, for example, a primary acidosis, a compensatory alkalosis, and another underlying acidosis.

BOX 6-12 Precipitants of Respiratory Acidosis

ACUTE

Pharmacologic CNS Depression

- Narcotics
- Benzodiazepines
- Alcohol abuse
- Gamma-hydroxybutyrate (GHB) toxicity

Lung Disease

- Interstitial edema
- Pneumonia

Airway Problems

- Foreign body
- Aspiration
- Bronchospasm
- Apnea

Hypoventilation

- Pneumothorax
- Flail chest
- Myasthenia gravis
- Guillain-Barré syndrome
- Primary CNS disorders
- Brain injury

CHRONIC

Lung Disease

- Chronic bronchitis
- COPD
- Pulmonary fibrosis

Neuromuscular Diseases

- Muscular dystrophy
- Myasthenia gravis

Obesity

- Sleep apnea

CNS, Central nervous system; *COPD*, chronic obstructive pulmonary disease.

Respiratory Acidosis

Respiratory acidosis is one of the most common acid-base problems encountered in the prehospital setting. Respiratory acidosis is characterized by a decline in pH as a result of CO_2 retention. Hypoventilation is the classic example of a clinical problem that leads to CO_2 retention. Respiratory acidosis may be classified as acute or chronic. The only way to distinguish between these states is to determine whether the body has begun to retain bicarbonate to compensate for the acidosis. During the acute phase, the serum bicarbonate level is normal. Once the body begins to retain bicarbonate, it has made the transition to chronic status.

Signs and Symptoms

You may encounter different clinical scenarios, depending on the severity of the primary problems. Common signs and symptoms include weakness, breathing difficulty, and altered LOC. Noting the LOC is critical when evaluating a patient with suspected respiratory acidosis because it may indicate the severity of the process and signal the need for advanced airway management. For instance, in a patient with COPD who has a diminished mental status, a high level of CO_2 is most likely responsible for the altered LOC. Such a patient has a higher risk of complications such as aspiration and therefore requires more aggressive intervention.

Pathophysiology

Any pathology that results in hypoventilation (e.g., primary pulmonary problems, airway obstruction, illnesses that depress the respiratory drive) will elicit respiratory acidosis. Precipitants of respiratory acidosis are summarized in Box 6-12.

Management

Standard monitoring equipment should be used according to your provider level, including ECG monitor, SpO_2, and $ETCO_2$. After your initial evaluation and stabilization of the patient's airway, breathing, and circulation (ABCs), therapy should focus on correcting minute ventilation to decrease CO_2 levels and thereby correct the acidosis. Depending on the etiology, you can accomplish this either by assisting ventilation or by providing pharmacologic intervention. Ventilatory assistance can range from airway positioning, bag-mask device with nasopharyngeal airway or oropharyngeal airway, continuous positive airway pressure (CPAP) or bilevel positive airway pressure (BiPAP) to endotracheal intubation with ventilator support. Pharmacologic intervention, such as naloxone administration, can reverse respiratory depression in patients whose hypoventilation can be attributed to the toxic effects of opiate overdose.

Although any hypoxic patient should be treated with supplemental oxygen, be cautious in providing high-flow oxygen to patients with chronic respiratory acidosis, because it can reduce their respiratory drive. You may wish to take a look back at this topic in Chapter 3 for details.

Respiratory Alkalosis

An increase in ventilation per minute is the cause of respiratory alkalosis, characterized by a decreased $PaCO_2$ and increased pH. The only way to differentiate between acute and chronic respiratory alkalosis is to measure serum bicarbonate. A patient with acute respiratory alkalosis will have a normal serum bicarbonate level. A patient with chronic respiratory alkalosis, on the other hand, will have a decrease in serum bicarbonate level.

Signs and Symptoms

The patient's clinical presentation depends on whether the respiratory alkalosis is chronic. Most signs and symptoms are nonspecific and are related to peripheral or CNS complaints such as paresthesia of the face or lips, lightheadedness, dizziness, and muscular pain or cramps.

Pathophysiology

Respiratory alkalosis is usually seen as a secondary compensatory mechanism to a primary metabolic problem, but it can be a primary derangement as well. Some causes of primary respiratory alkalosis include aspirin overdose, anxiety reaction, and pulmonary embolism. On occasion, it may be a normal physiologic response. The classic example is alkalemia of pregnancy, in which pH status is 7.46 to 7.5. This condition is primarily respiratory in origin and is characterized by a $P{CO_2}$ of 31 to 35 mm Hg.

Diagnosis

The diagnosis of respiratory alkalosis may not be obvious, since some of its signs and symptoms are almost identical to those of certain electrolyte emergencies such as hypocalcemia. A thorough history and physical exam will yield clues to the underlying cause of the respiratory alkalosis, which may guide management strategies. Be careful not to overlook life-threatening toxicologic etiologies like aspirin intoxication. Precipitants of respiratory alkalosis are summarized in Box 6-13.

Management

Administer oxygen to patients with hypoxemia without delay, and take steps to stabilize and support airway, breathing, and circulation. For hyperventilation caused by anxiety, use coaching techniques to calm the patient. Instruct him or her to use pursed-lip breathing. To avoid precipitating hypoxia, do not use a paper bag or a nonrebreather mask without oxygen attached.

Metabolic Acidosis

Metabolic acidosis is caused by the accumulation of acids in excess of the body's buffering capabilities. In the acute state, the body's physiologic response is to hyperventilate and compensate by reducing $Pa{CO_2}$. Chronic status is reached when the renal system begins to reabsorb bicarbonate in an effort to compensate for the metabolic acidosis.

Signs and Symptoms

The clinical manifestations of metabolic acidosis are directly related to the severity of the metabolic problem. Most patients have nausea, vomiting, abdominal pain, a rapid and deep respiratory pattern (Kussmaul's respiration), and in more severe cases, altered LOC and shock.

Pathophysiology

Metabolic acidosis is generated by three mechanisms: decreased renal excretion of acids, increased production or ingestion of acids, and loss of buffering mechanisms in the body.

Diagnosis

Metabolic acidosis is classified as either non–anion-gap acidosis or anion-gap acidosis. The anion gap is calculated using the following formula (see Chapter 1 for a complete review):

$$AG = Na^+ - (Cl^- + HCO_3^-)$$

This information gives the clinician an estimate of unmeasured anions in the plasma. An anion gap of 12 to 15 is

BOX 6-13 Precipitants of Respiratory Alkalosis

PULMONARY

- Pulmonary embolism
- Pneumonia (bacterial or viral)
- Acute pulmonary edema
- Atelectasis
- Assisted hyperventilation

INFECTIOUS

- Septicemia

DRUG INDUCED

- Vasopressors
- Thyroxine
- Aspirin or caffeine toxicity

HYPOXIA

- Ventilation/perfusion mismatch
- Altitude changes
- Severe anemia

HYPERVENTILATION

- Hysteria/anxiety
- Psychogenic disorders
- Central nervous system tumor
- Stroke

METABOLIC AND ELECTROLYTE DISTURBANCES

- Hepatic insufficiency
- Encephalopathy
- Hyponatremia

considered normal. An elevated gap points to conditions that may cause acidosis. The mnemonic CAT MUDPILES, expanded in the nearby Rapid Recall box, can help you remember the precipitants of high-anion-gap metabolic acidosis. The mnemonic F-USED CARS, detailed in the other Rapid Recall box, will help bring to mind the causes of normal-anion-gap metabolic acidosis.

RAPID RECALL

Cat Mudpiles

Mnemonic for Precipitants of High-Anion-Gap Metabolic Acidosis

C Carbon monoxide or cyanide intoxication
A Alcohol intoxication or alcoholic ketoacidosis
T Toluene exposure

M Methanol exposure
U Uremia
D Diabetic ketoacidosis
P Paraldehyde ingestion
I Isoniazid or iron intoxication
L Lactic acidosis
E Ethylene glycol intoxication
S Salicylate (ASA) intoxication

ASA, Acetylsalicylic acid.
Adapted from Marx JA, Hockberger RS, Walls RM: Rosen's emergency medicine, ed 7, St Louis, Mosby, 2009.

RAPID RECALL

F-Used Cars

Mnemonic for Precipitants of Normal-Anion-Gap Metabolic Acidosis

F Fistulae, pancreatic

U Ureteroenteric conduits
S Saline administration (0.9% normal saline)
E Endocrine dysfunction
D Diarrhea

C Carbonic anhydrase inhibitor ingestion
A Arginine, lysine (parenteral nutrition)
R Renal tubular acidosis
S Spironolactone (diuretic) ingestion

Adapted from Marx JA, Hockberger RS, Walls RM: Rosen's emergency medicine, ed 7, St Louis, Mosby, 2009.

You may not have access to the laboratory information necessary to calculate the anion gap. If that's the case, make your management decisions on the basis of sound clinical judgment, a thorough history, and physical exam findings. A specialty-care transport provider conducting a hospital transfer may have laboratory values for calculating the anion gap and can adjust the differential diagnosis accordingly. Capnometry can also provide key information. A patient with tachypnea and a low PCO_2 should be considered to have metabolic acidosis.

Every time you encounter a patient with clinical signs of acidosis, you must consider the following five conditions:

1. Diabetic ketoacidosis: as discussed earlier in the chapter, DKA is caused by inadequate use of insulin as a result of poor compliance or increased need. Patients with diabetes sometimes require higher insulin doses during periods of infection, after trauma, or in other circumstances that increase metabolic demand. DKA sets in when glucose utilization is impaired and fatty acids are metabolized, causing the formation of ketone bodies that generate hydrogen ions. If more acids are produced than the body's buffering system is able to tolerate, acidosis ensues. See earlier details regarding the management of DKA.
2. Renal failure: the kidneys are vital in maintaining an optimal acid-base balance. Most patients with renal failure have uremia because the kidneys are unable to secrete acid byproducts. The renal tubules have the primary responsibility for eliminating hydrogen ions. This function is directly related to the filtration rate of the kidneys, known as the *glomerular filtration rate (GFR)*. Any pathology that alters this process will increase the concentration of hydrogen ions, especially in the form of hydrogen sulfate (HSO_4) and HPO, increasing the anion gap. Patients with chronic renal failure will have some degree of anion gap acidosis, but the gap rarely exceeds 25. Patients with acute renal failure, on the other hand, more often have hyperchloremic non–anion-gap acidosis.
3. Lactic acidosis: lactic acid is largely generated when a significant number of cells in the body are inadequately perfused. Hypoperfusion shifts the cellular metabolism from aerobic (with oxygen) to anaerobic (without oxygen). Anaerobic metabolism produces lactic acid as its most important end product. This occurs in time-sensitive medical conditions associated with hypoperfusion (e.g., sepsis, ischemia, extreme physical exertion states, prolonged seizures, circulatory shock). Lactic acidosis is the result when lactic acid accumulates in larger amounts than the body can buffer.
4. Toxin ingestion: toxic metabolites that cause metabolic acidosis may be a byproduct of ingestion of toxins such as acetylsalicylic acid (ASA), ethylene glycol, methanol, and isoniazid. It's characteristic for patients with toxin-induced metabolic acidosis to evidence some degree of respiratory compensation. The toxin must be identified as soon as possible, because an antidote may be available to prevent further adverse effects.

5. Alcohol ketoacidosis: caused by abrupt cessation of intake after a prolonged period of ingesting a considerable amount of alcohol. The main problem—accumulation of ketoacids—is precipitated by dehydration, hormone imbalance, and chronic malnutrition. Although the condition is similar in presentation to DKA, blood sugar is normal or low. These patients often have mixed acid-base disorders associated with the vomiting that accompanies alcohol withdrawal.

Management

Most patients with metabolic acidosis will require a significant amount of volume resuscitation. Rapidly establish intravascular access to replenish volume status. Support airway, breathing, and circulation with oxygen as appropriate, and ensure adequate ventilation. In patients with history of renal failure or CHF, use caution to avoid causing pulmonary edema when administering IV fluids. If the patient needs ventilator support, be sure to maintain hyperventilation. A patient with metabolic acidosis is hyperventilating as a respiratory compensatory mechanism, and if he or she is sedated or paralyzed for intubation, metabolic acidosis will worsen. Initiate adjunct treatments on the basis of primary etiology. For instance, a patient with high-anion-gap metabolic acidosis due to DKA can be started on insulin.

The use of sodium bicarbonate may be necessary for certain conditions that elicit acute metabolic acidosis, but administration of bicarbonate can be fraught with complications, including hypocalcemia, volume overload, CNS acidosis, hypokalemia, and impaired oxygen delivery. Despite the controversy that surrounds it, rapid administration of sodium bicarbonate is nevertheless useful in treating certain life-threatening conditions. Clinicians use arterial blood gas and plasma electrolyte values to guide the decision of whether to administer bicarbonate. Of course, it's unlikely that such information will be available to you, yet you must consider administering bicarbonate in the following circumstances:

1. Cardiac arrest caused by acidosis associated with hyperkalemia
2. Overdose with tricyclic antidepressants (ECG shows QRS widening > 0.10 sec)
3. Hyperkalemia (presumptive diagnosis made on the basis of history and ECG findings)

Metabolic Alkalosis

Metabolic alkalosis is produced by illnesses that raise the level of serum bicarbonate or reduce the level of hydrogen in the body, such as those that cause volume, potassium, and chloride loss. Box 6-14 provides a list of specific conditions that may precipitate metabolic alkalosis.

Signs and Symptoms

Common findings in patients affected by metabolic alkalosis are anorexia, nausea, vomiting, confusion, hypotension, paresthesia, and weakness. A thorough assessment may reveal the use of antacids (e.g., sodium and calcium bicarbonates), loop diuretics such as thiazide, and corticosteroids. Underlying medical illnesses such as Cushing's and kidney and renal disease are common.

The patient will present with slow, shallow respirations. ECG changes with depressed T waves that merge with P waves indicate hypocalcemia and hypokalemia. Hypotension is also present. Many patients present with muscle twitching and loss of reflexes, numbness and tingling in extremities; a thorough neurologic exam should be performed. Arterial blood gas analysis reveals a blood pH above 7.45 and an HCO_3^- of 26 mEq/L. If respiratory compensation is occurring, the $Pa{CO_2}$ level may be above 45 mm Hg.

Pathophysiology

Metabolic alkalosis occurs by one of two mechanisms: either the body retains bicarbonate in response to hydrogen and chloride loss, or renal impairment precludes the excretion of bicarbonate.

Diagnosis

To make a definitive diagnosis of metabolic alkalosis, you need to know the serum bicarbonate level and the arterial CO_2 level, since a rise in the serum bicarbonate level may be a renal compensatory response to chronic respiratory

BOX 6-14 Precipitants of Metabolic Alkalosis

NORMAL SALINE–RESPONSIVE METABOLIC ALKALOSIS

Volume Depletion

- Vomiting
- Nasogastric suction
- Diuretics
- Low chloride ingestion

NORMAL SALINE–UNRESPONSIVE METABOLIC ALKALOSIS

- Mineralocorticoid excess
- Exogenous ingestions:
  - Chewing tobacco
  - Licorice
- Primary aldosteronism
- Cushing's syndrome
- Bartter's syndrome

acidosis. Unfortunately, this information is only available if blood gas testing can be performed.

Management

Management of metabolic alkalosis is directed toward correcting the underlying cause. A comprehensive history and physical exam are vital. Administration of IV fluids is essential if the primary cause is volume depletion. Isotonic solutions are the fluids of choice. Hypokalemia may need to be corrected with potassium replacement.

Mixed Disorders

Patients often have mixed acid-base disturbances, the diagnosis of which may be confounding even to an experienced emergency physician or intensivist. Mixed disturbances are identified on the basis of clinical history combined with blood gas analysis. Your initial clinical impression of whether the patient is sick or not sick is especially important. As always, take any immediate steps necessary to support airway, breathing, and circulation.

ELECTROLYTE DISTURBANCES

Electrolyte imbalances are common findings in patients with medical emergencies. A healthy electrolyte balance is fundamental to carrying out cellular functions. Electrolyte disturbances generally can't be diagnosed on the basis of clinical examination alone. Severe electrolyte disturbances can be fatal. Most patients have only nonspecific chief complaints until life-threatening manifestations appear. In the following section, we'll discuss the most important electrolyte problems you're likely to encounter in the field.

Hyponatremia

Sodium is the most important electrolyte responsible for maintaining a healthy water balance in the body. As the principal cation in the extracellular fluid, sodium together with chloride and bicarbonate regulates osmotic forces (the flow of water in and out of cells). Water balance is maintained by hormonal regulation controlled by the brain and kidneys.

Hyponatremia is defined as a serum sodium concentration below 135 mEq/L. To guide management, hyponatremia is classified into three categories, depending on volume status:

1. Hypovolemic hyponatremia is caused by the loss of water and sodium, with a higher degree of sodium loss relative to the amount of water loss. Common precipitants include vomiting, diarrhea, GI problems, nasogastric tubes, and third-spacing of fluids. Third-spacing (movement of intravascular and intracellular water into interstitial spaces) is a phenomenon that may occur in patients with burns, pancreatitis, and sepsis and in those who take certain medications such as diuretics.
2. Hypervolemic hyponatremia occurs when an excessive amount of water is retained relative to the amount of sodium. The condition classically occurs in a patient with an edematous condition such as CHF.
3. Euvolemic hyponatremia occurs when the serum osmolality is low despite the presence of concentrated urine.

Signs and Symptoms

The clinical presentation of hyponatremia depends on how quickly the sodium concentration declines. A patient with chronic hyponatremia may tolerate a level below 120 mEq/L. Clinical manifestations usually appear when the sodium level falls below this threshold. Conversely, a patient who suffers an acute drop in serum sodium may exhibit clinical symptoms at a much higher sodium level, perhaps in the range of about 125 mEq/L.

Most signs and symptoms of hyponatremia are related to CNS manifestations, such as agitation, hallucinations, weakness, lethargy, and seizures. Other complaints include abdominal pain, cramps, and headache. Patients with severe hyponatremia appear to be very ill and may have seizures or exhibit an altered mental status.

Athletic events like marathons and triathlons can precipitate exercise-induced hyponatremia. Although the mechanisms that cause this phenomenon aren't completely understood, persistent increased vasopressin levels and a decrease in glomerular function in sweat-induced dehydration may be implicated. Exercise-induced hyponatremia can cause loss of coordination, pulmonary edema, and changes in intracranial pressure that result in seizure and coma.

Differential Diagnosis

A possible cause of low sodium is pseudohyponatremia, a condition in which high glucose levels or excessive amounts of lipids or proteins in the blood plasma cause the measured sodium level to be lower than the actual serum sodium level.

Management

Try to determine the type of hyponatremia on the basis of history and physical exam. Patients who have a history of nausea and vomiting or decreased oral intake for any other reason may be dehydrated or have other signs and symptoms of low sodium. When needed, provide fluid resuscitation with 0.9% normal saline.

You will rarely have serum sodium measurements to guide management, although point-of-care testing is available in some circumstances. As a general rule, hyponatremia should be corrected at the rate at which it occurred unless the patient has seizures or severe altered mental status. Hyponatremia must be corrected not faster than a rate of 1 to 2 mEq/L/h. Patients with symptomatic hyponatremia who have severe signs and symptoms such as seizures and altered mental status may require administration of 3% sodium chloride (hypertonic saline). Administer this fluid carefully under the close supervision of Medical Control. Correcting the sodium too aggressively can cause severe neurologic complications as a result of central pontine myelinolysis.

Hypokalemia

Potassium is responsible for many vital functions in the body:

- Maintaining a normal electrical and osmotic gradient in all cells
- Facilitating neuronal transmission and cardiac impulse conduction
- Serving as a buffering mechanism in the cell membranes to help maintain acid-base homeostasis

Normal serum potassium levels range from 3.5 to 5 mEq/L but do not accurately reflect total body stores of the cation, since most potassium is stored within cells. Hypokalemia is an abnormally low serum level of potassium, usually < 3.5 mEq/L. Hypokalemia is fairly common and usually occurs secondary to decreased intake or increased excretion.

Signs and Symptoms

Hypokalemia often manifests no signs or symptoms initially. As it progresses and the level falls below 2.5 mEq/L, signs and symptoms of hypokalemia become apparent in multiple organ systems, including the neurologic, GI, and cardiovascular systems. Common symptoms include weakness, nausea, vomiting, lethargy, confusion, and paresthesia of the extremities.

A patient with severe hypokalemia (<2 mEq/L) will appear to be very ill and may also have cardiac dysrhythmias and muscular paralysis. Frequent cardiovascular manifestations include palpitations, low blood pressure, and cardiac electrical disturbances such as heart blocks, premature ventricular contractions, and supraventricular tachycardia. Fatal types of dysrhythmia, such as ventricular fibrillation and asystole, can also occur (Figure 6-12).

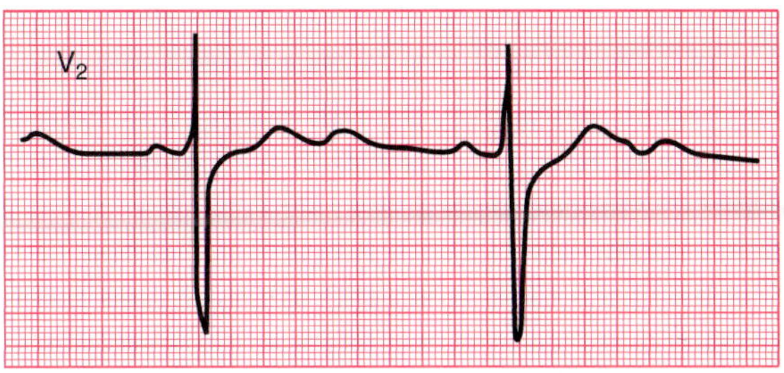

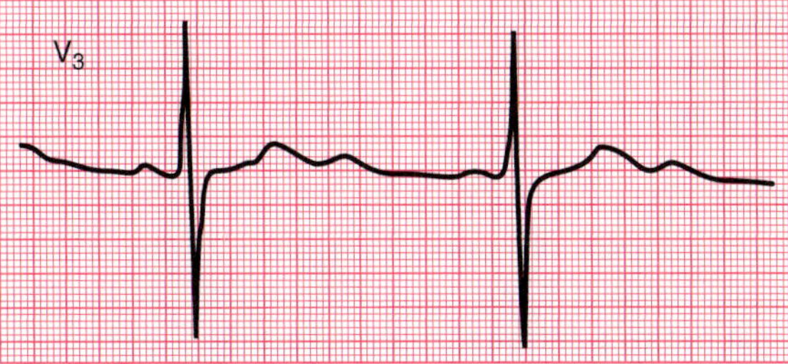

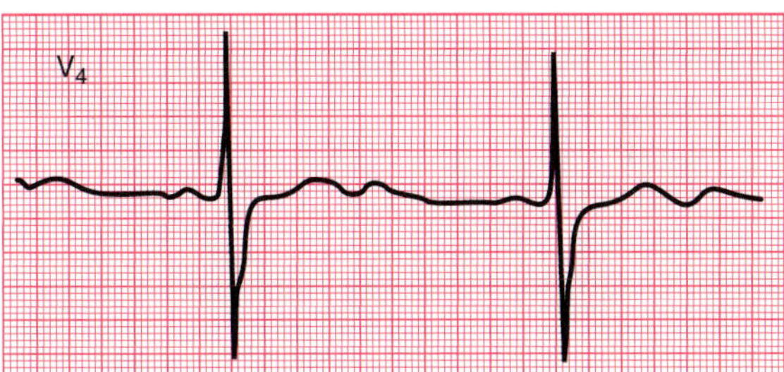

Figure 6-12 Electrocardiographic manifestations of hypokalemia. Serum potassium concentration was 2.2 mEq/L. ST segment is prolonged, primarily because of a U wave following the T wave, and T wave is flattened. (From Goldman L, Ausiello D: Cecil textbook of medicine, ed 23, Philadelphia, 2007, Saunders.)

Diagnosis

Signs of hypokalemia apparent on a 12-lead ECG include flattened T waves, U waves, and ST-segment depression.

Management

Treatment of hypokalemia may require IV fluids for dehydration. Oral intake (20 to 40 mEq per dose) is preferred over IV administration because of the potential side effects of IV potassium, namely cardiac arrest. Patients who are unable to take oral replacement or are critically ill will require IV potassium administered at a rate of 10 to 20 mEq/L. Critically ill patients (those with respiratory muscle weakness) can receive higher doses, but they should be given through a central venous catheter. A common complaint during IV administration is burning at the site of infusion, which you can usually resolve by slowing the rate of infusion. The most feared complication of potassium administration, of course, is hyperkalemia, which is especially likely in patients with kidney disease. It's critical, then, to know the patient's renal function status before you administer potassium.

Hyperkalemia

Hyperkalemia, a level of serum potassium > 5.5 mEq/L, is an electrolyte disorder that can be caused by ingestion of potassium supplements, acute or chronic renal failure, blood transfusion, sepsis, Addison's disease, acidosis, and crush syndrome (from rhabdomyolysis).

Signs and Symptoms

Hyperkalemia manifests primarily as neurologic and cardiovascular dysfunction. The patient may have generalized weakness, muscle cramps, tetany, paralysis, or cardiac palpitations or arrhythmias.

Diagnosis

In the prehospital setting, the only diagnostic study available to guide you toward a diagnosis of hyperkalemia is the ECG, which can help you determine whether the patient has an associated arrhythmia. The first change detected on the ECG of a patient with hyperkalemia is the development of peaked T waves. As serum potassium continues to increase, P waves disappear and the QRS complex widens. If hyperkalemia is not corrected, the ECG will progress to bradycardia and then terminate in a sine wave pattern or asystole.

Management

Assess and treat the underlying cause of hyperkalemia, institute rapid and appropriate treatment, and transport the patient to a hospital facility. Treatment of hyperkalemia has three goals:

1. Cellular membrane stabilization and decreased cardiac irritability. Maintain the patient on a cardiac monitor at all times. If the patient has hypotension or arrhythmias, administer calcium chloride 5 mL of 10% solution.
2. Elimination of potassium from the body. To help eliminate potassium from the body, the use of exchange resins is warranted. An oral dose of 20 g sodium polystyrene sulfonate can be used. Be careful using exchange resins in a cardiac patient, however, since they can produce fluid overload.
3. Potassium shift into cells. You can administer nebulized albuterol (5 to 20 mg) to lower the serum potassium level by shifting potassium into cells. The combined administration of 10 units of insulin and IV dextrose also produces a shift of potassium into the cells. Another treatment aimed at decreasing potassium is 44 mEq/L sodium bicarbonate IV administered over 5 to 15 minutes.

Hypocalcemia

As we discussed in the section on hypoparathyroidism earlier in this chapter, calcium is essential for a number of body functions, including muscular contraction, neuronal transmission, hormone secretion, organ growth, and immunologic and hematologic response. Most calcium in an adult is stored as a mineral component of bone.

Signs and Symptoms

Patients with symptomatic hypocalcemia may have seizures, hypotension, tetany, or cardiac dysrhythmias.

Management

Treatment of hypocalcemia is guided principally by laboratory results, but when hypocalcemia is presumed to be the cause of the patient's symptoms, it's reasonable to begin empirical treatment. Parenteral calcium is the primary treatment in patients with symptomatic hypocalcemia. Use one of the following two options:

1. 10 mL 10% calcium chloride, which contains 360 mg elemental calcium
2. 10 mL 10% calcium gluconate, which contains 93 mg elemental calcium

In an adult patient, the recommended dose is 100 to 300 mg elemental calcium. In a pediatric patient, administer 0.5 to 1 mL/kg of a 10% calcium gluconate solution over 5 minutes. To avoid significant side effects, dilution in normal saline or D_5W is highly recommended. You must make sure the peripheral catheter is working properly before administering calcium, since extravasation may cause tissue necrosis. Calcium administration will increase the serum concentration of calcium for only a short period of time, so you may need to give repeated doses, especially during a long transport or interfacility transfer.

Patients whose signs and symptoms persist after adequate treatment may have concomitant electrolyte problems such as hypomagnesemia.

Hypomagnesemia

Magnesium is the second most abundant intracellular bivalent cation in the human body. It is a cofactor in the activation of numerous enzymatic reactions. Its physiologic effects on the CNS are similar to those of calcium. Magnesium is distributed throughout the body in a unique way. Half of the total amount of magnesium (2000 mEq/L) is stored as a mineral component of bone, and 40% to 50% is intracellular. Only 1% to 2% of magnesium in the body is in extracellular fluid; thus the serum magnesium level is a poor reflection of the body's total magnesium content.

Signs and Symptoms

Patients usually become symptomatic at levels of 1.2 mg/dL (0.06 mmol/L) or less. Common signs and symptoms include:

- Tremors
- Hyperreflexia
- Tetany
- Nausea or vomiting
- Altered mental status and confusion
- Seizures
- Cardiac dysrhythmias, including torsades des pointes, polymorphic ventricular tachycardia, and cardiac arrest

Pathophysiology

Hypomagnesemia is one of the most common electrolyte disturbances you will see in clinical practice. It often accompanies conditions that involve malnutrition, alcoholism, dehydration, diarrhea, kidney disease, diuresis, or starvation and tends to coexist with diseases that cause hypokalemia and hypocalcemia.

Management

Take immediate steps to maintain airway, breathing, and circulation. It's reasonable to start magnesium replacement therapy when you suspect a diagnosis of hypomagnesemia. In patients with no history of renal problems, administer a dose of 2 to 4 grams of 50% magnesium sulfate. It must be given with normal saline or dextrose, ideally administered over 30 to 60 minutes per gram. However, in a patient with severe signs and symptoms, including dysrhythmias, you may need to give a rapid infusion over the course of 5 or 10 minutes. Do not give magnesium sulfate as a bolus, because doing so has been associated with severe side effects, including bradycardia, heart block, and hypotension.

RHABDOMYOLYSIS

Rhabdomyolysis is a skeletal muscle injury characterized by release of cellular contents, specifically myoglobin, leading to acute renal failure and other renal complications. Patients who are immobilized for prolonged periods, including those being transported a great distance and those trapped for long periods of time before they can be extricated, are at risk of rhabdomyolysis as a result of muscle destruction.

Signs and Symptoms

Patients with rhabdomyolysis complain of diffuse or localized weakness and muscle pain. Once the process of rhabdomyolysis has begun, patients may report having dark-colored urine.

Pathophysiology

Rather than being a primary problem, rhabdomyolysis occurs as a consequence of another insult. Common precipitants of rhabdomyolysis include:

- Metabolic problems
- Heatstroke and other severe heat-related emergencies
- Trauma
- Crush injuries
- Drugs of abuse
- Toxic ingestion/overdose
- Infections (rarely)
- Electrolyte abnormalities

Dysfunction of the Na^+/ K^+-ATPase pump allows uncontrolled calcium influx into skeletal muscle cells. The increased intracellular calcium content leads to cellular necrosis and release of myoglobin, potassium, and intracellular enzymes, such as creatinine phosphokinase. Once myoglobin enters the plasma, it is filtered and excreted through the kidneys. An excess of myoglobin can be directly toxic to the renal tubules or can obstruct them, especially if the patient is hypovolemic or acidotic as a result of the primary problem. If not treated aggressively with IV fluids, rhabdomyolysis can cause severe kidney damage and renal failure.

Diagnosis

Rhabdomyolysis is diagnosed in the ED by noting myoglobinuria and an elevated creatinine kinase level. However, you should suspect this diagnosis on the basis of a comprehensive history (including that of the primary condition) and physical exam findings. The patient may not have rhabdomyolysis initially, but an emergent condition may induce the condition later. A thorough physical exam is the key to identifying potential causes. For example, you may discover cola-colored urine, a strong indicator of the presence of rhabdomyolysis.

Management

Aggressive fluid hydration is crucial. IV fluids should be given (taking care to avoid hypothermia) in an effort to mitigate the complications of rhabdomyolysis. In addition to routine medical care, consider the following:

- Saline infusion is vital in the treatment of rhabdomyolysis. Consider aggressive saline infusion early, especially in patients with trauma or crush injuries.
- Titrate saline infusions to obtain a urine output of 200 to 300 mL/L. Be aware of potential electrolyte complications (such as hyperkalemia with hypocalcemia) that may elicit malignant cardiac dysrhythmias. If they occur, you must treat them aggressively.
- Consider administering mannitol for osmotic diuresis.
- If you already know the patient's primary diagnosis (e.g., when carrying out an interfacility transfer), you may initiate a bicarbonate infusion to begin alkalinizing the urine.

ENVIRONMENTAL DISORDERS

You may encounter environmental emergencies frequently or rarely, depending on your practice environment (i.e., wilderness or urban). In this chapter, we'll confine our discussion to hypo- and hyperthermic emergencies. Chapter 3 offers a discussion of pressure-related emergencies such as diving barotrauma, and Chapter 9 details the toxicology and treatment of envenomation.

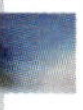

Temperature Regulation and Related Disorders

Most heat- and cold-related emergencies occur during seasonal exposure to significant temperature changes. You may associate such environmental emergencies with outdoor activities, but such problems are also common among special populations in urban areas, such as homeless patients who lack shelter.

Body temperature is regulated by neural feedback mechanisms that operate primarily through the hypothalamus. Normal body temperature has a diurnal fluctuation between 36°C and 37.5°C (96.8°F to 99.5°F). The hypothalamus contains not only the control mechanisms (which maintain a temperature set point) but also the sensory mechanisms necessary to detect and respond to temperature changes. For instance, sweating begins almost precisely at a skin temperature of 37°C (98.6°F) and increases quickly as skin temperature rises. In warm conditions, heat production in the body remains almost constant as the skin temperature increases. It's important to use a thermometer to quantify such changes and correlate them with clinical signs and symptoms. Oral, axillary, forehead surface, tympanic, rectal, or esophageal temperature measurements can be obtained using electronic (digital) or analog thermometers. Core temperature, which can be measured at the esophageal or rectal sites, is the most accurate.

If skin temperature falls below 35°C (95°F), the body attempts to retain body heat and increase body temperature using a range of mechanisms, some of which are:

- Vasoconstriction to decrease radiant heat loss from the skin
- Cessation of sweating
- Shivering to increase heat production in the muscles
- Secretion of norepinephrine, epinephrine, and thyroxine to increase heat production

COLD INJURIES

Frostbite

Local cold injury sets in at extremely cold temperatures, usually below the freezing point. Frostbite is the formation of ice crystals within local tissue in exposed areas. It commonly occurs in distal extremities, particularly the toes and feet, but it can affect the upper extremities or other areas as well. Factors that can increase an individual's chance of developing cold injury include prolonged time of exposure, exposure to wind, wearing wet clothing, inactivity or immobility, alcohol ingestion, and preexisting conditions involving decreased peripheral circulation. The areas of the body that are most at risk are the nose, ears, and penis.

BOX 6-15 Classification of Frostbite

Degree	Characteristics
First	No blisters, anesthesia, erythema
Second	Clear blisters, edema, erythema
Third	Hemorrhagic blisters, subcutaneous involvement, dead skin, and tissue loss
Fourth	Full-thickness (bone and muscle) tissue loss, necrosis, and deformity

Frostbite injury can be divided into several clinical stages. Frostnip is the first and least severe manifestation of frostbite. For the purpose of management, we classify frostbite as either superficial or deep. However, like burns, frostbite has been classified into degrees of injury after rewarming, because most frostbite injuries are similar initially (Box 6-15).

Signs and Symptoms

Frostbite can initially have a deceptively benign appearance, but it's important not to confuse frostbite with frostnip, a superficial cold insult. The patient may complain of clumsiness or heaviness in an extremity and will probably report coldness and numbness of the affected area, with pain and sensitivity to light touch. The patient may also complain of tingling, throbbing, and transient numbness that resolves fairly rapidly with rewarming. Complete anesthesia in a painful, cold extremity is a red flag for severe injury.

Your initial clinical examination will help you determine the extent and severity of frostbite. Frostbitten tissue will look white or blue-white, will be cool to the touch, and may be hard if still frozen. The skin may lack sensation. Signs and symptoms of superficial and deep frostbite are given in Box 6-16.

Pathophysiology

The pathophysiology of frostbite is complex and involves several stages of cold injury. The amount of tissue destruction is directly related to the extent of cold exposure. The formation of ice crystals in vulnerable tissues touches off an inflammatory reaction that culminates in cellular death. The crystals tend to form in extracellular areas, altering the local electrolyte balance as the crystals draw water out of adjacent cells. If the affected areas continue to be exposed to cold, the crystals may grow, causing a local mechanical obstruction of blood vessels.

One of the most important concepts in the pathophysiology of frostbite is thawing. When a frozen tissue thaws, the supply of blood to local capillaries is temporarily restored. The blood supply rapidly dwindles, however, as local arterioles and venules release small emboli, inducing hypoxia and thrombosis within the local vasculature. Starved of nutrients, local tissues begin to die. The process

BOX 6-16 Comparison of Superficial and Deep Frostbite

SUPERFICIAL FROSTBITE	DEEP FROSTBITE
• Numbness	• Hemorrhagic blisters
• Paresthesia (extreme pain during rewarming)	• Diminished range of motion
• Poor fine motor control (clumsiness)	• Necrosis, gangrene
• Pruritus	• Cold, mottled, gray area (after rewarming)
• Edema (usually after rewarming)	• Immobile tissue (lost elasticity)
• Coldness	

of thawing and refreezing, then, is more dangerous and damaging than the initial cold insult.

Management

Prehospital intervention is primarily limited to supporting vital functions and protecting affected extremities. Treat any systemic hypothermia first. If frostbite involves the lower extremities, do not allow the person to walk. Remove any jewelry or clothing that may compress the tissue, and remove wet or cold clothing. Apply constant warmth with blankets or towels. Friction or massage is ineffective and can damage injured tissue. The most effective therapy is rapid rewarming of the frozen area by immersion in warm water (40°C [104°F]). This treatment is not recommended, however, if there is any risk of refreezing. Transport the patient to an appropriate facility.

Systemic Hypothermia

Systemic **hypothermia**, defined as a core body temperature below 35°C (95°F), is a common environmental emergency. Hypothermia is caused by heat loss, decreased heat production, or a combination of the two. The condition can be attributed to a range of metabolic, traumatic, environmental, and infectious causes, but it occurs most often in patients who are exposed to cold environments. It's important to remember that in the presence of certain risk factors (prolonged time of exposure, exposure to wind, wearing wet clothing, inactivity or immobility, alcohol ingestion), hypothermia can be precipitated at temperatures well above freezing. To decrease morbidity and mortality, you must be able to recognize the signs and symptoms of systemic hypothermia.

Signs and Symptoms

To diagnose hypothermia, you must have a high degree of suspicion. In some cases, when the patient has been exposed to the elements, the diagnosis is obvious. In other cases, the clinical findings may be subtle. Nonspecific symptoms—chills, nausea, hunger, vomiting, dyspnea, dizziness—may be early signs.

A rapid determination of body temperature is necessary to diagnose hypothermia. In the prehospital environment, the most common and reliable method available is a tympanic measurement, which is closest to the hypothalamic temperature. Specialty-care transport providers may have other devices available for temperature measurement, such as bladder and esophageal thermometers. These devices yield more reliable core temperature readings than tympanic thermometers.

Depending on its clinical manifestations, systemic hypothermia is classified as mild, moderate, or severe. Certain clinical findings are characteristic of each stage, although signs and symptoms are variable, and the stages often overlap.

Mild Hypothermia (32°C to 36°C [89.6°F to 96.8°F]) In mild hypothermia, most people will shiver vigorously. This can be accompanied by nonspecific symptoms such as dizziness, lethargy, nausea, and weakness. An increased metabolic rate occurs in this range as the body tries to produce more heat. More severe neurologic signs such as ataxia (uncoordinated movement) appear once temperature drops to 33°C (91.4°F). Other signs include:

- Hyperventilation
- Tachypnea
- Tachycardia

Moderate Hypothermia (30°C to 32°C [86°F to 89.6°F]) As moderate hypothermia develops, clinical signs of deterioration become apparent. Breathing and heart rate slow, and mental status declines. At 32°C (89.6°F), the patient will become stuporous. As core temperature approaches 31°C (87.8°F), the patient will lose the shivering reflex. Other signs and symptoms of moderate hypothermia include:

- Poor judgment
- Atrial fibrillation
- Bradycardia, bradypnea
- Diuresis (increased urinary output)

Severe Hypothermia (<30°C [<86°F]) Life-threatening cardiovascular problems appear at 30°C (86°F). Hypotension and ventricular arrhythmias become apparent, and a J wave may be seen on the cardiac monitor. The patient is usually unconscious, with dilated and minimally responsive pupils. At this stage, the patient is near cardiac arrest and very susceptible to ventricular fibrillation from even minimal physical manipulation.

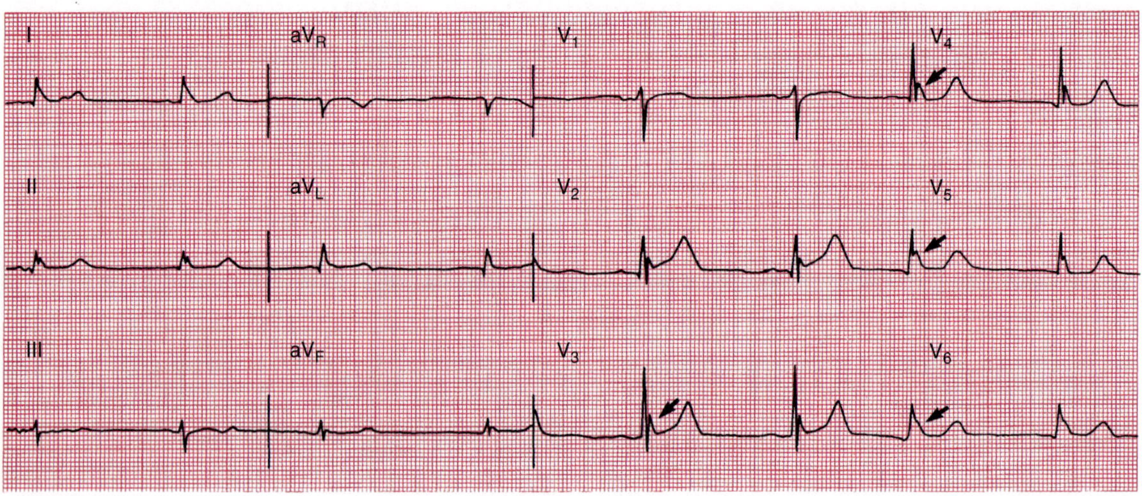

■ **Figure 6-13** Systemic hypothermia is associated with distinctive bulging of the J point (very beginning of ST segment). Prominent J waves *(arrows)* with hypothermia are referred to as *Osborne waves.* (From Goldberger A: Clinical electrocardiography: a simplified approach, ed 7, St Louis, 2006, Mosby.)

Pathophysiology

The pathophysiology of hypothermia is complex and involves the cardiovascular, renal, neurologic, and respiratory systems. As the core temperature drops, each of these systems responds with the aim of preserving heat:

- Vasoconstriction: first, peripheral blood vessels constrict in an effort to shift more blood to vital organs. Nevertheless, in severe hypothermia, blood flow to the kidneys drops by 50%, threatening renal function and upsetting electrolyte balance.
- Diuresis: vasoconstriction increases urinary output, a menacing development in a volume-depleted patient. Interestingly, the urinary output is up to 3.5 times higher if the patient is immersed in cold water. Alcohol intake further increases diuresis.
- Respiratory acidosis: respiratory rate decreases, followed by a drop in minute ventilation as a result of diminished metabolism. In severe hypothermia, CO_2 retention causes respiratory acidosis.
- Tachycardia and bradycardia: sinus tachycardia predominates during the initial phases of hypothermia. You must consider other conditions, however, if the tachycardia appears to be unrelated to the temperature decrease. Later, as hypothermia becomes more severe, bradycardia ensues as a result of diminished depolarization in the pacemaker cells. In this type of bradydysrhythmia, atropine is often ineffective and is not needed because overall metabolism is diminished.
- Ventricular fibrillation and asystole: in mild to moderate hypothermia, patients can develop atrial or ventricular dysrhythmias as a result of conduction changes that decrease transmembrane resting potential. As hypothermia worsens, the risk of ventricular fibrillation and asystole increases.
- Electrocardiographic anomalies: several unique electrocardiographic manifestations can point to a diagnosis of hypothermia. The classic Osborne (J) wave appears at the junction between the QRS complex and the ST segment (Figure 6-13). Osborne waves usually become evident at temperatures below 33°C (91.4°F). As the condition worsens, all intervals—particularly the QT interval—become prolonged. You may have trouble analyzing the ECG because of artifacts generated by the patient's shivering.

Management

Your prehospital management will have to be guided by where the patient is and the severity of his hypothermia. A patient in a cold, remote setting obviously needs immediate extrication. Rewarm the patient, prevent further heat loss, and avoid actions that may precipitate complications. For example, rough handling of a severely hypothermic patient can precipitate a cardiac arrhythmia.

Regardless of severity, you must focus on supporting airway, breathing, and circulation as needed and remove any cold, wet clothing to prevent a further drop in core temperature. In addition, nearly all hypothermic patients are volume depleted. Before administering fluids, warm them to 40°C to 42°C (104°F to 107.6°F). EMS systems that regularly respond to patients with hypothermia should have access to fluid warmers, but if such equipment is unavailable, a microwave may be used to warm fluids. A 1 L bag of crystalloid fluids can be warmed in a plastic container for 2 minutes on high power.

BOX 6-17 Key Considerations in the Management of Severe Hypothermia

- Dependent lividity and fixed, dilated pupils are not dependable criteria for withholding CPR in a hypothermic patient.
- Evaluation of vital signs and ECG tracings may be difficult, since the patient may have an undetectable pulse. Spend a longer time than usual (30-45 seconds) to check for signs of circulation. If there is any doubt or you are unable to detect a pulse, start CPR immediately.
- Patients with severe hypothermia often have bradycardia. This may be a protective mechanism, since a slow heart rhythm can deliver sufficient oxygen under hypothermic conditions. The use of pacing is rarely indicated.
- A patient with severe hypothermia will have a significantly reduced metabolic rate, resulting in a toxic buildup of cardiac resuscitation agents. Consider withholding drugs in a patient with a core temperature < 30°C (<86°F), since the heart is unlikely to respond to drugs at this temperature.
- Consider early endotracheal intubation for ventilation with warm humidified oxygen when available.
- Defibrillation may be unlikely to be effective at core temperatures < 30°C (<86°F). Consider withholding repeated defibrillation attempts until the core temperature can be increased above this point.
- Gastric dilation and decreased gastric motility can occur in severe hypothermia. Physical examination of the abdomen is unreliable because of rectus muscle rigidity, so after tracheal intubation, you should place a nasogastric tube in patients with moderate and severe hypothermia.

CPR, Cardiopulmonary resuscitation; *ECG*, electrocardiogram.

Mild Hypothermia (32°C to 36°C [89.6°F to 96.8°F]) Most cases of mild hypothermia will resolve with passive rewarming techniques (e.g., using blankets to help contain the patient's own body heat). In addition to the above general management instructions, provide warm oral fluids if there are no airway concerns. Avoid caffeinated beverages, however, because they can encourage diuresis. Reassess the patient frequently to evaluate for improvement or decline. Mildly hypothermic patients can quickly deteriorate to become moderately or severely hypothermic.

Moderate Hypothermia (30°C to 32°C [86°F to 89.6°F]) Mental status changes become more apparent in patients with moderate hypothermia. Management begins with immediate stabilization of airway, breathing, circulation, and core temperature. Start passive rewarming techniques and initiate active rewarming as well, such as forced warm air and administration of warm IV fluids. Do not permit the patient to ambulate, because the condition can evolve into a cardiac arrhythmia. Transport the patient rapidly and gently to an ED for continuous rewarming and observation.

Severe Hypothermia (<30°C [<86°F]) Patients with severe hypothermia are usually unconscious. Stabilization of airway, breathing, and circulation is essential to prevent further deterioration. If there is a palpable pulse, handle the patient gently and avoid abrupt movements. If the patient is in cardiac arrest, begin CPR immediately. The priority will be to provide quality compressions during active rewarming. Intravenous medications and defibrillation will have limited benefit at these temperatures. Active rewarming techniques include warming blankets, warm IV fluids, and bladder irrigation. More invasive active rewarming techniques include warm fluid irrigation through tube thoracostomy and extracorporeal membrane oxygenation (ECMO). In some remote regions, resuscitation efforts for hypothermic patients who are found in cardiac arrest are terminated in the field. However, in most jurisdictions, hypothermia is a contraindication to field termination of resuscitation. Key considerations in treating severe hypothermia are described in Box 6-17.

HEAT ILLNESS

Heat illness is a unique set of disorders brought on when the body is exposed to heat for extended periods; it's often triggered by exercising too much and not staying adequately hydrated in hot conditions. An inappropriate amount of exercise for one's age or physical condition is a risk factor for developing a heat-related illness. Certain groups—the very old, the very young, and those with obesity—are at higher risk.

Heat Cramps

Heat cramps are a common heat-related emergency among people who work or exercise in hot temperatures. These painful muscle contractions usually occur after physical activity has stopped. The classic history is that of a person who has been working in a hot environment and develops cramps after stopping to rest.

Signs and Symptoms

Cramps can occur all over the body, but the legs and abdomen are the most common sites. Patients will be sweaty and sometimes nauseated.

Pathophysiology

Heat cramps cause painful muscular spasms attributable to dehydration and electrolyte imbalances such as hyponatremia and hypokalemia. Such imbalances are characteristic of muscles that are fatigued after engaging in strenuous work. A direct correlation exists between heat cramps and salt depletion. The typical patient is someone who has been working or exercising in a hot, dry environment and losing salt by sweating but drinking hypotonic fluids that replenish fluids but don't replace salt.

Differential Diagnosis

Heat cramps must not be confused with athletic cramps, which occur during athletic activity and resolve with massage. Heat cramps most often involve several different muscles, whereas athletic cramps typically occur in one muscle due to overexertion or stretching.

Management

Heat cramps unaccompanied by associated heat-related illnesses are not a life-threatening emergency. Commercially available oral salt solutions, such as Gatorade or PowerAde, are useful in the treatment of mild heat cramps. Oral hydration is best (if the patient isn't vomiting). Patients with more severe heat cramps accompanied by vomiting will require IV fluids (0.9% normal saline). Salt tablets are not recommended alone, as they can induce nausea and don't address the issue of volume depletion.

Heat Exhaustion

Heat exhaustion is caused by volume depletion from excessive sweating in hot temperatures. People who work in hot environments, such as laborers, athletes, and military personnel, are at risk if they do not drink enough water. If left untreated, heat exhaustion can progress to heatstroke.

Signs and Symptoms

The clinical manifestations of heat exhaustion are nonspecific, but the condition should not be diagnosed if the patient exhibits CNS abnormalities such as seizures, coma, confusion, delirium, or severe hyperthermia (>40.5°C [>104.9°F]). These findings suggest heatstroke rather than heat exhaustion. Signs and symptoms of heat exhaustion include:

- Weakness, malaise, and lethargy
- Headache
- Vertigo
- Nausea and vomiting
- Core temperature often normal or less than 40°C (<104°F)
- Normal LOC
- Tachycardia, sweating
- Abdominal pain
- Muscle cramps

Pathophysiology

Heat exhaustion is characterized by water depletion and salt depletion in the setting of exercise. Core temperature may be normal or elevated up to 40°C (<104°F). Typically these patients are volume depleted and hemoconcentrated.

Management

Most patients with heat exhaustion have both water and salt depletion. The principal problem you will encounter is volume deficit. Mild cases can be managed with oral fluid replacement with salt-containing solutions. IV fluid replacement is often necessary, especially if there are any signs of hemodynamic instability. The fluid of choice is 0.9% normal saline, although determination of the patient's electrolyte status should be used to guide treatment if available. In addition, the patient should be moved to a cool, shady, or indoor environment.

Heatstroke

Heatstroke is a syndrome in which the body loses its ability to regulate temperature, resulting in altered mental status, elevated core body temperature, and multiorgan failure. Core body temperature can climb to 42°C (108°F) or even higher. Consequent damage will depend on how high the body temperature is and how long it stays elevated.

An almost universal finding in patients with heatstroke is neurologic dysfunction, including altered mental status, headache, seizures, and cerebral edema. During heatstroke, remarkably increased demands are made on the cardiovascular system, which can be a principal contributor to the ultimate collapse of bodily functions. Continued heat exposure produces peripheral vasodilatation with subsequent splanchnic and renal circulatory vasoconstriction, sometimes accompanied by hepatic dysfunction. Continued heat exposure will cause hemodynamic instability, poor skin perfusion, a further elevation of core temperature, and multiorgan failure.

Classification

Heatstroke is classified as either classic heatstroke or exertional heatstroke. It's not critical to differentiate these conditions in the field, since treatment is similar, but we will do so here for the purpose of discussion.

Classic Heatstroke Classic heatstroke is associated with prolonged exposure to even a moderately high environmental temperature and humidity level. It is classically associated with the chronically ill, bedridden, elderly, or psychiatric patient who lacks air conditioning or is using medications that impair tolerance to heat stress, such as diuretic, anticholinergic, and neuroleptic agents. Anhidrosis (lack of perspiration) is caused by extreme dehydration, skin disorders, or medication side effects.

Exertional Heatstroke In contrast, exertional heatstroke is associated with young people, such as athletes who train in conditions of high temperature and humidity, in whom core temperature rises faster than the body can dissipate heat. About 50% of such patients will continue to sweat even as heatstroke becomes imminent.

Signs and Symptoms

The patient with either type of heatstroke will have similar signs and symptoms:

- Altered mental status
- Hyperventilation
- Tachycardia
- Hypotension
- High-output cardiac failure (hypotension and tachycardia are warning signs)
- GI bleeding
- Pulmonary edema
- Electrolyte imbalance
- Hepatic dysfunction

Management

The first step in management is to recognize this potentially lethal condition. Maintain airway, ventilation, and circulation, initiate immediate cooling measures, and transport the patient rapidly to the ED. Place the patient on a cardiac monitor, establish two peripheral IV lines, and initiate supplemental oxygen therapy.

The patient's clothes must be removed. Check and record core temperature, preferably with a rectal probe, every 5 minutes. Once core body temperature drops to 39°C (102.2°F), cooling measures should be stopped to avoid inducing shivering. You can lower temperature by spraying the skin with lukewarm water and fanning. Using cold water is counterproductive because it induces shivering, which elevates core body temperature.

If evidence of hypovolemic shock is present, rehydrate the patient with a 500- to 1000-mL fluid bolus every 20 minutes. Cold IV fluids can be used. Reassess hemodynamic stability, and maintain a mean arterial pressure of 60 mm Hg. Avoid fluid overload, since the patient is at risk of developing high-output cardiac failure and pulmonary edema, as described previously.

If seizures are present, treat them with lorazepam or diazepam under medical direction or according to local protocol.

Heat Syncope and Exercise-Associated Syncope

Heat exposure combined with underlying physiologic problems that alter blood return can cause a transient loss of consciousness. This condition is more common among older adults, who are more susceptible to dehydration during heat exposure.

Signs and Symptoms

Patients with heat syncope have dizziness, lightheadedness, and signs of volume depletion. Those with exercise-associated syncope have these signs after cessation of exercise.

Pathophysiology

When a person is exposed to heat for a significant period, the body responds by dilating cutaneous vessels. Blood tends to pool in peripheral vessels. If a person stands for a prolonged period or suddenly rises from a sitting position in the heat, poor central venous return can cause inadequate cerebral perfusion, manifested as heat syncope.

Exercise-associated syncope has a similar pathophysiology but occurs in different circumstances. This condition usually occurs among endurance athletes whose muscles are hyperperfused with blood. The pumping action of the lower extremities facilitates venous return to the central circulation. On cessation of exercise, blood is still disproportionately distributed to skeletal muscle, but its return is no longer aided by the pumping of the legs. Blood quickly pools in the lower extremities, leading to syncope. This mechanism is much different from that of syncope during exercise, which suggests a more ominous diagnosis, such as acute coronary syndrome or arrhythmia.

Management

As with any heat-related illness, the patient should be moved to a cooler environment. Most cases are self-limiting, and lying down offers some relief of symptoms. Monitor the patient for signs of deterioration. People at risk for heat syncope should move frequently. Athletes, for instance, should be educated to continue walking after cessation of vigorous activity and to recognize warning symptoms such as lightheadedness or weakness so they can move out of the hot environment. This could help avoid potential traumatic injuries or medical sequelae that can occur after syncope .

Exercise-Associated Hyponatremia

Discussed briefly earlier in this chapter under the general heading Electrolyte Disturbances, a disorder that has come to light over the past several years is that of exercise-associated hyponatremia. This is one of the most common causes of death in young healthy athletes who are involved in endurance sports such as marathon running.

Signs and Symptoms

Patients should be categorized based on symptoms rather than measured serum sodium concentrations, but relative values are given in parentheses:

- Mild: dizziness, nausea, vomiting, headache (sodium 135-130 mmol/L)
- Moderate: mental status changes (confusion, disorientation) (sodium 130-125 mmol/L)
- Severe: altered consciousness, lethargy, pulmonary edema, seizures, coma (sodium < 125 mmol/L)

Pathophysiology

The most common cause of exercise-associated hyponatremia is overhydration with hypotonic fluids. Athletes lose both water and sodium through perspiration at a significant rate during exercise. If water is used as a replacement without an adequate sodium ingestion, the patient's serum sodium level is driven down. This can lead to CNS edema, neurologic symptoms, and death. Risk factors which have been shown to increase the risk of exercise-associated hyponatremia in the setting of marathons include excessive hydration, NSAID use, female gender, finishing time over 4 hours, and low body mass index.

Management

As with most conditions, prevention through education of persons at risk is the best course. Athletes should be instructed to avoid excessive ingestion of hypotonic fluids during exercise. Even commercially available sports drinks do not contain enough sodium to prevent hyponatremia. Salty snacks should be eaten along with fluids.

For patients with mild to moderate symptoms, fluid restriction should be initiated, and salty snacks or broth should be administered while a sodium level is obtained. IV fluids are generally contraindicated. For patients with severe symptoms, first address the ABCs. In addition, treatment with hypertonic (3%) saline is indicated. This must be done under extremely controlled conditions, as rapid correction of serum sodium concentration may result in central pontine myelinolysis, an irreversible injury to the CNS. These patients should be transported to a facility with ICU capabilities.

Neuroleptic-Malignant Syndrome

Neuroleptic-malignant syndrome is a hyperthermic medical emergency unrelated to heat exposure. Rather, it occurs as an adverse effect of taking neuroleptic antipsychotic medications such as lithium. It is considered the most serious of extrapyramidal effects. This relatively rare but often lethal syndrome is characterized by muscular rigidity, severe dyskinesia, tachycardia, and hyperthermia.

Signs and Symptoms

Most patients with neuroleptic-malignant syndrome have altered mental status, muscular rigidity, autonomic instability, and high temperatures. Signs of neuroleptic-malignant syndrome develop gradually up to a level where patients are too ill to seek help. Be cautious, since a patient with neuroleptic-malignant syndrome can become agitated, which could be confused with worsening psychosis in a psychiatric patient.

Pathophysiology

Neuroleptic-malignant syndrome usually occurs during the first 1 or 2 weeks of taking an antipsychotic medication. Rapid drug loading, an increase in dosage, and the addition of a new medication are known risk factors. Patients who are dehydrated or have previously had neuroleptic-malignant syndrome are at higher risk as well. The muscular rigidity that characterizes neuroleptic-malignant syndrome is attributable to dopaminergic receptor blockage.

Differential Diagnosis

Neuroleptic-malignant syndrome can be confused with malignant hyperthermia because they have in common muscular rigidity and elevated body temperature.

Management

When you suspect this syndrome, provide supportive care. If the patient is agitated or has psychomotor hyperactivity or muscular rigidity, benzodiazepines (lorazepam, 1 to 2 mg every 3 minutes, up to 10 mg) given intravenously can be considered until muscular rigidity improves (as dictated by local EMS protocol and Medical Control orders). Bromocriptine and dantrolene are alternative agents. Monitor the patient continually for possible complications, such as respiratory depression and seizures. Frequent reevaluation of hemodynamic status is essential, because rapid deterioration can occur. Undertake active cooling measures to treat hyperthermia. Transport the patient to a hospital with ICU capabilities.

Putting It All Together

Assisting patients with endocrine, metabolic, and environmental emergencies can be some of the most challenging problems a healthcare provider faces. Similarities and differences in cardinal presentations are sometimes subtle, and your ability to determine the underlying diagnosis can be obscured, delaying appropriate interventions. Utilizing the AMLS assessment philosophy will assist you in obtaining a comprehensive history and focused physical exam. This assessment-based approach supports putting your knowledge of anatomy, physiology, and pathophysiology to work to figure out both the common and uncommon etiologies of these diverse disease processes. The use of pattern recognition can help you compare your patient's clinical presentation to their chief complaint and formulate a working diagnosis. Becoming proficient in analyzing and synthesizing information to safely, efficiently, and effectively care for these patients will be well worth the effort it takes. Your contributions as an EMS team member are always a vital link in helping improve patient outcomes.

SCENARIO SOLUTION

1 **Differential diagnoses may include electrolyte imbalance such as hypokalemia or hypernatremia, metabolic alkalosis (related to Cushing's syndrome) or metabolic acidosis (related to treatment with metformin), hyperglycemia or hypoglycemia, digoxin toxicity, sepsis, or heart failure.**

2 **To narrow your differential diagnosis, you'll need to complete the history of past and present illness. Perform a physical examination that includes assessment for dehydration, assessment of heart and breath sounds, and mental status. Diagnostic testing should include blood glucose, ECG monitoring and 12-lead ECG, Sao_2, $ETCO_2$, and blood chemistry if available.**

3 **The patient has signs that may indicate shock, infection, or electrolyte imbalance. Signs of shock may be masked by prednisone treatment, and her treatment with digoxin will prevent the increase in heart rate to compensate for shock. Administer oxygen. Establish vascular access, and administer IV fluids. Continue to monitor ECG, and transport to the closest appropriate hospital.**

SUMMARY

- The endocrine system is responsible for hormone regulation, including homeostasis, reproduction, growth, development and metabolism, and is composed of the pituitary, thyroid, parathyroid, and adrenal glands, as well as the pancreas, ovaries, and testes.
- Hormones stimulate growth and development throughout the body, regulate the flow of water in and out of cells, help muscles contract, control blood pressure and appetite, modulate the sleep cycle, and much more.
- Endocrine glands are interdependent on one another.
- Parathyroid glands are composed of three types of cells, responsible for producing parathyroid hormone (PTH), detecting changes in extracellular calcium concentration, and inhibiting calcitonin secretion.
- Hypoparathyroidism is characterized by low serum levels of PTH, with the hallmark of this condition being hypocalcemia.
- The thyroid gland is composed of secretory cells, follicular cells, and C cells.
- Hyperthyroidism can result in thyrotoxicosis and, potentially, thyroid storm.
- A patient with hyperthyroidism is prone to arrhythmias such as sinus tachycardia, atrial fibrillation, atrial flutter, and premature ventricular contractions.
- The adrenal gland secretes glucocorticoids, mineralocorticoids, and supplemental sex hormones.
- Addison's disease, or primary adrenal insufficiency, is a metabolic and endocrine ailment caused by direct insult to or malfunction of the adrenal cortex.
- Acute adrenal insufficiency is a condition in which the body's need for glucocorticoids and mineralocorticoids exceeds the delivery of these hormones by the adrenal glands.
- Hyperadrenalism, or Cushing's syndrome, is caused by long-standing exposure to excessive circulating serum levels of glucocorticoids, particularly cortisol, as a result of overproduction in the adrenal cortex.
- Glucose is a vital fuel for key metabolic processes in organs, especially those in the central nervous system (CNS).
- Cellular survival depends on preserving a balanced serum glucose concentration; the body is able to maintain serum glucose through three metabolic processes:
  - Gluconeogenesis: the formation of new glucose from precursors, including pyruvate, glycerol, lactate, and amino acids
  - Glycogenolysis: glucose produced as glycogen breakdown occurs in the liver
  - Gastrointestinal absorption: direct intestinal absorption of glucose through the intestine
- Diabetes is the most common endocrine disorder, and hypoglycemia, a frequent complication of the treatment

of diabetes, is thus the most common endocrine emergency.

- Diabetes mellitus is characterized by defective insulin production or utilization, a high level of blood glucose, and unbalanced lipid and carbohydrate metabolism; left untreated, diabetes results in hyperglycemia.
- Hypoglycemia among diabetics is the result of a disruption in the delicate balance between the interdependent factors of exogenously administered insulin, glucose metabolism, and glucose intake.
- Hypoglycemia may occur in patients only taking oral hypoglycemic agents but should alert the healthcare provider to the potential presence of an underlying pathophysiologic state such as new-onset renal failure.
- Type 1 diabetes is characterized by pancreatic beta cell destruction, which renders the body incapable of producing the insulin necessary to carry out cell metabolism.
- Type 2 diabetes is characterized by cellular insulin resistance and a gradual failure of pancreatic insulin production.
- Gestational diabetes is a form of glucose intolerance that can occur among pregnant women.
- Healthy cellular function is directly related to a precise acid-base balance in the body, with the kidneys and lungs maintaining this balance, and measured by pH.
- Glucose is the principal fuel for metabolism in the body and its organs, especially the brain.
- Hypoglycemia results in a decrease in insulin secretion and secretion of counterregulatory hormones such as epinephrine. Symptoms include impaired cognition and, if untreated, can lead to significant morbidity and mortality.
- Hypoglycemia in nondiabetic patients is characterized by alimentary hyperinsulinism, commonly seen in patients who have undergone gastric surgery, or the result of an imbalance between glucose utilization and production.
- Diabetic ketoacidosis is an acute endocrine emergency in which insulin deficiency and an excessive glucagon level combine to create a hyperglycemic, acidotic, volume-depleted state.
- Hyperosmolar hyperglycemic nonketotic syndrome (HHNS) is a serious diabetic emergency, carrying a mortality rate of 10% to 50%.
- Respiratory acidosis is characterized by a decline in pH as a result of CO_2 retention.
- An increase in ventilation per minute is the cause of respiratory alkalosis, characterized by a decreased $PaCO_2$ and increased pH.
- Metabolic acidosis is caused by the accumulation of acids in excess of the body's buffering capabilities.
- The most common serious causes of metabolic acidosis are diabetic ketoacidosis, renal failure, lactic acidosis, toxic ingestion, and alcoholic ketoacidosis.
- Metabolic alkalosis is produced by illnesses that raise the level of serum bicarbonate or reduce the level of hydrogen in the body, such as those that cause volume, potassium, and chloride loss.
- A healthy electrolyte balance is fundamental to carrying out cellular functions; electrolyte imbalances include hyponatremia, hypokalemia, hyperkalemia, hypocalcemia, and hypomagnesemia.
- Rhabdomyolysis is a skeletal muscle injury characterized by release of cellular contents, specifically myoglobin, potentially leading to acute renal failure and hyperkalemia.
- Body temperature is regulated by neural feedback mechanisms that operate primarily through the hypothalamus; the hypothalamus contains not only the control mechanisms (which maintain a temperature set point) but also the sensory mechanisms necessary to detect and respond to body temperature changes.
- Cold emergencies include frost nip, frostbite, and systemic hypothermia.
- Heat illnesses include heatstroke, heat cramps, heat exhaustion, heat syncope and exercise-associated syncope, and neuroleptic-malignant syndrome.

BIBLIOGRAPHY

Hamilton GC, Sanders AB, Strange GR: Emergency medicine, ed 2, St Louis, 2003, Saunders.

Kumar G, Sng BL, Kumar S: Correlation of capillary and venous blood glucometry with laboratory determination, Prehosp Emerg Care 8(4):378, 2004.

Marx JA, Hockberger RS, Walls RM: Rosen's emergency medicine, ed 7, St Louis, 2009, Mosby.

Mistovich JJ, Krost WS, Limmer DD: Beyond the basics: endocrine emergencies, EMS Mag 36(10):123–127, 2007.

Mistovich JJ, Krost WS, Limmer DD: Beyond the basics: endocrine emergencies, Part II, EMS Mag 36(11):66–69, 2007.

Pagan KD, Pagana TJ: Mosby's manual of diagnostic and laboratory tests, ed 4, St Louis, 2010, Mosby.

Sanders MJ: Mosby's paramedic textbook, ed 3, St Louis, 2005, Mosby.

U.S. Department of Transportation National Highway Traffic Safety Administration: EMT-paramedic national standard curriculum, Washington, DC, 1998, The Department.

U.S. Department of Transportation National Highway Traffic Safety Administration: National EMS education standards, Draft 3.0, Washington, DC, 2008, The Department.

Chapter Review Questions

1. Your patient complains of discomfort in his hand as you inflate the cuff to assess the blood pressure. You note flexion of the wrist and adduction of his fingers. What endocrine disorder do you suspect?
   - **a.** Addison's disease
   - **b.** Cushing's syndrome
   - **c.** Hypoparathyroidism
   - **d.** Myxedema

2. A 47-year-old female is anxious and complaining of heart palpitations. She reports a recent diagnosis of "thyroid problems." On exam you note exophthalmos. Her vital signs are BP 108/72 mm Hg, P 128 bpm, R 20/min. Interventions should include administration of:
   - **a.** Amiodarone
   - **b.** Aspirin
   - **c.** Intravenous fluids
   - **d.** Methylprednisolone

3. Which assessment finding(s) should you anticipate in a patient who has myxedema?
   - **a.** Chvostek's sign
   - **b.** Dry, yellow skin
   - **c.** Exophthalmos
   - **d.** Hyperactive reflexes

4. What treatment should you anticipate in a patient with a history of Addison's disease who has the following vital signs: BP 94/58 mm Hg, P 124 bpm, R 20/min?
   - **a.** Blood products
   - **b.** Catecholamines
   - **c.** Potassium
   - **d.** Hydrocortisone

5. What finding should you anticipate on the physical examination of a patient with Cushing's syndrome?
   - **a.** Blood glucose 180 mg/dL (10 mmol/L)
   - **b.** Blood pressure 94/54 mm Hg
   - **c.** Heart rate 50 bpm
   - **d.** Thin face and body profile

6. When serum glucose drops below 70 mg/dL (3.9 mmol/L), which of the following occurs?
   - **a.** Epinephrine secretion increases.
   - **b.** Glucagon secretion decreases.
   - **c.** Growth hormone secretion increases.
   - **d.** Insulin production increases.

7. A 22-year-old male complains of a 2-day history of abdominal pain. His skin is flushed, and he has a fruity odor on his breath. Assessment reveals BP 106/54 mm Hg, P 128, R 28, glucose 568 mg/dL. Your highest priority intervention would be to:
   - **a.** Administer glucagon IM
   - **b.** Intubate his trachea
   - **c.** Infuse normal saline rapid IV
   - **d.** Perform a 12-lead electrocardiogram

8. Which patient would be an appropriate candidate for immediate intravenous administration of sodium bicarbonate?
   - **a.** 22-year-old who is unresponsive and breathing 8 per minute after heroin overdose
   - **b.** 22-year-old with anxiety, racing heart rate, and tachypnea
   - **c.** 34-year-old with 4 days of nausea, vomiting, and diarrhea, who has shallow respirations and mild confusion
   - **d.** 45-year-old who complained of chest pain and is now in cardiac arrest and unresponsive to treatment

9. A 72-year-old complains of a headache and being depressed, intermittent twitching in the facial muscles, and general weakness over the past 2 weeks. She has a medical history of hypoparathyroidism. The ECG reveals a prolonged QT segment. During transport she has a seizure. Which electrolyte imbalance is most likely?
   - **a.** Hypocalcemia
   - **b.** Hyperkalemia
   - **c.** Hypercalcemia
   - **d.** Hyponatremia

10. A 62-year-old hunter was lost in a swampy area. When you begin to care for him, he is lethargic, disoriented, and has a body temperature of 31°C (87.8°F). His ECG shows bradycardia. What should be your treatment priority?
    - **a.** Atropine 0.5 mg IV
    - **b.** Epinephrine drip at 2 to 10 mcg/min
    - **c.** Rapid rewarming
    - **d.** Transcutaneous pacing

CHAPTER 7

Abdominal Discomfort: Gastrointestinal, Genitourinary, and Reproductive Disorders

DIAGNOSING AND TREATING ABDOMINAL DISCOMFORT requires you to draw on all your skills as a provider. Since patients with abdominal complaints exhibit a wide range of signs and symptoms, formulating a broad differential diagnosis and then narrowing it down to arrive at a working diagnosis is challenging for the most expert of clinicians. This chapter will assist you to increase your expertise by examining the clues that add up to an accurate diagnosis, beginning with a review of the gastrointestinal system and the functions of the digestive organs. Then we'll discuss signs, symptoms, and treatment of various sources of abdominal discomfort you're likely to encounter most often in the field. Finally, we'll review common causes of abdominal discomfort that originate in body systems other than the gastrointestinal system.

Learning Objectives *At the conclusion of this chapter, you will be able to:*

1. Describe the anatomy and physiology of the cardiovascular, respiratory, gastrointestinal, genitourinary, reproductive, neurologic, and endocrine systems as they relate to abdominal discomfort.
2. Correlate the finding of pain based on location, referral, and type—visceral or somatic—with OPQRST findings as they relate to abdominal discomfort.
3. Demonstrate the ability to formulate a differential diagnosis, apply sound clinical reasoning skills, and use advanced clinical decision making in caring for the patient presenting with abdominal discomfort and the associated cardinal presentations of:
   a. Unstable vital signs
   b. Gastrointestinal bleeding
   c. Nausea and vomiting
   d. Diarrhea
   e. Jaundice
   f. Vaginal bleeding
4. Evaluate the patient for life-threatening conditions during the primary, secondary, and ongoing assessments.
5. List effective ways of discovering a patient's allergies, list of medications, incident and past medical history, and last oral intake, and determine how this information will affect patient care.
6. Apply appropriate treatment modalities for the management, monitoring, and continuing care of the patient with abdominal discomfort.

Key Terms

antiemetic A substance that prevents or alleviates nausea and vomiting

fulminant hepatic failure A rare condition that occurs when hepatitis progresses to hepatic necrosis (death of the liver cells); classic symptoms include anorexia, vomiting, jaundice, abdominal pain, and asterixis ("flapping").

gastrointestinal (GI) Pertaining to the organs of the GI tract. The GI tract links the organs involved in consumption, processing, and elimination of nutrients. It begins at the mouth, moves to the esophagus, travels through the chest cavity into the abdomen, and terminates in the pelvic girdle at the rectum.

hematemesis Vomiting of bright red blood, indicating upper GI bleeding

hematochezia Passage of red blood through the rectum

intussusception Prolapse of one segment of the bowel into the lumen of another segment. This kind of intestinal obstruction may involve segments of the small intestine, colon, or terminal ileum and cecum.

melena Abnormal black, tarry stool that has a distinctive odor and contains digested blood

referred pain Pain felt at a site different from that of an injured or diseased organ or body part

somatic (parietal) pain Generally well-localized pain caused by an irritation of the nerve fibers in the parietal peritoneum or other deep tissues (e.g., musculoskeletal system). Physical findings include sharp, discrete, localized pain accompanied by tenderness to palpation, guarding of the affected area, and rebound tenderness.

visceral pain Poorly localized pain that occurs when the walls of the hollow organs are stretched, thereby activating the stretch receptors. This kind of pain is characterized by a deep, persistent ache ranging from mild to intolerable and commonly described as cramping, burning, and gnawing.

viscus (*pl.* viscera) The internal organs enclosed within a body cavity, including the abdominal, thoracic, pelvic, and endocrine organs

volvulus A condition in which the stomach rotates more than 180 degrees; this twisting seals the stomach on both ends, blocking the flow of blood and the passage of fluid and food. The condition is characterized by an acute onset of abdominal pain, severe vomiting, and shock.

SCENARIO

YOU ARE DISPATCHED to a local tavern for a sick call. When you arrive, your 40-year-old female patient is curled in the fetal position on the floor. Chunky yellow vomitus is pooled beside her and has sprayed onto the nearby wall. Her medical history includes sickle cell disease, hypertension, and high cholesterol. The bartender and other patrons call her by name and say she wasn't herself this evening, but she hates to miss coming in each day. The patient tells you "this is the worst pain I've ever had." As you roll her to her back, she moans loudly and holds her abdomen. Her vital signs are BP 98/50 mm Hg, P 124 bpm, R 24/min. You note that she is pale, and small beads of sweat have welled up on her forehead.

1. ***What differential diagnoses are you considering based on the information you have now?***
2. ***What additional information will you need to narrow your differential diagnosis?***
3. ***What are your initial treatment priorities as you continue your patient care?***

German philosopher Friedrich Nietzsche—whose midlife was plagued by gastric problems—once observed, "The abdomen is the reason why man does not easily take himself for a god." From an episode of garden-variety stomach flu to a sudden attack of appendicitis, anyone who has suffered an abdominal disorder knows precisely what Nietzsche meant. But abdominal ailments are more than just a nuisance. In fact, they've actually changed the course of history and undoubtedly robbed us of great masterpieces of art and literature. French emperor Louis Napoleon, for example, is said to have been captured during the Franco-Prussian War because he was distracted by painful kidney stones. Novelist James Joyce died at age 58 of a perforated ulcer. Composer Lili Boulanger, winner of the prestigious Prix de Rome, was struck down by Crohn's disease before her 25th birthday.

We may have come a long way in treating abdominal complaints since the Napoleonic era, but abdominal pain is still one of the most often-cited reasons for seeking medical care. In 2006, the National Health Statistics Report from the U.S. Centers for Disease Control and Prevention (the most recent report available at the time of this printing) found that abdominal complaints were second only to chest pain in patients aged 15 and older. In children younger than age 15, abdominal complaints are less frequent. Given the varied anatomy and physiology of the **gastrointestinal (GI)** system, the causes of abdominal signs and symptoms are extremely diverse. We'll explore them in this chapter.

Anatomy and Physiology

The GI tract links the organs involved in the consumption, processing, and elimination of nutrients. It begins at the mouth, moves to the esophagus, travels through the chest cavity into the abdomen, and terminates in the pelvic girdle at the rectum. Figure 7-1 shows the location of the abdominal organs. Along this lengthy path, myriad problems can arise. Patients' complaints are often nonspecific, so arriving at a diagnosis can be challenging even with advanced diagnostic tools at your disposal.

Upper Gastrointestinal Tract

The GI system begins in the mouth with the tongue and salivary glands. The process of digestion starts with

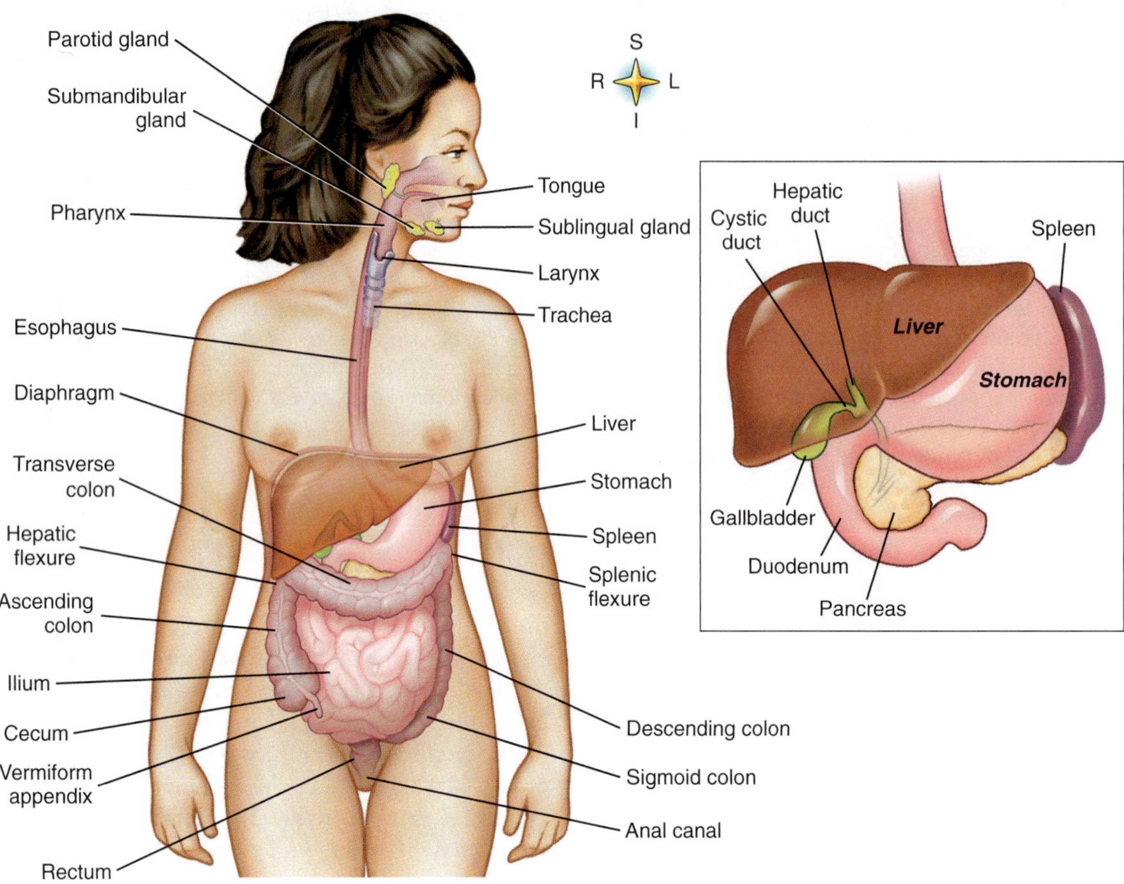

Figure 7-1 Location of digestive organs. (From Sanders MJ: Mosby's paramedic textbook, revised ed 3, St Louis, 2007, Mosby.)

mastication, or chewing. Mastication is the process by which the teeth and saliva break down solid food to facilitate its passage into the esophagus. The next step in digestion takes place in the esophagus, a hollow, muscular organ posterior to the trachea that passes distally through the chest, progresses through the diaphragm, and terminates at the stomach. The muscular wall of the esophagus propels food toward the stomach from the mouth. Since the esophagus lacks a rigid framework, it's easily compressible. At the termination of the esophagus is the lower esophageal sphincter, a muscular band that prevents the reflux of gastric contents from the stomach into the esophagus.

The stomach lies inferior to the diaphragm, just below the left lobe of the liver. It's protected by the rib cage. When empty, the stomach has numerous folds, or rugae, that allow it to expand to accommodate 1 to 1.5 liters of food and fluid. Three layers of smooth muscle enhance its expansion and the processing of food. Glands within the stomach produce digestive enzymes to aid digestion and protect the body from potentially harmful microorganisms that enter with the food. The speed at which the stomach empties its contents into the lower digestive tract, known as the *rate of gastric emptying*, depends on the type and amount of food ingested and on other factors such as the person's age and medical condition.

Lower Gastrointestinal Tract

Digestion continues from the stomach into the small intestine, the first structure in the lower GI tract. When stretched out, the small intestine is about 22 feet long, but in the body it's looped tightly within the relatively small abdominal cavity. The duodenum, the jejunum, and the ileum are the three sections of the small intestine. The duodenum extends from the stomach. At just a foot in length, it's the shortest portion of the small intestine. The duodenum receives the semifluid, partially digested stomach contents, or chyme, as well as exocrine secretions from the liver and pancreas. The jejunum is about 8 feet long and is responsible for most of the chemical digestion and absorption of nutrients. The ileum is the final section of the small bowel and is the longest section at 13 feet. It's responsible for nutrient absorption as well. The large intestine includes the cecum, colon, and rectum. The cecum is a pouch that receives the products of digestion from the small intestine. The vermiform appendix attaches to the cecum. The large intestine is primarily responsible

TABLE 7-1 Functions of the Liver

Metabolic	Hematologic	Other Major Functions
Extraction of nutrients from blood	Removal of aged or damaged red blood cells	Secretion of bile
Extraction of toxins from blood	Synthesis of plasma proteins	Absorption and breakdown of hormones
Removal and storage of excess nutrients such as glucose	Synthesis of clotting factors	
Maintenance of normal glucose levels		
Storage of vitamins		

for the reabsorption of water and absorption of vitamins. The rectum is responsible for expelling stool.

Accessory Organs

Liver The liver lies in the right upper quadrant of the abdominal cavity distal to the diaphragm. The specific functions of the liver are broad and include bile production and metabolic and hematologic regulation. The liver performs more than 200 functions in the body, several of which are listed in Table 7-1.

The liver is a dense, heavy organ, weighing about 1.5 kg (3.3 lb). It's divided into left and right lobes made up of lobules, masses of cells that comprise the basic structural units of the liver. The liver contains about 100,000 lobules. It's an extremely vascular organ. In fact, as the largest reservoir of blood in the body, even a small laceration can cause extensive blood loss.

Gallbladder The gallbladder is a pear-shaped organ housed below the liver. Its function is to modify and store bile. Excessive precipitation of bile salts can cause painful gallstones to form.

Pancreas The pancreas lies posterior to the stomach between the first part of the duodenum and the spleen in the midepigastric area, joining the common bile duct and emptying into the duodenum. It functions in digestion as an exocrine organ, secreting digestive enzymes, bicarbonate, electrolytes, and water. The pancreas performs an endocrine function that is not directly involved in digestion by secreting:

- Glucagon, to raise glucose levels
- Insulin, to promote movement of glucose into the tissues
- Somatostatin, to regulate other endocrine cells in the pancreatic islets

Functions of the Gastrointestinal System

To process or digest nutrients effectively, the four chief functions of the GI system—motility, secretion, digestion, and absorption—must be intact. These functions require a complex interaction among the nervous system, the endocrine system, the musculoskeletal system, and the cardiovascular system.

Motility

Food progresses through the GI tract by a process called *motility*. This process also mixes food components and reduces particle size so food can be digested and nutrients absorbed. A structured, coordinated muscular response known as *peristalsis* is required for the process to be successful. The neurologic system—specifically, the sympathetic and parasympathetic nervous systems—orchestrates this effort.

The vagus nerve, part of the parasympathetic nervous system, innervates the GI tract to the level of the transverse colon. This nerve plays a pivotal role in gastric emptying by affecting the motility of the GI tract. It does so by controlling the contraction and dilation of sphincters and smooth muscle. In addition, the nerve has a secretory function and helps stimulate vomiting. (Since the vagus nerve also helps regulate the heart rate, bradycardia is often present when a person retches or vomits.) The pelvic nerve stimulates the descending colon, sigmoid colon, rectum, and anal canal. The vagus and pelvic nerves innervate the striated muscle in the upper third of the esophagus and the external anal sphincter (Figure 7-2).

The sympathetic nervous system focuses on the major ganglia (celiac, superior mesenteric, inferior mesenteric, and hypogastric), the secretory and endocrine cells.

Secretion

The digestive tract is lined with cells that secrete fluids to aid in motility and digestion. These cells secrete up to 9 liters of water, acids, buffers, electrolytes, and enzymes in a 24-hour period. A majority of this fluid is reabsorbed, but when diarrhea occurs and is severe or extended, significant fluid loss can occur, and dehydration and shock may ensue.

Digestion

Digestion is the process of breaking down food into components to be used for nutrition for the body at the cellular level. Digestion involves the mechanical and chemical breakdown of the food we ingest.

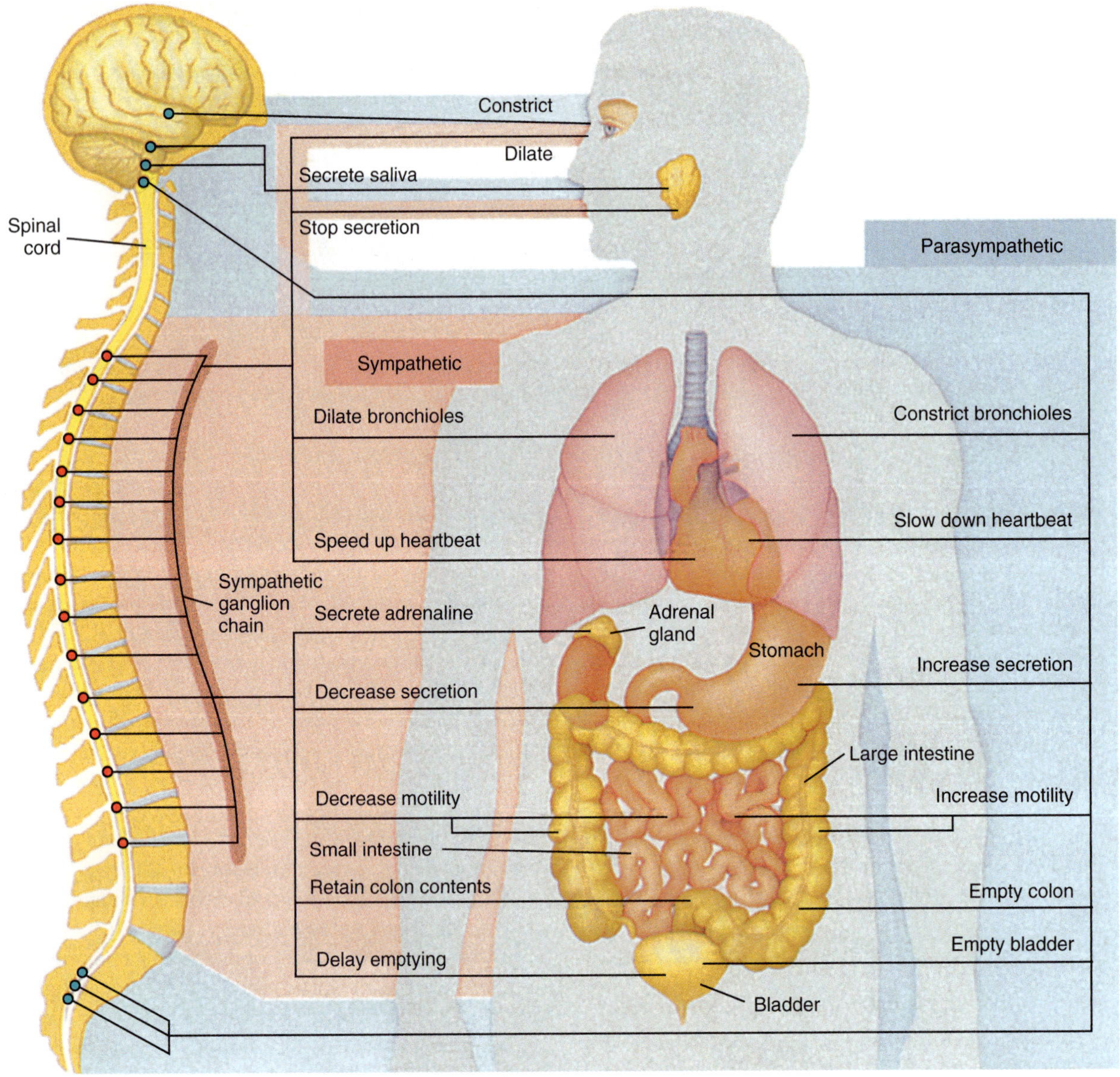

■ **Figure 7-2** Innervation of major target organs by the autonomic nervous system. Sympathetic fibers are highlighted with red, parasympathetic are highlighted with blue. (From Sanders MJ: Mosby's paramedic textbook, revised ed 3, St Louis, 2007, Mosby.)

Absorption

The small intestine is the primary site for absorption of fluid and nutrients, and the large intestine is the primary site of absorption of water and salts.

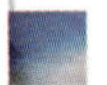

Pain

The most common GI complaint is abdominal pain. Despite or perhaps because of the frequency of the complaint, determining its cause can challenge even a seasoned healthcare provider. Often the complaint of abdominal pain is vague and ill defined. To obtain the necessary information from the patient and arrive at a diagnosis, you must know GI system pathophysiology and understand how to take a history and perform an assessment in a reassuring and supportive way. Because an accurate diagnosis is not always immediately apparent, patients can become frustrated and feel as if you don't believe them. Establishing an environment of trust can allow you to acquire much-needed information, including precipitating factors and a description of additional symptoms that may point to a probable diagnosis.

The very young and the elderly may have difficulty relaying pain to clinicians. Both have a different perception of pain, and both localize pain differently. Older adult patients may get confused about where pain actually originates and often live with chronic pain that may affect their perception of pain. Pediatric patients poorly localize the exact pain location and may have difficulty verbalizing their pain.

One complicating factor in the diagnosis of abdominal pain is that the perception of discomfort varies widely, depending on its cause and the patient's individual level of tolerance. In addition, abdominal pain often evolves over time, becoming better defined as the disease process progresses. Abdominal pain can be divided into three categories: visceral pain, parietal pain, and referred pain. Let's take a look at each of them.

Visceral Pain

Visceral pain occurs when the walls of the hollow organs are stretched, thereby activating the stretch receptors. This kind of pain is characterized by a deep, persistent ache ranging from mild to intolerable. Common descriptors include cramping, burning, and gnawing.

Visceral pain is difficult to localize, since the abdominal organs transmit pain signals to both sides of the spinal cord, but it's typically felt in the epigastric, periumbilical, or suprapubic region. Epigastric visceral pain typically comes from the stomach, gallbladder, liver, duodenum, or pancreas. Periumbilical pain tends to be related to the appendix, small bowel, or cecum, while suprapubic pain arises from the kidneys, ureters, bladder, colon, uterus, or ovaries (Figure 7-3).

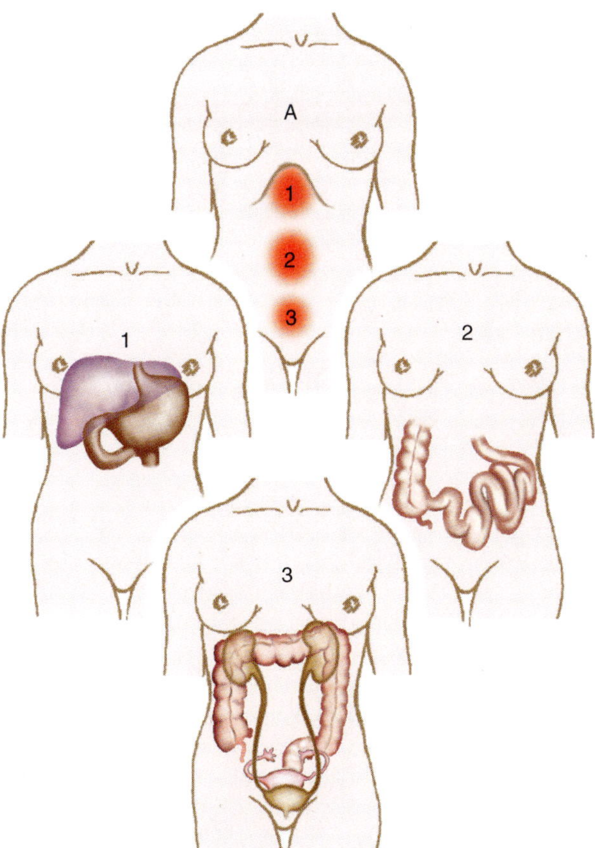

Figure 7-3 Localization of visceral pain. Pain arising from organ areas depicted in 1, 2, and 3 is felt in the epigastrium, midabdomen, and hypogastrium, respectively, as shown in A. (From Feldman M, Friedman LS, Brandt LJ: Sleisenger & Fordtran's gastrointestinal and liver disease pathophysiology/diagnosis/management, Philadelphia, Saunders, 2006.)

The patient may have trouble finding a comfortable position, so he or she will shift frequently or need to be adjusted during transport. Depending on the cause, diaphoresis, nausea, vomiting, restlessness, or pallor may be present. Table 7-2 outlines the differential diagnosis of abdominal discomfort in patients with nausea and vomiting. Table 7-3 lists **antiemetic** agents used in patients with nausea and vomiting.

Somatic (Parietal) Pain

Somatic (parietal) pain is caused by an irritation of the nerve fibers in the parietal peritoneum or other deep tissues, such as those of the musculoskeletal system. The origin of somatic pain is easier to pinpoint than visceral pain. Physical findings include sharp, discrete, localized pain accompanied by tenderness to palpation, guarding of the affected area, and rebound tenderness.

Somatic pain usually emerges later in the disease process. Since the parietal peritoneum surrounds the organs involved, it takes longer for the affected structures to become irritated and painful. The dorsal root ganglia in the spine activate peritoneal pain, so the pain is typically on the same side and in the same dermatome as the affected organ. Dermatomes represent the relationship between the spinal nerve and portion of the body they innervate (Figure 7-4).

Referred Pain

When pain emanates from a site other than that of its origin, it is said to be **referred pain.** In other words, the pain is "referred" from its origin to another location. Overlapping neural pathways are responsible for this phenomenon. For example, referred pain often accompanies cholecystitis, in which the patient usually feels pain in the right scapular area. It's also common in myocardial infarction, in which pain is referred to the neck, jaw, or arm (see Figure 1-18 in Chapter 1).

Assessment

Initial Observation

During initial observation, you form your first impression of the patient. The Advanced Medical Life Support (AMLS) pathway advises letting this initial observation guide much of your patient care.

Your initial observation actually begins when you receive the dispatch information related to an abdominal complaint. When you arrive on scene, you'll be able to determine how well that information squares with your own impressions. Next, look for clues that might indicate a life-threatening emergency. If one is apparent, initiate support of airway, breathing, and circulation as you continue your assessment. If no life threat is present, focus

TABLE 7-2 Differential Diagnosis of Abdominal Discomfort with Nausea and Vomiting

Disorder	Definition	History	Assessment	Assessment Tools	Interventions
NEUROLOGIC					
Intracerebral bleeding	Bleeding within the brain tissue	Trauma, stroke, hypertension, smoking, alcohol abuse	Hemiparesis, hemiplegia, nausea, headache, altered level of consciousness, Cushing's triad	CTA, CBC, coagulation studies, electrolytes, glucose	Maintain airway. Administer oxygen. Establish IV access. Place a 12-lead ECG.
Meningitis	Bacterial, viral, or fungal infection of the meninges	—	High fever, headache, stiff neck, seizures Resembles flu Can progress over several days	CBC, electrolytes, blood cultures, lumbar puncture	Maintain airway. Administer oxygen. Place a 12-Lead ECG. Establish IV access. Administer isotonic fluid. Give antibiotics if the infection is bacterial.
CARDIAC					
Acute MI	Necrosis of the heart muscle	Coronary artery disease, smoking, high cholesterol, history of MI	Chest, midepigastric, back, and neck pain Nausea Difficulty breathing	12-lead ECG, x-ray, CBC, coagulation studies, electrolytes	Administer oxygen. Establish IV access. Administer nitroglycerin, ASA, and anticoagulants. Angiography will be performed at the receiving facility.
GASTROINTESTINAL					
Boerhaave's syndrome	Spontaneous rupture of the esophagus	Explosive vomiting, coughing, seizures, childbirth, status asthmaticus	Pain in the chest, neck, back, or abdomen Difficulty breathing, tachycardia, hematemesis, fever, subcutaneous emphysema	CBC, coagulation studies, type and cross-match	Treat airway compromise, hypoxia, and shock. Surgery will be performed at the receiving facility.

Mallory-Weiss tear	Longitudinal tears in the esophageal mucosa, causing severe arterial bleeding	Severe, protracted vomiting, bleeding	Severe, protracted vomiting Bleeding	Bronchoscopy, CBC, coagulation studies, type and cross-match	Treat airway compromise and shock, administer oxygen, and establish IV access. Gastric lavage and possibly surgery will be performed at the receiving facility.
Upper GI bleeding	Bleeding proximal to the junction of the duodenum and jejunum	Hematemesis (vomiting blood that is bright red or resembles coffee grounds), alcohol abuse, use of NSAIDs, liver disease, varices	Abdominal pain Red or coffee-colored vomitus or stool	Chest and abdominal x-rays, angiography CBC, Hct, Hb, PTT, platelets, coagulation studies, type and cross-match, etc.) Nasogastric tube, endoscopy	Administer oxygen. Perform an ECG. Establish IV access. Treat shock. Administer blood products.
Ischemic bowel	Necrosis of the GI tract	Severe abdominal pain, sick appearance, hypercoagulability, recent surgery, shock	Abdominal pain, tachycardia, hypotension, fever, restlessness	CBC, coagulation studies, electrolytes, type and cross-match	Administer oxygen. Perform an ECG. Establish IV access. Treat shock. X-ray and CT imaging and surgery will be performed at the receiving facility.
ENDOCRINE					
Diabetic ketoacidosis	Hyperglycemia, ketosis, and acidosis	Diabetes, especially type 1, but can occur in patients with type 2 diabetes who are ill	Nausea, vomiting, polydipsia, polyuria, abdominal pain, metabolic acidosis	Blood glucose, serum electrolytes, arterial blood gas analysis, CBC	Administer oxygen. Establish IV access. Administer isotonic fluids and insulin as indicated.

ASA, Acetylsalicylic acid; *CBC,* complete blood count; *CT,* computed tomography; *CTA,* computed tomography angiography; *ECG,* electrocardiogram; *GI,* gastrointestinal; *Hb,* hemoglobin; *Hct,* hematocrit; *IV,* intravenous; *MI,* myocardial infarction; *NSAIDs,* nonsteroidal antiinflammatory drugs; PTT, partial thromboplastin time.

TABLE 7-3 Antiemetic Agents

Drug	Dosage	Side Effects
ondansetron (Zofran)	8 mg PO 3 times/day or 0.15 mg/kg IV over 15 min	Hypersensitivity, hypertension, tachycardia, anxiety, dizziness, headache
prochlorperazine (Compazine)	5–10 mg (PO, IM, IV) 3–4 times per day PRN	Extrapyramidal reaction, sedation, neuroleptic malignant syndrome
promethazine (Phenergan)	12.5–25 mg (PO, IM, or IV) every 4–6 h; slow IV infusion	Dry mouth, blurred vision, sedation, respiratory depression
metoclopramide (Reglan)	20–40 mg PO	Sedation, extrapyramidal reaction
meclizine (Antivert)	25–50 mg PO every 24 h PRN	Sedation, dry mouth, blurred vision

IM, Intramuscular; *IV*, intravenous; *PO*, per os (by mouth); *PRN*, as needed.

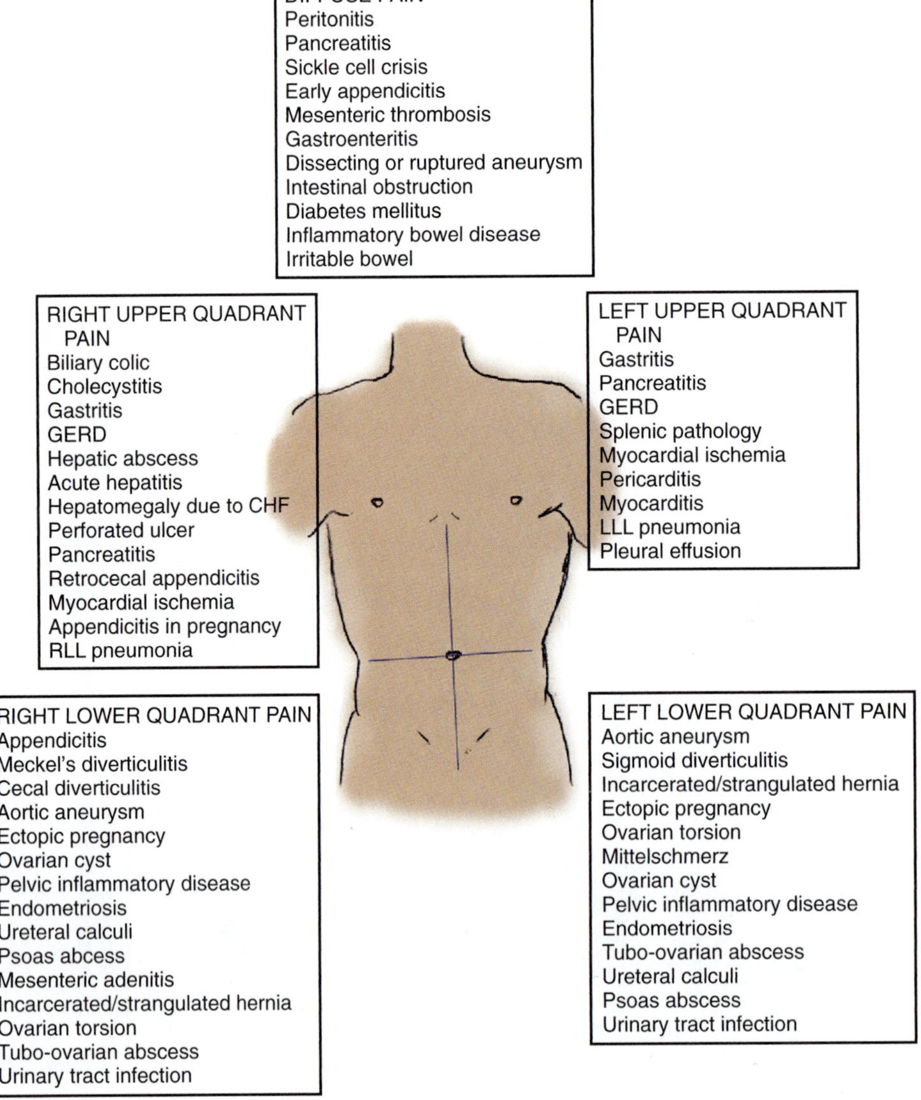

DIFFUSE PAIN
Peritonitis
Pancreatitis
Sickle cell crisis
Early appendicitis
Mesenteric thrombosis
Gastroenteritis
Dissecting or ruptured aneurysm
Intestinal obstruction
Diabetes mellitus
Inflammatory bowel disease
Irritable bowel
RIGHT UPPER QUADRANT PAIN
Biliary colic
Cholecystitis
Gastritis
GERD
Hepatic abscess
Acute hepatitis
Hepatomegaly due to CHF
Perforated ulcer
Pancreatitis
Retrocecal appendicitis
Myocardial ischemia
Appendicitis in pregnancy
RLL pneumonia
LEFT UPPER QUADRANT PAIN
Gastritis
Pancreatitis
GERD
Splenic pathology
Myocardial ischemia
Pericarditis
Myocarditis
LLL pneumonia
Pleural effusion
RIGHT LOWER QUADRANT PAIN
Appendicitis
Meckel's diverticulitis
Cecal diverticulitis
Aortic aneurysm
Ectopic pregnancy
Ovarian cyst
Pelvic inflammatory disease
Endometriosis
Ureteral calculi
Psoas abscess
Mesenteric adenitis
Incarcerated/strangulated hernia
Ovarian torsion
Tubo-ovarian abscess
Urinary tract infection
LEFT LOWER QUADRANT PAIN
Aortic aneurysm
Sigmoid diverticulitis
Incarcerated/strangulated hernia
Ectopic pregnancy
Ovarian torsion
Mittelschmerz
Ovarian cyst
Pelvic inflammatory disease
Endometriosis
Tubo-ovarian abscess
Ureteral calculi
Psoas abscess
Urinary tract infection

■ **Figure 7-4** Differential diagnosis of acute abdominal pain. *CHF,* Congestive heart failure; *GERD*, gastroesophageal reflux disease; *LLL*, left lower lobe; *RLL*, right lower lobe. (From Marx JA, Hockberger RS, Walls RM, et al: Rosen's emergency medicine, ed 7, St Louis, Mosby, 2009.)

your assessment on identifying the cardinal presentation and formulating a list of differential diagnoses associated with abdominal discomfort. Consider critical conditions first, and progress to emergent disorders. Signs associated with a range of critical, emergent, and nonemergent abdominal complaints are summarized in Table 7-4.

Your job is to gather assessment clues and combine them to build a differential diagnosis. As you look for clues, be sure to keep an eye out for the medical devices described in Box 7-1. You will need to rule in or rule out possible diagnoses on the basis of your own observations of the scene and the patient's history, physical exam

TABLE 7-4 Critical, Emergent, and Nonemergent Disorders with Abdominal Signs and Symptoms

Disorder	Pain	Nausea/ Vomiting	Bleeding	Constipation	Diarrhea	Jaundice	Vaginal Bleeding
CRITICAL							
Gastrointestinal							
Boerhaave's syndrome	Y	Y	Y				
Ischemic bowel	Y	Y			Y		
Mallory-Weiss tear	Y	Y	Y				
Upper GI bleeding	Y	Y	Y				
Fulminant hepatic failure	Y	Y				Y	
Cholangitis	Y	Y				Y	
Neurologic							
Intracerebral bleeding		Y					
Meningitis		Y					
Cardiac							
Acute myocardial infarction	Y	Y					
Budd-Chiari syndrome	Y	Y				Y	
Severe congestive heart failure						Y	
Obstructing aortic aneurysm						Y	
Endocrine							
Diabetic ketoacidosis	Y	Y					
Reproductive							
Preeclampsia/HELLP						Y	
Abruptio placentae	Y						Y
Placenta previa							Y
EMERGENT							
Gastrointestinal							
Gastric outlet obstruction	Y	Y					
Mesenteric ischemia	Y	Y			Y		
Intestinal obstruction	Y	Y		Y	Y		
Bowel perforation	Y	Y		Y			
Perforated viscus	Y	Y	Y				
Pancreatitis	Y	Y					
Ruptured appendix	Y	Y					
Peritonitis	Y	Y					
Crohn's disease	Y	Y			Y		
Ulcerative colitis	Y	Y			Y		
Cholelithiasis	Y	Y					
Neurologic							
Migraine		Y					
CNS tumor		Y					
Endocrine							
Adrenal insufficiency	Y	Y			Y		
Reproductive							
Hyperemesis gravidarum		Y					

Continued

TABLE 7-4 Critical, Emergent, and Nonemergent Disorders with Abdominal Signs and Symptoms—*Cont'd*

Disorder	Pain	Nausea/ Vomiting	Bleeding	Constipation	Diarrhea	Jaundice	Vaginal Bleeding
Genitourinary							
Testicular torsion	Y	Y					
NONEMERGENT							
Gastrointestinal							
Hepatitis	Y	Y			Y	Y	
Gastroenteritis	Y	Y			Y		
Irritable bowel syndrome	Y	Y		Y	Y		
Diverticulitis/diverticulosis	Y		Y	Y	Y		
Inflammatory bowel disease	Y	Y	Y		Y		

CNS, Central nervous system *GI,* gastrointestinal.

BOX 7-1 Home Medical Devices Used by Patients with Abdominal Disorders

As medical technology advances, prehospital medical providers are encountering a wider variety of medical devices in the home environment. Let's review a few of the devices you're likely to see most often.

- **Nasogastric and nasointestinal feeding tubes.** Nasogastric and nasointestinal feeding tubes are typically small-diameter, flexible tubes that travel from the nose to the stomach or intestines. They're used for food intake or fluid administration in patients who can't consume sufficient amounts of food or water by mouth, and they're used for medication infusion. Those who use such devices might include patients with a history of cancer, gastric bypass surgery, or stroke. Many complications can occur, including:
  - The tube can become displaced, causing the patient to aspirate fluid into the lungs. A dislodged tube can actually go into the lungs. Suspect either of these if the patient begins coughing or choking, is unable to speak, or air bubbles appear when the proximal end of the tube is placed in water.
  - The walls of the tube are typically thin and can easily develop a small leak.
  - An occlusion can form if the tube is not irrigated sufficiently after food or medication administration.

  If any abnormalities occur, use of the tube should be discontinued.
- **Transabdominal feeding tubes.** Transabdominal feeding tubes are tubes placed surgically to provide a route for direct feeding into the stomach (gastrostomy tube; see illustrations), jejunum (jejunostomy tube), or both (gastrojejunostomy tube). They are used when food, fluid, or medication must be administered for a longer term than would be suitable for a nasally placed tube.

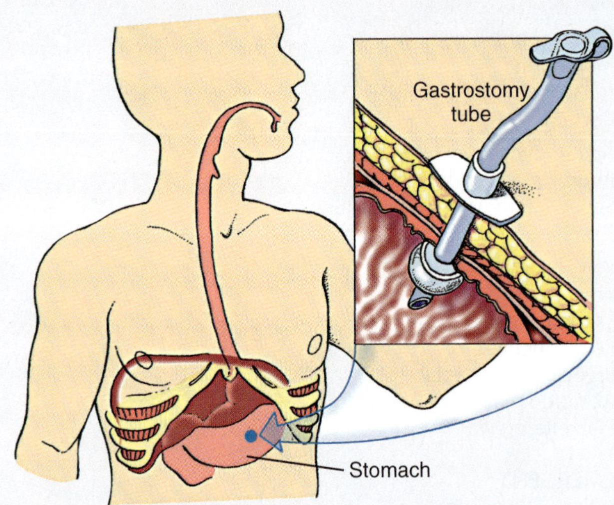

A gastrostomy tube is surgically placed into the stomach through the abdominal wall. (From American College of Emergency Physicians, Pons P, Carson D, editors: Paramedic field care: a complaint-based approach, St Louis, 1997, Mosby.)

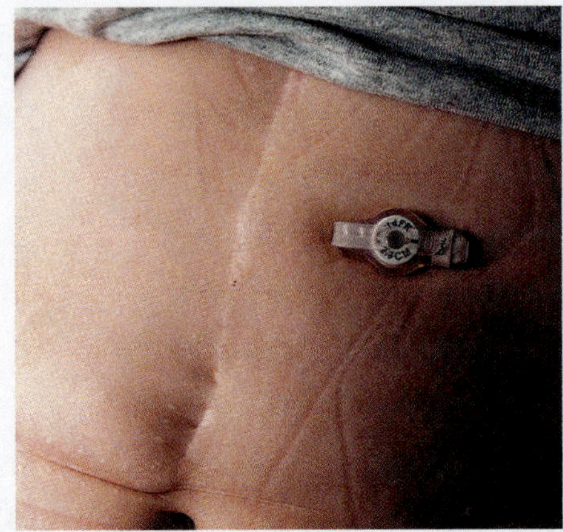

Gastrostomy button. (From Chaudhry B, Harvey D: Mosby's color atlas and text of pediatrics and child health, London, 2001, Mosby.)

BOX 7-1 Home Medical Devices Used by Patients with Abdominal Disorders—*Cont'd*

Transabdominal feeding tubes are often used in patients who have difficulty swallowing, esophageal atresia, esophageal burns or strictures, chronic malabsorption, or severe failure to thrive. Potential complications include:

- The stoma site can become infected. Look for drainage at the site and redness and inflammation of the surrounding skin.
- Leakage from the stoma can occur if the tube is too small.
- The feeding tube can become occluded or dislodged.
- The patient can develop peritonitis or gastric or colonic perforation.

If any abnormalities are apparent, feedings should be discontinued.

- **Bowel ostomy.** A bowel ostomy is a surgically created opening to eliminate waste from the bowel. It can be placed temporarily or permanently in patients with congenital bowel abnormalities, cancer, severe Crohn's disease, ulcerative colitis, or abdominal trauma. Any portion of the intestine can be rerouted through the abdominal wall. If the intestinal opening is closer to the stomach in the ileum, the patient is likely to have diarrhea, since stools cannot be formed. A bag placed over the ostomy to collect waste must be emptied regularly to minimize tissue degradation caused by prolonged contact with stool.
- **Hemodialysis access devices.** Hemodialysis is the process of passing the patient's blood through a machine called a *dialyzer* to remove waste products and stabilize the patient's fluid and electrolyte balance. Multiple sites and devices are used to gain vascular access so the blood can be cleaned and returned to the body during dialysis:
  - A shunt is a temporary synthetic connection between an artery and a vein.
  - A fistula is a permanent surgical connection between an artery and a vein.
  - A catheter placed in the subclavian artery may also be used to gain vascular access.
  - A button-shaped port (Hemasite) may be placed at the entry site.

Assess for a thrill or bruit to verify the patency of a shunt or fistula, which is usually found in the arm but may be located in the leg. It's important not to take blood pressure in the extremities when a shunt or fistula is in place.

- Peritoneal dialysis access devices. A peritoneal dialysis access device is a catheter that allows fluids to be infused into and then drained out of the abdomen. This process removes waste products and temporarily stabilizes the electrolyte and fluid balance.

BOX 7-2 Initial Assessment of Abdominal Complaints

- Follow Standard Precautions. Bleeding, nausea, and vomiting are hazards associated with abdominal pain and require you to use personal protective equipment to shield yourself from exposure to body fluids.
- What complaint was reported? Is the chief complaint associated with abdominal discomfort such as nausea, vomiting, or diarrhea? If so, use these signs and symptoms to rule out the conditions most likely to destabilize the patient, and progress to non–life-threatening signs and symptoms.
- Use your senses. You can glean a great deal of information from keen observation using your eyes, ears, and even your sense of smell:
  - How does the scene appear? Is the house clean? Do dirty bottles, dishes, or other items suggest a diagnosis such as gastroenteritis or food poisoning?
  - What does the patient look like? Is the skin color normal, or is the patient pale (suggesting shock) or yellowish (jaundiced, suggesting liver involvement)?
  - Is the patient pacing or curled on her side on the bed? Assessing the patient's ambulation or posture should direct you to possible diagnoses.
  - What odors are present? The smell of a gastrointestinal bleed would direct you to a possible life threat.
  - Do you hear retching or vomiting? If so, assess for GI bleeding, and be prepared to treat the patient for shock associated with hemorrhage or dehydration.
- Does any of this information suggest the cause of the abdominal discomfort? If so, initiate appropriate interventions, and continue your assessment on the basis of your initial observations.

findings, and lab results. Considerations for the initial assessment of the patient with an abdominal complaint are listed in Box 7-2. For a detailed description of general initial assessment considerations, a look back at Chapter 1 will help you review. Laboratory parameters often measured in patients with abdominal complaints are summarized in Table 7-5.

Patient Presentation

The primary life threat associated with abdominal discomfort is shock caused by hemorrhage, dehydration, or sepsis, as in the following circumstances:

- Internal bleeding due to a ruptured aneurysm, GI bleeding, or ectopic pregnancy

TABLE 7-5 Laboratory Studies for the Diagnosis of Abdominal Complaints

Component or Parameter	Normal Values	Interpretation	Indications
Glucose	70–110 mg/dL	↑ Indicates DKA, steroid use, stress ↓ Indicates decreased reserves, increased insulin	All types of shock
Hemoglobin/ hematocrit	Hb in men: 14–18 g/dL (8.7–11.2 mmol/L) Hb in women: 12–16 g/dL (7.4–9.9 mmol/L) Hct in men: 42%–52% (0.42–0.52 SI) Hct in women: 37%–47% (0.37–0.47 SI)	↓ Indicates severe blood loss ↑ Indicates plasma loss, dehydration	All types of shock
Gastric/stool hemoglobin	Negative	Positive indicates GI bleeding	Suspected GI bleeding
Lactic acid	Venous: 5–20 mg/dL (0.6–2.2 mmol/L)	↑ Indicates tissue hypoperfusion and acidosis, as occurs with prolonged use of a tourniquet	All types of shock
Complete blood cell count	Total white blood cell count 5000–10,000/mm^3 ($5–10 \times 10^9$/L)	↑ White blood cells indicates sepsis.	More important in septic shock
Arterial blood gases	pH 7.35–7.45 $PaCO_2$ 35–45 mm Hg PaO_2 80–100 mm Hg HCO_3 21–28 mEq/L	↑ pH indicates alkalosis. ↓ pH indicates acidosis, impaired perfusion. ↓ O_2 indicates hypoxia. ↓ HCO_3 indicates metabolic acidosis.	All types of shock
Serum electrolytes	Na 136–145 mEq/L (136–145 mmol/L) K 3.5–5 mEq/L (3.5–5 mmol/L)	↓ Na may be present with osmotic diuresis. ↓ K common with vomiting, diarrhea, diuretic use ↑ K common in acidosis, DKA High or low K may have an abnormal ECG.	All types of shock
Renal function	BUN 10–20 mg/dL (3.6–7.1 mmol/L) Creatinine W: 0.5–1.1 mg/dL M: 0.6–1.2 mg/dL (44–97 μmol/L)	↑ BUN indicates severe dehydration, shock, sepsis. ↑ Serum creatinine indicates impaired renal function.	All types of shock
Blood/urine cultures	Negative	Positive result indicates infection.	Septic shock
Bilirubin	Total: 0.3 mg/dL (5.1–17 μmol/L) Indirect: 0.2–0.8 mg/dL (3.4–12 μmol/L) Direct: 0.1–0.3 mg/dL (1.7–5.1 μmol/L)	↑ Indicates liver dysfunction and jaundice, gallstones, liver metastases, large-volume transfusion, hepatitis, sepsis, cirrhosis, sickle cell anemia. Can also be caused by certain drugs, such as allopurinol, anabolic steroids, dextran, diuretics, and many others.	Septic shock
Alkaline phosphatase	30–120 units/L (0.5–2 μmol/L)	↑ Can indicate cirrhosis, biliary obstruction, liver tumor, hyperparathyroidism	↓ Can indicate hypothyroidism, malnutrition, pernicious anemia, celiac disease, hypophosphatemia
Amylase	60–120 Somogyi units/dL (30–220 units/L)	↑ Can indicate pancreatitis, penetrating or perforated peptic ulcer, necrotic or perforated bowel, acute cholecystitis, ectopic pregnancy, DKA, duodenal obstruction	—
Ammonia	10–80 μg/dL (6–47 μmol/L)	↑ Indicates hepatocellular disease, Reye syndrome, portal hypertension, GI bleeding or obstruction with mild liver disease, hepatic encephalopathy or coma, genetic metabolic disorder	—

BUN, Blood urea nitrogen; *DKA*, diabetic ketoacidosis; *GI*, gastrointestinal; *Hb*, hemoglobin; *HCO_3*, bicarbonate; *Hct*, hematocrit; *K*, potassium, *Na*, sodium; *$PaCO_2$*, partial pressure of carbon dioxide; *PaO_2*, partial pressure of oxygen.

- Dehydration caused by vomiting or diarrhea from a wide range of causes
- Sepsis secondary to a ruptured appendix, an infection from an indwelling catheter, or perforated bowel

Once you have addressed airway, breathing, and circulation, begin to narrow down your list of potential diagnoses, and continue your assessment. The patient presentation will dictate your next actions. If you have the resources to perform a more detailed assessment as you stabilize the patient, then do so, but further assessment should not preclude stabilization of airway, breathing, and circulation.

Addressing Life Threats

Diagnosis of specific causes of abdominal pain is complex even with the most advanced laboratory and radiologic techniques. The fundamental determination you must make in the field is whether the patient's condition is life threatening, as evidenced by abnormal vital signs or respiratory distress. Patients who exhibit either one must be rapidly treated and transported to an appropriate facility. Management of life-threatening abdominal complaints is reviewed in Box 7-3. Table 7-6 outlines selected abdominal disorders with emergent presentations, including their treatment in the field and in the hospital. Table 7-7 summarizes radiologic studies used to diagnose abdominal disorders.

Gathering the Patient History

Gathering an accurate, detailed history is essential with any patient but especially important when attending those with GI complaints. It can be challenging to obtain useful information, but keeping in mind the SAMPLER mnemonic will help you remember to ask the right questions (see the Rapid Recall box in Chapter 1). Demonstrating patience and taking a genuine interest in the patient will improve your rapport with him or her. Box 7-4 includes a list of points to consider as you care for a patient with abdominal discomfort. Table 7-8 lists clinical signs associated with selected abdominal disorders. Any abdominal complaint should also prompt you to ask about appetite, bowel regimen, urine, menstrual history, and discharge from reproductive organs as you gather the patient's history.

Pain Assessment

In evaluating GI complaints, your assessment must include a detailed appraisal of the patient's pain. Abdominal pain is often diffuse and difficult to categorize, and documenting it methodically can help you reach a refined diagnosis. The initial task is to ascertain the origin of the pain and determine its referral sites (Figure 7-5; also see Figures 7-3 and 7-4). Knowing the time of onset will help you assess how the pain has evolved, which may indicate the severity of the illness. Be alert for any signs that typically accompany pain, such as vomiting. For signs associated with selected abdominal pain syndromes, see Table 7-4.

Document pain in the patient's own words, since they may be more revealing than the words a healthcare professional might use. Open-ended questions—What does your pain feel like? Can you describe your pain?—encourage candid disclosure. Answers may range from "It hurts" to

BOX 7-3 Management of Life-Threatening Abdominal Complaints

When a patient has abdominal discomfort with abnormal vital signs, follow these steps for effective management:

- Ensure scene safety.
- Follow Standard Precautions, including use of a mask, gown, gloves, and protective eyewear, as indicated.
- Manage the airway as necessary using appropriate basic life support techniques. Maintain the patient's oxygen saturation at >95% by administering additional oxygen through a nonrebreather mask or by assisting ventilation as necessary.
- Apply a cardiac monitor (consistent with your level of training), and consider placing a 12-lead ECG if appropriate.
- Control obvious hemorrhage. Use gastric suctioning if indicated.
- Establish IV access and administer crystalloid fluid. Use care, however, since aggressive fluid administration can dilute the concentration of red blood cells and impede clot formation if bleeding is present. Blood pressure should be maintained at a level vigorous enough to perfuse vital organs. Use a target systolic pressure of 80–90 mm Hg. Use mental status as a gauge to assess whether perfusion is adequate.
- Administer medications per local protocol.
- Monitor the patient closely, and reassess frequently to determine the response.
- Be prepared to administer blood products if the patient shows evidence of uncontrolled bleeding or an inability to maintain adequate perfusion.
- Consider placing a Foley catheter.
- A nasogastric tube should be placed if GI bleeding is suspected. Although an aspirate that does not contain blood does not conclusively rule out upper GI bleeding, placement is still necessary. The majority of the patients require only supportive care.
- At the hospital, specific laboratory tests performed will include a complete blood count (hematocrit, coagulation studies, BUN, creatine, electrolytes, glucose, liver function tests, and type and cross-match). Imaging studies will include CT and perhaps endoscopy. For a critically ill patient, however, resuscitation takes precedence.

TABLE 7-6 Differential Diagnosis of Abdominal Disorders with Emergent Presentations

Disorder	Causes	History	Findings	Prehospital Treatment	Hospital Testing/Treatment
Mesenteric ischemia	Myocardial infarction, valvular heart disease, arrhythmia, peripheral vascular disease, hypercoagulability, oral contraceptive use, aortic dissection, trauma	Acute onset of severe midabdominal pain, nausea, vomiting, and diarrhea	Severe midabdominal pain, nausea, vomiting, diarrhea Pain out of proportion to tenderness	Administer oxygen. Place patient in a comfortable position. Establish IV access.	Surgical consult
Intestinal obstruction	Obstruction can be due to stool, foreign body, intussusception, adhesions, polyps, volvulus, tumors, ulcerative colitis, or diverticulitis	Abrupt onset: suspect small-bowel obstruction Onset over 1–2 days: suspect distal obstruction History of bowel obstruction, abdominal surgery, cancer, radiation therapy, chemotherapy, hernia, or abdominal illness	Crampy abdominal pain, constipation, diarrhea, inability to pass flatus, distended abdomen Absent or high-pitched bowel sounds	Administer oxygen. Place patient in a comfortable position. Establish IV access. Give nothing by mouth.	Laboratory and x-ray to determine location and extent of obstruction
Perforated viscus	Peptic ulcer disease, diverticula, trauma, use of NSAIDs, advancing age	Acute onset of epigastric pain Vomiting	Epigastric pain, vomiting, fever, shock, sepsis Elevated WBCs and amylase	Administer oxygen. Place patient in a comfortable position. Establish IV access. Give nothing by mouth.	Laboratory, x-ray, and CT to determine location and extent of perforation
Acute pancreatitis	Alcohol, cholelithiasis, trauma, infection, inflammation	Alcohol use, use of certain drugs, recent trauma, cholelithiasis	Midepigastric abdominal pain, low-grade fever, nausea, vomiting	Place patient in a comfortable position. Establish IV access. Give nothing by mouth.	Amylase/lipase levels and CT
Ruptured appendix	Obstruction, infection	Initially patient feels diffuse pain, especially in umbilical area. Later, pain settles in the right lower quadrant or lower back.	Nausea, vomiting, fever, positive Rovsing's sign	Place patient in a comfortable position. Establish IV access. Give nothing by mouth.	Laboratory, CT/ultrasound, antibiotics, and surgical consult

CT, Computed tomography; *IV,* intravenous; *NSAIDs,* nonsteroidal antiinflammatory drugs; *WBCs,* white blood cells.

TABLE 7-7 Radiologic Studies for the Diagnosis of Abdominal Disorders

Test	Description	Indications	Advantages and Disadvantages
Plain-film x-ray	An upright abdominal film displays air-fluid levels. A supine abdominal film detects fluid or blood in the peritoneum or gas in bowel.	First test typically performed Can show free air, small-bowel obstruction, bowel ischemia, and foreign bodies	Inexpensive Easy to perform Causes minimal discomfort
Computed tomography (CT)	Images solid organs to detect scarring, tumors, metastasized cancers	First test performed for suspected diverticulitis, pancreatitis, appendicitis, aortic aneurysm, blunt trauma, and pancreatic cyst	Unlike x-ray, a good image can be obtained no matter what the level of air or gas in the bowel Rapid test Causes minimal discomfort Not available 24 hours a day at some hospitals
Ultrasonography	Reflects and refracts sound waves as they strike fluid, air, and solid tissues in the body, allowing imaging of organs, tissues, and body cavities	First test performed for right upper quadrant pain Can detect cholelithiasis, cholecystitis, pancreatic masses, and biliary duct dilation Used in trauma when abdominal injury is suspected	Noninvasive and inexpensive Can be performed at the bedside Accurate reading depends on operator skill

BOX 7-4 Selected System Considerations for Assessment of Abdominal Complaints

System	History, Differential Diagnosis, and Other Assessment Considerations
Neurologic	Ask about recent accidents or trauma, particularly if the patient has an altered level of consciousness or nausea and vomiting.
Respiratory	Explore any evidence of breathing problems. Pneumonia may be associated with upper abdominal discomfort. Esophageal ruptures may present with respiratory signs and symptoms.
Cardiovascular	Indigestion and upper abdominal discomfort should prompt you to evaluate the patient for acute coronary syndrome.
Gastrointestinal, genitourinary, and reproductive	Explore any history of chronic or acute diagnoses. Question the patient about any changes in eating, bowel, or urinary habits that may suggest a diagnosis. Vaginal discharge, bleeding, and menstrual changes suggest specific disease processes.
Musculoskeletal and skin	Observe the skin for pallor, jaundice, uremia, and other changes that may suggest the cause of abdominal pain. Look for any scars, ostomies, or external devices (such as drains, tubes, and pumps) that may indicate the cause of the patient's abdominal symptoms.
Endocrine, metabolic, and environmental	Collect past medical history. Assess blood glucose. Assess the scene or thoroughly question the patient, family, and bystanders if you are unable to observe the conditions to which the patient was subjected.
Infectious disease and hematologic	The patient's history, a foul smell, and the presence of a Foley catheter or other invasive drain may point to an infectious process. Take the patient's temperature to evaluate for fever. Assess the patient for damage to the bowel, which is associated with peritonitis and possibly sepsis. Analyze lab values that may be useful in making a hematologic diagnosis, such as white blood cell count, hemoglobin and hematocrit, prothrombin time, and partial thromboplastin time.
Toxicologic (nuclear, biological, and chemical)	Explore exposure problems. Many toxidromes have a GI component. Being familiar with a range of toxidromes and maintaining a high index of suspicion will prevent your overlooking them in your differential diagnosis.

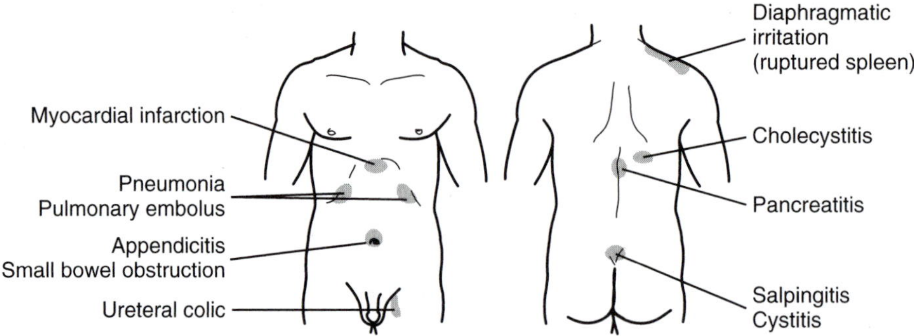

Figure 7-5 Referred pain patterns. Pain or discomfort in these areas often provide clues to underlying disease processes. (From Hamilton GC, Sanders AB, Trott AT, et al: Emergency medicine: an approach to clinical problem solving, ed 2, Philadelphia, 2002, Saunders.)

TABLE 7-8 Clinical Signs Associated with Selected Abdominal Disorders

Sign	Description	Differential Diagnosis
Hematemesis	Blood in vomitus	Upper GI bleeding
Coffee-ground emesis	Vomiting of partially digested blood	GI bleeding
Feculent vomiting	Foul-smelling vomit with a feculent odor	Bowel obstruction
Hematochezia	Red blood passed through the rectum	Lower GI bleeding
Melena	Black, tarry stool that contains digested blood	Upper GI bleeding
Hemoccult blood in stool	Laboratory identification of blood in the stool that's not obvious to the naked eye	Lower GI bleeding
White stools	White, chalky stool	Liver or gallbladder disease
Hematuria	Blood in the urine	Bladder infection Kidney disease Trauma

GI, Gastrointestinal.

"It feels like I'm being shredded apart." If the person is unable to describe the pain at all, offer a few key prompts: is it sharp, tearing, hot, burning, dull? Ask what activities or movements worsen or improve the pain, noting any home remedies or corrective measures that were attempted even if they were ineffective.

Using a pain scale allows you to compare the patient's pain over time. People have widely disparate levels of pain tolerance depending on cultural norms and their own pain thresholds. If each of us could experience identical pain, no doubt we would individually perceive it very differently. So the best use of a pain scale is not in determining the severity of pain, which is largely subjective, but in tracking any improvements or worrisome trends. Ask the patient frequently to reassess the pain, taking care to document the response, and trust the patient's statements about his or her symptoms.

Physical Assessment

One of the primary goals of the overall assessment of an abdominal complaint is to determine whether the patient will require surgery. (You may wish to review the comprehensive patient assessment in Chapter 1.) Note the patient's general appearance. Observing the level of consciousness (LOC) and color, temperature, and moisture level of the skin can help you gauge the severity of the problem. Patients who are confused, pale, and diaphoretic are more critically ill than others. Pain causes some patients to pace and show other signs of agitation. Again, once the airway, breathing, and circulation have been secured, you can carry out an examination more specific to the abdominal complaint.

Analysis of the patient's vital signs is critical to making a reliable diagnosis. Fever, for instance, tips you off that an infection may be present; typically, a temperature of 100.3°F (38°C) or greater is considered significant. This rule does not apply, however, to older adults or to patients with compromised immune systems. In such patients, a serious infection may be present even if the patient's body temperature is normal. Low blood pressure and a rapid heart rate can point to hypovolemia. The heart rate may accelerate as body temperature rises, except in patients who take beta-blockers, since such agents reduce the heart rate. An elevated respiratory rate can be a red flag portending serious illness such as pneumonia, myocardial infarction, sepsis, or hypoperfusion.

To obtain an adequate, effective physical examination, you must be systematic and thorough. Being subjected to an examination, though, can be a difficult experience for the patient. No one likes to be poked and prodded, but discomfort or unpleasantness is magnified in the face of the anxiety often associated with illness and injury. An already uncomfortable patient may worry that the exam will be painful. Preparing the patient by explaining the procedure first may diminish uncertainty and improve cooperation.

Physical examination skills include inspection, auscultation, percussion, and palpation. Let's discuss them briefly. (See Chapter 1 for a more detailed discussion of each skill.)

Inspection Examination of the abdomen should always begin with inspection, since any palpation can alter the abdomen's general appearance and perhaps provoke the patient's pain, after which further palpation may be hampered by guarding. Look for distention, pulsation, ecchymosis, asymmetry, pregnancy, scars, masses, and anything else unusual.

Auscultation Auscultation is the second step in the general physical examination. Palpating the abdomen before listening to it can alter the findings by stirring bowel sounds. If time and circumstances allow, auscultate each quadrant of the abdomen for about 30 seconds. Normal bowel sounds sound like water gurgling. Without experience, it's difficult to tell whether these sounds are normal or abnormal. Hyperactive bowel sounds may signal gastroenteritis or early bowel obstruction. Hypoactive or silent bowel sounds in one quadrant can indicate an ileus. It may be impossible, however, to hear abdominal sounds in a noisy environment like the back of an ambulance. To thoroughly assess bowel sounds, an extended auscultation time period of up to 2 to 5 minutes in each quadrant is required. Since this is usually impractical in the field, a shortened time is often used, or the sounds are not auscultated at all. If this shortened auscultation is used, it doesn't mean bowel sounds are absent, but just not heard at this time.

Percussion Abdominal percussion indicates whether certain areas contain more gas or liquid. Borders of organs and masses may also be determined using percussion. Like auscultation, percussion requires practice. Before you perform any palpation or percussion of the abdomen, make sure the patient understands what you're doing. The procedure is easier for the patient to tolerate and produces less anxiety if you begin with the unaffected side and then progress to the areas of discomfort. Pain and tenderness may present with percussion and should be noted.

Palpation It's important that the patient be relaxed during palpation, since abdominal rigidity and guarding caused by anxiety can make the findings less reliable. Encourage your patient to relax. During palpation of each quadrant, watch the reaction on the patient's face, and ask how it feels. Ideally, the patient will be distracted, and you can watch for signs of discomfort. Grimacing or tears may reveal more than verbal complaints. Attempt to elicit differences in pain before, during, and after palpation. Pain when the pressure is released, known as *rebound tenderness,* is a classic sign of peritoneal irritation, but it's present in up to 25% of patients with nonspecific abdominal complaints. In some areas, clinicians may be discouraged in eliciting rebound tenderness, as the patient may be resistant to further abdominal assessment. Tapping on the heel or coughing may elicit similar pain. Each of these activities jars or stimulates the irritated peritoneum and can help to isolate the pain.

Causes of Abdominal Discomfort

The causes of abdominal discomfort can have origins in any system of the human body. The severity of a given illness can range from innocuous to dire, yet limited treatment is available in the field. It's essential to identify patients who are critically ill as soon as possible. Recognizing that a patient is critically ill does not require advanced diagnostic equipment.

Upper Gastrointestinal or Esophageal Bleeding

Acute upper GI bleeding has a fairly high incidence, affecting 50 to 150 people per 100,000 population and leading to 250,000 admissions per year. Men and persons of advanced age are at much higher risk for the disorder. Lower GI bleeding is less common overall but has a higher incidence among women.

When assessing abdominal bleeding, you must ascertain whether the bleeding stems from an acute or chronic condition. Did the bleeding and pain begin suddenly, or did it have a delayed onset? Acute-onset GI bleeding is characterized by massive sudden hemorrhage and signs of hypovolemic shock. Chronic bleeding is more common in older adult patients and in those with chronic conditions such as renal failure. Fatigue and weakness will gradually exhaust the patient, and blood will appear in the stool. If the bleeding lasts long enough, signs of anemia may become evident. There are several questions specific to GI bleeding complaints (Box 7-5). Even if the patient does not complain of pain, the OPQRST mnemonic is helpful (see the Rapid Recall box in Chapter 1).

Many patients do report bleeding, but others have more ambiguous initial signs and symptoms such as tachycardia, syncope, hypotension, angina, weakness, confusion, or cardiac arrest. Taking a good history may be the only way to determine the cause of such complaints.

The possible causes of an upper GI bleed are extensive and include peptic ulcer disease, erosive gastritis and esophagitis, esophageal and gastric varices, and Mallory-Weiss syndrome. Factors that heighten the risk of mortality include hemodynamic instability, repeated **hematemesis** or **hematochezia,** failure to clear blood despite gastric lavage, age older than 60, and existence of an additional organ system disease, such as cardiovascular or pulmonary disease.

BOX 7-5 Gastrointestinal Bleeding

Onset	What was the onset of the bleeding? Was it gradual or sudden?
Provocation/palliation	Does anything make it better or worse? Has anything caused an increase—for example, vomiting?
Quality	What does it look like? What color is it? How much are you bleeding?
Region	From where are you bleeding? Question about upper and lower GI bleeds.
Severity	On a scale of 0–10, how do you rank the bleeding? Is it increasing or decreasing in severity?
Timing	How long have the symptoms been present? Are they continuous or intermittent?

TABLE 7-9 Antiulcer Drugs

Antisecretory Agents	Specific Drugs	Mechanism of Action
H_2 receptor antagonists	cimetidine (Tagamet) famotidine (Pepcid) nizatidine (Axid) ranitidine (Zantac)	Suppress acid secretion by blocking H_2 receptors on parietal cells
Proton-pump inhibitors	esomeprazole (Nexium) lansoprazole (Prevacid) omeprazole (Prilosec, Zegerid) pantoprazole (Protonix) rabeprazole (AcipHex)	Suppress acid secretion by inhibiting H, K-ATPase
Muscarinic antagonists	pirenzepine (Gastrozepin)	Suppress acid secretion by blocking muscarinic cholinergic receptors
Mucosal protectants	sucralfate (Carafate)	Form a barrier over ulcer

H, K-ATPase, Hydrogen, potassium, adenosine triphosphatase; *H_2,* histamine-2.

Peptic Ulcer Disease

Peptic ulcer disease affects about 5 million people in the United States and is the most common cause of GI bleeding, representing about 60% of cases. *Helicobacter pylori* has been found to be the cause of 60% to 70% of peptic ulcers over the last decade, so peptic ulcer is no longer considered a chronic disease.

Duodenal, gastric, and stomal ulcers are all types of peptic ulcer disease. Because the gastric mucosa secretes hydrochloric acid and pepsinogen, the stomach is an acidic environment. This acidity is necessary for the proper digestion of protein. A delicate balance is maintained by secretion of sodium bicarbonate in the duodenum. Peptic ulcers form when this balance is upset and the acidic environment is allowed to predominate. A few of the factors that may irritate or contribute to ulcers include nonsteroidal antiinflammatory drugs (NSAIDs), smoking, excessive alcohol ingestion, and stress.

Bleeding in peptic ulcer disease can be severe, and initial treatment calls for stabilization of life threats. Observe the patient for signs of shock, pallor, hypotension, and tachycardia, which should be quickly documented and treated. In rare incidents, the ulcer perforates (eats through the lining of the stomach or bowel), causing severe pain and a rigid, board-like abdomen. Swelling of the ulcerated tissue may cause an acute obstruction. As part of the history, ask about previous ulcers, whether the pain of the ulcer occurs prior to or after eating, and previous episodes of bleeding.

After you stabilize the patient, initiate proton pump inhibitors if the patient is not already taking them. Proton pump inhibitors (PPIs) diminish bleeding by reducing the amount of acid in the stomach. These medications can be given as an intravenous (IV) bolus followed by an IV drip. For more chronic treatment, in addition to PPIs, the patient should avoid NSAIDs, since their prostaglandin inhibition can cause gastric and duodenal ulcers by hindering blood flow to the submucosa, minimizing the secretion of mucus, bicarbonate, and gastric acid. Patients should also avoid aspirin, caffeine, and alcohol. Treatment of documented *H. pylori* infection with antibiotics has been shown to promote healing and diminish the chance of recurrence, whereas smoking exacerbates the disease and slows healing time. In order to treat the *H. pylori* infection, a combination of antibiotics may be required. Antiulcer drugs are used to suppress acid secretion and to form a barrier over the ulcer. These medications are summarized in Table 7-9.

Erosive Gastritis and Esophagitis

Erosive gastritis and esophagitis, as its name suggests, is due to erosion and inflammation of the gastric and esophageal mucosa. The condition can have an acute or chronic onset, and its potential causes are numerous. Nonspecific causes include alcohol, NSAIDs, corrosives, and radiation.

Erosive gastritis and esophagitis typically causes less bleeding than peptic ulcer disease, and the condition is self-limiting. The chief signs and symptoms include indigestion, heartburn, dyspepsia, and belching. A few patients also have nausea and vomiting. The severity of symptoms does not accurately indicate the severity of the lesions.

Little can be done for this condition in the prehospital setting. Maintain airway, breathing, and circulation, and offer comfort measures such as proper positioning, analgesics, and antiemetics. Gastric lavage can be performed to assess for active bleeding. If the patient has no active bleeding, a mixture of viscous lidocaine and an antacid may provide relief. For long-term care, as with peptic ulcer disease, the patient may be placed on a PPI and should be advised to avoid aspirin, NSAIDs, caffeine, and alcohol.

Esophageal and Gastric Varices

Esophageal and gastric varices are veins that have become dilated as a result of mounting pressure that damages the veins and weakens the venous structure. Varices occur when blood flow through the liver is restricted (portal hypertension). This causes the blood to back up into the veins in the wall of the esophagus, causing the vessels to dilate. Portal hypertension, most often associated with chronic excessive alcohol use, is the most common cause of the increasing pressure. Varices are typically asymptomatic until they rupture and bleed, causing massive blood loss. Patients who have bled from their varices have a 70% chance of bleeding again. If they do bleed a second time, 30% of the cases result in death.

Treatment centers on controlling bleeding by promoting clot formation. If hemorrhage is uncontrolled, balloon tamponade may be performed using a Sengstaken-Blakemore tube to apply pressure directly to the bleeding varices. This is a temporary solution that requires frequent monitoring. Pressure within the two balloons must be maintained at appropriate levels in order to apply the proper amount of pressure to the varices. Tension of 1 to 3 lb is applied to the tube by connecting it to a helmet the patient wears. Low intermittent suction is connected to both the gastric and esophageal ports (Figure 7-6). The patient must be intubated before this procedure is performed. If transportation to another facility is necessary, special precautions should be taken to protect the patient from changes in barometric pressure at higher elevations or during flight. Typically the balloons are deflated within 24 hours to diminish the risk of necrosis, but occasionally they are left in place for up to 72 hours.

Endoscopy may be performed to inject a sclerosing agent (a strong irritating solution) to promote clot formation, a procedure known as *sclerotherapy*. Octreotide may be administered, but its effectiveness for variceal bleeding is limited. Vasopressin infusion is an additional pharmacologic option. Another option to promote clot formation is band therapy using rubber bands on the varices. Varices resemble polyps, and banding can prevent bleeding (Figure 7-7).

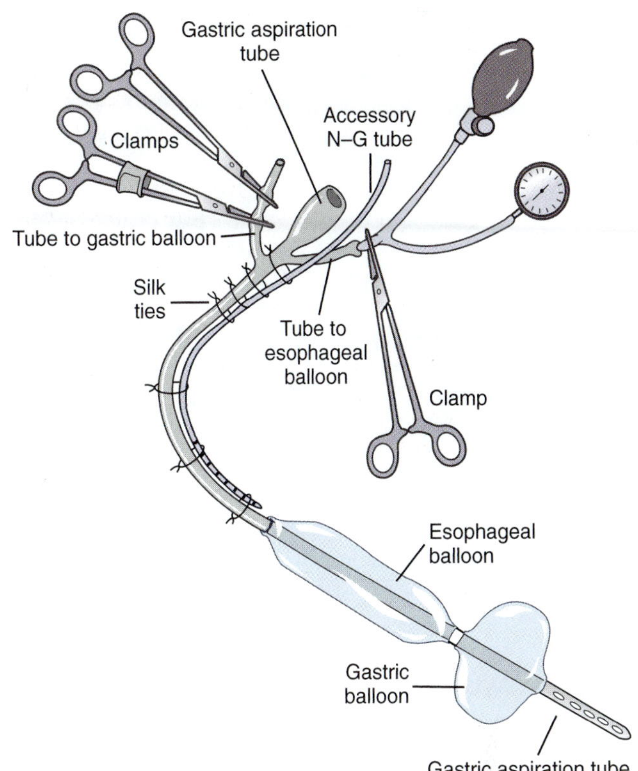

■ **Figure 7-6** Modified Sengstaken-Blakemore tube. Note accessory nasogastric (NG) tube for suctioning of secretions above esophageal balloon, and two clamps (one secured with tape) to prevent inadvertent decompression of gastric balloon. (From Townsend CM, Beauchamp RD, Evers BM, et al: Sabiston textbook of surgery: the biological basis of modern surgical practice, ed 18, Philadelphia, 2007, Saunders.)

Mallory-Weiss Syndrome

Mallory-Weiss syndrome is a form of GI bleeding stemming from longitudinal tears of the mucosa at the gastroesophageal junction, primarily at the level of the stomach. Severe, protracted vomiting can cause the tears, which then lead to arterial bleeding. This can range in severity from mild and self-limited to severe and life threatening. In serious cases, more vomiting is triggered as the person swallows blood. The initial symptom is often the severe bleeding itself; hematemesis occurs in 85% of patients with Mallory-Weiss syndrome. Aspirin use, excessive alcohol use, and bulimia (an eating disorder associated with episodes of binge eating followed by self-induced vomiting) are associated with the syndrome as well. The mortality rate is less than 10%.

Primary management is supportive, since the bleeding usually resolves spontaneously. Gastric lavage should be performed until the bleeding has ceased. If it continues, endoscopy may be necessary. If the patient is still nauseated or vomiting, antiemetics should be considered. If the bleeding cannot be controlled, the patient must be hospitalized.

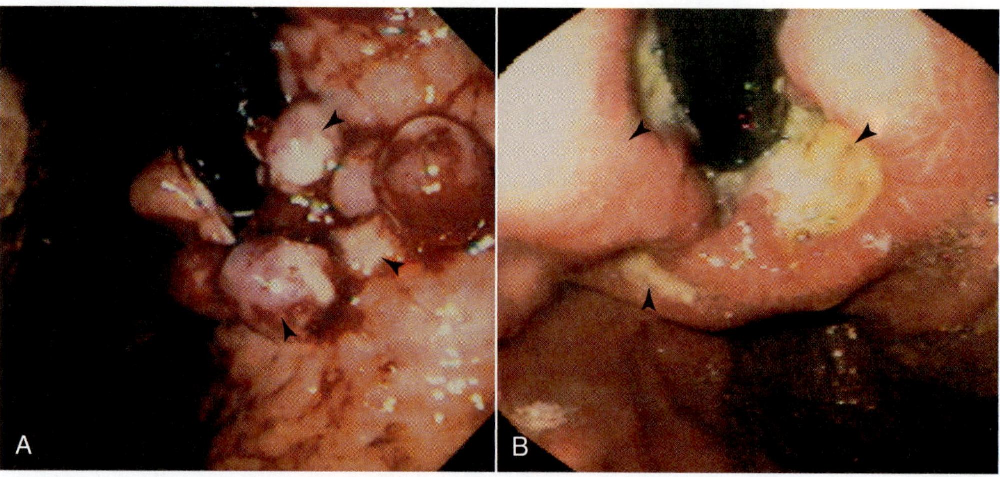

■ **Figure 7-7** Endoscopic view of variceal ligation–related ulcers. **A**, Gastroesophageal junction is seen on a retroflexed view following ligation of multiple gastric varices *(arrowheads)*, which resemble polyps. **B**, Upper endoscopy in same patient 4 weeks later demonstrates multiple ulcers at sites of prior ligation *(arrowheads)*. (From Feldman M, Friedman LS, Brandt LJ: Sleisenger & Fordtran's gastrointestinal and liver disease pathophysiology/diagnosis/management, Philadelphia, 2006, Saunders.)

Perforated Viscus

A perforated or ruptured **viscus** (*pl.* **viscera**) is an emergent event. It often occurs when a duodenal ulcer erodes the serosa (the outermost layer of the bowel). Peritonitis ensues when the intestinal contents spill into the abdominal cavity. As the time between perforation and diagnosis lengthens, the mortality rate climbs. Rupture of the large intestine, small intestine, colonic diverticula, or gallbladder is possible but constitutes a rare event. Risk factors include advanced age, diverticular disease, use of NSAIDs, and a history of peptic ulcer disease.

Perforation usually causes an acute onset of epigastric pain; however, older adult patients may not have significant pain. The pain may be diffuse, with guarding and rebound tenderness. A rigid abdomen is a late sign. About half of patients have vomiting. A low-grade fever, attributable to the peritonitis, may also be a late sign. Bowel sounds are diminished, tachycardia is common, and shock may develop with massive bleeding and sepsis. Establishment of IV access and support of airway, breathing, and circulation are essential.

In the emergency department (ED), preoperative labs and diagnostic imaging should be performed. An elevated white blood cell count may be seen due to the peritonitis. In 70% to 80% of patients, an upright x-ray will show free air if an ulcer perforates. Computed tomography (CT) will reveal more information about the extent of the perforation.

Boerhaave's Syndrome

Boerhaave's syndrome is a spontaneous rupture of the esophagus as a consequence of hyperemesis gravidarum, childbirth, violent coughing, seizures, status asthmaticus, weight lifting, certain neurologic disorders, or explosive vomiting after overindulgence in food and drink. The patient typically has diffuse, severe, distracting pain in the chest, neck, back, and abdomen, as well as difficulty breathing, tachycardia, vomiting blood, and fever. If the rupture occurs in the neck, subcutaneous emphysema may be present. Assist oxygenation, and prepare the patient for immediate surgery, since the mortality rate is as high as 50% without early surgical intervention.

Acute Pancreatitis

Diabetes is the most common disorder related to the pancreas, but pancreatitis is also common. Acute pancreatitis is an inflammatory process in which premature activation of pancreatic enzymes causes the pancreas to begin to digest itself, resulting in pain and necrosis as the inflammation spreads. The disease is thought to be caused by cholelithiasis or alcohol abuse in more than 90% of cases. Alcoholic pancreatitis is more common in men between the ages of 35 and 45. Urban EDs tend to be more familiar with the condition. In addition, certain medications, such as amiodarone (an antidysrhythmic), carbamazepine (an antiseizure medication), metronidazole (an antifungal), and quinolones (a class of antibiotics), can cause drug-induced pancreatitis.

The typical patient has constant, severe midepigastric pain that radiates to the back. It is generally not exacerbated by eating. Cullen sign, a blue discoloration around the umbilicus, and Grey Turner sign, a blue discoloration around the flanks, may be present. Other symptoms may include low-grade fever, nausea, and vomiting. A systemic inflammatory response can develop, leading to shock and multiorgan failure.

Definitive diagnosis can be made only in pathologic analysis. CT, serum amylase, and lipase can assist in the diagnosis. No single laboratory test can diagnose pancreatitis, but lipase is thought to be more sensitive and specific than amylase. Amylase is less sensitive 36 hours after the onset of pain, since it stays elevated for only a short time. Lipase, on the other hand, is more specific to the pancreas and stays elevated for several days.

Treat patients with known or suspected pancreatitis by establishing IV access, giving nothing by mouth, providing fluid resuscitation, and administering analgesics and antiemetics. If the patient is unable to tolerate oral fluids in the ED, he or she will most likely be admitted. Complications can include pancreatic hemorrhage or necrosis. The treatment of chronic pancreatitis is similar and is generally supportive.

Appendicitis

The appendix is a small tubular structure that lies adjacent to the colon near the cecum, and appendicitis is typically caused by an infection or the buildup of fluid. As the appendix becomes distended and inflamed, it may rupture, spilling toxins into the abdomen and touching off peritonitis. Bacteria can also enter the bloodstream, causing sepsis. Even if the appendix does not rupture, gangrene is a possibility and constitutes a surgical emergency. Despite a 7% incidence among the general population, there is no way of predicting who will develop appendicitis, although the condition is most common in persons aged 20 to 40.

Patients with appendicitis have pain localized to the right lower quadrant or right lower back. The pain classically begins in the periumbilical region, then becomes more localized in the right lower quadrant as inflammation worsens. Other signs and symptoms include fever, nausea and vomiting, and a positive psoas sign, which is quite specific to appendicitis. To assess for this sign, place the patient in the left lateral decubitus position and extend the right leg at the hip. Exacerbation of pain in the right lower quadrant is a positive psoas sign. Physical examination findings suggestive of other abdominal disorders are summarized in Table 7-10.

To treat a patient with suspected appendicitis, establish IV access, administer analgesics and antiemetics, and transport the patient in a comfortable position. At the receiving facility, a definitive diagnosis will be made using ultrasound or CT. Laboratory studies such as a complete blood cell count and a urinalysis will be evaluated. CT is the most useful study because it can also reveal an alternative diagnosis if the patient does not have appendicitis. In fact, use of CT has been shown to reduce the number of unnecessary appendectomies in women. If appendicitis is confirmed, surgery to remove the appendix is required. Prophylactic antibiotics will be given before surgery in case the appendix ruptures.

Young children, older adult patients, pregnant women, and patients who have human immunodeficiency virus/acquired immunodeficiency syndrome (HIV/AIDS) may have an abnormal presentation of appendicitis and be at higher risk of complications. In young children, the onset of appendicitis may be delayed and nonspecific. Misdiagnosis is common because of the limitations in communicating with preverbal patients and because of the atypical presentation. As you might expect, misdiagnosis elevates the risk of perforation. In patients older than 70, the rate of misdiagnosis is as high as 50%, and early rupture is common. Since appendicitis is the most common cause of extrauterine abdominal pain during pregnancy, it must be suspected with GI complaints in pregnant women. However, a gravid uterus makes appendicitis difficult to diagnose. Since it's preferable to avoid CT in pregnant women because of the radiation exposure, ultrasound or MRI can aid in diagnosis. Patients with HIV/AIDS have the same symptoms as other patients, but they have a much higher risk of complications. They are also more likely to delay seeking treatment for appendicitis because of the frequency of other GI problems.

Mesenteric Ischemia

Mesenteric ischemia is caused by an occlusion of the mesenteric artery or vein. Symptoms typically include an acute onset of nausea, vomiting, diarrhea, and severe

TABLE 7-10 Physical Examination Findings Associated with Selected Abdominal Disorders

Sign	Description	Implication
Cullen's sign	Discoloration or bruising around the umbilicus	Intraabdominal bleeding Pancreatitis
Kehr's sign	Abdominal pain that radiates to the left shoulder	Irritation of the diaphragm is often associated with spleen involvement.
Murphy's sign	Press firmly upward into right upper quadrant and ask patient to take a deep breath. Arrest of inspiration because of pain is a positive finding.	Commonly associated with gallbladder or hepatic involvement Suggestive of cholecystitis
Psoas sign	Place patient in the left lateral decubitus position, and extend the right leg at the hip. An increase of pain in the right lower quadrant is a positive finding.	Commonly associated with appendicitis
Rovsing's sign	Palpate the left lower quadrant of the abdomen. Pain or tenderness elicited in the right lower quadrant is a positive finding.	Suggests appendicitis

midabdominal pain that appears to be out of proportion to abdominal tenderness and physical findings.

The condition is more common in older adult patients and in those with a history of myocardial infarction, arrhythmia, valvular heart disease, or peripheral vascular disease. Use of oral contraceptives, hypercoagulability, aortic dissection, and trauma can also precipitate an ischemic event. No laboratory studies are specifically diagnostic, although elevated serum lactate can be a clue. Abnormal radiologic findings are a late sign, so you should suspect mesenteric ischemia in patients with other risk factors and no other cause for the abdominal pain. An angiogram should be performed. Newer-generation CT scanners offer improved resolution, and computed tomography angiography (CTA) of the abdomen will probably be the initial imaging choice. Mesenteric ischemia can progress to infarction if not identified early and may result in gangrenous bowel, perforation, and death.

Intestinal Obstruction

Intestinal obstruction is an emergent event in which stool, a foreign body, or a mechanical process obstructs passage of intestinal contents. Mounting pressure in the intestine diminishes blood flow, leading to septicemia and intestinal necrosis. The mortality rate rises dramatically as shock develops. Patients with a history of bowel obstruction, abdominal surgery, recent abdominal illness, cancer, radiation, chemotherapy, or hernia are at greater risk of developing an intestinal obstruction.

Patients with intestinal obstruction have nausea, vomiting, and abdominal pain. In addition, they may be unable to pass flatus (bowel gas) and may have constipation and a distended abdomen. The natural peristalsis of the intestines continues despite the obstruction, causing intermittent pain the patient may describe as being crampy or feeling like a knot. Mechanical causes of small-bowel obstruction are intussusception, adhesions, polyps, volvulus, and tumors. Gastric **volvulus**, a condition in which the stomach rotates more than 180 degrees, is a rare event that has been documented in only 400 cases in the United States. This twisting seals the stomach on both ends, blocking the flow of blood and the passage of fluid and food. The condition is characterized by an acute onset of abdominal pain, severe vomiting, and shock. The patient is likely to die in the absence of timely intervention.

Intussusception occurs when a portion of the bowel telescopes into an adjacent portion of the intestine, thereby occluding passage of intestinal contents and diminishing blood flow to the area. Intussusception accounts for 7% of all intestinal obstructions. The condition is more common in children than among adults. About 80% of intussusceptions in adults occur in the small intestine.

Large-bowel obstruction is less common than small-bowel obstruction because of the colon's greater diameter. When such an obstruction does develop, it's usually caused by cancer, fecal impaction, ulcerative colitis, volvulus, diverticulitis, or intussusception.

Any abdominal complaint should prompt you to ask about appetite and bowel regimen as you gather the patient's history. In a patient with an obstruction, auscultation of the bowel will reveal high-pitched or absent sounds. The sounds can be difficult to hear because sound may be referred from one portion of the abdomen to the other, so be sure to auscultate each quadrant for several minutes. Percussion may reveal a hollow sound. Palpation may provoke the pain, and a distended, firm abdomen indicates a severe obstruction.

It's impossible to make a definitive diagnosis of intestinal obstruction in the field, but you can still treat the patient if you suspect the condition. Begin by stabilizing the patient if you identify any life threats. Then establish IV access and administer medications for nausea and pain per local protocol. Give nothing by mouth, since the patient may need to undergo immediate surgery. Transport the patient in a comfortable position.

In the ED, both flat and upright x-rays of the abdomen and chest will be taken to confirm the obstruction. A complete blood count and a check of electrolytes will be performed. An elevated white blood cell count may indicate ischemia and impending bowel necrosis. A nasogastric tube may be placed to remove excess pressure pending surgical intervention.

Abdominal Compartment Syndrome

Abdominal compartment syndrome is caused by intraabdominal hypertension and is a critical presentation for patients with abdominal discomfort. The patient may have a tense, tender, distended abdomen, respiratory distress, metabolic acidosis, declining urine output, and dwindling cardiac output. The drop in cardiac output occurs as the pressure builds up in the abdomen, restricting venous return to the heart.

The condition is more common among trauma patients, but it may be seen in medical patients as well. Since these signs and symptoms are often associated with other critical events such as hypovolemia, compartment syndrome may be missed, usually to the patient's detriment. Awareness is essential, since you can worsen the condition by placing equipment on a patient's abdomen during transport.

Treatment in the field for this condition is limited to loosening restrictive clothing, avoiding excessive fluid administration, and perhaps administering diuretics. In the ED, the abdomen may be decompressed by removing fluid.

Viral Gastroenteritis

Viral gastroenteritis, the second leading cause of illness in the United States, is characterized by watery diarrhea, nausea and vomiting, mild abdominal pain, and low-grade

TABLE 7-11 Causes of Abdominal Discomfort with Jaundice

Critical	Emergent	Nonemergent
HEPATIC		
Fulminant hepatic failure	Hepatitis with abnormal mental status Primary biliary cirrhosis Drug induced	Hepatitis with normal mental status
CARDIOVASCULAR		
Abdominal aortic aneurysm Budd-Chiari syndrome Severe congestive heart failure	Right-sided congestive heart failure Veno-occlusive disease	
BILIARY		
Cholangitis	Bile duct obstruction	
SYSTEMIC		
Sepsis Heatstroke	Sarcoidosis Amyloidosis Graft-versus-host disease	Posttraumatic hematoma reabsorption Total parenteral nutrition
HEMATOLOGIC		
Transfusion reaction	Hemolytic anemia Massive malignant infiltration Pancreatic head tumor	Gilbert's syndrome Physiologic neonatal jaundice
REPRODUCTIVE		
Preeclampsia/HELLP syndrome Acute fatty liver of pregnancy	Hyperemesis gravidarum	Cholestasis of pregnancy

fever. Many viruses cause viral gastroenteritis, but *Norovirus* is most often the culprit. Viral gastroenteritis is easily transmissible and can cause large outbreaks. These outbreaks are usually sporadic and tend to flourish in the winter months. Gastroenteritis can be caused by bacteria and parasites as well. Treatment is symptomatic and consists of administering antiemetics and providing IV fluid replacement.

Abdominal Pain with Jaundice

Jaundice

Jaundice is a condition in which excess (unconjugated) serum bilirubin binds to albumin, yellowing the eyes and skin and causing fatigue, fever, anorexia, and confusion. To be eliminated from the body, bilirubin must be conjugated by the liver. As the excess unconjugated bilirubin crosses the blood-brain barrier, encephalopathy and death can ensue. Jaundice is often associated with premature infants, but the condition can befall patients of any age. Physical examination may show an enlarged liver, an aggravation of pain with palpation of the right upper quadrant, and ascites. Diagnostic tests include CT or ultrasound and laboratory studies such as a complete blood count, serum bilirubin, alkaline phosphatase, prothrombin time/partial thromboplastin time (PT/PTT), serum amylase, ammonia level, a pregnancy test, and a toxicology screening.

Patient history may include recent trauma, blood transfusion, viral illness, chronic alcohol use, acetaminophen overdose, hepatitis, pregnancy, malignancy, high fever, or encephalopathy. Causes of abdominal pain with jaundice are given in Table 7-11.

Fulminant Hepatic Failure

Fulminant hepatic failure sets in when hepatitis progresses to hepatic necrosis (death of the liver cells). Classic symptoms include anorexia, vomiting, jaundice, abdominal pain, and asterixis, or "flapping." The mechanism causing asterixis is unknown. To test for it, ask the patient to extend the arms, flex the wrists, and spread the fingers, and then observe for flapping. Extensive hepatic necrosis is irreversible and can be treated only with a liver transplant. Hepatitis B and C are most often responsible, but drug toxicity (acetaminophen overdose) and metabolic disorders can also be to blame. Liver function tests will be elevated.

Treatment is merely supportive. In the case of acetaminophen overdose, if the patient is seen soon after ingestion, an antidote of *N*-acetylcysteine can be given with excellent results. Time of ingestion of the acetaminophen is key to determining whether the patient meets treatment criteria. First, support the patient's airway, breathing, and circulation. Then establish IV access, and administer antiemetics and pain medication as necessary.

Budd-Chiari Syndrome

Budd-Chiari syndrome is an extremely rare cardiovascular disorder resulting from occlusion of the major hepatic veins or inferior vena cava. The venous thrombosis that characterizes this syndrome can be due to hematologic disease, coagulopathy, pregnancy, use of oral contraceptives, abdominal trauma, or a congenital disorder. Signs and symptoms include acute or chronic fulminant liver failure, emergent abdominal pain, hepatomegaly, ascites, and jaundice. Diagnosis is usually made by ultrasound. The treatment selected depends on the cause of the occlusion, but anticoagulants and supportive therapy are typically given.

Cholelithiasis, Cholecystitis, and Cholangitis

Cholangitis and cholelithiasis are diseases that affect the gallbladder, a structure that produces bile to aid digestion of fats and fat-soluble nutrients. In cholelithiasis, an elevated level of cholesterol that cannot be converted by bile acids leads to the formation of gallstones. This condition is more prevalent among older adults and women and in people with morbid obesity, those who have lost weight rapidly, those with a familial predisposition to the disorder, and those who have taken certain drugs. The four F's are often cited to characterize patients at risk for developing gallstones: female, fat, over forty, and fertile.

Stones are asymptomatic in some people. In others, they provoke severe pain in the right upper quadrant, sometimes referred to the right shoulder, accompanied by nausea and vomiting. This pain, called *biliary colic,* is typically cyclic and tends to be aggravated by eating fatty foods. Murphy's sign may also be present and can be elicited by pressing firmly upward into the right upper quadrant and asking the patient to take a deep breath. Arrest of inspiration because of pain is a positive finding. Biliary colic can be treated with outpatient elective cholecystectomy.

Cholecystitis is a complete obstruction of the bile duct caused by gallstones, a stricture, or a malignancy. Signs and symptoms include persistent right upper quadrant pain, nausea, vomiting, and fever. The condition will be treated urgently with antibiotics and cholecystectomy (gallbladder removal).

Cholangitis, an ascending infection of the biliary tract, has the same symptoms as cholecystitis, but with jaundice. Sepsis will develop if the condition is left untreated. Treatment centers on maintaining hemodynamic stability, controlling pain and nausea, administering antibiotics, and decompressing the biliary tract.

Hepatitis

Hepatitis simply means an inflammation of the liver. Despite its simple name, the etiology of hepatitis is often complex. Causes include viral, bacterial, fungal, and parasitic infections, exposure to toxic substances, adverse drug reactions, and immunologic disorders. The symptoms of hepatitis vary but tend to be nonspecific. They include malaise, fever, and anorexia, followed by nausea and vomiting, abdominal pain, diarrhea, and jaundice later in the course of the disease.

Alcohol is one of the toxic substances that can cause severe liver disease and hepatitis, since the liver is responsible for degrading alcohol. Chronic alcohol abuse leads to liver disease, malnutrition, accumulation of toxic metabolites, and enzyme alteration. The interaction of these mechanisms is thought to cause hepatitis, although researchers do not yet understand precisely how. The liver disease is typically asymptomatic until it evolves into alcoholic hepatitis, at which time signs and symptoms may include nausea and vomiting, abdominal pain, tachycardia, fever, ascites, and orthostatic hypotension.

Viruses are among the most frequent causes of hepatitis. Viral hepatitis is classified as type A, type B, or type C. Although the incidence of all types is declining, these infectious diseases still pose a threat.

Hepatitis A Hepatitis A virus (HAV) is typically spread from person to person through the fecal-oral route. It thrives in areas with poor sanitation, particularly in unsanitary cooking facilities. HAV exposure is widespread. In fact, in some regions of the world, 100% of the population has been exposed. In the United States, the rate of exposure is as high as 50%. However, very few of those who have been exposed actually become ill. A vaccination can be given to prevent HAV. HAV is not a chronic illness.

Hepatitis B In infected people, hepatitis B virus (HBV) can be found in most bodily secretions, including saliva, semen, stool, tears, urine, and vaginal secretions. The virus is usually spread through exposure to infected blood or by sexual activity. The highest rates, then, are among IV drug users and men who have sex with men. Historically, blood transfusions were a frequent cause of HBV, but careful screening of blood products has virtually eliminated the risk of exposure. Unlike HAV, once infected with HBV, a person is always a carrier and can always transmit the disease. A vaccine for HBV is also available.

Hepatitis C Hepatitis C is commonplace in the United States and is linked to blood transfusions. Other possible causes are unsafe needle-sharing practices and exposure of healthcare workers to the blood of infected patients. The cause of infection is never found in 40% to 57% of cases.

Abdominal Discomfort Associated with Diarrhea or Constipation

The large intestine is the origin of several disorders that cause diarrhea or constipation. We've already discussed large-bowel obstruction, volvulus, intussusception, and ischemia. Now let's take a look at irritable bowel syndrome, diverticulosis, diverticulitis, and inflammatory bowel disease.

Irritable Bowel Syndrome

Irritable bowel syndrome is a chronic disorder that affects 10% to 15% of the U.S. population. Although not life threatening, it causes abdominal pain, diarrhea, constipation, and nausea that can greatly impair the quality of life. Because lab findings and radiologic studies are normal in patients with irritable bowel syndrome, the disorder was originally thought to be psychiatric in nature. Current physiologic research, however, suggests that the condition is due to an error of gut motility and sensation. It does arise more often in those with a history of depression or anxiety and worsens when the patient is under stress. The condition also appears to be predominant among women. Dietary modification is advised, and behavioral therapy and supportive care are typically given.

Diverticular Disease

Diverticular disease is characterized by small, saclike appendages called *diverticula* that form when the lining of the colon herniates through the mucosal wall. Diverticular disease was first described as recently as the 20th century and is thought to be attributable to a lack of fiber in the modern diet. Researchers believe that the formation of smaller stools containing little fiber raises pressure in the colon, and small outpouchings form in weakened areas of the intestinal wall. The disease is far more likely to appear in those over age 50 than among younger adults.

Diverticulosis is a precursor to diverticulitis. Diverticulosis is often asymptomatic. When the disorder does generate symptoms, they include abdominal bloating, crampy pain, and changes in bowel habits. Diverticulitis sets in when the diverticula become infected, precipitating bleeding, persistent left lower quadrant pain, diffuse tenderness, vomiting, and abdominal distention.

Patients are generally treated symptomatically, given antibiotics, and placed on a high-fiber diet. Potential complications include bowel perforation and consequent sepsis. Patients with severe diverticulitis may require surgical colectomy or abscess drainage.

Inflammatory Bowel Syndrome

Inflammatory bowel disease is characterized by chronic, unpredictable inflammation of the GI tract. More than 1 million people in the United States live with this debilitating disorder. The two types of inflammatory bowel disease are Crohn's disease and ulcerative colitis. Treatment is complicated and may include medications and multiple abdominal surgeries.

Unfortunately, the inflammation in Crohn's disease is very deep and may involve the entire colonic wall, causing intestinal strictures and forming fissures with adjacent organs. In ulcerative colitis, inflammation and ulceration are found throughout the colon and rectum. Both diseases cause severe crampy abdominal pain and loose, sometimes bloody stools or diarrhea. Patients are often treated with long-term prednisone or other immunosuppressive therapy. Complications include intraabdominal abscess and fistula formation.

Neurologic Causes of Abdominal Discomfort

A broad range of mechanisms not directly related to a GI diagnosis can cause nausea and vomiting. These mechanisms include neurologic complaints such as migraines, tumors, and increased intracranial pressure. If such a diagnosis is suspected, you should perform a more in-depth neurologic assessment. Table 7-12 outlines emergent causes of abdominal discomfort in patients with nausea and vomiting. In addition, Chapter 2 contains detailed information on neurologic complaints.

Intracerebral Bleeding

Although intracerebral bleeding does not cause abdominal pain, you should consider it when nausea and vomiting are present. In cases of acute onset of nausea and vomiting, you should undertake further assessment to confirm or eliminate this diagnosis. A history of recent head trauma, hemiparesis, hemiplegia, and difficulty speaking or swallowing, especially when accompanied by risk factors such as hypertension or advanced age, boosts the likelihood of intracerebral bleeding. See Chapter 2 for more information.

Meningitis

Meningitis is a bacterial, viral, or fungal infection of the meninges of the brain. Although meningitis is not a GI disorder, you should consider this diagnosis when the patient has nausea or vomiting. Bacterial meningitis has a 25% to 50% mortality rate, is highly contagious, and requires aggressive antibiotic treatment. Viral meningitis calls for supportive care. Since it's virtually impossible to know in the prehospital setting which type of meningitis a patient might have, it's critical to wear personal protective equipment, including a mask. See Chapter 2 for more information.

Vertigo

Vertigo is dizziness associated with a variety of conditions, trauma, infection, and intracranial bleeding, to name several. Although not an abdominal illness, vertigo can cause nausea and vomiting and may be peripheral or central. For peripheral vertigo (e.g., labyrinthitis, benign paroxysmal positional vertigo, vestibular neuronitis), provide supportive care. If the patient has other neurologic symptoms such as headache or confusion, you should suspect intracranial bleeding. See Chapter 2 for more information about vertigo.

TABLE 7-12 Emergent Causes of Abdominal Discomfort with Nausea and Vomiting

	Description	Symptoms	Treatment
NEUROLOGIC			
Migraine	Recurrent headache, sometimes accompanied by an aura Lasts 3–72 hours	Unilateral or bilateral throbbing or sharp headache Photophobia Nausea and vomiting	Provide supportive care. Dim the ambulance lights. Establish IV access. Administer antiemetics. Apply ice or heat packs.
CNS tumor	Primary tumor: begins in the brain Secondary tumor: spreads from another cancerous site More common among people over age 65, in those who have had radiation to the head, and in those who smoke or are HIV+	Recurrent, severe headaches Nausea and vomiting Dizziness and lack of coordination Vision alterations Seizures	Provide supportive care to reduce nausea and vomiting, ease pain, and prevent or control seizures.
Increased ICP	Can be caused by obstruction or by increase of CSF in ventricles	Headache Photophobia Nausea and vomiting Seizures	Provide comfort care. Position the patient lying flat. Administer antiemetics and antiseizure medications.
GASTROINTESTINAL			
Gastric outlet obstruction	Complication of peptic ulcer disease in which the abdominal contents are unable to drain from the stomach Diagnosed by endoscopy	Vomiting Bloating and abdominal pain Weight loss	Gastric decompression
Pancreatitis	Inflammation of the pancreas Pancreatic enzymes autodigest the pancreas Major causes are alcohol abuse and gallbladder disease	Constant, severe midepigastric pain Nausea and vomiting Fever	Provide supportive care. Establish IV access. Administer antiemetics and analgesics. Give nothing by mouth.
Cholecystitis	Inflamed gallbladder usually caused by gallstone obstruction	Fever Abdominal pain Nausea and vomiting	Give IV fluids. Administer antiemetics and pain medications.
Bowel obstruction/ ileus	History of bowel obstruction, abdominal surgery, cancer, radiation therapy, chemotherapy, hernia, or abdominal illness Obstruction can be attributable to stool, foreign body, intussusception, adhesions, polyps, volvulus, tumors, ulcerative colitis, or diverticulitis Diagnosed by laboratory and x-ray studies	Crampy abdominal pain Constipation or diarrhea Inability to pass flatus Distended abdomen Absent or high-pitched bowel sounds	Administer oxygen. Place patient in a comfortable position. Establish IV access. Give nothing by mouth.
Ruptured viscus	Possible causes include peptic ulcer disease, diverticula, trauma, NSAIDs, and advancing age. Diagnosed by laboratory, x-ray, and CT studies	Acute onset of epigastric pain Vomiting	Administer oxygen. Place patient in a comfortable position. Establish IV access. Give nothing by mouth.
Appendicitis	Inflammation of the appendix Diagnosed by CT Surgery required for definitive treatment	Periumbilical pain Nausea and vomiting Fever Positive psoas sign	Place patient in a comfortable position. Establish IV access and administer analgesics and antiemetics.
Peritonitis	Inflammation of the peritoneal membrane caused by infection, trauma, or bowel rupture	Fever Nausea and vomiting Diffuse abdominal pain	Place patient in a comfortable position. Establish IV access and administer antiemetics, analgesics, and antibiotics.

TABLE 7-12 Emergent Causes of Abdominal Discomfort with Nausea and Vomiting—*Cont'd*

	Description	Symptoms	Treatment
ENDOCRINE			
Adrenal insufficiency	Addison's disease Inability of the adrenal cortex to produce aldosterone or cortisol or both Can be caused by autoimmune disease, infectious disease, or a genetic disorder	Weakness and fatigue Darkening of the skin Anorexia Hypoglycemia Nausea and vomiting Abdominal pain Diarrhea	Support airway, breathing, and circulation. Give IV fluids. Treat electrolyte imbalance as indicated.
REPRODUCTIVE			
Hyperemesis gravidarum	Severe vomiting that can occur throughout pregnancy Hospitalization may be required	Nausea and vomiting Weight loss Electrolyte imbalance	Establish IV access. Administer antiemetics.
GENITOURINARY			
Testicular torsion	Twisting of the spermatic cord inside the scrotum More common in infants <12 months Can be caused by blunt trauma, but cause is often unknown Without prompt surgical intervention, the testicle will become necrotic.	Acute onset of severe pain in one testis Edema on one side of the scrotum A lump on the testis Blood in the semen Nausea and vomiting Lightheadedness	Offer comfort care. Promptly transport to the ED. Administer analgesics.
METABOLIC			
Electrolyte disturbance	Specific disturbances include hyponatremia, hypernatremia, hypokalemia, hyperkalemia, hypercalcemia, hypermagnesemia, Diagnosis is made on the basis of laboratory and ECG studies	Nausea and vomiting	Offer comfort care. Administer IV antiemetics.

CNS, Central nervous system; *CSF,* cerebrospinal fluid; *CT,* computed tomography; *ECG,* electrocardiogram; *ED,* emergency department; *HIV,* human immunodeficiency virus; *ICP,* intracranial pressure; *IV,* intravenous; *NSAIDs,* nonsteroidal antiinflammatory drugs.

Cardiopulmonary Causes of Abdominal Discomfort

When abdominal discomfort is accompanied by respiratory distress, you must consider extraabdominal diagnoses. Frequent signs and symptoms of an acute myocardial infarction, for instance, may include abdominal or epigastric pain and nausea and/or vomiting. Pulmonary embolism and pneumonia are other possible causes of abdominal pain with shortness of breath. Consider obtaining a 12-lead electrocardiogram (ECG) if you suspect the patient's signs and symptoms have a cardiopulmonary cause.

Abdominal Aortic Aneurysm

Abdominal aortic aneurysm is an enlargement of part of the aorta caused by a weakness in the vascular wall. These bulges in the arterial wall typically begin small and become larger over the course of several months to years. Most such aneurysms do not rupture, leak, or dissect. Less than half of patients with an abdominal aortic aneurysm exhibit the classic triad of symptoms: hypotension, abdominal or back pain, and a pulsatile abdominal mass. Be sure to consider this diagnosis in patients with syncope or any one of the triad of symptoms.

Because of the large size of the aorta, rupture causes massive blood loss, and survival depends primarily on the body's ability to spontaneously contain the bleeding. Any patient suspected of having a ruptured abdominal aortic aneurysm should be treated as a critical patient. Fluid resuscitation may be necessary. Consider immediate transport to the operating room if the patient has a known ruptured aneurysm. If the patient is older than 50 and is complaining of abdominal or back pain, an abdominal aneurysm should be considered, even if hypotension or a pulsatile mass are not present. Consider a bedside sonogram as the first evaluative tool, followed by CT if necessary. A stable patient may proceed to CT, since a sonogram cannot always detect retroperitoneal leakage or rupture. It's important to remember that even with a stable patient, deterioration can happen suddenly at any time. Even patients who have had a repair are at risk for an aneurysm rupture.

Acute Coronary Syndrome

Myocardial infarction can be accompanied by midepigastric pain and nausea that cause it to mimic an abdominal complaint such as peptic ulcer disease or gastritis. Since it may be difficult to distinguish between GI and cardiac causes, assess the patient for acute coronary syndrome and initiate care as appropriate. A look back at Chapter 5 will help you review the diagnosis and treatment of acute coronary syndrome and myocardial infarction.

Pulmonary Embolism

As with acute coronary syndrome, pulmonary embolism should be suspected in patients who have upper abdominal pain. A pulmonary embolism is a life-threatening condition that occurs when a thrombus (a blood clot, cholesterol plaque, or air bubble) travels through the bloodstream and becomes lodged in a pulmonary artery. The area of the lung perfused by that portion of the pulmonary artery no longer receives oxygenated blood, causing pain and shortness of breath.

You should suspect pulmonary embolism in patients with hip or long-bone fractures, people who are sedentary or have recently taken a long flight or car trip, those who smoke, use oral contraceptives, have a history of deep vein thrombosis or cancer, and women who are pregnant or were recently pregnant. See Chapter 3 for more information about pulmonary embolism.

Lobar Pneumonia

Lobar pneumonia causes upper abdominal pain in some patients. The pain tends to be more focal than in bronchopneumonia, which causes inflammation of the entire lung. Lobar pneumonia is usually accompanied by a fever, chest pain, and respiratory distress. Chapter 3 addresses pneumonia at greater length.

Genitourinary Causes of Abdominal Discomfort

Vaginal Bleeding

Abruptio Placentae During the second half of pregnancy, about 4% of women have vaginal bleeding. Bleeding during the second trimester signals imminent fetal distress and should be considered an emergency. Abruptio placentae, the premature separation of the placenta from the uterine wall, is responsible for about 30% of all cases of bleeding during the second half of pregnancy. Trauma, maternal hypertension, or preeclampsia typically precipitates abruption. Other risk factors include patients younger than 20, advanced maternal age, multiparity or a history of smoking, prior miscarriage, prior abruptio placentae, or cocaine use.

Abruptio placentae should be considered in patients with vaginal bleeding, contractions, uterine or abdominal tenderness, and a decrease in fetal movement. The majority (80%) of patients with abruptio placentae report vaginal bleeding. The blood is usually dark in color. With small abruptions, bleeding may not be noted until delivery. The volume of blood loss can vary from minimal to life threatening. These patients can progress from stable to unstable in a short period of time. Fetal distress or death ensues in about 15% of patients. Assessment should include evaluation of vaginal bleeding, contractions, and uterine tenderness and assessment of fundal height and fetal heart tones. Fetal heart tones may vary from absent to fetal bradycardia to decelerations. Short-term variability may be decreased as well if the fetus is compromised. Vaginal exams should not be performed until an ultrasound can be completed to rule out placenta previa. Management is based on the severity of the blood loss. The following may be indicated: oxygen, fluid support with two large-bore IVs, blood administration, and administering Rh globulin if the patient is Rh negative.

Placenta Previa In some pregnancies, the placenta becomes implanted over the cervical os (opening). This anomaly is one of the leading causes of vaginal bleeding in the second and third trimesters. It may be identified early in the pregnancy but may resolve as the uterus expands. The patient is at risk of significant bleeding, however, if the condition does not resolve and the placenta completely occludes the cervix. Ultrasound is used to localize the placenta. Advanced maternal age, multiparity, and a history of smoking and prior cesarean section predispose a woman to placenta previa. The patient will usually present with bright red bleeding. The bleeding is usually painless, but some patients (20%) will have uterine irritability as well. Ask for a history of bleeding; many patients may have an initial episode of bleeding that spontaneously stops and then have additional episodes of bleeding later in the pregnancy. In addition to bleeding, monitor for signs and symptoms of shock, uterine tone (usually soft and nontender), and fetal heart tones. Do not perform vaginal or rectal examinations. Speculum exam can trigger hemorrhage if the condition is present (see Chapter 1 for additional assessment information). Monitor for disseminated intravascular coagulopathy (DIC), as maternal deaths with placenta previa are associated with blood loss or DIC. Care is directed at supporting the patient's hemodynamic status to include oxygen, two large-bore IVs, fluids, and blood as needed.

- **Whereas abruptio placentae tends to present with abdominal pain and vaginal bleeding, placenta previa tends to present with painless vaginal bleeding.**

Abdominal Pain

Preeclampsia/HELLP Preeclampsia with HELLP syndrome (H = hemolysis, EL = elevated liver enzymes, LP = low platelet count) is a particularly devastating complication of pregnancy. Preeclampsia, which occurs in 6% to

8% of pregnancies, is characterized by hypertension and protein in the urine. The risk of preeclampsia is higher among women younger than age 20 and in those with first or multifetal pregnancies, gestational diabetes, obesity, or a family history of gestational hypertension. Gestational hypertension typically resolves within 6 weeks postpartum. Right upper quadrant pain, midepigastric pain, nausea and vomiting, and visual disturbances are the chief symptoms of preeclampsia. Patients should also be monitored for hyperreflexia or clonus. Seizures occur in eclampsia. Magnesium sulfate should be considered in these patients for management.

HELLP syndrome is considered by some authorities to be a severe and rare form of preeclampsia; others suggest that it may be a syndrome of its own. The precise cause of HELLP syndrome has not been established. It is often misdiagnosed or found later in the course of the syndrome, so your awareness of the signs and symptoms is vitally important. HELLP syndrome usually occurs antepartum, but it may also present during the postpartum period (approximately one-third of cases appear postpartum). Most patients complain of malaise, epigastric pain, nausea and vomiting, and headache. The key to identification is a low platelet count. An elevated D-dimer may also help identify HELLP syndrome. Prehospital treatment is supportive and aimed at blood pressure control, fluid replacement, blood product replacement, and monitoring for DIC development. Pharmacologic interventions may include corticosteroids (for fetal lung development), magnesium sulfate, Apresoline, or labetalol (to address hypertension). Delivery may have to be induced to protect both the fetus and mother.

Ectopic Pregnancy Ectopic pregnancy, implantation of the fertilized ovum (egg) outside of the uterus, is a life-threatening condition. The characteristic site of implantation in an ectopic pregnancy is the fallopian tube, but the ovum may also implant in the abdominal cavity or elsewhere. If the fertilized ovum implants in the fallopian tube, the tube will begin to stretch as the embryo divides, causing pain and bleeding. The bleeding may be internal or vaginal.

Risk factors for ectopic pregnancy include scarring or inflammation of the pelvis from previous surgeries or ectopic pregnancies, pelvic inflammatory disease, tubal ligation, and placement of an intrauterine device. Because symptoms become apparent within 5 to 10 weeks of implantation, many women are not yet aware that they are pregnant. Consider ectopic pregnancy in any woman of childbearing age who has vaginal bleeding with or without abdominal pain. Especially after an ectopic rupture, the bleeding can be severe, placing the patient at risk of shock.

Your initial goals for this patient will be to ensure that the airway and breathing are secure and to establish IV access. In the ED, a urine or serum pregnancy test can be obtained to establish whether the patient is pregnant. If a pregnancy is confirmed, a quantitative beta-hCG (human chorionic gonadotropin) should be obtained to help determine the stage of the pregnancy. The level of beta-hCG rises as the pregnancy progresses through the early stages. The next step will be transvaginal ultrasound to determine whether the pregnancy has been established in the uterus or in an extrauterine location. If the latter is confirmed, surgical intervention will be required.

Hyperemesis Hyperemesis occurs early in pregnancy, usually in the first trimester, and can result in dehydration and fluid and electrolyte imbalance. It is defined by weight loss, starvation metabolism, and prolonged ketosis. Once other causes of vomiting are ruled out, management includes fluid therapy, electrolyte replacement, and antiemetics.

Renal Failure

Patients with renal disease often have nausea and vomiting. Assessment to identify any life-threatening symptoms should be performed immediately. Warning signals include altered LOC, signs of congestive heart failure, dysrhythmia, and electrolyte imbalance. There are many myths and misconceptions surrounding renal patients. Box 7-6 reviews them.

Renal failure is typically classified as acute or chronic. In acute renal failure, the kidneys suddenly stop working, and waste products quickly begin to accumulate. If the condition is not corrected, it will progress to chronic renal failure.

Acute Renal Failure Acute renal failure has three phases: oliguric, diuretic, and recovery. These phases are summarized in Table 7-13. Oliguric acute renal failure can be due to one of three causes: prerenal failure, intrinsic renal failure, or postrenal failure. In prerenal failure, the kidney responds to inadequate perfusion by retaining fluids, which retards the glomerular filtration rate and encourages the reabsorption of sodium and water. This process is usually reversible if caught within 24 hours of onset. If you're called to assist a patient in acute renal failure, you must know how to identify the most feared complications of acute renal failure: pulmonary edema and hyperkalemia. Aggressive treatment of the cause of acute renal failure—hemorrhage, sepsis, congestive heart failure, or shock of any kind—is the best way to arrest prerenal acute renal failure in the field. If not managed properly, prerenal failure will progress to chronic renal failure, in which the renal tissue itself is damaged.

Intrinsic acute renal failure is commonly caused by autoimmune disease, chronic uncontrolled hypertension, or diabetes mellitus. Heavy metals, poisons, and nephrotoxic medications may also be responsible for intrinsic acute renal failure. Under certain conditions, a heat emergency or crush injury may lead to rhabdomyolysis, in which myoglobin released from damaged muscles obstructs the tubular portion of the nephrons, causing

BOX 7-6 Myths and Misconceptions

- Fluid administration: fluids should not be withheld from a renal failure patient in need of fluid resuscitation, but consult with Medical Control before initiating aggressive fluid resuscitation. Hypovolemic or hypotensive patients should receive a fluid bolus when indicated. Be careful to limit fluids in patients who do not need fluids. Typically, renal failure patients are difficult to obtain IV access on. If IV access is indicated, it shouldn't be deferred simply because a patient has renal failure.
- Diuretic administration: some end-stage renal failure patients continue to have some degree of residual kidney function. These patients may retain up to 20% of normal renal function, so a patient who presents in pulmonary edema may respond to a large dose of a loop diuretic like furosemide (Lasix). Patients themselves will be able to tell you whether they still make urine, which will indicate whether diuretics will be effective in increasing urine output. Renal failure patients often require large doses of diuretics, so consult Medical Control if necessary. It's important to note that in addition to decreasing fluid volume through increased renal excretion, furosemide causes venodilation and has a secondary therapeutic effect in fluid overload.
- Morphine administration: pain is undertreated in 75% of the renal failure population, and yet pain medication administration in renal patients is extremely controversial. Codeine, meperidine (Demerol), propoxyphene (Darvon), and morphine are renally excreted. The metabolites build up in patients with chronic kidney disease and can cause neurotoxicity. According to the World Health Organization, the preferred pain medication is fentanyl. It has been proven safe and effective in patients with chronic kidney disease. Hydromorphone (Dilaudid) may also be used but with caution. The World Health Organization recommends that codeine, meperidine, propoxyphene, and morphine not be used. Other opinions are that in the emergency setting (i.e., pulmonary edema, AMI), it's safe to administer morphine. When in doubt, always consult with your Medical Control physician.
- Succinylcholine (an RSI medication) should be avoided in patients with known renal disease.

A good thing to remember is that all dialysis patients require special consideration regarding ANY medication because of their altered pharmacokinetic and pharmacodynamic issues and increased potential for adverse reactions. They are at high risk for medication-related problems.

TABLE 7-13 Phases of Acute Renal Failure

Phase	Description and Characteristics	Treatment
Oliguric phase	Usually lasts 10–20 days, with urine output decreasing by 50–400 mL/day Protein spill Hyponatremia Hyperkalemia Metabolic acidosis	Monitor ECG for peaked T waves and a widened QRS (hyperkalemia). Order a laboratory potassium study, since a lethal level may exist. Be prepared to administer sodium bicarbonate and calcium until dialysis can be initiated. CHF may also develop, so monitor for signs of left- and right-sided heart failure.
Diuretic phase	Occurs when urine output exceeds 500 mL in 24 hours Causes sodium and potassium loss in the urine May cause hypovolemia, since the patient may lose up to 3000 mL in 24 hours through diuresis	Monitor for electrolyte disturbances and signs of hypovolemia. Be prepared to administer fluids and electrolytes to replace as much as 75% of the previous day's volume loss. Be prepared to treat GI bleeding and respiratory failure.
Recovery phase	May last weeks to months	Prevent fluid overload. Closely monitor electrolyte and fluid balance.

CHF, Congestive heart failure; *ECG*, electrocardiogram; *GI*, gastrointestinal.

permanent damage if not caught early. Myoglobin in the urine turns it tea colored, and this may be an early clue.

Postrenal failure commences when urine flow is obstructed, causing a backflow of urine into the ureters and kidneys and causing the kidneys to dilate. This process disrupts kidney function, ultimately causing necrosis. If the backflow is not resolved, chronic renal failure may be the result.

Laboratory tests that indicate renal function include blood urea nitrogen (BUN) and serum creatinine. If either level is elevated, the patient should be evaluated for renal insufficiency or failure. The normal ratio of BUN to creatinine is less than 20:1. A ratio of greater than 20:1 suggests a prerenal cause of the failure. A ratio of less than 20:1 indicates intrinsic renal failure.

Chronic Renal Failure Chronic renal failure is the permanent loss of renal function. The threshold for such metabolic disruption is reached when 80% of the estimated 1 million nephrons in the kidney are damaged or destroyed. At that point, dialysis or a kidney transplant is required for survival. In caring for the patient with chronic renal failure, you must know how the disease is typically managed and be aware of the complications associated with the disease and its treatment, especially dialysis.

Fluid imbalances may lead to hypertension, pulmonary edema, or hypotension. Vascular overload caused by retention of fluid and sodium may be responsible for hypertension or congestive heart failure. Be cautious administering fluids, and in patients with hypertension, consider giving non–potassium sparing diuretics, ACE inhibitors, or peripheral vasodilators.

Patients with acute congestive heart failure may have pulmonary edema, crackles, shortness of breath, jugular venous distention, an enlarged liver, or pitting edema. The mainstay of treatment is administration of nitrates and positive-pressure ventilation using a continuous positive airway pressure (CPAP) or bilevel positive airway pressure (BiPAP) device (see Chapter 3). Support respiration, place the patient in a comfortable position, monitor cardiac status, and assess for cardiac damage by obtaining a 12-lead ECG. If the patient becomes hypotensive, administer small fluid boluses of 200 to 300 mL if indicated. *Lactated Ringer's solution should not be used, because it contains potassium.*

A patient with renal complaints may also have chest discomfort or acute coronary syndrome. It's important to remember that many renal patients have diabetes, so any coronary symptoms may be masked or silent. Be sure to place a 12-lead ECG and initiate cardiac monitoring. If you suspect myocardial infarction or if the patient has premature ventricular contractions, administer oxygen. Fluids and antianginal medications may be indicated. Administration of antiarrhythmics may also be required. Consult Medical Control when administering medications to renal patients because of the complexity of their fluid and electrolyte imbalances and the potential for multisystem involvement.

Don't overlook the possibility of hyperkalemia, which is a life threat. It can develop rapidly in the renal patient, and weakness may be the only sign or symptom present. Patients may remain asymptomatic until a fatal arrhythmia occurs. Cardiac monitoring and early lab work will help you identify this complication in time to treat it. If you suspect hyperkalemia, calcium, insulin, albuterol, furosemide, and Kayexalate should be administered. Calcium gluconate protects the myocardium, insulin and albuterol shift potassium into the cells, furosemide increases renal excretion of potassium, and Kayexalate removes potassium from the gut. If acidosis is present, sodium bicarbonate may be used as well. Further discussion of hyperkalemia is found in Chapter 6. Acidosis stemming from an electrolyte imbalance, hypoperfusion, or diabetic complications may be identified if the patient exhibits an altered LOC, Kussmaul's respiration, or abnormal arterial blood gas levels. Management may include support of ventilation, fluid administration, and perhaps administration of sodium bicarbonate to address the electrolyte imbalance.

Anticoagulant administration during dialysis may cause hemorrhage. This bleeding is complicated by anemia caused by dwindling erythropoietin secretion, which reduces red cell production. You should have a high index of suspicion for bleeding if the patient has shortness of breath or angina. Blood loss may be obvious, as in trauma to a vascular access site, or not so obvious, as in a patient with occult blood loss through GI bleeding. Prehospital priorities should be to control bleeding, ensure adequate oxygenation, and provide fluid support.

Sudden onset of dyspnea, respiratory distress, chest pain, cyanosis, and hypotension indicates an air embolism. If this clinical picture becomes evident during dialysis, administer high-flow oxygen, and position the patient on his or her left side. Maintain IV access, and be prepared to support blood pressure. Consider placing the patient in a modified Trendelenburg position. This position is used to trap air in the right ventricle.

Disequilibrium syndrome is a neurologic problem patients sometimes experience during or immediately after hemodialysis. Researchers believe the syndrome is caused by cerebral edema that develops when the BUN is lowered too quickly. In mild cases, the patient may complain of headache, restlessness, nausea, muscle twitching, and fatigue. In severe cases, signs and symptoms include hypertension, confusion, seizures, and coma. The event can be fatal. In most cases, however, the episode is self-limiting and will resolve over a few hours. If the patient does have a seizure, consider administering anticonvulsant medications. Prevention is the priority in these patients. Disequilibrium syndrome can be prevented by slowing the rate at which urea is removed from the body during hemodialysis. Other assessment considerations are given in Box 7-7.

Kidney Stones

Kidney stones, or renal calculi, form as a result of metabolic abnormalities, primarily calcium buildup. Those at greater risk are men, individuals with a family history of kidney stones, those who abuse laxatives, and patients with primary hyperparathyroidism, Crohn's disease, renal tubular acidosis, or recurrent urinary tract infection.

Although complete renal obstruction by kidney stones is an anomaly, it is possible and can precipitate renal failure. The size and location of the stone determines its ability to pass through the ureter. Patients typically have constant dull flank pain that radiates to the abdomen, punctuated by bouts of sharp, colicky pain during hyperperistalsis of the smooth muscle of the ureter. Nausea, vomiting, and hematuria may be present. Fever indicates an infection but is an infrequent finding.

Prehospital treatment is supportive. Transport the patient in a position of comfort, establish IV access, and administer pain medications and antiemetics. At the

BOX 7-7 Assessment Considerations for Chronic Renal Failure Patients

Patients with chronic renal failure will be some of the most challenging patients you'll encounter. These patients usually will have a multitude of problems, many of which are unique to chronic renal failure and end-stage renal disease. Medical history is often extensive, with many comorbidities. It's impossible to cover all the presentations you may see in these patients, but some of the more common problems and possible causes are:

- Volume overload—may cause CHF and pulmonary edema
- Hypertension
- Hypotension—complication of fluid shifts or sepsis. Blood pressure usually drops during dialysis.
- Uremia—may lead to pericardial effusion and in rare cases pericardial tamponade. LISTEN TO THOSE HEART TONES!
- Electrolyte imbalances—hyperkalemia (usually asymptomatic; consider hyperkalemia in EVERY patient that has CRF or ESRD), hyponatremia (mental status changes and seizures), hypocalcemia (tetany, paresthesia), hypermagnesemia (weakness, loss of reflexes, dysrhythmias)
- Acidosis—may present with shortness of breath due to the work of breathing from compensatory hyperpnea
- Chest pain—can be pleuritic or otherwise; may be caused by pericardial effusion (common in end-stage renal disease patients), MI
- ECG changes—MI, peaked T waves, widening of the QRS, low-voltage or absent P waves, flattened T wave, ST-segment depression, prominent U wave
- Infections—infected catheters, fistulas, diabetic ulcers, etc.
- GI problems—appendicitis, pancreatitis, diverticulitis
- Extremity pain—distal limb ischemia from clotted fistulas and arteriovenous (AV) grafts
- Bleeding tendency—usually from heparin use during dialysis
- Neurologic disorders—dizziness, headache, and in severe cases, mental status changes (Dialysis dysequilibrium syndrome is a common neurologic complication.)

Assessment of the renal failure patient is similar to the assessment of any other medical patient, but extra attention should be paid to certain areas. Your index of suspicion should be raised for problems such as cardiac arrhythmias, internal bleeding, hypoglycemia, altered mental status, and seizures. When assessing and evaluating the dialysis patient, information that may be crucial to your treatment is:

Dialysis schedule:

- In-center (typically 3 days a week) or home dialysis (typically 6 days a week or peritoneal dialysis)
- Last time dialysis was received and the next scheduled day
- Length of dialysis (When did the patient start receiving dialysis, and how long do they usually run?)

Dry weight (estimated weight of the patient in normal fluid balance)

Does the patient still produce urine?

Weight today—beneficial in determining if patient has fluid overload (1 L equals 1 kg)

Where is their access site, and are there any signs of infection?

If the patient missed a dialysis appointment, do they have any shortness of breath, edema, chest pain, or hypertension?

Peripheral edema, HJR, JVD (not always CHF), murmurs, rubs, bruits

- On exam, pay very close attention to heart tones, lung sounds, and any sign of edema.

Because of the many complications that arise in the treatment of renal failure patients, consulting online Medical Control is strongly encouraged. When discussing treatment with advising physicians, it's imperative they know you're dealing with a renal failure patient and whether or not that patient is receiving dialysis.

CHF, Congestive heart failure; *CRF*, chronic renal failure; *ECG*, electrocardiogram; *ESRD*, end-stage renal disease; *GI*, gastrointestinal; *HJR*, hepatojugular reflux; *JVD*, jugular venous distention; *MI*, myocardial infarction.

hospital, a urinalysis will be ordered to look for blood in the urine. BUN and creatinine will be checked, and CT or ultrasound studies will be performed.

Endocrine Causes of Abdominal Discomfort

Diabetic Ketoacidosis

Diabetic ketoacidosis is a life-threatening complication of diabetes. It is often characterized by nausea, vomiting, and abdominal pain in addition to polyuria, polydipsia, hyperglycemia, polyphagia, and metabolic acidosis. Although it's possible for people with type 2 diabetes to develop diabetic ketoacidosis, especially in the presence of an infection, the condition is far more characteristic of type 1 diabetes. More information is available in Chapter 6. Additional endocrine causes of abdominal discomfort and nausea and vomiting are addressed in Chapter 6 as well.

Infectious Causes of Abdominal Discomfort

Sepsis

Abdominal pain is not a typical presentation of sepsis, but some patients do have nausea and vomiting. Sepsis is discussed further in Chapter 4 relative to shock.

 Special Considerations

Transporting Patients

Choosing the appropriate method of transport for a patient with a GI complaint can be complicated. First you must decide whether the patient is critically ill and determine which modes of transportation the patient can tolerate. Altitude changes during flight can cause severe pain unless the pressure is relieved. The GI system contains a large amount of air. Under normal circumstances, the pressure in the GI system is equal to the pressure in the external environment. At an elevation of 25,000 feet or higher, however, these gases expand as the barometric pressure decreases. The expanding gases in turn put pressure on the diaphragm, thereby diminishing the ability of the lungs to expand.

In a patient who has had recent abdominal surgery and is being transported by air at a high elevation, place a gastric tube or an ileus to release pressure. Empty any ostomy bags, and monitor the patient closely so the new bag does not rupture from an excessive buildup of gas. See Chapter 1 for a detailed discussion of transport and flight safety considerations.

Older Adult Patients

Caring for the older adult population presents special challenges for prehospital providers. Because of diminishing cardiac and pulmonary reserves, altered gastric motility, and inadequate nutrition, older adult patients may become ill more quickly and be more vulnerable to conditions such as abdominal aortic aneurysm, ischemic colitis, pancreatitis, cholecystitis, and large-bowel obstruction.

Many abdominal complaints that become more common with advanced age have ambiguous symptoms. In fact, in diagnosing abdominal pain in patients over age 50, the rate of accuracy is less than 50%. The rate drops to less than 30% in patients over age 80. Further confounding the diagnosis is the fact that many medications frequently prescribed to older adults can mask signs of critical illness. Finally, obtaining a reliable and complete history may be complicated by memory deficits, dementia, hearing impairment, or anxiety.

Obese Patients

Morbid obesity is defined as having a body mass index (BMI) of 40 or higher or, alternatively, being 100 pounds or more overweight. This condition has become more prevalent in the United States. Two surgical options are available to facilitate weight loss in patients with morbid obesity. Restrictive procedures shrink the size of the stomach or the bowel circumference. Gastric banding, for example, reduces the amount of food the patient can eat by restricting the size of the opening from the esophagus to the stomach. These bands are sometimes adjustable, allowing the bariatric surgeon to enlarge or reduce the capacity of the stomach as indicated. The second option is gastric bypass surgery, in which food is diverted around the stomach and upper small bowel through a pouch about the size of an egg. Unlike gastric banding, this procedure is not reversible.

The problems clinicians should be concerned with in bariatric patients are dependent on when the procedures were performed. As with all surgeries, both procedures carry the risk of complications, including infection, bleeding, abdominal pain, abdominal hernia, and lower-extremity deep vein thrombosis secondary to inactivity during recovery from surgery. Potential complications specific to patients who have had bariatric surgery include nausea, vomiting, diarrhea, electrolyte imbalance, and malnutrition, especially if the patient does not take vitamins as advised. These complications are ongoing and not only associated with the surgery itself.

Pregnant Patients

When you assess any woman of childbearing age for an abdominal complaint, you should assume she is pregnant until proven otherwise. Many complications of pregnancy can be mistaken for abdominal complaints, and abdominal complaints can be exacerbated by pregnancy. Keep in mind that medications administered to treat abdominal symptoms may be harmful to the fetus.

While caring for a pregnant patient, you must recognize that the survival of two patients depends on maintaining adequate perfusion. As the fetus grows, it places increasing pressure on the internal organs, diaphragm, and venae cavae. Because of the boost in cardiac output and expansion of intravascular volume during pregnancy, signs of hypoperfusion may be delayed. During the second half of pregnancy, you should position the patient carefully to avoid triggering hypotension by putting pressure on the venae cavae. Tilt or wedge the patient on her left side, and transport. Consider transport to a facility that cares for high-risk obstetric patients as appropriate.

 Putting It All Together

Assessment of the patient with abdominal discomfort begins with the initial observation to determine whether the patient is sick or not sick (see Chapter 1). Let this initial impression tell you whether to intervene immediately or proceed to a more detailed assessment. Assess the patient for critical or emergent diagnoses first, and then consider less menacing conditions. The rule of thumb is to consider the more common or likely diagnosis and work toward the less common. To confirm or rule out conditions that make up your differential diagnosis, use tools such as SAMPLER, OPQRST, physical examination findings, and lab results. If the patient becomes unstable, support of airway, breathing, and circulation always takes precedence. Once the patient has been stabilized, return to your assessment. Because the possible causes of abdominal discomfort are so numerous, it's important to recognize that you may not be able to make a definitive diagnosis in the field. Offering supportive care, managing signs and symptoms, and providing quick transport is the best strategy for many patients with abdominal discomfort.

SCENARIO SOLUTION

1 **There are many possible causes of this patient's abdominal pain. She is still of childbearing age so it's possible she has a gynecologic problem such as ectopic pregnancy. She's the right age for cholecystitis. If she's a frequent drinker, she could have pancreatitis. It's also possible she's having a sickle cell crisis, or she could have an ulcer.**

2 **To narrow your differential diagnosis, you'll need to complete a past history as well as the history of the present illness. Perform a physical examination of her abdomen. Assess her oxygen saturation. Consider obtaining a 12-lead ECG. Palpate for tenderness, masses, guarding, or pulsatile mass.**

3 **The patient has signs of impending shock. You should administer oxygen. Prepare to suction her airway if she vomits again. Establish vascular access, and deliver IV fluids. Consider medication for nausea or pain if her blood pressure improves. Transport her to the closest appropriate hospital for further diagnostic tests and definitive intervention.**

SUMMARY

- The causes of abdominal discomfort are innumerable and may seem overwhelming when you try to make a diagnosis.
- It's important to identify life threats first and then progress toward making a diagnosis as time and the patient's condition allow.
- Patient presentation, history, physical examination, and lab results will be the keys to arriving at an accurate diagnosis of abdominal discomfort.
- The abdomen contains multiple systems, each of which—alone or in combination—may be responsible for abdominal discomfort.
- Abdominal discomfort may be associated with other cardinal symptoms, such as nausea and vomiting, constipation, diarrhea, GI bleeding, jaundice, and vaginal bleeding. Taking into account these cardinal symptoms may assist pinpointing a diagnosis.
- Making a diagnosis should not take precedence over intervention in a patient with abdominal discomfort.

BIBLIOGRAPHY

Aehlert B: Paramedic practice today: above and beyond, St Louis, 2009, Mosby.

Azer A: Esophageal varicies. http://emedicine.medscape.com/article/175248-overview. Accessed January 29, 2010.

Becker S, Dietrich TR, McDevitt MJ, Roy L: Advanced skills: providing expert care for the acutely ill, Springhouse, PA, 1994, Springhouse.

Burcurescu G: Uremic encephalopathy. http://www.medscapecrm.com/article/1135651-overview. Accessed December 18, 2009.

Chronic kidney disease. www.kidney.org/kidneydisease/ckd/index.cfm.

Chronic renal failure. www.nephrologychannel.com/crf/index.shtml. Original date of publication: May 2001.

Dean M: Opioids in renal failure and dialysis patients, J Pain Symptom Manage 28:497–504, 2004.

Deering SH: Abruptio placentae. http://emedicine.medscape.com/article/252810-overview. Accessed May 1, 2010.

Gould BE: Pathophysiology for health care professionals, ed 3, Philadelphia, 2006, Saunders.

Hamilton GC: Emergency medicine: an approach to clinical problem-solving, ed 2, Philadelphia, 2003, Saunders.

Holander-Rodriguez JC, Calvert JF Jr: Hyperkalemia, Am Fam Physician 73:283–290, 2006.

Holleran RS: Air and surface patient transport: principles and practice, ed 3, St Louis, 2003, Mosby.

Johnson LR, Byrne JH: Essential medical physiology, ed 3, Amsterdam, Boston, 2003, Elsevier Academic Press.

Kidney failure. www.mayoclinic.com/healty/kidney failure/ds00280. Accessed May 13, 2008.

Ko P, Yoon Y: Placenta previa. http://emedicine.medscape.com/article/796182-overview. Accessed May 1, 2010.

Krause R: Renal failure, chronic and dialysis complications: multimedia. http://emedicine.medscape.com/article/777957-media. Accessed December 18, 2009.

Lehne RA: Pharmacology for nursing care, ed 6, St Louis, 2007, Saunders.

McCance KL, Huether SE: Pathophysiology: the biologic basis for disease in adults and children, ed 6, St Louis, 2009, Mosby.

Mosby: Mosby's dictionary of medicine, nursing & health professions, ed 8, St Louis, 2009, Mosby.

National Institutes of Health: Bariatric surgery for severe obesity, publication No. 08-4006. 2009. Weight Control Information Network. www.win.niddk.nih.gov/publications/gastric.htm#whataresurg. Accessed June 14, 2009.

Padden MO: HELLP syndrome: recognition and perinatal management. Am Fam Physician, 30:829–836, 1999.

Paula R: Compartment syndrome, abdominal: differential diagnosis & workup. Updated February 23, 2009. http://emedicine.medscape.com/article/829008-diagnosis. Accessed June 30, 2009.

Pitts SR, Niska RW, Xu J, et al: National hospital ambulatory medical care survey: 2006 emergency department summary, national health statistics reports no. 7, Hyattsville, MD, 2008, National Center for Health Statistics.

Rosen P, Marx JA, Hockberger RS, et al: Rosen's emergency medicine: concepts and clinical practice, ed 6, St Louis, 2006, Mosby.

Sanders M: Mosby's paramedic textbook, rev ed 3, St Louis, 2007, Mosby.

Silen W, Cope Z: Cope's early diagnosis of the acute abdomen, Oxford, 2000, Oxford University Press.

Song L-M, Wong KS: Mallory-Weiss tear. Updated April 16, 2008. http://emedicine.medscape.com/article/187134-overview. Accessed February 10, 2010.

Taylor MB: Gastrointestinal emergencies, ed 2, Baltimore, 1997, Williams & Wilkins.

Treatment methods for kidney failure hemodialysis. http://kidney.niddk.nih.gov 07-4666. Accessed December 2006.

Wagner J, McKinney WP, Carpenter JL: Does this patient have appendicitis? JAMA 276:1589, 1996.

Wingfield WE: ACE SAT: The Aeromedical Certification Examinations Self-Assessment Test, 2008, The ResQ Shop Publishers.

Chapter Review Questions

1. A 33-year-old male has right lower quadrant abdominal pain and vomiting. Five minutes after you administer a dose of ondansetron, he vomits forcefully. His vital signs are now BP 102/72, P 52, R 20. The alteration in his vital signs is likely related to:
a. Cardiac conduction defect
b. Fluid loss
c. Medication side effects
d. Vagal stimulation

2. Your patient is complaining of a cramping pain around her umbilical area that "won't let up." This is most suggestive of disease involving the:
a. Appendix
b. Gallbladder
c. Liver
d. Ovary

3. A 43-year-old male with diffuse abdominal pain and vomiting has a yellowish discoloration of his sclera. This indicates he has excess serum:
a. Amylase
b. Bilirubin
c. Fibrinogen
d. Protein

4. A 42-year-old male complains of a gnawing, severe pain in the epigastric area that radiates to his back. His vital signs are T 102°F, BP 94/68, P 128, R 24. Your highest-priority intervention would be to administer:
a. Metoclopramide, 5 mg IV
b. Morphine, 2 mg IV
c. Normal saline, 250 mL bolus
d. Thiamine, 100 mg IV

5. A 22-year-old patient at a restaurant is complaining of abdominal pain and diarrhea. Her skin is flushed, and she feels faint. Her vital signs are: BP 98/50, P 124, R 24. Which finding in her SAMPLER history is most likely to guide your differential diagnosis for this patient?
a. Medical history includes endometriosis.
b. Home medicines include Tegretol and Keppra.
c. Illness began about 10 minutes after eating.
d. She had a normal menstrual period 3 weeks ago.

6. A 45-year-old female complains of right upper quadrant abdominal pain. To help confirm your differential if you suspect cholecystitis you should:
a. Ask her to take a deep breath as you press upward into her right upper quadrant.
b. Auscultate her bowel sounds.
c. Percuss her abdomen.
d. Tap her heel.

7. An 18-year-old, 35-kg female is vomiting copious amounts of bright red blood. The most likely diagnosis would be:
a. Crohn's disease
b. Esophageal varices
c. Mallory-Weiss syndrome
d. Peptic ulcer disease

8. An 88-year-old female complains of nausea, vomiting, and constipation. Her abdomen is tender to palpation and appears distended. Her lungs are clear, and her vital signs are: BP 104/76, P 120, R 20. An appropriate action would be to:
a. Administer sodium bicarbonate, 1 mEq/kg IV.
b. Ask her to contact her personal physician in the morning.
c. Infuse normal saline at 250 mL/h.
d. Suggest an enema to relieve the pressure of her stool.

9. A 45-year-old male complains of severe epigastric pain radiating to his back. He has vomited several times. His history is significant for alcohol abuse and hypertension. You suspect an inflammatory condition of a gastric accessory organ. To confirm your differential on physical exam you should assess for:

a. Blood in the stool
b. Psoas sign
c. Grey Turner sign
d. Pain when the leg is extended

10. When assessing your patient's medication history, which would indicate the patient may have a preexisting ulcer?

a. Atropine
b. Diphenhydramine
c. Famotidine
d. Tegretol

CHAPTER

8 Infectious Disease

AS A HEALTHCARE PROVIDER, you come into daily contact with patients who have a wide range of illnesses and infectious processes. Patients may or may not know they have a communicable disease, may have an altered level of consciousness that prevents disclosure, or may choose not to reveal such information to you. This chapter is designed to give you more expertise in recognizing and understanding the nature and communicability of the infectious diseases you're most likely to encounter in the field. Safe practice and Standard Precautions will be reviewed, as will the signs, symptoms, and treatment of a number of infectious diseases. It's beyond the scope of this chapter to give you more than an overview of such a broad, ever-changing topic, so you're encouraged to do some further reading and keep up to date. Start with the Bibliography at the end of the chapter, which informed the content that follows, and take advantage of websites like www.cdc.gov, always a great source for current trends.

Learning Objectives ***At the conclusion of this chapter, you will be able to:***

1. Define specific terminology associated with infectious diseases.
2. Explain how healthcare providers and the general public are protected from communicable and infectious diseases through regulations developed by federal, state, and various local governmental agencies.
3. Identify the links in the chain of infection, and describe how bacteria, fungi, parasites, and viruses cause disease.
4. Explain how an exposure to a pathogen may evolve into an infection, and describe how each body system responds.
5. Describe the cell-mediated and humoral immunity defense processes of the immune system.
6. Discuss infection with bloodborne viruses such as human immunodeficiency virus and hepatitis B, including the causative agents, organs and systems affected, signs and symptoms, patient management strategies, and prevention measures.
7. Identify and discuss the epidemiologic and psychosocial aspects, pathophysiology, methods of transmission, clinical manifestations, and treatment and prevention protocols and strategies for the following bloodborne pathogenic microorganisms: human immunodeficiency virus (HIV), hepatitis B, hepatitis C, hepatitis D, as well as non-bloodborne viruses such as hepatitis A and hepatitis E—including the causative agents, organs and systems affected, signs and symptoms, patient management strategies, and prevention measures.
8. Compare and contrast the epidemiology, pathophysiology, methods of transmission, clinical manifestations, and treatment and prevention protocols and strategies for the following childhood diseases: rubeola (measles), mumps, rubella, pertussis, varicella zoster, and respiratory syncytial virus.
9. Identify and discuss the epidemiology, psychosocial aspects, pathophysiology, clinical manifestations, and treatment and prevention protocols for the following diseases transmitted by droplet transmission: viral meningitis and bacterial meningitis.

10 Compare and contrast diseases passed by droplet transmission (e.g., severe acute respiratory syndrome, meningitis) with those transmitted by the airborne route (e.g., novel H1N1 influenza tuberculosis).

11 Compare and contrast the pathophysiology, clinical manifestations, and treatment and prevention strategies for *Haemophilus influenzae* type B (Hib), pneumococcal, and meningococcal meningitis.

12 Identify and describe the pathophysiology, clinical manifestations, and treatment and prevention strategies for several types of herpesvirus infections.

13 Explore the problem of emerging multidrug-resistant organisms. Identify and describe the pathophysiology, clinical manifestations, and treatment and prevention strategies for these pathogens, including tuberculosis.

14 Explain the rationale for the various types of personal protective equipment, and describe proper disinfection of patient care equipment.

15 Describe the healthcare provider's responsibilities in prevention of communicable and infectious diseases and maintaining patients' confidentiality.

16 Identify and describe the pathophysiology, clinical manifestations, and treatment and prevention strategies for the following sexually transmitted infections: gonorrhea, syphilis, genital herpes, and papillomavirus.

17 Identify and describe the pathophysiology, clinical manifestations, and treatment and prevention strategies for the following zoonotic diseases: rabies and hantavirus.

18 Analyze your local protocol for reporting and documenting a communicable disease.

19 Identify and describe the pathophysiology, clinical manifestations, and treatment and prevention strategies for the following vector-borne diseases: Lyme disease, West Nile virus, and Rocky Mountain spotted fever.

20 Identify and describe the pathophysiology, clinical manifestations, and treatment and prevention strategies for the following multidrug-resistant organisms: MRSA, enterococcus, and pseudomembranous colitis.

Key Terms

antibodies Immunoglobulins produced by lymphocytes in response to bacteria, viruses, or other antigenic substances

antigens Substances, usually proteins, that the body recognizes as foreign and that can evoke an immune response

bloodborne pathogens Pathogenic microorganisms that are transmitted via human blood and cause disease in humans; some examples include hepatitis B virus (HBV) and human immunodeficiency virus (HIV).

communicable diseases Any disease transmitted from one person or animal to another either directly, by contact with excreta or other discharges from the body; or indirectly, by means of substances or inanimate objects such as contaminated drinking glasses, toys, water, or by vectors such as flies, mosquitoes, ticks, or other insects

contaminated A condition of being soiled, stained, touched, or otherwise exposed to harmful agents, making an object potentially unsafe for use as intended or without barrier techniques. An example is entry of infectious or toxic materials into a previously clean or sterile environment.

decontamination The process of removing foreign material such as blood, body fluids, or radioactivity. It does not eliminate microorganisms but is a necessary step preceding disinfection or sterilization.

epidemic A disease that affects a significantly large number of people at the same time and spreads rapidly through a demographic segment of the human population

epidemiology The study of the determinants of disease events in populations

exposure incident A state of being in the presence of or subjected to a force or influence (e.g., viral exposure, heat exposure)

hospital-acquired infection (HAI)/healthcare-associated infections An infection acquired from exposure to an infectious agent at a healthcare facility, defined as at least 72 hours after hospitalization

infectious diseases Diseases caused by another living organism or virus; may or may not be transmissible to another person.

nosocomial infection See hospital-acquired infection (HAI).

pandemic A disease occurring throughout the population of a large part of the world

parenteral Pertaining to treatment other than through the digestive system

retrovirus Any of a family of ribonucleic acid (RNA) viruses containing the enzyme, reverse transcriptase, in the virion. Examples of retroviruses include human immunodeficiency virus (HIV1, HIV2) and human T-cell lymphotropic virus (HTLV).

Standard Precautions Guidelines recommended by the Centers for Disease Control and Prevention for reducing the risk of transmission of bloodborne and other pathogens in hospitals. Standard precautions apply to (1) blood; (2) all body fluids, secretions, and excretions except sweat, regardless of whether or not they contain blood; (3) nonintact skin; and (4) mucous membranes.

virulence The power of a microorganism to produce disease

SCENARIO

PARAMEDICS ARRIVE AT AN ASSISTED-LIVING FACILITY to find a 45-year-old male seeking care for weakness and cough. He is found supine in his bed in a multiresident unit. He is jaundiced, his abdomen is distended, and he has swollen, edematous feet. He says he is recovering from heroin addiction. His cough has been persistent for a month, and his chest hurts when he coughs. You note a tremor of both hands. His vital signs are: BP 96/54, P 118, R 24. His SpO_2 is 90% on RA.

1 *Based on the information you have now, what differential diagnoses are you considering?*

2 *What additional historical and physical exam information will you need to narrow your differential diagnosis?*

3 *What are your initial treatment priorities as you continue your patient care?*

4 *How can you decrease your risk of acquiring infection if you are exposed to blood or bodily fluids during your care of this patient?*

The incidence of infectious and communicable disease is on the rise because of globalization and the reemergence of diseases once thought to have been eradicated. Healthcare providers must maintain awareness of the risks of disease transmission when assessing the patient and his or her environment. When we respond to a call for emergency medical services (EMS), we typically arrive to an uncontrolled environment. Be mindful that transmission of a communicable disease is more likely in situations where people live in close proximity to each other.

Our cautiousness, however, must be tempered by the obligation we have as providers to give the best possible care, without prejudice, to all who request our services. In the words of the early 20th century essayist Randolph Bourne, "We can easily become as much slaves to precaution as we can to fear." Having a fundamental knowledge of disease processes, understanding the communicability of infectious organisms, and observing Standard Precautions will allow us to administer care without undue concern about transmission of infectious disease to ourselves, our co-workers, or others.

Infectious diseases are illnesses caused by pathogenic organisms such as bacteria, viruses, fungi, protozoa, and parasites. Most infectious diseases—the common cold and otitis media, for example—are not life threatening. **Communicable diseases** constitute a subset of infectious diseases made up of illnesses that can be transmitted from person to person. Communicable diseases, then, are those that pose a threat to the healthcare provider. Not all infectious diseases are communicable. Rabies, for example, can be transmitted to humans only by infected animals. A case of human-to-human transmission has never been documented. Thus rabies is an infectious disease but not a communicable one. Infectious agents such as human immunodeficiency virus (HIV), hepatitis types B and C, tuberculosis (TB), and meningitis are both infectious and communicable and may be responsible for occupationally acquired illness.

Infection control always centers on early recognition through proficient assessment. As a healthcare provider, you must strike a careful balance between caring for patients and limiting the spread of infectious agents to others, including yourself, other healthcare workers, and the public. When dealing with communicable diseases, always consider the impact of the disease process not only on the infected patient but also on the community. The risk of transmission can be limited by taking the following simple precautions:

- Receiving immunizations/vaccinations
- Using personal protective equipment (PPE) consistent with the signs and symptoms of infectious disease
- Pursuing postexposure medical reporting and follow-up
- Gaining a broad comprehension of typical disease progression and recommended supportive management of the conditions for which patients seek care

Public Health and Safety Regulation

The public health and safety system is responsible for ensuring the general health of the population by means of education, disease reduction and surveillance, sanitation, and pollution control. An important segment of public health is **epidemiology**, the branch of medicine concerned with studying the causes, distribution, and control of disease in a population. Applied epidemiology also helps public health officials prevent or identify and control trends in the spread of infectious diseases.

Protecting public health is a multifaceted process:

- Instituting preventive measures, such as establishing immunization programs
- Overseeing health-related environmental matters, such as ensuring clean food, air, and water
- Pursuing educational initiatives, such as smoking cessation and obesity reduction programs

Local Agencies

At the local level, agencies including fire departments, EMS providers and agencies, health departments, healthcare facilities, and laboratories are the first line of defense in disease surveillance, outbreak identification, and pandemic planning.

Local agencies also support efforts to reduce the incidence and prevent the spread of infectious diseases by collecting and sharing data related to illness and injury; organizing it according to geographical region, race, age, sexual orientation, and ethnicity; and implementing priority initiatives.

Federal Agencies

At the international level, the United Nations World Health Organization (WHO) coordinates worldwide disease prevention efforts for members of the United Nations by providing leadership on global health issues and technical and logistical support for health research. WHO also establishes evidence-based standards related to health trends.

In the United States, public health and safety initiatives at the national level are executed primarily by the Department of Health and Human Services. The following agencies operate under its auspices:

- The Centers for Disease Control and Prevention (CDC) in Atlanta, Georgia, is the chief agency responsible for tracking and preventing morbidity and mortality associated with infectious disease. It's the most visible epidemiologic agency in the international medical community. The CDC monitors national infectious disease data and distributes this information liberally to all healthcare providers and to the community through the internet (www.cdc.gov) and in publications such as *Morbidity and Mortality Weekly Report (MMWR)* and *Emerging Infectious Diseases*.
- The Office of the Surgeon General oversees the U.S. Public Health Service and spearheads risk reduction activities, such as promoting childhood immunization, ensuring public preparedness for bioterrorist attacks, and addressing disparities in rates of infectious disease and access to treatment among various racial, ethnic, and socioeconomic patient population groups.
- The Food and Drug Administration (FDA) is responsible for ensuring the safety of prescription and over-the-counter drugs and medical devices, including those associated with transmission of infectious disease, such as indwelling catheters.

In addition, The Department of Homeland Security's Federal Emergency Management Agency (FEMA) works with the CDC, the Office of the Surgeon General, and other agencies to coordinate emergency preparedness for hurricanes, earthquakes, and other natural disasters that foster outbreaks of a variety of diseases. Infectious diseases are associated with floodwater, sewer line breaks, and crowded living conditions in shelters.

Standards, Guidelines, and Statutes

The Department of Labor's Occupational Safety and Health Administration (OSHA) oversees compliance, enforcement, inspection, tracking, and reporting related to infection control practice in the workplace. This is the agency that establishes guidelines for preventing transmission of airborne and **bloodborne pathogens** and develops postexposure protocols for use in occupational settings. OSHA standard 1910.120 specifies which personal protective equipment (PPE) must be available in given occupational settings and dictates how employees must be educated on its use to protect themselves from the hazards they're likely to encounter during the normal course of their work.

One of the OSHA regulations most important to healthcare workers is 29 CFR 1910.1030, which is intended to reduce the number of **exposure incidents**, defined as the transmission of bloodborne pathogens through **parenteral** contact with blood or other potentially infectious materials and the eyes, mouth, or other mucous membranes or nonintact skin during the performance of an employee's duties.

The Ryan White Care Act, passed by the U.S. Congress in 1990 and reappropriated in September 2009, constitutes Part G of the law. It contains a provision requiring that each emergency response agency have a designated infection control officer (DICO) who is notified in the event of an exposure. The DICO acts as a liaison between the exposed employee and the medical facility to ensure proper notification, testing, and reporting of results.

Epidemics and Pandemics

An **epidemic** is a disease outbreak in which many people in a community or region become infected with the same disease, either because the disease has been brought into the community by an outside source, such as an infected traveler, or because a pathogen (in this case, a bacterium or virus) has mutated in a way that either has enabled it to evade the immune system or has made it more virulent. Some epidemics occur when an entirely new disease emerges, as occurred with HIV and severe acute respiratory syndrome (SARS). Others begin when a new version of an old disease reemerges, as was the case with influenza A strains H1N1 and H5N1.

A **pandemic**, such as the devastating 1918 influenza pandemic, is an epidemic that sweeps the globe, reaching all seven continents. As might be expected, a pandemic usually results in a high death toll. As with an epidemic, a pandemic may arise from an old disease, such as smallpox or the bubonic plague, or from the development of a new disease or a new form of an old disease.

If the source of the pandemic is a virulent new pathogen or a new form of a pernicious old pathogen, very few people if any will have antibodies that make them resistant to the disease. Consequently, the rates of illness and death

TABLE 8-1 Biological Threats and National Security Issues

Diseases that spread across borders, crossing countries and continents (e.g., cholera, bacterial meningitis and measles)
The emergence of new and antibiotic-resistant diseases that arise in one region and spread throughout the world (e.g., AIDS and drug-resistant TB)
Environmental issues that may have global effects (e.g., pollution, loss of biodiversity, and global warming, which may affect the growth rate of insect vectors of disease)
Population overgrowth that may lead to disease, war, famine, and political instability
Bioterrorism: the deliberate release of infectious agents by a terrorist or rogue nation

Adapted from Goldberg J: Our Africa problem, New York Times, March 2, 1997.

may be catastrophic unless effective prevention strategies are rapidly developed and implemented. Although immunization is often an effective prevention strategy, developing a vaccine and ensuring its safety and efficacy in humans is a protracted process. The purpose of a vaccination is to induce a long-lasting protective immune response to prevent disease in a healthy individual receiving the vaccine. An immunization schedule recommended by the Department of Health and Human Services and the CDC can be obtained by accessing www.cdc.gov. Evolving technology has begun to compress the amount of time necessary to develop, manufacture, and distribute new vaccines. Table 8-1 lists some of the biological national security issues we are faced with today.

The Chain of Infection

Microorganisms that ordinarily reside in the human body without causing disease are part of the body's normal flora and constitute one layer of the host's defenses. Normal flora help keep the host disease free by creating environmental conditions inhospitable to pathogens, which are disease-causing microorganisms that rely on a host to supply their nutritional needs. The state of balance maintained by normal flora, in which conditions are favorable to the host and unfavorable to pathogens, is known as *homeostasis*.

Reservoir/Host

Pathogens may live and reproduce on and within humans, animal hosts, or other organic substances. Once infected, the human host may show clinical signs of illness or may become an asymptomatic carrier who has no knowledge of the infection but is nevertheless capable of transmitting the pathogen to another person. The life cycle of the pathogen depends on several factors: demographics of the host (e.g., age), genetic factors, temperature, and the efficacy of any therapeutic measures taken once the infection has been recognized.

Portal of Exit

A portal of exit is necessary if a pathogenic agent is to leave one host to invade another. The organism may exit the body by a single portal or several, such as the genitourinary tract, intestinal tract, oral cavity, respiratory tract, or an open lesion.

Transmission

Direct or indirect transmission may occur through the portal of exit and the portal of entry. Direct transmission results from physical contact between the source (reservoir) and the newly infected host. Indirect transmission takes place when the organism survives in or on an animate object, such as a healthcare provider's hands, or on an inanimate object (called a *fomite*), such as an ATM keypad or bed sheet. When indirect transmission occurs, the organism survives for at least a brief period of time outside the human host. Modes of direct and indirect transmission and examples of each are listed in Table 8-2.

Portal of Entry

The portal of entry is the site at which the pathogenic agent enters a new host. The organism may be ingested, inhaled, or injected through the skin, or it may cross a mucous membrane, the placenta, or nonintact skin. The amount of time it takes for the infectious process to begin in a new host after the pathogen enters varies with the organism and the host's susceptibility. In fact, exposure to an infectious agent usually does not produce illness in a healthy person, since the immune system is able to destroy it before it can multiply to cause an infection. The duration of exposure and the quantity of pathogens required to produce infection in the host differ for each pathogen.

Host Susceptibility

For an organism to produce illness, the host must be susceptible to infection by the pathogen—that is, he or she must be in an unhealthy or weakened state. If the host is healthy, the immune system subdues the pathogen and protects the host from infection (Figure 8-1). However, certain factors can impair the host's ability to do so. These factors are summarized in Box 8-1.

Natural Defenses of the Body

The body is equipped with an arsenal of clever defenses that inhibit pathogen invasion. The arrival of a pathogen through a portal of entry (see earlier) touches off a complex cascade of immune system responses. First, a nonspecific inflammatory response occurs involving migration of neutrophils and release of inflammatory substances in an

TABLE 8-2 Modes of Transmission of Infectious Diseases

Mode	Examples of How Contact Might Occur	Selected Infectious Diseases Transmitted by this Mode
DIRECT TRANSMISSION		
Touching an infected person	Shaking hands	Influenza, chickenpox
	Wrestling	Scabies
Oral transmission	Kissing or drinking after an infected person	Mumps, pertussis, infectious mononucleosis, herpes simplex virus type 1
Droplet transmission	Source coughs or sneezes, and new host inhales airborne mucus particles	Rubeola, mumps, pertussis, chickenpox, respiratory syncytial virus, SARS, bacterial meningitis, H1N1 influenza
Fecal contamination	Contact with feces at a daycare center	Viral meningitis, CMV
Sexual contact	Having intercourse without a condom	HIV, herpes simplex virus type 2, gonorrhea, CMV, syphilis, HPV
INDIRECT TRANSMISSION		
Food	Consumption of raw shellfish	Hepatitis A
Water	Drinking from a contaminated municipal water supply	*Escherichia coli*
Biological matter	Needle sharing, needlestick injuries, tattooing, and body piercing	HIV, hepatitis B, hepatitis C
	Touching an infected surface such as a bed rail	Rubeola, respiratory syncytial virus, HA-MRSA
	Contact with fomites such as towels and linens	Scabies
	Healthcare provider who has had contact with an infected patient touches another patient without washing his or her hands	*Clostridium difficile*
Soil/ground surfaces	Puncture wound	Tetanus
	Contact of nonintact skin with field turf	CA-MRSA
Air	Cleaning a basement or barn that contains infected rodent feces	Hantavirus

CA-MRSA, Community-acquired methicillin-resistant *Staphylococcus aureus*; *CMV,* cytomegalovirus; *HA-MRSA,* hospital-acquired methicillin-resistant *Staphylococcus aureus*; *HIV,* human immunodeficiency virus; *HPV,* human papillomavirus; *SARS,* severe acute respiratory syndrome coronavirus.

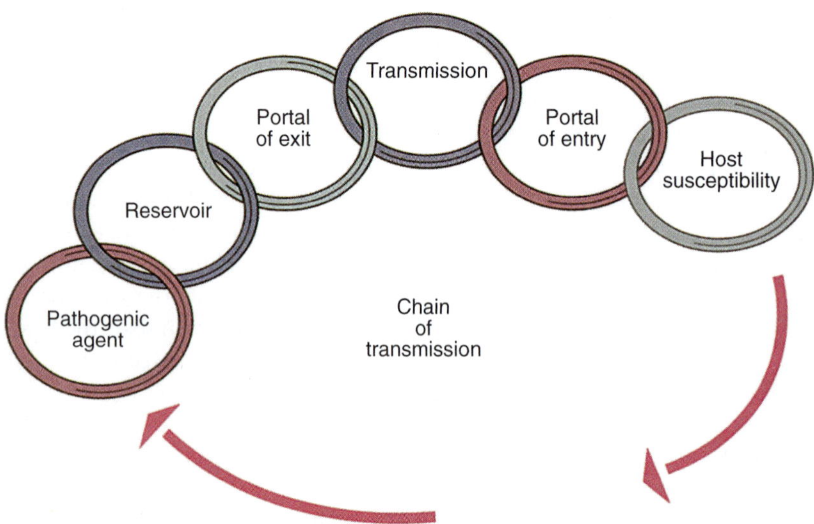

■ **Figure 8-1** Chain of transmission for infection. The chain must be intact for an infection to be transmitted to another host. Transmission can be controlled by breaking any link in the chain. (From Sanders M: Mosby's paramedic textbook, revised ed 3, St Louis, 2007, Mosby.)

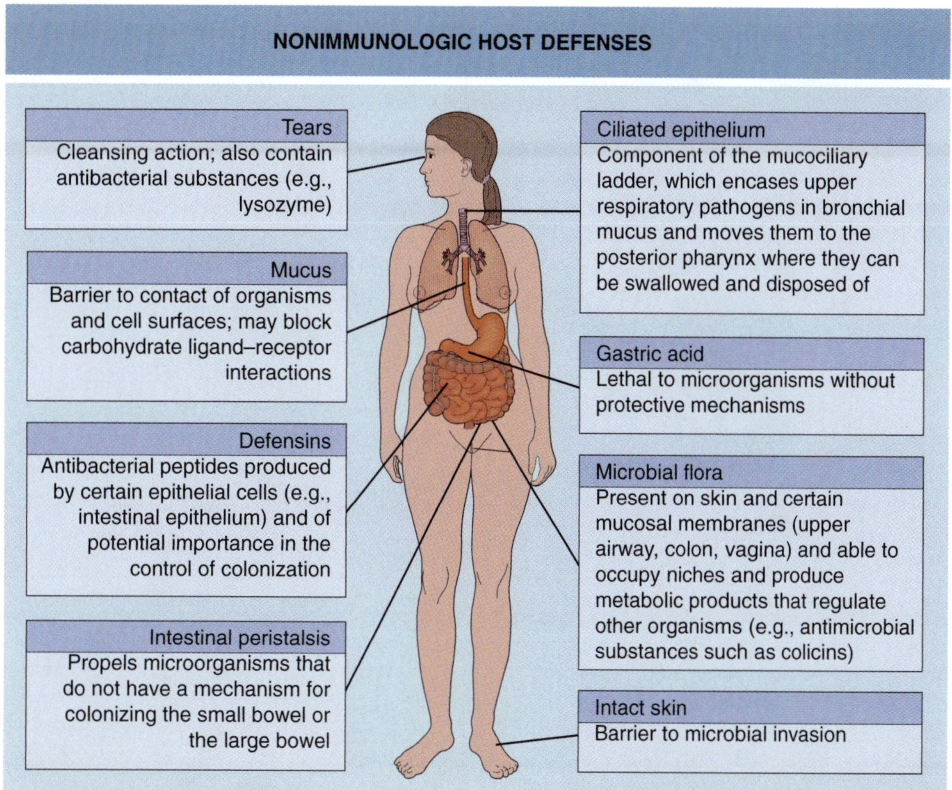
NONIMMUNOLOGIC HOST DEFENSES
Tears
Cleansing action; also contain antibacterial substances (e.g., lysozyme)
Mucus
Barrier to contact of organisms and cell surfaces; may block carbohydrate ligand–receptor interactions
Defensins
Antibacterial peptides produced by certain epithelial cells (e.g., intestinal epithelium) and of potential importance in the control of colonization
Intestinal peristalsis
Propels microorganisms that do not have a mechanism for colonizing the small bowel or the large bowel
Ciliated epithelium
Component of the mucociliary ladder, which encases upper respiratory pathogens in bronchial mucus and moves them to the posterior pharynx where they can be swallowed and disposed of
Gastric acid
Lethal to microorganisms without protective mechanisms
Microbial flora
Present on skin and certain mucosal membranes (upper airway, colon, vagina) and able to occupy niches and produce metabolic products that regulate other organisms (e.g., antimicrobial substances such as colicins)
Intact skin
Barrier to microbial invasion

Figure 8-2 Host defenses. (From Cohen J, Powderly W: Infectious diseases, ed 2, St Louis, 2004, Mosby.)

BOX 8-1 Factors That Increase Host Susceptibility to Infection

- **Age.** The very young and the very old are more at risk of contracting an infectious disease.
- **Use of drugs.** Taking immunosuppressive medications, steroids, or other drugs may affect immune response.
- **Malnutrition.** Poor nutrition weakens the immune system.
- **Chronic disease.** Chronic disease, such as diabetes and heart disease, gradually saps the body of its ability to defend itself.
- **Shock/trauma.** When a person is in shock or has been injured, body defenses are mobilized to restore organ function and to recover from injury, leaving him or her in a weak position to fight infection.
- **Smoking.** Use of tobacco products has been shown to impair the body's immune response.

effort to contain and inactivate the pathogen. Then a more specific response is initiated in which T lymphocytes develop receptors for a specific antigen on the pathogen. This allows the T cells to attach to and ingest the pathogen. B lymphocytes are activated and begin to produce **antibodies** (free-floating proteins) that have an affinity for the specific antigen as well. These circulating antibodies then bind to the antigen on the pathogen, either rendering the pathogen ineffective or allowing other body defenses to inactivate or destroy it. An antigen might be a component of a pathogen such as a virus, parasite, dust mite, or a blood product transfused into the body. The **antigen** is a molecule the immune system doesn't recognize as its own. The immune system sometimes reacts to components within the body, known as *self-antigens,* but it's activated primarily in response to exogenous antigens—that is, those introduced into the body from an external source. The immune system's capacity to distinguish between "self" and "other" is essential. Without it, the body would indiscriminately lay siege to its own cells.

Some cloned B cells become memory cells, which generate specific antibodies quickly in the event of a reexposure. This supports immunity to certain diseases by zeroing in on specific antigens and disabling them when they make a reappearance.

The human body has many other nonspecific protective mechanisms such as barriers like the skin, mucus, and cilia that trap organisms (Figures 8-2 and 8-3). Acidic secretions, such as those in the intestinal tract, inhibit organism growth. Several body systems also have mechanisms that affect immunity. A few are further explained in Box 8-2.

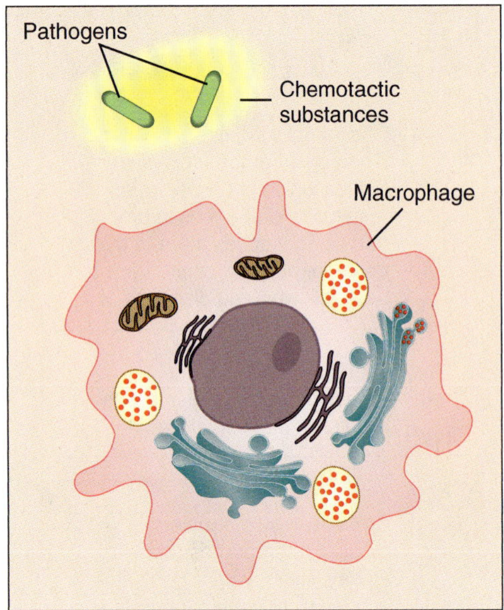

1. Injured area produces chemotactic exudate that attracts macrophages in area.

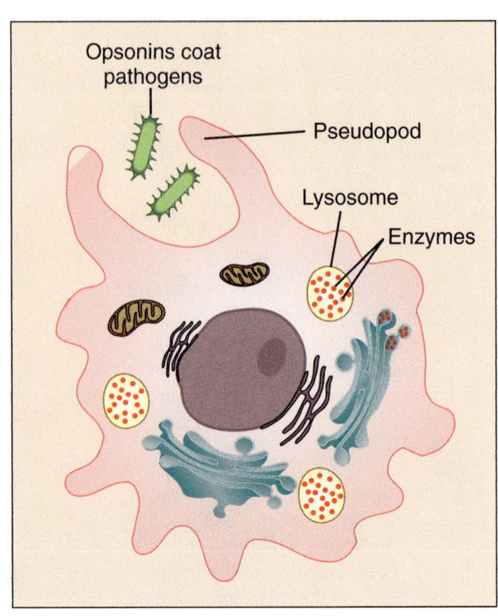

2. Opsonins facilitate phagocytosis.

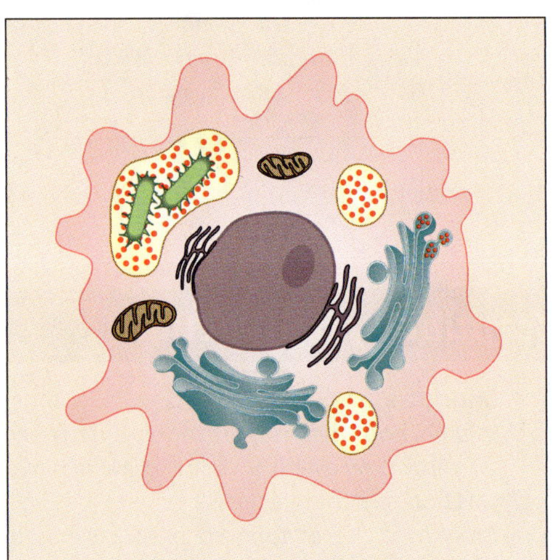
3. The engulfed pathogen becomes digested by enzymes in the lysosomes.

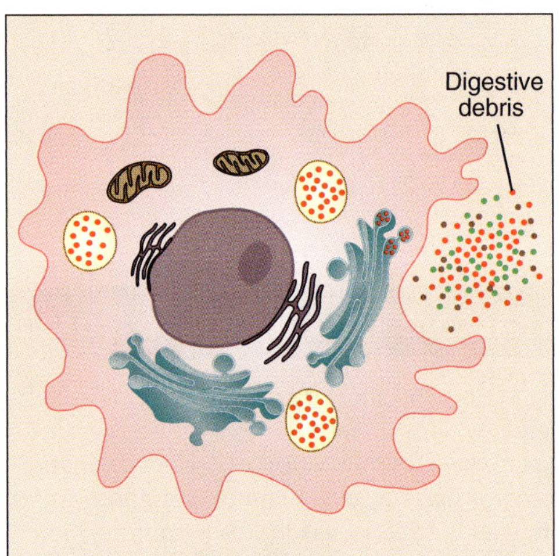

4. The macrophage expels debris after digestion is complete, including prostaglandins, interferon, and complement components. These elements continue the immune response.

■ **Figure 8-3** Second line of defense: inflammatory response. (From Sanders M: Mosby's paramedic textbook, revised ed 3, St Louis, 2007, Mosby.)

INFECTION

Infectious Agents

Bacteria

Bacteria are single-celled microorganisms that live in water, inside the human body, in organic matter, and on inorganic surfaces (fomites). Antibiotics are effective against most bacterial infections. Aerobic bacteria, such as TB and plague, can survive only in the presence of oxygen, whereas anaerobic bacteria, such as *Clostridium* strains (botulism and tetanus), carry out their cellular functions without oxygen.

Most bacteria are surprisingly fastidious, requiring specific conditions in order to grow, reproduce, and flourish. Certain bacteria, for example, must be confined to a narrow temperature range and must be supplied with particular nutrients to survive.

Viruses

Viruses, one of the smallest disease agents, must grow and multiply inside the living cells of a host. Viruses can cause minor illnesses, such as the common cold, or grave diseases, including acquired immunodeficiency syndrome (AIDS) and smallpox.

Only supportive care is required to treat most viral illnesses. In general, viruses are not vulnerable to

BOX 8-2 Role of Body Systems in Immunity

System	Role
Integumentary system	The immune system's first line of defense is intact skin. Organisms are unable to pass through intact skin, and the normal secretions of the skin are bacteriocidal, killing off many would-be invaders. Nonintact skin, on the other hand, serves as a portal of entry for pathogens.
Ocular system	The conjunctiva are protected in two ways. First, blinking sweeps away pathogens before they can enter the eye. Second, tear film dilutes the concentration of organisms present.
Respiratory system	Built-in protections in the lungs include moist mucous membranes and cilia that trap organisms that enter during inhalation. Then the cough reflex expels the pathogens from the body.
Gastrointestinal tract	Gastric acids and juices, along with helpful microorganisms that live in the GI tract, serve as another line of defense. Phagocytes assist in the ingestion and digestion of bacteria.
Genitourinary system	The genitourinary system is protected by a thick layer of cells and by the acidic secretions of the mucous membranes that line the genitourinary tract.
Immunologic system	Chemical properties of the immune system include properdin, a protein that acts with the complement system to protect against viruses and bacteria. The viricidal protein, interferon, is stimulated when viruses are present in tissue cells. Leukocytes initiate a nonspecific inflammatory response, then T and B lymphocytes generate cellular and humoral response specific to the invading organism.

antibiotics. Antiviral drugs have been formulated, and many more vaccines are being developed to prevent lethal viral infections or to moderate the severity of symptoms and reduce the length of illness.

Fungi

Fungi are plantlike microorganisms, most of which are not pathogenic. Yeast, mold, mildew, and mushrooms are types of fungi. Those of particular importance to humans and the illnesses they cause are:

- Dermatophytes (skin infections such as tinea corporis, also called *ringworm*)
- *Aspergillus* spp. (pulmonary aspergillosis and infections of the external ear, sinuses, and subcutaneous tissue)
- *Blastomyces dermatitidis* (blastomycosis, which causes abscesses of skin and subcutaneous tissue)
- *Histoplasma capsulatum* (histoplasmosis)
- *Candida* spp. (vaginal candidiasis and oral candidiasis, also called *thrush*)

Antifungal agents have been developed to treat most of these infections.

Parasites

Parasites are a common cause of disease where sanitation is poor, generally in developing countries, although cases are still found in the United States. Unlike viruses, parasites are living organisms. Like viruses, however, they must have a living host in order to survive and reproduce. Parasites live in or on the host and feed on it or consume some of the host's supply of nutrients at the host's expense.

Depending on the parasite, irritation and infection can be topical or systemic. Treatment is focused on agents that will relieve the irritating symptoms as well as eradicate developing eggs and live parasites. Antihistamines may be prescribed to relieve urticaria. Insecticides, acetylcholinesterase inhibitors, ovicidals, and pediculicides can be effective (Tables 8-3 and 8-4).

Formula for Infection

Disease progression varies greatly depending on the pathogen dose (the number of organisms present), the **virulence** of the organism, and the susceptibility of the host. Several conditions must be met for infection to occur.

A key concept in infection control is that exposure to a pathogen is not tantamount to infection. It simply means that the pathogen entered the host. Whether infection occurs depends on the above-mentioned factors. Postexposure prophylaxis can also decrease likelihood of infection. Hepatitis C constitutes one exception to this rule of thumb. It will be discussed later in this chapter.

Communicable diseases have stages, or periods, that identify the components of the infectious process. Let's explore each of them briefly.

Latent Period

The latent period begins when the pathogen enters the body by evading the host's outermost layers of defense, such as skin or acidic mucous secretions. During this period, the infection is not communicable, and the person exhibits no symptoms. This period may be protracted, lasting for months or years, or it may be as brief as a single day. This latent period is not the same as a latent infection or a latent disease. A latent infection is an

TABLE 8-3 Mechanisms of Cell and Tissue Damage Produced by Microorganisms

	Mechanism	Examples
Direct damage by *Shigella* toxin microorganisms	Production of toxins	*Escherichia coli* enterotoxin,
	Production of enzymes	Proteases, coagulase, DNAses produced by *Staphylococcus aureus*
	Apoptosis	HIV (CD41 T cells); *Shigella flexneri* (macrophages)
	Virus-induced cytopathic effects:	
	Cell lysis	Cytomegalovirus
	Formation of syncytium	Respiratory syncytial virus
	Inclusion bodies:	
	Intracytoplasmic	Rabies
	Nuclear	Herpesviruses
	Transformation	Human papillomaviruses type 16
Damage via the host immune response	Cytotoxic T cells and natural killer lymphocytes	Production of the measles rash
	Autoimmunity	Acute rheumatic fever
	Immediate hypersensitivity	Rashes associated with helminthic infections
	Cytotoxic hypersensitivity	Cell necrosis induced by hepatitis B
	Immune complexes	Glomerulonephritis in malaria
	Delayed-type hypersensitivity	Tuberculous granuloma

Adapted From Cohen J, Powderly WG: Infectious diseases, ed 2, St Louis, 2004, Mosby.

TABLE 8-4 Commonly Used Topical Preparations for the Treatment of Ectoparasite Infestations

Class	Agent	Uses	Toxicity	Efficacy
Acetylcholinesterase inhibitors	Malathion	Scabies Head lice Pubic lice		Good residual protection Recommended for pubic lice Infestation of eyelashes; safe in pregnancy
	Carbaryl	Head lice Pubic lice	Carcinogenic in animals; minimal risk to humans in therapeutic doses	Prescription-only in the UK
Organochlorines	Lindane	Head lice Pubic lice	Neurotoxic (potential for systemic absorption)	Increasing resistance; no longer available in the UK
Natural pyrethroids	Pyrethrin Phenothrin	Head lice Pubic lice		Less evidence of efficacy than synthetic pyrethroids
Synthetic pyrethroids	Permethrin	Scabies Head lice Pubic lice	Rarely rash and local edema	Probably safe in pregnancy and breastfeeding (limited data)
Others	Benzyl benzoate	Scabies	Skin irritation	Limited safety data in pregnancy; avoid in breastfeeding
	Ivermectin	Head lice Scabies		Available for topical and systemic use
	Crotamiton	Head lice Scabies		Relatively poor efficacy Avoid in pregnancy
	Mercury preparations	Head lice	Contact dermatitis Systemic toxicity	Available over the counter in some European countries
	Monosulfiram	Scabies	"Antabuse" effect (alcohol should be avoided)	No longer available in the UK
	Sulfur ointment	Scabies	Skin irritation	Cheap, safe, reasonably effective

inactive yet communicable infection that may become symptomatic at some future time. A disease is said to be latent when signs and symptoms wane between flare-ups. The herpesvirus family is an example of a pathogen that often enters a period of latency. During this stage, symptoms disappear; they reappear when the pathogen is reactivated.

Incubation Period

The incubation period is the interval between exposure to the pathogen and the onset of symptoms. Like the length of the latent stage, the length of the incubation period varies from one organism to another, ranging from hours to years. The difference is that during the incubation

TABLE 8-5 Infection Control Concept

Stage	Begins	Ends
Latent period	With invasion	When the agent can be shed
Incubation period	With invasion	When the disease process begins
Communicability period	When the latent period ends	Continues as long as the agent is present and can spread to others
Disease period	Follows incubation period	Variable duration

period, the pathogen reproduces in the host, mobilizing the body's immune system to produce specific disease antibodies. At this point, seroconversion may occur, which means that the antibodies reach a detectable level, and the infected person's blood begins to test positive for exposure to the pathogen. After infection, a window may occur during which no disease-specific antibodies can be detected in the blood despite the pathogen's still being present in the body in modest numbers.

Communicability Period

A period of communicability follows the latent stage. This stage lasts as long as the agent remains in the body and can be spread to other people. This period varies in length and is dependent on the virulence, number of organisms that are transmitted, mode of transportation, and the host's resistance. The age and general health status of the individual prior to exposure affects the susceptibility and risk factors of contracting the infectious disease.

Disease Period

A period of disease follows the incubation period. Its duration depends on the particular pathogen (Table 8-5). This stage may be symptom free or may produce obvious symptoms such as skin lesions or a cough. The body may eventually be able destroy the pathogen and thus eliminate the disease. Some tenacious pathogens, however, cannot be evicted from their new surroundings despite the immune system's best efforts to do so. They may lie low for a while, causing a latent infection, but pathogens such as HIV and herpesviruses remain in the body indefinitely once an infection has occurred.

THE AMLS ASSESSMENT

In assessing any patient, you must maintain a keen awareness of the risk for transmission of an infectious disease, not only from patient to provider but also from provider to patient. As you begin to assess the patient and the scene and situation, note the character and severity of the patient's signs and symptoms as clues to the possible presence of an infectious process. At the start of your assessment, consider the implications of such a diagnosis for your treatment strategy and for the infection control precautions you choose to implement.

The AMLS assessment process for a patient suspected of having an infectious disease rests on a thorough, comprehensive, efficient approach to diagnosing and managing associated medical emergencies. You must ensure that the patient has a patent airway, efficient work of breathing, and adequate perfusion, while simultaneously minimizing the risk of disease transmission through selection of proper PPE and other infection control strategies.

Evaluate the quality and regularity of the patient's pulse and the color, temperature, and moisture of the skin. Assess the patient's alertness using the AVPU mnemonic. Determine whether his or her condition is urgent or emergent, and identify and manage promptly any diagnoses of immediate concern. Initiate early treatment on the basis of these initial findings and your determination of how sick the patient appears to be.

Your differential diagnosis and subsequent working diagnosis should be made on the following basis:

- Incident and past medical history taken with the help of the OPQRST and SAMPLER mnemonics
- A focused physical examination
- Interpretation of diagnostic findings

Clinical reasoning and the patient's response to treatment will guide you as you select identifying laboratory or radiographic diagnostic tools that can confirm or rule out potential infectious disease processes in order to arrive at a definitive diagnosis. It's essential to be able to recognize the cardinal presentation of a wide variety of infectious diseases and to know how they are most effectively treated or prevented. In the following sections, we'll help you do just that by exploring signs and symptoms, diagnostic studies, and assessment and management strategies for the infectious diseases you're likely to encounter most often in the prehospital setting.

Infection Control

Universal Precautions/Standard Precautions

Transmission of bloodborne viruses occurs through exposure incidents (see earlier discussion). The prevention of

BOX 8-3 Elements of an Agency Exposure Control Plan

- Policy for health maintenance and surveillance
- Appointment of a designated officer (DICO) to serve as a liaison between the agency and healthcare facilities
- Identification of work functions when a risk of exposure to pathogens exists
- Policy for use of personal protective equipment (PPE) and availability of PPE to healthcare workers
- Procedure for identifying and evaluating exposures and a strategy for postexposure counseling, medical care, and documentation (as required by the Ryan White Emergency Response Notification Act, Part G)
- Effective plan for decontaminating personnel and for disinfecting and storing equipment
- Education regarding disease transmission, cleaning and disinfection procedures, use of PPE, and the purpose of immunization
- Steps for complying with medical waste regulations
- Strategy for compliance monitoring
- Recordkeeping policies and procedures

such incidents has always been an element of Universal Precautions, now called **Standard Precautions**, for routine patient care. Prevention efforts in the healthcare setting are now subject to OSHA's Bloodborne Pathogens Standard (which has retained use of the term Universal Precautions).

In addition to using PPE, safe work practices can help to protect mucous membranes and nonintact skin from exposure. These include keeping gloved and ungloved hands that may be **contaminated** from touching your mouth, nose, eyes, or face, and positioning patients to direct sprays and splatter away from your face. Carefully selecting and gathering PPE before direct patient contact will help you avoid the need to make PPE adjustments, reduce the likelihood of face or mucous membrane contamination during use, and reduce the possibility of contaminating gloves before you have contact with the patient. In areas where the need for resuscitation is unpredictable, mouthpieces, pocket resuscitation masks with one-way valves, and other ventilation devices provide an alternative to mouth-to-mouth ventilation, preventing exposure of your nose and mouth to the patient's oral and respiratory secretions during the procedure.

Preventing Sharps Injuries

Sharps injuries have been associated with transmission of hepatitis B and C viruses (HBV, HCV) and HIV to healthcare personnel. The prevention of sharps injuries has always been an essential element of Universal and now Standard Precautions. Needles and other sharp devices must be handled in a way that will prevent injury to the user and to others who may encounter the device during or after a procedure.

Since 1991, when OSHA first issued its Bloodborne Pathogens Standard to protect healthcare personnel from blood exposure, the focus of regulatory and legislative activity has been on implementing such control measures, including removing sharps hazards by developing and using engineering controls. The federal Needlestick Safety and Prevention Act, signed into law in November 2000, authorized OSHA to revise its Bloodborne Pathogens Standard to require more explicitly the use of safety-engineered sharps devices.

After a needlestick exposure, your risk of infection depends on the pathogen involved, your immune status, the severity of the needlestick injury, the amount of circulating virus in the source patient, and the availability and use of appropriate postexposure prophylaxis. Since 1991, each fire/rescue department has been required to formulate a comprehensive plan to address these issues. Exposure control plans are summarized in Box 8-3.

Healthcare Providers' Responsibilities

Employers are required to establish specific policies and procedures to protect personnel during the course of their duties. However, employees and volunteers play a role in protecting themselves as well. Employee self-protection responsibilities include:

- Giving full consideration to participation in vaccination/immunization programs
- Attending required education and training programs
- Using PPE properly
- Promptly reporting exposures
- Complying with all aspects of the department's Exposure Control Plan

Proper Use of Standard Precautions and Personal Protective Equipment

Handwashing The best means of preventing transmission of infectious agents remains the most basic one: effective handwashing. Since no barrier is 100% effective, hands should be washed before and after caring for each patient and after removing gloves. Alcohol-based antimicrobial products may be used when no gross contamination is visible or when conventional soap and water are not available.

Personal Protective Equipment Protective barriers offer a second line of defense to block entry of pathogens. These barriers include gloves, gowns, masks and other protective eyewear, sharps containers, and engineering controls that limit needlesticks. Gloves reduce contamination of hands but do not prevent penetrating injuries by needles or other sharp objects. Gowns prevent saturation of clothing and contact of skin with body fluids during procedures and patient care. Masks, face shields, and other protective eyewear reduce the likelihood of contamination of mucous membranes of the eyes, nose, and mouth.

PPE selection should be task specific. For example, gloves are not required for giving IM or subcutaneous injections. Table 8-6 shows the PPE necessary to perform various tasks when caring for a patient infected with HIV or HBV. Local protocols, policies, and procedures should be followed.

Needlesafe Devices Historically, most needlesticks have occurred during recapping procedures. The passage of the Needlestick Safety and Prevention Act of 2000 prompted the development of many engineering controls, including self-capping IV catheter needles, needleless IV tubing, resheathing scalpels, and safety syringes for medication administration. OSHA requires that sharps and other disposal containers be easily accessible at their sites of use.

Cleaning and Decontamination Procedures Decontaminate infected equipment according to the CDC guidelines and in keeping with local requirements. **Decontamination** of equipment should be performed only in marked, designated areas. Each area should have an appropriate ventilation system and adequate drainage. Always wear gloves, a cover gown if your uniform might become contaminated, and protective eyewear or a full face mask if blood or other potentially infectious materials might be splashed when decontaminating equipment.

Begin decontamination by removing gross dirt and debris with soap and a copious amount of water. Then disinfect as appropriate. It's important to follow the manufacturer's recommendations for each piece of equipment so as not to void the warranty.

Post Exposure In the event you experience an exposure to a communicable or infectious disease while on duty, report the occurrence without delay to your supervisor per protocol. Many agencies and institutions have designated faculty to recommend immediate and follow-up testing and evaluation.

Patient care should continue as appropriate. Washing hands and proper disposal of contaminated items should continue.

TABLE 8-6 Guidelines for Prevention of Transmission of HIV and HBV to Healthcare and Public Safety Workers

EXAMPLES OF RECOMMENDED PERSONAL PROTECTIVE EQUIPMENT FOR WORKER PROTECTION AGAINST HIV AND HBV TRANSMISSION[1] IN PREHOSPITAL[2] SETTINGS

Task or Activity	Disposable Gloves	Gown	Mask[3]	Protective Eyewear
Bleeding control with spurting blood	Yes	Yes	Yes	Yes
Bleeding control with minimal blood	Yes	No	No	No
Emergency childbirth	Yes	Yes	Yes, if splashing is likely	Yes, if splashing is likely
Blood drawing	At certain times	No	No	No
Starting an intravenous (IV) line	Yes	No	No	No
Endotracheal intubation, esophageal obturator use	Yes	No	No, unless splashing is likely	No, unless splashing is likely
Oral/nasal suctioning, manually cleaning airway	Yes[4]	No	No, unless splashing is likely	No, unless splashing is likely
Handling and cleaning instruments with microbial contamination	Yes	No, unless soiling is likely	No	No
Measuring blood pressure	No	No	No	No
Measuring temperature	No	No	No	No
Giving an injection	No	No	No	No

[1]The examples provided in this table are based on application of universal precautions. Universal precautions are intended to supplement rather than replace recommendations for routine infection control, such as handwashing and using gloves to prevent gross microbial contamination of hands (e.g., contact with urine or feces).

[2]Defined as setting where delivery of emergency health care takes place away from a hospital or other healthcare facility.

[3]Refers to protective masks to prevent exposure of mucous membranes to blood or other potentially contaminated body fluids.

[4]While not clearly necessary to prevent human immunodeficiency virus (HIV) or hepatitis B virus (HBV) transmission unless blood is present, gloves are recommended to prevent transmission of other agents (e.g., herpes simplex).

Physiologic Response to Infections by Body System

Respiratory

A variety of infectious organisms can infect the respiratory system. Respiratory infections such as the common cold, pharyngitis, tonsillitis, sinusitis, laryngitis, epiglottitis, and croup are principal causes of illness in the United States. Nevertheless, the healthy human body is generally able to stay free of serious infection.

Upper respiratory illnesses comprise infections of the nose, throat, sinuses, and larynx. Signs and symptoms of upper respiratory infection include sore throat, fever, chills, nasal drainage, and painful swallowing or speaking. One of the most common reasons for seeking medical care is pharyngitis, an inflammatory syndrome of the oropharynx, often localized to the lymphatic tissue and producing swelling of the tonsils, fever, and occasional secondary otitis media from blockage of the pharyngotympanic tube.

Lower respiratory infections, including pneumonia, often require antibiotic therapy. For patients with compromised immune function, respiratory infections may exacerbate underlying pulmonary conditions and progress to significant infection. Management should focus on supporting ventilation and hydration and on preventing spread of the pathogen.

Cardiovascular

Significant increases in pulse rate may occur as infection sets in and body temperature rises. Fever increases metabolic needs, necessitating more oxygen and nutrients to carry out physiologic functions. Hypotension may also occur because of dehydration, vasodilation, or both, as happens with septic shock. In rare cases, infection of the heart valves (endocarditis) may lower cardiac output, resulting in cardiogenic shock.

Identify and aggressively treat hypotension promptly. The treatment you select depends on its etiology. If the patient's lungs are clear and you suspect hypovolemia due to dehydration, vomiting, or diarrhea, aggressive use of IV fluids may be indicated.

Most patients with bacterial endocarditis have one of three predisposing factors: rheumatic or congenital heart disease, a history of endocarditis, or IV drug use. The most common site of infection in endocarditis is the mitral valve. Patients often have tachycardia, tachypnea, hyper- or hypothermia, and in severe cases, profound hypotension. Release of inflammatory mediators causes vasodilation and hyperdynamic cardiovascular effects. The patient will appear flushed, with warm extremities and adequate capillary refill. Prevention of septic and/or cardiogenic shock are emergent care priorities.

Depending on the type and virulence of the infectious organism, aggressive antibiotic therapy is the general course of treatment. In cases where the infection has damaged heart valves, surgical intervention to replace the valves may be necessary.

Genitourinary

Indwelling catheters are a major source of infection, especially among older adults. Decreased renal function, loss of muscle strength for urination, bladder obstruction, and lack of sphincter control are factors that often necessitate placement of an indwelling catheter. You should suspect infection when the patient has fever, chills, dysuria, back pain, difficulty voiding, an unusual color or odor of urine, or hematuria.

Integumentary

The skin serves as a barrier to pathogens, ultraviolet radiation, and loss of body fluids. It also helps regulate body temperature and maintain an internal homeostatic environment.

Wounds such as burns and even IV punctures can predispose a person to skin infection by breaking the continuity of the skin structures and allowing a portal for infection. Local infection such as cellulitis is easily recognized and treated. Signs of infection include redness, tenderness, warmth, drainage, and induration. Infection also makes skin vulnerable to parasites such as scabies and lice, which can be diagnosed on the basis of a visual inspection and the patient's report of intense itching, especially at night.

Special Circumstances

Older Adults

Because of diminished functioning of the immune system as they age, the elderly are more vulnerable to infection than younger patients and suffer greater morbidity and a higher rate of mortality from infectious disease. Aging lowers primary antibody response and cellular immunity and increases susceptibility to infection and autoimmune disorders. A number of other factors increase the risk of infection among older adults:

- The frequent existence of comorbid conditions, such as diabetes and neurologic diseases
- The living conditions inherent to group living situations such as nursing care facilities
- The higher rate of hospitalization among this population, which significantly increases the risk of contracting a **hospital-acquired infection/healthcare-associated infection (HAI)** (formerly called **nosocomial infections**)
- An increased incidence of malnutrition, which directly impairs the immune response

Assessment of older adults with infections may be challenging because of the difficulty in taking a thorough, accurate history and the absence of fever in nearly half of older adults with bacterial infections. The older patient may not exhibit the typical signs and symptoms of infection because of difficulties regulating body temperature and a depressed immune system. Invasive instrumentation (e.g., IV therapy, tracheal intubation, Foley catheterization) is often associated with infection. The benefits should outweigh the risks of doing so. Pneumonia, urinary tract infections, and sepsis occur more often in older adult patients, and pneumonia is one of the leading causes of death and hospitalization in this patient population.

Patients with Obesity

The branch of medicine that focuses on the treatment of patients who are obese is known as *bariatric medicine*. Obesity is defined as being 30% or more above ideal body weight. It affects nearly a third of the U.S. population (approximately 72 million people). The complications of obesity, such as hypertension, stroke, heart disease, and diabetes, can impact the immune system and increase serious illness when they contract an infection.

Patients Who Are Technology Dependent

Today many patients are cared for at home and are dependent on medical technology for their care, comfort, and survival. Care of such patients in the home setting is growing because of burdensome hospital costs, insurance limitations placed on length of hospital stay, and the goal of reducing risk of HAIs. These patients' medical needs, most of which are attributable to neuromuscular and respiratory disorders, include mechanical ventilation, tracheostomy care, administration of IV medications, maintenance of feeding tubes, administration of oxygen, and wound care. Decubitus ulcers are more prevalent in patients who are immobile and have compromised immune systems and increase the patient's risk factors for acquiring an infection.

Patients in Hospice Care

Out-of-hospital end-of-life care is becoming a more popular option across the country. Hospice care can be rendered in the patient's home or in a hospice care center. Vascular access devices, Foley catheters, and a compromised immune system from treatments such as chemotherapy diminish these patients' resistance to common viral and bacterial infections. Measures to reduce fever and control pain may be taken, and every effort will be made to promote the dying patient's comfort. When caring for such patients, you must consider the patient's and family's wishes with respect to advance directives for health care regarding resuscitation. Supportive care or comfort care is essential, especially for pain management.

Bloodborne Viruses

Human Immunodeficiency Virus and Acquired Immunodeficiency Syndrome

HIV, the virus that causes AIDS, was first identified in the United States in the late 1970s. It is a double-stranded RNA **retrovirus** that attacks the immune system, rendering a reduction in the ability to fight off infection. A person is generally considered able to transmit the HIV virus once he or she has tested positive for it. However, some people who are HIV positive can't transmit the virus to others because they have inherited a mutated gene (CCR5) that protects them either from developing active disease or from transmitting the virus to others. Such patients, called *nonprogressors,* comprise about 10% of the HIV-positive Caucasian population and an unknown percentage of the nonwhite HIV-positive population. People exposed to HIV who have not inherited this mutation may go on to develop AIDS.

Signs and Symptoms

HIV allows attacks on any body system (Figure 8-4)—cardiovascular, respiratory, or musculoskeletal. Signs and symptoms of HIV/AIDS are summarized in Box 8-4.

Pathophysiology

An uninfected HIV-negative person has a normal count of CD4 cells (500–1500 cells/mm^3), also called *T-helper cells*. These specialized lymphocytes are an important component of the body's cellular immune system. A person's CD4 count is reduced during the first 6 weeks after transmission of HIV because of uncontrolled replication of the virus. This is called the *initial phase* of the disease process, and the flulike condition associated with it is sometimes referred to as *acute retroviral syndrome*. This phase is followed by mobilization of a cellular and humoral response to the presence of the HIV virus. Nevertheless, the CD4

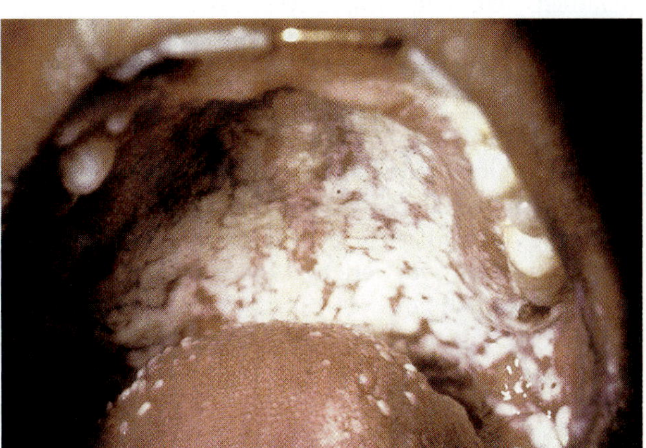

Figure 8-4 Oral candidiasis (thrush). (From Mandell G, Bennett J, Dolin R: Mandell, Douglas, and Bennett's principles and practice of infectious disease, ed 7, Philadelphia, 2010, Churchill Livingstone.)

BOX 8-4 Selected Signs and Symptoms of HIV/AIDS

GENERAL

- Enlarged lymph nodes, liver, spleen
- Vision loss, which may indicate cytomegalovirus infection of the retina
- Muscle wasting
- Weight loss

NEUROLOGIC

- Encephalopathy
- Peripheral neuropathy
- Increased intracranial pressure
- Behavioral changes
- Rapid eye movements
- Tremors or seizures

RESPIRATORY

- Low oxygen saturation
- Signs of pneumonia, such as:
  - Difficulty breathing
  - Rapid respiration
  - Persistent cough
  - Chest pain
  - Coughing up blood

CARDIOVASCULAR

- Chest pain
- Pale, ashen skin

INTEGUMENTARY

- Purplish lesions (Kaposi's sarcoma)
- Thrush (candidiasis of the mouth)
- Herpes lesions

level fails to return to normal because, over time, the virus slowly chokes off the body's supply of CD4 cells as it uses them to replicate itself.

By the third year after infection, the count may fall to a level of 500 cells/mm^3 or lower. This milestone represents the beginning of the second phase of the illness, known as the *asymptomatic phase* because the person still has no detectable signs or symptoms.

Finally, the infected person reaches the symptomatic phase, during which he or she begins to have signs and symptoms such as fever and weight loss (see Box 8-4). The HIV-positive patient is said to have AIDS when the CD4 count slumps to less than 200 cells/mm^3. During this phase, the patient becomes vulnerable to opportunistic infections because of the low CD4 count. The low CD4 count continues with progression of the disease as CD4 cells are destroyed more rapidly, therefore more readily identified, than other lymphocyte cells.

Treatment

Antiretroviral agents halt replication of the HIV virus and prevent damage to the immune system. These drugs are so effective that many individuals begin to test negative for the virus in their circulating blood. People who are HIV positive live as active members of their communities, participating fully in work and other aspects of normal life. Once started, however, antiretroviral treatment must be taken every day for the remainder of the patient's life. Every missed dose increases the risk that the drugs will become ineffective.

Antiretroviral drugs include Ziagen, Videx, Emtriva, Epivir, Zerit, and AZT. They may be prescribed individually, but combination medications pack two or three agents into a single pill. These compound agents include Combivir, Trizivir, Epzicom, and Truvada. Laboratory testing of viral load and CD4 cell count is essential in gauging how well the patient is responding to drug treatment.

Adverse drug reactions associated with antiretroviral agents may include headache, diarrhea, nausea, hypersensitivity reaction, and peripheral neuropathy (nerve damage). Since many of these symptoms are also symptoms of HIV disease itself, it's important to assess when they began relative to the start of antiretroviral therapy.

Prevention

HIV cannot survive outside the human host. Transmission occurs primarily during sexual contact or inoculation of infected blood directly into the bloodstream of an uninfected person, as occurs when IV drug users share needles. To protect yourself from HIV infection, use gloves when you're in contact with a patient's nonintact skin, mucous membranes, blood, or other potentially infectious materials. Use needlesafe devices and wear eye, nose, and mouth protection when you intubate a patient or suction the airway.

Routine use of a mask is not necessary. Good handwashing, however, is an important part of risk reduction. If an exposure to a patient's blood occurs, the medical facility must perform rapid HIV testing on the source patient. Such testing produces results in less than 1 hour. Rapid testing is accurate, since it identifies proteins present during the beginning of the life cycle of the HIV virus.

The use of postexposure rapid HIV testing is enforced by OSHA. If the source patient tests negative for HIV, no testing of the exposed provider is needed or recommended. If the source patient tests positive, the provider may be offered antiretroviral drugs as a preventive measure. However, because these agents have substantial side effects, such treatment is given only to patients who meet certain risk criteria established by the CDC. The exposed

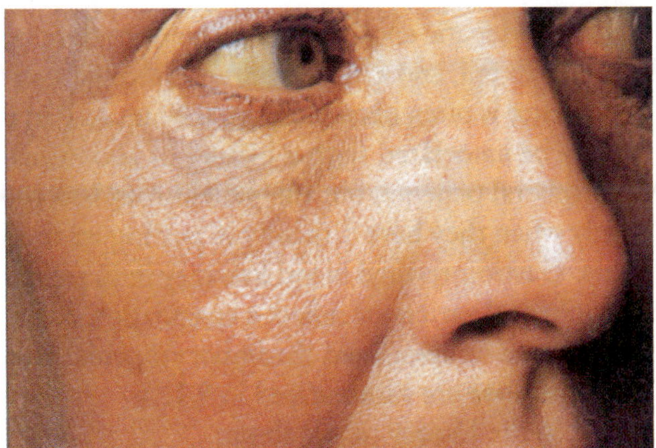

■ **Figure 8-5** Cholestatic jaundice in a patient with primary biliary cirrhosis. The high level of conjugated bilirubin, maintained over a long period, gives a characteristic dark brown-orange pigmentation to the skin and sclerae. Large xanthelasmas and corneal arcus usually develop in patients with primary biliary cirrhosis as a consequence of disordered lipid metabolism. (From Forbes CD, Jackson WF: Color atlas and text of clinical medicine, ed 3, London, 2003, Mosby.)

provider should be counseled regarding the risks and benefits of its use.

HEPATITIS

Hepatitis B

Hepatitis B virus (HBV) is a small DNA virus that overproduces envelope proteins called *HBV surface antigens,* which are easily detected by testing serum. HBV core antigens (HBcAg) and e antigens (HBeAg) are markers of infectivity and viral load. Testing for these markers is used to identify and monitor acute and chronic infection.

Signs and Symptoms

Signs and symptoms of HBV infection occur in two phases. During the first phase, the patient has flulike symptoms including fever, nausea, diarrhea, and abdominal pain. A large amount of virus is present in circulating blood. During the second phase, the patient's skin and eyes become jaundiced (Figure 8-5), the stools become whitish, and the urine becomes almost brown. The viral load drops, and antibodies appear in the blood. About 10% of those with HBV infection will become chronically infected, and the disease may progress to liver failure or liver cancer (Figure 8-6).

For both stages of infection, assessment is primarily visual but also depends on taking a thorough history. Ask the patient when symptoms began, and instruct him or her to describe the character of any pain and to identify its location.

Pathophysiology

Transmission of HBV occurs primarily through exposure to blood and blood products, sexual contact, or perinatal exposure. Risk activities for HBV infection include IV drug use and multiple sexual contacts. The incubation period for HBV ranges from 30 to 200 days. Five to 10% of adults have fever, arthritis, and a rash during the prodromal phase of the illness.

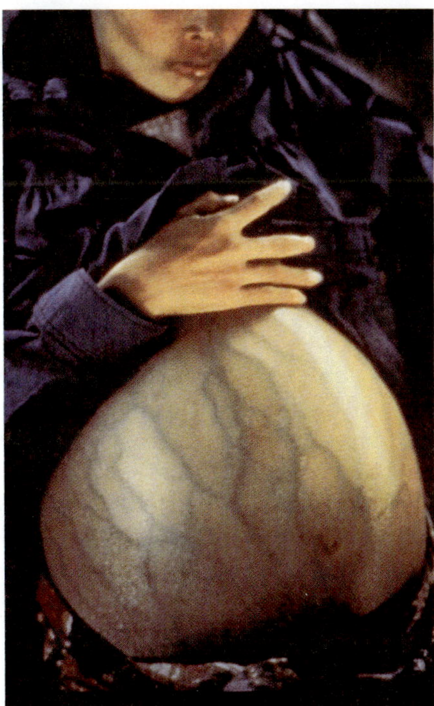

■ **Figure 8-6** A female patient with a distended abdomen caused by a liver tumor resulting from chronic hepatitis B infection. (Courtesy Centers for Disease Control and Prevention, Patricia Walker, Regions Hospital, Minnesota.)

Diagnosis

Laboratory markers for HBV infection (HBcAg and HBeAg) may be present for 2 to 7 weeks before symptoms appear. The appearance of symptoms coincides with a rise in levels of alanine aminotransferase (ALT), bilirubin, and aspartate aminotransferase (AST). These markers will decrease over about the next 6 months.

Treatment

Pharmacologic treatment is available for patients with chronic infection. Check the patient's medication list for interferon drugs, which may cause flulike symptoms, depression, and anxiety. Other drugs used for treatment, such as adefovir and tenofovir, may cause kidney dysfunction.

Prevention

You can protect yourself from HBV infection by following Standard Precautions when you must be in contact with blood or blood-tinged fluids. However, HBV vaccination is the primary method of protection for all people in the United States, where immunization is universal. Since 1991, all newborns have been vaccinated within 12 hours of birth. As of 2000, all middle school, high school, and college students were required to have been vaccinated before enrolling in school. Most healthcare personnel have been vaccinated since 1982. Thus the risk for and incidence of HBV has declined precipitously nationwide. Vaccination confers lifetime protection from the illness, so no booster or routine titer testing is required or recommended.

Hepatitis C

The hepatitis C virus (HCV) was first identified only very recently, in 1988. Testing became available in 1992. HCV is a single-stranded RNA virus that infects an estimated 1.5% of the U.S. population. In 2008, however, only 877 new cases of HCV infection were reported in the United States, and the incidence has continued to tumble.

Signs and Symptoms

Early signs and symptoms of HCV infection include fatigue, abdominal pain, and hepatomegaly (an enlarged liver). Palpate the abdomen and check for fever. Only 20% of patients with HCV infection develop symptoms associated with the second phase of hepatitis: jaundice, whitish stools, and dark urine. About 20% of such patients develop chronic infection, and 30% become carriers of the illness.

Pathophysiology

HCV has at least six genotypes and more than 50 subtypes, and it's difficult to culture. Genotype 1 is the most common and the least responsive to treatment. Transmission occurs through injection of contaminated blood, chiefly among IV drug users who share needles but occasionally in the following other ways:

- Tattooing or body piercing
- Needlestick injury
- Organ transplantation
- Transfusion of blood or blood products
- Sexual contact

The incubation period is 6 or 7 weeks but appears to be shorter when exposure occurs through transfusion.

Diagnosis

Laboratory testing has improved in recent years, and the actual viral protein, HCV-RNA, can now be detected. In 2003, the CDC began requiring that laboratories at all medical facilities be equipped to perform HCV-RNA testing, which can detect HCV infection in the exposed person 4 to 6 weeks after the event. Testing by reverse transcription–polymerase chain reaction (RT-PCR) is even faster, yielding results only 1 to 2 weeks after the exposure. The enzyme immunoassay method produces a high rate of false positives, however, and the results must be confirmed with a recombinant immunoblot assay (RIBA). Checking for antibodies with HCV-RNA testing can detect infection after exposure.

Treatment

People found to be infected with HCV receive a 24-week course of medication. The administration of interferon A, often in combination with antiviral drugs is a consideration for treatment.

Prevention

You can reduce your risk of contracting HCV by following Standard Precautions, including good handwashing practices, when in contact with a patient's blood or other potentially infectious materials. Promptly report any exposure so that the source patient can be tested. If the source patient tests positive for HCV, you should have an HCV-RNA test performed 4 weeks postexposure.

Currently, no medication can be given for postexposure prophylaxis, and no HCV vaccine has been developed. If you test positive for HCV at 4 weeks post exposure, a course of pegylated interferon plus ribavirin (PegaSys) will clear the blood of the virus.

Hepatitis D

Hepatitis D virus (HDV), or delta agent, was first identified in 1977. HDV is an RNA virus that depends on HBV for transmission. Consequently, it's often referred to as a *parasite of HBV*. This virus is most often seen in IV drug users, but the HDV infection rate in the United States is extremely low because of universal vaccination against HBV.

Signs and Symptoms

Assess for signs and symptoms of HBV infection, which include fever, abdominal pain, nausea, and vomiting. Often, behavioral factors such as anorexia can occur.

Pathophysiology

Transmission occurs by percutaneous exposure and, in addition, inefficient transmission occurs by sexual contact. The incubation period for this disease is 30 to 180 days.

Diagnosis

Serologic studies are done to evaluate the presence of the HDV antigen and HDV IgM antibody as a sign of active infection. The HDV has two properties which are both hepatitis D antigens. These antigens are identified early in the infectious process and involved in inhibiting the replication of the virus.

Treatment

Treatment consists of supportive care, since research does not support the use of antiviral medications for HDV.

Prevention

HDV can be prevented with vaccination against HBV. Always follow Standard Precautions, including good handwashing practices, when in direct contact with a patient's blood or other potentially infectious materials.

Non–Bloodborne Hepatitis Viruses

Hepatitis A

Hepatitis A virus (HAV) is a single-stranded RNA virus found in the feces of infected people. This virus replicates in the liver, but it usually does not directly damage the liver. In fact, this illness is often said to be benign.

Infection rates in the United States have declined about 90% since a vaccine for HAV became available in 1995. In 2008, 2585 cases were reported in the United States, the lowest rate ever reported in this country.

Signs and Symptoms

Patients with HAV may initially have malaise, fatigue, anorexia, nausea, vomiting, diarrhea, fever, or abdominal discomfort. Signs and symptoms during the second phase of the illness are the same as those for any type of hepatitis: jaundice, dark urine, and whitish stools. Ask the patient about any recent travel outside the United States, and inquire about possible dietary intake of contaminated water or food, such as raw shellfish.

Pathophysiology

Transmission of HAV occurs by the fecal-oral route. HAV colonizes the gastrointestinal (GI) tract and is detectable in the blood 4 weeks before symptoms occur. The incubation period is 2 to 4 weeks. Chronic infection with HAV does not occur, and the development of antibodies confers lifelong immunity.

Diagnosis

Laboratory tests can detect the presence of anti-HAV and immunoglobulin M (IgM) antibodies within 3 weeks of exposure.

Treatment

Treatment is supportive and centers on providing good nutrition and administering IV fluids.

Prevention

Follow Standard Precautions, including good handwashing practices, when you're in direct contact with a patient's stool. HAV vaccination is not recommended for healthcare providers.

Hepatitis E

Hepatitis E virus (HEV), which is often termed *enterically transmitted non-A, non-B hepatitis (ET-NANBH),* is a small RNA virus that multiplies in the liver cells and in peripheral blood mononuclear cells. Only one genotype has been identified. This virus is the leading cause of hepatitis in developing countries and elsewhere in the world, including Russia, South Asia, Africa, Mexico, and Central America, but it's extremely rare in the United States.

Signs and Symptoms

When assessing a patient suspected of having HEV, begin by asking about country of origin and travel history. Evaluate the patient for abdominal pain or tenderness, fever, nausea, and malaise.

Pathophysiology

The reservoirs for this virus are believed to be swine, chickens, and rats. The incubation period is 2 to 9 weeks.

Diagnosis

Low prevalence areas, such as in the United States, test for HEV-specific immunoglobulin M (IgM) to indicate infection.

Treatment

Treatment of HEV is limited to supportive care.

Prevention

Observe Standard Precautions, and use good handwashing practices when you're in direct contact with a patient's stool.

Airborne/Droplet-Transmitted Childhood Diseases

Immunizations have dramatically reduced the incidence of communicable diseases in children and adults, but they still occur. It's important to understand the clinical presentations of these diseases to implement appropriate PPE and interventions.

RUBEOLA, MUMPS, AND RUBELLA

The measles, mumps, and rubella (MMR and MMRV) vaccine uses live, weakened viral strains to confer immunity to these three childhood diseases. First licensed as a combined vaccine in 1971, MMR contains the safest and most effective forms of each vaccine. Consideration for administration of the appropriate vaccine is determined by the patient's specific health history and underlying health factors. Vaccination is recommended for all healthcare providers who do not have proof of immunity. It's not, however, recommended for pregnant women, and women of childbearing age who are offered MMR vaccine must be counseled not to become pregnant for 3 months after being vaccinated.

Rubeola

Rubeola is an illness caused by the measles virus, which can be found in an infected person's blood, urine, and pharyngeal secretions.

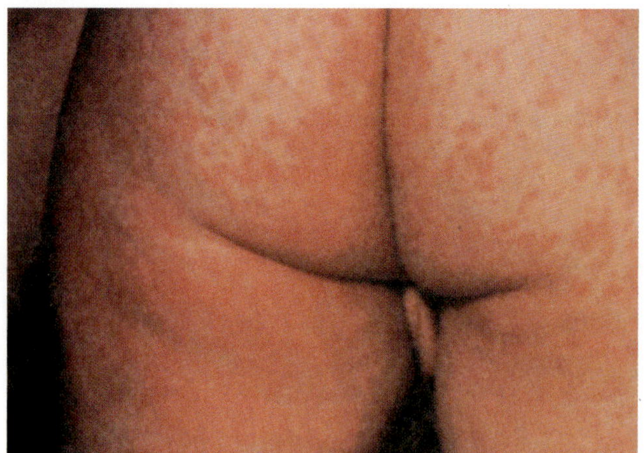

■ **Figure 8-7** Rubeola (measles) rash on the third day. (Courtesy Centers for Disease Control and Prevention, 1990.)

Signs and Symptoms

A key sign of measles is the presence of Koplik spots (whitish-gray spots visible on the buccal mucosa). Other signs and symptoms of rubeola include diarrhea, fever, conjunctivitis, cough, coryza (nasal congestion and discharge), and a blotchy red rash (Figure 8-7). Complications such as otitis media, pneumonia, myocarditis, and encephalitis occur in about 20% of reported measles cases.

Pathophysiology

The rubeola virus resides in the mucus of the nose and throat of the infected person. When the person sneezes or coughs, droplets spray into the air. The virus remains active and contagious on infected surfaces for up to 2 hours. The illness lasts for about 9 days. It usually is passed directly or indirectly through contact with infected respiratory secretions. In severe cases, seizures may occur, or the illness may prove fatal. Serious complications are more common among children under age 5 years and in adults over age 20.

Diagnosis

Serologic testing for the measles virus and antigens is helpful for diagnosis and treatment. If an IgM blood test is positive, viral cultures are performed. IgM is an antibody that's first produced in an immune response.

Prevention

If you're giving care to a patient with rubeola and you haven't been vaccinated or aren't immune to rubeola, place a surgical mask on the patient. If you're unsure whether you're immune, a serologic blood test should be performed. If results indicate nonimmunity, consider being vaccinated.

Rubella

Rubella, or German measles, is also caused by a virus found in respiratory secretions. This illness lasts for about 3 days. Rubella contracted during pregnancy may cause miscarriage, premature birth, or a low-birth-weight infant. If rubella is passed from the mother to fetus during the first trimester of pregnancy, anomalies in fetal development can occur, including mental retardation, deafness, and an increased risk of congenital heart disease and sepsis during the first 6 months of life. Collectively, these developmental anomalies are known as *congenital rubella syndrome*.

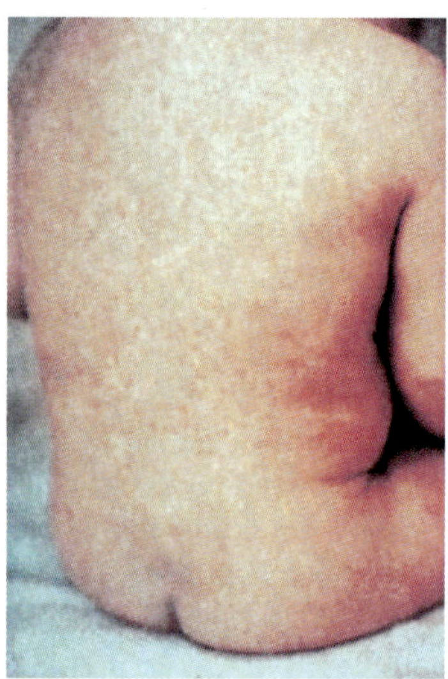

■ **Figure 8-8** Child with rubella. (Courtesy Centers for Disease Control and Prevention, 1990.)

Signs and Symptoms

Signs and symptoms of rubella include low-grade fever, rash, and swollen lymph glands behind the ears and at the base of the skull (Figure 8-8).

Pathophysiology

Rubella is highly contagious and can be transmitted from 4 days before the onset of the rash to 4 days after its onset.

Diagnosis

Serologic tests are performed to identify antibodies. PCR identification is done to isolate the virus.

Treatment

Supportive care is central to the management of patients with rubella.

Prevention

You can reduce your risk of contracting rubella by taking respiratory precautions such as placing a surgical mask on the patient, but vaccination is the key to risk reduction for healthcare personnel.

Mumps

Mumps, or infectious parotitis, is an acute, communicable, systemic illness caused by the mumps virus.

Signs and Symptoms

Mumps is characterized by swelling and tenderness of the parotid salivary glands affecting one or both sides of the neck. The patient will also have a fever. Rare complications include hydrocephalus, hearing loss, Guillain-Barré syndrome, pancreatitis, and myocarditis.

Pathophysiology

The mumps virus is transmitted by inhaling the saliva droplets of an infected person. This occurs most often in older children during winter and spring. The virus has an incubation period of 12 to 26 days and a communicable period ranging from 1 week to 9 days after the onset of symptoms.

Diagnosis

Assessment for parotid swelling is performed. Serologic tests are not necessarily done for measles and mumps.

Treatment

Treatment is supportive and includes analgesic and antipyretic medications.

Prevention

Take respiratory droplet precautions (place a surgical mask on the patient) when you transport a patient suspected of having mumps. Vaccination is the key to risk reduction among healthcare personnel.

Pertussis (Whooping Cough)

According to the WHO, in 2005, 50 million cases of pertussis occurred worldwide, with 300,000 deaths attributable to the disease. In developing countries as well as in the United States, pertussis is a reemerging problem. The incidence of the disease has increased every year since the 1980s.

Signs and Symptoms

Ask about the patient's exposure to patients with known cases of pertussis. Signs and symptoms during the first stage of whooping cough, known as the *catarrhal phase,* include fever, malaise, sneezing, and anorexia. This stage lasts several days. The second stage of the illness, the paroxysmal coughing phase, is the key to identifying the disease. The patient may have 50 or more episodes of spasmodic coughing per day. When each convulsive cough subsides, a whooping sound emerges. Assess for vomiting, low oxygen saturation, convulsions, and coma. During the third stage, the convalescent phase, the coughing begins to subside, becoming less frequent and intense. The illness may last several weeks.

Pathophysiology

The causative organism in whooping cough is the gram-negative bacterium *Bordetella pertussis*. The organism can survive outside the respiratory tract for only a short period of time. When it does gain entry to the respiratory tract, it attaches to cilia, immobilizing them. The bacteria produce toxins that can cause systemic illness. The incubation period is 7 to 10 days, and transmission occurs by direct contact with oral or nasal secretions. The primary risk group is children and adolescents; however, a worrisome rise has been reported in the incidence of pertussis among adults.

Diagnosis

Diagnosis consists of laboratory testing for rising antibody titers.

Treatment

Treatment centers on antibiotic therapy, usually with erythromycin.

Prevention

A pertussis vaccine became available in 1940, and childhood vaccination remains the primary means of prevention and control. Take droplet precautions when caring for a patient suspected of having whooping cough. Place a surgical mask or an oxygen mask on the patient and follow Standard Precautions.

Vaccination may not confer lifetime immunity to pertussis as previously believed, so healthcare providers should receive a one-time booster dose of Tdap (tetanus, diphtheria, acellular pertussis). Report any exposure as soon as possible so that a 14-day course of antibiotics can be given.

Varicella-Zoster Virus (Chickenpox)

Chickenpox is a highly contagious disease caused by the varicella-zoster virus (Figure 8-9), a member of the herpesvirus family. Chickenpox occurs worldwide, affecting people of all races, ages, and both sexes. However, it's largely a childhood disease, with most cases occurring

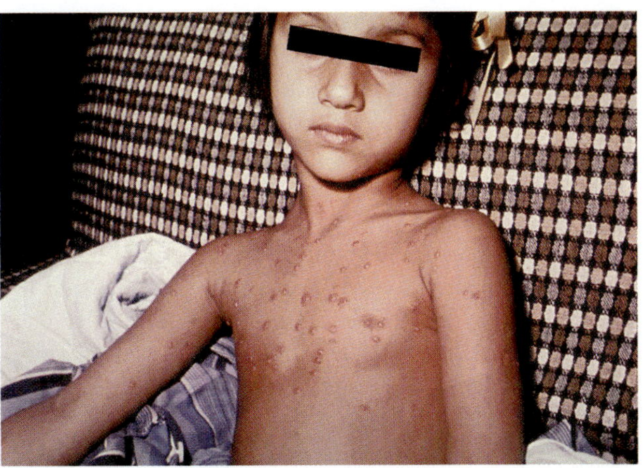

Figure 8-9 Chickenpox. (From Marx J, Hockberger R, Walls R: Rosen's emergency medicine, ed 7, St Louis, 2009, Mosby.)

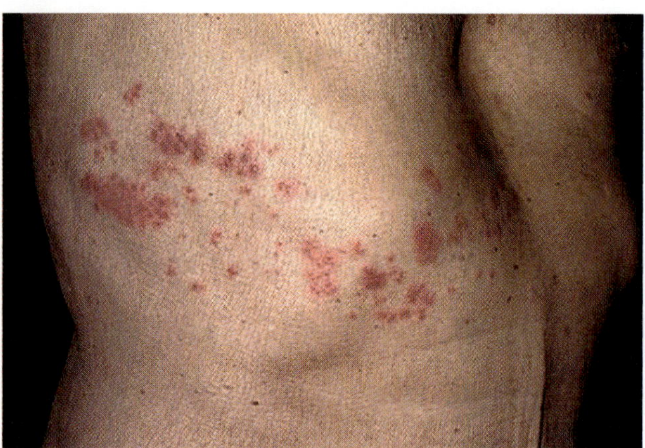

■ **Figure 8-10** Herpes zoster (shingles). (From Marx J, Hockberger R, Walls R: Rosen's emergency medicine, ed 7, St Louis, 2009, Mosby.)

before age 10. An estimated 60 million cases occur worldwide each year.

Once a person has had chickenpox, he or she is unlikely to contract the illness again, since infection is thought to confer lifelong immunity in most people. However, those with compromised immune systems are susceptible to the virus regardless of their history, and measures should be taken to either prevent or modify the course of the disease if the person is exposed to the virus.

Generally, varicella-zoster is eliminated from the body after infection. In some people, however, the virus is retained in the spinal dorsal nerve root ganglia, reappearing later in life as herpes zoster (shingles) infection (Figure 8-10). This reactivation of the virus may occur during a period of physical or emotional stress. The herpes zoster lesions drain live virus and are extraordinarily painful.

Signs and Symptoms

Prodromal symptoms of chickenpox include fever, malaise, anorexia, and headache. Next, the patient will develop itchy blisters or a rash. Assess for signs of superinfection, including impetigo, cellulitis, necrotizing fasciitis, and arthritis. Question the patient about any recent exposure to others, especially children who are known to have the illness. If the patient is an adult, ask about their immunodeficiency status.

Pathophysiology

Transmission of this virus may occur in one of two ways: inhalation of airborne respiratory droplets or contact with drainage from vesicles. The portal of entry is usually the conjunctival or upper respiratory mucosa. Viral replication takes place in regional lymph nodes during the next 2 to 4 days, after which a primary viremia occurs (4 to 6 days after inoculation). The virus then replicates in the liver, spleen, and possibly in other organs. This secondary viremia occurs 14 to 16 days after initial exposure. It's characterized by the spread of viral particles to the skin, which causes the typical vesicular rash. The rash initially appears on the covered areas of the body and spreads to the face, scalp, and sometimes the mucous membranes of the mouth or genitals. The shallow vesicles progress to become deeper pustules. As they heal, the lesions dry up and crust over. The usual incubation period of varicella-zoster is 10 to 21 days. The patient is contagious for 1 to 2 days before the rash appears until all the lesions are dry and crusted.

Diagnosis

Laboratory testing is generally not performed. Diagnosis is made on the basis of clinical presentation.

Treatment

Treatment for patients with chickenpox is symptomatic. Oral antihistamines or lotion can be prescribed to relieve itching. In children, fever should be reduced without the use of aspirin, to avoid the risk of developing Reye's syndrome. Fingernails should be trimmed to prevent skin excoriation from scratching. Antiviral medications and corticosteroids may be prescribed to shorten the duration of symptoms.

Prevention

Vaccination is the primary means of protection from varicella-zoster for both patients and healthcare providers. If possible, take droplet precautions by placing a surgical mask on the patient. If you are unable to do so, place a surgical mask on yourself. Wear gloves when in direct contact with draining lesions. Routine cleaning of the vehicle is adequate, and no airing of the vehicle is needed. If an exposure occurs, contact your DICO, since postexposure medical treatment may be indicated. If you are vaccinated after exposure, you must be on work restriction from day 10 to day 28 after exposure.

Respiratory Syncytial Virus

Respiratory syncytial virus is an RNA respiratory virus that infects the lungs and breathing passages. In the United States, it's seasonal, occurring in the late fall, winter, and early spring. In countries near the equator, the virus is present year round.

Most healthy adults recover from respiratory syncytial virus infection in 1 to 2 weeks, but in infants, young children, and older adults, the virus is one of the leading causes of respiratory illness. In the United States, it's the most common cause of bronchiolitis (inflammation of the small airways in the lungs) and pneumonia in children under age 1.

Signs and Symptoms

Symptoms of respiratory syncytial virus include fever, sneezing, wheezing, cough, decreased appetite, and nasal congestion. Hypoxemia and apnea are common in infants with respiratory syncytial virus and constitute the primary reason for hospitalization. Assess the patient for a history of exposure to the virus, and evaluate the patient's ventilation and breath sounds.

Pathophysiology

Transmission of respiratory syncytial virus occurs by airborne droplets or by contact with contaminated surfaces. The portal of entry is usually the eyes, nose, or mouth. Respiratory syncytial virus is a large-particle virus that travels only about 3 feet. It may have a limited range, but it compensates by surviving well on fomites; for example, virus can be cultured more than 5 hours after it's transferred to an impervious surface such as a bed rail. The virus has an incubation period of 2 to 8 days.

Diagnosis

Testing is usually used during the respiratory syncytial virus season to help diagnose the illness in patients who have moderate to severe symptoms and lower respiratory tract involvement. Testing is ordered primarily on infants between age 6 months and 2 years, elderly patients, and those with compromised immune systems, such as those with preexisting lung disease and recipients of organ transplants.

Treatment

Treatment is limited to the administration of beta-agonists and supportive care and may include administering oxygen, hydrating the patient, and providing suctioning, ventilation assistance, or intubation as necessary.

Prevention requires following Standard Precautions, including frequent handwashing. Clean surfaces with a disinfectant registered with the Environmental Protection Agency (EPA).

Prevention

Respiratory syncytial virus immune globulin intravenous (RSV-IGIV) is an FDA-approved treatment for prevention of lower respiratory tract infections in infants at high risk of contracting respiratory syncytial virus.

Diseases Transmitted by Droplet Transmission

Droplet transmission of a communicable disease occurs when the droplets of an infected person, which can travel only 3 to 6 feet, are spread during close person-to-person contact: kissing, hugging, or otherwise touching someone, sharing eating or drinking utensils, or talking to someone within a 3-foot radius. In contrast to airborne transmission, the particles passed by droplet transmission are larger and do not travel as far. The heavy particles do not become aerosolized, so they can't hang suspended in the air for any appreciable length of time.

Exposure to a disease communicable by droplet transmission is defined as direct contact with a patient's oronasal secretions, which may occur, for example, during unprotected mouth-to-mouth ventilation, suctioning, or spraying of secretions with no facial protection during intubation.

Severe Acute Respiratory Syndrome

The severe acute respiratory syndrome coronavirus (SARS-CoV) has a brief and puzzling history. It was first identified in 2003. From its point of origin somewhere in China, an outbreak of this new virus swept through Asia and quickly made its way around the world. The virus vanished, however, almost as quickly as it had appeared. Panicky predictions of global calamity failed to materialize, and not a single case of SARS has been reported since 2003.

During its brief appearance, the disease was spread through close person-to-person contact by means of large-particle respiratory droplets. The virus was also spread by contact with contaminated surfaces.

Viral Meningitis

More than 90% of meningitis cases have a viral etiology. This illness occurs worldwide. Viral meningitis, or aseptic meningitis, is not a risk to the healthcare provider. It does, however, pose a threat to the patient.

Signs and Symptoms

Signs and symptoms include the sudden onset of a headache, sensitivity to light, fever, stiff neck, and vomiting. Some strains of viral meningitis cause a rash, which may cover most of the body or just the arms and legs. The rash is red and mostly flat, although it may be raised in some areas. It's not the same as the rash seen in meningococcal meningitis, which is characterized by small, bright-red pinpoint spots covering most of the body.

The clinical presentation of viral meningitis can seem benign. Patients typically have fever, headache, and nausea and vomiting. Photophobia and nuchal rigidity are less common and are not definitive signs of CNS infection. Alterations in mentation indicate the need for emergent intervention and stabilization. You must identify increased intracranial pressure and signs of seizure activity early in the assessment process. Monitor the patient continually for seizures, disseminated intravascular coagulation, arrhythmias, and increased intracranial pressure.

Pathophysiology

Viral meningitis is a common and relatively mild illness spread by direct contact with infected feces or nose and throat secretions. The incubation period is 2 to 10 days.

The virus spreads most rapidly among young children and among those in group living situations. It usually strikes in the summer and early autumn. High schools and colleges are common sites of seasonal outbreaks. Most children and adults recover completely from viral meningitis within 10 to 14 days. Anyone can contract the disease, but most people older than age 40 have developed immunity to it.

Diagnosis

A recent history of travel may point to a specific cause. Patients who have headaches that worsen when they lean forward, sneeze, or cough may have increased intracranial pressure.

A thorough neurologic exam, including cranial nerves, is also performed. Bacteria that form neurotoxins, such as *Staphylococcus* and *Streptococcus,* can cause changes in mentation similar to those observed in patients with viral meningitis, so they must be included in your differential diagnosis. In addition, inflammation of the meninges can also be caused by fungi such as *Candida albicans* and *Cryptococcus neoformans* and by tumors and subarachnoid hemorrhage.

Blood and cerebrospinal fluid (CSF) cultures must be drawn to distinguish viral from bacterial or fungal causes. A cloudy appearance of the CSF indicates an increased white blood cell (WBC) count. The presence of a large concentration of WBCs in the CSF points to bacterial meningitis or a cerebral abscess. Gram stain analysis can identify the causative organism and allow antibiotic therapy to be targeted more precisely.

Before a spinal tap is performed, the plasma glucose level is determined. This level is a diagnostic clue because when the number of bacteria in the CSF cells rises, more glucose is utilized during cell metabolism. A low CSF glucose level (<60% mg/dL [<3.3 mmol/L] of blood glucose) suggests meningitis. In addition, diagnostic studies such as an electroencephalogram (EEG), computed tomography (CT) scan, or magnetic resonance imaging (MRI) study may provide valuable diagnostic information about potentially serious complications.

Treatment

Identifying underlying treatable causes of the meningitis improves outcomes. The earlier you can pinpoint such conditions, the sooner effective management strategies can be initiated. Stabilizing airway, breathing, and circulation and obtaining a thorough history and physical exam are the keys to identifying any latent disease process that may be causing the meningitis.

Antimicrobial medications such as antibiotics, antifungals, and antivirals usually offer definitive treatment. Supportive therapy includes ensuring adequate hydration and administering antipyretics and analgesics. If seizure activity is present, initiate anticonvulsant therapy. Observe local protocol regarding notifying the public health department in order to assist in early identification of any uptick in the incidence of meningitis in the area. In severe cases, the patient may require rehabilitation and physical therapy during recovery from the illness.

Prevention

Prevention through vaccination is the ideal way to prevent meningitis. Follow Standard Precautions, including practicing scrupulous hand hygiene. Use proper PPE when treating a patient suspected of having viral meningitis.

BACTERIAL MENINGITIS

Bacterial meningitis is a serious infection of the fluid that surrounds the brain and spinal cord. Cases of bacterial meningitis occur worldwide. Bacterial meningitis is usually caused by one of three types of bacteria: *Haemophilus influenzae* type b (Hib), *Neisseria meningitidis,* or *Streptococcus pneumoniae.*

Bacterial meningitis from Hib and *S. pneumoniae* can be prevented by vaccination. Since these bacteria were common causes of meningitis, the incidence of bacterial meningitis has greatly diminished because of immunization programs for children, especially in the United States.

Haemophilus influenzae Type B Meningitis

H. influenzae appears to be an exclusively human pathogen. In infants and young children, Hib causes bacteremia, pneumonia, acute bacterial meningitis, and sometimes cellulitis, osteomyelitis, epiglottitis, and joint infections. Before 1985 when a vaccine became available, 1 in 200 children was believed to have had Hib meningitis by 2 months of age. The worldwide incidence of Hib was 2 million cases annually, resulting in 300,000 deaths. Immunization programs are now available in North America, Western Europe, Japan, and some Latin American countries.

Signs and Symptoms

Hib meningitis is similar to other types of meningitis. Signs include:

- Fever
- Severe headache
- Stiff neck
- Irritability and crying
- Tiredness, drowsiness, or difficulty waking up
- Vomiting
- Refusing food and drink
- Convulsions or seizures
- Loss of consciousness

Hib epiglottitis, a dangerous infection that may accompany meningitis, causes noisy, labored breathing and is often misdiagnosed as croup in children between the ages of 6 and 8.

Pathophysiology

The incubation period for Hib meningitis is unknown, but it may be about 2 to 4 days.

Diagnosis

Laboratory confirmation of Hib meningitis is made by isolating the organism in a culture of blood or CSF.

Treatment

Support oxygenation, and administer IV drugs to control seizure activity or treat shock if present. Antibiotics should be administered intravenously as early as possible.

Prevention

Children are immunized against Hib in a series, beginning at 2 months of age. Doses are given at 2, 4, and 6 months, followed by another dose at age 12 to 15 months, depending on the vaccine used. When treating a child suspected of having bacterial meningitis, use good hand hygiene practices. No postexposure treatment is needed or recommended for adults.

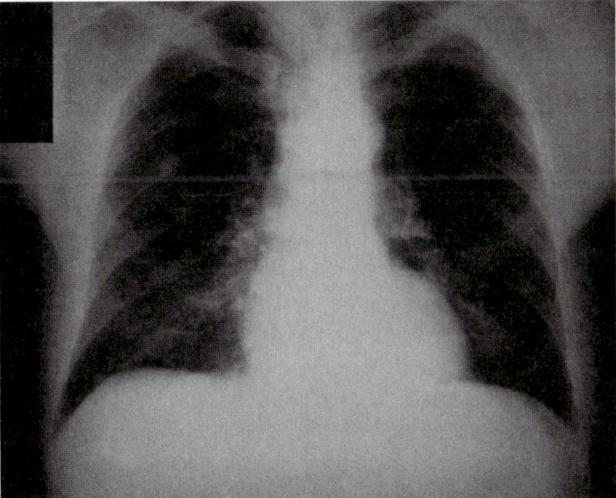

■ **Figure 8-11** A patient with pneumonia in the upper right lobe. (Courtesy Centers for Disease Control and Prevention, Thomas Hooten.)

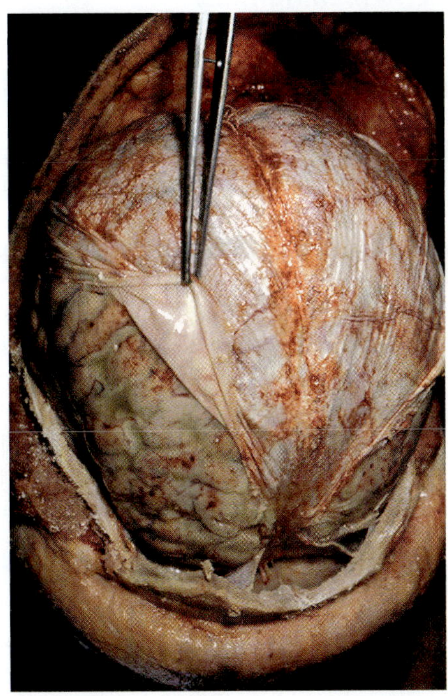

■ **Figure 8-12** Pneumococcal meningitis. (Courtesy Centers for Disease Control and Prevention, Edwin P. Ewing, Jr.)

■ *Streptococcus pneumoniae* (Pneumococcal) Meningitis

Streptococcus pneumoniae (often called *pneumococcus*) is a bacterium that can be cultured from the nasopharynx of most healthy people. The presence of pneumococcus in the nasopharynx is referred to as *carriage*. Most people have been carriers of *S. pneumoniae* at some point in their lives. Carriage is more common in young children and generally causes no illness.

Worldwide, *S. pneumoniae* is the most common cause of bacterial meningitis, community-acquired pneumonia, bacteremia, and otitis media. More than 90 serotypes of *S. pneumoniae* have been identified. Certain populations in the United States, including Alaska Natives, have high rates of pneumococcal disease (Figures 8-11 and 8-12).

Signs and Symptoms

Signs and symptoms of pneumococcal meningitis may include difficulty breathing, abnormal breath sounds, fever, irritability, and ear infection.

Pathophysiology

S. pneumoniae is an exclusively human pathogen spread from person to person by respiratory droplet transmission (see earlier discussion). Carriers of *S. pneumoniae*, while generally healthy themselves, often infect others. *S. pneumoniae* sometimes causes disease by spreading from the nasopharynx of a colonized person to other parts of the body, such as the middle ear (otitis media), nasal sinuses (sinusitis), and lungs. Meningitis is the result when the bacteria colonize the brain and spinal cord. If the bacteria reach the bloodstream, bacteremia may result.

Diagnosis

Sensitive, rapid diagnostic tests are not available for most types of pneumococcal infection, although a new urinary antigen test may be useful in adults. Sputum culture can be performed, but a Gram stain is the quickest way to diagnosis the infection.

Treatment

Penicillins, cephalosporin, and macrolides (e.g., azithromycin) are the first-choice antibiotics for treating pneumococcal infection, but many strains of pneumococcal bacteria resist commonly prescribed antibiotics.

Prevention

When treating a patient suspected of having pneumococcal meningitis, mask the patient or wear a surgical mask. Observe Standard Precautions, including good handwashing practices. The polyvalent pneumococcal polysaccharide (PPS) vaccine used today for older children and adults is "23-valent"—that is, it's effective against 23 types of pneumococci. Consequently, it protects against 85% to 90% of the strains of pneumococcus that cause serious infection. Adults aged 65 and older and those younger than 65 who have a chronic illness should receive this PPS 23-valent (PPSV23) vaccine, manufactured under the proprietary name Pneumovax.

For infants, the pneumococcal conjugate 7-valent (PCV7) vaccine (Prevnar) is given as a series of four vaccinations at 2, 4, 6, and 12 to 15 months of age.

Neisseria meningitidis (Meningococcal Meningitis)

Neisseria meningitidis is a gram-negative organism that's part of the normal flora of the nasopharynx in many people. In certain circumstances, such as weakened host resistance, the bacteria enter the bloodstream and gain access to the CNS, including the meninges, causing meningococcal meningitis. This illness is seasonal and tends to occur in the early spring and fall. It occurs worldwide, especially in sub-Saharan Africa. Each year in the United States, 2500 to 3500 cases of *N. meningitidis* infection are diagnosed, 10% to 14% of which are fatal. Those at increased risk of contracting meningococcal meningitis include infants and young children, refugees living in crowded or unsanitary conditions, military recruits, college freshmen living in a dormitory for the first time, high school students, and the household contacts of those who have the illness.

Signs and Symptoms

The classic symptom of meningococcal meningitis is a petechial rash that rapidly develops into purpura, accompanied by high fever, headache, and meningismus. Leg pain, cold hands and feet, and pallor may indicate that the condition has progressed to septic shock. Neurologic symptoms of meningococcal meningitis, which can occur within 24 to 48 hours of the onset of the illness, include mental status changes, seizures, and coma. Ask the patient or his or her family about vaccination status. Check for evidence of an earlier infection, such as aches, rash, and flulike symptoms.

Pathophysiology

Transmission of meningococcal meningitis occurs by direct contact with droplets from the oronasal secretions of an infected person. This pathogen is not passed by airborne transmission. It has five primary serotypes: A, B, C, Y, and W-135. Types A and C appear primarily in Asia and Africa.

Diagnosis

Gram stain analysis of CSF is diagnostic and should be available in less than 30 minutes. A culture of CSF takes 24 to 72 hours.

Treatment

Antibiotics are administered to patients infected with *N. meningitidis*. Third-generation cephalosporins, such as cefotaxime (Claforan) and ceftriaxone (Rocephin), are tried initially. Strains resistant to ciprofloxacin (Cipro and Ciloxan) have been documented in several states in the United States. Some strains of *Neisseria* are susceptible to penicillin G (Bicillin and Wycillin).

Prevention

Vaccination is recommended for those in high-risk groups: children aged 2–18, first-year college students living in a dormitory, and military recruits. Postexposure treatment consists of either oral rifampin for 2 days or one dose of oral Cipro. Prophylaxis should be started within 24 hours of the exposure.

Novel H1N1 Influenza

The H1N1 virus is a resurgence of an influenza A virus, with the highest concentration of cases occurring in Mexico. The illness spread from this suspected point of origin and was declared a pandemic by the WHO in May 2009. However, the WHO qualified this declaration by noting that the H1N1 pandemic has not been particularly severe. In fact, H1N1 has acted much like a normal seasonal flu virus, except that children, young adults, and pregnant women, rather than older adults, have been most vulnerable to the illness.

Signs and Symptoms

Signs and symptoms initially resemble those of a regular seasonal flu, except that the patient also has diarrhea. Severe signs and symptoms include:

Children:
- Respiratory distress
- Fever with rash
- Low fluid intake
- Bluish skin color
- Irritability
- Drowsiness and lethargy

Adults:
- Shortness of breath
- Chest pain or pressure
- Dizziness
- Confusion
- Persistent vomiting

These signs and symptoms could lead to respiratory distress and the need for ventilatory assistance.

Pathophysiology

H1N1 is a large-particle virus passed by the droplet route. The incubation period is 1 to 7 days, and the illness is thought to be transmissible for up to 24 hours after fever has subsided.

Diagnosis

Specific serologic testing is used to determine infection. A rapid influenza diagnostic test (RIDT) may be ordered to detect the novel influenza A (H1N1).

Treatment

Treatment is supportive unless the patient shows signs of respiratory distress, in which case ventilation assistance may be needed. Be sure to obtain a travel history for all patients who have respiratory difficulties. Hospitalized patients will receive antiviral drug treatment (Tamiflu or Relenza).

Prevention

If possible, place a surgical mask on the patient. If you cannot do so, you should wear a mask. Currently, scientific data do not support the use of N95 respirators for droplet-transmitted infectious diseases. WHO guidelines for H1N1 patient care do not call for such equipment. Immunization is the key to slowing the spread of H1N1. Postexposure treatment with antivirals is not indicated.

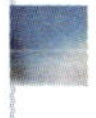

Diseases Transmitted by Airborne Pathogens

A common transmission of communicable pulmonary diseases occurs during inhalation of airborne pathogens. Patients with compromised immune systems and those living and working in densely populated areas are at risk of acquiring these types of diseases. Healthcare providers must maintain a vigilant awareness of the potential risk of these types of diseases and ensure appropriate PPE and work in well ventilated areas.

Mycobacterium Pulmonary Tuberculosis

Tuberculosis is caused by the bacterium *Mycobacterium tuberculosis*. TB has plagued humankind for centuries and remains a significant source of suffering in the world. Historically, the incidence of the disease has surged every 30 or 40 years. The WHO has published a plan, the Stop TB Global Strategy, to reduce the worldwide incidence of TB. TB rates are highest in Africa and Southeast Asia, and at least 2 million deaths worldwide are attributed to TB every year. In contrast, the lowest rate ever reported occurred in 2008 in the United States.

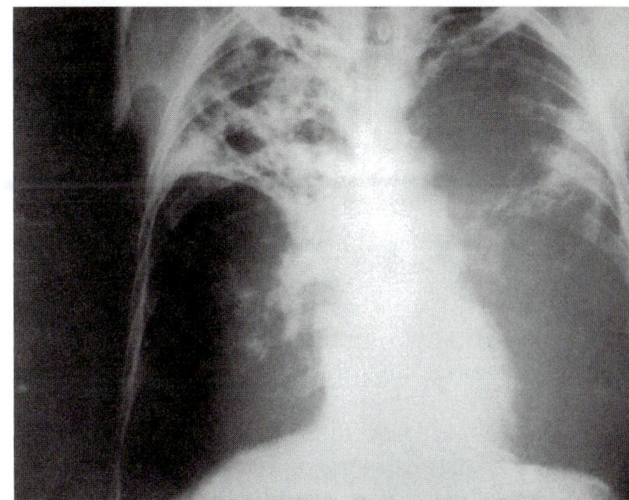

Figure 8-13 Radiograph of a patient with bilateral tuberculosis. (Courtesy Centers for Disease Control and Prevention.)

In discussing this illness, a distinction must be made between TB infection and TB disease. *TB infection* means only that exposure to TB has occurred. The exposed person does not have active disease, and may never develop it. People with TB infection do not pose a threat to others. Depending on the exposure, nature of infection, and drug-resistant profile, individuals may be prescribed one medication, such as isoniazid (INH) or multidrug regimens, such as INH and rifampin. *TB disease* refers to active TB illness verified by laboratory testing and a positive chest x-ray (Figure 8-13). Patients with active TB disease will be prescribed several medications.

Multidrug-Resistant Tuberculosis Multidrug-resistant tuberculosis (MDR-TB) was first identified in the United States in 1985, and it continues to occur in small numbers. In MDR-TB, *M. tuberculosis* is resistant to two of the first-line oral medications used to treat the illness. Since many other oral medications, including isoniazid and rifampin, are effective against the bacterium, MDR-TB is a treatable disease. MDR-TB is no more easily communicable than non–drug-resistant TB.

Resistance to medications used to treat TB is either primary or acquired. Acquired resistance is more common and occurs in patients who have undergone prior TB treatment. These are called *retreatment cases*. Primary resistance occurs when a patient is resistant to medications used to treat TB without having had any previous exposure to them.

Most cases of MDR-TB are identified in foreign-born people, and the WHO reports a growing global trend in MDR-TB.

In an effort to reduce the incidence of MDR-TB, the United States and the WHO are instituting direct observed therapy, a strategy intended to ensure full compliance with drug therapy. In this instance, the healthcare provider physically watches the patient ingest the medication. In some cases, the patient may be required to come to a clinic on a daily basis for drug administration. In assisted living environments, providers witness and document ingestion. In the United States, this program is overseen by local public health departments.

Extensively Drug-Resistant TB (XDR-TB) In 2006, another emerging global problem was identified in KwaZulu-Natal, South Africa. In extensively drug-resistant TB (XDR-TB), *M. tuberculosis* is resistant to isoniazid, rifampin, and at least three of the six main classes of second-line drugs (aminoglycosides, polypeptides, fluoroquinolones, thioamides, cycloserine, and para-aminosalicylic acid).

XDR-TB is not more communicable than TB or MDR-TB, and it's treatable in this country. It is seen in immunocompromised hosts, especially patients who are HIV positive, and carries nearly a 100% mortality rate because of the lack of treatment options. The prevalence of XDR-TB is lower than that of MDR-TB, but for the first time, the former is being reported by the WHO. In 2007, two cases of XDR-TB were reported in the United States.

Signs and Symptoms

Signs and symptoms of TB disease (including the drug-resistant types) include a persistent cough for 2 to 3 weeks, night sweats, headache, weight loss, hemoptysis, and chest pain. If the patient has signs and symptoms of TB, ask about his or her history of TB treatment, and check breath sounds. Oxygen administration may be necessary. Place a surgical mask on the patient for transport. Check medications; if the patient has been receiving treatment, the infection may no longer be communicable.

Pathophysiology

Tuberculosis is not a highly contagious disease. Transmission occurs by passage of airborne particles when a person with active untreated disease coughs. In general, such exposure occurs among people who have continuous intimate exposure to the infected individual, chiefly those living in the same household. For the healthcare provider working in the field, such intense exposure is likely to occur only if mouth-to-mouth ventilation is given to a patient with active untreated TB. Ten percent of people no longer have communicable disease after 2 days of treatment with new medications. The rest are no longer communicable after 14 days of treatment even though they continue taking medication for 12 months. The incubation period for TB is 4 to 12 weeks. There are three types of TB: atypical and extrapulmonary (TB of the bone, kidney, or lymph glands, for example), which are not communicable, and typical, which is communicable.

Diagnosis

The Mantoux skin test is the most common screening done to determine exposure to TB. Induration of less than 5 mm is regarded as negative to exposure. Sputum cultures and chest x-rays are indicated if the test is positive.

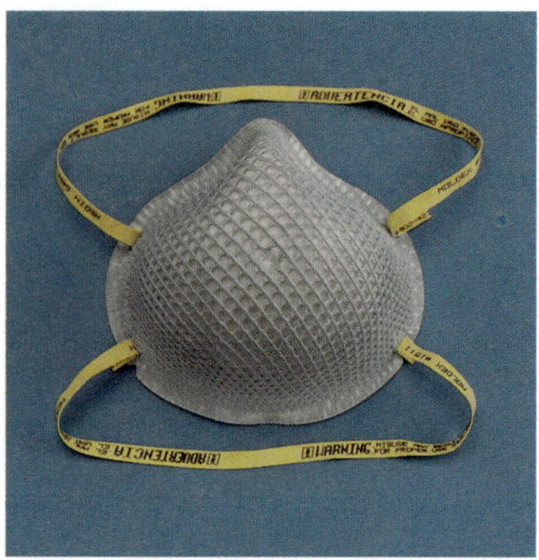

■ **Figure 8-14** High-efficiency particulate air (HEPA) respirator. (From Sanders M: Mosby's paramedic textbook, revised ed 3, St Louis, 2007, Mosby.)

TB testing for healthcare providers depends on risk assessment in the workplace. If a given place of employment has not had contact with three or more patients with active untreated TB during the previous year, annual testing is to be discontinued. Testing is then carried out only on newly hired employees and in healthcare providers known to have been exposed to TB. However, in emergency care settings, annual testing is often mandated.

Treatment

Patients with TB may need supplemental oxygen when oxygen saturation levels are diminished and there are signs of dyspnea. Initial treatment with antimycobacterial drugs such as isoniazid (INH) and rifampin are indicated. Patient isolation should be implemented for infectious patients.

Prevention

Place a surgical mask on the patient. If one is not available or the patient cannot be masked, mask yourself (Figure 8-14). An N95 respirator may be worn but is not required, since vehicles have rapid air exchange systems and exhaust fans, and transport times are generally short.

No special cleaning methods or solutions are required, and no airing of the vehicle is necessary after transporting a patient suspected of having active TB.

Herpesvirus Infections

Infectious Mononucleosis

Mononucleosis ("mono") is caused by a herpesvirus known as *Epstein-Barr virus*. Epstein-Barr virus is also suspected of causing a disease called *chronic fatigue syndrome,* which produces similar signs and symptoms, but this etiology has not been well established. The Epstein-Barr virus grows in the epithelium of the oropharynx and sheds into saliva, which explains why it's often referred to as the "kissing disease."

Signs and Symptoms

Signs and symptoms include sore throat, fever, pharyngeal secretions, and swollen lymph glands, with or without malaise, anorexia, headache, muscle pain, and an enlarged liver and spleen.

Pathophysiology

Transmission occurs by direct contact with the saliva of an infected person. Cases of transmission have also been linked to transfusion of contaminated blood or blood products. The incubation period is 4 to 6 weeks. The period of communicability is prolonged. Pharyngeal shedding may persist for a year or more after infection.

Diagnosis

For patients with classic symptoms, a positive heterophile antibody test (Monospot) is diagnostic, but this test may not become positive until the second or third week of illness. If this test is negative, and infectious mononucleosis strongly suspected, specific antibody testing for Epstein-Barr virus can be performed. DNA testing for Epstein-Barr virus is also available.

Treatment

Treatment is supportive in most cases. Antiviral agents may be prescribed for patients with compromised immune systems.

Prevention

When you're in direct contact with a patient's oral secretions, follow Standard Precautions, including the use of gloves and good hand hygiene. No special cleaning solution is required or recommended after transporting a patient suspected of having mononucleosis. No postexposure treatment is needed or recommended.

Herpes Simplex Type 1

Herpes simplex type 1 (HSV-1) is usually referred to as *oral herpes, cold sores,* or *fever blisters* (Figure 8-15). This disease occurs worldwide. In children aged 6 months to 5 years, HSV-1 appears as herpes gingivostomatitis. This can be a serious infection accompanied by high fever, sore throat, and swollen lymph glands. In adolescents and young adults, the infection may present as herpes pharyngitis.

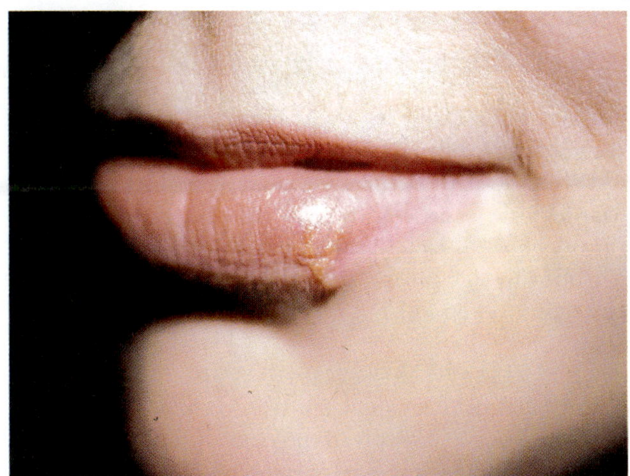

Figure 8-15 Herpes simplex 1. (From Rakel R: Textbook of family medicine, ed 7, Philadelphia, 2007, Saunders.)

Signs and Symptoms

The patient may complain of itching or burning and report the appearance of a vesicle. Ask about any previous history of oral lesions, and evaluate the patient's stress level, since the onset of HSV-1 has been associated with stress.

Pathophysiology

HSV-1 begins with a prodromal stage characterized by tingling and itching, followed by the appearance of a vesicle within 6 to 24 hours. The lesion may last 2 to 10 days. Recurrent outbreaks of HSV-1 lesions are common. The virus can be transmitted to other areas of the body if good hand hygiene is not performed after contact with draining vesicles, a process called *autoinfection*. Healthcare providers have acquired herpesvirus infections of the finger(s), a condition called *herpetic whitlow*, from not wearing gloves over nonintact skin when suctioning patients who are shedding virus.

Diagnosis

HSV-1 can be diagnosed rapidly by performing indirect immunofluorescent staining of a specimen taken by swabbing the lesion.

Treatment

Antiviral medications such as acyclovir or valacyclovir are typically prescribed for initial outbreaks and recurrences. A topical form is also available.

Prevention

Follow Standard Precautions and good handwashing practices. Cover open wounds when providing patient care.

Cytomegalovirus

Human cytomegalovirus (CMV) is classified taxonomically as a beta-herpesvirus, and it's one of the largest human herpesviruses. Many strains of CMV exist, and it's thought to be one of the leading causes of mental retardation in the United States. CMV is a leading cause of blindness in people with HIV/AIDS.

Signs and Symptoms

Most healthy children and adults infected with CMV have no symptoms and may not even know they've been infected. In assessing a patient suspected of having CMV, ask about any infections that were present at birth, since CMV can lead to permanent medical problems such as hearing or vision loss, mental disability, a small head (microcephaly), lack of coordination, and seizures. In a person with HIV infection or AIDS, ask the patient about any recent vision loss.

Pathophysiology

Nearly 60% of pregnant women infected with CMV are seropositive and may spread the virus from the cervix and in breast milk, passing the infection to their infants. CMV is transmitted sexually. CMV can also be transmitted in transfused blood or blood products, and it can contaminate donor organs. Patients who are immunocompromised are at greater risk of infection.

Diagnosis

It's not currently recommended that pregnant women be routinely tested for CMV, but an immunoglobulin G (IgG) antibody test can establish whether a woman has ever been infected with CMV.

Treatment

No treatment is currently available for CMV infection.

Prevention

Antiviral drugs may be given preemptively to fend off CMV infection. Preliminary research into a vaccine for CMV is under way. The virus is not deemed to be an occupational health risk for healthcare providers, but observe Standard Precautions when caring for infected patients.

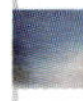

Sexually Transmitted Infections

Gonorrhea

Gonorrhea is the second most commonly reported disease in the United States. Worldwide, more than 60 million cases are reported annually. Gonorrhea is caused by *Neisseria gonorrhoeae,* a spore-forming, gram-negative diplococcus bacterium.

Signs and Symptoms

Gonorrhea has a different clinical presentation in men than in women. In assessing a patient suspected of having gonorrhea, ask him or her about the presence of vaginal or urethral discharge or burning on urination.

Men In men, gonorrhea is localized to the penis (Figure 8-16). It causes discomfort and/or a thick white, yellow, or greenish discharge from the tip of the penis. Infection in men can spread to the prostate, seminal vesicles, testes, and bladder, perhaps leading to abscess, difficulty urinating, and swollen testicles.

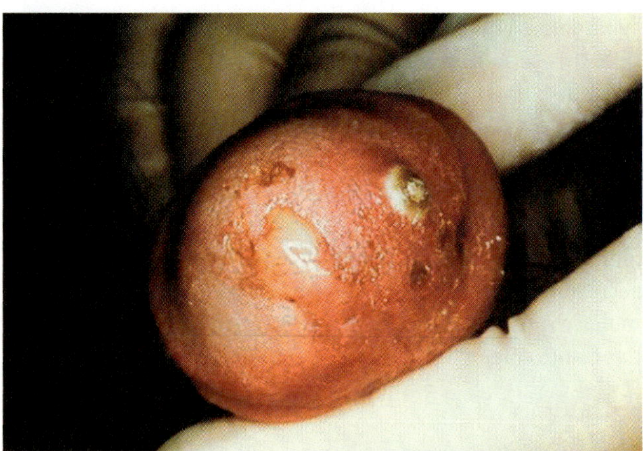

Figure 8-16 Male with a purulent penile discharge from gonorrhea and an overlying penile pyodermal lesion. Pyoderma involves the formation of a purulent skin lesion, as in this case located on the glans penis and overlying the sexually transmitted disease, gonorrhea. (From Goldman L, Ausiello D: Cecil medicine, ed 23, Philadelphia, 2007, Saunders.)

Women More than 50% of women infected with gonorrhea have no symptoms, especially in the early stages of infection. Symptoms include burning or frequent urination, a yellowish vaginal discharge, redness and swelling of the genitals, and vaginal burning or itching. If untreated, gonorrhea can cause a severe pelvic infection, with inflammation of the fallopian tubes and ovaries. Gonorrheal infection of the fallopian tubes can lead in turn to a dangerous, painful infection of the pelvis known as *pelvic inflammatory disease (PID)*. PID may cause a puslike discharge from the vagina. To assess for pelvic infection, evaluate the patient for abdominal pain or tenderness.

Pathophysiology

Anorectal and oral gonorrhea are common. Perinatal transmission also occurs, but the primary mode of transmission is intimate sexual contact with an infected partner. The incubation period for *N. gonorrhoeae* ranges from 2 to 10 days.

Diagnosis

Diagnosis is made by testing drainage from the site. In men, a Gram stain of urethral drainage may also be performed to screen for the disease.

Treatment

In uncomplicated cases, oral cefixime (Suprax) is prescribed or ceftriaxone (Rocephin) intramuscular (IM) is given in a single dose.

Prevention

Follow Standard Precautions, including good handwashing practices, when in contact with drainage or lesions.

No special cleaning is needed for vehicles or equipment. For patients, partner notification is essential. Educate patients about the disease and its prevention, including the use of condoms.

Syphilis

Syphilis has been increasing in the U.S. population, especially in the southern states, for the past decade or so. Internationally, the incidence of the disease has been increasing at a fast pace. The disease tends to strike young people aged 20 to 35, with an especially high prevalence in urban areas. About 60% of new cases occur in men who have sex with men. In May 2006, the CDC published guidelines with the goal of eliminating syphilis in the United States by 2015, using evidence-based practices and targeted surveillance activities.

Many people infected with HIV or HCV are co-infected with syphilis. OSHA requires that healthcare providers be given education and training on syphilis and that this disease be part of any postexposure evaluation and medical follow-up.

Signs and Symptoms

Initial infection with syphilis produces a chancre, a painless ulcerative lesion of the skin or mucous membranes at the site of infection (Figure 8-17). The site of infection is usually the genital region, so suspected syphilis may not be noted during routine physical assessment. Tertiary signs and symptoms of syphilis include:

- Rash
- Patchy hair loss
- Swollen lymph glands
- Cardiac, ophthalmic, auditory, or CNS complications
- Lesions of the tissues or bone

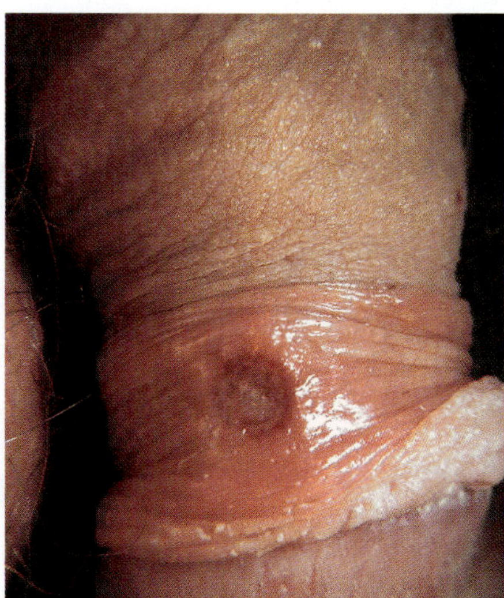

Figure 8-17 Primary syphilis. Syphilitic chancre is an ulcer with a clean, nonpurulent base and smooth, regular, sharply defined border. (From Habif T: Clinical dermatology, ed 5, St Louis, 2009, Mosby.)

If signs and symptoms are observed, question the patient regarding high-risk activities.

Pathophysiology

Syphilis is caused by the spiral-shaped bacterium *Treponema pallidum*. Infection can be either acute or chronic. Transmission generally occurs by direct contact, such as sexual contact, with the draining primary lesion(s). Syphilis can also be transmitted across the placenta from an infected mother to her fetus. In some cases, transmission has occurred by blood transfusion. The incubation period of *T. pallidum* is 10 days to 3 months. The communicable period is variable and has not been well established.

Diagnosis

A diagnosis of syphilis is confirmed by performing a rapid plasma reagin (RPR) test or the classic Venereal Disease Research Laboratory (VDRL) test.

Treatment

Routine treatment for syphilis includes administration of penicillin G. If the patient is pregnant, a second dose should be given 1 week later. If the patient is allergic to penicillin, give oral doxycycline or oral tetracycline, prescribed daily for 28 days.

Prevention

Observe Standard Precautions, including good handwashing practices. No special cleaning precautions are needed or recommended. If you sustain a needlestick injury with a contaminated needle, notify your DICO. The source patient should be tested if an actual exposure occurred. People who receive syphilis treatment must abstain from sexual contact with new partners until the lesions have healed completely. Sexual partners must be notified so they can be tested for the infection.

Genital Herpes

Genital herpes is a chronic recurrent illness produced by HSV type 2 (HSV-2). This disease is characterized by vesicular lesions.

Signs and Symptoms

In women, the vesicles may also appear on the vulva, legs, or buttocks. In men, lesions are most common on the penis, as well as around the anus in men who have sex with men. Lesions may also be present on the mouth as a result of oral sex. In assessing a patient suspected of having genital herpes, ask the patient about localized pain, burning, and tenderness, fever, and headache.

Pathophysiology

The incubation period for HSV-2 is 3 to 14 days.

Diagnosis

Testing for HSV-2 is the same as for HSV-1 (see earlier heading).

Treatment

Antiviral drugs may be prescribed, the most common of which is oral acyclovir (Zovirax), taken daily.

Prevention

Counsel patients that transmission of genital herpes can be prevented by using condoms to prevent contact with viral particles on the genitals of an infected person.

Papillomaviruses

Worldwide, human papillomavirus (HPV) is the most common sexually transmitted infection (STI) in adults. Epidemiologists estimate, for example, that more than 80% of American women will have contracted at least one strain of HPV by age 50.

Papillomaviruses were first identified in the early 20th century, when it was shown that skin warts, or papillomas, are communicable from person to person. HPV has been identified as a precursor of cervical cancer. Public health officials in Australia, Canada, Europe, and the United States recommend that young women be immunized against HPV to prevent cervical cancer and genital warts and to reduce the need for painful and costly treatment for cervical dysplasia, a precancerous condition often caused by HPV.

Signs and Symptoms

HPV cannot be identified on visual inspection unless it's associated with genital warts. If no warts are present, pathologic examination must be done to confirm the presence of the virus. To assess a patient suspected of having HPV, ask about sexual history and, if the patient is a woman, ask her whether she has been vaccinated against HPV.

Pathophysiology

The papillomavirus genome is composed of genetically stable, double-stranded DNA. Papillomaviruses replicate almost exclusively in the outermost layers of the skin, as well as in some mucosal surfaces, such as on the inside of the cheek and on the vaginal walls.

Diagnosis

Papanicolaou (Pap) smears and HPV DNA testing are useful in identifying HPV in women, but no testing is available for men.

Treatment

Chemoprevention can be implemented to assist in stopping aggressive neoplastic cell growth. Interferon therapy can also be introduced. Cryosurgery (cold), laser (heat) surgery, and invasive surgery (e.g., hysterectomy) are appropriate interventions.

Prevention

Women Vaccination prevents infection with certain species of HPV associated with the development of cervical cancer, genital warts, and some less common cancers. Two HPV vaccines are currently available: Gardasil and Cervarix. These vaccines protect against two types of HPV that can cause cervical cancer (HPV-16 and HPV-18) and prevent some other genital cancers as well. Gardasil also protects against two of the HPV types that cause genital warts.

Men Men with penile cancer may increase their female sexual partner's risk of cervical cancer.

Scabies

Scabies, caused by the parasitic mite *Sarcoptes scabiei,* can be described as a sexually transmitted infection. However, scabies "infection" is actually an infestation with the organism itself; the scabies mite is not a vector for transmission of other infectious agents.

The incidence of scabies infection in the United States and Europe has increased during the past few years. Scabies infestation can affect families and children, sexual partners, patients who have chronic illnesses or are hospitalized, and people who live in group homes.

Signs and Symptoms

Signs and symptoms of scabies infestation include nocturnal itching and the presence of a rash (Figure 8-18) in any of the following areas:

- Hands and interdigits
- Flexor aspects of the wrists
- Axillary folds

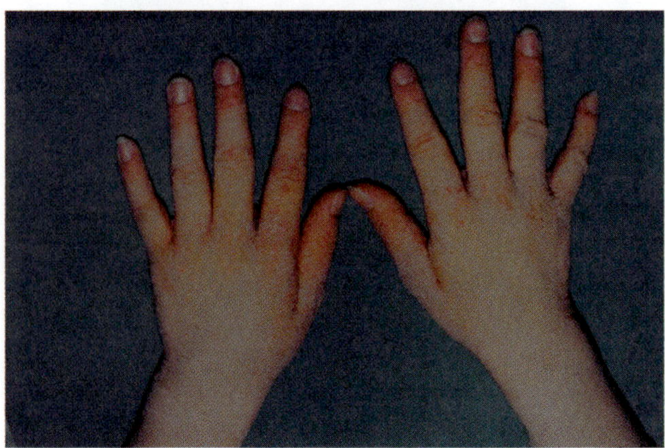

Figure 8-18 Scabies. (From Marx J, Hockberger R, Walls R: Rosen's emergency medicine, ed 7, St Louis, 2009, Mosby.)

- Ankles or toes
- Genital area
- Buttocks
- Abdomen

Pathophysiology

Transmission occurs by direct skin-to-skin contact during activities such as wrestling and sexual intercourse. It can also occur when an uninfected person has contact with fomites such as undergarments, towels, and linens. The incubation period for people with no previous exposure is 2 to 6 weeks. The disease is communicable until the mites and their eggs have been destroyed by treatment.

Diagnosis

Diagnosis is made by microscopic examination of the mite. Specimens are taken using a needle or scalpel to remove mites that have burrowed into the skin.

Treatment

Permethrin (Elimite) is a topical treatment for scabies. Reapplication may be required to treat the infestation effectively in children. This cream should be applied carefully, according to the instructions on the package insert. Lindane (Kwell) lotion may be prescribed as a second-line treatment, but lindane toxicity has been reported with overuse.

Prevention

Prevention requires wearing gloves and following good handwashing practices. Vehicle linens require only routine washing in hot water (10 min at 122°F). Routine cleaning of the vehicle after patient transport is sufficient. If you are concerned you may have been exposed, contact your supervisor to establish whether an exposure occurred. If so, treatment will be ordered, and work restriction from patient care may be necessary.

Pediculosis (Lice)

Pubic lice, *Phthirus pubis* is a grayish parasite that, like scabies, causes an infestation rather than a true infection (Figure 8-19). Lice are common in people who live in group homes, have poor hygiene, or have multiple sexual partners.

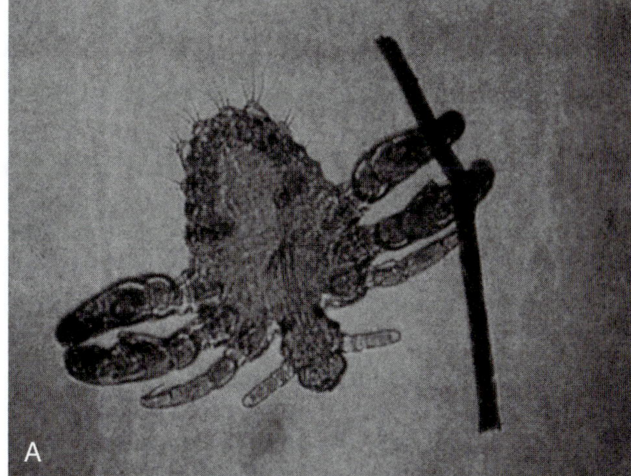

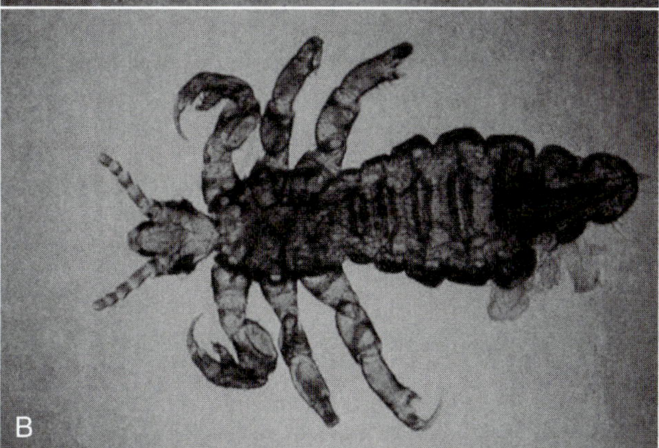

Figure 8-19 A, The pubic, or crab, louse. B, Male of the human head louse. (From Sanders M: Mosby's paramedic textbook, revised ed 3, St Louis, 2007, Mosby.)

Signs and Symptoms

Signs and symptoms of pubic lice include mild to severe itching and visible nits clinging to hair in the pubic, perianal, or perineal areas. Pubic lice can also infest eyelashes, eyebrows, axillae, scalp, and other hair-covered body areas.

Pathophysiology

Transmission occurs through physical or sexual contact. The incubation period is about 8 to 10 days after the eggs hatch. The lice are communicable until all mites and their eggs, including those in infested clothing, are destroyed by treatment. Humans are the only reservoir for lice.

Diagnosis

Diagnosis is made by a visual observation of nits (white eggs) attached to hair shafts.

Treatment

Manual removal of the nits and application of pediculicides is the treatment. 1% Lindane shampoo is applied for 7 to 10 days to kill any hatching nymphs. These shampoos can be toxic if not used according to the directions, so for young children, a 1% permethrin cream rinse, such as Nix, is used. The cream kills both the lice and nits with one application.

Prevention

Prevention requires wearing gloves and practicing good handwashing techniques. Routine cleaning of the vehicle post transport is sufficient. If an actual exposure occurred, treatment may be ordered with permethrin cream, and restriction from patient care may be indicated.

Neurologic Infections

Neurologic infections can be caused by either viruses or bacteria, and their severity ranges from virtually innocuous to life threatening. Symptoms of CNS viral infections can be mild and self-limiting, as seen in the mumps, or they can cause significant brain tissue injury, as in encephalopathies that accompany rabies and HSV. Since the brain tissue injury may cause permanent neurologic deficits, early diagnosis and management are essential if the patient is to have a favorable outcome.

Clostridium tetani Infection (Tetanus)

Tetanus (lockjaw) is a disease caused by the gram-positive anaerobic bacterium *Clostridium tetani*. Tetanus occurs worldwide and affects all age groups, with the highest prevalence found in neonates and young people. Tetanus is one of the target diseases of the WHO Expanded Program on Immunization. Overall, the annual incidence of tetanus is 500,000 to 1 million cases. About 60% of the cases occur in people older than 60. They are usually isolated to rural areas where contact with animal waste is common, and immunization is inadequate. The tetanus bacillus is found in the intestines of horses and other animals and in contaminated soil. Some cases of tetanus have been linked to IV drug use.

Signs and Symptoms

Signs and symptoms begin at the site of the wound, followed by painful muscle contractions in the neck and trunk muscles. The cardinal sign of tetanus is abdominal rigidity; however, rigidity may be confined to the location of the injury.

Pathophysiology

Transmission occurs when tetanus spores enter the body by way of a puncture wound contaminated with animal feces, street dust, or soil, or by the injection of contaminated street drugs. Occasionally, cases have occurred postoperatively or after minor injuries that were left untreated. The incubation period is thought to be about 14 days from the exposure, but a period of as little as 3 days has been reported. A short incubation period is associated with a higher level of contamination. Tetanus is not transmitted person to person, so there is no period of communicability.

Diagnosis

Diagnosis is made on the basis of signs and symptoms; no laboratory testing for tetanus has been developed.

Treatment

The wound must be cleaned and surgically débrided. The antibiotic metronidazole (Flagyl) may be prescribed. Anyone infected with tetanus should be vaccinated against it, since having had the illness does not confer immunity to future infection with the bacterium.

Prevention

Wear gloves when handling any patient who has a draining wound. Prevention of tetanus requires vaccination during childhood and booster doses every 10 years. No special cleaning of the vehicle is necessary after transporting a patient with tetanus.

Zoonotic (Animal-Borne) Diseases

Rabies

The rabies virus is a bullet-shaped, single-stranded RNA virus that reaches the CNS by way of the peripheral nerves. The infection causes a progressive encephalomyelitis that is almost always fatal. In the United States, rabies is common in wild and domesticated animals—skunks, raccoons, bats, foxes, dogs, and cats (Figure 8-20). However, animal immunization programs have reduced the incidence of rabies and the number of deaths attributable to the disease to one or two per year. Hawaii is the only state whose animal population is free of rabies. Worldwide, most rabies deaths occur in countries with inadequate public health resources, limited access to preventive treatment, few diagnostic facilities, and virtually nonexistent rabies surveillance programs.

Signs and Symptoms

Humans are very susceptible to rabies virus infection after exposure to saliva in a bite or scratch from an infected animal. The lethality of the infection depends on several

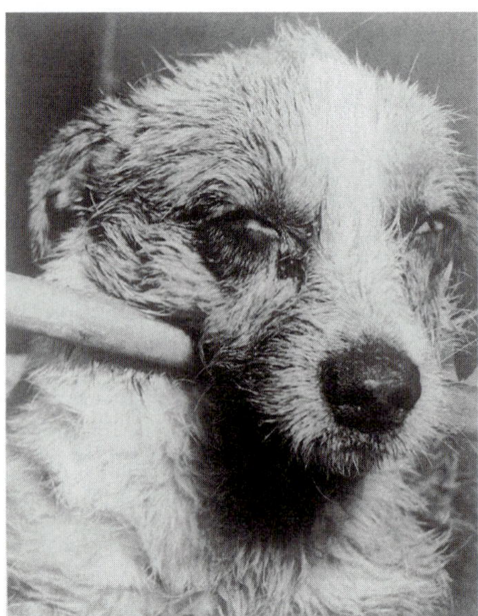

■ **Figure 8-20** Close-up of a dog's face during late-stage "dumb" paralytic rabies. (Courtesy Centers for Disease Control and Prevention, Barbara Andrews.)

factors, including severity and location of the wound and the virulence of the strain. Ask the patient about any recent history of contact with animals. Early symptoms are nonspecific, consisting of fever, headache, and general malaise. As the disease progresses, neurologic symptoms appear, including insomnia, anxiety, confusion, slight or partial paralysis, excitation, hallucinations, agitation, hypersalivation, and difficulty swallowing. Contrary to popular belief, rabies does not make the infected person afraid of water. The patient will, however, be averse to drinking water, because doing so induces agonizing throat spasms. This condition is called *hydrophobia,* a term formerly synonymous with rabies itself. Death may occur within days of the onset of symptoms.

Pathophysiology

Rabies is an acute viral infection of the CNS primarily affecting animals; however, it can be transmitted to humans through the virus-laden saliva of an infected animal. Transmission from person to person has never been documented. All animals found outside their natural habitat or behaving abnormally or aggressively should be presumed to be infected.

Diagnosis

Diagnosis is based on the patient's medical history, history of the exposure, and clinical presentation.

Treatment

Clean the wound area thoroughly. Begin rabies vaccination in accordance with current guidelines. Usually, a series of IM injections is given starting on the day of injury or within 10 days, with follow-up injections on days 3, 7, 14, and 28. Rabies immunoglobulin (HRIG) is also given with first dose of vaccine. Dosage is determined on the basis of body weight.

Prevention

The incubation period of the rabies virus ranges from 9 days to 7 years. Vaccination of domestic animals is essential. When treating a patient suspected of having been exposed to rabies, observe Standard Precautions, including wearing gloves and using good hand hygiene. Rabies vaccination is available through local public health departments. Criteria for administering this vaccine have changed because of reduced availability. Vaccination of healthcare providers as a preventive measure is not recommended.

Hantavirus

The *Hantavirus* genus of rodent-borne viruses is distributed worldwide and causes a group of related hantavirus diseases, including hantavirus pulmonary syndrome and hemorrhagic fever with renal syndrome. The virus is spread by the deer mouse, the white-footed mouse, and the cotton rat, as well as by garden-variety city rats.

Hantavirus occurs in Asia, western Russia, Europe, the United States, and South and Central America. Worldwide, approximately 150,000 to 200,000 cases are reported annually. The disease was first described in Korea in the early 1950s. There are two seasonal peaks for almost all outbreaks of hantavirus disease: a small outbreak appears in the spring, and a more substantial spike occurs in fall. Epidemiologists suspect that these upturns correspond with farming cycles and with seasonal increases in the infection rate of the rodents who carry the disease.

Signs and Symptoms

Signs and symptoms begin with the sudden onset of fever, which lasts 3 to 8 days. The fever is accompanied by headache, abdominal pain, loss of appetite, and vomiting. Facial flushing is characteristic, and a petechial rash usually appears (generally limited to the axillae). Sudden and extreme albuminuria on about day 4 is a cardinal sign of severe hantavirus. The patient may also have ecchymosis and scleral injection (bloodshot eyes). Additional symptoms include hypotension, shock, respiratory distress or failure, and renal impairment or failure. The characteristic damage to the renal medulla is unique to hantaviruses.

Hantavirus pulmonary syndrome is a febrile illness. It is characterized by flulike symptoms including fever, myalgia, headache, cough, chills, abdominal pain, diarrhea, and malaise. Subsequent symptoms may include shortness of breath, tachypnea, tachycardia, dizziness, arthralgia, sweating, and back or chest pain. Ask the patient about exposure to mice or other rodent droppings if you observe symptoms consistent with hantavirus.

Pathophysiology

Transmission occurs by inhalation of aerosolized rodent waste. The virus is shed into the urine, feces, and saliva of chronically infected rodents. The incubation period is usually about 12 to 16 days, but it may be as little as 5 days or extend to 42 days. Although human-to-human transmission of hantavirus has been reported in Argentina and Chile, this disease is rarely transmitted from person to person, so there is no period of communicability.

Diagnosis

Diagnosis is confirmed by IgM antibody response or a rising IgG titer, or by PCR testing. The differential diagnosis for hantavirus pulmonary syndrome includes severe generalized pneumonia, interstitial pneumonia, and eosinophilic pneumonia. Chest x-rays may reveal a diffuse interstitial infiltrate.

Treatment

No specific treatment is available other than supportive measures, including oxygen administration, monitoring of respiratory status, maintenance of fluid and electrolyte balances, and support of blood pressure.

Prevention

Follow normal Standard Precautions, since hantavirus is not transmitted from person to person. Routine cleaning of the vehicle is sufficient. Public health officials will assess the need for cleaning out areas of rodent infestation.

Vector-Borne Diseases

A disease vector is an organism that transmits disease to another species without itself suffering any ill effects from carrying the pathogen.

Lyme Disease

Lyme disease is the most common tickborne disease in the United States. The number of reported cases has increased since 1982, when a national reporting system was established. This disease is limited primarily to the Atlantic coast, the upper Midwest, and the Pacific coast. However, Lyme disease is found worldwide, with most cases occurring in the temperate regions of the globe. This disease is not caused by a virus but by a bacterium, the spirochete *Borrelia burgdorferi*. The disease occurs most often in children younger than 10 and middle-aged adults.

Signs and Symptoms

Lyme disease primarily affects the skin, heart, joints, and nervous system. Some patients are asymptomatic. The disease is usually divided into three stages:

1. Early localized. In the early localized stage, a round, slightly irregular red skin lesion called *erythema migrans* appears 3 to 32 days after the tick bite. This lesion is often described as a bull's-eye rash, since it consists of a central necrotic spot surrounded by an area of clearing, around which a dark-red ring appears, with lighter erythema around the periphery. The rash is more than 5 cm in diameter. It usually appears on the skin of the groin, thigh, or axilla and is easy to miss. The skin is warm to the touch and may be blistered or covered with a scab.
2. Early disseminated. The second, early disseminated stage may develop within days. This stage is characterized by secondary lesions and flulike symptoms such as fever, chills, headache, malaise, and muscle pain. The patient may also have a nonproductive cough, sore throat, enlarged spleen, or enlarged lymph nodes. Men may have testicular swelling. Neurologic involvement occurs in 15% to 20% of untreated patient within 2 to 8 weeks (Figure 8-21). Cardiac involvement appears in about 10% of untreated patients.
3. Late manifestations. In the final phase of the illness, which may begin days or years after the second phase, arthritis occurs in about 60% of untreated patients. Intermittent joint pain lasting days or months occurs in about half of patients. Chronic neurologic symptoms are uncommon. In the United States, memory impairment, depressed mood, and severe fatigue are the most frequent symptoms.

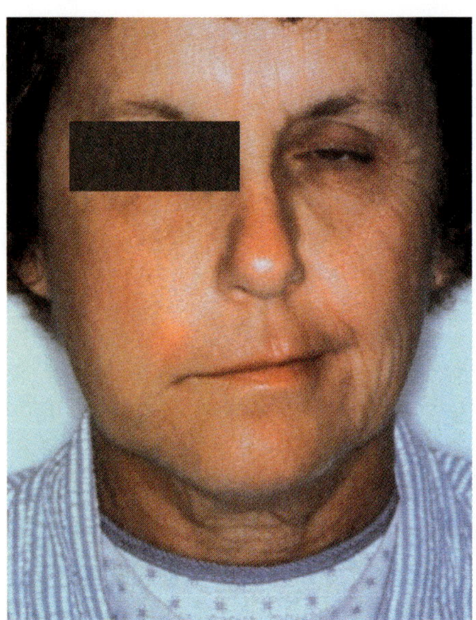

Figure 8-21 Patient with facial palsy caused by Lyme disease. (Courtesy Centers for Disease Control and Prevention.)

Pathophysiology

Lyme disease is transmitted by the tick bite. Adult ticks are not as likely to transmit disease to humans because they prefer deer as hosts. The peak season is between June and August, with the incidence of the disease receding in early fall. The incubation period ranges from 3 to 32 days. The disease has no period of communicability because it's not transmitted person to person.

Diagnosis

Diagnosis can be made by culturing the skin lesion for *B. burgdorferi*. More commonly, antibody titers are obtained. However, a thorough history and observation of the lesions and associated patient complaints are essential.

Treatment

The patient may receive oral doxycycline or amoxicillin for 10 to 21 days.

Prevention

As always, good handwashing is important, but Lyme disease is not transmitted person to person. Wear long sleeves and trousers when you must work in tick-infested areas. Repellents such as diethyltoluamide (DEET) can deter these insects, but such chemicals can be toxic and must be used judiciously, especially around young children. Postexposure treatment with antibiotics is not warranted or recommended.

West Nile Virus

West Nile virus is a *Flavivirus*, a genus of diseases relatively new to the United States. This disease derives its name from the place of its origin, along the Nile River. West Nile virus was first discovered in Uganda in the 1930s but made its first appearance in the Western Hemisphere when it was identified in New York City in 1999, marking the beginning of the largest outbreak of mosquito-borne illness in United States history. Other outbreaks of West Nile virus have been reported in Russia, Israel, and Romania. In most cases, the disease is mild and uneventful. In fact, about 80% of those infected are not aware that they've acquired the disease.

Signs and Symptoms

About 80% of those infected with West Nile virus are asymptomatic. The remaining 20% have mild signs and symptoms such as fever, headache, body rash, and swollen lymph glands. About 1 in 150 will go on to develop severe signs and symptoms, such as encephalitis and meningitis which can lead to neurologic complications and death.

Question the patient about recent mosquito bites if cases have been reported in the area. Ask about risks for exposure, such as work and travel history. Observe for severe signs and symptoms that suggest meningitis or encephalitis, such as loss of consciousness, confusion, stiff neck, and muscle weakness.

Pathophysiology

Transmission occurs when a person is bitten by a mosquito carrying the West Nile virus. Only about 1% of mosquitoes are vectors for this pathogen. The disease is not transmitted from person to person. West Nile virus has been transmitted by donor blood, organ transplantation, and by needlestick injury among laboratory workers handling the virus. The incubation period is 2 to 14 days after the bite, during which time the virus multiplies in the lymph nodes before entering the bloodstream. Symptoms typically last 3 to 6 days.

Diagnosis

Keen observation of signs and symptoms is the key to making a preliminary diagnosis. Recent and convalescent testing are accomplished by enzyme immunoassay and IgM antibody testing.

Treatment

Supportive treatment is offered. No prescribed treatment is available for West Nile virus.

Prevention

Use needlesafe device systems to avoid a contaminated sharps injury. No particular medical follow-up treatment is recommended if a needle exposure occurs. In addition, no special cleaning of the vehicle or equipment is needed or recommended after transporting a patient suspected of having West Nile virus.

The public can assist in controlling the spread of this infection by draining standing pools of water, using insect repellent, and wearing long sleeves after dusk. These precautions will reduce reproduction capabilities and risk of exposure.

Rocky Mountain Spotted Fever

Rocky Mountain spotted fever is a tickborne illness caused by *Rickettsia rickettsii,* a small bacterium that grows inside the cells of its hosts. The disease was first recognized in 1896, in the Snake River Valley of Idaho. It was originally given the foreboding name "black measles." Rocky Mountain spotted fever has been a reportable disease in the United States since the 1920s. Despite its name, the disease can be found throughout most of the country, including the District of Columbia and states in the south Atlantic (Delaware, Maryland, Virginia, West Virginia, North Carolina, South Carolina, Georgia, and Florida), Pacific (Washington, Oregon, and California), and west south-central (Arkansas, Louisiana, Oklahoma, and Texas) regions. Worldwide, infection with *R. rickettsii* has been documented in Argentina, Brazil, Colombia, Costa Rica, Mexico, and Panama.

About two-thirds of Rocky Mountain spotted fever cases occur in children younger than 15, with a peak at ages 5 to 9. People who are often around dogs or who live close to wooded areas or patches of tall grass are also at increased risk of infection. Only about 60% of people diagnosed with Rocky Mountain spotted fever recall having had a tick bite.

Signs and Symptoms

Initial symptoms of Rocky Mountain spotted fever may include fever, nausea, vomiting, severe headache, muscle pain, and lack of appetite. A rash appears 2 to 5 days after the onset of fever (Figure 8-22). It often appears initially as a smattering of small, flat, pink, non-itchy spots (macules) on the wrists, forearms, and ankles.

Rocky Mountain spotted fever can be a life-threatening illness, because *R. rickettsii* infects the cells that line blood vessels throughout the body. Severe manifestations of this disease may involve the respiratory or renal system, the CNS, or the GI tract. Those with illness severe enough to require hospital care may have the following long-term effects:

- Partial paralysis of the lower extremities
- Gangrene requiring amputation of fingers, toes, arms, or legs
- Hearing loss
- Loss of bowel or bladder control
- Movement or language disorders

Question any patient with a rash about possible tick bites. Check the patient for fever as well.

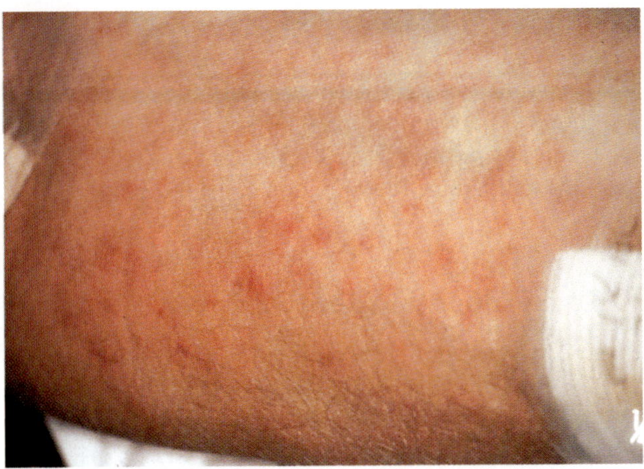

Figure 8-22 Late acute stage of Rocky Mountain spotted fever. Lower portion of the arm shows a florid petechial rash. (From Mandell G, Bennett J, Dolin R: Mandell, Douglas, and Bennett's principles and practice of infectious disease, ed 7, Philadelphia, 2010, Churchill Livingstone.)

Pathophysiology

More than 20 species are currently classified in the genus *Rickettsia,* but not all are known to cause disease in humans. The rickettsiae that cause spotted fever grow in the cytoplasm or in the nuclei of host cells. The organisms multiply, damaging or destroying those cells and causing blood to leak through tiny holes in vessel walls into adjacent tissues. This mechanism is responsible for the characteristic rash associated with the disease. The incubation period is 3 to 14 days after the tick bite. The illness is not transmissible from person to person.

Diagnosis

Diagnosis is often made on the basis of signs and symptoms, but indirect immunofluorescence assay can be used to detect IgG or IgM antibodies. IgG antibodies are more specific and reliable, since other bacterial infections can also cause elevations in rickettsial IgM antibody titers.

Treatment

Doxycycline (100 mg every 12 hours for adults or 4 mg/kg body weight per day in two divided doses for children under 45 kg [100 lbs]) is the drug of choice for patients with Rocky Mountain spotted fever. Therapy is continued for at least 3 days after fever subsides and until there is unequivocal evidence of clinical improvement, generally for a minimum total course of 5 to 10 days. Severe or complicated disease may require a longer course of treatment.

Prevention

Good handwashing is essential for healthcare providers. Risk of contracting the disease can be limited by reducing your exposure to ticks. In those who are exposed to ticks, careful inspection and removal of crawling or attached ticks is a simple but important way of preventing disease.

When the presence of ticks is recognized, they should be removed. Ticks are easily removed with tweezers or forceps by identifying and grabbing the tick's mouth, very close to the person or animal's skin. The entire tick should be gently removed. In order to prevent further contamination, the body of the tick should not be squeezed. The area should be cleaned and an antiseptic applied.

Gastrointestinal Diseases

Acute Gastroenteritis

Gastroenteritis may be caused by bacterial or viral pathogens, parasites, chemical toxins, allergies, or immune disorders. The inflammation may cause hemorrhage and erosion of the mucosal layers of the GI tract, affecting absorption of water and nutrients.

What is typically called *acute gastroenteritis,* or a "stomach flu," is a viral infection of the stomach and intestines, leading to abdominal cramping, vomiting, and diarrhea. This is the most common cause of gastroenteritis and is self-limiting, with strains causing symptoms for 1 to 3 days. The most important treatment is maintenance of hydration.

Escherichia coli Infection

Most strains of *Escherichia coli (E. coli)* are harmless, but other strains cause foodborne illnesses. *E. coli* has been recognized as a major cause of colonization and infection in cattle, which can contaminate food. The first serious outbreak caused by the O157:H7 subtype occurred in a fast-food restaurant in Washington State in 1993. Epidemiologists estimate that this bacterium is the cause of more than 75,000 cases of illness each year, resulting in more than 3000 hospital stays and 60 deaths. Illness occurs mostly in young children and in older adults.

Signs and Symptoms

Infection with *E. coli* O157:H7 begins with abdominal pain and tenderness, myalgia, and headache. Vomiting may also occur, followed by hemorrhagic colitis, which causes visible blood in the stool. This stage may last 3 to 7 days and occurs mostly in people aged 65 or older. A grave complication of this illness is hemolytic uremic syndrome, a life-threatening condition that occurs in about 10% of those infected with *E. coli* O157:H7. As a result, hemolytic uremic syndrome is now recognized as the most common cause of acute kidney failure in infants and young children. Adolescents and adults are also susceptible, and older adults often succumb to the disease.

Ask the patient whether he or she might have eaten any uncooked or undercooked meat. Question the patient about the appearance of his or her stool. Watery, yellow-green, or bloody stool, or stool that contains pus, is a clue to this illness. Check for signs of dehydration or shock.

Pathophysiology

E. coli is a gram-negative bacterium belonging to the Enterobacteriaceae family. More than 30 serotypes of *E. coli* have been identified. Of these, *E. coli* O157:H7 has been the most notable in recent years. This organism has been found in improperly cooked meat, municipal water supplies, milk, raw vegetables, unpasteurized apple cider, lettuce, and products contaminated by cattle waste. The organism has an incubation period of 1 to 9 days. *E. coli* interacts with DNA from a Shiga toxin–producing bacterium known as *Shigella dysenteriae type 1. S. dysenteriae* is transferred to *E. coli* by a bacteriophage (a bacterium infected with a virus) to form *E. coli* O157:H7, giving an otherwise mild-mannered germ the souped-up genes necessary to produce one of the most potent toxins known to man.

Diagnosis

Diagnosis is made on the basis of a stool culture. Ninety percent of bloody stools culture positive for *E. coli* bacteria.

Treatment

Supportive treatment is offered, since antibiotics have not been effective against the O157:H7 strain of *E. coli*. Transfusion may be indicated if the patient becomes severely anemic. Dialysis may be indicated for acute renal failure.

Prevention

Standard Precautions, including the use of gowns to protect clothing are recommended. As always, follow thorough handwashing practices. Vehicles and care equipment must be cleaned thoroughly per local protocols.

Shigellosis

Shigellosis is a highly infectious acute bacterial enteritis that affects the large and small intestines. Only a small dose of bacteria—possibly as few as 10 to 100 organisms—is needed to cause infection. The disease is believed to be responsible for more than 600,000 deaths each year worldwide. Most infections and deaths occur in children younger than age 10.

Signs and Symptoms

Shigella strains can produce three different enterotoxins which have enterotoxic, cytotoxic, and neurotoxic effects. Patients infected with this illness have watery diarrhea, fever, vomiting, and cramps. Rehydration may be necessary. Convulsions are a complication sometimes seen in young children. Illness lasts about 4 to 7 days. In mild infection, the only sign may be watery diarrhea. Other symptoms may include nausea, high fever, and abdominal tenderness and cramping.

Pathophysiology

Shigella is a genus of gram-negative, non–spore-forming, rod-shaped bacteria closely related to *E. coli* and *Salmonella.*

Shigella spp. are transmitted by the fecal-oral route. Failing to wash hands or not doing so properly after defecation is an easy way to spread this infection. The incubation period may be as brief as 12 hours but can extend to 96 hours. A person can harbor this disease for up to 4 weeks.

Diagnosis

Diagnosis is made by history, signs and symptoms, and culturing a stool sample.

Treatment

The patient will show improvement after 3 days of rehydration and antibiotic therapy.

Prevention

Following Standard Precautions, including good handwashing practices, can reduce the risk of contracting shigellosis. Ensure that the water supply is safe and that appropriate facilities are available for disposal of feces. Chlorination of the water supply also reduces risk.

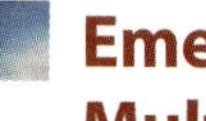

Emerging Infectious Diseases: Multidrug-Resistant Organisms

Methicillin-Resistant *Staphylococcus aureus* (MRSA)

Methicillin-resistant *Staphylococcus aureus* (MRSA) has emerged as an organism that can be community acquired (CA), not just a healthcare-associated infection. MRSA infection usually affects several body systems and is resistant to multiple antibiotics, including nafcillin (Unipen), oxacillin (Bactocill and Prostaphlin), cephalosporins, erythromycins, and aminoglycosides.

Signs and Symptoms

The patient may have fever, redness, localized pain, small red bumps, or deep abscesses that can affect bones, joints, heart valves, and the bloodstream. CA-MRSA has a different genetic makeup and is chiefly associated with soft-tissue infections such as abscesses and cellulitis. Abscesses are treated with incision and drainage and usually do not require antibiotics.

Pathophysiology

HA-MRSA and CA-MRSA are caused by different organisms. CA-MRSA can be acquired from household pets, contaminated gym equipment, contact between field turf and nonintact skin, and improper handwashing or failure to wash hands.

Diagnosis

Diagnosis of MRSA is confirmed by Gram stain and/or culture. A rapid test for MRSA produces results in 2 hours. A culture takes 48 to 72 hours.

Treatment

Use gloves and follow meticulous handwashing practices when in direct contact with draining wounds. No medical treatment is recommended after exposure to MRSA. Notify your DICO and document the event. Medications used for treating difficult MRSA infections include vancomycin (Vancocin), clindamycin (Cleocin), cotrimoxazole (Bactrim), quinupristin and dalfopristin injection (Synercid), and tigecycline (Tygacil).

Prevention

MRSA is a slow-growing bacterium and is easily destroyed by routine EPA-approved cleaning solutions. Clean the vehicle and patient care equipment after each use. Shower after physical activity and clean exercise equipment before use. Cover open skin areas with a dressing.

Vancomycin-Resistant *Enterococcus*

Enterococcus is a common organism that constitutes part of the normal flora of the GI tract, urinary tract, and genitourinary tract. This genus comprises more than 400 species, many of which are often resistant to antibiotics. A cagey organism, it flourishes equally well under conditions of scarce or abundant oxygen. When this organism becomes resistant to vancomycin (Vancocin), the primary drug used to treat *Enterococcus* infection, the patient is said to have vancomycin-resistant enterococcus (VRE). This is primarily an HAI.

Signs and Symptoms

Ask the patient about his or her medical history, particularly any hospital stay for surgery and any prolonged antibiotic treatment. Other signs and symptoms include wound infection, redness, tenderness, fever or chills, and urinary tract infection (indicated by an unusual urine color or odor and pain on urination).

Pathophysiology

This organism may be found in patients with urinary tract or bloodstream infections. VRE has also been found in livestock waste and improperly prepared chicken. Those who work on farms or in processing plants are at higher risk of exposure. Patients identified with VRE outside the hospital setting often reside in nursing homes or spend time at hemodialysis centers. VRE can live on surfaces for long periods of time, so thorough cleaning of devices used in healthcare settings is important.

Transmission occurs by direct contact with contaminated surfaces or equipment, or by direct contact of an open cut or sore with a draining wound. This illness can be treated with a new synthetic antibiotic, linezolid (Zyvox), which belongs to a novel antibiotic class called *oxazolidinones*.

Diagnosis

Diagnosis is made by culturing a wound, urine, blood, or stool.

Treatment

Antibiotic treatment is given using linezolid or another drug to which the organism demonstrates susceptibility on culture.

Prevention

Follow Standard Precautions, including wearing gloves and using good handwashing techniques, when you are in contact with wound drainage. A gown is needed only if wound drainage may come in contact with your uniform. Clean all areas with which the patient had contact; no special cleaning solution is needed. Direct contact between an open wound and VRE-infected body fluids should be reported to your supervisor. An exposure report will be completed, but no postexposure medical treatment is indicated.

It's important to note that patients with MRSA and VRE may be protected by the Americans with Disabilities Act (ADA), so it's important to exercise sensitivity and not go overboard with the use of unnecessary PPE; doing so may be considered discriminatory.

Clostridium difficile (Pseudomembranous Colitis)

Clostridium difficile (C. diff, for short) is not a multidrug-resistant organism but is treated like one. Rates of C. diff infection in the United States have tripled since 2000, and mortality has increased. Toxic variant strains are now widespread in North America and Europe.

This illness is the direct result of antibiotic therapy, which suppresses the normal flora in the GI tract and allows C. diff to predominate. Therefore, it's classified as an HAI but is also associated with outpatient antibiotic therapy. High-risk environments include acute and long-term facilities.

Signs and Symptoms

Patients with this illness have diarrhea that's not bloody but has a characteristic foul odor. Abdominal pain and cramping are present in about 22% of patients. If these signs are present, ask the patient about any recent hospital stays or antibiotic therapy. Check the odor of stool, and assess for the presence of fever.

Pathophysiology

Clostridium difficile is a gram-negative, spore-forming anaerobic bacillus that produces two large toxins, A and

B. Spore production causes heavy contamination of environmental surfaces. As a result, healthcare providers' unwashed hands are a major means of transmission of C. diff.

Diagnosis

Diagnosis is made on the basis of a thorough history, focused physical exam, and the patient's cardinal presentation. In addition, an increased WBC count, a positive stool culture, and an enzyme immunoassay assist in identifying which toxin is present.

Treatment

Stopping any unnecessary antibiotic treatment may be enough to resolve the infection, but treatment with oral metronidazole (Flagyl) or vancomycin (Vancocin) for 10 days is usually required. In some cases, symptoms will return within 30 days, generally caused by the same strain of C. diff.

Prevention

Follow Standard Precautions, including good handwashing practices with soap and vigorous rubbing. Use of just alcohol-based gels does not eradicate the spores. A chlorine-based solution must be used to clean equipment, since C. diff is a spore-forming organism. Avoiding the use of unnecessary antibiotics is essential and calls for a worldwide education program.

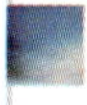

Prevention and Risk-Reduction Measures

Prevention and risk-reduction practices include being vaccinated, taking antiseptic measures, living in more sanitary conditions, pursuing a healthier lifestyle, and using good handwashing techniques. Preventing the transmission of infectious agents requires selecting infection control measures consistent with the way in which each disease is transmitted.

Department members are to be updated annually on new information about diseases, technology, equipment modifications, department exposure rates, and number of infectious disease transmissions and TB contacts during the previous year. This information serves to place risk in a proper perspective. Risk of disease transmission is present, but the risk is low when proper protective measures are followed by healthcare providers. OSHA has framed such risk-reduction and education requirements as a "right to know" issue.

Putting It All Together

Understanding the epidemiology and pathophysiology of a variety of infectious disease processes is essential in early identification of the cause of an illness. In addition, becoming aware of an abrupt increase in the incidence of patients with a similar cardinal presentation will help you and your public health colleagues pinpoint geographic trends that might need to be reported to the appropriate local, state, and federal authorities.

Identification of the patient's cardinal presentation, a thorough history, focused physical exam, and evaluation of diagnostic findings will all help you recognize a communicable or infectious disease. Early recognition will support prevention of the spread of the disease by choosing the appropriate PPE early in patient contact. The healthcare team's assessment and early interventions are critical strategies in preventing transmission of infectious diseases. However, the healthcare environment is often unpredictable, and disease identification may not occur until after you have rendered care. Fortunately, research endeavors continue to make progress in identifying communicable and infectious diseases and developing new vaccines, medications, and treatment protocols.

SCENARIO SOLUTION

1 **Differential diagnoses may include: alcoholic cirrhosis, hepatitis, or HIV infection. You worry about secondary lung infection from opportunistic infection, pneumonia, or tuberculosis or the presence of congestive heart failure.**

2 **To narrow your differential diagnosis you will need to complete the history of past and present illness. Assess his temperature. Perform a physical examination to include examination of the oral cavity for opportunistic infection or signs of dehydration; his neck for JVD; his breath sounds for equality and for the presence of adventitious sounds; his abdomen for the presence of hepatomegaly or splenomegaly; and his extremities for pulses and the presence of edema.**

3 **The patient has signs of liver failure and hypoxia. Administer high flow oxygen. Initiate an IV and titrate fluids based on your other physical findings. Transport to the appropriate facility.**

4 **Use Standard Precautions on all patients. If you are exposed to blood or bloody body fluids on this patient, follow the same actions you would on any exposure. Report it immediately to the healthcare provider receiving facility. Notify your designated officer for infection control. Complete the necessary reports and follow-up. This patient is high risk for HIV, hepatitis B, and hepatitis C because of his former IV drug use.**

SUMMARY

- Exposure to an infectious agent does not mean that a person has acquired the disease and can pass it on to others.
- PPE is a secondary barrier to the protection the body already offers.
- The Ryan White Notification Law was reinstated on September 30, 2009.
- Vaccination is essential for risk reduction in the healthcare setting.
- PPE should be selected with an understanding of the mode of transmission of the diseases to which you expect to be exposed.
- Meningitis is usually spread by inhalation of droplets and by direct contact with an infected person's respiratory or nasal secretions. Only exposure to meningococcal meningitis requires prophylactic antibiotics.
- Healthcare providers decrease the risk of exposure to infectious diseases by using Standard Precautions and thorough handwashing techniques.
- Local and federal governmental agencies establish standards and guidelines to reduce the risk of infection for the healthcare provider and the communities in which they serve.
- Prevention of transmission of infectious diseases can result from an understanding of the pathophysiology, clinical manifestations, and treatment strategies for communicable and infectious diseases.

BIBLIOGRAPHY

2007 Guideline for isolation precautions: preventing transmission of infectious agents in healthcare settings.

29 CFR 1910.1020 Medical records standard.

29 CFR 1910.1300 Bloodborne pathogens standard.

Aehlert B: Paramedic practice today: above and beyond, ed 1, St Louis, 2009, Mosby.

Alter MJ, Kuhnert WL, Finelli L, et al: Guidelines for laboratory testing and result reporting of antibody to hepatitis C virus, MMWR Recomm Rep 52(RR-3):1–13, 2003.

American Academy of Pediatrics Committee on Infectious Diseases and Committee on Fetus and Newborn: Revised indications for the use of palivizumab and respiratory syncytial virus immune globulin intravenous for the prevention of respiratory syncytial virus infection, Pediatrics 112(6Pt1): 1442–1446, 2003.

Association for Professionals in Infection Control and Epidemiology, Inc: APIC text of infection control and epidemiology, Washington, DC, 2009, APIC.

CDC Division of Bacterial and Mycotic Diseases: *Streptococcus pneumoniae* disease prevention and control of meningococcal disease: recommendations of the Advisory Committee on Immunization Practices (ACIP), MMWR, Morb Mortal Wkly Rep, May 27, 2005.

Centers for Disease Control and Prevention: Controlling tuberculosis in the United States, 2005. http://www.cdc.gov/mmwr/preview/mmwrhtml/rr5412a1.htm. Accessed December 24, 2009.

Centers for Disease Control and Prevention: Fight the bite! www.cdc.gov/ncidod/dvbid/westnile/index.htm. Accessed December 24, 2009.

Centers for Disease Control and Prevention: Guidance on H1N1 influenza A. www.cdc.gov/h1n1. Accessed December 24, 2009.

Centers for Disease Control and Prevention: Guideline for hand hygiene in health-care settings: recommendations of the Healthcare Infection Control Practices Committee and the HICPAC/SHEA/APIC/IDSA Hand Hygiene Task Force, 2002. http://www.cdc.gov/Handhygiene. Accessed December 24, 2009.

Centers for Disease Control and Prevention: The national plan to eliminate syphilis from the United States, May 2006. http://www.cdc.gov/stopsyphilis/SEEPlan2006.pdf. Accessed December 24, 2009.

Centers for Disease Control and Prevention: Rabies. www.cdc.gov/ncidod/dvrd/rabies.http. Accessed January 12, 2010.

Centers for Disease Control and Prevention: Updated U.S. public health service guidelines for the management of occupational exposures to HBC, HCV, and HIV, recommendations for postexposure prophylaxis, 2005. http://www.cdc.gov/mmwr/preview/mmwrhtml/rr5011a1.htm. Accessed December 24, 2009.

Cohen J, Powderly WG: Infectious diseases, ed 2, St Louis, Mosby, 2004.

CPL 2-2.69, Enforcement procedures for the occupational exposure to bloodborne pathogens, Occupational Safety and Health Administration, November 27, 2001.

Cross JR, West KH: Clarifying HIPAA and disclosure of disease information, JEMS, August, 2007.

Global tuberculosis control, WHO Report, 2008. http://data.unaids.org/pub/Report/2008/who2008globaltbreport_en.pdf. Accessed December 24, 2009.

Centers for Disease Control and Prevention: HPV vaccination. http://www.cdc.gov/vaccines/vpd-vac/hpv/default.htm. Accessed January 12, 2010.

Kretsinger K, Broder KR, Cortese MM, et al: Preventing tetanus, diphtheria, and pertussis among adults: use of tetanus toxoid, reduced diphtheria toxoid, and acellular pertussis vaccine: recommendations of the Advisory Committee on Immunization Practices (ACIP) and recommendation of ACIP, supported by the Healthcare Infection Control Practices Advisory Committee (HICPAC), for use of Tdap among health-care personnel, MMWR Recomm Rep Dec 15;55(RR-17):1–37, 2006.

Mast EE, Weinbaum CM, Fiore AE, et al: A comprehensive immunization strategy to eliminate transmission of hepatitis B virus infection in the United States: recommendations of the Advisory Committee on Immunization Practices (ACIP) part II: immunization of adults, MMWR Morb Mortal Wkly Rep 56(42):1114, 2007.

McCance KL, Huether SE: Pathophysiology: the biologic basis for disease in adults and children, ed 5, St Louis, 2006, Elsevier.

Needlestick Prevention Act, U.S. Congress, March 2000.

Patient care checklist for H1N1, World Health Organization, August 2009.

Personal communication, Dr. Paul Jensen, CDC, January, 2006; no need for N95s for TB in fire/EMS setting.

Recommended antimicrobial agents for treatment and postexposure prophylaxis of pertussis, MMWR Recomm Rep 54(RR-14):1–16, 2005.

Respiratory protection for healthcare workers in the workplace against novel H1N1 influenza A: a letter report, Institute of Medicine, 2009. http://www.iom.edu/Reports/2009/RespProtH1N1.aspx. Accessed December 24, 2009.

Roome AJ, Hadler JL, Thomas AL, et al: Hepatitis C virus infection among firefighters, emergency medical technicians, and paramedics—selected locations, United States, 1991–2000, MMWR Morb Mortal Wkly Rep 49(29):660–665, 2000.

Ryan White CARE Act, S. 1793, part G, section 2695, notification of possible exposure to infectious diseases, September 30, 2009—reauthorization.

Sanders MJ: Mosby's paramedic textbook, ed 3 revised, St Louis, 2007, Mosby.

Siegel JD, Rhinehart E, Jackson M, et al: 2007 Guideline for isolation precautions: preventing transmission of infectious agents in healthcare settings, www.cdc.gov/ncidod/dhqp/pdf/guidelines/Isolation2007.pdf. Accessed December 24, 2009.

Trends in tuberculosis–United States, 2008, MMWR Morb Mortal Wkly Rep 58(10):249–253, 2009.

U.S. Department of Transportation National Highway Traffic Safety Administration: EMT-Paramedic National Standard Curriculum, Washington, DC, 1998, The Department.

U.S. Department of Transportation National Highway Traffic Safety Administration: National EMS Education Standards, Draft 3.0, Washington, DC, 2008, The Department.

West KH: Infectious disease handbook for emergency care personnel, ed 3, Cincinnati, 2001, ACGIH.

Workowski KA, Berman SM: Sexually transmitted diseases treatment guidelines, CDC, 2006. http://www.cdc.gov/mmwr/preview/mmwrhtml/rr5511a1.htm. Accessed December 24, 2009.

Chapter Review Questions

1. Which agency oversees the compliance, tracking and reporting, and guidelines for preventing transmission of bloodborne pathogens in the workplace?
   a. Department of Public Health
   b. Food and Drug Administration
   c. The Center for Disease Control and Prevention (CDC)
   d. Department of Labor's Occupational Safety and Health Administration (OSHA)

2. You are treating a patient who has been diagnosed with herpes simplex type 1. He exhibits no signs or symptoms at this time. He is in which stage of the communicable disease?
   a. Latent disease
   b. Incubation period
   c. Communicability period
   d. Disease period

3. Which of the following is an occupational exposure incident?
   a. You notice blood spattered on the intact skin of your forearm after a call.
   b. You stick your finger on a contaminated lancet at your brother's house.
   c. Blood sprays in your face when a child with a face laceration sneezes.
   d. A patient you cared for is reported to be HIV positive.

4. Antibodies that are produced from lymphocytes are known as what kind of immunity?
   a. Humoral
   b. Cell-mediated
   c. Autoimmunity
   d. Artificial

5. Hepatitis A (HAV) is transmitted by which route?
   a. Airborne
   b. Droplet
   c. Oral-fecal
   d. Bloodborne

6. The best measures you can take to reduce your risk of acquiring hepatitis C from an occupational exposure is to:
   a. Be vaccinated.
   b. Get immune globulin if you have an exposure.
   c. Take postexposure drugs as prescribed.
   d. Use Standard Precautions.

7. Which sign or symptom can help diagnose headache from meningococcal meningitis?
   a. Fever
   b. Light sensitivity
   c. Petechial rash
   d. Stiff neck

8. A patient infected with which disease should be assessed for pneumonia, encephalitis, and myocarditis?
   a. Infectious parotitis
   b. Pertussis
   c. Rubella
   d. Rubeola

9. While treating a trauma patient, you lacerate your hand. Your bleeding hand comes in contact with the blood of the patient. What action is most important to increase your chance of appropriate follow-up?

a. Ask the patient if they are infected with HIV, hepatitis B, or hepatitis C.
b. Complete an incident report, and contact your chief officer on the next business day.
c. Make an appointment to see occupational health within 1 week.
d. Notify the receiving facility and your designated infection control officer immediately.

10. Your adolescent patient presents with fever, malaise, sneezing, and paroxysmal spasmodic coughing phases. Which infectious disease would you suspect?

a. Tuberculosis
b. Rubella
c. Pneumonia
d. Pertussis

CHAPTER

9 Toxicology, Hazardous Materials, and Weapons of Mass Destruction

THIS CHAPTER EXPLORES the devastating effects of natural and manmade toxins on the human body. As always, what you'll learn rests on the methodical AMLS approach, at the heart of which is a thorough scene survey, skillful assessment, and rapid stabilization of life threats. We'll begin with land and marine environmental toxicology, which includes arthropod and snake envenomation and plant toxins. Medicines as toxins and drugs of abuse will be examined in detail. Then we'll talk about toxins in the home and workplace and cover the essentials of how to recognize and respond safely and effectively to hazardous materials exposure. We'll discuss regulatory agency notification, setting up staging areas, decontamination, and personal protective equipment. Finally, we'll address biological, chemical, and radiologic contamination by weapons of terrorism, including incendiary devices and their attendant fire and chemical dangers.

Learning Objectives ***At the conclusion of this chapter, you will be able to:***

1. Understand the basic approach to a patient who has been poisoned or taken an overdose.
2. Identify and describe the most common toxidromes.
3. Recognize which patients are at risk of respiratory depression and arrhythmia from poisoning.
4. Discuss the cardinal presentation, assessment, and treatment of patients with toxicologic medical emergencies.
5. Describe the value of poison control in the treatment of toxicologic emergencies.
6. Outline general principles of assessment and management for patients exposed to a variety of hazardous materials and weapons of mass destruction.
7. Understand the treatment of toxin-induced arrhythmias.
8. Describe the signs and symptoms, assessment, and treatment of patients who encounter chemical, biological, and radiologic agents.
9. Specify safety concerns for healthcare providers and patients who are at risk of exposure to hazardous materials or weapons of mass destruction.
10. Describe general decontamination procedures for patients and healthcare providers who have been exposed to a toxic agent.

Key Terms

biological agent Disease-causing pathogen or toxin that may be used as a weapon to cause disease or injury to humans

cold (green) zone A support zone for general triage, stabilization, and management of illness or injuries. Patients and uncontaminated personnel are given access to this zone, but healthcare personnel must wear protective clothing while in the green zone and properly discard it in predetermined areas on exiting.

contamination Condition of being soiled, stained, touched, or otherwise exposed to harmful agents, making an object potentially unsafe for use as intended or without barrier techniques. An example is entry of infectious or toxic materials into a previously clean or sterile environment.

delirium An acute mental disorder characterized by confusion, disorientation, restlessness, clouding of consciousness, incoherence, fear, anxiety, excitement, and often illusions

dirty bomb A conventional explosive device used to disperse radiologic agents

emergency decontamination Process of decontaminating people exposed to and potentially contaminated with hazardous materials; focuses on rapidly removing the contamination to reduce their exposure and save lives, with secondary regard for completeness of decontamination

fulminant Describes a sudden intense occurrence that creates a hazardous environment

gastrointestinal decontamination Any attempt to limit absorption or hasten elimination of a toxin from a patient's gastrointestinal tract. Examples include activated charcoal, gastric lavage, and whole-bowel irrigation. While these methods do have a small role in toxicology, their use is not routinely recommended and should be discussed with a poison control center or medical toxicologist.

hot (red) zone An area where the hazardous material is located and contamination has occurred. Access to this zone is limited so as to protect rescuers and patients from further exposure. Specific protective gear worn by trained personnel is required for access.

huffing The act of pouring an inhalant onto a cloth or into a bag and inhaling the substance, usually in an attempt to alter one's mental status

intoxication The state of being poisoned by a drug or other toxic substance; the state of being inebriated as a result of excessive alcohol consumption

lethal concentration 50% (LC50) The air concentration of an agent that kills 50% of the exposed animal population. This denotes the concentration and the length of exposure time of that population.

lethal dose 50% (LD50) The oral or dermal exposure dose that kills 50% of an exposed animal population in 2 weeks

methemoglobinemia The presence of methemoglobin in the blood, which prevents the ability of hemoglobin to carry and transport oxygen to the tissues. Hemoglobin is converted to methemoglobin by nitrogen oxides and sulfa drugs.

National Fire Protection Association (NFPA) A national and international voluntary membership organization that promotes improved fire protection and prevention and establishes safeguards against loss of life and property by fire. The NFPA writes and publishes national voluntary consensus standards.

North American Emergency Response Guidebook A book published by the U.S. Government Printing Office that provides a quick reference to hazardous materials emergencies for first responders

Occupational Safety and Health Administration (OSHA) The U.S. federal agency that regulates worker safety

packer A person who ingests a large quantity of well-packed drugs for the purpose of smuggling. These carefully prepared packages are less likely to rupture than those ingested by stuffers, but toxicity can be severe if they do because of the large amount of drug present.

placards Diamond-shaped signs placed on containers that identify hazardous materials

prodromal Early symptoms that mark the onset of a disease

psychosis Any major mental disorder characterized by a gross impairment in reality testing, in which the individual incorrectly evaluates the accuracy of perceptions and thoughts and makes incorrect references about external reality. It is often characterized by regressive behavior, inappropriate mood and affect, and diminished impulse control. Symptoms include hallucinations and delusions.

pulmonary agent An industrial chemical used as a weapon to kill those who inhale the vapor or gas; lung damage causes asphyxiation. Also known as a *choking agent*.

radioactive Giving off radiation as the result of the disintegration of atomic nuclei

Standard on Hazardous Waste Operations and Emergency Response (HAZWOPER) (CFR 1910.120) Occupational Safety and Health Administration (OSHA) and Environmental Protection Agency (EPA) regulation intended to protect the safety of employees who respond to emergency incidents related to storage and disposal of hazardous materials

stuffer A person who hastily ingests small packets of poorly packaged drugs to avoid apprehension and drug confiscation. The dose is much lower than that seen with packers, but the likelihood of toxicity is much greater because the packages, meant for distribution, are likely to open in the patient's stomach or bowel.

toxidrome A specific syndrome-like group of symptoms associated with exposure to a given poison

warm (yellow) zone The area surrounding a contaminated hot zone. Properly protected healthcare providers are allowed to access this zone for rapid assessment and management of emergent or life-threatening conditions. Decontamination occurs in this zone.

SCENARIO

A 24-YEAR-OLD QUADRIPLEGIC MALE is anxious and slightly combative. His vital signs are BP 188/104, P 136, R 28. He was found this way when his roommate returned from work.

1 ***What differential diagnoses are you considering based on the information you have now? (Include any toxidrome or specific drugs you may be considering.)***

2 ***What additional information will you need to narrow your differential diagnosis?***

3 ***What treatments would you consider for this patient?***

Toxicologic emergencies are an important and ever prevalent spectrum of illnesses faced by prehospital and other healthcare providers. They include intentional overdose, unintentional poisoning, occupational exposure, environmental hazards, envenomation, biological and chemical warfare, and radiation illness. Early recognition of toxicity and identification of the causative agent can help you initiate appropriate management, maintain safe conditions for yourself, the patient, and the public, and provide essential information to your colleagues at all levels.

Such emergencies cause a broad spectrum of illness, yet regardless of the offending agent, early recognition and management of dangerous environments and life-threatening patient presentations necessitates following an orderly, unwavering set of fundamental principles. To diagnose and treat toxicologic disorders efficiently, you must have a solid grasp of nervous system, cardiac, and respiratory physiology. In this chapter, then, we've chosen to focus on the body's response to classes of drugs and toxins (toxidromes) rather than analyze scores of particular agents. In addition, we'll discuss hazardous materials that pose a threat to you and your patients. When appropriate, we'll recommend symptomatic therapy, since the causative agent in any given exposure is often unknown. We'll review intoxications you'll encounter frequently, as well as those you'll treat rarely or perhaps never—but for which you must be well prepared nonetheless. We'll emphasize the following areas:

- Obtaining historical information
- Identifying toxins
- Understanding the pathophysiology of toxicity
- Making a preliminary evaluation
- Applying general treatment concepts
- Selecting specific therapy

Appropriate early management of patients exposed to a variety of toxins and hazardous materials remains a fundamental aspect of emergency care.

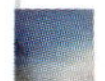

Overview

Toxicologic emergencies caused by accidental and intentional exposures are a principal cause of morbidity and mortality in the United States. In 2006, The CDC's National Center for Injury Prevention and Control reported 23,618 unintentional poisonings; 37,286 deaths were attributed to poisoning. Unintentional poisoning was second only to motor vehicle crashes for injury deaths reported in the 2005 data. In 2006, the American Association of Poison Control Centers National Poison Data System indicated that 83% of poisonings were unintentional, and more than 50% of those involved children younger than 6 years of age. In 2007, nearly 2.5 million poison and drug exposures were reported to U.S. poison control centers.

As in any emergent medical or traumatic illness, diagnosing and treating toxicologic emergencies calls for a consistent, reliable approach. The safety of prehospital and first-response personnel is the initial concern. During every emergency response, even for a suspected medical emergency, you arrive at the scene knowing you have to be aware of the potential for toxic and hazardous materials exposure. But it becomes critically important to follow a systematic process for safe emergency response when the patient has been exposed to chemical, biological, or radiologic toxins.

The AMLS survey guides you through an efficient but comprehensive assessment of the poisoned patient. In some cases, preventing life-threatening sequelae means immediate initiation of therapy, such as stabilizing the airway or administering cardioactive drugs. After first addressing your patient's critical needs, performing a more detailed history, scene survey, and examination often narrows the diagnosis significantly, allowing you to institute potentially life-saving treatment measures without delay.

AMLS Approach

History Taking

Historical information is often critical in the diagnosis and treatment of toxicity. Interviewing family members and witnesses, particularly when treating a child or a patient with altered mental status, can be crucial. When the offending agent has been identified, you must consider and ask about co-ingestions and verify the following:

- Timing of ingestion
- Suspected dose
- Patient's access to the drug or chemical
- Situational information like the patient's position and location and the presence or absence of nearby drug paraphernalia or other intoxicated patients

As a provider who responds on scene, you're often in a position to gather the most accurate information. Unfortunately, for a variety of reasons, historical information is often untrustworthy. Clues revealed during physical examination may be more reliable, and here in particular is where the AMLS survey helps you organize a swift and detailed evaluation of the patient who has had a toxicologic exposure.

Initial Observation

You must verify that the scene is safe before entering it (see Chapter 1 and the discussion later in this chapter). A number of gases and toxins have the capacity to injure or incapacitate medical personnel. The dispatchers should ask thorough questions about scene safety and relay the answers to all responding providers. This information is particularly important when multiple patients are affected. In fact, the involvement of more than one patient suggests that toxicity may be related to a gas, which can rapidly induce symptoms. The causative agent in an exposure is often unknown. When a hazardous material is suspected, consider requesting a hazardous materials (HazMat) response team. Resources to help you identify toxic materials and handle them safely are given in the Hazardous Materials section of this chapter.

Once you arrive on scene, you can gather a great deal of useful information at the outset of the encounter. The patient's physical location may lead you to consider toxicity as the primary cause of the illness. For instance, finding a patient with altered mental status in a house where heroin abuse has been known to occur can guide appropriate management of that patient. In addition, the position and circumstances in which you find the patient offer clues to the underlying toxicity and prognosis. Finding pill bottles in the room or easily accessible in the house, for example, can give you useful information even before you begin your examination.

As in any emergency situation, evaluation of airway, breathing, circulation, and perfusion forms the backbone of your assessment. The Rapid Recall box offers a review of the ABCDEE mnemonic.

First Impression

For each patient, you'll form a first impression of whether the person is sick or not sick. In this context, "sick" means that the patient's illness is likely to become life threatening if you don't intervene immediately. Weak or erratic vital signs and a poor mental status evaluation generally contribute to this impression. In patients with toxicologic emergencies, mental status changes can range from agitation and **psychosis** to coma. Either extreme is profoundly dangerous. Coma is associated with respiratory depression and an inability to protect the airway. Agitation and **delirium** may indicate significant metabolic derangements and can provoke dangerous behavior or trigger acute, severe cardiovascular disorders that may be fatal.

The adage "Vital signs are vital" holds true in toxicologic emergencies. Assessing and stabilizing abnormal vital signs is critical in early management. Frequent ongoing evaluation can help you gauge the nature and severity of toxicity in a poisoned patient. Initiate airway support and advanced cardiac life support (ACLS) protocols in sick patients without delay.

RAPID RECALL

ABCDEE Assessment Mnemonic

A Airway
B Breathing
C Circulation
D Disability
E Exposure
E Environment

In addition to checking the ABCs of airway, breathing, and circulation, be sure to remember D for disability, which refers to perfusion related to altered mental status. Changes in mentation might be caused by a serum glucose derangement, so it's vitally important to take a serum glucose reading in patients who exhibit neurologic symptoms. Also keep in mind E for exposure, which necessitates visualizing your patient for any abnormal skin lesions such as rashes, bumps, or needle marks. In addition, E should prompt you to ensure that the environment is not making your patient too cold (hypothermic) or too hot (hyperthermic).

Differential Diagnosis and Interventions

The primary and secondary survey focus on identifying and managing life-threatening emergencies related to the specific toxin exposure. Interventions are aimed at treating the patient's mental status changes and perfusion abnormalities. The range of toxic agents and specific therapies is vast, but the AMLS assessment pathway will help you narrow the differential diagnosis to a working diagnosis so emergent treatment can begin right away. Continual monitoring of the patient's response to therapy is essential, and as always, early communication with the receiving facility can ensure a fluid continuum of care.

Coma

Coma, a state of unconsciousness or deep sedation from which the patient cannot be aroused by any external stimulus, is a common presentation after intoxication. The term **intoxication** simply refers to the presence of a poison or toxin in the body, with no specific implication of altered consciousness, but it's often used to describe patients who have an impaired or depressed mental status.

Because historical information cannot be obtained from an unconscious patient, bystanders, family, and a physical examination may provide the only data for arriving at a prehospital diagnosis. Therefore, it's essential that you be proficient in recognizing environmental variables, mechanisms of injury, patient posturing, and odors that may offer insight regarding the patient's condition.

Treatment of the comatose patient is primarily supportive and may include advanced airway support. Most current recommendations suggest first supporting airway, breathing, and circulation and then considering drug therapy. Therapeutic agents used to reverse coma include thiamine, glucose, naloxone (Narcan), and occasionally flumazenil (Romazicon), a benzodiazepine reversal agent.

Naloxone

Naloxone has a key role in the management of comatose patients. Naloxone is a μ-opioid receptor antagonist which reverses the effects of opioids. The primary indication for its use is respiratory depression as evidenced by a decreased respiratory rate, hypercapnia, or hypoxemia, a late finding. The endpoints of naloxone therapy are restoration of adequate oxygenation and ventilation. Excessive dosing of naloxone causes acute opioid withdrawal in opioid-dependent patients. Naloxone has also been associated with hypertension and acute lung injury, presumably from catecholamine release associated with abrupt withdrawal. Patients who are known or thought likely to be opioid dependent should be given smaller doses of naloxone to avoid inducing these complications. If the initial dose is ineffective, however, rapid escalation of dosing is recommended.

Flumazenil

Flumazenil is a γ-aminobutyric acid (GABA) benzodiazepine receptor antagonist that effectively reverses sedation; however, you should be aware of the danger associated with its use. Many patients being treated for overdose have taken benzodiazepines in combination with other drugs. Benzodiazepines are often protective in this scenario, particularly when the patient has also ingested a tricyclic antidepressant. In such cases, reversal with flumazenil may worsen toxicity and patient outcome. Withdrawal from GABA-agonist medications is associated with severe vital sign abnormalities, seizures, delirium, and death. Many patients who overdose on benzodiazepines take them chronically, and administering flumazenil to such patients may precipitate an acute withdrawal syndrome.

Hypoglycemia

Hypoglycemia is a rapidly reversible, life-threatening cause of altered mental status. Availability of bedside glucose testing using rapid reagent strips allows you to test quickly for hypoglycemia before administering glucose. Intravenous (IV) administration of a 50% dextrose in water solution (D_{50}) is safe and advisable.

Thiamine Deficiency

Thiamine deficiency may lead to Wernicke encephalopathy in patients who are chronically malnourished, primarily those who are alcohol dependent (see Chapter 2 for more information on Wernicke-Korsakoff syndrome). Although this condition is uncommon, a single dose of thiamine may provide some benefit and poses no risk at the standard dose of 100 mg administered intravenously (IV) or intramuscularly (IM). Despite widely propagated concerns, it's not necessary to give thiamine before dextrose. Although encephalopathy due to thiamine deficiency can be exacerbated by chronic hypoglycemia, administration of dextrose in an acute situation has not been shown to induce Wernicke-Korsakoff syndrome in a previously healthy person. You should not delay treatment of hypoglycemia because of concern about thiamine deficiency.

Agitation

Many drugs and toxins can cause central nervous system (CNS) excitation, agitation, or psychosis. Regardless of the cause, however, initial management is the same. The goal of treatment in an agitated patient is to depress the CNS to protect the patient from metabolic derangements associated with agitation, tissue injury from cardiovascular toxicity, and self-injurious behavior.

Benzodiazepines

Benzodiazepines are a mainstay of therapy for the agitated patient. Because benzodiazepines have a benign safety profile and a wide therapeutic index, this class of medications is widely used to prevent injury to intoxicated patients and the providers who care for them. Benzodiazepines also have the benefit of preventing seizure activity, attenuating sympathetic hyperactivity, and reducing other causes of morbidity often associated with severe agitation (e.g., rhabdomyolysis).

Benzodiazepines depress the CNS, but physical restraint may be necessary in order to administer them. You should take great care to minimize physical restraint in favor of chemical restraint, however, since the former is associated with worsening metabolic acidosis, rhabdomyolysis, and occasionally respiratory compromise.

The benzodiazepines most commonly used for sedation of the acutely agitated patient in the emergency care setting are lorazepam (Ativan) and diazepam (Valium). Midazolam (Versed) is available in IV, IM, and oral formulations; diazepam is available in IV, oral, and rectal formulations. The amount of the agent required to adequately sedate a patient varies significantly with body size, degree of agitation, history of benzodiazepine tolerance, and amount of stimulant ingested. Benzodiazepines can cause respiratory depression, blunting the patient's reflex to protect the airway, so don't administer them unless you can closely monitor the patient and provide airway support if necessary.

Antipsychotics

Antipsychotic medications, especially haloperidol (Haldol) and ziprasidone (Geodon), are also commonly used in emergency care to treat agitated patients. Haloperidol is an antipsychotic agent that potently antagonizes dopamine D_2 receptors. A desired side effect of administration is sedation. Ziprasidone is approved for acute agitation in schizophrenic patients. It's mechanism of action is unknown, but it's been theorized that ziprasidone's antipsychotic activity, like haloperidol's, is mediated primarily by antagonism at dopamine D_2 receptors.

If benzodiazepines are not immediately available, use of an antipsychotic agent is preferable to physical restraint. Despite the potential for adverse effects, use of antipsychotics after administration of benzodiazepines has a central role in the treatment of agitated patients. Intoxicated patients suffering from excess dopaminergic stimulation exhibit acute psychosis, often manifested by visual and tactile hallucinations or choreoathetoid movements, so-called crack dancing. Once benzodiazepines have been given to improve agitation and cardiovascular instability, haloperidol is effective in treating these specific toxic effects.

Seizures

CNS excitation can also lead to seizures. Most toxin-induced seizures are generalized tonic-clonic seizures that rarely progress to status epilepticus, although exceptions do occur (e.g., isoniazid toxicity). Seizure activity should always prompt you to evaluate the patient's blood glucose level or to administer dextrose prophylactically. Otherwise, benzodiazepines are used in both the prevention and treatment of seizures. If a patient shows evidence of tremor, especially if it's accompanied by tachycardia and anxiety, you should administer benzodiazepines in an effort to prevent seizure activity. Once a seizure has occurred, administration of high-dose benzodiazepines is indicated.

If benzodiazepines are ineffective for seizure activity, you should administer barbiturates, typically phenobarbital (Luminal), 20 mg/kg. Be prepared to address airway concerns and correct hypotension in patients who require barbiturate loading doses, although in some extremely agitated patients, intubation may not be necessary. Propofol (Diprivan), a GABA agonist and *N*-methyl-D-aspartate (NMDA) antagonist, is another potent sedative that can be titrated quickly but requires intubation for administration. Phenytoin (Dilantin) and other typical anticonvulsants are ineffective in the treatment of toxin-induced seizures.

Finally, consider pyridoxine (vitamin B_6) in the treatment of refractory seizures. Classically, pyridoxine has been used as an antidote for seizures caused by isoniazid (Nydrazid) toxicity, but it can be used as an adjunct agent in status epilepticus due to any cause. Empirical dosing of at least 1 g IV is generally recommended, with a maximum dose of 70 mg/kg. Consider continuous electroencephalogram (EEG) monitoring if seizures continue despite an apparent halt in motor activity.

Temperature Alteration

Although often overlooked, particularly in the prehospital setting, getting an accurate body temperature is crucial in managing toxicologic emergencies. Stimulant intoxication or poisoning is associated with increased mortality when accompanied by hyperthermia. Temperature alteration is a cardinal feature of some toxicologic diagnoses such as serotonin syndrome, neuroleptic malignant syndrome, and malignant hyperthermia. The therapeutic goal for such patients is rapid normalization of temperature through external cooling techniques and medication administration.

Hypothermia can occur after ingestion of sedative-hypnotic agents or opioids. Whether the patient's temperature has climbed or fallen, you should initiate treatment of any severe temperature alteration as soon as you discover it.

Heart Rate Abnormalities

The pulse irregularities and arrhythmias that often occur during toxicologic emergencies can help you diagnose the patient's condition and select initial therapy. Although the patient's pulse rate may deviate significantly from the norm, however, you must concentrate on the patient as a whole, rather than focus on treating the number. In many patients, mild tachycardia or bradycardia need not be treated aggressively if no evidence suggests end-organ injury as a result of the rhythm disturbance.

Tachycardia

In a toxicologic emergency, tachycardia may be caused directly by the drug effect, rather than by volume depletion. A variety of pharmacologic mechanisms may accelerate the heart rate, including sympathomimetic toxicity, dopamine receptor agonism, and calcium channel blockade, which causes vasodilation and reflex tachycardia (Table 9-1). Many toxins are active at more than one receptor site, which may complicate treatment algorithms. In addition to these pharmacologic effects, toxicity from drugs, plants, or chemicals causes volume depletion as a result of reduced oral intake, prolonged immobilization, vomiting, diarrhea, or a combination of such factors.

Regardless of the etiology, initial treatment with isotonic IV fluids is indicated and may be all that's required.

TABLE 9-1 Mechanisms of Toxin-Induced Tachycardia

Mechanism of Toxicity	Examples	Treatment
Sympathomimetic toxicity	Cocaine, amphetamine, ephedrine, phencyclidine	IV fluids, benzodiazepines
Peripheral α-blockade	Antipsychotics, tricyclic antidepressants, doxazosin	IV fluids, phenylephrine
Peripheral calcium channel blockade	Dihydropyridine calcium channel blockers (nifedipine, amlodipine)	IV fluids, phenylephrine
Muscarinic receptor blockade	Tricyclic antidepressants, diphenhydramine, cyclobenzaprine, antipsychotics	IV fluids, benzodiazepines, +/− physostigmine
Nicotinic receptor activation	Tobacco, poison hemlock, betel nut, carbamates, organophosphates	IV fluids, benzodiazepines
Serotonin receptor stimulation	Selective serotonin reuptake inhibitors (SSRIs), tricyclic antidepressants, cocaine, tramadol, meperidine	IV fluids, benzodiazepines, +/− cyproheptadine
Dopamine receptor agonism	Amantadine, bupropion, bromocriptine, amphetamine, cocaine	IV fluids, benzodiazepines, +/− haloperidol
GABA agonist withdrawal/GABA antagonism	Ethyl alcohol or benzodiazepine withdrawal, water hemlock, flumazenil	IV fluids, benzodiazepines, barbiturates
Adenosine receptor antagonism	Methylxanthines (e.g., theophylline, caffeine)	IV fluids, benzodiazepines, esmolol
β-Receptor agonism	Albuterol, clenbuterol, terbutaline	IV fluids, esmolol

TABLE 9-2 Mechanisms of Toxin-Induced Bradycardia

Mechanism of Toxicity	Examples	Treatment
Cardiac sodium channel opening	Veratrum alkaloids, aconite, grayanotoxin, ciguatera	Atropine, dopamine
Cardiac sodium channel blockade	Tricyclic antidepressants, carbamazepine, yew plant, propranolol	Sodium bicarbonate, hypertonic saline, pressors
β-Adrenergic receptor blockade	Atenolol, propranolol, metoprolol	Atropine, glucagon, epinephrine, insulin
Calcium channel antagonism	Verapamil, diltiazem	Atropine, calcium salts, epinephrine, insulin
Na^+/K^+-ATPase inactivation	Digoxin, foxglove, oleander, lily of the valley	Atropine, digoxin-specific antibody fragments (Fab)
Muscarinic and nicotinic activation	Carbamates, *Clitocybe* mushrooms, organophosphates	Atropine, pressors, +/− pralidoxime
Peripheral α-receptor agonists	Imidazolines (e.g., clonidine initial activity)	Supportive care, +/− phentolamine vs. nitroprusside
Central α-receptor agonists	Imidazolines (e.g., clonidine secondary activity)	Atropine, dopamine
Opioids	Oxycodone, heroin, fentanyl	Rarely required; supportive care, +/− pressors

ATPase, Adenosine triphosphatase; *K^+,* potassium; *Na^+,* sodium.

In many patients, tachycardia is accompanied by agitation and tremulousness. Administration of benzodiazepines in these patients provides sympatholysis, helping to moderate vital signs and quell agitation. Otherwise, treatment depends on assessment of heart rate, blood pressure, and specific drug activity. For instance, beta-blockers such as esmolol (Brevibloc) may be used to treat β-adrenergic toxicity but can worsen hypotension or coronary artery vasospasm in patients with cocaine toxicity.

A degree of tachycardia is acceptable if the patient's blood pressure is controlled and intensive supportive care has been instituted, but give special consideration to patients with underlying coronary artery disease or evidence of myocardial ischemia. More aggressive control of heart rate and blood pressure is required in this patient population.

Bradycardia

A variety of plant and drug toxicities and chemical exposures can cause bradycardia (Table 9-2). Many patients require no treatment. In those who do, the goal is to maintain end-organ perfusion. Patients must be closely monitored, often using invasive techniques like placement of central venous or pulmonary artery catheters. Urine output, mental status, renal function, and acid-base status serve as markers of perfusion.

Management of toxin-induced bradycardia can be complex. Atropine has little downside but inconsistent success, depending on the toxin, and its effects are often transient. Glucagon is a reasonable option, particularly when treating known beta-blocker toxicity, but its effectiveness is limited. Cardioactive vasopressors such as dopamine and epinephrine are often required. These agents will be discussed in greater detail later. In patients with bradycardia accompanied by hypertension, boosting the heart rate may precipitate a further spike in blood pressure, causing secondary organ injury by mechanisms such as intracranial hemorrhage.

Heart Rhythm Abnormalities

In addition to monitoring the patient's heart rate, recognizing rhythm and interval changes is also critically important to accurate diagnosis and initial stabilization of an intoxicated patient. Toxin-induced ventricular dysrhythmias can be the result of excess sympathetic activation, increased myocardial sensitivity, or alterations in myocardial action potential and ion channel activity.

Fast-acting sodium channel influx is responsible for rapid depolarization of myocardial cells. This depolarization corresponds to the QRS interval on an electrocardiogram (ECG). The opening of potassium channels allows potassium efflux and repolarization, which is represented on ECG by T waves. Sodium channel blockade results in QRS prolongation, which can eventually devolve into bradycardia, hypotension, ventricular dysrhythmia, and death. A number of drugs and toxins, including tricyclic antidepressants, induce sodium channel blockade. Some of these agents are listed in Table 9-2.

Indications for treatment include a widened QRS complex (>100 ms, new right bundle branch block) or evidence of significant cardiovascular toxicity. Treatment consists of serum alkalinization, which is accomplished by administering a bolus of sodium bicarbonate and hypertonic saline (1-2 mEq/kg) over several minutes. Monitoring strips often show a decrease in QRS duration, but repeat boluses may be necessary. Once the necessity of administering sodium bicarbonate has been established, a sodium bicarbonate infusion is generally necessary.

Potassium chloride may also be given to counter potassium shifts and extracellular hypokalemia caused by alkalinization (Figure 9-1). Many drugs and toxins have potassium channel–blocking properties. Inhibition of potassium influx causes prolongation of the QT interval corrected for heart rate (the QTc interval), eventually leading to polymorphic ventricular tachycardia (*torsades*

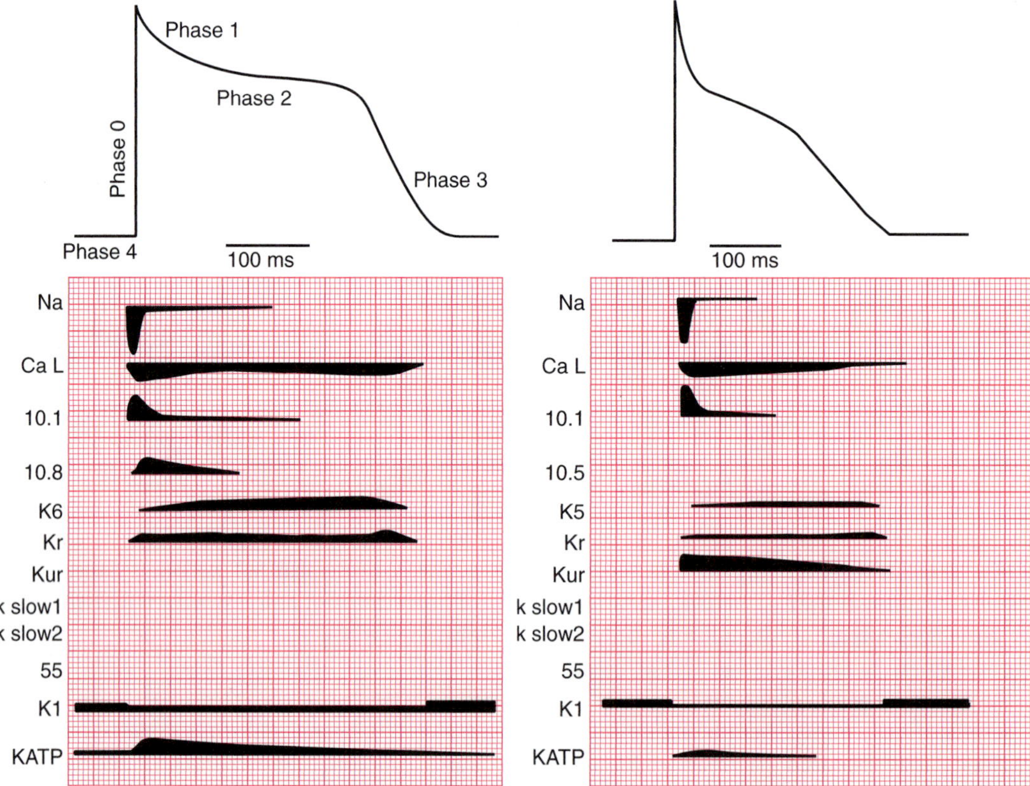

■ **Figure 9-1** Cardiac action potential waveforms and underlying ionic currents in adult human ventricular *(left)* and atrial *(right)* myocytes. Time- and voltage-dependent properties of voltage-gated inward Na^+ (Nav) and Ca^{2+} (Cav) currents expressed in human atrial and ventricular myocytes are similar. In contrast, multiple types of K^+ currents, particularly Kv currents, contribute to atrial and ventricular action potential repolarization. Properties of various Kv currents are distinct, and in contrast to inward currents, multiple Kv currents are expressed in individual myocytes throughout the myocardium. (From Nerbonne JM, Kass RS: Molecular physiology of cardiac repolarization, Physiol Rev 85:1207, 2005.)

de pointes). Consider preventive treatment with IV magnesium sulfate when the QTc interval is >500 ms. If the patient has unstable *torsades de pointes*, perform defibrillation in addition to administering magnesium sulfate. In patients with recurrent *torsades de pointes*, overdrive pacing with isoproterenol (Isuprel) or a mechanical pacemaker (transvenous or transcutaneous) is indicated, since the QTc interval shortens as heart rate accelerates.

Evaluation of QRS and QTc intervals in the intoxicated patient, particularly in those with evidence of cardiovascular instability, is critical. If the patient has QTc interval prolongation, administer magnesium sulfate to induce tachycardia. Administer sodium bicarbonate liberally to a patient with any kind of toxin-induced ventricular dysrhythmia, since standard therapies alone are unlikely to be effective. Otherwise, follow ACLS protocol.

Notable exceptions to ACLS guidelines within the scope of toxicology are the avoidance of amiodarone (Cordarone) in toxin-induced ventricular dysrhythmia, and the avoidance of epinephrine in patients suspected of **huffing**, or abusing, inhalants. Among other mechanisms of action, amiodarone is a potassium channel blocker. As such, it can further prolong the QTc interval, exacerbating dysrhythmias in toxicology patients, since many toxins affect potassium channels. Therefore, lidocaine is recommended as an alternative.

Inhaled halogenated hydrocarbons enhance myocardial sensitivity to catecholamines and can provoke sudden sniffing death syndrome. In this syndrome, the cause of death is ventricular dysrhythmia induced by release of the patient's endogenous catecholamines. Such a dysrhythmia would probably be exacerbated by exogenous administration of epinephrine, and the patient might benefit from administration of a beta-blocker. However, accurate diagnosis of this cause of cardiovascular toxicity is fraught with difficulty. Unless you have overwhelming evidence of inhalant use, you should perform cardiovascular stabilization according to standard ACLS protocol.

Blood Pressure Abnormalities

Because of significant baseline variation in normal blood pressure, as well as the possibility of underlying hypertension, blood pressure variation can be a misleading parameter by which to judge acute toxicity. Nevertheless, blood pressure extremes are of pivotal importance in identifying intoxication and guiding management. Depending on the agent, a toxic exposure may induce extreme hypotension or hypertension. In some cases (e.g., alpha-2 agonists), both hypertension and hypotension may be seen, depending on how long ago the ingestion occurred. The degree of blood pressure derangement dictates care.

Hypertension

Toxin-induced hypertension may be due to a variety of agents. Toxicity of a sympathomimetic agent like cocaine or amphetamines is most often responsible. These agents induce hypertension by stimulating peripheral alpha receptors, both the alpha-1 and alpha-2 subtypes. They also tend to step up cardiac output and increase systemic vascular resistance, further elevating blood pressure.

Isolated alpha-receptor stimulation results in hypertension and reflex bradycardia, as seen early in the course of alpha-2 agonist toxicity (e.g., in clonidine [Catapres] and oxymetazoline [Afrin] ingestions). Other agents, such as anticholinergic agents and hallucinogens, can cause mild hypertension but are rarely responsible for severe hypertension.

The treatment of toxin-induced hypertension depends on both the severity and the mechanism of hypertension. Mild hypertension frequently responds to supportive care, including the benzodiazepines that are often administered to agitated patients with sympathomimetic toxicity. However, if the patient has significantly increased blood pressure, further treatment with vasoactive drugs may be necessary.

The precise blood pressure at which treatment is required is unknown but is different for each patient. Many patients can tolerate significant blood pressure elevation without adverse effects, but older patients and patients with underlying hypertension may lack autoregulatory mechanisms at high pressures. Such patients can have significant adverse sequelae, including intracranial hemorrhage, ischemic stroke, myocardial or intestinal ischemia, and arrhythmia. Evidence of end-organ damage due to hypertension is an indication for rapid initiation of treatment. Arbitrarily, a systolic blood pressure above 180 mm Hg or a diastolic blood pressure above 110 mm Hg is considered a relative indication for treatment and should, at the very least, prompt you to consider taking steps to lower blood pressure.

In general, β-adrenergic antagonists are a poor choice in the treatment of toxin-induced hypertension, because these medications can generate unopposed alpha-adrenergic stimulation, which can worsen hypertension and result in end-organ injury. Short-acting vasodilators with alpha-1 antagonist properties, dihydropyridine calcium channel–blocking activity (e.g., nicardipine [Cardene]), or direct vasodilation properties (e.g., nitroglycerin [Nitro-Dur, Nitrol] or nitroprusside [Nipride]) are typically preferred. Such medications can be titrated as needed to control blood pressure without exacerbating the underlying toxicity. Although it can usually be well controlled with supportive care and adequate sedation, toxin-induced hypertension can cause severe tissue injury and should be addressed with short-acting, titratable vasodilators (Table 9-3).

Hypotension

Treating toxin-induced hypotension is often complicated. The condition can be caused by any of several discrete toxicologic mechanisms or by a combination of several (Table 9-4). Although toxin-directed antidotal therapy is

TABLE 9-3 Toxin-Induced Hypertension

Drug Class	Examples	Clinical Presentation	Treatment
Sympathomimetics	Cocaine, amphetamines, ephedrine, monoamine oxidase inhibitors, methylphenidate, phentermine	Tachycardia, mydriasis, diaphoresis, hypertension, agitation, tremors, seizure, delirium	Benzodiazepines, barbiturates, phentolamine, nitrates, calcium channel blockers
α_1-Agonists	Ergot alkaloids, phenylephrine	Hypertension, reflex tachycardia, limb ischemia	Phentolamine, nitrates, calcium channel blockers
α_2-Agonists	Clonidine, oxymetazoline, tetrahydrozoline	Mental status depression, pinpoint pupils, bradycardia with hypertension initially, followed by bradycardia and hypotension	Nitroprusside or nitroglycerin for initial hypertension if needed
α_2-Antagonists	Yohimbine	Tachycardia, hypertension, mydriasis, diaphoresis, lacrimation, salivation, nausea, vomiting, and flushing	Benzodiazepines, clonidine, nitrates
Anticholinergic	Diphenhydramine, cyclobenzaprine, benztropine, doxylamine	Tachycardia, flushing, mydriasis, dry, urinary retention, delirium	Supportive care; vasodilators rarely required
Hallucinogens	Dextromethorphan, lysergic acid diethylamide (LSD), mescaline	Mydriasis, tachycardia, mild hypertension, hallucinations	Supportive care; vasodilators rarely required

often the preferred approach to treating toxin-induced hypotension, general therapeutic principles are applicable as well.

A common cause of hypotension in the toxicology patient is volume depletion associated with a variety of mechanisms, including decreased oral intake, gastrointestinal (GI) losses from vomiting and diarrhea, excessive insensible losses from diaphoresis, and tachypnea or osmotic diuresis, as is seen in alcohol toxicity. Before you resort to vasopressor administration, aggressive resuscitation with isotonic fluids like normal saline is an important first step in treating hypotension. Even in patients with toxin-induced heart failure, an initial trial of crystalloid fluids is reasonable. However, you must carefully consider the total volume administered and the risk of exacerbating pulmonary edema, particularly in patients with bradycardia and hypotension. Patients with tachycardia and hypotension can generally tolerate a much larger fluid volume.

Norepinephrine (Levophed) and phenylephrine (Neo-Synephrine) are the agents of choice for the treatment of toxin-induced hypotension. Phenylephrine is preferable in patients with significant tachycardia and hypotension, whereas norepinephrine may be used in patients with low to normal heart rates. Patients with significant bradycardia and associated hypotension may be treated with epinephrine (Adrenalin) infusions.

A common pitfall with the use of vasopressors is underdosing. In toxin-induced hypotension, high doses of vasopressors are often required to compete with the toxic effects of the drug the patient has overdosed on. This may entail administering more than the stated maximum dose of these drugs. Don't consider vasopressor treatment to have failed if you administer the so-called maximum dose without achieving the anticipated clinical response. Continue to titrate the original drug rather than making the mistake of switching to an alternative agent.

Another common pitfall is the use of dopamine monotherapy. Dopamine is a mixed-acting sympathomimetic agent whose vasopressor activity depends primarily on presynaptic uptake and subsequent release of endogenous norepinephrine. At low doses, dopamine receptor activation does boost heart rate and contractility but may result in splanchnic vasodilation and worsening hypotension. This is particularly true in the setting of overdose, since many drugs (e.g., tricyclic antidepressants) block presynaptic uptake channels. Dopamine may be effective in the setting of mild hypotension and bradycardia associated with a sodium channel opener and alpha-2 agonist toxicity or as an adjunctive treatment in combination with a more potent vasopressor after beta-blocker or calcium channel blocker–induced heart failure.

Respiratory Rate Abnormalities

One vital sign that's often overlooked or inaccurately recorded is respiratory rate. This sign can be an important clue in diagnosing the intoxicated patient and guiding therapy. Bradypnea (decreased respiratory rate) or hypopnea (decreased tidal volume) can complicate exposure to several different toxins. Opioids, for example, are typically associated with respiratory depression; however, beta-blocker toxicity, severe sedative-hypnotic toxicity, and alpha-2 agonist toxicity have also been associated with respiratory depression. Early recognition of hypoventilation by physical examination, blood gas analysis, or capnography is critical in the appropriate treatment of the intoxicated patient. Reversal of the effects of opioids was

TABLE 9-4 Toxin-Induced Hypotension

Drug Class	Examples	Clinical Presentation	Treatment
Sodium channel openers	Veratrum alkaloids, grayanotoxin, aconite	Nausea, vomiting, bradycardia, hypotension, paresthesias, dysesthesias, mental status depression, paralysis, seizures	IV fluids Atropine Dopamine, epinephrine, or norepinephrine
Sodium channel blockers	Tricyclic antidepressants, diphenhydramine, carbamazepine, quinine, taxine	Nausea, vomiting, bradycardia, QRS prolongation, hypotension, coma, seizures (many are also anticholinergic)	IV fluids Sodium bicarbonate Hypertonic saline Epinephrine, norepinephrine, or phenylephrine
α_1-Antagonists	Prazosin, doxazosin, tricyclic antidepressants, antipsychotics	Mental status depression, hypotension, reflex tachycardia	IV fluids Norepinephrine or phenylephrine
α_2-Agonists	Clonidine, tetrahydrozoline, oxymetazoline	Mental status depression, pinpoint pupils, bradycardia with hypertension initially followed by bradycardia and hypotension	IV fluids, atropine, dopamine, epinephrine, or norepinephrine Case reports of benefit with yohimbine and naloxone
Beta-blockers	Metoprolol, atenolol, sotalol, labetalol, propranolol	Mental status depression, bradycardia, hypotension	Atropine, glucagon, epinephrine, or insulin
β-Agonists	Albuterol, terbutaline, clenbuterol	Supraventricular tachycardia, hypotension	Esmolol +/– phenylephrine
Adenosine antagonists	Theophylline, caffeine	Supraventricular tachycardia, hypotension, altered mental status, tremor, seizure	Benzodiazepines, esmolol +/– phenylephrine, hemodialysis
Calcium channel blockers	Diltiazem, verapamil, nifedipine, amlodipine, felodipine	Hypotension with bradycardia (diltiazem, verapamil, high-dose -pines) or reflex tachycardia (-pines)	IV fluids Atropine Calcium salts Epinephrine, norepinephrine, or insulin
Sedative hypnotics and opioids	Heroin, morphine, barbiturates	Sedation, pinpoint pupils (with opioids), respiratory depression	IV fluids, supportive care, vasopressors rarely required
Na^+/K^+-ATPase inhibitors	Digoxin, foxglove, oleander, lily of the valley, Bufo toads, Chan su	Nausea, vomiting, atrioventricular node block, premature ventricular contractions, ventricular dysrhythmias	Atropine or digoxin-specific antibody fragments (Fab)
Electron transport chain toxins	Cyanide, cyanogenic glycosides (e.g., amygdalin), carbon monoxide, salicylate	Hypotension, reflex tachycardia, severe metabolic acidosis, hyperthermia (uncouplers), altered mental status, seizures	Dextrose, IV fluids, sodium bicarbonate, amyl nitrite + sodium nitrite + sodium thiosulfate vs. hydroxocobalamin (CN), hyperbaric oxygen (CO), epinephrine vs. norepinephrine vs. phenylephrine
Agents that cause endothelial disruption/ distributive shock	Surfactant-containing herbicides (e.g., glufosinate [Basta]), phenol, caustic agents	Hypotension, tachycardia, pulmonary edema, third spacing of fluid, altered mental status, seizures	IV fluids Benzodiazepines Norepinephrine or phenylephrine

discussed earlier in the chapter. In addition, supportive care such as ventilatory assistance or endotracheal intubation may be necessary.

Arterial or venous blood gas measurements can be used to differentiate metabolic acidosis with respiratory compensation from a combined metabolic acidosis and respiratory alkalosis. Toxin-induced metabolic acidosis typically creates an anion gap. Although medications such as carbonic anhydrase inhibitors (e.g., acetazolamide [Diamox] and topiramate [Topamax]) do cause non–anion gap metabolic acidosis, the presence of a high–anion gap metabolic acidosis is more common and carries a broad differential diagnosis that can typically be narrowed rapidly by careful history and further laboratory testing. The classic mnemonic for this differential diagnosis is "MUDPILES," which can be expanded to "CAT MUDPILES" to include a broader range of possible toxicologic causes. A look back at the Rapid Recall box in Chapter 6 will help you review.

Tachypnea

Tachypnea may be an indicator of a significant metabolic acidosis or acute respiratory disease like pneumonia or pneumonitis. In metabolic acidosis, the exaggerated respiratory rate is a compensatory mechanism that allows the body to decrease the partial pressure of carbon dioxide (PCO_2), thereby raising systemic pH. In some patients, the actual rate of respiration may not accelerate significantly, but an uptick in tidal volume and minute ventilation has the same effect.

Hyperpnea

An increase in the depth of breathing is referred to as *hyperpnea*. Any underlying metabolic acidosis can result in tachypnea, hyperpnea, or both. Patients might or might not be aware of the change in their breathing pattern, depending on the severity of the alteration. Another cause of hyperventilation is direct activation of a patient's respiratory center. Classically, salicylate toxicity may cause tachypnea or hyperpnea in the absence of metabolic acidosis. In fact, early toxicity may be accompanied by an isolated respiratory alkalosis.

Oxygen Saturation Abnormalities

Oxygen saturation should be measured in any acutely ill patient. A normal oxygen saturation is reassuring but does not rule out the possibility of lung disease, hemoglobin dysfunction, or impaired oxygen delivery to body tissues. For example, oxygen saturation measured by noninvasive pulse oximetry may remain normal despite severe carbon monoxide toxicity that prevents delivery of oxygen to tissues. Aspiration often occurs when treating patients with toxicologic emergencies. Toxic emergencies related to ingestion can be accompanied by a high incidence of vomiting, which is a risk factor for aspiration. Noncardiogenic pulmonary edema and pneumonitis can also complicate the course of opioid toxicity and withdrawal, salicylate toxicity, and toxin inhalation, all of which may cause hypoxemia and diffuse alveolar disease. Pneumothorax has also been reported in patients who smoke or inhale toxins. However, oxygen saturation and, more important, partial pressure of oxygen (PO_2), can be helpful metrics in sick intoxicated patients.

Abnormal pulse oximetry readings sometimes accompany hemoglobinopathies such as methemoglobinemia and sulfhemoglobinemia. Of these two derangements, the former is the more common. It's generally caused by oxidative stress, which converts the ferrous iron (Fe^{2+}) in hemoglobin into the ferric state (Fe^{3+}), curtailing the oxygen-carrying capacity of hemoglobin and resulting in poor oxygen delivery to tissues. Cyanosis, or blue discoloration of the skin, is a common finding. Pulse oximetry typically reveals an oxygen saturation in the high 80s to low 90s regardless of the amount of supplemental oxygen delivered. Treatment with the reducing agent, methylene blue, allows reduction of ferric iron and consequent restoration of oxygen-carrying capacity and tissue-delivery capability. See Carbon Monoxide later in the chapter for more information on the use of methylene blue in patients with methemoglobinemia.

Various toxins may also produce a relative tissue hypoxia without inducing a significant change in hemoglobin binding. Uncouplers and oxidative phosphorylation inhibitors impede the proper functioning of the electron transport chain, which is responsible for using oxygen during adenosine triphosphate (ATP) synthesis. The result is constrained energy production and cellular injury. Uncouplers such as salicylate invigorate this process with increased oxygen consumption, but they prohibit ATP synthesis. Therefore, the energy created is dissipated as heat. Hyperthermia is a late finding in uncoupler toxicity. Arterial oxygen saturation is generally normal, but venous oxygen content is significantly diminished as a result of the escalating cellular demand for oxygen. Oxidative phosphorylation inhibitors such as cyanide, on the other hand, suppress cellular oxygen demand, raise venous oxygen content, and decrease ATP production. Both classes of toxins cause metabolic acidosis, altered mental status, seizures, and eventual cardiovascular collapse. In either scenario, treat the patient with sodium bicarbonate to buffer acidosis and, in the case of salicylates, to decrease tissue distribution and toxicity.

Cyanide toxicity is treated with a cyanide antidote kit. Historically, the patient is given a series of treatments. Inhaled amyl nitrite and intravenous sodium nitrite induce methemoglobinemia, which draws cyanide out of cells. This is followed by IV sodium thiosulfate, creating thiocyanate, which is renally excreted. More recently, hydroxocobalamin, a vitamin B_{12} precursor, has been approved for the treatment of cyanide toxicity. Cobalt within the hydroxocobalamin moiety binds cyanide to form cyanocobalamin, which is then excreted by the kidneys. See Chemical Asphyxiants for a detailed look at cyanide toxicity.

Measured by conventional pulse oximetry and blood gas evaluation, arterial and venous oxygen content can be altered by various anatomic and physiologic changes in the intoxicated patient. Recognizing and identifying the underlying cause and rapidly reversing decreased blood oxygen content and tissue oxygen delivery are critical in the effective treatment of toxicity. Administer high-flow oxygen to any patient with respiratory compromise and abnormal oxygen saturation.

Toxidromes

You'll be more likely to identify a poisoned patient early if you're aware of a broad range of specific toxidromes. A **toxidrome** (an abridgement of "toxin" and "syndrome") is the constellation of symptoms, vital signs, and exam findings typically associated with exposure to a particular toxin. Taken together, a patient's history and toxidrome can often help you identify the class of drug or, in some instances, the specific toxin responsible for the patient's illness. In general, if the class of toxin is known, the

TABLE 9-5 Selected Common Toxidromes

	Sympathomimetic	Anticholinergic	Cholinergic	Opioid	Sedative-Hypnotic
Findings	Tachycardia Hypertension Mydriasis Diaphoresis Agitation Tremor Delirium	Tachycardia Mydriasis Agitation Delirium Mumbling speech Dry axillae/ membranes	**DUMBELS:** **D**iarrhea **U**rination **M**iosis **B**ronchorrhea/ bradycardia **E**mesis **L**acrimation **S**alivation/seizures	**CPR:** **C**oma **P**inpoint pupils **R**espiratory depression	Depressed mental status Normal vitals
Examples of responsible agents	Cocaine Amphetamine/ methamphetamine Ephedrine Monoamine oxidase inhibitors (MAOIs) Withdrawal (e.g., ethyl alcohol, benzodiazepines)	Antihistamines Tricyclic antidepressants GI antispasmodics OTC sleep aids Some muscle relaxants (e.g., Flexeril)	Organophosphates Carbamates Nicotine Pilocarpine Mestinon (pyridostigmine)	Heroin Hydromorphone (Dilaudid) Fentanyl Oxycodone Hydrocodone Diphenoxylate/ atropine (Lomotil) Tramadol	Benzodiazepines Barbiturates Alcohols Some muscle relaxants (e.g., carisoprodol [Soma]) Gamma hydroxybutyrate (GHB)
Prehospital treatment strategies	Benzodiazepines IV fluids	Benzodiazepines IV fluids	Atropine Airway management	Supplemental oxygen Naloxone (0.4 mg IV/IM per dose)	Elevate head of bed Nasal or oral airway Supplemental oxygen

specific agent is unimportant, since the treatment will be the same. Descriptions of various toxidromes are outlined in Table 9-5.

Gastrointestinal Decontamination

After completing your initial evaluation and stabilization of the patient, you must consider treatment strategies to attempt to limit GI absorption of an ingested toxin. The issue of **gastrointestinal decontamination** with syrup of ipecac and activated charcoal has been researched and debated for decades. The current standard of care does not call for administration of ipecac in any patient and rarely indicates administration of activated charcoal. Activated charcoal is recommended only when less than 1 hour has elapsed between the confirmed time of *potentially toxic* exposure and the time of administration. Even then, activated charcoal is contraindicated in patients with any alteration in mental status or with nausea or vomiting, because of the significant documented risk of aspiration (see Oxygen Saturation section).

Body stuffers represent one notable exception to these contraindications to the use of activated charcoal. If good mentation exists after ingestion of a poorly wrapped packet of drugs, administration of single-dose activated charcoal is recommended. Activated charcoal continues to play a role in the treatment of some ingestions (e.g., salicylate), but the risks associated with its use may outweigh the benefits of treatment. Multiple-dose activated charcoal may also be considered in some cases; you should consult with a medical toxicologist or poison control center before initiating such therapy. Whole-bowel irrigation is used in the treatment of body packers, as well as in patients with a proven residual intraluminal toxin (e.g., lithium, lead, or other heavy metals).

Environmental Toxicology

A wide variety of environmental toxins and envenomations can have adverse effects in humans. Many of the cardiovascular and neurologic effects of natural toxins are treated in ways similar to those used to treat other toxic exposures, as we've outlined in the preceding sections. However, several specific toxic mechanisms and clinical manifestations require directed therapy.

ARTHROPOD ENVENOMATION

In the United States, you may treat patients for envenomation by *Latrodectus* (black widow spider), *Loxosceles* (brown recluse spider), or *Buthidae* (scorpion). Although envenomation by any of these arthropods can be painful, death is rare. The linchpins of treatment are supportive care and symptomatic management with opioids and anxiolytics. Table 9-6 summarizes toxicity, mechanism of action, and recommended treatment for each type of arthropod envenomation.

Black Widow

The black widow spider lives in all parts of the continental United States. It's usually found outdoors in woodpiles, brush, sheds, or garages, and it may hitchhike into the

TABLE 9-6 Arthropod Toxicity

Arthropod	Toxin	Toxic Mechanism	Clinical Manifestations	Treatment
Latrodectus mactans (black widow)	Alpha-latrotoxin	Presynaptic calcium channel opening with release of multiple vasoactive and myoactive neurotransmitters	Nausea, vomiting, sweating, tachycardia, hypertension, muscle cramping	Diazepam, fentanyl Consider antivenin for severe toxicity
Loxosceles recluse (brown recluse)	Sphingomyelinase-D Hyaluronidase	Sphingomyelinase-D: Local tissue destruction, intravascular clotting Hyaluronidase: promotes tissue penetration	Local: tissue necrosis and ulcer formation Systemic: loxoscelism, including fever, vomiting, rhabdomyolysis, disseminated intravascular coagulation, hemolysis	Local wound care, tetanus prophylaxis, and analgesia Supportive care for systemic toxicity
Centruroides exilicauda (bark scorpion)	Neurotoxin I-IV	Sodium channel opening with repeated depolarization and neurotransmitter release	Local paresthesias, tachycardia, hypertension, salivation, diaphoresis, muscle fasciculations, opsoclonus, roving eye movements	Tetanus prophylaxis, wound care, anxiolysis, analgesia Severe toxicity may be treated with antivenin where available

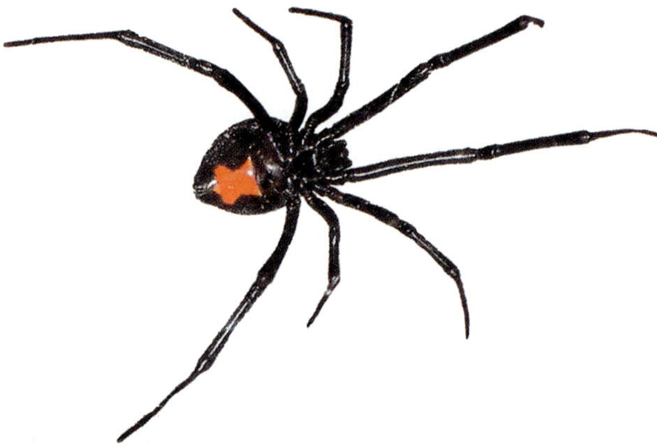

■ **Figure 9-2** Female black widow spider with red hourglass marking on underside of abdomen. (From Habif TP: Clinical dermatology: a color guide to diagnosis and therapy, ed 5, St Louis, 2009, Mosby.)

home on outdoor-stored items like firewood or Christmas trees.

Identification

The female black widow is recognizable by its bulbous, shiny black abdomen and red hourglass marking on the ventral side (Figure 9-2). The spider is usually an inch or less in length. Its venom is a potent neurotoxin. The male black widow is brown, about half the size of the female, and nonvenomous.

Signs and Symptoms

Signs and symptoms of black widow envenomation include muscle spasms, nontender abdominal rigidity, and immediate severe localized pain, redness, and swelling with papule formation at the site. The patient may describe the bite as a bee sting–like sensation. You might observe two small fang marks spaced 1 mm apart. Systemic effects of envenomation may include nausea and vomiting, diaphoresis (sweating), a decreased level of consciousness, seizures, and paralysis.

Treatment

Prehospital Prehospital treatment is mainly supportive. Treat muscle spasms with muscle relaxants such as diazepam (Valium) or calcium gluconate. Monitor and treat hypertension aggressively to prevent hypertensive crisis. Antivenin is available for black widow envenomation, making identification of the spider and rapid transport to the facility important.

Emergency Department Antivenin may be administered in the emergency department (ED).

Brown Recluse

The brown recluse spider lives in dark, dry locations, including inside houses, in relatively warm climates. In the United States, the recluse is found in Hawaii and in the South, the Midwest, and the Southwest. Most envenomations occur in states in the south-central part of the country.

Identification

The recluse is tan to brown, with a distinctive violin-shaped marking on its back (hence it's also known as the "violin spider" or the "fiddle-back spider"; Figure 9-3). Its body can be up to three quarters of an inch long. Another identifying feature is its six eyes, rather than the usual eight eyes with which most spiders are endowed. These eyes are arranged in a semicircle in pairs of three.

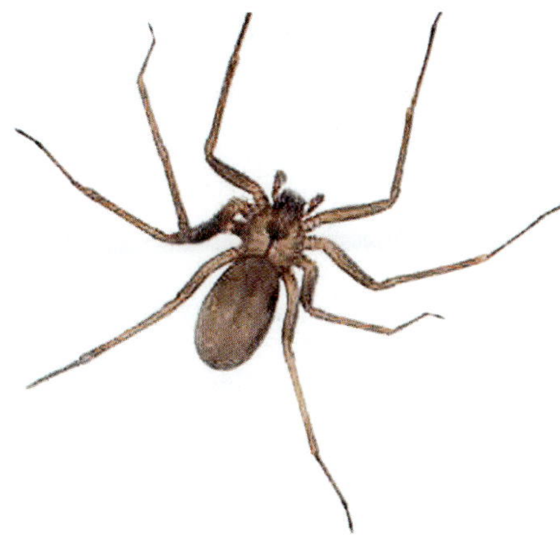

■ **Figure 9-3** Brown recluse spider. Note dark, violin-shaped marking on spider's back. (From Habif TP: Clinical dermatology: a color guide to diagnosis and therapy, ed 5, St Louis, 2009, Mosby.)

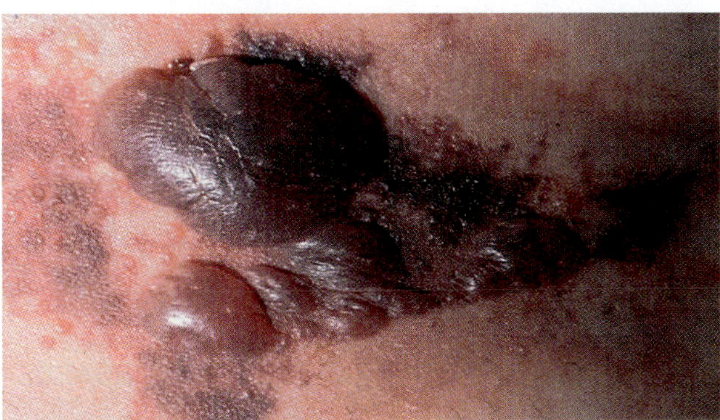

■ **Figure 9-4** Brown recluse spider bite. A severe reaction in which infarction, bleeding, and blistering have occurred. (From Habif TP: Clinical dermatology: a color guide to diagnosis and therapy, ed 5, St Louis, 2009, Mosby.)

Signs and Symptoms

Systemic symptoms of brown recluse envenomation include malaise, chills, fever, nausea and vomiting, and joint pain. Life-threatening symptoms may include bleeding disorders such as disseminated intravascular coagulation and hemolytic anemia. Treatment is supportive, since no approved antivenin is available. Clean and dress the wound, apply a cold compress to the envenomation site, and transport the patient for medical evaluation.

Pathophysiology

The venom of the brown recluse is a pernicious cocktail of at least 11 peptides that possess a variety of cytotoxic properties. The necrotic venom produces a classic bull's-eye lesion at the injection site. Many envenomations occur at night while the patient is asleep. The bite is painless and initially begins as a small blister (papule), sometimes surrounded by a white halo. Over the next 24 hours, localized pain, redness, and swelling develop (Figure 9-4). During the next few days or weeks, tissue necrosis develops at the site, and the redness and swelling begin to spread. The necrosis makes the wound slow to heal, and it may be visible months after the bite.

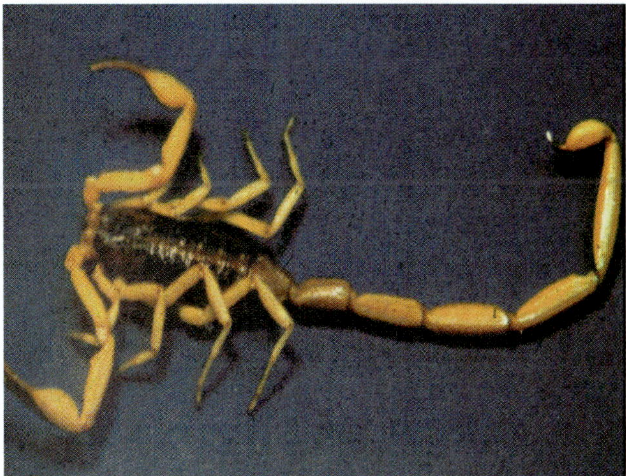

■ **Figure 9-5** Arizona bark scorpion (*Centruroides exilicauda*). (From Marx JA, Hockberger RS, Walls RM, et al: Rosen's emergency medicine, ed 7, St Louis, 2009, Mosby.)

Treatment

Prehospital care should focus on airway management and pain control. Fentanyl is the opioid of choice in the treatment of envenomation because it does not produce the histamine release associated with other opioids. Specific antidotes to brown recluse envenomation have been investigated, but because of serious potential adverse effects like serum sickness are routinely recommended only in severe envenomation.

Scorpion Stings

More than 14,000 scorpion exposures were reported in 2003, with no fatalities. In excess of 600 scorpion species are found in the United States, but only the bark or sculptured scorpion of the desert Southwest is dangerous to humans. Scorpions are nocturnal and hide beneath objects and buildings during the day. They may wander into dwellings, especially at night.

Identification

Scorpions are yellowish-brown, may be striped, and are about 1 to 3 inches long (Figure 9-5). The scorpion injects venom stored in a bulb at the base of a stinger on the end of its tail. It usually injects only a small amount of poison. The sculptured scorpion is active from April to August and hibernates during the winter.

Signs and Symptoms

Systemic effects can include slurred speech, restlessness, salivation, abdominal cramping, nausea and vomiting, muscle fasciculations (twitching), and seizures. Symptoms typically peak within 5 hours of injection. If redness and swelling are present at the injection site, a bark scorpion is probably not responsible for the sting, because its venom does not induce localized inflammation.

Pathophysiology

The venom of the bark scorpion is a neurotoxin that initially produces a burning or tingling sensation followed by numbness. The toxin is a mixture of proteins and polypeptides that affect voltage-dependent ion channels, especially the sodium channels involved in nerve signaling. A secondary effect of envenomation is CNS stimulation through sympathetic neurons.

Treatment

Prehospital Begin treatment by managing airway, breathing, and circulation and by calming the patient. Offer supportive care for respiratory depression. Clean the wound, apply a cold compress, and immobilize the appendage, including the fingers and toes. Place a constricting band over the site of envenomation to restrict lymphatic flow if transport time is expected to be long. The band should be at least 2 inches wide and not tighter than a watch band. The amount of pressure should be similar to that of an elastic bandage used for a sprained ankle. Be aware that this technique is controversial, however. It should *not* be confused with application of a tourniquet.

Avoid giving analgesics, because they may exacerbate respiratory symptoms. Provide rapid transport to the hospital.

Emergency Department Antivenin may be available for scorpion stings, especially in Arizona.

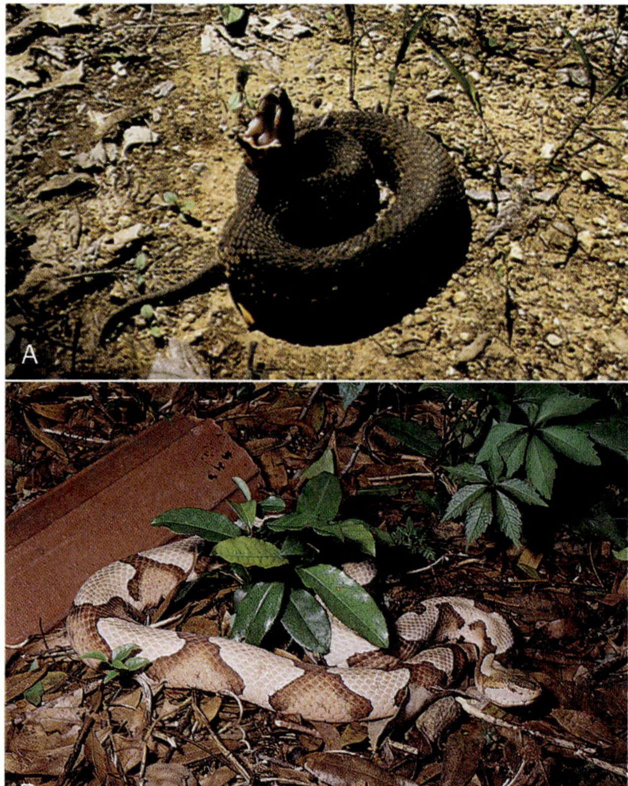

Figure 9-6 A, Water moccasin (cottonmouth) snake. B, Southern copperhead *(Agkistrodon contortrix contortrix)* has markings that make it almost invisible when lying in leaf litter. (**A** courtesy Michael Cardwell and Carl Barden, Venom Laboratory. **B** courtesy Sherman Minton, MD.)

SNAKE ENVENOMATION

There are thousands of snakebite exposures annually, many of which are fatal. Poisonous snakes can be found throughout the continental United States and Alaska (Figure 9-6). There are two families of poisonous snakes:

1. The *Crotalidae* (pit vipers), a family that comprises rattlesnakes (including the pygmy and Massasauga varieties), cottonmouths (water moccasins), and copperheads
2. The *Elapidae* (coral snakes)

Snake venom toxicity and mode of action vary between the families. To see how, let's take a closer look.

Crotalids (Pit Vipers)

In the United States, nearly all snake envenomations can be blamed on the *Crotalidae* family of snakes, the pit vipers. Crotalids are native to every state in the continental United States except Maine.

Identification

Pit vipers are named for the distinctive pits that form grooves in the maxillary bone on each side of their triangular heads. They have vertical elliptical pupils and large fangs.

Signs and Symptoms

Signs and symptoms of crotalid envenomation include distinctive fang marks at the injection site, accompanied by redness, pain, and swelling that may precede compartment syndrome. Systemic effects can include:

- Thirst
- Sweating
- Chills
- Weakness
- Dizziness
- Tachycardia
- Nausea and vomiting
- Diarrhea
- Hypotension
- Hypovolemic shock due to clotting defects
- Respiratory distress
- Numbness and tingling around the head

Because pit viper venom is designed to paralyze and digest small prey, difficulty breathing and a prickling sensation about the head are classic symptoms of pit viper envenomation.

Pathophysiology

Crotalid venom contains a complex cocktail of enzymes and hemotoxins that produces tissue necrosis at the site of envenomation. The venom can also touch off a cascade of systemic effects such as red blood cell destruction (hemolysis), clotting defects, intravascular coagulation, and renal failure. The more venom injected, the more severe the symptoms. Serious bites can kill the victim within 30 minutes, primarily as a result of septic shock. However, about 20% to 25% of bites are considered dry, meaning that little or no venom is delivered with the bite.

Treatment

Treatment consists of supporting airway, breathing, and circulation and slowing absorption of the venom.

Prehospital Option #1 Position the affected extremity below the heart, and keep the patient quiet and still. Immobilize the limb with a splint, but do *not* suction, incise, or apply cold packs to the wound. As noted earlier for scorpion bites, prehospital intervention includes placing a constricting band over the site of envenomation to restrict lymphatic flow if transport time is expected to be long. Remember, the band should be at least 2 inches wide, not tighter than a watch band, and the amount of pressure should be similar to that of an elastic bandage used for a sprained ankle. To reiterate, this technique is controversial. It should *not* be confused with application of a tourniquet.

Antivenin is available for crotalid envenomation, so rapid transport to an appropriate medical facility is critical.

Prehospital Option #2 The primary goal of treatment option 2 is to limit local tissue injury that may cause long-term disability. First aid consists of elevating and immobilizing the bite site to allow lymphatic drainage of the venom to larger compartments like the proximal limbs and trunk. Do not apply a constricting band or tourniquet, because application of pressure exacerbates local tissue injury.

Using snakebite kits or attempting to "suck out" the venom has never been proved beneficial. Give fentanyl as needed for analgesia.

Emergency Department Once at a healthcare facility, antivenin may be administered in consultation with a medical toxicologist if evidence of local or systemic toxicity is apparent. The patient must be closely observed for a possible allergic reaction to the antivenin.

Tissue injury and limb dysfunction may take weeks or months to resolve, and physical therapy may be necessary.

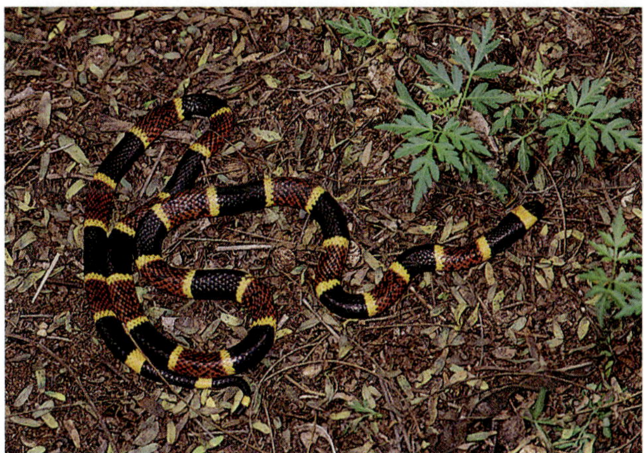

Figure 9-7 Texas coral snake (*Micrurus tener,* formerly *M. fulvius tenere*) has a highly potent venom but is secretive, and bites are uncommon. (Courtesy Michael Cardwell and the Gladys Porter Zoo.)

In rare cases, surgical intervention and fasciotomy may also be necessary to treat compartment syndrome or other complications.

Elapids

In the United States, snakes of the elapid genus *Micrurus*, the coral snakes, are found in the Southeast (Eastern variety) and Southwest (Arizona variety).

Identification

Coral snakes are smaller than pit vipers and have round pupils, a narrow head, small fixed fangs, and no pits on the head (Figure 9-7). They can be identified by their distinctive alternating horizontal bands of black, pale yellow or white, and deep orange or red. Some nonpoisonous snakes (such as the king snake) mimic this color pattern, but imperfectly. The old saying "Red on yellow, kill a fellow; red on black, venom lacks" can be helpful in distinguishing between the coral snake and its imposters. However, the rhyme applies only to coral snakes native to the United States.

Signs and Symptoms

Coral snake envenomation is uncommon because of the snake's docile nature, its short fixed teeth, and its small size, but severe envenomations can cause respiratory and skeletal muscle paralysis. Signs and symptoms include fang marks and swelling, redness, and localized numbness at the injection site. Systemic effects, some of which may be delayed for 12 to 24 hours, include:

- Weakness
- Drowsiness
- Slurred speech or salivation
- Ataxia
- Paralysis of the tongue and larynx

- Drooping eyelids
- Dilated pupils
- Abdominal pain
- Nausea and vomiting
- Seizures
- Respiratory distress
- Hypotension

Pathophysiology

The venom of a coral snake contains a mixture of hydrolytic toxins and a neurotoxin that blocks acetylcholine receptor sites. It has more noxious neurologic effects than pit viper venom and may induce paralysis and respiratory failure, but only 40% of bites cause envenomation.

Treatment

Prehospital Initial management of elapid envenomation differs from that of crotalid envenomation. The primary concern after elapid envenomation is systemic neurotoxicity rather than local limb injury, so pressure immobilization to prevent lymphatic drainage is recommended. Do *not* apply a tourniquet, however, because of the risk of limb ischemia. Decontaminate the wound with water or normal saline, keep the affected extremity below the heart, and encourage the patient to remain quiet and still. Immobilize the limb with a splint, apply a loose-fitting constricting band (see earlier description), and start an IV with a volume-expanding crystalloid fluid. Do not incise or apply cold packs to the wound. Antivenin is available, so rapid transport to an appropriate medical facility is critical.

Emergency Department Because of the severity of toxicity and the lack of distinctive symptoms associated with coral snake envenomation, treatment consists of specific antivenin therapy if there is any evidence of skin penetration. Alternatively, the patient may be admitted to the hospital and observed for 24 hours for any sign of delayed neurologic toxicity, which may last days or weeks if it develops.

MARINE TOXICOLOGY

Many marine creatures deliver venom by means of bites or stings, producing intense pain at the site of envenomation (Figure 9-8). Some of these organisms—jellyfish, fire coral, and sea anemones—inject toxin with stinging cells called *nematocysts*. Other organisms like sea urchins and stingrays have spines that inject venom deeper into the tissue, causing trauma as well as envenomation.

Envenomation by Jellyfish

Many jellyfish stings cause only minor local dermal irritation and pain, but some species, such as *Chironex fleckeri* (the "box jellyfish"), produce more severe symptoms and systemic toxicity. Drowning deaths have been reported when victims incapacitated by severe pain have been unable to swim to shore.

Signs and Symptoms

Jellyfish envenomation can cause the following signs and symptoms:

- Intense localized pain
- Swelling and skin discoloration along the line of tentacle contact
- Nausea and vomiting
- Respiratory difficulty
- Cardiovascular toxicity that infrequently results in cardiac dysrhythmia and death

Pathophysiology

Jellyfish have long tentacles equipped with nematocysts that discharge and deposit venom on contact with skin.

Treatment

The primary recommendations for treating jellyfish stings are to administer opioids and antihistamines, apply salt water, and place the affected area in warm (110°F to 113°F) water.

Researchers have studied various methods of removing nematocysts, including flushing the area with water, vinegar, urine, or ethanol and applying commercially available products such as StingEze. Do not use fresh water, because the difference in osmolarity (compared with salt water) causes embedded nematocysts to fire. Vinegar is beneficial in some species but intensifies symptoms in others. Antivenin is of uncertain benefit and, in any case, is available only for box jellyfish stings and only in Australia.

Envenomation by Spinous Sea Creatures

Many species of fish and echinoderms have venomous spines. Venom from such spinous sea animals produces similar symptoms of varying severity, but the treatment of envenomation is standard.

Signs and Symptoms

Toxicity from spinous marine animals causes severe local irritation and pain that may radiate proximally. Systemic symptoms can include nausea, vomiting, and cardiovascular instability. Envenomations are occasionally fatal.

Pathophysiology

A stingray tail is armed with a serrated spine within an integumentary sheath that not only delivers venom but can also deliver significant traumatic injuries. The tail reflexively whips dorsally and may penetrate deeply into tissue, causing intrathoracic and intraabdominal injuries that have sometimes proved fatal to divers.

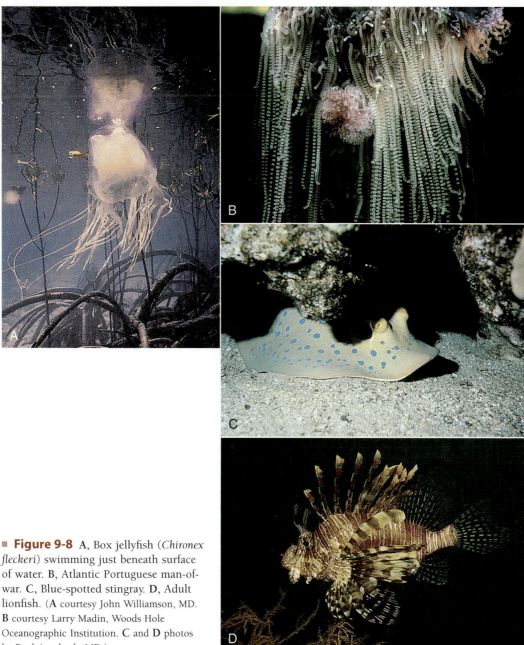

■ **Figure 9-8** A, Box jellyfish (*Chironex fleckeri*) swimming just beneath surface of water. B, Atlantic Portuguese man-of-war. C, Blue-spotted stingray. D, Adult lionfish. (A courtesy John Williamson, MD. B courtesy Larry Madin, Woods Hole Oceanographic Institution. C and D photos by Paul Auerbach, MD.)

Sea urchins and other echinoderms have spines of varying lengths that typically envenomate us when we step on them. Fish of the Scorpionida family have venomous spines as well. This family includes the scorpionfish, the lionfish, and the stonefish, which is responsible for the most severe toxicity.

Treatment

All venom from spinous creatures is heat labile, which means that it's neutralized by heat. Prolonged immersion in hot water is associated with improvement in toxicity. The water temperature and the duration of immersion should be limited only by the patient's tolerance. Surgical intervention may be required to repair traumatic damage after stingray impalement.

The spines and stingers of all these fish and rays are brittle, often breaking off during exposure and attempted removal. Plain radiography is generally suggested to ensure that all fragments have been completely removed. Treat lacerations from spines. Update tetanus prophylaxis, and consider giving antibiotic therapy covering normal skin flora and selected marine bacteria (e.g., *Vibrio parahaemolyticus*). Antivenin therapy is available and recommended for only a few species, including the stonefish, because of the potency of its venom.

■ Envenomation by Biting Sea Creatures

Sea snakes, cone snails, and the blue-ring octopus are all capable of delivering venom through bites. Sea snake

TABLE 9-7 Mechanisms of Marine Food-Borne Intoxication

Toxin	Source	Mechanism	Description	Clinical Manifestations	Treatment
Brevetoxin	Shellfish	Neuromuscular sodium channel opening	Neurotoxic shellfish poisoning	GI upset, paresthesias, hot/cold reversal	Supportive
Ciguatoxin	Reef fish (e.g., amberjack, barracuda, grouper, snapper)	Neuromuscular sodium channel opening	Seafood poisoning from ingestion of fish that ingested other fish that were toxic (dinoflagellates)	Paresthesias, GI upset, hot/cold reversal, bradycardia, hypotension	Supportive (?)mannitol Tricyclic antidepressants for prolonged neuropathy
Saxitoxin	Shellfish	Neuromuscular sodium channel blockade	Paralytic shellfish poisoning	Numbness, paresthesia, muscle weakness, paralysis, respiratory failure	Supportive
Tetrodotoxin	Puffer fish (fugu), blowfish	Neuromuscular sodium channel blockade	Neurotoxin that blocks nerve cell action potential	GI upset, paresthesia, numbness, ascending paralysis, respiratory failure	Supportive
Domoic acid	Mussels	Glutamate and kainic acid analogues	Amnestic shellfish poisoning	GI upset, memory loss, coma, seizures	Supportive
Histidine	Tuna, mackerel, skipjack	Histamine production due to improper cooling	Scombroid fish poisoning	Upper body erythema, pruritus, bronchospasm, angioedema	Antihistamines

venom contains several toxins that primarily produce myotoxicity and neurotoxicity. Severe rhabdomyolysis and paralysis may occur.

Supportive care and antivenin administration are the primary therapies recommended for marine envenomation. Since the venom is chiefly neurotoxic, pressure immobilization may be advisable, as with elapids. Following are specific recommendations:

- Blue-ring octopus venom consists of tetrodotoxin, a peripheral nervous system sodium channel blocker that causes paresthesia, paralysis, and respiratory depression in severe toxicity. Treatment is supportive.
- Cone snail bites may cause severe local pain and systemic sequelae of muscle weakness, coma, and cardiovascular collapse. Again, supportive therapy is indicated.
- Ingestion of certain fish may cause systemic toxicity. Table 9-7 summarizes marine food-borne toxicity.

Plant Toxicity

Most plants and mushrooms are nontoxic or only slightly toxic, but plant ingestion can cause GI, cardiovascular, and neurologic toxicity through various mechanisms. Of the thousands of exposures annually, fatalities blamed on plants or mushrooms are rare.

Most plant poisonings are accidental and involve household plants or ornamentals ingested by children. The categories of plant poisonings are GI irritants, dermatitis inducers, and oxalate-containing plant ingestions. The specific toxins involved include cyanogenic glycosides, cardiac glycosides, and solanine.

It's impossible for you to become familiar with all the different poisonous plants and mushrooms in North America or with the mosaic of signs and symptoms they cause, but it's helpful to know how to approach a patient suspected of having ingested a toxic plant or mushroom. Irritating chemicals in the plant may produce redness or irritation at the site of contact, so begin by examining the patient's oropharynx for redness, irritation, swelling, or blistering. Excessive salivation, lacrimation, and diaphoresis may also be present. Abdominal effects of toxicity may include nausea and vomiting, cramps, and diarrhea. Severe exposures may diminish the patient's level of consciousness or induce a coma.

In any toxic plant or mushroom ingestion, it's critical to gather a good patient history and collect a sample of the ingested material for later identification or laboratory analysis. Poison control centers and wilderness medicine resources can help you identify specific species and gauge their level of toxicity.

Treatment of plant ingestions is mainly supportive. GI toxicity is managed with fluid resuscitation, antiemetics, and electrolyte repletion as needed. Cardiovascular and neurologic toxicity is mediated by altering the activity of neurotransmitters, receptors, and ion channels. Clinical presentation and management will depend on the toxin's specific activity and are summarized in detail in the following pages.

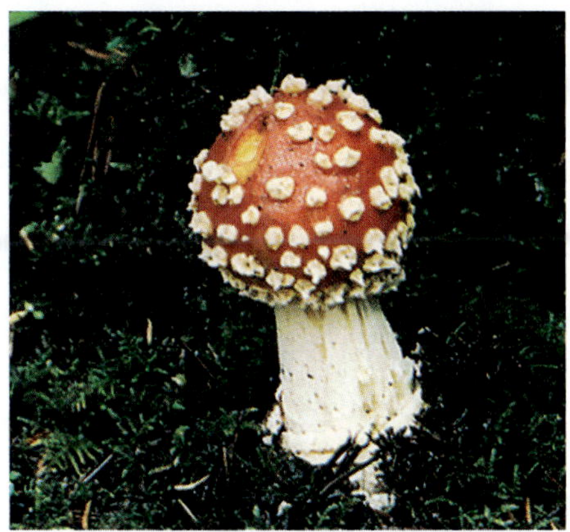

■ **Figure 9-9** *Amanita muscaria* mushroom. (From Auerbach P: Wilderness medicine, ed 5, St Louis, 2007, Mosby.)

Mushrooms

Mushroom poisonings can be either accidental or intentional. Children sometimes ingest unknown mushrooms, and adults who forage for mushrooms for food can make mistakes. Hallucinogenic mushrooms may be ingested accidentally or intentionally; the age group most often affected seems to be children and young adults between the ages of 6 and 19. The cyclopeptide group of mushrooms, which includes the *Amanita* and *Galerina* genera, contains potent hepatotoxins (liver toxins) and accounts for most lethal exposures (Figure 9-9).

Cardiac Glycoside Plants and Digitalis Toxicity

Cardiac glycoside plants contain naturally occurring toxins similar to digoxin (also known as *digitoxin* or *digitalis* and sold under the proprietary names Digitek and Lanoxin). Toxicity after ingestion of these plants is similar to toxicity after acute digoxin ingestion.

The incidence of plant-induced cardiac glycoside toxicity is low, with only 1% of plant exposures attributable to cardiac glycoside plants. Mortality from plant cardiac glycoside toxicity is rare, and the rate is much lower than that associated with pharmaceutical digitalis toxicity.

Identification

Following are examples of common plants that contain digoxin-like glycoside toxins (Figure 9-10):

- Foxglove (*Digitalis purpurea*)
- Lily of the valley (*Convallaria majalis*)
- Oleander (*Nerium oleander*)
- Red squill (*Urginea maritima*)
- Yellow oleander (*Thevetia peruviana*)

Signs and Symptoms

Acute toxicity from plants containing cardiac glycosides often causes nonspecific GI symptoms like abdominal pain, nausea, and vomiting within a few hours. It may also induce hyperkalemia and nonspecific neurologic symptoms such as altered mental status and weakness. Chronic toxicity likewise manifests with nonspecific GI symptoms but can also cause weight loss, diarrhea, anorexia, hypokalemia, and hypomagnesemia.

In both acute and chronic exposures, the patient usually reports a variety of cardiac symptoms, including palpitations, lightheadedness, dizziness, shortness of breath, and chest pressure. Almost any type of dysrhythmia may occur and can rapidly evolve into a life-threatening ventricular tachycardia.

Pathophysiology

Digitalis is a cardiac glycoside heart medication derived from the foxglove plant. Plants containing cardiac glycosides, such as the lily of the valley, are popular as ornamental flowers and sometimes accidentally ingested, especially by children. The digoxin-like property of these plants increases the force of myocardial contraction and decreases the conduction rate of the atrioventricular (AV) node.

Diagnosis

Diagnosis of cardiac glycoside toxicity depends on gathering accurate information from the scene and the patient. The presence of cardiac glycoside plants in the environment should arouse suspicion if you detect a cardiac dysrhythmia during the physical exam. Ask whether the exposure was accidental or intentional and whether other people were also exposed. The poisoning may represent a suicide attempt, which may make the patient history unreliable.

On physical exam, you may find the patient to be bradycardic or tachycardic, with a weak, irregular pulse. The skin is usually pale, cold, and clammy (diaphoretic). Lung sounds are typically normal. Examination of emesis may reveal plant material. The neurologic exam reveals altered mental status.

Treatment

The general steps in treating cardiac glycoside plant toxicity include providing supportive care, minimizing further toxin absorption, neutralizing absorbed toxin using an antidote, and treating any complications.

Prehospital Management of cardiac glycoside toxicity in the prehospital setting consists primarily of supportive care and transportation to the hospital for further evaluation and testing. Administer atropine to patients with bradycardia. Consider initiating gastric decontamination with activated charcoal in an alert patient with a protected airway.

Emergency Department ACLS procedures for support of airway, breathing, and circulation should be followed. Further exposure and absorption should be prevented

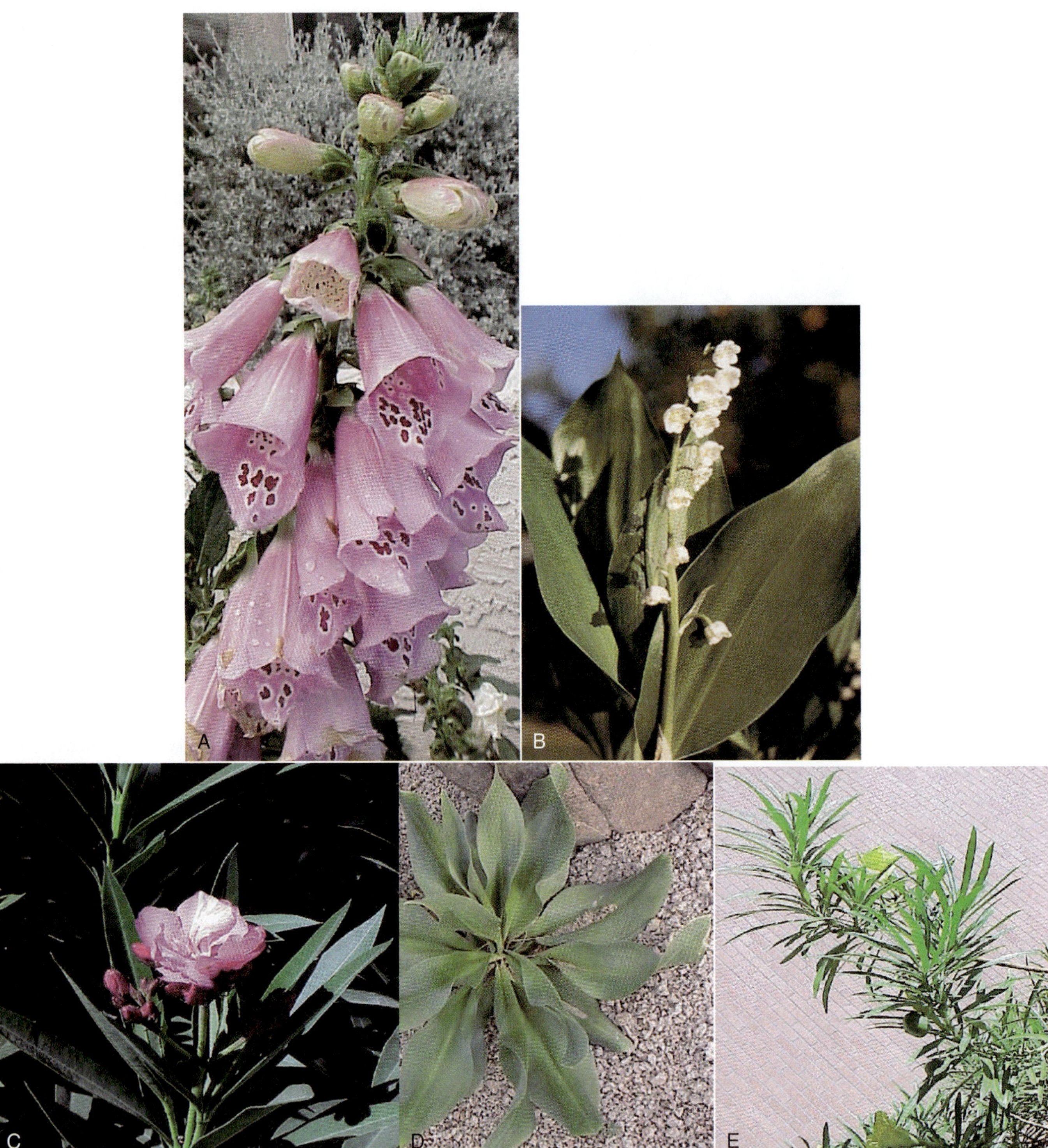

■ **Figure 9-10** A, *Digitalis purpurea* (foxglove). B, Lilly of the valley (*Convallaria majalis*). C, *Nerium oleander* (common oleander) plants have white or pink flowers and long, narrow seedpods. D, *Urginea* species (squill or sea onion) have broad leaves and a red underground bulb (some varieties have a white bulb). E, *Thevetia peruviana* (yellow oleander) has yellow flowers with smooth seedpods known as "lucky nuts," which are composed of green flesh surrounding a hard brown seed. (**A** courtesy Kimberlie Graeme, MD. **B** courtesy Donald Kunkel, MD. **C**, **D**, and **E** courtesy Kimberlie Graeme, MD.)

using activated charcoal, gastric lavage, and enhanced elimination. Cardiac glycoside toxicity can be treated with a digoxin-specific antibody Fab fragment (antigen binding fragment).

Medicines as Toxins

A number of prescription medications and over-the-counter (OTC) products can have toxic effects if used improperly, especially by vulnerable individuals like the very young and those with reduced drug clearance due to renal or liver impairment (Table 9-8).

Acetaminophen

Acetaminophen (*N*-acetyl-*p*-aminophenol [APAP], or Tylenol) is a commonly used OTC antipyretic and analgesic. The drug's benign safety profile at therapeutic doses has led to its inclusion in a variety of combination medications, including prescription and OTC pain relievers, cough and cold preparations, and allergy medications. The drug is widely available and easy to obtain.

Although it's safe at therapeutic levels, overdose ingestions of acetaminophen carry significant risk. The primary threat is hepatotoxicity. In fact, acetaminophen-related liver injury is the leading cause of acute liver failure in the United States, making it a far more common cause of liver failure than acute viral hepatitis. Questions about possible acetaminophen toxicity accounted for nearly 100,000 calls to poison control centers in 2007.

Signs and Symptoms

The clinical presentation of APAP toxicity can vary significantly, depending on the dose and timing of ingestion.

Text to be continued on page 357

TABLE 9-8 Drugs and Toxins

Drug or Toxin	Clinical Presentation of Intoxication	Specific Collaborative Management
Acetaminophen	*Mild/early stage* May be asymptomatic Anorexia, nausea, vomiting Diaphoresis Hypotension Pallor *12 hours to 4 days later* Signs of hepatotoxicity may occur: liver enzymes, bilirubin, PT increased; right upper quadrant pain Gradual return to normal may occur *Late: indications of hepatic failure* Anorexia, nausea, vomiting Jaundice Hepatosplenomegaly Clinical indications of hepatic encephalopathy: confusion to coma Bleeding Hypoglycemia Acute renal failure may develop Dysrhythmias and shock may occur	Gastric lavage only if within 2 hours of ingestion Activated charcoal if patient arrives within 4-6 hours after ingestion (although activated charcoal does adsorb *N*-acetylcysteine and reduces its peak serum levels, the loading dose of *N*-acetylcysteine does not need to be increased) *N*-acetylcysteine (Mucomyst) 140 mg/kg initially, then 70 mg/kg every 4 hours × 17 doses to total of 1330 mg/kg If given PO, dilute in juice or carbonated beverage; if given via nasogastric or duodenal tube, dilute with water May cause anorexia, nausea, vomiting; repeat dose if vomiting occurs within 1 hour Vitamin K may be prescribed, especially if hepatic failure occurs Dextrose (e.g., $D_{50}W$) may be needed Antidysrhythmics may be needed
Amphetamines	Tachycardia Hypertension Tachypnea Dysrhythmias Hyperthermia, diaphoresis Dilated but reactive pupils Dry mouth Urinary retention Headache Paranoid-type psychotic behavior Hallucinations Hyperactivity, anxiety Hyperactive deep tendon reflexes, tremor, seizures Confusion, stupor, coma	Calm, quiet environment Avoid overstimulation of patient Do not speak loudly or move quickly Do not approach from behind Avoid touching the patient unless you speak to the patient first or are sure it is safe Gastric lavage, activated charcoal Diazepam (Valium) for agitation Phentolamine (Regitine) for hypertension Anticonvulsants (e.g., diazepam, phenytoin, phenobarbital) for seizures Antidysrhythmics (e.g., lidocaine) for ventricular dysrhythmias Haloperidol (Haldol) for acute psychotic reactions Hypothermia blanket, ice packs, icewater sponge baths for hyperthermia Dantrolene (Dantrium) may be prescribed for malignant hyperthermia

Continued

TABLE 9-8 Drugs and Toxins—*Cont'd*

Drug or Toxin	Clinical Presentation of Intoxication	Specific Collaborative Management
Barbiturates, sedatives, hypnotics, tranquilizers	Bradycardia, cardiac dysrhythmias Hypotension Hypothermia Respiratory depression to respiratory arrest Headache Nystagmus, disconjugate eye movements Dysarthria Ataxia Depressed deep tendon reflexes Confusion, stupor, coma Hemorrhagic blisters Gastric irritation (chloral hydrate) Pulmonary edema (meprobamate) Hypertonicity, hyperreflexia, myoclonus seizures (methaqualone)	Gastric lavage, multiple-dose activated charcoal, cathartics Phenobarbital: sodium bicarbonate to alkalinize the urine and increase rate of barbiturate excretion; maintain urine pH > 7.50 Monitor potassium, calcium, and magnesium levels Anticonvulsants (e.g., diazepam, phenytoin, phenobarbital) for seizures Hemodialysis or hemoperfusion may be required
Benzodiazepines	Hypotension Respiratory depression Diminished or absent bowel sounds Decreased deep tendon reflexes (DTR) Confusion, drowsiness, stupor, coma	Gastric lavage, multiple-dose activated charcoal, cathartics Flumazenil (Romazicon), a benzodiazepine receptor antagonist may be prescribed Contraindicated if patient has co-ingested tricyclic antidepressants; use cautiously if patient has history of long-term use of benzodiazepines Monitor for seizures, agitation, flushing, nausea, and vomiting as side effects of flumazenil Intubation and mechanical ventilation may be necessary
Beta-blockers	Sinus bradycardia, arrest, block Junctional escape rhythm, AV nodal block Bundle branch block (usually right) Hypotension Heart failure Cardiogenic shock Cardiac arrest Decreased LOC Seizures Respiratory depression, apnea Bronchospasm Hyperglycemia or hypoglycemia	Gastric lavage, activated charcoal, cathartic Bowel irrigation if sustained-release preparations ingested Glucagon 3-5 mg IV, IM, or SQ, followed by infusion of 1-5 mg/h Epinephrine, dopamine, isoproterenol, or atropine for bradycardia and hypotension; temporary pacing may be required $D_{50}W$ for hypoglycemia Anticonvulsants (e.g., diazepam, phenobarbital) for seizures; phenytoin is contraindicated
Calcium channel blockers	Sinus bradycardia, arrest, block SA blocks (diltiazem) AV blocks (verapamil) Hypotension Heart failure Confusion, agitation, dizziness, lethargy, slurred speech Seizures Nausea, vomiting Paralytic ileus Hyperglycemia	Gastric lavage, activated charcoal, cathartic Bowel irrigation if sustained-release preparations ingested Calcium chloride 5 (500 mg) to 10 (1 g) mL of 10% solution Glucagon 3-5 mg IV, IM, or SQ, followed by infusion of 1-5 mg/h Anticonvulsants (e.g., diazepam, phenytoin, phenobarbital) for seizures Atropine, isoproterenol, temporary pacing for bradycardia
Carbon monoxide NOTE: the affinity between carbon monoxide and hemoglobin is approximately 200 times the affinity between oxygen and hemoglobin	Dysrhythmias Impaired hearing or vision Pallor; cherry-red skin coloring may be seen 10%-20%: mild headache, flushing, dyspnea or angina on vigorous exertion, nausea, dizziness 20%-30%: throbbing headache, nausea, vomiting, weakness, dyspnea on moderate exertion, ST-segment depression 30%-40%: severe headache, visual disturbances, syncope, vomiting 40%-50%: tachypnea, tachycardia, chest pain, worsening syncope 50%-60%: chest pain, respiratory failure, shock, seizures, coma 60%-70%: respiratory failure, shock, coma, death	Removal from contaminated area Oxygenation: 100% oxygen via mask initially; CPAP by mask may be utilized Intubation and mechanical ventilation until COHb level <5%; PEEP may be utilized Hyperbaric oxygen (at 2-3 atmospheres) as soon as available if: COHb > 25% COHb > 15% if history of cardiovascular disease, acute ECG changes, or CNS symptoms Fluids, diuretics, urine alkalinization to treat myoglobinuria if present Anticonvulsants (e.g., diazepam, phenytoin, phenobarbital) for seizures

TABLE 9-8 Drugs and Toxins—*Cont'd*

Drug or Toxin	Clinical Presentation of Intoxication	Specific Collaborative Management
Caustic poisoning Acids (e.g., battery acid, drain cleaners, hydrochloric acid) Alkalis (e.g., drain cleaners, refrigerants, fertilizers, photographic developers)	Burning sensation in the oral cavity, pharynx, esophageal area Dysphagia Respiratory distress: dyspnea, stridor, tachypnea, hoarseness Soapy-white mucous membrane Acid: Oral ulcerations and/or blisters May have signs of shock Alkali: May have signs of esophageal perforation (e.g., chest pain, subcutaneous emphysema)	Diluent: flush mouth with copious volumes of water; drink water or milk (approximately 250 mL) Do not induce vomiting or perform gastric lavage Activated charcoal Esophagogastroscopy to assess damage Corticosteroids may be prescribed for alkali poisoning
Cocaine, including "crack" cocaine	Tachycardia, dysrhythmias Hypertension or hypotension Tachypnea or hyperpnea Cocaine-induced MI Pallor or cyanosis Hyperexcitability, anxiety Headache Hyperthermia, diaphoresis Nausea, vomiting, abdominal pain Dilated but reactive pupils Confusion, delirium, hallucinations Seizures Coma Respiratory arrest	Swabbing of inside of nose to remove any residual drug if cocaine was snorted Gastric lavage, multiple-dose activated charcoal if ingested Bowel irrigation for "body packers" Anticonvulsants (e.g., diazepam, phenytoin, phenobarbital) for seizures Antidysrhythmics, usually lidocaine; calcium channel blockers may also be used (they may also help with coronary artery spasm) Antihypertensives: alpha-blockers (e.g., phentolamine), alpha- and beta-blockers (e.g., labetalol [Normodyne]), or vasodilators (e.g., nitroprusside [Nipride]) Hypothermia blanket, ice packs, icewater sponge baths for hyperthermia Dantrolene (Dantrium) may be prescribed for malignant hyperthermia Fluids, diuretics, urine alkalinization to treat myoglobinuria if present
Cyanide	Anxiety, restlessness, hyperventilation initially Bradycardia followed by tachycardia Hypertension followed by hypotension Dysrhythmias Bitter almond odor to breath Cherry-red mucous membranes Nausea Dyspnea Headache Dizziness Pupil dilation Confusion Stupor, seizures, coma, death	100% oxygen initially by mask Hyperbaric oxygen may be needed Intubation and mechanical ventilation is frequently necessary Supportive care if only anxiety, restlessness, hyperventilation Discontinuance of causative agent (e.g., nitroprusside) Antidotes for more serious symptoms Amyl nitrite by inhalation Sodium nitrite IV Sodium thiosulfate IV Gastric lavage, activated charcoal if cyanide was ingested Flushing of eyes and/or skin with water if dermal contamination; removal and isolation of clothing Fluids, vasopressors for BP support Anticonvulsants (e.g., diazepam, phenytoin, phenobarbital) for seizures Antidysrhythmics (e.g., lidocaine) for ventricular dysrhythmia, atropine for bradydysrhythmias Vitamin B_{12} may be prescribed

Continued

TABLE 9-8 Drugs and Toxins—*Cont'd*

Drug or Toxin	Clinical Presentation of Intoxication	Specific Collaborative Management
Digitalis preparations	Anorexia Nausea Vomiting Headache Restlessness Visual changes Sinus bradycardia, block, or arrest PAT with AV block Junctional tachycardia AV blocks: 1st, 2nd type I, 3rd PVCs: bigeminy, trigeminy, quadrigeminy Ventricular tachycardia: especially bidirectional Ventricular fibrillation	Activated charcoal, cholestyramine Correction of hypoxia, electrolyte imbalance (especially potassium) Treatment of dysrhythmias For symptomatic bradydysrhythmias and blocks Atropine External pacemaker For symptomatic tachydysrhythmias Lidocaine Phenytoin Magnesium if hypomagnesemia or hyperkalemia present Cardioversion at lowest effective voltage and only if life-threatening dysrhythmias exist Defibrillation for ventricular fibrillation Verapamil if SVT Digoxin immune Fab (Digibind) if >10 mg ingested (adult), serum digoxin >10 mg/mL or serum potassium >5.0 mEq/L Monitor closely for exacerbation of condition if digitalis was being used for (i.e., increase in heart rate, heart failure)
Ethanol	Ethanol concentration (mg/dL) <25: sense of warmth and well-being, talkativeness, self-confidence, mild incoordination 25-50: euphoria, decreased judgment and control 50-100: decreased sensorium, worsened coordination, ataxia, decreased reflexes and reaction time 100-250: nausea, vomiting, ataxia, diplopia, slurred speech, visual impairment, nystagmus, emotional lability, confusion, stupor 250-400: stupor or coma, incontinence, respiratory depression >400: respiratory paralysis, loss of protective reflexes, hypothermia, death NOTE: These signs/symptoms and blood ethanol levels vary widely; these signs/symptoms are for a non-alcohol-dependent person *Also:* Alcohol odor to breath Hypoglycemia Seizures Metabolic acidosis	Gastric lavage if within 1 hour of ingestion Fluid and electrolyte replacement (potassium, magnesium, calcium may be needed) Anticonvulsants (e.g., diazepam, phenytoin, phenobarbital) for seizures Glucose for hypoglycemia along with multivitamins including thiamine and folic acid NOTE: Thiamine is necessary for the brain to utilize glucose; thiamine deficiency in alcoholic patients may cause Wernicke encephalopathy Hemodialysis may be necessary
Ethylene glycol	*First 12 hours after ingestion* Appears "drunk" without the odor of ethanol on breath Nausea, vomiting, hematemesis Focal seizures, coma Nystagmus, depressed reflexes, tetany Metabolic acidosis with increased anion gap *12-24 hours after ingestion* Tachycardia Mild hypertension Pulmonary edema Heart failure 24-72 hours after ingestion Flank pain, costovertebral tenderness Acute renal failure	Gastric lavage (especially helpful if within 2 hours of ingestion) 10% ethanol in D_5W IV to maintain serum ethanol level at 100-200 mg/dL Fomepizole (Antizol) may be used instead of ethanol Fluid and electrolyte replacement (particularly calcium, but potassium and magnesium may also be needed) Sodium bicarbonate for severe metabolic acidosis Glucose for hypoglycemia and multivitamins, including thiamine, folic acid, and pyridoxine NOTE: Thiamine is necessary for the brain to utilize glucose; thiamine deficiency in alcoholic patients may cause Wernicke encephalopathy Anticonvulsants (e.g., diazepam, phenytoin, phenobarbital) for seizures Hemodialysis may be needed

TABLE 9-8 Drugs and Toxins—*Cont'd*

Drug or Toxin	Clinical Presentation of Intoxication	Specific Collaborative Management
Hallucinogens (e.g., D-lysergic acid diethylamide [LSD])	Tachycardia, hypertension Hyperthermia Anorexia, nausea Headaches Dizziness Agitation, anxiety Impaired judgment Distortion and intensification of sensory perception Toxic psychosis Dilated pupils Rambling speech Polyuria	Reassurance Quiet environment with soft lighting If ingested orally: charcoal may be used Benzodiazepines (e.g., diazepam) for anxiety and agitation Anticonvulsants (e.g., diazepam, phenytoin, phenobarbital) for seizures Restraints only if necessary to protect patient
Isopropyl alcohol	Gastrointestinal distress (e.g., nausea, vomiting, abdominal pain) Headache CNS depression, areflexia, ataxia Respiratory depression Hypothermia, hypotension	Gastric lavage (especially helpful if within 2 hours of ingestion), activated charcoal Fluids and vasopressors for hypoperfusion Hemodialysis may be needed
Lithium	*Mild* Vomiting, diarrhea Lethargy, weakness Polyuria, polydipsia Nystagmus Fine tremors *Severe* Hypotension Severe thirst Tinnitus Hyperreflexia Coarse tremors Ataxia Seizures Confusion Coma Dilute urine, renal failure Heart failure	Gastric lavage Hydration Anticonvulsants (e.g., diazepam, phenytoin, phenobarbital) for seizures Hemodialysis may be necessary
Methanol	Nausea and vomiting Hyperpnea, dyspnea Visual disturbances ranging from blurring to blindness Speech difficulty Headache CNS depression Motor dysfunction with rigidity, spasticity, and hypokinesis Metabolic acidosis with anion gap	Gastric lavage (especially helpful if within 2 hours of ingestion) 10% ethanol in D_5W IV to maintain serum ethanol level at 100-200 mg/dL Sodium bicarbonate for severe metabolic acidosis Hemodialysis if visual impairment, base deficit >15, renal insufficiency, or blood methanol concentration >30 mmol/L
Methemoglobinemia caused by nitrites, nitrate, sulfa drugs, and others	Tachycardia Fatigue Nausea Dizziness Cyanosis in the presence of a normal PaO_2; failure of cyanosis to resolve with oxygen therapy Dark red or brown blood Elevated methemoglobin levels Headache, weakness, dyspnea (30%-40%) Stupor, respiratory depression (60%)	Oxygen Removal of cause Stop nitroglycerin, nitroprusside, sulfa drugs, anesthetic agents, or other causative agent Gastric lavage, activated charcoal, cathartic if agent ingested Methylene blue If stupor, coma, angina, or respiratory depression or if level 30%-40% or more Administered at 2 mg/kg over 5 min; repeated at 1 mg/kg if patient still symptomatic after 30-60 min Ascorbic acid may be administered in large doses

Continued

TABLE 9-8 Drugs and Toxins—*Cont'd*

Drug or Toxin	Clinical Presentation of Intoxication	Specific Collaborative Management
Opioids and opiates	Bradycardia Hypotension Decreased level of consciousness Respiratory depression to respiratory arrest Hypothermia Miosis Diminished bowel sounds Needle tracks, abscesses Seizures Pulmonary edema (especially with heroin)	Gastric lavage, activated charcoal, cathartics if ingested Bowel irrigation for "body packers" Naloxone (Narcan) 0.4-2 mg IV, IM, or transtracheally or nalmefene (Revex) 0.5 mg IV Duration of action of naloxone is 1-2 hours, whereas nalmefene has a duration of action of 4-8 hours (heroin and morphine 4-6 hours, meperidine 2-4 hours) Anticonvulsants (e.g., diazepam, phenytoin, phenobarbital) for seizures Intubation and mechanical ventilation may be required; PEEP may be needed for pulmonary edema
Organophosphate and carbamate (cholinesterase inhibitors)	Bradycardia Nausea, vomiting, diarrhea Abdominal pain and cramping Increased oral secretions Dyspnea Slurred speech Constricted pupils Visual changes Unsteady gait Urinary incontinence Poor motor control Twitching Change in level of consciousness Seizures	Gastric lavage, activated charcoal, cathartic if ingested Removal and isolation of clothing Washing of skin with ethyl alcohol and then soap and water if dermal contamination Atropine 1-2 mg IV or IM; repeated as required Pralidoxime chloride (Protopam) 1-2 grams IV over 15-30 min followed by infusion of 10-20 mg/kg may be used for organophosphates Anticonvulsants (e.g., diazepam, phenytoin, phenobarbital) for seizures
Petroleum distillates	Flushed skin Hyperthermia Vomiting Diarrhea Abdominal pain Tachypnea Dyspnea Cyanosis Coughing Breath sound changes: crackles, rhonchi, diminished breath sounds Staggering gait Confusion CNS depression or excitation	Gastric lavage, activated charcoal, cathartic may be indicated; endotracheal tube should be inserted prior to gastric lavage if patient's LOC diminished Washing of skin with soap and water if dermal contamination; removal and isolation of clothing Oxygen, mechanical ventilation my be required
Phencyclidine (PCP)	Tachycardia Hypertensive crisis Hyperthermia Agitation, hyperactivity Nystagmus Blank stare Hypoglycemia Violent, psychotic behavior Ataxia Seizures Myoglobinuria, renal failure Lethargy, coma Cardiac arrest	Quiet environment Gastric lavage if within 1 hour of ingestion, multiple-dose activated charcoal, cathartic Gastric suction Benzodiazepines (e.g., diazepam) for anxiety and agitation Haloperidol (Haldol) to improve schizophrenic symptoms Fluids and diuretics for forced diuresis Beta-blockers for dysrhythmias Antihypertensives: vasodilators (e.g., nitroprusside [Nipride]) Hypothermia blanket, ice packs, icewater sponge baths for hyperthermia Dantrolene (Dantrium) may be prescribed for malignant hyperthermia Anticonvulsants (e.g., diazepam, phenytoin, phenobarbital) for seizures Haloperidol (Haldol) for acute psychotic reactions Fluids and diuretics for myoglobinuria; urinary alkalinization interferes with urinary elimination of PCP, so sodium bicarbonate contraindicated

TABLE 9-8 Drugs and Toxins—*Cont'd*

Drug or Toxin	Clinical Presentation of Intoxication	Specific Collaborative Management
Salicylates	*Initial:* Hyperthermia Burning sensation in mouth or throat Change in level of consciousness Petechiae, rash, hives *Later:* Hyperventilation (respiratory alkalosis) Nausea, vomiting Thirst Tinnitus Diaphoresis *Late:* Hearing loss Motor weakness Vasodilation and hypotension Respiratory depression to respiratory arrest Metabolic acidosis	Gastric lavage, activated charcoal, cathartic Bowel irrigation if enteric-coated salicylates ingested Fluids with dextrose (e.g., D_5-1/2 NS) Hypothermia blanket, ice packs, icewater sponge baths for hyperthermia Dantrolene (Dantrium) may be prescribed for malignant hyperthermia Sodium bicarbonate to alkalinize the urine and increase rate of salicylate excretion; maintain urine pH >7.50 Monitor potassium, calcium, and magnesium levels Vitamin K may be needed Anticonvulsants (e.g., diazepam, phenytoin, phenobarbital) for seizures Hemodialysis may be necessary
Tricyclic antidepressants (TCA)	*Anticholinergic* Tachycardia, palpitations Dysrhythmias Hyperthermia Headache Restlessness Mydriasis Dry mouth Nausea, vomiting Dysphagia Decreased bowel sounds Urinary retention Decreased deep tendon reflexes Restlessness, euphoria Hallucinations Seizures Coma *Anti–alpha adrenergic* Hypotension QT prolongation and quinidine-like dysrhythmias (including torsades de pointes) AV and bundle branch blocks Clinical indications of heart failure	Gastric lavage, multiple-dose activated charcoal, cathartic Sodium bicarbonate to alkalinize the urine and increase rate of TCA excretion; maintain urine pH > 7.50 Monitor potassium, calcium, magnesium levels Hyperventilation may be used to produce alkalosis Physostigmine (Antilirium) may be prescribed Cardioversion, defibrillation, pacemaker as needed for dysrhythmias; avoid quinidine, lidocaine, digitalis; phenytoin or beta-blockers may be used to shorten QRS duration; overdrive pacing for torsades de pointes Anticonvulsants (e.g., diazepam, phenytoin, phenobarbital) for seizures Fluids and vasopressors for hypotension Bethanechol (Urecholine) for urinary retention

From Dennisson RD: Pass CCRN, St Louis, 2007, Mosby.

Single doses of over 150 mg/kg are considered toxic, but dosage history in overdose scenarios is notoriously unreliable, and the dosage threshold fails to account for staggered ingestions or for unintentional repeated supratherapeutic ingestions. Nonetheless, it does give us some idea of what constitutes a worrisome single dose. In a 70-kg person, ingestion of 10.5 g of APAP, or 21 extra-strength tablets, would be enough to confer toxicity. The time of the ingestion is also critical, both for evaluation of symptoms and interpretation of serum levels, which is discussed in the next section. Clinical manifestations, summarized in Box 9-1, can be loosely divided into stages on the basis of the amount of time elapsed since ingestion.

Nephrotoxicity (kidney damage) may occur with or without liver injury. Renal failure requiring hemodialysis generally occurs only in patients who have also suffered significant hepatotoxicity, but otherwise, renal injury improves with IV fluids and time. Long-term renal dysfunction is not an expected sequela of acute acetaminophen toxicity.

Another variable that may confound the clinical picture is the presence of a co-ingestion. APAP is often combined with anticholinergic and opioid medications (e.g., hydrocodone [Vicodin]). The toxicity of the other drug may obscure signs of acetaminophen-induced toxicity. Moreover, in an overdose scenario, acetaminophen ingestion must always be considered and specifically queried because of its wide availability and the relative absence of early symptoms. In cases of unintentional overdose, the patient may have taken repeated supratherapeutic doses in an attempt to relieve unremitting pain. Obtaining a thorough, accurate history is vitally important in preventing advanced hepatotoxicity.

BOX 9-1 Clinical Manifestations of APAP Toxicity

Stage I (<24 hours): Symptoms are nonspecific and may include nausea, vomiting, and malaise. In severe overdose, patients may have an altered level of consciousness and acidosis. Patients may also have very mild or no symptoms, even after toxic ingestions.

Stage II (24–36 hours): This stage is marked by the onset of hepatic injury, characterized by abdominal pain, worsening nausea and vomiting, and elevated liver enzymes and coagulation studies.

Stage III (48–96 hours): Peak liver injury, perhaps progressing to fulminant hepatic failure, occurs during this period. Liver enzyme tests typically become significantly elevated, but of greater clinical relevance are the patient's coagulation studies, mental status, acidosis, and renal function. A systemic inflammatory response syndrome (SIRS) resembling septic shock can occur. Death may occur as a result of multiorgan failure, acute respiratory distress syndrome (ARDS), sepsis, or cerebral edema (Makin, 1994).

Stage IV (>96 hours): If the patient survives, the liver regenerates quickly and is unlikely to evidence any chronic damage.

Pathophysiology

Acetaminophen is metabolized through several pathways, and most of its metabolites are nontoxic. However, after supratherapeutic dosing, the major metabolic pathways become saturated, resulting in excessive formation of the toxic metabolite N-acetyl-*p*-benzoquinoneimine (NAPQI). When insufficient glutathione (<30% of normal stores) is present, NAPQI induces a series of reactions that lead to cell death. Cells with cytochrome P450 enzyme systems (e.g., hepatic and renal cells) are primarily affected, resulting in hepatic centrilobular necrosis and renal proximal tubular necrosis.

Diagnosis

On arrival to the ED, diagnostic tests include acetaminophen level, liver function tests, coagulation (PT/INR) studies, and measurement of electrolytes, blood urea nitrogen (BUN), and creatinine. In the setting of severe toxicity, arterial or venous blood gases may also be analyzed, since acidemia due to metabolic acidosis is a reliable predictor of morbidity and mortality.

Interpretation of serum acetaminophen level hinges on the time of ingestion. The Rumack-Matthew nomogram can be used to predict which patients will develop serious hepatic injury, defined as an aspartate aminotransferase [AST] level above 1000 IU/L. The nomogram has an established treatment line. On the basis of time since ingestion and serum level, you can plot an individual patient's data on the graph. If the patient's mark is above the line, he or she requires treatment. If it falls below this threshold, no further treatment is required. The gold standard is to initiate treatment at a 4-hour level above 150 μg/mL. Note, however, that this boundary is valid only for assessment of a single, all-at-one-time ingestion. It's not valid for chronic or multiple-dose ingestions.

Treatment

Treatment decisions center primarily on the time of ingestion and obtaining a thorough, accurate history.

Prehospital Offer intensive supportive care, including airway management as needed on the basis of mental status. Provide aggressive IV fluid resuscitation. In rare cases in which your evaluation takes place within 1 hour of ingestion and the patient is awake and oriented without nausea, you may consider using activated charcoal. An IV antiemetic may be administered for symptomatic control.

Emergency Department Treatment of acetaminophen toxicity consists of either IV or oral administration of N-acetylcysteine (NAC). NAC acts in a variety of ways to detoxify NAPQI, replenish glutathione stores, decrease inflammatory toxicity, and encourage metabolism of APAP to nontoxic metabolites. If given within 8 hours of ingestion, before glutathione stores have been depleted, severe hepatic injury can be avoided. Once again, this demonstrates the importance of accurately determining the time of ingestion. Regardless of how much time has elapsed, however, NAC does offer benefit compared with placebo. NAC therapy should be continued until one of three endpoints is reached:

1. Symptomatic and laboratory improvement occurs.
2. A liver transplant is performed.
3. The patient dies.

In patients without progression of toxicity, treatment protocols generally unfold over a minimum of 20 hours. Side effects of NAC therapy are generally minor, uncommon, and easily treated. Oral NAC is associated with a high incidence of nausea and vomiting because it has an odor of rotten eggs. Intravenous NAC has been associated with anaphylactoid reactions, which aren't true immunoglobulin E (IgE)-mediated allergic reactions. Symptoms generally include rash, pruritus, and occasionally wheezing and upper airway edema. According to the package insert, the incidence of pruritus is 10%, hypotension 4%, bronchospasm 6%, and angioedema 8%. When these symptoms occur, treatment must be temporarily discontinued while the patient is treated with antihistamines, bronchodilators, and epinephrine if necessary. Infusion may then be continued at a slower rate. If symptoms recur, oral NAC may be used.

Special Populations Pediatric patients are actually somewhat protected from acetaminophen toxicity compared with adults because they have an increased capacity for nontoxic metabolism of acetaminophen. Diagnosis and treatment of pregnant women does not differ from standard treatment. Patients with chronic alcohol abuse or malnutrition (who probably have decreased glutathione stores) may be at increased risk of hepatotoxicity. Nevertheless, the Rumack-Matthew nomogram and NAC therapy remain the same in these groups of patients, as no evidence exists to support alteration of treatment.

Salicylates

Salicylates such as aspirin (acetylsalicylic acid) are common OTC analgesics. They are also involved in many toxicologic emergencies, although their toxicity threshold (300 mg/kg) is twice as high as that of acetaminophen. Salicylate overdose is complicated by the fact that other medications are often co-ingested.

Signs and Symptoms

Early symptoms of acute salicylate poisoning include gastric irritation and pain. Chronic poisoning can occur with aspirin, because it's an extremely effective analgesic and is now being prescribed at low doses as a daily preventive agent for cardiac care. Symptoms of chronic poisoning, such as gastric irritation and pain, are similar to the early symptoms of acute poisoning. The prevailing thought behind aspirin misuse seems to be if a little is good, a lot must be better.

Pathophysiology

Salicylates act therapeutically by inhibiting prostaglandin synthesis by acetylating cyclooxygenases (COX-1 and COX-2). In larger doses, salicylates uncouple oxidative phosphorylates. This upsets the body's acid-base balance and can lead to anion-gap metabolic acidosis.

Diagnosis

A blood workup should be done to determine the baseline serum salicylate level; levels should be measured at least every 6 hours afterward. In this manner, the serum salicylate half-life can be determined to aid treatment. Results can be plotted on the Done nomogram to yield approximate guidelines for management of an acute toxicologic emergency, but it's important to note that the Done nomogram is not accurate for chronic toxicity.

Treatment

Salicylate poisoning has no antidote. The most effective treatment is activated charcoal, which must be given within 1 hour of ingestion.

Prehospital Administration of IV fluids is essential. If metabolic acidosis develops, treat it aggressively with sodium bicarbonate. Supportive care, especially airway management, is of primary importance. Rule out hypoglycemia using a blood glucose test.

Emergency Department Renal excretion can be enhanced using alkaline diuresis (IV sodium bicarbonate and D_5W). Potassium therapy can be useful. Hemodialysis is indicated by renal failure, serum salicylate assays, severe metabolic acidosis, severe CNS depression, and cardiac dysfunction.

Beta-Blockers

Beta-blockers are frequently prescribed for the treatment of hypertension, coronary artery disease, congestive heart failure, arrhythmias, migraine headache prophylaxis, and anxiety disorders. Commonly prescribed beta-blockers include metoprolol (Lopressor, Toprol), carvedilol (Coreg), propranolol (Inderal), and atenolol (Tenormin). Topical ophthalmic preparations, including timolol (Timoptic), may be prescribed for glaucoma. Systemic toxicity has been reported with ingestion and use of these preparations.

Both intentional and unintentional ingestions leading to beta-blocker toxicity are frequently reported. In 2007, beta-blocker ingestions accounted for nearly 20,000 calls to poison control centers, resulting in more than 3600 visits to healthcare facilities (Bronstein, 2008). Despite this large number of ingestions, only three deaths were attributed to beta-blocker toxicity in 2007. Nevertheless, beta-blocker ingestion is a dangerous condition seen frequently in the prehospital setting.

Signs and Symptoms

As with all ingestions, in patients with suspected beta-blocker toxicity, you must obtain a detailed history of drug exposure, approximate dose, and time of ingestion, as well as possible co-ingestions. In patients who have ingested beta-blockers prescribed to them, obtaining information about the underlying disorder that necessitated the prescription may aid in eventual treatment of the toxic ingestion. A history of severe coronary artery disease, congestive heart failure, or dysrhythmia, for example, can affect decisions about the patient's long-term management. Remember to ask about previous pulmonary diseases like asthma and COPD.

Patients typically present with bradycardia and hypotension after ingesting β-adrenergic antagonists. The bradycardia may be a sinus bradycardia or, uncommonly, it may represent a first-, second-, or third-degree heart block. Mental status depression may or may not be present, depending on the specific drug ingested and its cardiovascular toxicity. If it occurs, the altered mental status may be caused by cerebral hypoperfusion or by the direct CNS depressive effects of the drug, particularly lipophilic drugs such as propranolol. Seizures occur in some patients, particularly in those with propranolol toxicity. Patients with CNS depression may also have respiratory depression.

Pathophysiology

Beta-blockers are often classified as β_1-specific agents or nonspecific agents on the basis of their respective pharmacologic structures. Examples of β_1-specific drugs include atenolol (Tenormin) and metoprolol (Lopressor, Toprol). Propranolol (Inderal) is a nonspecific beta-blocker. In general, β_1 receptor inhibition decreases chronotropy and inotropy by modulating G protein–linked second-messenger systems. These receptors are primarily found in cardiac tissue. Peripheral β_2 receptor agonist action causes vasodilation. Beta blockade may cause respiratory distress in patients with a predisposition to bronchoconstriction, such as those with asthma or COPD.

Diagnosis

In a patient with suspected beta-blocker toxicity, focused physical examination of the cardiovascular system may reveal a decreased respiratory rate, bilateral crackles secondary to acute pulmonary edema, or wheezing. Evaluation of capillary refill serves as an adjunctive measure to assess tissue perfusion. Beta-blocker toxicity can also cause metabolic derangements like mild hypoglycemia or slightly elevated potassium levels, which may be clinically significant in children. The presence of either mild hypoglycemia or normoglycemia can help you differentiate beta-blocker toxicity from bradycardia and hypotension due to calcium channel blocker toxicity. As discussed in the next section, calcium channel blocker toxicity is usually accompanied by hyperglycemia.

Evaluation of patients with suspected beta-blocker toxicity focuses on identifying end-organ dysfunction and hypoperfusion. Beyond physical examination of mental status, cardiopulmonary function, capillary refill response, and urine output, several ancillary tests are often performed. Arterial or venous blood gases may be obtained as a rapid measure of gas exchange and a possible indicator of metabolic acidosis secondary to tissue hypoperfusion and hypoxia. Electrocardiography is used to evaluate heart rhythm and rule out myocardial ischemia. Elevated cardiac enzymes (troponins) indicate myocardial injury due to hypotension and inadequate myocardial oxygen delivery.

Decreased serum bicarbonate levels and elevated BUN and creatinine are markers of poor tissue perfusion. Foley catheter insertion and subsequent documentation of urine output often yields the best real-time measurement of perfusion. Invasive hemodynamic monitoring, including placement of an arterial line, central venous pressure monitor, or Swan-Ganz catheter, may be initiated as well, depending on the severity of toxicity.

Treatment

Prehospital After managing the airway and establishing IV access, consider giving activated charcoal if less than 1 hour has elapsed since the beta-blocker ingestion, and the patient is alert and free of nausea or vomiting. Inhaled β-agonists like albuterol (Proventil, Ventolin) are indicated in patients with wheezing. Use caution when giving normal saline IV boluses in hypotensive patients because of the negative inotropic effects of β-adrenergic antagonists. Aggressive volume resuscitation can cause pulmonary edema. If the patient remains underperfused, as indicated by altered mental status, decreased capillary refill, or evidence of ischemia, provide pharmacologic support. Atropine is an option for bradycardia associated with hypoperfusion, but its effects may be minimal and transient. Additional therapy is often required. Calcium administration has demonstrated some benefit in animal studies, and you can consider it, although it rarely offers definitive treatment.

Glucagon is often referred to as the "antidote" for β-adrenergic antagonist toxicity. Cardiac glucagon receptors, like β-adrenergic receptors, are coupled to G proteins, increasing intracellular cyclic adenosine monophosphate (cAMP). At the same time, glucagon inhibits phosphodiesterase. In animal models, this combination of activity increases cardiac contractility, cardiac output, and heart rate. Glucagon itself is a vasodilator and therefore may not produce a corresponding increase in blood pressure. Human data regarding glucagon efficacy are limited to case reports and a case series. Adverse effects may include vomiting, hyperglycemia, and mild hypoglycemia.

If these therapies fail, progress to administering catecholamine vasopressors and other experimental therapies. Cardiac pacing is rarely effective in these patients.

Emergency Department Initial ED treatment of patients with beta-blocker toxicity follows the same algorithm as prehospital management. Failure of first-line treatment strategies necessitates administration of vasoactive medications. Pure β-adrenergic agonists such as isoproterenol (Isuprel) can be effective, but their β-agonist action may cause peripheral vasodilation and deteriorating hypotension. Dobutamine (Dobutrex), another β-agonist, also improves cardiac function and stimulates less peripheral vasodilation than isoproterenol. Epinephrine (Adrenalin) infusions can result in improved cardiac function and peripheral vasopressor effects. Primary vasoconstrictors like norepinephrine (Levophed) and phenylephrine (Neo-Synephrine) may be less beneficial because they increase afterload but produce relatively little improvement in cardiac function. This intervention poses a risk of worsened heart failure and pulmonary edema. Regardless of the catecholamine used, providers must be aware that very high doses—often higher than the recommended "maximum" dosage—may be required to compete with the ingested drug.

A newer therapy gaining popularity (on the basis of encouraging animal data but limited human experience) is high-dose insulin infusion. Referred to as *hyperinsulinemia-euglycemia (HIE) therapy,* exactly how it acts to reverse toxicity is unclear. Researchers hypothesize that the therapy may improve glucose utilization and energy production by the poisoned myocardium, or it may alter fatty acid metabolism or calcium sensitivity. HIE therapy in humans has been studied primarily in the setting of calcium channel blocker toxicity, but animal studies have also demonstrated its benefit in beta-blocker toxicity. As the infusion is administered, blood glucose levels must be checked and corrected every 30 minutes initially, and then at less frequent intervals depending on the patient's response.

Special Treatment Considerations Although the basic therapeutic concepts in managing beta-blocker toxicity can be generalized to all beta-blockers, several agents have special properties and thus require customized management strategies. Propranolol (Inderal), for instance, possesses the most potent membrane-stabilizing properties among beta-blockers. As a result, toxicity may lead to sodium channel blockade, QRS prolongation, and ventricular dysrhythmia. (Sodium channel blockade is discussed later in more detail in the Tricyclic Antidepressants section.) In addition to standard therapy, then, sodium bicarbonate administration may be required in the treatment of propranolol toxicity. Propranolol is the most lipophilic beta-blocker, so it causes more significant CNS toxicity than other beta-blockers, including seizures. Benzodiazepines are first-line treatment for propranolol-induced seizures.

Calcium Channel Blockers

Calcium channel blockers account for about 40% of cardiovascular drug exposures reported to the American Association of Poison Control Centers and more than 65% of deaths from cardiovascular medications. There are three commonly prescribed classes of calcium channel blockers in the United States:

1. Phenylalkylamines (e.g., verapamil [Calan, Isoptin])
2. Benzothiazepines (e.g., diltiazem [Cardizem, Cartia, Dilacor])
3. Dihydropyridines (e.g., amlodipine [Norvasc] and felodipine [Plendil])

Verapamil and diltiazem are often lumped together and referred to as *nondihydropyridines* because their characteristic cardiovascular activity differs from that of dihydropyridines.

Signs and Symptoms

Signs and symptoms of calcium channel blocker–induced toxicity may include chest pain, shortness of breath, lightheadedness, syncope, hypotension, and bradycardia or tachycardia, depending on the class of calcium channel blocker ingested. First-, second-, or third-degree heart block may also be present. As discussed in the previous section, hyperglycemia typically accompanies calcium channel blocker toxicity, differentiating it from beta-blocker toxicity.

Pathophysiology

Calcium channels are found on cardiac cells, vascular smooth muscle, and pancreatic beta islet cells. Opening of calcium channels contributes to myocardial contractility and vascular smooth muscle constriction. In pancreatic cells, calcium influx triggers insulin release. Reduction of intracellular calcium in cardiac muscle, smooth coronary muscle, and peripheral vessels depresses both chronotropy and inotropy and suppresses peripheral vasodilation. Because of differences in resting membrane potentials, dihydropyridine calcium channel blockers act preferentially on peripheral vascular calcium channels, decreasing peripheral vascular resistance but having little or no effect on cardiac calcium channels at therapeutic doses. This class of calcium channel blocker typically reduces blood pressure by inducing vasodilation with reflex tachycardia.

Diagnosis

The history obtained and physical examination performed after calcium channel blocker ingestion are similar to the history and exam that follow beta-blocker ingestion. It's important to obtain a detailed medical history, particularly regarding cardiovascular disease, and an incident history of dose, time of ingestion, and possible co-ingestions.

After evaluation and stabilization of the patient's airway and breathing, cardiovascular evaluation begins with close, often invasive monitoring of the patient's blood pressure and perfusion status, which may be accomplished with the aid of an arterial line or Swan-Ganz catheter (Figure 9-11). In patients with altered mental status or diminished airway reflexes, a chest x-ray is routinely performed to evaluate for pulmonary edema and aspiration pneumonitis. Acute pulmonary edema may cause bilateral crackles on auscultation and a decreased pulse oximetry measurement on room air. Mental status is not usually affected directly by calcium channel blockers, but cerebral hypoperfusion may alter the patient's level of consciousness. Extremity capillary refill examination, as in beta-blocker toxicity, provides a clue to perfusion status. In patients with evidence of toxicity, a Foley catheter is placed and urine output documented as a surrogate marker of renal perfusion. An ECG is obtained to evaluate for rhythm abnormalities and evidence of ischemia. Serial electrolyte, BUN, creatinine, and cardiac enzyme studies provide further indicators of possible organ hypoperfusion with resulting kidney injury, metabolic acidosis, and ischemic myocardial injury. Arterial or venous blood gas measurement can also aid in rapid evaluation of acid-base status, but is often not necessary. Patients who are found unresponsive or are known to have been immobile for prolonged periods are evaluated for rhabdomyolysis by serum CPK studies and muscle compartment examination.

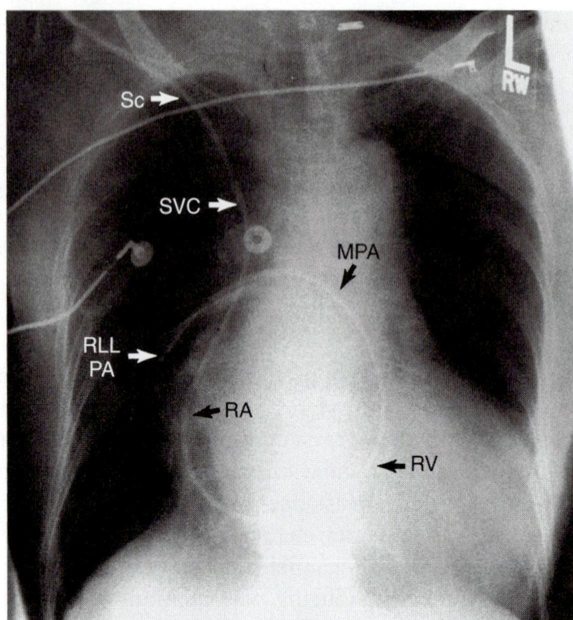

■ **Figure 9-11** Normal course of a Swan-Ganz catheter. A Swan-Ganz catheter inserted on the right goes into the subclavian vein (Sc), into the superior vena cava (SVC), right atrium (RA), right ventricle (RV), main pulmonary artery (MPA), and in this case, the right lower lobe pulmonary artery (RLL PA). (From Mettler F: Essentials of radiology, ed 2, Philadelphia, 2005, Saunders.)

Treatment

Prehospital As in beta-blocker poisoning, initial management of calcium channel blocker toxicity centers on controlling the patient's airway and breathing. In appropriate patients, consider using activated charcoal. You may administer IV boluses of normal saline for hypotension, but their effect may be limited by the negative inotropic effects and resultant pulmonary edema associated with calcium channel blockers. You should administer atropine in patients with symptomatic bradycardia, but it's often ineffective or only transiently effective. IV glucagon at doses similar to those studied in beta-blocker toxicity has been used but with less consistent effects. Administration of calcium salts can improve outcomes, but the use of this therapy may be limited by symptomatic hypercalcemia. Administration of IV calcium gluconate poses little risk to the patient and may be beneficial, especially when given in doses of several ampules. Calcium chloride contains more than three times as much elemental calcium as calcium gluconate, but it may provoke more peripheral venous irritation and other adverse effects. For patients taking digoxin, use of calcium salts is contraindicated because of the presumed risk of potentiating digoxin toxicity.

Emergency Department After administration of IV fluid boluses, calcium salts, and atropine or glucagon, patients typically receive IV vasopressors. As in beta-blocker toxicity, the choice of vasopressor has been widely debated, with reports of success and failure of multiple agents. Dopamine remains a poor choice because of its indirect sympathomimetic activity.

As already noted, in animal studies, HIE therapy has demonstrated promising results compared to administration of vasopressors, calcium, and glucagon. Although human data remain limited, several reports of successful treatment of calcium channel blocker toxicity with HIE have been published. On the basis of the available data, insulin therapy with maintenance of euglycemia is recommended in patients with severe calcium channel blocker toxicity resistant to vasopressor therapy.

Although severe dihydropyridine calcium channel blocker toxicity can cause bradycardia and hypotension, as with nondihydropyridine calcium channel blockers, toxic ingestions typically lead to peripheral vasodilation and hypotension with reflex tachycardia. As a result, after administration of IV fluids, the treatment of choice is a peripheral vasoconstrictor such as norepinephrine (Levophed) or phenylephrine (Neo-Synephrine).

When standard therapies fail, an intraaortic balloon pump (IABP) or cardiopulmonary bypass may be considered as temporizing measures. Limited success has been reported.

■ Tricyclic Antidepressants

Tricyclic antidepressants have historically been a leading cause of toxicologic emergencies, especially intentional overdoses. These medications have a narrow therapeutic index, which means there's a fine line between an ineffectually low dose and an overdose. Ironically, giving too low a dose may lead to an intentional overdose (a suicide attempt), and too high a dose could lead to an accidental overdose. The use of tricyclic antidepressants has declined recently as newer, safer alternatives have been introduced.

Signs and Symptoms

Tricyclic antidepressant toxicity is a result of potassium efflux inhibition and sodium channel inhibition in the myocardium. Early signs and symptoms include classic anticholinergic toxidrome effects like dry mouth, urinary retention, constipation, and blurred vision. Late signs and symptoms include respiratory depression, confusion, hallucinations, hyperthermia, cardiac dysrhythmias (such as *torsades de pointes* and wide QRS complexes), and seizures.

Pathophysiology

Tricyclic antidepressants act therapeutically by increasing the amount of norepinephrine and serotonin available in the CNS. They do so by blocking the reuptake of these neurotransmitters, extending the duration of their action. This has the effect of blocking cellular ion channels and α-adrenergic, muscarinic, and histaminergic receptors.

Cardiac toxicity is the hallmark of tricyclic antidepressant poisoning.

Diagnosis

Serum levels of tricyclic antidepressants are not well correlated with the severity of intoxication, but a drug screen should be performed to detect possible co-ingestants like acetaminophen. This is especially crucial in intentional poisonings. Other lab studies that are indicated include measurement of electrolyte, BUN, and creatinine levels, anion-gap analysis, a complete blood cell count (CBC), and evaluation of arterial blood gases (ABGs). Qualitative urine immunoassays are also available, although cyclobenzaprine is cross-reactive. Chest imaging may be indicated if aspiration has occurred or other respiratory symptoms are noted.

Treatment

Cardiac monitoring is critical in patients with suspected tricyclic antidepressant overdose, because cardiac complications are the primary cause of death. Sudden cardiac arrest may occur days after the overdose. There is no antidote for tricyclic antidepressant poisoning, but activated charcoal is usually effective if administered within an hour of ingestion.

Prehospital Provide supportive care, especially cardiac monitoring. Establish IV access, and administer sodium bicarbonate bolus and infusion.

Emergency Department The patient should be observed for at least 6 hours to rule out sequelae. Maintaining alkaline serum (pH 7.50 to 7.55) by bicarbonate infusion counteracts cardiac conduction effects. This treatment should be given if QRS widening, significant tachycardia, or ventricular ectopy occurs.

Lithium

Lithium is an agent used to treat bipolar disorder, also known as *manic-depressive illness*. Although lithium is an effective treatment, it has a narrow therapeutic index, increasing the likelihood of both accidental and intentional poisonings. To avoid accidental therapeutic poisoning, frequent blood tests are necessary to fine tune the patient's lithium dosage.

Several variables affect the drug's toxicity, including acute versus chronic ingestion, dose relative to existing serum levels, and overdose amount. Since lithium is an antidepressant, it's not surprising that lithium poisoning is common in suicide attempts. Toxicity is exacerbated by dehydration, diuretic use, and renal dysfunction.

Signs and Symptoms

Signs and symptoms of lithium poisoning depend heavily on the dose. Low serum levels (<1.5 mEq/L) tend to produce nonspecific GI signs and symptoms like nausea, vomiting, and diarrhea. Intermediate serum levels (1.5 to 3 mEq/L) produce more severe signs and symptoms that affect not only the GI system but also the CNS. GI effects include polyuria, resulting in urinary and fecal incontinence. The patient may have muscle weakness that eventually progresses to myoclonic twitching and muscle rigidity. Neurologic effects include restlessness, slurred speech, blurred vision, and vertigo. High serum levels (> 3 mEq/L) induce hypotension, seizures, cardiac dysrhythmia, and coma.

Pathophysiology

Lithium is a small cation (positively charged ion). It's similar to sodium and acts in place of it but has different effects. The precise mechanism by which lithium produces its medicinal benefit is still unknown, although the drug is thought to alter neuronal cell membrane function, cellular sodium and energy balance, and hormonal response. These effects may cause permanent CNS damage. Lithium decreases kidney function and is eliminated almost entirely by the kidneys. This property of the drug sometimes causes inadvertent lithium reabsorption.

Diagnosis

The lab workup of a patient with suspected lithium toxicity should include a urinalysis and periodic monitoring of serum lithium levels until symptoms resolve. Cardiac monitoring may be indicated, since chronic lithium toxicity is associated with depressed ST segments on ECG. To yield accurate results, the blood sample must be sent in a lithium-free tube. A thyroid function panel, analysis of acetaminophen level, and a lumbar puncture can be useful in eliminating alternative etiologies. Toxic co-ingestion must always be considered as a possibility.

Treatment

Prehospital In the field, treatment is mainly supportive. Maintain airway, breathing, and circulation. Establish IV access, since fluid administration is especially important in patients with lithium poisoning because of the effects of volume depletion on the cardiovascular and renal systems. Some reports indicate that sodium therapy encourages elimination of lithium by the kidneys.

Emergency Department Volume replacement may take several hours. Gastric decontamination, including both gastric lavage and whole-bowel irrigation, is indicated when less than 1 hour has elapsed since the ingestion. Hemodialysis is indicated in cases of severe intoxication (as evidenced by high serum lithium levels), renal failure, severe cardiovascular effects, or severe neurologic symptoms.

Amphetamines

Amphetamines are a diverse class of commonly abused legal and illicit drugs that can cause significant toxicity.

TABLE 9-9 Names of Common Street Drugs

Drug	Street Name
Methamphetamine	Crank, speed (oral or injected form) Ice, crystal meth (smoked form)
Methylenedioxymethamphetamine (MDMA)	Ecstasy, E, X, XTC, Adam, 007, B-bomb, care bear, Deb, go Jerry Garcia, love pill, playboy, wafer, white diamond
Methcathinone	Cat, khat, Jeff, ephedrine

Abuse of these drugs, particularly medications used to treat attention deficit hyperactivity disorder (ADHD), is common, partly because they are being prescribed to an increasing number of adolescents. Since the 1980s, the number of stimulant prescriptions for ADHD has increased fourfold. In one anonymous survey, 15% of 12th-grade students in the United States admitted to having abused prescription amphetamines.

Individuals who ingest packets of drugs while evading police, known colloquially as **stuffers**, may develop severe toxicity because of the relatively large amount of drug ingested and because its packaging was not designed to traverse the GI tract. They are often identified early by police, who may see them swallow the packets. Administration of activated charcoal is recommended in such patients in order to attenuate potential toxicity. Toxic effects don't always develop, but these patients must undergo extended observation in the ED because of the risk of delayed absorption and toxicity. Otherwise, evaluation and treatment remain the same as for any toxic ingestion.

Packers, people who smuggle large amounts of drugs by ingesting them, require admission to the intensive care unit (ICU) when they are identified. Although the risk of packaging failure is relatively low, such a large amount of drug is present in the GI tract that release of the drug would unleash a torrent of severe toxicity, GI ischemia, and death regardless of treatment. In fact, surgical removal of drug packages is indicated after any sign of toxicity in such patients.

Another concern with illicit amphetamine use and trafficking is the possibility of drug contamination. Many amphetamines are produced by generating chemical reactions that may in themselves be injurious. For example, outbreaks of lead and mercury toxicity have been traced to methamphetamine contamination. Amphetamines are also used in combination with other drugs, such as cocaine, heroin, and marijuana, which may alter their toxicity and clinical presentation.

Identification

Prescription amphetamines include methylphenidate (Ritalin, Concerta), amphetamine/dextroamphetamine (Adderall), phentermine (Adipex-P), atomoxetine (Strattera), and dexmethylphenidate (Focalin). These medications are generally used to treat ADHD but in some cases are used as diet pills. In addition, selegiline (Eldepryl), an agent used to treat Parkinson's disease, is metabolized to l-methamphetamine.

A wide variety of illicit amphetamines is abused, including amphetamine, methamphetamine, methylenedioxymethamphetamine (MDMA, or "ecstasy"), and methcathinone ("cat" or "Jeff"). Most users are simply trying to get high, but some users take the drugs as physical performance enhancers. Methamphetamine abuse is particularly dangerous because of the drug's astonishing potency. Between 2002 and 2005, roughly 1.4 million people older than age 12 had used methamphetamine during the previous year. Methamphetamine abuse is predominant in the Southwest.

Methcathinone is a derivative of cathinone, the active compound in khat leaves, which are commonly chewed by people in Eastern Africa for their stimulant effects. The potency of methcathinone is similar to that of methamphetamine. It's primarily abused in Eastern Europe, but its use has been reported in the Midwestern United States.

Both prescription and illicit amphetamines are abused in a variety of ways. They can be taken orally or they can be crushed and then snorted, injected, or smoked if sufficiently pure. Street names of some of these drugs are listed in Table 9-9.

Signs and Symptoms

Amphetamine abuse results in sympathomimetic toxicity. Tachycardia, hypertension, agitation, and tremor are typical. Severe toxicity may cause seizures, intracranial hemorrhage, myocardial infarction, ventricular dysrhythmia, or death. Patients may exhibit a marked increase in strength as well as blunted pain perception. Because of excessive dopamine release, amphetamine toxicity may induce psychosis and choreoathetoid movements.

Pathophysiology

Amphetamines are structurally similar to endogenous catecholamines. They act at presynaptic nerve terminals to prevent reuptake of biogenic amines (norepinephrine, dopamine, and serotonin) from the synaptic cleft and to promote release of these neurotransmitters. The consequent excessive postsynaptic stimulation leads to the clinical manifestations of toxicity as well as to the euphoria associated with use of these drugs. Chemical substitutions alter the potency of amphetamines and confer slight alterations in toxicity. For example, MDMA has predominantly serotonergic properties, which are responsible for the drug's characteristic clinical effects.

Diagnosis

Although obtaining a history of the dose or time of ingestion may be helpful, this information probably will not affect management significantly. Identification of the drug is the most important component of the history. Knowing the street names of drugs may help you do so (see Table 9-9). Gathering additional information about past medical history of cardiovascular disease, seizure disorder, or stroke also aids in management.

Physical examination often reveals mydriasis and diaphoresis, which are a result of sympathetic overstimulation. In patients who have taken MDMA, you may observe bruxism (jaw clenching or chewing). MDMA use, especially in the setting of raves, has also been associated with hyponatremia, which can manifest as altered mental status or seizures. With any amphetamine overdose, hyperreflexia and excessive motor activity can cause muscle breakdown and rhabdomyolysis, raising the specter of possible myoglobinuric renal failure. Hyperthermia is a late and ominous sign. In fact, of all the vital signs, hyperthermia is the most predictive of significant morbidity and mortality in patients with amphetamine overdose.

Treatment

Benzodiazepine administration, IV fluid hydration, and external cooling are the mainstays of treatment in amphetamine toxicity.

Prehospital Prehospital treatment of patients with sympathomimetic toxicity begins with appropriate airway management and continuous cardiac monitoring. Measurement of blood glucose is critical to rule out hypoglycemia as the cause of altered mental status and tachycardia. Otherwise, initiate IV access and administer fluid boluses. Owing to diaphoresis, increased activity, and insensible fluid losses, these patients are often dehydrated and in need of volume resuscitation. In addition, administering IV fluids may protect patients from kidney injury as a result of rhabdomyolysis.

In patients who are agitated and combative, administer benzodiazepines. The dose required to achieve sedation varies among individual patients, but the goal of therapy is to achieve sedation and suppress excessive motor activity. Benzodiazepines also act as sympatholytics, thereby treating tachycardia and hypertension. Occasionally, despite adequate sedation, patients may demonstrate rhythmic or choreoathetoid movements as a result of excessive dopaminergic stimulation. Haloperidol (Haldol) may be used to treat this movement disorder, but you should reserve haloperidol treatment until after you administer benzodiazepines whenever possible, because of the risk of seizures.

Perform a 12-lead ECG in patients who complain of chest pain or have evidence of significant toxicity. You can consider giving aspirin or nitroglycerin, but in patients with altered mental status, withhold aspirin until computed tomography (CT) of the brain can be performed to rule out intracranial hemorrhage. Treating the underlying toxicity with benzodiazepines also treats cardiovascular sequelae. Myocardial ischemia is more commonly related to vasospasm than to vasoocclusive disease. Finally, in patients who are hyperthermic, institute external cooling measures.

Emergency Department After initial stabilization, ED evaluation focuses on identifying end-organ injury from amphetamine toxicity. Most commonly affected are the CNS and cardiovascular system. CT scanning of the brain without IV contrast is often performed to evaluate for hemorrhage, cerebral edema, or early evidence of ischemia. ECG and cardiac enzyme testing may be ordered because of the risk of myocardial ischemia and ventricular dysrhythmia.

Blood tests include a CBC, kidney function tests, and measurement of electrolyte levels and total creatine phosphokinase (CPK). Arterial or venous blood gas measurement is obtained in sick patients, since metabolic acidosis is common in severe sympathomimetic toxicity, primarily as a result of increased psychomotor activity. Further testing may be required on the basis of clinical presentation.

Urine drug testing may confirm the presence of amphetamine but should not guide acute management. The patient's clinical presentation, consistent with a sympathomimetic toxidrome, should be a sufficient basis on which to initiate management. Moreover, prescription and OTC medications (e.g., pseudoephedrine [Sudafed]) may cause false-positive results on standard urine drug screens.

ED management is similar to prehospital management. In severe cases, intubation and sedation with propofol (Diprivan) or phenobarbital (Luminal) may be required. In patients with active myocardial ischemia, including ST-segment elevation myocardial infarction (STEMI), cardiology consultation may be obtained, but the decision to perform cardiac catheterization in these patients is not supported by evidence. Generally, acute drug toxicity is treated with follow-up cardiac evaluation once the patient is hemodynamically stable. Because of vascular toxicity, hypertension, and lack of evidence to support thrombosis, thrombolytics are not administered to patients with sympathomimetic toxicity. Patients may require ICU care after initial stabilization.

Barbiturates

Barbiturates have been commercially available since 1903. Phenobarbital (Luminal) was used extensively to treat seizure disorders before the advent of newer anticonvulsants, and it's still used to treat refractory seizure disorders. Some patients are treated successfully with phenobarbital for years. Primidone (Mysoline), which is metabolized to phenobarbital, is also used as an anticonvulsant. Butalbital combined with caffeine and either aspirin (Fiorinal) or acetaminophen (Fioricet) is a barbiturate used as a pain reliever, primarily in the treatment of migraine headaches. Other barbiturates, or "barbs" as they are commonly known, are available but rarely prescribed. Barbiturates have a narrow therapeutic index and are responsible for the highest risk of morbidity and mortality of all sedative-hypnotic agents (Baltarowich, 1985).

Signs and Symptoms

Sedation is the primary clinical effect of barbiturate intoxication. Signs of significant barbiturate overdose may include hypothermia, bradycardia, hypotension, and coma. Unlike benzodiazepines, which are discussed in the next section, barbiturates alone do induce hypoventilation, respiratory depression, and sometimes apnea. Co-ingestion of other sedative-hypnotic agents, alcohol, or opioids causes synergistic inhibition of the respiratory drive.

Secondary injury after barbiturate ingestion often occurs as a result of hypoxemia, hypotension, and tissue hypoperfusion. Renal injury and elevated liver enzymes are common laboratory abnormalities. Hypoxic brain injury may also occur. Another common effect of barbiturate toxicity is loss of airway reflexes and aspiration pneumonia, which in severe cases can precipitate acute respiratory distress syndrome (ARDS). In addition, prolonged immobilization while comatose can lead to skin breakdown, rhabdomyolysis, and compartment syndrome, depending on the patient's position. Pressure ulcers found in comatose patients are often still referred to as "barb blisters" because of the historical prevalence of this complication among patients with barbiturate overdose, but the nickname is misleading. These fluid-filled bullae are the indirect effect of protracted pressure on skin during immobilization and can occur in patients immobilized for any reason; they're not a direct result of barbiturate toxicity.

Pathophysiology

Barbiturates act primarily through $GABA_A$ receptor binding. $GABA_A$ receptor agonist action prolongs the duration of chloride influx and hyperpolarizes the cell membrane. Therefore, $GABA_A$ agonists cause neuroinhibition and sedation. This mechanism is primarily responsible for the therapeutic and toxic effects of barbiturates. Sedative activity is further potentiated by inhibition of the excitatory neurotransmitter glutamate at the NMDA receptor.

Diagnosis

Associated mental status depression often makes an accurate history difficult to obtain in a patient with barbiturate overdose. In patients who are found unresponsive, the position of the patient on discovery and an estimate of the duration of toxicity may be helpful in guiding treatment and predicting outcome. This information can usually be obtained from friends or family.

After your initial evaluation of airway, breathing, and vital signs, conduct a thorough neurologic exam, including assessment of cranial nerves and deep tendon reflexes. The absence of these reflexes indicates severe toxicity. The patient may also have decreased bowel sounds and abdominal distention. Pulmonary exam may reveal bradypnea with or without rales, but this exam can be normal in patients with only mild toxicity. Pay special attention to skin bullae during the musculoskeletal exam, and palpate the muscle compartments of the upper and lower extremities. Early identification of compartment syndrome can significantly improve the patient's overall outcome.

Treatment

Prehospital Management of barbiturate toxicity in the prehospital setting consists primarily of supportive care. Ventilatory assistance and airway management are required in patients with significant respiratory depression, refractory hypoxemia despite high-flow oxygen delivery, evidence of hypercapnia on end-tidal carbon dioxide detectors, or inability to protect the airway. If airway patency and ventilatory effort are adequate, give the patient supplemental oxygen, elevate the head to prevent aspiration, and use a nasal trumpet if upper airway soft-tissue obstruction is present and the patient tolerates placement. Establish IV access and give IV fluid boluses with normal saline to treat volume depletion from decreased oral intake, mild hypotension, and possible rhabdomyolysis.

Emergency Department Evaluation of barbiturate-intoxicated patients in the ED begins with assessment of airway and breathing, which may include testing of arterial or venous blood gases for hypercapnia and acidosis and a chest x-ray to rule out aspiration pneumonitis. After stabilization of respiratory status, urine drug screening may confirm barbiturate exposure. Quantitative evaluation of serum phenobarbital levels is available in most hospitals, but results won't necessarily correlate with toxicity. Differences in chronicity of use and patient tolerance will mean the clinical status of the patient, not the drug level, should dictate care. In general, phenobarbital levels above 80 mg/L are considered lethal.

Evaluation of secondary toxicity includes renal and liver function tests, an ECG, analysis of cardiac enzymes, and brain imaging to check for evidence of hypoxic injury. Muscle breakdown and consequent rhabdomyolysis, which often complicates toxicity, is indicated by elevated CPK with or without renal injury. Serial CPK measurements and renal function tests are frequently obtained to follow progression and resolution of the condition. Electroencephalogram tracings may be severely inhibited, resembling findings consistent with the profound sedation of brain death. Evaluation for brain death should not be performed, however, until barbiturate toxicity has resolved.

Airway management, including endotracheal intubation, is often required in significant toxicity, but mild to moderate toxicity may necessitate only supplemental oxygen and continuous pulse oximetry. Hypotension is treated initially with IV boluses of normal saline; refractory hypotension warrants vasopressor administration. The choice of vasopressor generally depends on the physician's preference. Norepinephrine and dopamine are most commonly used, but no randomized controlled study shows benefit of any one pressor compared with others in patients with barbiturate toxicity. Beyond respiratory and circulatory support, general supportive care (hydration, elevation of the head, wound care, prevention of recurrence) is the mainstay of treatment.

Accelerated elimination of barbiturates has been demonstrated with urinary alkalinization, achieved with a sodium bicarbonate infusion. The infusion is prepared by adding 100 to 150 mEq of sodium bicarbonate (2 or 3 ampules) to 1 L of a 5% dextrose in water solution (D_5W). Addition of 30 mEq of potassium chloride helps prevent severe hypokalemia associated with bicarbonate administration. The endpoint of treatment is improvement in mental status rather than a specific serum drug level. In severe cases of toxicity that fail to respond sufficiently to standard therapy, hemodialysis has been effectively employed to hasten recovery.

Special Populations You must also be cognizant of the effect of barbiturate withdrawal in an agitated patient. As with all GABA-agonist withdrawal syndromes, the patient may have tachycardia, hypertension, tremor, seizure, or delirium. Treatment is the same regardless of the offending agent. Long-acting barbiturates (e.g., phenobarbital [Luminal]) or benzodiazepines (e.g., diazepam [Valium] or lorazepam [Ativan]) are used to prevent and treat withdrawal. Withdrawal from long-acting barbiturates is uncommon because of their long half-life.

Benzodiazepines, Sedative-Hypnotics, and Tranquilizers

Sedative-hypnotic medications include a variety of drug classes in addition to barbiturates. Because of the similarities among these drugs, we'll use the term *benzodiazepines* to include all sedative-hypnotics.

Benzodiazepines were introduced in the 1960s, largely replacing barbiturates because of their improved safety profile and lower potential for addiction. As a group, these medications are frequently prescribed, overdose toxicity is common, but significant morbidity or death due to benzodiazepine ingestion alone is rare. The risk of morbidity and mortality is greater when a benzodiazepine is co-ingested with another CNS depressant such as alcohol, an opioid, or a barbiturate. Benzodiazepines do not cause respiratory depression on their own, but they may be responsible for a decreased ability to protect the airway. The other agents just mentioned have similar effects on respiration.

TABLE 9-10 Duration and Half-Life of Selected Benzodiazepines

Estimated Duration	Benzodiazepine/ Benzodiazepine-like Drug	Half-Life (hours)
Short	zolpidem (Ambien)	1.4–4.5
	triazolam (Halcion)	1.5–5.5
Intermediate	oxazepam (Serax)	3–25
	temazepam (Restoril)	5–20
	alprazolam (Xanax)	6.3–26.9
	lorazepam (Ativan)	10–20
Long	chlordiazepoxide (Librium)	5–48
	clonazepam (Klonopin)	18–50
	diazepam (Valium)	20–80

Benzodiazepines are differentiated from one another by half-life of the parent compound, estimated duration of action, and presence of active metabolites. Table 9-10 lists this information for selected common benzodiazepines, as well as for the benzodiazepine-like drug zolpidem (Ambien).

Signs and Symptoms

Patients with benzodiazepine overdose exhibit a variable clinical picture. Perhaps most notable is the fact that depression of the respiratory rate typically does not occur after benzodiazepine ingestion alone, even with massive overdoses. Some patients display mild bradycardia but rarely develop clinically significant hypotension. Hypoxemia may be present, however, in cases of aspiration pneumonitis or concomitant ingestion of another sedative or opioid. Underlying respiratory disease, such as COPD, may also cause respiratory complications. Pressure ulcers may occur after protracted immobilization, but as with "barb blisters" are not specific to benzodiazepines. Firmness of muscle compartments indicates muscle injury and possible compartment syndrome.

Neurologic signs and symptoms vary with the degree of sedation. Mild intoxication with benzodiazepines causes ataxia, slurred speech, somnolence, and nystagmus. Severe toxicity induces deep sedation, but the patient exhibits essentially normal vital signs. Patients may display hyporeflexia and sluggish cranial nerve reflexes. They often arouse slightly with noxious stimuli, but some have no response.

Pathophysiology

Benzodiazepines affect $GABA_A$ receptors, allowing increased frequency of chloride channel opening. This mechanism has CNS depressant effects and produces anxiolysis. More recently, nonbenzodiazepine sleep aids like zolpidem, zaleplon, and eszopiclone (Ambien, Sonata, and Lunesta, respectively) have surpassed benzodiazepines in popularity for treatment of sleep disorders, but they are less potent anxiolytics. The primary activity of all these drugs is $GABA_A$ agonism.

Diagnosis

As with barbiturate toxicity, history is usually difficult to obtain from a patient suffering from benzodiazepine-induced toxicity. History of medication availability and a scene survey may aid in your diagnosis. Obviously, the patient's having a current prescription for a benzodiazepine boosts the likelihood of ingestion simply because it confirms that the drug was available to him or her.

If the cause of altered mental status is unknown, a broad workup is performed, frequently including CT of the brain, measurement of ammonia level, liver function tests, CBC, and urine drug screen. Most urine drug screens include benzodiazepine testing, but they may yield false-negative results. For confirmation, the provider must often rely on a history of exposure and a clinical course consistent with benzodiazepine toxicity in the absence of other sedating drugs.

Treatment

Treatment of benzodiazepine toxicity consists primarily of supportive care. Administration of IV fluids, electrolyte repletion, head elevation, supplemental oxygen, and serial evaluation of CPK and kidney function result in favorable outcomes for most patients.

Prehospital The most important prehospital intervention is to protect the patient from aspiration by positioning him or her properly. You should also administer supplemental oxygen. It may be necessary to place an oral airway or nasal trumpet if the patient has evidence of upper airway obstruction like snoring or elevated end-tidal carbon dioxide, but many patients will not tolerate this intervention.

Establishing IV access and infusing normal saline may be helpful, particularly in patients with borderline blood pressure or evidence of prolonged down time. Patients occasionally have mild hypotension, but it's generally fluid responsive; administration of vasopressors will not likely be required. Give activated charcoal only after careful consideration. It's not usually recommended after benzodiazepine ingestion because of progressive mental status deterioration and the accompanying risk of aspiration. If the patient already shows evidence of mental status changes, activated charcoal is contraindicated.

Emergency Department After addressing the airway and the patient's cardiovascular status, ED evaluation consists of identifying potential co-ingestions, particularly acetaminophen and salicylate, and assessing secondary organ injury due to toxicity. As with all sedatives, kidney injury caused by rhabdomyolysis is a concern. Total CPK, electrolytes, BUN, and creatinine are usually obtained. Arterial or venous blood gases may be measured if hypoventilation is of concern.

Endotracheal intubation to protect the airway is occasionally required, but patients rarely need prolonged ventilation. The routine use of the GABA antagonist, flumazenil, is not recommended (see earlier discussion of the drug).

Special Considerations

Benzodiazepine withdrawal is an important syndrome for prehospital providers to recognize. Signs and symptoms are similar to alcohol withdrawal and include tachycardia, hypertension, diaphoresis, tremor, seizure, and delirium. This syndrome is most often seen in patients who are chronically dependent on short- or intermediate-acting benzodiazepines, especially alprazolam (Xanax). Administration of long-acting benzodiazepines followed by tapering doses is the treatment of choice for this disorder.

Toxicity of older nonbenzodiazepine sedative-hypnotics may have unusual features. Carisoprodol (Soma) is prescribed as a centrally acting muscle relaxant. In addition to producing sedation from GABA agonist effects, toxicity may produce sinus tachycardia and myoclonic jerking (Roth, 1998). The exact mechanism of toxicity is unclear. Chloral hydrate can cause myocardial sensitization to endogenous catecholamines, as can all halogenated hydrocarbons. As a result, patients are at risk for ventricular dysrhythmia that may respond to beta-blocker therapy. Zolpidem, zaleplon, and eszopiclone (Ambien, Sonata, and Lunesta, respectively) are GABA agonists but not benzodiazepines. Nevertheless, their toxic effects are similar, and they are likewise reversible with flumazenil. Overall, these drugs are associated with less severe toxicity and withdrawal.

Opioids and Opiates

Opiates and opioids (synthetic opiates) are CNS depressants. Fentanyl (Duragesic, Sublimaze), morphine (Duramorph, MS Contin), methadone (Dolophine), oxycodone (Percodan), meperidine (Demerol), propoxyphene (Darvon), heroin, codeine, and opium are included in this drug class. Heroin is a bitter-tasting, white or off-white powder. It has usually been adulterated, or cut, with various substances like sugar, baking soda, or starch. The depressant effect of these drugs increases the risk of respiratory failure when an overdose occurs.

Opioids may be administered orally, intranasally (snorting), intradermally (skin popping), intravenously (mainlining), or by inhalation (smoking). A "speed ball" is a bolus of heroin and cocaine injected IV. Injection "track marks" can often be seen in abusers who "mainline," but the absence of obvious injection sites does not rule out a possible heroin or opioid overdose.

Signs and Symptoms

Signs and symptoms of opioid overdose may include:

- Euphoria or irritability
- Diaphoresis
- Tremors
- Miosis (pupil constriction)
- Abdominal cramps
- Nausea and vomiting
- Hyperthermia
- CNS depression
- Respiratory depression
- Hypotension
- Bradycardia or tachycardia
- Pulmonary edema

These signs and symptoms can generally be treated with supportive care. CNS depression, pinpoint pupils, and respiratory depression—the so-called opiate triad—are classic signs. Severe intoxication can cause respiratory arrest, seizures, and coma. Opioid intoxication is distinguished from other causes of toxicity on the basis of euphoria, pinpoint pupils, and hypotension.

Pathophysiology

Opiates and opioids act on the opiate receptors in the brain and cause CNS depression. Their effects can be agonistic or antagonistic, depending on the opioid in question.

Diagnosis

A thorough physical exam and patient history are necessary to determine the etiology of the toxicity. It's especially important to determine the type of opiate, the quantity ingested, the time of ingestion, and whether any other toxins were co-ingested. Lab studies are dictated by these findings. Drug screens are not particularly useful in simple intoxications, but they may be helpful in identifying the offending agent in more complicated poisonings. In severe intoxications, a metabolic panel, CBC, creatine kinase level, and ABG analysis are indicated. Imaging is useful if the patient is suspected of having swallowed drug packages, either for transport or for evasion of law enforcement.

Treatment

Treatment of opiate and opioid overdose consists of supportive care and administration of the antidote agent, naloxone (Narcan). This drug is structurally similar to opioids but has only antagonistic properties. It displaces the opioid molecules from the opiate receptors, reducing the effective opiate dose. This process reverses miosis, respiratory depression, altered mental status, and even coma. Naloxone is useful in overdose of almost all opioids and opioid-like chemicals. Responsiveness to naloxone is indicative of opioid or other narcotic poisoning. The drug is typically given in small doses. The aim is to relieve respiratory depression, yet leave the patient in a responsive but lethargic state. Users sometimes become agitated or violent when their "high" wears off unexpectedly, and they are faced with people in uniform. Seizure activity is a possible side effect, so naloxone should be reserved for patients with respiratory depression.

Prehospital Supportive care, including management of airway, breathing, and circulation, is of primary importance. Airway management is of special concern because of the CNS depressive effects of opiates. Administer naloxone early if significant CNS depression is evident, but be cautious when doing so. Increased patient alertness may also lead to escalating combativeness. Consider applying restraints before administration and summoning law enforcement to accompany you during treatment and transport.

Emergency Department In the hospital, supportive care and monitoring are vital to preventing unexpected CNS depression after opiate antagonist treatment wears off. Naloxone acts for 30 to 120 minutes, whereas opioids typically act for 3 to 6 hours. Cardiac monitoring is important, especially for severe intoxication.

Drugs of Abuse

Although many legally prescribed drugs with legitimate medical uses (e.g., opiates, benzodiazepines) are subject to diversion and intentional misuse or abuse, in the following sections we'll discuss drugs that have few or no legitimate medical uses. For purposes of classification, they can be considered primarily drugs of abuse; ethanol is included in this section. Of course, alcoholic beverages are enjoyed responsibly by many people, but alcohol is undeniably subject to widespread abuse as well. The toxic alcohols—ethylene glycol, isopropyl alcohol, and methanol—are discussed later in the section on home and workplace toxins.

Methamphetamine Laboratories

Methamphetamine laboratories pose a particular danger to emergency medical services (EMS) healthcare providers. The chemicals used to manufacture methamphetamine are extremely volatile, and toxic gases such as phosphine can be generated as a byproduct of meth production. Exposure to such chemicals can cause mucous membrane irritation, headaches, burns, and death. Of even greater concern is the risk of explosion of improvised explosive devices (IEDs). Meth manufacturers often place IED booby traps in and around their makeshift labs to deter thieves and law enforcement personnel from entering. Never enter such a facility without law enforcement support. If you inadvertently enter a meth lab, exit immediately using the same route by which you entered. If you should come upon a patient while exiting, you should remove him or her as quickly as possible.

Cocaine

Cocaine is derived from the coca plant, which is native to South America. Cocaine is a strong CNS stimulant, causing robust sympathetic discharge that results in increased catecholamine release. The lethal dose in the average adult is estimated to be about 1200 mg. Most fatalities occur from cardiac dysrhythmia, which can occur at a much lower dose in a susceptible person.

Two forms of cocaine are in common use today:

1. Powdered cocaine, a fine white crystalline substance that is cocaine in its pure form. It's typically inhaled, or snorted, through the nose.
2. Freebase ("crack") cocaine, which takes the form of solid white or off-white lumps, crystals, or rocks. In this form, the drug is much more potent than in its powdered form. The rocks of cocaine are heated and their fumes inhaled in a fashion similar to that of smoking a cigarette.

Signs and Symptoms

Cocaine produces a high that users say makes them feel euphoric and energetic. Because cocaine is a CNS stimulant, people high on cocaine often appear mentally alert and talkative. Unlike opiates, cocaine stimulates the sympathetic nervous system, causing dilated but sluggish pupils, tachycardia, vasoconstriction, and hypertension. Vasoconstriction and increased motor activity may in turn cause hyperthermia. Because dopamine reuptake is limited, seizures may occur. The risk of stroke is significantly increased. For many reasons, chief among them cardiac stimulation and hypertension, sudden death is not uncommon among people who use cocaine.

Pathophysiology

Cocaine has a wide variety of effects on the body. It acts as a local anesthetic by reversibly inhibiting sodium channels, blocking nerve conduction. In the myocardium, it decreases the rate of depolarization and the amplitude of the action potential. Cocaine also inhibits the reuptake of norepinephrine and dopamine at the preganglionic sympathetic nerve endings, causing central and peripheral adrenergic stimulation (activation of the brain's pleasure center). It causes catecholamine to accumulate at the postsynaptic membranes by preventing reuptake. This increases intracellular calcium levels and sustains the action potential of neurotransmitters, resulting in vasoconstriction, hypertension, tachycardia, and increased myocardial oxygen consumption. Taken together, these effects stress the heart, sometimes inducing ventricular fibrillation.

Diagnosis

Diagnosis of any suspected cocaine overdose should begin with a good patient history that includes what substance was used, how it was administered, in what quantity, and how long ago. When a patient has an unremarkable history and mild symptoms, a lab workup is generally not needed. If a history is unavailable or if clinically significant toxicity is noted, however, appropriate lab studies may include a CBC, measurement of glucose, calcium, BUN, creatinine, electrolytes, and troponin (or creatine kinase), a pregnancy test, a urinalysis, and a toxicology screen. The creatine kinase screen may help eliminate rhabdomyolysis as a cause of the patient's signs and symptoms. Serum cocaine levels are unreliable and thus not clinically useful because the drug has a short half-life (30 to 45 minutes). Standard cardiac diagnostic protocols should be followed in patients with chest pain.

Imaging studies may be useful to rule out head injuries and respiratory issues, and they may reveal signs of drug abuse (such as granulomatous changes caused by parenteral abuse) or show whether the patient has swallowed packets of drugs (see earlier discussion of "packers").

Treatment

Supportive care, including support of airway, breathing, and circulation, is the primary treatment for cocaine intoxication. Supplemental oxygen, establishing IV access, cardiac monitoring, and pulse oximetry are usually indicated.

Because its cardiovascular effects are similar to those of cocaine, epinephrine should be avoided if possible in patients with cocaine intoxication. Vasopressin is often a better alternative. Some evidence also indicates that nonselective beta-blockers should be avoided in these patients.

Prehospital Cocaine users, especially after consuming large doses, can exhibit erratic or violent behavior. Your safety is of paramount importance. Summon help from law enforcement early, and monitor the patient's body language and behavior carefully.

Rule out hypoglycemia by performing a serum glucose. Patients with dysrhythmias require aggressive cardiac care. Initiate cardiac monitoring with a 12-lead ECG to look for cardiac ischemia due to coronary vasospasm. Use benzodiazepines as necessary to calm the patient, reduce CNS stimulation, and treat seizures.

Emergency Department Hyperpyrexia must be treated aggressively. Hypoglycemia, cardiac symptoms, and trauma should be treated per standard protocols. The effects of cocaine are generally short lived, so the patient can usually be discharged after 2 to 6 hours of uneventful observation.

Ethanol

Ethanol is not a particularly toxic chemical at low doses, as evidenced by its legal use in beer, wine, and distilled spirits, but chronic overuse causes significant morbidity, including cirrhosis and different types of cancer. Because of its wide availability and classification as a food, ethanol causes more toxicologic emergencies than any other kind of alcohol. Most cases are classified as intentional because they involve alcoholic beverages. Ethanol is also used in industrial solvents.

Signs and Symptoms

Signs and symptoms of ethanol intoxication vary by blood alcohol level and may include euphoria, inebriation, confusion, lethargy, CNS depression, ataxia (and associated injuries from falls), stupor, respiratory depression, hypothermia, hypotension, coma, and cardiovascular collapse (Table 9-11).

Extreme intoxication can lead to decreased levels of consciousness, severe respiratory difficulties, or death. Preexisting conditions are often exacerbated by the effects of ethanol. Vasodilation may lead to hypotension and hypothermia. The latter may be severe, depending on the patient and the ambient conditions. Vasodilation may also dangerously reduce cardiac output in predisposed individuals.

Pathophysiology

Ethanol is readily absorbed into the bloodstream through the GI tract, primarily in the small intestine and stomach. Most of the alcohol consumed is absorbed within an hour. Ethanol passes easily through the blood-brain barrier. This property is responsible for the intoxicating effects of ethanol on the CNS. Although the exact mechanism by which ethanol produces these effects is unclear, the chemical is believed to affect the function of neurotransmitters, probably including GABA.

TABLE 9-11 Effects of Ethanol Related to BAC

BAC (%)	Effects
0.02	Few obvious effects, slight intensification of mood
0.05	Loss of emotional restraint, feeling of warmth, flushing of skin, mild impairment of judgment
0.10	Slight slurring of speech, loss of fine motor control, unstable emotions, inappropriate laughter
0.12	Coordination and balance difficult, distinct impairment of mentation and judgment
0.20	Responsive to verbal stimuli, very slurred speech, staggering gait, diplopia (double vision), difficulty standing upright, memory loss
0.30	Briefly aroused by painful stimuli; deep, snoring respirations
0.40	Unresponsiveness, incontinence, hypotension, irregular respirations
0.50	Death possible from apnea, hypotension, or aspiration of vomitus

BAC, Blood alcohol concentration.
From Aehlert B: Paramedic practice today: above and beyond, St Louis, 2009, Mosby.

Diagnosis

The laboratory workup of a patient with suspected ethanol intoxication should include:

- Serum glucose level to rule out hypoglycemia
- Serum ethanol level
- Serum electrolytes (e.g., calcium, magnesium)
- Serum osmolality to calculate the osmolar gap
- Electrolyte levels to determine the size of the anion gap
- Pregnancy testing
- Testing for toxic levels of drugs that may have been co-ingested, such as acetaminophen, salicylates, and methanol
- Imaging studies in patients with severely altered mental status or possible trauma suggested by history or physical exam

Treatment

A good patient history must be obtained to determine the type and amount of alcohol consumed and the time of consumption. Treatment is mainly supportive: maintaining airway, breathing, and circulation and establishing IV access. Cardiac monitoring is especially indicated if the patient has a preexisting heart condition. Opiate ingestion and hypoglycemia should be ruled out by administering naloxone (Narcan) and performing a serum glucose test, respectively. Thiamine, a cofactor needed to process ethanol, may be indicated after heavy alcohol use, and hemodialysis may be considered in significant ethanol toxicity.

Prehospital The airway is vulnerable because of the CNS depressive effects of ethanol. As a result, airway management may be necessary if the patient is severely intoxicated.

Emergency Department In the ED, body temperature should be monitored. Endotracheal intubation is often necessary in severely intoxicated patients. Gastric lavage is indicated if less than 1 hour has elapsed since the exposure. Activated charcoal is not effective for ethanol but may be helpful if other toxins like acetaminophen were co-ingested. Emetics are not recommended because of the risks associated with CNS depression.

Hallucinogens

Hallucinogens cause visual disturbances (hallucinations) and alter the user's perception of reality. They include substances such as L-lysergic acid diethylamide (LSD), peyote, mescaline, and psychedelic mushrooms. Hallucinogens can be grouped into four major classes:

1. Indole alkaloids (e.g., LSD, lysergic acid amide [LSA], psilocin, and psilocybin)
2. Piperidines (e.g., PCP and ketamine)

3. Phenylethylamines (e.g., mescaline, MDMA, methylenedioxyamphetamine [MDA], and methoxymethylenedioxyamphetamine [MMDA])
4. Cannabinoids (e.g., marijuana or tetrahydrocannabinol [THC])

Signs and Symptoms

Patients who have ingested hallucinogens can exhibit dangerous and sometimes bizarre behavior. They have altered mental status, perhaps including behavioral disturbances such as aggressiveness, delusional or paranoid thinking, and visual illusions (hallucinations). CNS effects of the drug can include stimulation or depression, depending on the causative agent, the dose, and the time elapsed since poisoning. Other possible effects include hypertension and tachycardia. Hallucinogen toxicity is distinguished from other possible causes on the basis of behavioral abnormalities and hallucinations.

Pathophysiology

The pathophysiology of hallucinogenic drugs is only imperfectly understood, but the principal effects of the drugs are concentrated in the CNS. It's generally believed that hallucinogens alter both serotonin and norepinephrine concentrations in the brain. Indole amine derivatives are thought to act on serotonin receptors. Piperidine derivatives are thought to block serotonin, dopamine, and norepinephrine reuptake. Phenylethylamine derivatives block serotonin and norepinephrine reuptake and even increase their presynaptic release.

In the case of cannabinoids, the component delta (9)-tetrahydrocannabinol (THC) is the source of pharmacologic effects. The chemical causes maximum plasma concentration within minutes and psychotropic effects in 2 to 3 hours.

Diagnosis

A lab workup is not particularly helpful for hallucinogen intoxication. Selected studies may be needed to differentiate it from other etiologies. A comprehensive drug screen may be indicated to rule out co-ingestion or to confirm a questionable diagnosis. Imaging studies are useful only to assess other possible causes of the patient's symptoms.

Treatment

A hallucinogen user may seek medical attention to treat traumatic injuries associated with hallucinogen use or to alleviate unpleasant or distressing psychotropic effects of the drug—a so-called bad trip. Hallucinogens typically have minimal acute side effects. Some patients become violent, and physical or chemical restraints and law enforcement assistance may be needed. Primary treatment consists of calming the patient and providing reassurance that the drug's effects are temporary.

LSD is skin absorptive, and every effort should be made to avoid cross-contamination. The job is interesting enough as it is.

Prehospital Manage traumatic injuries per protocol. Acquire a thorough patient history to help determine the correct etiology and ultimately to identify the hallucinogen.

Emergency Department After thorough evaluation, LSD-intoxicated patients should be isolated to help them remain calm. They may require sedation with benzodiazepines. In severe psychotic episodes, haloperidol may be indicated. LSD intoxication lasts about 8 to 12 hours, but the psychotic effects of the drug may persist for days.

Phencyclidine

The most common hallucinogen is phencyclidine (PCP), which was originally developed as a general anesthetic and later used as a veterinary tranquilizer. When its potential for abuse was discovered, it was replaced with safer alternatives. PCP has CNS stimulatory and depressant properties. It's available as a white crystalline powder, a liquid, or a tablet.

Signs and Symptoms

At low doses (10 mg or less), PCP produces a combination of psychoactive effects, including euphoria, disorientation and confusion, and sudden mood swings (such as rage). Signs of PCP use may include flushing, diaphoresis, hypersalivation, and vomiting. The pupils generally remain reactive. Facial grimacing and nystagmus, or involuntary eye movement, are identifiable effects of low-dose PCP use.

PCP users are much less sensitive to pain, which may give them the appearance of having superhuman strength as they overexert themselves. In fact, at low doses, mortality is associated with self-destructive behavior related to the analgesic and CNS depressant effects of PCP. Remember, patients under the influence of hallucinogens pose a threat to themselves and others, including the providers on scene.

High doses of PCP (>10 mg) may produce extreme CNS depression, including coma. Respiratory depression, hypertension, and tachycardia are common. The hypertension may cause cardiac difficulties, encephalopathy, intracerebral hemorrhage, and seizure. High-dose overdoses may require management of respiratory arrest, cardiac arrest, and status epilepticus. Such patients must be rapidly transported to the hospital.

Acute onset of PCP psychosis may occur even at low doses. This condition is a true psychiatric emergency that may persist for days or weeks after the exposure. Behavior can range from unresponsiveness (a catatonic state) to violent and enraged. Such patients can be extremely dangerous, and law enforcement should accompany you as you transport the patient to an appropriate medical facility.

Pathophysiology

PCP is a dissociative anesthetic with hallucinogenic properties. It has both stimulant and depressant effects on the CNS. Its sympathomimetic effects are probably due to dopamine and norepinephrine reuptake inhibition. The drug also acts at nicotinic and opioid receptors, has cholinergic and anticholinergic effects, is a glutamate antagonist at NDMA receptors, and affects the dopamine pathway. Clearly, PCP produces some very complicated interactions that researchers are still attempting to delineate fully. PCP is metabolized in the liver and has a half-life of about 15 to 20 hours.

Diagnosis

Patient history is critical to making a diagnosis of PCP intoxication. The lab workup should include urine toxicology screening, a metabolic panel, measurement of serum glucose level, a CBC, and analysis of ABGs. An elevated WBC count and increased BUN and creatinine levels are often seen in patients with PCP intoxication. Rhabdomyolysis can be assessed by monitoring serum creatine kinase and urine myoglobin levels.

Treatment

Primary treatment consists of calming the patient and providing reassurance that the drug's effects are temporary. You must obtain a thorough patient history to determine the correct etiology of the patient's signs and symptoms and to identify the hallucinogen ingested. The history should include the type and amount of drug ingested and the time at which the ingestion occurred. Endotracheal intubation will probably be necessary in severely intoxicated patients.

Prehospital Treatment is mainly supportive, including maintaining airway, breathing, and circulation and establishing IV access. Manage traumatic injuries per protocol.

Emergency Department Cardiac monitoring is indicated in any patient with a suspected PCP overdose who has a preexisting heart condition. The patient should be kept calm, and abrupt movements, bright lights, and noise should be avoided. Physical or chemical restraints may be necessary if the patient becomes erratic or violent. Benzodiazepines work well for this purpose. Antipsychotic agents such as haloperidol should not be given to patients with PCP intoxication, because they may induce cardiac dysrhythmia or seizure. Opiate use and hypoglycemia should be ruled out.

Toxins in the Home and Workplace

In the following sections, we'll explore common causes of toxic exposure in the home and workplace. Some poisons, such as carbon monoxide, are inhaled. Others, such as antifreeze, are swallowed. Toxins such as pesticides and corrosives are absorbed through the skin or cause dermal irritation and burns. Of course, many of the poisons we'll discuss have important industrial uses and may even be capable of causing mass-casualty disasters (e.g., during a train derailment). But on a day-to-day basis, as a prehospital provider you're most likely to encounter these toxins in patient's home or workplace.

THE TOXIC ALCOHOLS

Ethylene Glycol

Ethylene glycol, one of the toxic alcohols, is found in automotive antifreeze, windshield-washer fluid, and deicers. It's used to prevent overheating and freezing of elements found in these substances. Because it tastes sweet, it's more likely to be ingested accidentally and in larger quantities by children and pets. However, 70% of cases of ethylene glycol poisoning occur in adults, and most such exposures are accidental. The toxicity results from conversion of the alcohol to metabolites. According to the annual 2007 report of the American Association of Poison Control Centers' National Poison Data System, almost 900 had minor outcomes from related toxicity, approximately 150 had severe outcomes, and 16 deaths occurred.

Ingestion is the primary route of exposure, since ethylene glycol is not readily absorbed through the skin and has a low vapor pressure that prevents its aerosolization during inhalation.

Signs and Symptoms

Ethylene glycol toxicity typically occurs in three stages:

- **Stage 1 (1 to 12 hours post ingestion)** is characterized by CNS effects, including signs of intoxication such as slurred speech, ataxia, sleepiness, nausea and vomiting, convulsions, hallucinations, stupor, and coma.
- **Stage 2 (12 to 36 hours post ingestion)** is characterized by cardiopulmonary effects, which may include tachypnea, cyanosis, pulmonary edema, or cardiac arrest.
- **Stage 3 (24 to 72 hours post ingestion)** affects the renal system and may include flank pain, oliguria, crystalluria, proteinuria, anuria, hematuria, or uremia.

Not all patients go through all stages. Depending on the patient's physiology, any preexisting conditions, and the quantity ingested, some patients develop life-threatening symptoms early. Life-threatening signs and symptoms include intoxication, headache, CNS depression, respiratory difficulty, metabolic acidosis, cardiovascular collapse, renal failure, seizures, and coma.

Pathophysiology

Ethylene glycol is metabolized into glycolic acid and oxalic acid by the enzyme, alcohol dehydrogenase, in the liver. These two metabolites cause most of the significant toxicity, acidosis, and kidney damage associated with ethylene glycol ingestion. The oxalic acid sequesters and binds calcium in the body to form calcium oxalate, which precipitates out and forms crystals. This process has two detrimental effects. First, it causes hypocalcemia, which increases the risk of cardiac dysrhythmia. Second, it causes severe joint pain at the sites of crystal deposition. These oxalic acid crystals can wreak havoc on the liver and kidneys, but the destruction usually doesn't become evident until a sufficient amount of the toxic metabolite has accumulated to cause damage. The threshold for ethylene glycol toxicity has been reported to be 1 to 2 mL/kg.

Diagnosis

Patients with ethylene glycol ingestion may initially have an unremarkable physical examination until enough toxic metabolites build up to cause signs and symptoms. Serum osmolality may be used to calculate the osmolar gap. Alternatively, a qualitative colorimetric test may be used to detect the presence of ethylene glycol in serum (Long, 2008). In addition, a urinalysis and measurement of serum calcium levels and ABGs are indicated. Urinalysis may reveal the presence of calcium oxalate crystals, a late-stage sign.

Treatment

Supportive care, antidote administration, and hemodialysis are the core treatments for ethylene glycol poisoning. Supportive care should focus on airway management. Either ethanol or fomepizole (Antizol) can be administered as an antidote. Both are competitive inhibitors of alcohol dehydrogenase. Cofactor therapy consisting of pyridoxine (vitamin B_6) and thiamine (vitamin B_1) administration may be given to boost the metabolism of ethylene glycol. However, hemodialysis is the definitive treatment for ethylene glycol poisoning.

Prehospital In addition to basic treatment, obtain a detailed patient history, especially regarding the time of ingestion. Establish IV access for rehydration and for antidote therapy in extreme cases. If less than 1 hour has elapsed since the ingestion, activated charcoal may be beneficial, assuming no contraindications exist. Administer sodium bicarbonate for metabolic acidosis and diazepam (Valium) for seizures as necessary. Transport the patient rapidly to a hospital for hemodialysis.

Emergency Department The antidote for ethylene glycol poisoning has traditionally been ethanol, which is usually administered intravenously but can also be delivered orally. A newer antidote is fomepizole (Antizol), which works in similar fashion to ethanol. Ethanol is a competitive inhibitor of alcohol dehydrogenase and prevents the formation of toxic metabolites. Ethylene glycol itself is harmlessly excreted by the kidneys. In the body, the half-life of ethylene glycol is normally 5 hours, but with ethanol treatment it's 17 hours. This allows prolonged excretion time. Serum ethanol levels should be monitored to maintain the appropriate ethanol dose.

Magnesium and pyridoxine are cofactors in the detoxification of ethylene glycol poisoning. Cofactor therapy has been reported to reduce morbidity associated with ethylene glycol toxicity by converting glyoxylic acid to the nontoxic amino acid, glycine.

Hypocalcemia may be present in severe poisoning and requires treatment because insoluble calcium oxalate forms when the toxic metabolite oxalic acid binds with free calcium in the body. Sodium bicarbonate administration is indicated for metabolic acidosis.

Hemodialysis, which offers definitive treatment by removing toxic metabolites from the blood, is indicated by renal failure, serum assays, and severe acidosis.

Isopropyl Alcohol

Isopropyl alcohol is one of the toxic alcohols, but it's significantly less toxic than either methanol or ethylene glycol. Isopropyl alcohol (isopropanol or rubbing alcohol) is a common household and industrial solvent and is involved in many toxic exposures. It's also a common household item, found in items such as mouthwash, skin lotion, and hand disinfectant. Annually, thousands of isopropyl alcohol exposures are reported, although few result in fatalities. Isopropyl alcohol is often abused as an alternative to ethanol. In high doses, it can cause severe hypotension and cardiac ischemia.

Signs and Symptoms

The typical route of entry is oral. Large ingestions can cause acetonemia (acetone buildup in the blood) and ketonuria (ketone buildup in the urine). Signs and symptoms include confusion, lethargy, CNS depression, respiratory depression, ketonemia, mild hypothermia, hypotension, and coma. As a result of acetone production, you may notice a fruity breath odor similar to that of a person with diabetes.

Pathophysiology

Isopropanol is quickly absorbed in the stomach and metabolized into acetone, which is not particularly toxic. Isopropyl alcohol toxicity is similar to that of ethanol toxicity. As such, it's twice as strong a CNS depressant as ethyl alcohol and is also a vasodilator. The hypotension caused by vasodilation is typically resistant to fluid and vasopressor administration.

Diagnosis

A thorough physical exam and patient history are necessary to determine the etiology of the toxicity. Lab studies are dictated by the findings, but in severe intoxication, the workup may include measurement of ABGs and analysis of electrolytes and serum alcohol and bicarbonate levels.

Treatment

As with other drug intoxications, a serum glucose test should be performed to rule out alternative etiologies. Consider administration of naloxone if the patient exhibits respiratory depression, which may be due to concurrent opiate ingestion. Because of the low toxicity of the metabolites of isopropyl alcohol, ethanol therapy is not indicated. In fact, such therapy may actually exacerbate CNS depression and hypotension, the primary life-threatening complications associated with isopropyl alcohol toxicity.

Prehospital In the field, treatment is mainly supportive. Maintain airway, breathing, and circulation, and establish IV access. Consider giving activated charcoal if the ingestion has occurred within the last hour.

Emergency Department Hospital treatment is similar to prehospital treatment. Supportive care is of primary importance, gastric decontamination may be initiated, vasopressor therapy may be attempted, and hemodialysis may be indicated in cases of extreme intoxication or severe, unresponsive hypotension.

Methanol

Methanol (methyl alcohol or wood alcohol), a common household solvent, is a component of windshield-washer fluid, paint, gasoline treatments, and canned tabletop fuels such as Sterno. Methanol is used extensively in industry as a solvent and reagent. Intoxication usually follows oral ingestion; just a mouthful can be highly toxic. Methanol has been intentionally ingested as an ethanol substitute, although most poisonings appear to be accidental. Methanol is also absorbed through the skin but not particularly well. In addition, because of its high volatility, it's readily inhaled.

Signs and Symptoms

Methanol initially causes inebriation but to a lesser degree than the other alcohols. Early signs and symptoms mimic ethanol intoxication, with slurred speech, ataxia, drowsiness, and nausea and vomiting. Signs and symptoms of more severe toxicity include sedation, ataxia, headache, vertigo, nausea and vomiting, abdominal pain, respiratory difficulty, seizures, and coma. Vision complaints like blurred vision and visual haziness are an initial hallmark of methanol poisoning. The initial onset of symptoms can be rapid, occurring in as little as 30 minutes, or delayed up to 30 hours, depending on the dose and route of entry. After the initial symptoms have passed, a second set of symptoms can occur 10 to 30 hours after exposure. Complete loss of vision and snow blindness–like symptoms, acidosis, and respiratory failure can occur, especially when ethanol is co-ingested. A long asymptomatic phase does not necessarily preclude later toxicity. Mortality is associated with severe acidosis and cerebral edema.

Visual impairment indicates the need for an eye exam. The pupils may be dilated, with little response. The optic disc may be inflamed, and blindness can ensue over several days as the optic disc bleaches.

Pathophysiology

Methanol is a protoxin that is readily excreted by the kidneys if it escapes liver conversion. In the liver, it's converted by the enzyme, alcohol dehydrogenase, into formaldehyde, a short-lived intermediate metabolite. Formaldehyde is then converted by the enzyme, aldehyde dehydrogenase, into formic acid, which causes most of the significant toxicity, including possible metabolic acidosis and blindness. Onset of symptoms of toxicity is usually delayed 12 to 24 hours until the toxic metabolites have accumulated.

Diagnosis

A thorough physical exam and patient history are necessary to determine the etiology of the toxicity. Lab studies are dictated by the findings. In severe methanol intoxication, analysis of serum alcohol level, electrolytes, ABGs, and serum bicarbonate level is indicated. The serum methanol level can be measured directly in many labs, or it can be estimated by calculating the osmolar gap and the anion gap.

Treatment

As with other drug intoxications, a serum glucose test should be performed to rule out alternative etiologies. Consider administration of naloxone if the patient exhibits respiratory depression, which may be due to concurrent opiate ingestion.

Prehospital Treatment consists of maintaining airway, breathing, and circulation. Airway management is particularly important. Activated charcoal does not absorb methanol significantly and should not be used.

Emergency Department Hospital treatment consists of supportive care, antidote administration, and hemodialysis as indicated. Supportive care should focus on maintaining an airway. IV ethanol or fomepizole (Antizol) are given to minimize further production of toxic metabolites. Ethanol and fomepizole are both competitive inhibitors of alcohol dehydrogenase. Cofactor therapy consisting of tetrahydrofolate should be given to encourage the elimination of formic acid. If the ingestion occurred within the last hour, gastric lavage may be helpful. Hemodialysis is indicated in severe exposures in which the patient complains of visual symptoms, severe acidosis is present, or serum methanol levels are found to be high. Folate is a cofactor in the enzymatic detoxification of toxic methanol metabolites, and folate therapy has been reported to reduce morbidity.

Carbon Monoxide

In the United States, carbon monoxide is the leading cause of morbidity and mortality from poisoning. The Centers for Disease Control and Prevention (CDC) report that more than 2500 Americans die each year from carbon monoxide poisoning. As many as 40,000 can seek medical attention annually. Carbon monoxide is a colorless, odorless gas produced by incomplete combustion of organic fuels. Sources include household furnaces, space heaters, generators, and gas stoves, motor vehicles, and smoke from house fires. Any gasoline- or propane-powered engine, not only vehicle engines, can produce carbon monoxide.

In addition, methylene chloride, a chemical used as a paint stripper, degreaser, and industrial solvent, is metabolized to carbon monoxide in the liver. Significant inhalation exposure to methylene chloride can thus cause delayed carbon monoxide toxicity.

Signs and Symptoms

Symptoms of carbon monoxide toxicity range from mild to fatal, depending on the concentration of the gas and the duration of exposure. Patients often have fatigue, headache, myalgia, nausea, and vomiting. Severe toxicity can cause chest pain, shortness of breath, syncope, ataxia, seizure, and coma. In high concentrations, carbon monoxide is considered a knockdown agent, meaning that it causes rapid toxicity and loss of consciousness. In addition to primary cellular toxicity, the combined toxic effects of carbon monoxide can induce myocardial ischemia, decreased contractility, vasodilation, and hypotension. Patients with underlying cardiovascular disease are at increased risk of these adverse effects, so it's important to obtain a detailed past medical history.

The vital signs of a patient with carbon monoxide toxicity may be normal. However, the patient may have tachycardia, tachypnea, or hypotension. Oxygen saturation is usually normal, since pulse oximetry cannot differentiate between carboxyhemoglobin and oxyhemoglobin (see Chapter 3). Blood pressure and peripheral perfusion can be gauged by capillary refill evaluation. Cherry-red skin, a classically described examination finding, is explained by the presence of oxygenated venous blood as a result of the combined inability of hemoglobin to unload oxygen and of tissue to extract it. This finding is rare, though, and is typically a late sign. Pallor is more common. Pulmonary exam may reveal pulmonary edema caused by either cardiogenic failure or primary pulmonary toxicity. Except for nausea and vomiting, the abdominal exam is generally unremarkable.

On neurologic examination, mild abnormalities in gait and balance indicate significant exposure, whereas altered mental status and seizure coincide with severe toxicity. The patient may have focal neurologic deficits attributable to carbon monoxide–induced stroke. In some patients with carbon monoxide poisoning, the cascade of cytotoxicity and delayed injury leads to delayed neurologic sequelae. In contrast to focal deficits caused by localized tissue hypoxia, these sequelae often involve memory, personality, and behavior. Symptoms may not develop for several weeks after recovery from the acute event. Patients who have lost consciousness or had periods of hypotension are at risk for such delayed adverse effects, but it's impossible to predict either their occurrence or severity.

Pathophysiology

Carbon monoxide induces toxicity in a variety of ways. The most obvious is its effect on the function of hemoglobin. Carbon monoxide has greater affinity than oxygen for heme's oxygen-binding sites. It also inhibits the release of oxygen from hemoglobin. This combination results in decreased oxygen delivery to tissues despite a normal partial pressure of dissolved oxygen in the blood. Mitochondrial cytochrome oxidase is also bound by carbon monoxide, decreasing cellular activity and thus impairing energy production by oxidative phosphorylation. The effects of carbon monoxide toxicity are similar to those of cyanide. Myocardial myoglobin binding by carbon monoxide decreases oxygen extraction by cardiac myocytes, contributing to cardiac toxicity. Finally, carbon monoxide toxicity unleashes a volley of tissue injury by free radical formation, inflammatory mediators, delayed lipid peroxidation, and cellular apoptosis (programmed cell death).

Diagnosis

Mild carbon monoxide toxicity is probably underrecognized because its symptoms are either nonspecific or resemble those of a flulike illness. The diagnosis may be further complicated by the fact that unintentional carbon monoxide exposures tend to occur in cold-weather months, when furnaces are in use and the incidence of viral illness increases. Because carbon monoxide has no color or odor, its presence often goes undetected.

Diagnosis of carbon monoxide toxicity, then, depends heavily on gathering accurate information from the scene. Obviously, a history of running a motor vehicle or other engine is telling. The patient may have been in an enclosed space like a garage, with a motor running from a space heater, power generator, or other appliance. Household poisoning from a faulty furnace can provoke symptoms in several family members at once. Another historical clue might be the resolution of symptoms when the patient leaves the exposure source and the return of symptoms on reentering. Animals are often affected by carbon monoxide poisoning earlier and more severely than humans who are exposed to the same source. The patient may report that a pet has been acting strangely. Most fire departments are now equipped with carbon monoxide meters, which can be used to detect elevated levels of the dangerous gas at the scene, thereby accelerating diagnosis and treatment (see Chapter 3). Newer technology is now available for EMS providers which allows field measurement of a patient's carbon monoxide levels using a noninvasive oximetry device.

In addition to physical examination, supplemental laboratory and radiographic data are used to evaluate patients with carbon monoxide toxicity. The patient's carboxyhemoglobin level can be measured with the oximetry device and confirmed with a venous or arterial blood sample. The documentation of an elevated carboxyhemoglobin level aids in diagnosis, but for a variety of reasons, the specific level does not necessarily predict toxicity or outcome. A patient with severe carbon monoxide toxicity who has been managed with high-flow oxygen for a prolonged period before evaluation could have a normal carboxyhemoglobin level, whereas a patient with only mild symptoms may have a significantly elevated level. In fact, patients who are habitual tobacco smokers can have levels as high as 10%. Normal carboxyhemoglobin levels in nonsmokers range from zero to 5%.

In patients with direct carbon monoxide exposure, carboxyhemoglobin is measured only once, since the level cannot increase after the patient is removed from the source of carbon monoxide. Patients with suspected exposure to methylene chloride, however, require prolonged observation and repeated testing to ensure that toxicity has peaked, since the carboxyhemoglobin level rises as the body metabolizes methylene chloride.

Supplemental evaluation of the patient with suspected carbon monoxide exposure includes assessment of acid-base status. Metabolic acidosis may be accompanied by an elevated serum lactate as a result of impaired oxygen delivery and anaerobic respiration. An ECG is performed to assess myocardial ischemia. Cardiac enzyme studies are obtained and followed serially in patients with demonstrated toxicity. Brain imaging with unenhanced CT or magnetic resonance imaging (MRI) may be obtained. Early changes, particularly on CT, portend a poor neurologic outcome. MRI is more sensitive than CT to cerebral changes after carbon monoxide toxicity and is useful in identifying areas of ischemia and infarct.

Treatment

Prehospital The most important treatment for the patient, as well as for the provider, is immediate removal from the source of carbon monoxide. Even a brief exposure can be toxic if the gas is sufficiently concentrated. After moving him to a safe location, place the patient on high-flow oxygen delivered through a nonrebreather mask. Increasing the fractional concentration of oxygen in inspired gas (FIO_2) decreases the half-life of carbon monoxide binding, allowing it to be exhaled. In room air, the average half-life of carbon monoxide on hemoglobin is roughly 5 hours, but at 100% FIO_2, the half-life drops to 1 to 2 hours.

Employ standard airway management. If endotracheal intubation is required, maintain the patient on 100% FIO_2. Treat cardiac arrhythmias as you normally would after administration of oxygen. Hypotension often responds to IV boluses of normal saline; however, you may need to administer vasopressors. Otherwise, provide supportive care and symptomatic treatment. Whenever practical, a patient who shows evidence of significant carbon monoxide toxicity (loss of consciousness, neurologic deficits, myocardial ischemia) should be transported to a medical center that can deliver hyperbaric oxygen.

Emergency Department In the ED, the administration of high-flow oxygen is continued to hasten the dissociation of carbon monoxide from hemoglobin. Support of airway, breathing, and circulation is continued.

After hemodynamic stabilization, hyperbaric oxygen therapy is indicated. Hyperbaric oxygen chambers are called either *monoplace* or *multiplace*, in reference to the number of patients each can accommodate. A monoplace chamber is roughly the size of a casket and can accommodate only one person at a time. A multiplace chamber is a small room in which several patients or providers can be treated at once. Oxygen is pumped into the room at increasing pressure. Because pressurized oxygen is used, patients are screened carefully to remove any flammable objects.

Hyperbaric oxygen further decreases the half-life of carbon monoxide to roughly 20 minutes. Animal models have also shown that such therapy prevents the cellular damage associated with carbon monoxide toxicity. Several limited human trials have been performed, with mixed results. In the most recent prospective randomized controlled study, patients showed a benefit in some areas of neuropsychological testing but no difference in their ability to perform activities of daily living. Other prospective studies have shown no significant benefit. All of these studies have had limitations, many of which cannot be controlled, such as a lack of baseline data. On the basis of the data that do exist, hyperbaric oxygen therapy for severe carbon monoxide toxicity is recommended, but its benefit in less severely poisoned patients is unclear.

Specific criteria for determining the need for hyperbaric oxygen have been poorly defined. Recommendations vary, depending on the source. Severe, persistent symptoms, including altered mental status, coma, seizure, focal neurologic deficits, and hypotension, are widely accepted indications for hyperbaric oxygen therapy; symptoms such as syncope are less obvious indications. In patients with milder toxicity, high-flow oxygen should be administered until symptoms resolve.

The most common complications of barotrauma are sinus pain and tympanic membrane irritation or rupture. Patients undergoing hyperbaric oxygen therapy who are unable to decompress their own tympanic membranes receive temporary bilateral myringotomy incisions.

Special Treatment Considerations In treating carbon monoxide exposure, pregnant women represent a special patient population. Fetal hemoglobin may bind carbon monoxide with more affinity than maternal hemoglobin, leading to a high concentration of carboxyhemoglobin in the fetus, which is compounded by decreased oxygen delivery from the mother. Maternal carboxyhemoglobin levels do not necessarily reflect fetal levels. Severe fetal toxicity, long-term neurologic deficits, and fetal demise have been reported with maternal exposure. These adverse outcomes seem to occur most frequently when the mother exhibits significant symptoms. Children born to mothers with mild carbon monoxide toxicity have done well.

Hyperbaric oxygen therapy presents a theoretical threat to the fetus, but the risk has not been substantiated. Pregnant women with carbon monoxide toxicity should undergo hyperbaric oxygen therapy if they develop significant symptoms. As with nonpregnant patients, the specific carboxyhemoglobin level at which therapy should be initiated is not known, but 20% has been suggested.

Corrosives

Corrosives are a broad category of chemicals that corrode metal and destroy tissue on contact. Several U.S. agencies, such as the Department of Transportation (DOT) and the Environmental Protection Agency (EPA), define precise parameters for corrosive solutions. The corrosivity of a solution—that is, its ability to oxidize and chemically disintegrate materials it comes into contact with—is measured by its pH. The standard pH scale runs from an acidic low of 0 to an alkaline high of 14. A neutral or normal pH is 7.0. Both acids and alkalis are corrosives. Acids have low pH: DOT defines a strong acid as a solution with a pH below 2. Bases have high pH: DOT defines a strong base as a solution with a pH above 12.5. These pH thresholds are, of course, approximate. A solution with a pH of 4 does not meet the definition of a strict acid but is nevertheless extremely destructive if it enters the eye and isn't flushed out immediately.

Acids and bases are incompatible. This means they react violently when concentrated acid and base solutions come into contact with each other. Usually heat is generated, but the reaction may also give rise to toxic gases. For example, mixing household bleach (hypochlorite) with an ammonia-based cleaner generates chlorine gas. Examples of acids and bases are given in Box 9-2.

Acids are a ubiquitous presence in our lives. At home, we use them to open clogged drains, treat swimming pools, polish metal, and clean everything from toilet bowls to wheel rims. Acids are also found in the foods we eat. Vinegar, for instance, is composed of about 5% to 10% acetic acid, and many soft drinks contain phosphoric acid.

In industry, acids are used as chemical reagents, catalysts, industrial cleaning agents, and neutralizing agents. Sulfuric acid is used in such great quantities that some countries set their gross domestic product (GDP) by the quantity of sulfuric acid produced and used each year.

BOX 9-2 Selected Acids and Bases

Acids	Alkalis (Bases)
Battery acid	Drain cleaners
Drain cleaners	Refrigerants
Hydrochloric acid	Fertilizers
Hydrofluoric acid	Anhydrous ammonia
Sulfuric acid	Lye
Nitric acid	Sodium hydroxide
Phosphoric acid	Bleach
Acetic acid	Sodium hypochlorite
Citric acid	Lime
Formic acid	Calcium oxide
Trichloroacetic acid	Sodium carbonate
Phenol	Lithium hydride

Alkaline solutions, also known as *caustics* and *bases*, are as ubiquitous as acids. At home and in industrial processes, they serve many of the same functions as acid solutions. They are used in toilet bowl cleaners, drain openers, household bleach, and ammonia-based cleaning solutions. In industry, they are used as reagents, neutralizing agents, and cleaning solutions.

Ammonia is a widely used and available corrosive and flammable chemical. It's used in agriculture as a fertilizer and in industry as a refrigerant (in the form of a liquefied gas) and chemical reagent. In addition to these legitimate uses, ammonia is a primary ingredient in methamphetamine production. An increasing number of injuries occur each year from the illicit possession and use of ammonia. Several people have died of chemical burns sustained when this flammable gas ignited while they were manufacturing ("cooking") meth. Utmost caution is required if you respond to an ammonia injury under suspicious circumstances. Examples of such calls may include a chemical-related injury in the middle of the night in a rural area, or a chemical-related injury in a primarily residential area. Allow law enforcement to secure the scene and rule out the presence of other chemical hazards before you proceed.

Signs and Symptoms

Hydrofluoric acid, or hydrogen fluoride, is considered to be the most dangerous acid because it's a strong acid that not only has corrosive properties but also induces acute and systemic toxicity. Burns caused by hydrofluoric acid penetrate much deeper than those of most acids. The fluoride ion (F^-) has a strong attraction to calcium and magnesium in the body. A white or yellowish-white precipitate of calcium fluoride salt may form beneath the skin in patients with hydrofluoric acid burns. Severe exposures can cause systemic hypocalcemia and hypomagnesemia. Most deaths from hydrofluoric acid poisoning are directly attributable to cardiac dysrhythmia caused by hypocalcemia of cardiac tissue.

Alkaline burns to the stomach in toxic ingestions are usually more severe than acid burns because the caustic dissolves the protective mucous lining of the stomach, increasing the likelihood of ulceration and perforation.

Pathophysiology

The pathophysiology of various acid and base exposures varies widely. First, acid burns and alkali burns are distinctly different. Acids tend to produce necrosis by denaturing proteins, forming an eschar that limits the penetration of the acid, a process called *coagulation necrosis*. Bases, on the other hand, tend to produce *liquefaction necrosis*. (Hydrofluoric acid, which tends to produce liquefaction necrosis like an alkali, is an exception to this rule.) Liquefaction necrosis is a more penetrating injury in which cell membranes break down and dissolve, essentially forming soap. Consequently, a hallmark of caustic exposure is that the skin feels slick or slimy. This process, called *saponification*, results in a deeper burn that's more difficult to decontaminate. Pain is often delayed in these types of exposures.

Second, the severity of the burn depends on a number of variables such as pH, surface area, contact time, concentration, and physical form (solid, liquid, or gas) of the corrosive. Ingestion of solid pellets of alkalis such as lye causes severe burns because the pellets remain in prolonged contact with the stomach. Full-thickness or circumferential esophageal burns can be complicated by strictures that form as the burns heal.

Diagnosis

Lab workups are necessary to confirm most corrosive exposures. The extent of the workup depends on the type of corrosive, the surface area of the burn, and the route of exposure. Localized burns don't typically require lab workups because of the circumscribed effects of the exposure. Severe burns, however, warrant a CBC including hemoglobin/hematocrit, blood glucose level , electrolytes, creatinine, BUN and CPK, a coagulation profile, and a urinalysis. Hydrofluoric acid burns require calcium, magnesium, and potassium workups to ascertain the extent of toxicity and identify any systemic effects, in addition to broader lab workups that may be dictated by the severity of the exposure. Phenol exposure requires a CBC, electrolyte studies, creatinine, liver function tests, and a urinalysis.

In addition, pulse oximetry and ABGs should be ordered if the patient has respiratory symptoms. Endoscopy (specifically, esophagoscopy and gastroscopy) should be performed for corrosive ingestions, since significant esophageal injury can occur even in the absence of visible oral burns. Finally, chest radiography is indicated in patients with respiratory symptoms, and abdominal radiography is indicated in those with signs of peritonitis.

Treatment

Prehospital An acid creates a chemical burn at the site of contact. The longer the acid remains in contact with the skin, eyes, or GI tract, the more severe the burn will be. External decontamination is effective in removing acids. Although acids are considered water reactive, the most effective decontaminating agents are plain soap and water or just water alone. This method of decontamination is safe because a relatively small quantity of acid is being washed away by a large quantity of water. The heat generated by the chemical reaction is absorbed by the cool water; take care to not induce hypothermia when decontaminating patients for more than a few minutes.

Carry out decontamination procedures in an area with good ventilation and adequate space. The amount of time to irrigate depends on the corrosive, its concentration, and the size of the body surface area affected. For ocular decontamination, there are two typical approaches that should be guided by the potential damage of the chemical agent: (1) irrigate the eyes for 15 minutes with water or normal saline, or (2) extend irrigation time to 30 to 60 minutes with a Morgan irrigation lens or IV tubing and topical anesthetic. Assess eye acuity after decontamination.

Flush the skin with water for at least 5 minutes. Flushing can continue during transport, so long as contaminated water is isolated in a reservoir such as an emesis basin. Testing the area with litmus paper (pH paper) is the best way to determine whether decontamination is complete.

Internal decontamination is more controversial. Never give emetics to a patient who has ingested a corrosive agent. After a toxic acid or alkali ingestion, emesis is corrosive and thus burns the esophagus and mouth if vomiting is induced. In addition, a significant risk exists that the patient will aspirate the corrosive fluid into the lungs. Activated charcoal does not absorb corrosives, and it could interfere with later endoscopy. Never attempt to neutralize a corrosive agent, since the resulting exothermic reaction will generate excessive heat. Medical Control may advise you to dilute the acid by giving the patient milk or water to drink. Gastric lavage may be indicated, but because this procedure is also associated with a risk of aspiration, it's rarely performed in the field.

If decontamination is not rapidly completed, the acid produces intense pain at the site of contact. This site becomes a necrotic sore, and eschar may or may not form, depending on the nature of the exposure. Eye exposures produce immediate and severe pain. The thin layer of cells of the corneal epithelium is rapidly destroyed, and the acid begins denaturing the proteins in the cornea, which may lead to permanent visual impairment. GI damage from ingestion of an acid may include burns of the mouth, esophagus, and stomach. Since their severity depends largely on contact time, the stomach is usually the most severely affected part of the GI tract. Injury ranges from local burns to ulceration or perforation of the stomach or esophagus, causing severe abdominal pain. The acid may be absorbed into the vasculature, inducing acidosis.

Hydrofluoric acid burns require special consideration. Fluoride ions can be bound by either calcium or magnesium, so for any hydrofluoric acid burns, administer calcium gluconate or calcium chloride and magnesium to forestall cardiac effects. The antidote for hydrofluoric acid skin burns is thorough decontamination with water, followed by application of topical calcium gluconate gel. Because of the penetrating nature of fluoride burns, you must apply calcium gluconate to the burn site repeatedly and continuously even after initial decontamination and treatment has been completed. Deeper burns may require subcutaneous injections of calcium gluconate. Cover burns and wounds with dry, sterile dressings.

For eye exposures involving hydrofluoric acid, irrigate the eyes with calcium gluconate dissolved in normal saline. Even patients with minor hydrofluoric acid burns or suspected burns should be transported to an appropriate medical facility for evaluation. Avoid administering pain medications to such patients, since resolution of pain is the endpoint of burn treatment with calcium.

In the case of alkali (base) burns, copious and continuous flushing en route to the emergency room is needed. Alkali exposures burn longer and deeper, causing greater tissue damage. Typical alkali substances are caustic, such as drain cleaners, lye ammonia, and household bleaches.

Emergency Department Thorough decontamination is the first order of business in any corrosive exposure (details in the Hazardous Materials section). In addition, because many corrosives are volatile, the airway may need to be secured. Endotracheal intubation may be indicated for ingestion or facial burns. Corrosive burns affecting a large body surface area require fluid therapy analogous to fluid resuscitation given after thermal burns. As with most skin injuries, infection can complicate long-term recovery.

Special Considerations

Elemental forms of lithium, potassium, sodium, and magnesium react with water to form alkalis. Therefore, *do not irrigate with water*. Instead, coat the area with mineral oil, and remove the caustic material manually with forceps.

Nitrites and Sulfa Drugs That Cause Methemoglobinemia

Compounds such as nitrites and nitrates, which can oxidize the iron in hemoglobin, cause the condition known as **methemoglobinemia**. These types of poisonings can be attributed to a number of different chemicals, some of which are listed in Box 9-3.

Overuse of certain medications like nitroprussides and benzocaine sprays can cause methemoglobinemia. In rural areas, biological processes such as fermentation can create nitrites after silos are filled with grain. Peak toxicity occurs about a week after filling. Agricultural groundwater contamination with fertilizers such as ammonium nitrate can cause methemoglobinemia cyanosis in infants, deemed "blue baby syndrome," in some Midwestern states.

BOX 9-3 Selected Chemicals That Cause Methemoglobinemia

Aniline dyes	Nitrites (such as butyl nitrite and isobutyl nitrite)
Aromatic amines	Nitroaniline
Arsine	Nitrobenzene
Chlorates	Nitrofurans
Chlorobenzene	Nitrophenol
Chromates	Nitrosobenzene
Combustion products	Nitrous oxides
Dimethyl toluidine	Resorcinol
Naphthalene	Silver nitrate
Nitric acid	Trinitrotoluene
Nitric oxides	

Signs and Symptoms

Patients with methemoglobinemia due to nitrate and nitrite poisoning have altered levels of consciousness, including anxiety, confusion, and stupor. They have a slate-gray cyanosis caused by methemoglobin production. Nausea and vomiting, dizziness, and headache are common. Severe signs and symptoms may include cerebral ischemia, hypotension, and respiratory distress, which can lead to cardiovascular collapse and asphyxiation.

Pathophysiology

The pathophysiology of methemoglobinemia can be inferred from its antidote, methylene blue, which was first used by Dr. Madison Cawein in the Appalachian mountains of Kentucky in the early 1960s. Oxygen and other oxidizers naturally convert a small percentage of hemoglobin to methemoglobin on a continuous basis. Diaphorase enzymes have evolved to dispatch this constant threat, and people with active enzymes do not suffer from even mild methemoglobinemia. The "Kentucky blue" people, as they are known, have a mutation in the enzyme diaphorase I, which converts ferric methemoglobin back to ferrous hemoglobin. Affected individuals have a blue skin tone that makes them appear cyanotic, but this bluish tinge isn't caused by oxygen-deprivation cyanosis but by methemoglobin, which is a dark bluish-brown color. Dr. Cawein empirically administered methylene blue to these patients, correctly surmising that it would eliminate their blue pallor by acting as an electron donor (reducing agent) to convert methemoglobin to hemoglobin.

Diagnosis

Recognition of methemoglobinemia can be challenging, since the patient may have only mild complaints. Pulse oximetry is inaccurate with methemoglobinemia because the methemoglobin interferes with measurement of oxyhemoglobin (the wavelengths are too close together). As noted in the earlier discussion of carbon monoxide poisoning, pulse oximeters sensitive to methemoglobin are available. A thorough history and physical assessment are crucial to discovering the correct etiology. Serum methemoglobinemia and ABG levels should be analyzed in serious exposures.

Methemoglobinemia can be diagnosed quickly in the field with a blood-drop test. Place a drop of blood on a 4 × 4 gauze pad. If it's chocolate brown and doesn't turn red in a few minutes with exposure to atmospheric oxygen, you can make a diagnosis of methemoglobinemia with confidence, since carboxyhemoglobin turns red when it oxidizes, whereas methemoglobin does not.

Treatment

As mentioned, the antidote to nitrate and nitrite poisoning is methylene blue, a thiazine dye that reduces methemoglobin to hemoglobin by boosting the action of a second enzyme, diaphorase II. Paradoxically, at high concentrations, methylene blue actually acts as an oxidizing agent. In the body, methylene blue must first be converted to its bioactive form, leukomethylene blue. At higher dosages, the body can't keep up with this conversion process.

Prehospital Provide supportive care, including maintenance of airway, breathing, and circulation. Administer supplemental oxygen, and support the airway. Ensure that the patient has been removed from the offending environment and thoroughly decontaminated. Decontamination is also important to prevent cross-contamination.

Emergency Department Treatment is selected on the basis of severity of symptoms. External and internal decontamination are extremely important to prevent continued intoxication and avoid cross-contamination of healthcare personnel and of the ED itself. Gastric lavage and activated charcoal are indicated for intoxication with most methemoglobinemia-inducing agents.

Mild exposures resolve on their own, whereas more severe exposures require intervention with supportive care and antidote therapy. Supplemental oxygen is crucial to ensure that the remaining hemoglobin becomes fully saturated with oxygen. Patients in whom methylene blue is contraindicated will benefit from hyperbaric oxygen therapy.

Cholinesterase Inhibitors (Organophosphates and Carbamates)

Organophosphates and carbamates, examples of which are given in Box 9-4, are classes of widely used pesticides. They are found in insect sprays as a liquid, in rose-dusting formulations as a solid, and in mist preparations for application over larger areas. The dangers these agents pose vary widely, depending on the chemical structure of the pesticide and the carrier in which the pesticide is dissolved. Most of these pesticides are not water soluble and are enveloped in a hydrocarbon solvent that acts as a carrier. These two characteristics make most of them highly skin absorbent. However, most organophosphate pesticides are designed to be toxic by ingestion or on contact, rather than poisonous by inhalation, to reduce the risk to the applicator. In addition, household formulations are typically more dilute, and the chemical agents they contain are often less potent. Pesticides intended for commercial use can be highly concentrated and deadly.

BOX 9-4 Selected Organophosphates and Carbamates

Organophosphates	Carbamates
Acephate	Sevin
Azinphos-methyl	Aldicarb
Chlorpyrifos	Carbaryl
Demeton	Carbofuran
Diazinon	Methomyl
Dichlorvos	Propoxur
Ethyl 4-nitrophenyl phenylphosphonothioate (EPN)	
Ethion	
Malathion	
Parathion	
Ronnel	
Tetraethyl pyrophosphate	

Organophosphates were first developed as nerve agents in Germany during World War II, so they were designed as agents of chemical warfare first and adapted for agricultural use as pesticides only later. Nerve agents have been optimized for human toxicity, whereas pesticides have been optimized for toxicity to targeted pests such as wasps or aphids. Some mushrooms also have these effects.

Signs and Symptoms

The signs and symptoms of organophosphate and carbamate poisoning are the same. The "wet" patient has symptoms that can be summarized using the mnemonic SLUDGE BBM, expanded in the Rapid Recall box. The *M* in this mnemonic, which stands for *miosis*, is specific to these pesticides and nerve agents. This is one of the stronger clues in narrowing the differential diagnosis. Other symptoms include early, nonspecific flulike symptoms, sweating, and muscle fasciculations (twitching). Severe poisoning can lead to respiratory arrest. The DUMBBELS mnemonic is used to describe muscarinic signs and symptoms brought on by these agents, and their nicotinic effects can be recalled by the mnemonic MTWtHF. Details of these two mnemonics also appear in the Rapid Recall box. Additional signs and symptoms include CNS depression, confusion, convulsions, seizures, and coma.

RAPID RECALL

Mnemonics for Signs and Symptoms of Organophosphate and Carbamate Poisoning

SLUDGE BBM:

S Salivation
L Lacrimation
U Urination
D Defecation
G Gastrointestinal distress
E Emesis

B Bradycardia
B Bronchoconstriction
M Miosis

DUMBBELS:

D Diarrhea
U Urination
M Miosis
B Bradycardia
B Bronchorrhea
E Emesis
L Lacrimation
S Salivation

MTWtHF:

M Muscle weakness and paralysis
T Tachycardia
W Weakness
tH Hypertension
F Fasciculations

Pathophysiology

Organophosphates and carbamates overstimulate the parasympathetic nervous system by interfering with its primary neurotransmitter, acetylcholine. The nerve signal travels along the neuron through an electrochemical channel and stops at synapses, the junctions between neurons, where a chemical neurotransmitter—in this case acetylcholine—must be released from the neuron for the signal to travel across the junction. At the target, acetylcholine binds to the cholinergic receptor. The electrochemical impulse continues in the next neuron, or contraction begins in the muscle.

Once the signal has been conducted, the neurotransmitter must be removed. Enzymes, proteins that carry out vital metabolic processes, are the workhorses of the cell. Acetylcholinesterase is the enzyme that breaks down acetylcholine into acetate and choline after impulse conduction. Organophosphates inhibit carboxyl ester hydrolases in general and the enzyme acetylcholinesterase specifically.

However, organophosphates and carbamates inhibit acetylcholinesterase in slightly different ways. Organophosphates and nerve agents contain an organic phosphate group, whereas carbamates do not. The phosphate portion of the pesticide binds to the acetylcholinesterase, preventing the enzyme from breaking the organophosphate in half. The phosphate portion gets stuck, putting acetylcholinesterase out of commission. Over a variable period of time, these two molecules form a permanent bond. The shorter the aging time, the faster the antidote, particularly pralidoxime, must be administered.

Diagnosis

Organophosphate and carbamate intoxication are recognizable primarily by signs and symptoms. Cholinesterase assays can aid diagnosis, but they're not always reflective of the severity of intoxication if preexisting conditions such as pernicious anemia and use of antimalarial drugs skew results. There are two types of cholinesterase assays: RBC and CNS. The RBC cholinesterase assay is more accurate, but it's difficult to perform. If possible, you should draw the blood for this assay before administering pralidoxime.

Treatment

When treating a patient with organophosphate poisoning, you must take great care to avoid cross-contamination from the victim (Box 9-5). The patient's clothing must be removed and isolated (bagged or removed from the immediate area). You must wear personal protective clothing, including gloves, a gown, and eye protection, while treating the patient. In addition, some organophosphates and carbamates are volatile, and respiratory protection may be required. Emesis may also contain significant amounts of poison and must be isolated and handled carefully.

Supportive care, including management of airway, breathing, and circulation, is of paramount importance. Airway management must be a priority because of the increased bronchial secretions and muscle paralysis associated with the cholinergic effects of these agents. Cardiac monitoring is also necessary. Gastric lavage and activated charcoal may be indicated if less than 1 hour has elapsed since the exposure.

Prehospital Prehospital treatment consists of supportive care and antidote administration. The antidotes for organophosphate poisoning are atropine and pralidoxime (2-PAM). Atropine treats the wet symptoms, while 2-PAM reactivates acetylcholinesterase. Atropine can be given in 1- to 5-mg doses every 5 minutes, depending on symptoms, up to 100 mg. Note that these doses are significantly higher than those used for cardiac conditions. As a cholinesterase antidote, the atropine binds to the acetylcholine receptor, inhibiting the parasympathetic stimulation caused by the organophosphate or carbamate. The endpoint of atropine administration is drying of the secretions and reversal of bradycardia.

To be most effective, 2-PAM should be administered before the aging process occurs. In contrast, carbamates (such as the pesticide Sevin) do not contain an organophosphate group but can still bind to the acetylcholinesterase enzyme. Because carbamates do not have an

BOX 9-5 Treatment of Pesticide (Organophosphate/Carbamate) Exposure

- Adequate decontamination is essential to limit the patient's exposure and the chance of secondary exposure to the caregiver.
- Establish an open airway. Consider orotracheal or nasotracheal intubation for airway control in the patient who is unconscious, has severe pulmonary edema, or is in severe respiratory distress.
- Ventilate as necessary. Positive-pressure ventilation with a bag-mask device may be beneficial.
- Monitor for pulmonary edema and treat as necessary.
- Monitor cardiac rhythm and treat dysrhythmias as necessary.
- Start an IV and infuse at 30 mL/h. For hypotension with signs of hypovolemia, administer fluid cautiously. Consider vasopressors if the patient is hypotensive with a normal fluid volume, per local protocol. Watch for signs of fluid overload.
- Administer atropine per local protocol. Correct hypoxia before giving atropine.
- Mydriasis should not be used to determine the endpoint of atropine administration; the endpoint for atropine administration is the drying of pulmonary secretions.
- Administer pralidoxime chloride per local protocol.
- Treat seizures with adequate atropinization and correction of hypoxia. In rare cases, diazepam (Valium) or lorazepam (Ativan) may be necessary per local protocol.
- Succinylcholine, other cholinergic agents, and aminophylline are contraindicated.
- For eye contamination, immediately flush eyes with water. Continuously irrigate each eye with normal saline during transport.

IV, Intravenous line.
Reprinted from Currance PL, Clements B, Bronstein AC: Emergency care for hazardous materials exposure, ed 3, St Louis, 2005, Mosby.

organophosphate group, they don't require 2-PAM as an antidote. Only atropine is given to dry out the patient's SLUDGE symptoms (see the Rapid Recall box). Routine medical care includes high flow oxygen and IV therapy.

Emergency Department If seizures occur, benzodiazepine therapy of 0.1 to 0.2 mg/kg IV is appropriate. A continuous infusion of 2-PAM at 8 mg/kg/h for adults is administered. After initial resuscitation, activated charcoal 1 g/kg (up to 50 g) is a consideration.

Petroleum Distillates

Hydrocarbons are a broad class of combustible or flammable liquids derived from oil. These liquids are not water soluble and generally float on water. Hydrocarbons are found in small quantities around the home and in large quantities in industry. At home, most of us have small quantities of gasoline, mineral spirits, paint thinner, and other solvents in the garage or shed. In industry, large quantities of hydrocarbons are used as fuels (including diesel fuel), solvents, and reagents for chemical processes (especially in the plastics industry). Examples of other petroleum distillates are toluene, xylene, benzene, and hexane.

Huffing is a recent phenomenon of chemical abuse in which abusers intentionally inhale various halogenated or aromatic hydrocarbons to produce a euphoric high. These effects, which can include severe CNS depression and respiratory depression, can have a rapid onset.

Signs and Symptoms

Signs and symptoms of petroleum distillate toxicity vary greatly depending on the specific properties of the hydrocarbon, the route of entry, and the quantity of the chemical ingested. Fortunately, most hydrocarbon poisonings are not serious, and fewer than 1% require medical intervention, but some hydrocarbons and hydrocarbon derivatives are extremely dangerous or deadly.

Pathophysiology

Hydrocarbons generally affect the CNS. They are readily absorbed through the skin and are thought to change the properties (such as fluidity) of cell membranes in CNS neurons as they dissolve. Some hydrocarbons cause cancer, whereas others are protoxins, and their metabolites are harmful. The volatility of a substance, which is a measure of vapor pressure, indicates the degree of threat it poses to the respiratory system. The higher the vapor pressure, the greater the concentration of the chemical in the air and the more volatile it's said to be. Higher volatility also equates with greater flammability.

The viscosity of a hydrocarbon affects the likelihood of aspiration during an ingestion. Thinner, less viscous hydrocarbons are more likely to be aspirated than thicker ones. For example, gasoline is more likely than motor oil to cause pulmonary damage. Some hydrocarbon derivatives such as phenol possess anesthetic properties. Phenol burns may therefore go unnoticed for longer periods, which will result in more severe burns with possible systemic effects.

A good scene size-up is critical in determining the level of risk associated with a particular exposure. Many hydrocarbons require specialized personal protective equipment (PPE) to approach the victim. The National Institute of Occupational Safety and Health (NIOSH) guide can be used to determine the degree of danger a particular hydrocarbon poses to both prehospital provider and victim.

Diagnosis

A lab workup is indicated in petroleum distillate intoxication. A CBC should be performed, since chronic benzene exposure leads to leukemia or aplastic anemia. A basic metabolic panel, including glucose level, BUN, creatinine, and electrolyte studies, is indicated. Hepatic transaminase studies and serum creatine kinase levels (to identify rhabdomyolysis) are also indicated. Chest imaging is necessary when aspiration of petroleum distillates is suspected.

Treatment

Prehospital A good patient history and thorough external decontamination are crucial. It's important to observe the patient to pinpoint which specific hydrocarbon has been ingested and in what quantity. Generally, the most pronounced effects of toxicity are on the CNS. Activated charcoal does not bind all hydrocarbons effectively, but studies have shown it's very capable of binding kerosene and turpentine. Gastric lavage may be indicated in patients who have ingested *c*amphor, ***h***alogenated hydrocarbons, *a*romatic hydrocarbons, heavy *m*etal–containing hydrocarbons, or *p*esticide-containing hydrocarbons (CHAMP).

Emergency Department A good patient history should be obtained to determine the type of hydrocarbon, the amount, and time of consumption. In addition, questions should focus on co-ingestants and the possibility of aspiration. Treatment is mainly supportive, including maintaining airway, breathing, and circulation, providing supplemental oxygen, and establishing IV access. The airway is vulnerable to aspiration.

The physical exam should include a thorough neurologic exam, including cranial nerves, to rule out any tramatic injury. Typically ethanol is rapidly absorbed from the gastrointestinal tract; therefore, the administration of activated charcoal may not be indicated.

Hazardous Materials

Exposure to hazardous materials poses a threat to all the communities we serve as healthcare providers. Hazardous materials are found, for example, in local refineries, factories, and industrial plants that produce a variety of chemicals. These dangerous goods pass along our highways and railways and through our airports as they are transported across the country. Hazardous materials are also manufactured in illicit neighborhood and rural meth labs.

We must maintain a keen awareness of these threats when we approach a perilous scene or situation or when a patient's cardinal presentation indicates he or she may have been exposed to a hazardous material. Continuing education will help you stay informed about the risks in your geographic area and keep up with local protocols and national management guidelines. The AMLS assessment provides a systematic approach to obtaining an efficient and thorough history so that life-threatening exposures and related diagnoses can be immediately identified and managed.

A hazardous material is any substance that poses an unreasonable threat to health, safety, or the environment. It includes corrosives, **radioactive** matter, and flammable materials. Hazardous substances can be inhaled, ingested, or absorbed through the skin. The cardinal presentation of an exposed patient is as varied as the myriad types of hazardous materials and their routes of exposure and levels of toxicity. Patients with underlying medical conditions, immunosuppression, or extremes of age are all at higher risk because of their perfusion challenges. Many patients sustain traumatic injuries in addition to the medical emergency associated with the exposure, providing daunting assessment and treatment challenges for us in the field.

An efficient primary survey that allows immediate identification and management of life threats is essential, not only to ensuring your safety but to reducing the likelihood of morbidity and mortality for the patient. Through the AMLS assessment process, emergent/critical and non–life threatening diagnoses are quickly revealed and decisively treated.

Regulatory Agency Notification

It's important to ensure that you notify receiving facilities and local, state, and national agencies of hazardous materials and possible weapons of mass destruction as soon as you recognize them. Chief among these agencies are the **Occupational Safety and Health Administration** (OSHA) and the Environmental Protection Agency (EPA). These agencies develop and mandate personnel training and local, state, and federal emergency plans. An OSHA regulation known as the **Standard on Hazardous Waste Operations and Emergency Response** (HAZWOPER) provides guidelines for the development of and compliance with safety protocols and procedures for governmental and nongovernmental personnel who make, store, or dispose of, or are first responders to cleanup of hazardous materials. For first-response personnel such as firefighters, EMTs, and paramedics, the **National Fire Protection Association** (NFPA) identifies standards for safety competency related to scene management.

Incident Recognition

In general, patients with medical emergencies often have subtle or nondescript clinical presentations for a variety of conditions. The occurrence of a hazardous materials incident can be equally difficult to identify. For prehospital providers, dispatch information regarding the number of patients and any similarities in the signs and symptoms they exhibit can indicate the need for immediate identification of appropriate safety precautions and additional resources.

At the scene, low-lying clouds, smoke, or unusual fog patterns or air density should heighten your awareness that a hazardous materials incident may have occurred.

Significant skin or eye irritation, respiratory difficulties, and unfamiliar odors are all descriptors that warrant taking special precautions. If you recognize an unsafe scene before making patient contact, view the area with binoculars to look for evidence of hazards. This practice allows you to avoid contamination and deploy resources efficiently.

Once you recognize that an area or patient may have been subject to a hazardous materials exposure, you must immediately don personal protection devices and notify the appropriate agencies. Transportation destinations may be altered, depending on the number of patients and available resources.

Identification and Labeling

The presence of a hazardous material is identified by the use of placards, shipping papers, labels, or pictographs that specify the type of hazardous agent present, the nature and degree of the medical compromise expected if an exposure were to occur, and the signs and symptoms of exposure. All healthcare providers must be able to interpret hazardous materials labeling or have immediate access to guides or agencies that can assist in identification. Providers who cannot recognize the labeling on hazardous products risk unintentionally entering a contaminated area or beginning treatment of an exposed patient without first completing proper decontamination procedures.

In the United States, the DOT regulates the transportation of hazardous materials, including the labeling of such materials during transport. The agency sets standards specifying:

- Which types of containers must be used to transport various kinds of hazardous materials
- How the containers must be labeled
- By which modes of transportation they may be moved
- What kind of documentation must accompany the transport container

First-response personnel must be available at the delivery destination, such as a laboratory, refinery, or factory, to take safety precautions before the shipment arrives. Appropriate PPE must be used by all personnel if the threat of a hazardous materials exposure incident exists.

A **placard** is a diamond-shaped sign affixed to a transport vehicle (Figure 9-12). It's color coded to identify the hazardous agent as being flammable, combustible, poisonous, radioactive, gaseous, explosive, oxidizing, infectious, or corrosive. Each placard carries a four-digit identification number that allows the agent to be looked up quickly in print and online reference sources.

OSHA requires chemical manufacturers to create Material Safety Data Sheets (MSDS) for every chemical developed, stored, and used in the United States. These sheets provide instructions for safe handling and storage of the chemical and outline emergency actions to take if an exposure occurs. These sheets must remain with the chemical at all times.

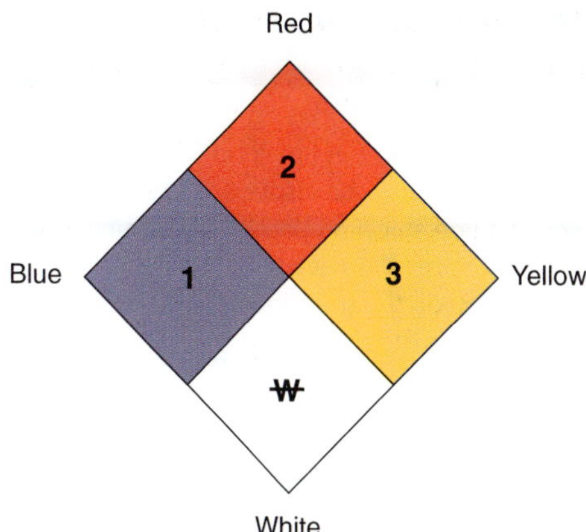

Figure 9-12 National Fire Protection Association placard consists of four diamonds within a larger diamond. Red (flammability) diamond is at "12 o'clock"; yellow (instability) diamond is at "3 o'clock"; white (special hazards) diamond is at "6 o'clock"; and blue (health) hazard diamond is at "9 o'clock." Degree of hazard severity is indicated by a numerical rating that ranges from 4, indicating the most severe hazard, to 0, indicating no hazard. Special hazards are indicated in the white section and refer to chemicals that react with water (W), and those that are oxidizers (OX). (From Shannon M, Borron S, Burns M: Haddad and Winchester's clinical management of poisoning and drug overdose, ed 4, Philadelphia, 2007, Saunders.)

A number of published guides and books offer detailed instructions regarding the safe handling and transport of various types of hazardous materials:

- The DOT publishes the **North American Emergency Response Guidebook**.
- A poison control center can be accessed by calling 1-800-222-1222. It can provide a list of toxic substances and appropriate medical interventions.
- The Chemical Manufacturers Association offers a public service known as the *CHEMical TRansportation Emergency Center (CHEMTREC)*, which provides scene advice on hazardous materials identification. CHEMTREC can be accessed by dialing 800-424-9300.
- Transport Canada's CANUTEC (1-613-996-6666) is a good resource.
- Web-based services such as the National Library of Medicine's Wireless Information System for Emergency Responders (WISER). WISER is available free of charge on the web, and the information can be downloaded to a laptop or PDA (www.webwiser.nlm.nih.gov).

Take advantage of these resources if you anticipate or have identified a hazardous materials incident. Box 9-6 and Table 9-12 present the Classification System for

BOX 9-6 International Classification System for Hazardous Materials

Class or division numbers may be displayed in the bottom of placards, or they may be displayed in the hazardous materials description on shipping papers. In certain cases, a class or division number may replace the written name of the hazard class description on the shipping paper. The class and division numbers have the following meanings:

Class 1	**Explosives**
Division 1.1	Explosives with a mass explosion hazard
Division 1.2	Explosives with a projection hazard
Division 1.3	Explosives with predominantly a fire hazard
Division 1.4	Explosives with no significant blast hazard
Division 1.5	Very insensitive explosives
Division 1.6	Extremely insensitive explosive articles
Class 2	**Gases**
Division 2.1	Flammable gases
Division 2.2	Nonflammable gases
Division 2.3	Poison gases
Division 2.4	Corrosive gases (Canadian)
Class 3	**Flammable Liquids**
Division 3.1	Flashpoint below −18°C (0°F)
Division 3.2	Flashpoint −18°C and above but less than 23°C (73°F)
Division 3.3	Flashpoint of 23°C and up to 61°C (141°F)
Class 4	**Flammable Solids, Spontaneously Combustible Materials, Materials That Are Dangerous When Wet**
Division 4.1	Flammable solids
Division 4.2	Spontaneously combustible materials
Division 4.3	Materials that are dangerous when wet
Class 5	**Oxidizers and Organic Peroxides**
Division 5.1	Oxidizers
Division 5.2	Organic peroxides
Class 6	**Poisonous and Etiological (Infectious) Materials**
Division 6.1	Poisonous materials
Division 6.2	Etiological (infectious) materials
Class 7	**Radioactive Materials**
Class 8	**Corrosives**
Class 9	**Miscellaneous Hazardous Materials**

From U.S. Department of Transportation, National Highway Traffic Safety Administration: EMT-Paramedic national standard curriculum, Washington DC, 1997, The Department.

Hazardous Materials, and Box 9-7 lists selected agencies that assist in hazardous material incidents.

Dispatch to Scene

At the time of dispatch and while en route to the scene of a hazardous materials incident, begin assessing information and taking stock of your resources:

- Note weather conditions and wind direction.
- Gauge the proximity of highly populated areas relative to the exposure area.
- Determine the number and location of receiving facilities.
- Review the type of hazardous material and the amount to which victims are thought to have been exposed.
- Estimate the number of people who have been exposed or are at risk of exposure.

Approach all external scenes uphill and upwind. Be sure the scene has been secured. Deploy the appropriate mutual aid agencies before accessing the scene.

Staging Areas

The incident command system will assume control of the incident and direct responders to the appropriate safe staging zones for decontamination and patient triage and care. These zones must be clearly marked and well circumscribed to prevent further contamination and maintain an organized approach to patient access. Safety zones are identified as follows:

- **Hot (red) zone.** This is where the hazardous material is located and contamination has occurred. Access to this zone is limited to protect rescuers and patients from further exposure. Specific protective gear worn by trained personnel is required for access.
- **Warm (yellow) zone.** This is usually the area surrounding the contaminated hot zone. Properly protected healthcare providers are allowed to access this zone for rapid assessment and management of emergent or life-threatening conditions. Decontamination occurs in this zone.
- **Cold (green) zone.** This is a support zone for general triage, stabilization, and management of illness or injuries. Patients and uncontaminated personnel are given access to this zone. However, healthcare personnel must wear protective clothing while in the green zone and properly discard it in predetermined areas on exiting.

Hazardous materials incidents can be emotionally and physically challenging for rescue personnel and healthcare providers. Your health history should be evaluated and

TABLE 9-12 Classes of Hazardous Materials

Class/Division	Notes
CLASS 1: EXPLOSIVES Division 1.1: Mass detonation hazard Division 1.2: Mass detonation hazard with fragments Division 1.3: Fire hazard with minor blast or projectile hazard Division 1.4: Explosive substances that present no significant hazard Division 1.5: Very insensitive explosives Division 1.6: Extremely insensitive explosives	Explosive placards and labels are orange and have a symbol showing an exploding ball with fragments on the top and a division number (1.1 to 1.6) on the bottom. The word "explosive" or a four-digit ID number appears in the center of the symbol.
CLASS 2: GASES Division 2.1: Flammable gases Division 2.2: Nonflammable gases Division 2.3: Poisonous gases	Compressed or liquefied gas placards and labels are red (flammable), green (nonflammable), or white (poison); have a fire symbol, gas cylinder symbol, or a skull and crossbones on the top; and have a division number (2.1 to 2.3) on the bottom. These symbols have "flammable gas," "nonflammable gas," or "poison gas" labeling or a four-digit ID number in the center.
CLASS 3: FLAMMABLE OR COMBUSTIBLE LIQUIDS Division 3.1: Liquids with flash points <0°F Division 3.2: Liquids with flash points from 0°F to 73°F Division 3.3: Liquids with flash points from 73°F to141°F Combustible liquids	Flammable or combustible liquids placards and labels are red, have a flame symbol on the top, and a division number (3.1 to 3.3) on the bottom. They have the wording "flammable liquid" or "combustible liquid" or a four-digit ID number in the center.
CLASS 4: FLAMMABLE SOLIDS Division 4.1: Flammable solids Division 4.2: Spontaneously combustible or pyrophoric solids and liquids Division 4.3: Dangerous when wet	Flammable solid placards and labels are red-and-white striped (flammable solids), red over white (spontaneously combustible solids and liquids), or blue (dangerous when wet); have a flame symbol on the top; and have a division number (4.1 to 4.3) on the bottom. They have the wording "flammable solid," "spontaneously combustible," or "dangerous when wet" or a four-digit ID number in the center.
CLASS 5: OXIDIZING SUBSTANCES Division 5.1: Oxidizing substances Division 5.2: Organic peroxides	Oxidizing substances placards and labels are yellow, have a symbol showing an "O" with flames on the top, and a division number (5.1 to 5.2) on the bottom. They have the wording "oxidizer" or "organic peroxide" or a four-digit ID number in the center.
CLASS 6: POISONOUS AND INFECTIOUS SUBSTANCES Division 6.1: Poisons Division 6.2: Infectious substances	Poison liquid and solid material and infectious material placards and labels are white; have either a skull and crossbones, biomedical symbol, or grain stock with an *X* through it (depending on material) on the top; and a division number (6.1 to 6.2) on the bottom. These symbols have the wording "poison," "infectious material," "keep away from foodstuffs" or a four-digit ID number in the center.
CLASS 7: RADIOACTIVE SUBSTANCES	Radioactive materials placards and labels are yellow over white, have the radioactive "propeller" symbol on the top, and the number 7 on the bottom. Labels must identify the radionuclide and the amount of activity in the package. They will have the Roman numerals I, II, or III in the center to identify the level of hazard and type of container and space to write in specific information. The I, II, or III numbering designates the amount of radiation detectable from outside the package. Labels have the wording "radioactive material" or a four-digit ID number in the center.
CLASS 8: CORROSIVE MATERIALS	Corrosive materials placards and labels are white over black, have a symbol showing a test tube spilling liquid onto a human thumb, and a piece of steel on the top and have the number 8 on the bottom. The word "corrosive" or a four-digit ID number appears in the center.
CLASS 9: MISCELLANEOUS HAZARDOUS MATERIALS	Miscellaneous hazardous materials placards and labels are black and white striped over white and have the number 9 on the bottom. They have a four-digit ID number in the center.

From Aehlert B: Paramedic practice today: above and beyond, St Louis, 2009, Mosby.

BOX 9-7 Agencies That Assist in Hazardous Materials Incidents*

FEDERAL AGENCIES

Centers for Disease Control and Prevention
Department of Transportation
Environmental Protection Agency
Federal Aviation Administration
National Response Center
U.S. Armed Forces (Army, Navy, Air Force, Marines)
U.S. Coast Guard
U.S. Department of Energy

REGIONAL AND STATE AGENCIES

National Guard
State emergency management agencies
State Environmental Protection Agency
State health departments
State police

LOCAL AGENCIES

Emergency management
Fire service (hazardous materials units)
Law enforcement agencies
Poison control center
Public utilities
Sewage and treatment facilities

COMMERCIAL AGENCIES

American Petroleum Institute
Association of American Railroads and Hazardous Materials Systems
Chemical Manufacturers Association
Chevron (provides assistance with Chevron products)
HELP (the Union Carbide Emergency Response System for company shipments)
Local industry
Local contractors
Local carriers and transporters
Railway industry

*This box lists only a sampling of the agencies; the list is not all-inclusive.
From Sanders MJ: Mosby's paramedic textbook, ed 3, St Louis, 2005, Mosby.

your vital signs assessed before you're allowed to enter staging areas. In events that involve many patients and resources, rescuers often remain at the scene or in transport vehicles for long hours while wearing heavy and constricting protective clothing. Rescuers can become drained by dehydration, heat or cold exposure, and exhaustion. All healthcare personnel should receive a medical evaluation and rehydration after the incident or after each shift.

Decontamination

A final safety component in management of hazardous materials incidents is the decontamination process. Staged decontamination areas should be clearly identified by incident command personnel at the scene and at all receiving facilities. Decontamination procedures should be implemented for patients, rescuers, and equipment.

Decontamination may be dry or wet. Dry decontamination procedures are appropriate for minimal exposures. These procedures call for careful and systematic removal and disposal of all clothing. For wet decontamination procedures, use copious amounts of warm (90°F to 95°F [32°C to 35°C]) water and mild soap to cleanse exposed equipment and clothing. Remove clothing and personal items, and place them in designated labeled bags. Contain runoff water to keep it from entering irrigation or sewer systems. Use small wading pools or commercially purchased containers to house runoff particles and water.

Take care during the primary decontamination process to ensure that the hazardous material has been completely removed. Secondary decontamination should be performed at the receiving facility if remnants of the contaminant remain in transport vehicles or on your clothing. After the incident, dispose properly of contaminated clothing. Thoroughly decontaminate rescue and transport vehicles. Box 9-8 explains measures of toxicity, and Box 9-9 lists levels indicating potentially dangerous exposure.

Personal Protective Equipment

OSHA and the EPA classify protective clothing on the basis of its ability to seal exposed skin. These agencies identify protection by levels:

- Level A is the highest level of skin and respiratory protection. It necessitates a fully encapsulating, airtight outer garment and self-contained breathing apparatus (SCBA), completely sealing off the wearer from the environment. A NIOSH-certified positive-pressure respirator must be worn. This level of protection is worn by first responders who enter the contaminated site.
- Level B provides the highest level of respiratory/breathing protection. It consists of an SCBA plus protective clothing. This level is typically worn by decontamination crews.
- Level C protection consists of an air-purifying respirator plus protective clothing.
- Level D for less worrisome exposures. This level requires standard work gear, gloves, and goggles or a facemask, as appropriate.

The proper sequence for donning PPE is outlined in Box 9-10, and the order in which you should remove PPE is summarized in Box 9-11.

Severity and Symptoms of Exposure

Several factors determine the severity of a hazardous materials exposure. The type of hazardous material, its chemical components, the route of entry, and the individual's general health all affect the severity of the signs and symptoms exhibited. Some symptoms appear immediately, whereas others may be delayed, making it difficult to obtain an accurate patient history. General symptoms of exposure to a hazardous material include:

- Dyspnea and chest tightness
- Nausea and vomiting
- Diarrhea
- Excessive salivation and drooling
- Tingling and numbness of the extremities
- Altered mentation
- Skin discoloration

BOX 9-8 Measures of Toxicity

Lethal dose 50% (LD50): The oral or dermal exposure dose that kills 50% of the exposed animal population in 2 weeks' time.

Lethal concentration 50% (LC50): The air concentration of a substance that kills 50% of the exposed animal population. This also is commonly noted as LCt50. This denotes the concentration and the length of exposure time that results in 50% fatality in the exposed animal population.

From Aehlert B: Paramedic practice today: above and beyond, St Louis, 2009, Mosby.

Types of Hazardous Materials Exposure

Oral and Inhalation

OSHA, along with the EPA and NIOSH, has used animal studies to ascertain the levels of exposure considered to be dangerous for each type of hazardous material. This level is expressed using metrics known as the **lethal dose**, 50% (LD50) and the **lethal concentration**, 50% (LC50). The LD50 is the level of oral or dermal exposure dose that kills 50% of an exposed animal population in 2 weeks.

BOX 9-9 Levels That Identify Potentially Dangerous Exposure

Threshold limit value: the airborne concentrations of a substance; represents conditions under which nearly all workers are believed to be repeatedly exposed day after day without adverse effects.

Permissible exposure limit: allowable air concentration of a substance in the workplace as established by OSHA. These values are legally enforceable.

Immediately dangerous to life or health concentrations (IDHLs): maximal environmental air concentration of a substance from which a person could escape within 30 minutes without symptoms of impairment or irreversible health effects.

OSHA, Occupational Safety and Health Administration.
From Aehlert B: Paramedic practice today: above and beyond, St Louis, 2009, Mosby.

BOX 9-10 Sequence for Donning Personal Protective Equipment

The type of PPE used will vary based on the level of precautions required (e.g., Standard Precautions and contact, droplet, or airborne infection isolation).

1. Gown:
   - Fully cover torso from neck to knees, arms to end of wrists, and wrap around the back.
   - Fasten in back of neck and waist.
2. Mask or respirator:
   - Secure ties or elastic bands at middle of head and neck.
   - Fit flexible band to nose bridge.
   - Fit snug to face and below chin.
   - Fit-check respirator.
3. Goggles or face shield:
   - Place over face and eyes and adjust to fit.
4. Gloves:
   - Extend to cover wrist of isolation gown.

Use safe work practices to protect yourself and limit the spread of contamination:

- Keep hands away from face.
- Limit surfaces touched.
- Change gloves when torn or heavily contaminated.
- Perform hand hygiene.

From Centers for Disease Control and Prevention, Atlanta. In Pons: PHTLS. Box 20-2.

BOX 9-11 Sequence for Removing Personal Protective Equipment

Except for the respirator, remove PPE at doorway or in an anteroom. Remove respirator after leaving patient room and closing door.

1. Gloves:
   - Outside of glove is contaminated!
   - Grasp outside of glove with opposite gloved hand; peel off.
   - Hold removed glove in gloved hand.
   - Slide fingers of ungloved hand under remaining glove at wrist.
   - Peel glove off over first glove.
   - Discard gloves in waste container.
2. Goggles:
   - Outside of goggles or face shield is contaminated!
   - To remove, handle by head band or ear pieces.
   - Place in designated receptacle for reprocessing or in waste container.
3. Gown:
   - Gown front and sleeves are contaminated!
   - Unfasten gown ties.
   - Pull away from neck and shoulders, touching inside of gown only.
   - Turn gown inside out.
   - Fold or roll into a bundle and discard.
4. Mask or respirator:
   - Front of mask/respirator is contaminated—do not touch!
   - Grasp bottom, then top ties or elastics, and remove.
   - Discard in waste container.

From Centers for Disease Control and Prevention, Atlanta. In Pons: PHTLS. Box 20-3.

The LC50 is the air concentration of an agent that kills 50% of the exposed animal population. LD50 applies to hazardous materials that are dangerous when swallowed or absorbed through the skin, whereas LC50 applies to agents that are toxic when inhaled.

Exposure to agents with low water solubility can seriously damage lung tissue, resulting in irreversible pulmonary edema and long-term chronic lung disease. Exposure to agents with high water solubility, such as ammonia, causes only benign symptoms in the upper airway, because such agents are absorbed in the mucous membranes before reaching the lungs. The patient will complain of eye irritation, skin burns, respiratory tract irritation, and a nonproductive cough.

On your initial physical assessment, identify and manage any increased work of breathing. If the patient is wheezing, administer bronchodilators such as albuterol (Proventil). Give fluids and vasopressors for hypotension. Because of the potential for pulmonary edema, monitor IV fluids closely to avert fluid overload. Once you've completed decontamination protocols, initiate routine supportive care.

Ingestion

Ingestion of hazardous materials is not common, but it can occur if decontamination is not thorough. If a hazardous material is still present and you or the patient places the hands near the mouth, as when drinking a cup of coffee, contamination can occur.

Injection

For medication administration, the IV route offers the fastest rate of absorption compared with intramuscular and subcutaneous routes. However, penetrating contaminated skin tissue can allow the toxic substance to be absorbed by the body where it may damage organs. Many injected substances are metabolized by the liver and are capable of causing debilitating damage. Identifying a patient or provider's risk for this route of exposure is essential in preventing contamination.

WEAPONS OF MASS DESTRUCTION

Acts of terrorism involving biological, chemical, or radiologic agents threaten military personnel and civilians alike. Response to these types of disasters poses a significant safety risk to healthcare providers and rescue personnel. Although providers often respond to natural disasters such as earthquakes, avalanches, and floods and to mass-casualty accidents such as building collapses and crashes involving mass-transportation vehicles, the focus of the following section is to increase your awareness of common Category A weapons of terrorism and the implications of such incidents for patients and healthcare providers.

Biological, chemical, or radiologic **contamination** by a terrorist attack results in a crime scene designation for the affected area. In addition, the Department of Homeland Security must be notified of all suspected terrorist attacks. As is the case with hazardous materials, weapons of mass destruction can be biological, chemical, incendiary, or explosive agents or devices. The difference is that when used by terrorists, these agents are released with the intent to destroy or to cause injury and death when inhaled, ingested, or absorbed. In 2000, the CDC established categories of bioterrorism agents to assist in identifying those that are lethal (Table 9-13).

TABLE 9-13 Critical Biological Agents for Public Health Preparedness

Biological Agent	Disease
CATEGORY A	
Variola major	Smallpox
Bacillus anthracis	Anthrax
Yersinia pestis	Plague
Clostridium botulinum (botulinum toxins)	Botulism
Francisella tularensis	Tularemia
Filoviruses and arenaviruses (e.g., Ebola, Lassa fever)	Viral hemorrhagic fevers
CATEGORY B	
Coxiella burnetii	Q fever
Brucella spp.	Brucellosis
Burkholderia mallei	Glanders
Burkholderia pseudomallei	Melioidosis
Alphaviruses (VEE, EEE, WEE)	Encephalitis
Rickettsia prowazekii	Typhus fever
Toxins (e.g., ricin, staphylococcal enterotoxin B)	Toxic syndromes
Chlamydia psittaci	Psittacosis
Food safety threats (e.g., *Salmonella* spp., *Escherichia coli* O157:H7)	
Water safety threats (e.g., *Vibrio cholerae, Cryptosporidium parvum*)	
CATEGORY C	
Emerging threat agents (e.g., Nipah virus, hantavirus)	

EEE, Eastern equine encephalomyelitis; *VEE,* Venezuelan equine encephalomyelitis; *WEE,* western equine encephalomyelitis.
Reprinted from Rotz L, Khan A, Lillibridge SR, et al: Public health assessment of potential biological terrorism agents (website). Published 2000. http://www.cdc.gov. Accessed August 9, 2008.

Biological Agents

Agents of bioterrorism do not call attention to themselves. There is no dramatic implosion, no blazing cone of fire, no hail of shrapnel to announce their presence. That insidious quality makes **biological agents** all the more threatening, because it gives them time to infect many people in a wide geographic area before health officials recognize a pattern of illness. Public health authorities eventually begin to notice a high incidence of certain signs and symptoms or similar chief complaints within a given geographic area. Perhaps they're tipped off by an unorthodox disease presentation, a heavy load of cases within a circumscribed area, or reports of unusual routes of exposure.

Regardless of how the incident finally comes to light, the recognition that a biological exposure has occurred is almost invariably delayed. Healthcare providers can help compress the time from exposure to awareness by promptly reporting any unexpected influx of patients or other atypical patient trend. Let's take a look at the biological agents of greatest concern.

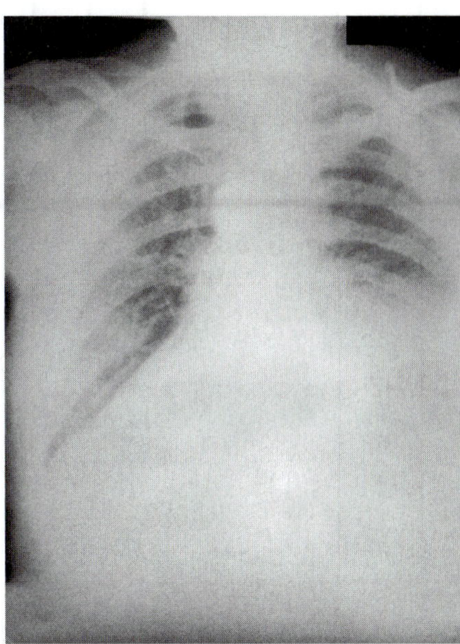

Figure 9-13 Respiratory distress and sepsis in anthrax. (From Habif TP: Clinical dermatology: a color guide to diagnosis and therapy, ed 5, St Louis, 2009, Mosby.)

Anthrax

Anthrax is an acute infectious disease caused by the gram-positive, spore-forming bacterium *Bacillus anthracis.* The most common route of entry is by direct skin contact and absorption of spores, which causes a localized red, itchy ulcer (cutaneous anthrax). Workers and farmers who are in frequent direct contact with animals are highly susceptible to this route of exposure. Within 2 weeks, skin begins to necrose, and a black eschar forms. Anthrax spores can also be inhaled (inhalation anthrax; Figure 9-13), which may initially cause apparently benign symptoms similar to those of the common cold. In the early **prodromal** stage, the patient complains of a nonproductive cough, fever, and nausea. The disease then progresses to the **fulminant** stage, which is characterized by high fever, cyanosis, shock, diaphoresis, and severe respiratory distress.

Treatment

Prehospital Supportive care with supplemental oxygen, IV therapy for fluid replacement, and application of dry, sterile dressing to wounds is appropriate. You must notify the receiving facility of the exposure. **Emergency decontamination** is not necessary unless the exposure has just occurred. You're at risk only if you have direct contact with lesions.

Emergency Department Care in the hospital includes blood cultures to identify the toxin and determine appropriate antibiotics. Scientists doing anthrax research and military personnel can receive vaccinations to prevent anthrax.

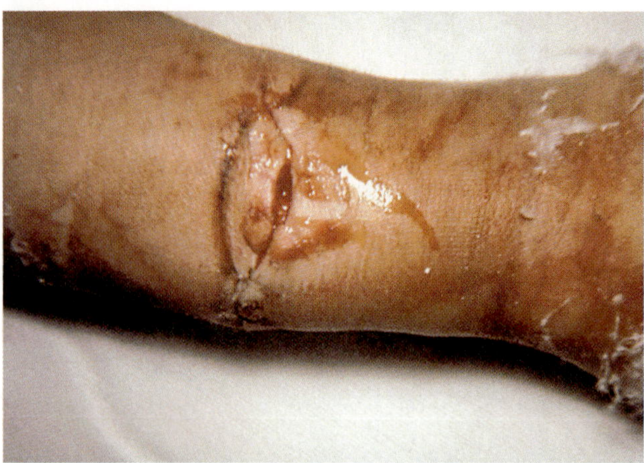

■ **Figure 9-14** Wound botulism. (From Sanders M: Mosby's paramedic textbook, revised ed 3, St Louis, 2005, Mosby.)

Botulism

Clostridium botulinum, the bacterial agent that causes botulism, produces a nerve toxin that causes paralysis. Types of exposure include ingestion of contaminated food and contamination of wounds with the bacterium (Figure 9-14). All forms are considered medical emergencies and can be lethal. In the case of bioterrorism, infiltration of food sources or the water supply can cause many people to become sick. Even small amounts of the bacteria can devastate large populated areas.

The patient with botulism usually has nausea, blurred vision, fatigue, slurred speech, muscle weakness, and paralysis. Symptoms can occur within hours or several days after exposure. Report any increase in patients with similar complaints to the appropriate receiving facilities and agencies.

Treatment

Prehospital Provide routine medical care, with continuous monitoring for signs of respiratory distress due to respiratory muscle paralysis. Cover wounds to prevent further infection.

Emergency Department Blood cultures to determine the type of toxin will allow the most effective antitoxin to be identified. Hospitals may not have antitoxin immediately available, so local protocols must include a process for obtaining the appropriate therapies. Mechanical ventilation may become necessary in patients with respiratory failure.

Plague

Yersinia pestis is the bacterium that causes plague. Transmission occurs through the bites of fleas from rodents such as mice, groundhogs, squirrels, and chipmunks. In terrorist attacks, the bacteria can be aerosolized, which is considered a pulmonic category of exposure (pneumonic plague). Assessment reveals difficulty breathing, productive cough, bloody sputum, and an associated complaint of chest pain. If not treated, these symptoms are followed by respiratory and cardiovascular collapse.

Bubonic plague occurs when a person is bitten by a flea infected by a rodent. Patients with this form of plague have enlarged lymph nodes, altered mentation, agitation, anuria, tachycardia, and hypotension. Untreated bubonic plague can progress to a third type of plague known as *septicemic plague*. Patients with this form of the illness have nausea and vomiting, diarrhea, necrotic skin lesions, and gangrene.

Treatment

Everyone who has come into contact with the patient should also be evaluated for symptoms.

Prehospital Initiate routine supportive medical care. Use PPE to avoid contact with airborne droplets.

Emergency Department Early intervention with antibiotics and antimicrobial agents is appropriate. Providers must take respiratory precautions, using N-95 respirators.

Ricin

Ricin is a cytotoxic protein derived from the bean of the castor plant (*Ricinus communis*). Terrorist applications include extracting this toxin into an aerosol, powder, or pellet form. Within 8 hours of inhalation, an exposed person will develop severe respiratory compromise. Hypoxia will become evident within 36 to 72 hours of exposure. Symptoms are flulike and vague but typically include nausea, vomiting, cough, weakness, fever, and hypotension. Trends in symptoms within a population can be easily overlooked because of the vagueness of their presentation, until high numbers of patients with similar symptoms indicate reason for concern and evaluation.

Treatment

Prehospital Remove contaminated clothing, and secure it in a bag. Decontaminate the patient, your equipment, and yourself if necessary. If exposure occurred by inhalation, the vehicle should remain well ventilated during transport. Continuous assessment and management of airway, breathing, and circulation is the initial intervention. Monitor the patient for respiratory and cardiovascular abnormalities.

Emergency Department Since there is no antidote for ricin exposure, hospital interventions are aimed at elimination of the toxin and avoidance of secondary contamination.

Viral Hemorrhagic Fevers

Filoviruses, flaviviruses, and arenaviruses can all be categorized as viral hemorrhagic fevers. Arthropods and other animals are common hosts for these highly infectious viruses. Contact with the urine, feces, or saliva of an infected rodent and bites from infected arthropods such as fleas or ticks are typical routes of transmission. The infected person will have fever, fatigue, and muscle aches. If exposure is undetected, severe symptoms such as bleeding from the ears, nose, and mouth and bleeding of internal organs develop. Altered mentation and collapse of the cardiovascular and renal systems may result.

Treatment

Prehospital Provide routine supportive medical care and continuous monitoring of airway, breathing, circulation, and perfusion status. Don appropriate PPE for infection control.

Emergency Department No vaccine or antidote is currently available unless there is a diagnosis of yellow fever. Initial and continuing interventions focus on support of vital organ function. Isolation rooms should be used for contaminated patients. Air-purifying respirators should be worn by all immediate caregivers.

Radiologic Weapons

Nuclear radiation comprises particles and energy released when atoms break up (fission) or combine (fusion). *Ionizing radiation* refers to radiation (alpha, beta, gamma, and neutrons) whose energy is sufficient to strip electrons from atoms or molecules. Essentially all types of radiation from the atomic nucleus are ionizing. Nonionizing radiation includes visible light, microwaves, radio waves, ultrasound, and so forth. We'll limit our discussion to ionizing radiation, which can be exploited as a weapon of mass destruction.

Types of Ionizing Radiation

Ionizing radiation can be classified as alpha, beta, gamma, or neutron particles. Let's take a look at each.

Alpha Radiation

Alpha particles (protons and neutrons) generally do not pass through the skin. In fact, they travel only a few feet and can be blocked by a simple barrier such as a piece of paper. They present a significant biohazard, then, only when radioactive material is inhaled or ingested.

Beta Radiation

Beta particles (electrons) are smaller and faster than alpha particles and thus can travel farther, penetrating tissue to a depth of about 8 mm. They can cause significant burns to the skin's surface, although these burns are not usually visible immediately after the exposure. Since clothing effectively shields covered areas, the primary danger is to exposed skin. Standard skin-cleansing procedures remove most of contamination from beta particles. The only means of detection is a radiation-sensing instrument called a *Geiger-Mueller counter*, which all hospitals should have. If exposure continues, significant exposure to gamma radiation can occur, because most radioisotopes decay by emitting beta radiation followed by gamma emission.

Gamma Rays

Gamma rays are photons emitted from the nucleus of the atom. They are electromagnetic waves that travel quickly and penetrate deeply through skin, soft tissue, and bone. Gamma rays are involved in nearly all accidents involving external irradiation. X-rays are relatively lower-energy photons that are occasionally involved in radiation accidents arising from improper use of industrial or medical equipment. Gamma rays are emitted from radioisotopes after beta decay and are the primary cause of acute radiation syndrome. Phases of this syndrome are outlined in Table 9-14. Delayed effects occur in symptom clusters (Table 9-15).

Neutrons

The fourth classification, neutron, easily penetrates surfaces and can cause significant damage to body systems (Figure 9-15). Neutrons are unique. When they are stopped, or "captured," after emission, they cause previously stable atoms to become radioactive. This is the source of radioactive fallout. The surface burst of a thermonuclear weapon instantly vaporizes tons of soil, transforming it by intense neutron bombardment into highly radioactive material. This cloud—the so-called mushroom cloud we associate with the nuclear bomb—rises with the fireball and is carried away by the prevailing winds at high altitudes. Its radioactive particles ultimately descend as fallout. A nuclear reactor harnesses this same powerful form of radiation by creating a controlled, sustained neutron chain reaction in order to generate energy.

Some gamma exposure also occurs with neutron exposure. Quantification of the radioactive material generated by neutron irradiation is helpful in estimating neutron exposure and, sometimes indirectly, the dose of gamma radiation. The radioactivity generated is primarily sodium-24, which can be detected by a Geiger-Mueller counter or in a blood sample. If neutron exposure is suspected, save and refrigerate all feces and urine. In addition, save all clothing, especially items containing metal parts such as belt buckles for analysis of neutron-induced radioisotopes.

Radiologic Exposure

Radioactive materials used by terrorists are easily accessible and can be found in research laboratories, hospitals, facilities with radiograph capabilities, and industrial complexes. Radioactive devices that are combined with explosives can be employed as terrorist weapons.

TABLE 9-14 Phases of Acute Radiation Syndrome

	EFFECTS OF WHOLE-BODY IRRADIATION FROM EXTERNAL RADIATION OR INTERNAL ABSORPTION BY DOSE RANGE IN RAD (1 Rad = 1 cGy; 100 Rad = 1 Gy)					
Feature	**0-100**	**100-200**	**200-600**	**600-800**	**800-3000**	**>3000**
PRODROMAL PHASE						
Nausea, vomiting	None	5%-50%	50%-100%	75%-100%	90%-100%	100%
Time of onset		3-6 h	2-4 h	1-2 h	<1 h	Minutes
Duration		<24 h	<24 h	<48 h	48 h	N/A
Lymphocyte count	Unaffected	Minimally decreased	<1000 at 24 h	<500 at 24 h	Decreases within hours	Decreases within hours
Central nervous system (CNS) function	No impairment	No impairment	Routine task performance Cognitive impairment for 6-20 h	Simple, routine task performance Cognitive impairment for >24 h	Rapid incapacitation May have a lucid interval of several hours	
LATENT PHASE						
No symptoms	>2 wk	7-15 days	0-7 days	0-2 days	None	None
MANIFEST ILLNESS						
Signs/symptoms	None	Moderate leukopenia	Severe leukopenia, purpura, hemorrhage, pneumonia Hair loss after 300 rad		Diarrhea, fever, electrolyte disturbance	Convulsions, ataxia, tremor, lethargy
Time of onset		>2 wk	2 days-4 wk			1-3 days
Critical period		None	4-6 wk; greatest potential for effective medical intervention		2-14 days	1-46 hr
Organ system	None		Hematopoietic; respiratory (mucosal) systems		GI tract Mucosal systems	CNS
Hospitalization duration	0%	<5% 45-60 days	90% 60-90 days	100% 100+ days	100% Weeks to months	100% Days to weeks
Mortality	None	Minimal	Low with aggressive therapy	High	Very high; significant neurologic symptoms indicate lethal dose	

Modified from Armed Forces Radiobiology Institute: Medical management of radiological casualties, Bethesda, Md, 2003.

TABLE 9-15 Symptom Clusters as Delayed Effects of Radiation Exposure

1	2	3	4
Headache Fatigue Weakness	Anorexia Nausea Vomiting Diarrhea	Partial-thickness and full-thickness skin damage Depilation (hair loss) Ulceration	Lymphopenia Neutropenia Thrombocytopenia Purpura Opportunistic infections

Time, Distance, and Shielding

The extent of injury and illness from the initial blast of a radioactive device is related to the duration (time) of exposure, distance from the explosion or blast, and the amount of shielding or protection the person had. The exposed person may then contaminate others if gas, liquid, or dust particles on their bodies or clothing are transferred to others. It's essential for first-response providers to ascertain accurate information regarding time, distance, and shielding. Box 9-12 offers additional important information for dealing with a terrorist attack involving ionizing radiation.

Dirty Bombs

A terrorist can intentionally detonate an explosive device such as a so-called **dirty bomb** in a highly populated area. Contamination of humans, animals, buildings, and the environment occurs when radioactive materials such as cobalt-60 and radium-226 are released. The initial blast will cause traumatic injury. If early recognition of the radiologic exposure does not occur, prolonged exposure can cause emergent medical problems. Inhalation of radioactive particles can provoke respiratory distress, and ingestion can induce GI discomfort.

TYPE OF RADIATION	SYMBOL	USUAL SOURCE	PENETRATION OF EXTERNAL RADIATION	PRINCIPAL TYPES OF INTERACTION
X-rays Gamma rays	x γ	X-ray machines and accelerators Most radioisotopes emit a gamma ray following beta decay	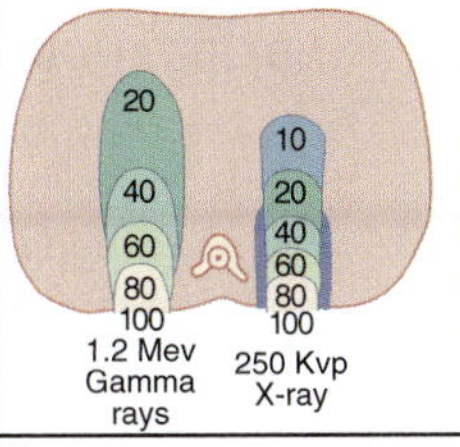 1.2 Mev Gamma rays; 250 Kvp X-ray X- and γ rays penetrate deeply, for only a fraction of the rays interact with each layer of tissue	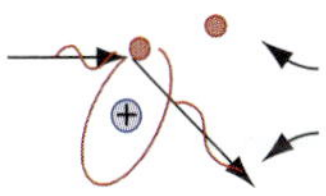 Ejected electron loses energy by causing additional ionization Deflected x- or γ ray may interact again some distance away Ionized atom formed after electron ejection
Neutrons	n	Neutrons are generally produced by critical assemblies, nuclear reactors, or accelerators	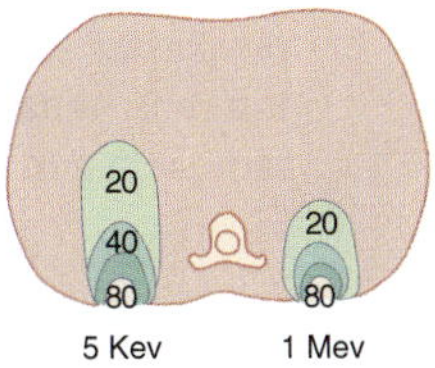 5 Kev; 1 Mev Neutrons penetrate deeply, for only a fraction of the neutrons interact with each layer of tissue	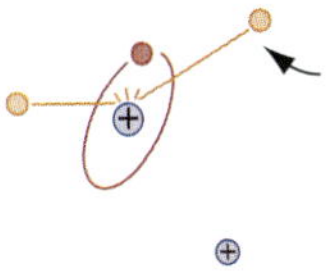 Deflected neutron may interact again some distance away Recoil proton loses energy by causing ionization
Beta particles	β	Most radioisotopes decay by beta emission, usually followed by gamma emission	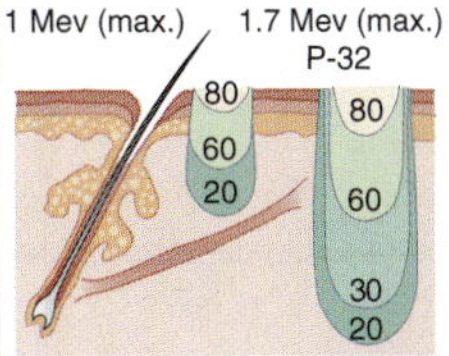 1 Mev (max.); 1.7 Mev (max.) P-32 Penetration depends on energy of beta but is usually limited to less than 8 mm in tissue	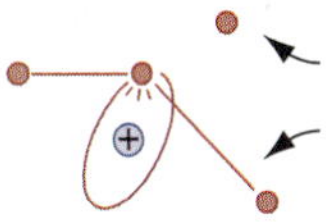 Ejected electron loses energy by causing additional ionization Deflected electron or beta particle causes additional ionization Ionized atom formed after electron ejection
Alpha particles	α	Many of the heavy radioactive elements such as plutonium decay by alpha particle emission	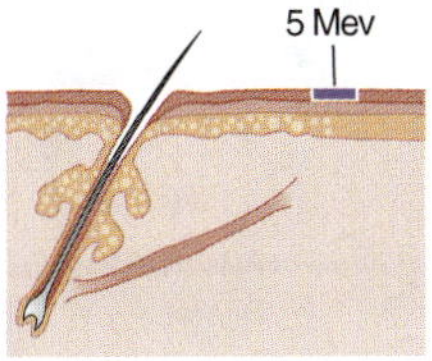 5 Mev Penetration is limited to about the thickness of the epidermis	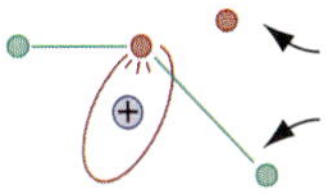 Ejected electron loses energy by causing additional ionization Deflected alpha goes on to cause additional ionization Ionized atom formed after electron ejection
Protons	p	Energetic protons are found only near particle accelerators	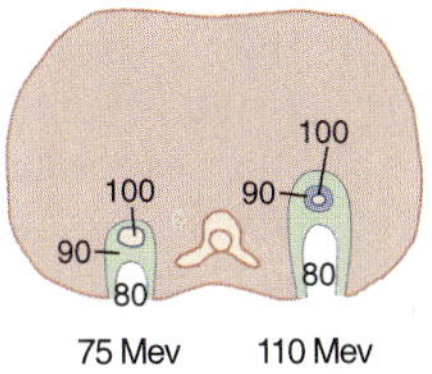 75 Mev; 110 Mev Penetration depends on energy of the proton	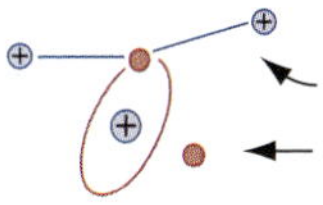 Deflected proton causes additional ionization Ejected electron loses energy by causing additional ionization Ionized atom formed after electron ejection

■ **Figure 9-15** Types of radiation and possible external hazards. (Redrawn from Gould A, Cloutier RJ: Arch Environ Health 10:499, 1965.)

Nuclear Weapons

The components necessary to construct an actual nuclear weapon of mass destruction—namely, plutonium and uranium—are much more difficult to obtain than the readily available components of a dirty bomb.

AMLS Assessment

Absorbed ionizing radiation is expressed in units called *rad*. One rad is equal to an absorbed dose of 0.01 gray (Gy). Assessment of a patient exposed to ionizing radiation requires determining the dose of rad he or she has absorbed. The greater the dose of rad absorbed, the greater the potential for serious illness and injury:

- 100 rad: nausea, vomiting, and abdominal cramping within hours of exposure
- 600 rad: dehydration and gastroenteritis; death within a few days
- 1000+ rad: cardiovascular and neurologic complications, altered mentation, ataxia, arrhythmia, cardiovascular collapse, and shock

In addition to obtaining a thorough AMLS history, a rapid head-to-toe examination must be performed to rule out associated injury. Management principles that can be implemented during a radiologic attack are given in Box 9-13.

Treatment

Prehospital Initial interventions center on ensuring scene safety and donning appropriate PPE (see Box 9-13). Avoid direct contact with radioactive materials.

BOX 9-12 Terrorism with Ionizing Radiation: General Guide

DIAGNOSIS

Be alert to the following:

1. The acute radiation syndrome follows a predictable pattern after substantial exposure or catastrophic events (see Table 9-14).
2. Individuals may become ill from contaminated sources in the community and may be identified over much longer periods based on specific syndromes (see Table 9-15).
3. Specific syndromes of concern, especially with a 2- to 3-week prior history of nausea and vomiting, are the following:
   - Thermal burn–like skin effects without documented thermal exposure
   - Immunologic dysfunction with secondary infections
   - Tendency to bleed (epistaxis, gingival bleeding, petechiae)
   - Marrow suppression (neutropenia, lymphopenia, and thrombocytopenia)
   - Depilation (hair loss)

UNDERSTANDING EXPOSURE

Exposure may be known and recognized or clandestine through the following mechanisms:

1. Large recognized exposures, such as a nuclear bomb or damage to a nuclear power station.
2. Small radiation source emitting continuous gamma radiation, producing group or individual chronic intermittent exposures (e.g., radiologic sources from medical treatment devices or environmental, water, or food contamination).
3. Internal radiation from absorbed, inhaled, or ingested radioactive material (internal contamination).

Modified from Department of Veterans Affairs pocket guide produced by Employee Education System for Office of Public Health and Environmental Hazards. This information is not meant to be complete but to be a quick guide; please consult other references and expert opinion. In Pons: PHTLS. Box 20-6.

BOX 9-13 Principles of Management of a Radiologic Disaster

1. Assess the scene for safety.
2. All patients should be medically stabilized from their traumatic injuries before radiation injuries are considered. Patients are then evaluated for their external radiation exposure and contamination.
3. An external source of radiation, if great enough, can cause tissue injury, but it does not make the patient radioactive. Patients with even lethal exposures to external radiation are not a threat to medical staff.
4. Patients can become contaminated with radioactive material deposited on their skin or clothing. More than 90% of surface contamination can be removed by removal of clothing. The remainder can be washed off with soap and water.
5. Protect yourself from radioactive contamination by observing, at a minimum, Standard Precautions, including protective clothing, gloves, and a mask.
6. Patients who develop nausea, vomiting, or skin erythema within 4 hours of exposure have probably received a high dose of external radiation.
7. Radioactive contamination in wounds should be treated as dirt and irrigated as soon as possible. Avoid handling any metallic foreign body.
8. Potassium iodide (KI) is of value only if there has been a release of radioactive iodine. KI is not a general radiation antidote.
9. The concept of time/distance/shielding is key in the prevention of untoward effects from radiation exposure. Radiation exposure is minimized by decreasing time in the affected area, increasing distance from a radiation source, and using metal or concrete shielding.

Modified from Department of Homeland Security Working Group on Radiological Dispersion Device Preparedness/Medical Preparedness and Response Subgroup, 2004, www1.va.gov/emshg/docs/Radiologic_Medical_Countermeasures_051403.pdf.

Decontaminate only patients who were exposed to liquids or gases that were combined with the explosive materials. If contamination is questionable or undetermined, wrap the patient in a blanket or sheet to minimize possible contamination of others. Notify the receiving facility of the contamination from the scene to allow for appropriate precautions on your arrival. Keep in mind the psychological effects of sustaining a sudden, violent injury and illness from the blast.

In mass-casualty situations, local medical and response-team resources can easily become overwhelmed. Verbal communication is an important part of the team effort to minimize contamination efficiently and to assess and manage multiple patients effectively.

Emergency Department Once decontamination and appropriate mass-casualty protocols have been implemented, initial patient interventions can proceed. Consider administration of sodium bicarbonate, calcium gluconate, or ammonium chloride. Administer the chelating agents and potassium iodide.

Incendiary Threats

Terrorists use incendiary threats such as firebombs to create panic in heavily populated areas. These types of devices produce large conflagrations.

Incendiary Devices

A typical example of an incendiary device is the Molotov cocktail, which consists of a fuel-soaked rag placed in a bottle or other container. The rag is ignited and the container thrown into a populated area or building. The explosion causes a fire, creating panic and injuries. As with any fire, cyanide poisoning is a medical emergency of concern (see earlier discussion).

Treatment

Prehospital Attention to scene safety, including use of the appropriate PPE, is essential in treating victims of incendiary devices. When safe to do so, notify receiving facilities from the scene that multiple patients will be arriving. Initial care consists of stabilizing airway, breathing, and circulation and treating related injuries.

Emergency Department Consider instituting internal protocols to prepare for a mass casualty.

Chemical Agents

Chemical Asphyxiants

Exposure to chemical asphyxiants can occur through inhalation, absorption, or ingestion. One of the most common asphyxiants is hydrogen cyanide, which carries the military designation *AC*. Notable for its almond-like odor when found in a solid form, cyanide can also take the form of a liquid or a colorless gas. It's often used to treat metals and is a byproduct of gas combustion. Another chemical asphyxiant used as an agent of warfare is cyanogen chloride, which carries the military designation *CK*. Once these chemicals enter the bloodstream, they decrease the ability of cells to absorb oxygen and manufacture ATP. Initial exposure causes respiratory distress, headaches, and tachycardia. If exposure is undetected or prolonged, seizures and respiratory failure result.

Carbon monoxide is an inhaled chemical asphyxiant that binds with hemoglobin, reducing the oxygen-carrying capacity of the red blood cells and inducing hypoxia. For a more detailed discussion, have a look back at the section on carbon monoxide exposure earlier in this chapter.

Treatment

Assessment of respiratory and cardiovascular status is the key to determining treatment interventions. Routine medical care includes providing supplemental oxygen, administering IV therapy, and monitoring for cardiac arrhythmias. Cyanide toxicity requires administration of a cyanide antidote kit or hydroxocobalamin. If seizure activity occurs, benzodiazepines are administered (Box 9-14). Remember that pulse oximetry readings will be inaccurate in patients with chemical asphyxiant exposure.

Prehospital If the contaminant is a known liquid, initiate the decontamination processes immediately. Stabilizing airway, breathing, and circulation and treating presenting signs and symptoms are the initial medical interventions. Use a cyanide antidote kit on each patient exposed to that chemical. These kits include amyl nitrite, sodium nitrite, and sodium thiosulfate. The first

BOX 9-14 Treatment of Chemical Asphyxiant Exposure

- Patients exposed to CO usually do not require decontamination. Because of cyanide's toxicity, patients should undergo decontamination. With liquid or solid cyanide exposure, adequate decontamination is essential.
- Establish an open airway. Consider orotracheal or nasotracheal intubation for airway control in the patient who is unconscious, has severe pulmonary edema, or is in severe respiratory distress.
- Ventilate as necessary. Positive-pressure ventilation with a bag-mask device may be beneficial.
- Do not induce vomiting or use emetics.
- Monitor for pulmonary edema, and treat as necessary.
- Monitor cardiac rhythm, and treat dysrhythmias as necessary.
- Start an IV, and infuse at 30 mL/h. For hypotension with signs of hypovolemia, give fluid cautiously. Consider vasopressors if the patient is hypotensive with a normal fluid volume, per local protocol. Watch for signs of fluid overload.
- Administer cyanide antidote kit per local protocol for symptomatic patients with cyanide exposure.
- Treat seizures with diazepam (Valium) or lorazepam (Ativan) per local protocol.
- For eye contamination, immediately flush eyes with water. Continuously irrigate each eye with normal saline during transport.
- Pulse oximetry readings may not be accurate in these exposures.
- Hyperbaric oxygen may be required for optimal treatment.

CO, Carbon monoxide; *IV*, intravenous line.
Reprinted from Currance PL, Clements B, Bronstein AC: Emergency care for hazardous materials exposure, ed 3, St Louis, 2005, Mosby.

two medications combine with hemoglobin to form methemoglobin. Methemoglobin attaches to cyanide ions and binds them to cyanmethemoglobin. The third medication, sodium thiosulfate, converts cyanmethemoglobin into thiocyanate, which is easily excreted by the kidneys. A recently approved and simpler therapeutic agent is hydroxocobalamin.

Emergency Department In the ED, the patient is observed and given continued supportive care.

Nerve Agents

The most toxic agents in chemical warfare are nerve agents. These agents disrupt nerve transmission in the central and peripheral nervous systems by inhibiting acetylcholinesterase release, exciting the cholinergic response and overstimulating the parasympathetic nervous system. Although minimal exposure has no long-term devastating results, high amounts and long duration of exposure are associated with high rates of mortality and morbidity. Nerve agents are similar to organophosphates (see Toxins in the Home and Workplace) but much more potent and destructive. Nerve agents can also be classified as G and V agents.

The G agents include tabun (GA), sarin (GB), soman (GD), and cyclohexyl methylphosphonofluoridate (GF). Developed in the United Kingdom, VX is the most common V agent. G agents are very volatile, limited-action, colorless liquids. When aerosolized or released into warm environments or closed buildings, they become more volatile. V liquids are usually not volatile and are longer acting.

Your initial response must be to secure scene safety. Since the nerve agent vapors are heavier than air, it's prudent to park vehicles uphill and upwind. Prevention of secondary contamination is essential; appropriate PPE is required. Removal of contaminants by decontamination procedures may be necessary, since chemicals can stay on clothing 30 to 40 minutes after exposure. It's essential that you move patients to a well-ventilated area. Use the SLUDGE BBM mnemonic shown in the Rapid Recall box to identify presenting symptoms. Supportive care for airway, breathing, and circulation are the initial medical interventions. Provide continual monitoring of blood pressure alterations. Manage cardiac arrhythmias per American Heart Association (AHA) ACLS protocols.

Use nerve agent autoinjector antidote kits, known as *Mark 1 antidote kits*, containing atropine and pralidoxime (Figure 9-16). Newer kits, known as *DuoDote kits*, combine the two medications in one autoinjector. A detailed explanation of how these agents work to reverse toxicity was given earlier. If seizures develop, administer diazepam (Valium) or lorazepam (Versed).

Sarin (GB)

In its liquid state, sarin is colorless, odorless, and tasteless. It can infiltrate into waterways and reach toxic levels in drinking water or water used for bathing. Sarin can also be converted to a gas and released as a vapor into the air, contaminating large geographic areas. People exposed to sarin complain of headache, increased salivation, abdominal cramping, and respiratory distress with wheezing. Symptoms begin minutes to hours after exposure.

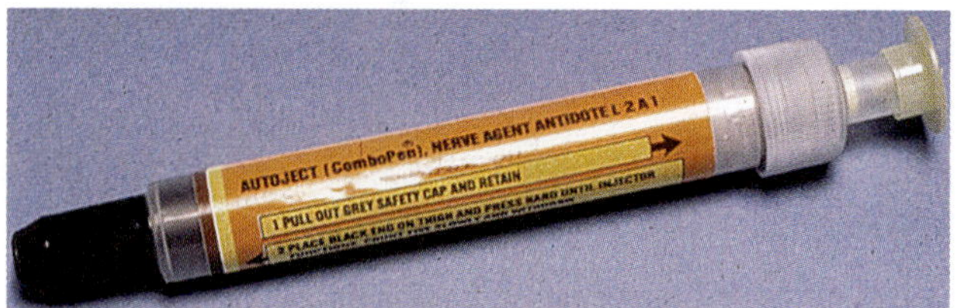

■ **Figure 9-16** Mark I antidote kit. (From Miller R, Eriksson L, Fleisher L, et al: Miller's anesthesia, ed 7, New York, 2009, Churchill Livingstone.)

Soman (GD)

Soman is also a clear, colorless, tasteless liquid, but it can have a camphor odor similar to mentholated rubs and cough drops. More volatile than sarin, this liquid provokes symptoms within seconds or minutes, rather than hours after exposure. Signs and symptoms are similar to those associated with sarin exposure.

Tabun (GA)

Tabun, also a clear, colorless, and tasteless liquid, has a minimal fruity odor. It can vaporize and thus be inhaled. Exposure can also occur through ingestion or absorption. Since the liquid mixes easily with water, it can be ingested, causing GI discomfort. Absorption can cause skin and eye irritation. If the liquid remains on clothing, it can cause secondary contamination of those who touch it. Symptoms begin within seconds when a person is exposed to the vapor and within several hours when a person is exposed to tabun in liquid form. Patients exhibit altered mentation, seizures, watery eyes, cough, and excessive sweating. Cardiac arrhythmia sometimes occurs.

VX

VX, a V agent, is an odorless, slightly amber liquid. This liquid is more toxic when inhaled or absorbed through the skin than when ingested. It mixes easily with water, causing abdominal discomfort when ingested. Signs and symptoms begin to appear within seconds or hours of exposure and are similar to those provoked by other nerve agents. Victims may have muscle twitching and miosis. Unrecognized and untreated, the twitching can progress to status epilepticus and can be difficult to stop.

Pulmonary Agents

Poisonous gases, known as **pulmonary agents**, pose a grave threat to the safety of first responders and prehospital personnel. These gases are easily obtained, and victims can be quickly contaminated by inhaling them.

Unfortunately, no antidote exists. Contaminated clothing must be removed and properly packaged per local protocol. Decontamination must be performed promptly by trained personnel.

Chlorine

Chlorine is a yellow-green gas that has a slight odor some describe as smelling like a combination of pepper and pineapple. It's commonly found in plastics and solvent manufacturing plants. When pressurized, chlorine easily vaporizes into a gas. Chlorine can be inhaled, absorbed through the skin, or ingested if water is contaminated. Signs and symptoms include eye and throat irritation, burns from skin exposure, and respiratory distress caused by inhalation. Severe respiratory complications such as pulmonary edema can become evident within 20 to 24 hours of exposure.

Phosgene (CG)

Phosgene appears in gaseous form as a gray-white cloud with the vague odor of freshly bailed hay. This agent is commonly found in pesticides, pharmaceuticals, and dyes. When cooled, it converts to a liquid. When released into the air, it vaporizes quickly. Signs and symptoms are similar to those that appear after chlorine exposure, but the agent can cause significant cardiovascular compromise and hypotension. If the exposure is not identified and managed, death can occur within a few days.

Anhydrous Ammonia

Anhydrous ammonia is a colorless gas commonly found in agricultural settings, where it's used as fertilizer. Industrial factories use this gas for cooling and freezing foods like meat and poultry. Anhydrous ammonia is considered volatile and, when present in high concentrations, forms a white cloud. Symptoms occur within several hours of exposure.

Putting It All Together

When you're a first responder to a patient with a toxicologic exposure or a situation involving hazardous materials or possible weapons of mass destruction, the initial scene and patient assessment challenges can be daunting. If you can maintain a heightened level of awareness for situations and patients that may present safety issues, your AMLS training and skills can then help you organize a methodical healthcare plan. First you have to know the extent of the threat of the toxic exposure to yourself and your patient, and then you have to be able to implement appropriate safety precautions in addition to treating your patient's medical emergency.

Get familiar with local, regional, state, and federal agencies that can offer support in these situations. If mutual aid is required, those agencies should be contacted immediately for activation. As always, the AMLS assessment pathway begins with the patient's cardinal presentation and uses step-by-step clinical reasoning to evaluate presenting signs and symptoms, determine a working diagnosis, and arrive at an effective treatment plan. In toxicologic emergencies in particular, the patient's historical information can provide key clues to medical management that will stabilize the patient and improve outcomes.

SCENARIO SOLUTION

1 **Differential diagnoses may include sympathomimetic intoxication (cocaine, amphetamine, ephedrine, phencyclidine), stroke, autonomic hyperreflexia, or alcohol withdrawal.**

2 **To narrow your differential diagnosis, you'll need to complete a more thorough history of past and present illness. Question his roommate about the use of alcohol or other drugs. Perform a physical examination that includes vital sign assessment, stroke scale, pupil assessment, evaluation of heart and breath sounds, ECG monitoring and a 12-lead ECG, Sao_2, capnography, and blood glucose analysis. If you suspect autonomic hyperreflexia, look for a trigger such as a full bladder that could be the source of the problem.**

3 **The patient has signs that indicate an exaggerated sympathetic response. Administer oxygen if indicated. Establish vascular access. Continue to monitor the ECG. Further treatment will depend on the rest of your assessment findings. If you suspect sympathomimetic overdose or alcohol withdrawal, treat with a benzodiazepine and IV fluid administration. If the patient has signs of stroke, transport him to the closest appropriate center. If his exam points to autonomic hyperreflexia, transport if the source of the problem is not immediately resolved.**

SUMMARY

- Ensure safety before entering any scene that may be contaminated, and consider airborne toxins that could be dangerous.
- Obtain a thorough history, including available drugs/toxins, time of ingestion, and dose. Ask bystanders and witnesses for additional information.
- Maintain supportive care for comatose patients, including airway management and administration of glucose, thiamine, and small doses of naloxone if necessary.
- Obtain an accurate core temperature, and institute temperature normalization strategies if necessary.

- Gauge perfusion status by monitoring mental status, urine output, blood pressure, capillary refill time, and acid-base status. Initiate invasive monitoring as time allows.
- Contact a poison control center early in the diagnosis, and treat any toxicologic disorder.
- Scene assessment of an environment compromised by a hazardous material or a biological, chemical, or radiologic agent is a key component in preserving the safety of healthcare personnel and patients.
- Incident command should establish hot, warm, and cold zones to maintain scene control and safety.
- Identification of the proper personal protective devices needed for unstable scenes and patient exposures is critical to ensuring the safety of personnel and patients and containing the spread of a toxin or hazardous material.
- Decontamination must occur before entering a hot zone, and it must be performed again before and after transport to the receiving facility.
- Understanding various procedures for responder, patient, and equipment decontamination is essential to maintaining the safety of all healthcare providers and patients and to preventing secondary contamination.
- The potential for exposure is reduced when providers make use of references for the identification of possible hazardous materials. These references also specify associated signs and symptoms and outline appropriate treatment modalities, should an exposure occur.
- Disaster response preparedness is essential in the emergent assessment and management of patients and scenes with possible exposure to toxic agents, hazardous materials, or chemical, biological, or radiologic weapons.
- Identifying chemical, biological, and radiologic agent cardinal presentations and safety and management strategies reduces morbidity and mortality in individuals and reduces the potential for exposure.
- Performing a thorough assessment and obtaining a complete history can help eliminate secondary exposure by identifying contamination early.
- Presentation of signs and symptoms of exposure varies with different contaminants, on the basis of volatility, duration, and route of exposure.
- Early recognition of hazardous materials and bioterrorist incidents can reduce exposure and promote timely implementation of treatment strategies for all involved agencies.
- Report all suspected hazardous materials and bioterrorist incidents to the appropriate local, state, and federal authorities so that disaster response protocols can be implemented.
- Weapons of mass destruction include biological, nuclear, incendiary, chemical, and radiologic agents.

BIBLIOGRAPHY

Auerbach P: Wilderness medicine, ed 5, St Louis, 2007, Mosby.

Bailey B: Glucagon in beta-blocker and calcium channel blocker overdoses: a systematic review, J Toxicol Clin Toxicol 41:595–602, 2003.

Baltarowich L: Barbiturates, Top Emerg Med 7:46–53, 1985.

Brent J, Wallace K, Bukhart K: Critical care toxicology, St Louis, 2004, Mosby.

Bronstein AC, et al: 2006 annual report of the American Association of Poison Control Centers National Poison Data System, Clin Toxicol 45:815–917, 2007.

Bronstein AC, et al: 2007 Annual Report of the American Association of Poison Control Centers National Poison Data System: 25th Annual Report. American Association of Poison Control Centers, Clin Toxicol 46:927–1057, 2008.

Buchanan JF, Brown CR: "Designer drugs": a problem in clinical toxicology, Med Toxicol 3:1–17, 1988.

Budisavljevic MN, et al: Hyponatremia associated with 3,4-methylenedioxy-methylamphetamine ("ecstasy") abuse, Am J Med Sci 326:89–93, 2003.

Cai Z, McCaslin PP: Acute, chronic, and differential effects of several anesthetic barbiturates on glutamate receptor activation in neuronal culture, Brain Res 611:181–186, 1993.

Campbell NR, Baylis B: Renal impairment associated with an acute paracetamol overdose in the absence of hepatotoxicity, Postgrad Med J 68:116–118, 1992.

Caravati EM: Hallucinogenic drugs. In Medical toxicology, ed 3, Philadelphia, 2004, Lippincott, pp 1103–1111.

Cater RE: The use of sodium and potassium to reduce toxicity and toxic side effects from lithium, Med Hypotheses 20:359–383, 1986.

Chan P, et al: Fatal and nonfatal methamphetamine intoxication in the intensive care unit, J Toxicol Clin Toxicol 32:147–155, 1994.

Chance BC, Erecinska M, Wagner M: Mitochondrial responses to carbon monoxide, Ann NY Acad Sci 174:193–203, 1970.

Chandler DB, Norton RL, Kauffman J: Lead poisoning associated with intravenous methamphetamine use—Oregon, 1988, MMWR Morb Mortal Wkly Rep 38:830–831, 1989.

Chyka PA, Seger D: Position statement: single-dose activated charcoal, J Toxicol Clin Toxicol 35:721–741, 1997.

Coburn RF, Mayers LB: Myoglobin oxygen tension determines from measurements of carboxyhemoglobin in skeletal muscle, Am J Physiol 220:66–74, 1971.

Coupey SM: Barbiturates, Pediatr Rev 18:260–264, 1997.

Cumberland Pharmaceuticals, Inc.: Acetadote package insert. Nashville, Tenn, March 2004.

DeWitt CR, Waksman JC: Pharmacology, pathophysiology, and management of calcium channel blocker and beta blocker toxicity, Toxicol Rev 23:223–238, 2004.

Doyon S, Roberts JR: The use of glucagon in a case of calcium channel blocker overdose, Ann Emerg Med 22:1229–1233, 1993.

Eddleston M, et al: Multiple-dose activated charcoal in acute self-poisoning: a randomised controlled trial, Lancet 371:579–587, 2008.

Emerson TS, Cisek JE: Methcathinone ("cat"): a Russian designer amphetamine infiltrates the rural Midwest, Ann Emerg Med 22:1897–1903, 1993.

Fingerhut LA, Cox CS: Poisoning mortality, 1985–1995, Public Health Rep 113:218–233, 1998.

Finkle BS, McCloskey KL, Goodman LS: Diazepam and drug-associated deaths. A survey in the United States and Canada, J Am Med Assoc 242:429–434, 1979.

Flomenbaum NE, Goldfrank LR, Hoffman RS, et al: Goldfrank's toxicologic emergencies, ed 8, New York, 2006, McGraw-Hill.

Frierson J, et al: Refractory cardiogenic shock and complete heart block after unsuspected verapamil—SR and atenolol overdose, Clin Cardiol 14:933–935, 1991.

Garnier R, et al: Acute zolpidem poisoning—analysis of 344 cases, J Toxicol Clin Toxicol 32:391–404, 1994.

Graham SR, et al: Overdose with chloral hydrate: a pharmacological and therapeutic review, Med J Aust 149:686–688, 1988.

Greenblatt DJ, et al: Acute overdosage with benzodiazepine derivatives, Clin Pharmacol Ther 21:497–514, 1977.

Hariman RJ, et al: Reversal of the cardiovascular effects of verapamil by calcium and sodium: differences between electrophysiologic and hemodynamic responses, Circulation 59:797–804, 1979.

Hendren WC, Schreiber RS, Garretson LK: Extracorporeal bypass for the treatment of verapamil poisoning, Ann Emerg Med 18:984–987, 1989.

Hesse B, Pedersen JT: Hypoglycaemia after propranolol in children, Acta Med Scand 193:551–552, 1973.

Hoegholm A, Clementson P: Hypertonic sodium chloride in severe antidepressant overdosage, J Toxicol Clin Toxicol 29:297–298, 1991.

Horowitz AL, Kaplan R, Sarpel G: Carbon monoxide toxicity: MR imaging in the brain, Radiology 162:787–788, 1987.

Kaim SC, Klett CJ, Rothfeld B: Treatment of the acute alcohol withdrawal state: a comparison of four drugs, Am J Psychiatry 125:1640–1646, 1969.

Kerns W II, et al: Insulin improves survival in a canine model of acute beta-blocker toxicity, Ann Emerg Med 29:748–757, 1997.

Kitchens CS, Van Mierop LHS: Envenomation by the eastern coral snake (*Micrurus fulvius fulvius*), J Am Med Assoc 258:1615–1618, 1987.

Kline JA, et al: Insulin is a superior antidote for cardiovascular toxicity induced by verapamil in the anesthetized canine, J Pharm Exp Ther 267:744–750, 1993.

Kunkel DB, et al: Reptile envenomations, J Toxicol Clin Toxicol 21:503–526, 1983–1984.

Lange RA, et al: Potentiation of cocaine-induced coronary vasoconstriction by beta-adrenergic blockade, Ann Intern Med 112:897–903, 1990.

Leonard LG, Scheulen JJ, Munster AM: Chemical burns: effect of prompt first aid, J Trauma 22:420–423, 1982.

Lindberg MC, Cunningham A, Lindberg NH: Acute phenobarbital intoxication, South Med J 85:803–806, 1992.

Long H, Nelson LS, Hoffman RS: A rapid qualitative test for suspected ethylene glycol poisoning, Acad Emerg Med 15:688–690, 2008.

Love JN, et al: A potential role for glucagon in the treatment of drug-induced symptomatic bradycardia, Chest 114:323–326, 1998.

Lundborg P: The effect of adrenergic blockade on potassium concentrations in different conditions, Acta Med Scand Suppl 672:121–126, 1983.

Makin AJ, Williams R: The current management of paracetamol overdosage, Br J Clin Pract 48:144–148, 1994.

Marques I, Gomes E, de Oliveira J: Treatment of calcium channel blocker intoxication with insulin infusion: case report and literature review, Resuscitation 57:211–213, 2003.

McCarron MM, et al: Acute phencyclidine intoxication: clinical patterns, complications, and treatment, Ann Emerg Med 10:290–297, 1981.

Mitchell JR, et al: Acetaminophen-induced hepatic necrosis. I. Role of drug metabolism, J Pharmacol Exp Ther 187:185–194, 1973.

Miura T, et al: CT of the brain in acute carbon monoxide intoxication: characteristic features and prognosis, AJNR Am J Neuroradiol 6:739–742, 1985.

Monitoring the Future: 2003 Data from in-school surveys of 8th, 10th, and 12th grade students. Drug and alcohol press release: trends in use of various drugs. Available from www.monitoringthefuture.org/data/03data/pr03t1.pdf. Accessed August 20, 2010.

Moon RE, DeLong E: Hyperbaric oxygen for carbon monoxide poisoning, Med J Aust 170:197–199, 1999.

NAEMT: PHTLS Prehospital trauma life support, ed 7, St Louis, 2010, Mosby.

Ostapowicz G, et al: Results of a prospective study of acute liver failure at 17 tertiary care centers in the United States, Ann Intern Med 137:947–954, 2002.

Palmer BF: Effectiveness of hemodialysis in the extracorporeal therapy of phenobarbital overdose, Am J Kidney Dis 36:640–643, 2000.

Pena BM, Krauss B: Adverse events of procedural sedation and analgesia in a pediatric emergency department, Ann Emerg Med 34:483–491, 1999.

Pentel PR, Benowitz NL: Tricyclic antidepressant poisoning—management of arrhythmias, Med Toxicol 1:101–121, 1986.

Peterson JE, Stewart RD: Absorption and elimination of carbon monoxide by inactive young men, Arch Environ Health 21:165–171, 1970.

Prescott LF: Paracetamol overdosage: pharmacological considerations and clinical management, Drugs 25:290–314, 1983.

Raphael JC, et al: Trial of normobaric and hyperbaric oxygen for acute carbon monoxide intoxication, Lancet 1989:414–419, 1989.

Reith DM, et al: Relative toxicity of beta blockers in overdose, J Toxicol Clin Toxicol 34:273–278, 1996.

Roth BA, Vinson DR, Kim S: Carisoprodol-induced myoclonic encephalopathy, J Toxicol Clin Toxicol 36:609–612, 1998.

Seger DL: Flumazenil—treatment or toxin? J Toxicol Clin Toxicol 42:209–216, 2004.

Sieghart W: Structure and pharmacology of gamma-aminobutyric $acid_A$ receptor subtypes, Pharmacol Rev 47:181–234, 1995.

Stewart R, et al: Carboxyhemoglobin levels in American blood donors, J Am Med Assoc 229:1187–1195, 1974.

Vale JA: Position statement: gastric lavage, J Toxicol Clin Toxicol 35:711, 1997.

Van Hoesen KB, et al: Should hyperbaric oxygen be used to treat the pregnant patient for acute carbon monoxide poisoning? A case report and literature review, J Am Med Assoc 261:1039–1043, 1989.

Vollenweider FX, et al: Psychological and cardiovascular effects and short-term sequelae of MDMA ("ecstasy") in MDMA-naive healthy volunteers, Neuropsychopharmacology 19:241–251, 1998.

Wason S, Lacouture PG, Lovejoy FH: Single high-dose pyridoxine treatment for isoniazid overdose, J Am Med Assoc 246:1102–1104, 1981.

Weaver LK, et al: Hyperbaric oxygen for acute carbon monoxide poisoning, N Engl J Med 347:1057–1067, 2002.

Wiley CC, Wiley JF II: Pediatric benzodiazepine ingestion resulting in hospitalization, J Toxicol Clin Toxicol 36:227–231, 1998.

Yildiz S, et al: Seizure incidence in 80,000 patient treatments with hyperbaric oxygen, Aviat Space Environ Med 75:992–994, 2004.

Zuvekas S, Vitiello B: Recent trends in stimulant medication use among U.S. children, Am J Psych 163:579–585, 2006.

Chapter Review Questions

1. Your patient is agitated and sweaty. Her vital signs are BP 170/108 mm Hg, P 132 bpm, and R 20/min. Her pupils are dilated, and her hands are trembling. These signs and symptoms may be associated with:
   a. Alcohol withdrawal
   b. Carbamates
   c. Diazepam
   d. Tramadol

2. Which source provides the most detailed information related to hazardous materials?
   a. Location of the emergency
   b. Material safety data sheets
   c. Pictographs
   d. Placards

3. A 2-year-old male is found chewing on berries from a lily of the valley plant. Predict his vital signs.
   a. BP 130/72, P 128 bpm
   b. BP 100/60, P 100 bpm
   c. BP 70/50, P 128 bpm
   d. BP 70/50 P 70 bpm

4. A 24-year-old female took 24 diphenhydramine tablets. Her vital signs are BP 86/54 mm Hg, P 110 bpm, R 20/min. What other sign or symptom should you anticipate?
   a. Drooling
   b. Pale skin
   c. Pinpoint pupils
   d. Seizures

5. The family of a 72-year-old male is worried about their father. His blood glucose is 80 mg/dL (4.4 mmol/L). His rate and depth of breathing are increased, and he is sleepy and weak. He takes metformin (Glucophage). You suspect his signs and symptoms may be related to:
   a. Diabetic ketoacidosis
   b. Hyperosmolar hyperglycemic nonketotic coma
   c. Lactic acidosis
   d. Pulmonary embolus

6. A farmer was spraying his barn when he became ill. His heart rate is 60 bpm, and his blood pressure is 88/50 mm Hg. Tears are streaming down his cheeks, and he is vomiting. What toxidrome does this clinical picture fit?
   a. Anticholinergic
   b. Cholinergic
   c. Opioid
   d. Sympathomimetic

7. Which of the following biological warfare agents causes serious neurologic symptoms that may include paralysis?
   a. Botulism
   b. Plague
   c. Ricin
   d. Viral hemorrhagic fever

8. A 22-year-old female is found at a party unresponsive and breathing approximately 8 breaths/min. Her skin is gray. Which of the following signs or symptoms will confirm your suspicion that the opioid toxidrome is causing her emergency?
   a. Blood pressure 170/110 mm Hg
   b. Pupils 2 mm and equal
   c. QRS duration is 0.24 sec.
   d. Tremors are present.

9. Your patient is reported to have taken an overdose. She has a history of anxiety disorder and depression. She is unresponsive, and vital signs are BP 100/70, P 128 bpm, R 20/min. Her ECG shows right bundle branch block. You expect she has taken:
   a. Amitriptyline
   b. Lorazepam
   c. Paroxetine
   d. Quetiapine

10. You respond to a warehouse for "multiple patients with difficulty breathing." From a hallway, you see your patient lying in a room with two other people who don't seem to be breathing. He calls out to you, saying he can't breathe. You should first:
    a. Administer oxygen by nonrebreather mask.
    b. Drag him out of the room.
    c. Examine the shipping papers.
    d. Stage at a safe distance.

APPENDIX

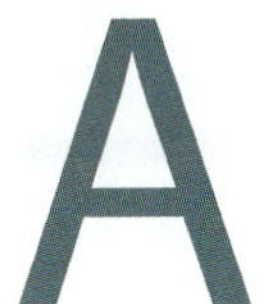

AMLS Assessment Pathway

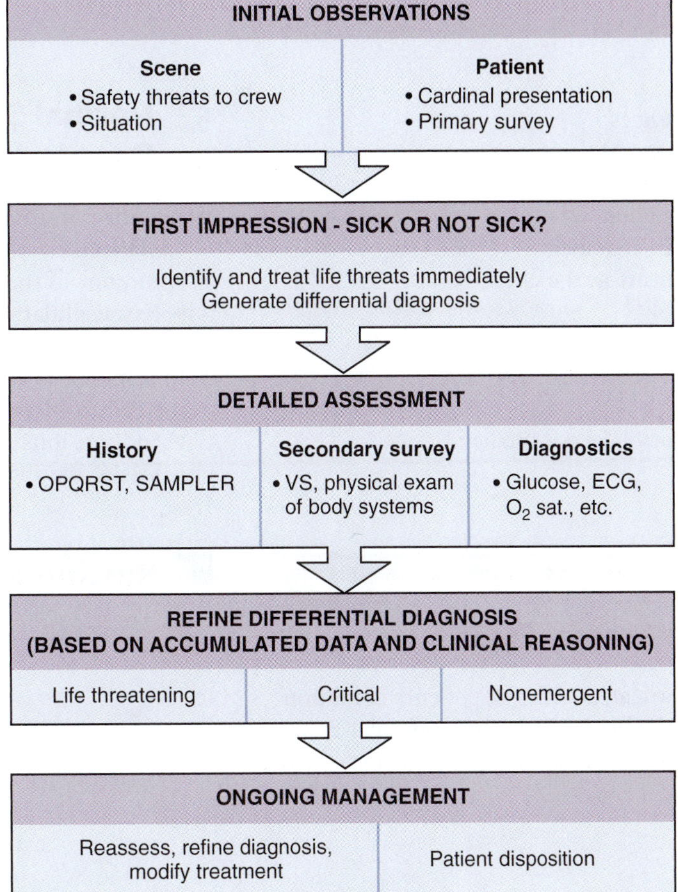

INITIAL OBSERVATIONS
Scene
• Safety threats to crew
• Situation
Patient
• Cardinal presentation
• Primary survey
FIRST IMPRESSION - SICK OR NOT SICK?
Identify and treat life threats immediately
Generate differential diagnosis
If new life threats identified, treat immediately
DETAILED ASSESSMENT
History
• OPQRST, SAMPLER
Secondary survey
• VS, physical exam of body systems
Diagnostics
• Glucose, ECG, O_2 sat., etc.
REFINE DIFFERENTIAL DIAGNOSIS
(BASED ON ACCUMULATED DATA AND CLINICAL REASONING)
Life threatening
Critical
Nonemergent
ONGOING MANAGEMENT
Reassess, refine diagnosis, modify treatment
Patient disposition

APPENDIX

B 12-Lead Electrocardiogram Review

 Know Your Electrocardiogram (ECG)

- Identifies:
  - Rhythm disturbances
  - Conduction abnormalities
  - Electrolyte disorders
- Contributes information about:
  - Size of the heart's chambers
  - Position of the heart in the chest
- As a diagnostic tool:
  - Myocardial infarctions (MIs)
  - Ischemia
  - Pericarditis
  - Functioning of artificial pacemakers
- Monitors:
  - Drug effects
  - Treatment effects

 The Limitations of ECGs

- Must always be correlated with the patient's condition
- Patients with healthy hearts may have abnormal ECGs, and patients with serious cardiac disease may have normal ECGs.
- An ECG represents electrical events in the heart—not mechanical.

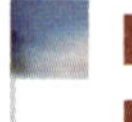 Normal Sequence of Cardiac Depolarization/Repolarization

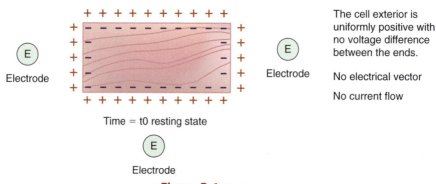

- In the resting state, the myocardial cells are "polarized."
  - Interior of the cells are negatively charged.
  - Extracellular: sodium ions
  - Intracellular: potassium ions
- In response to various stimuli, movements of ions cause the cell to "depolarize."
  - Sodium ions rapidly enter the cell, causing a rapid loss of the internal negative charge.

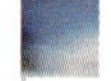 Resting State

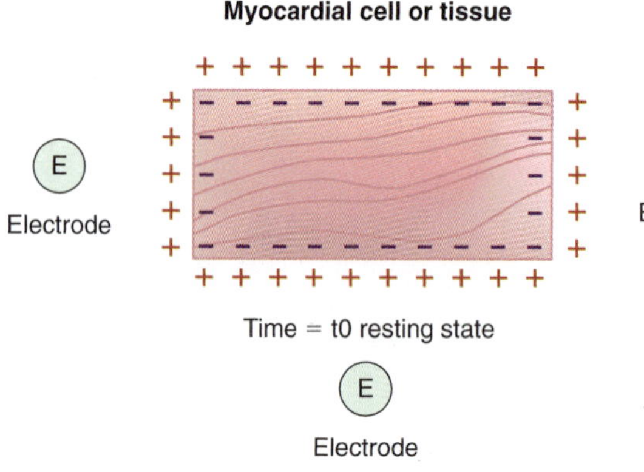

Figure B-1 Resting state.

Depolarization Complete

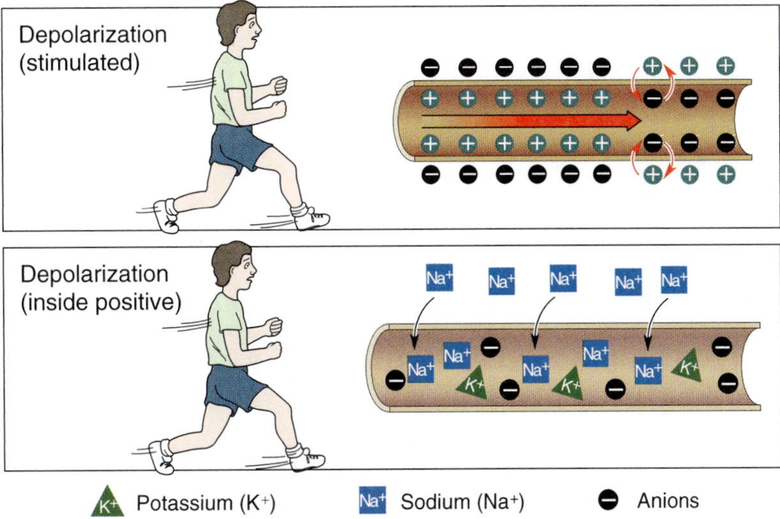

■ **Figure B-2** *Depolarization* is movement of ions across a cell membrane, causing inside of cell to become more positive. (From Aehlert B: ECGs made easy, ed 3, St Louis, 2006, Mosby.)

Repolarization Complete

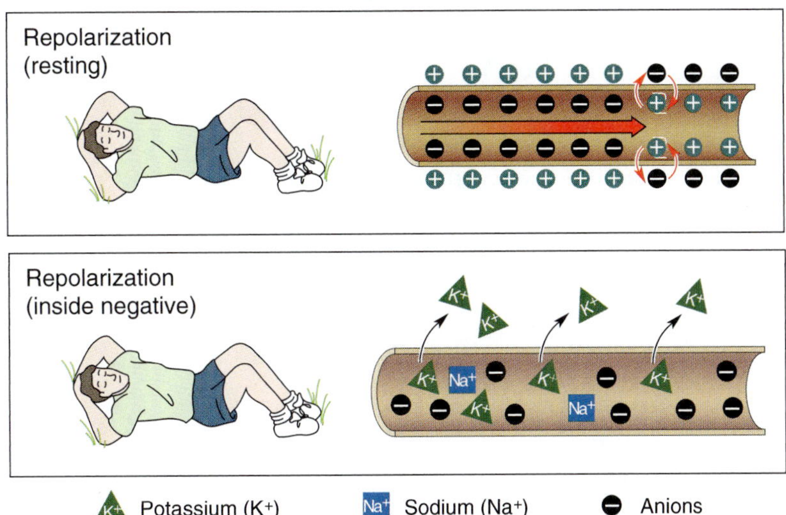

■ **Figure B-3** *Repolarization* is movement of charged particles across cell membrane, causing inside of cell to be restored to its negative charge. (From Aehlert B: ECGs made easy, ed 3, St Louis, 2006, Mosby.)

The Conduction System

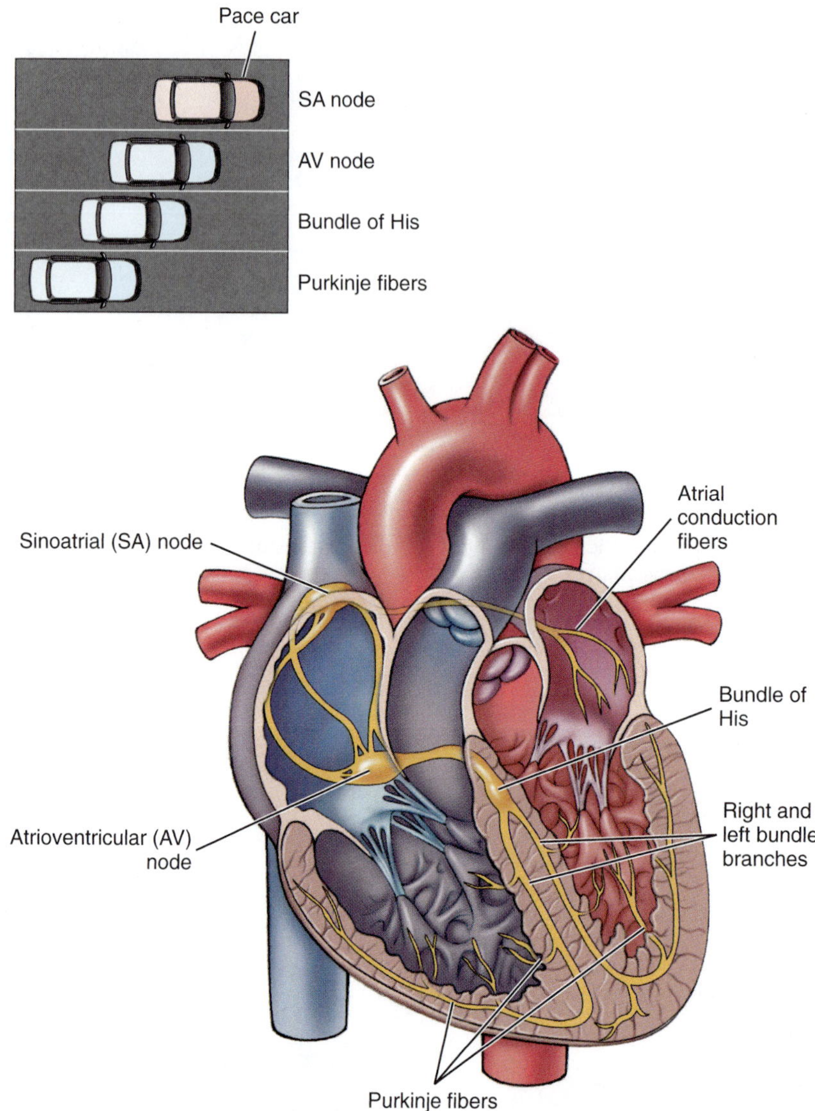

Figure B-4 Cardiac conduction system. (From Aehlert B: ECGs made easy, ed 3, St Louis, 2006, Mosby.)

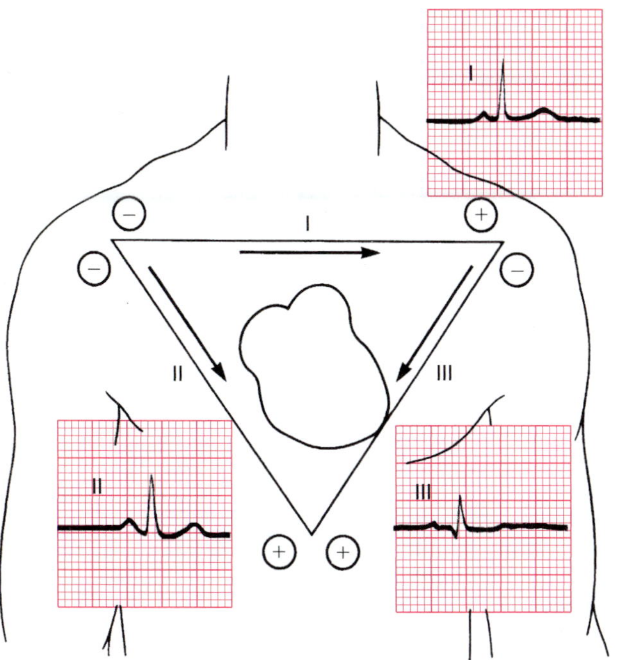

■ **Figure B-5** Comparison of waveforms recorded in standard limb leads. (From Aehlert B: ECGs made easy, ed 3, St Louis, 2006, Mosby.)

ECG Lead Placement

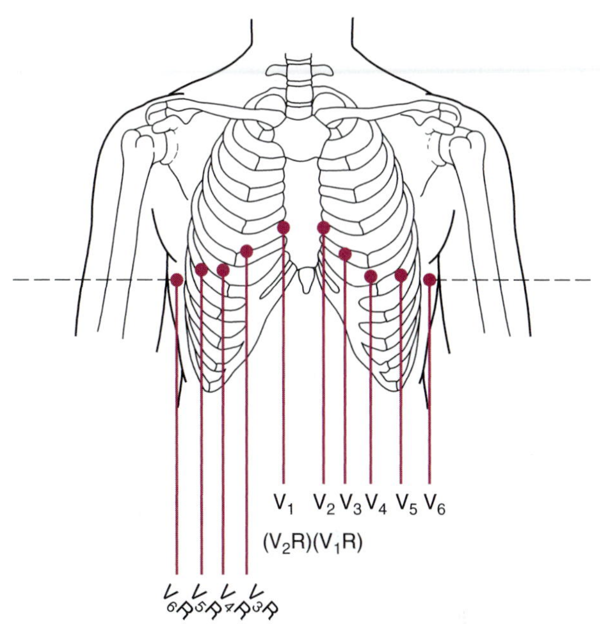

■ **Figure B-6** Anatomic placement of left and right chest leads. (From Aehlert B: ECGs made easy, ed 3, St Louis, 2006, Mosby.)

- V_1: right fourth intercostal space
- V_2: left fourth intercostal space
- V_3: halfway between V_2 and V_4
- V_4: left fifth intercostal space, midclavicular line
- V_5: horizontal to V_4, anterior axillary line
- V_6: horizontal to V_5, midaxillary line

Standard ECG

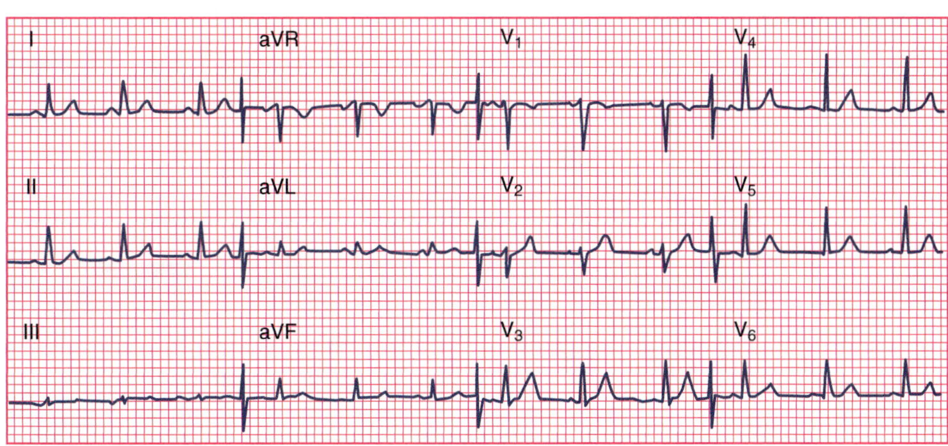

■ **Figure B-7** Example of normal 12-lead electrocardiogram. (From Zipes DP, Libby P, Bonow R, Braunwald E: Braunwald's heart disease: a textbook of cardiovascular medicine, ed 7, Philadelphia, 2005, Saunders.)

ECG Paper and Recording

- Standard graphing
  - Small box (1 mm) = 0.04 second
  - Large box = 0.2 second
- Check voltage
  - Standard is 1 mV = 10 mm
- Check paper speed
  - Standard is 25 mm/sec
- Location of the 12 "leads"

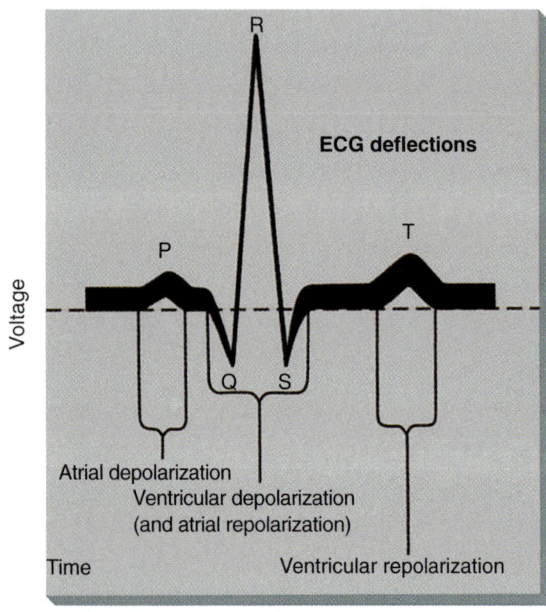

■ **Figure B-8** Electrocardiogram waveforms: P, QRS, and T. (From Aehlert B: ECGs made easy, ed 3, St Louis, 2006, Mosby.)

The Normal P Wave

- Represents atrial depolarization
- Precedes the QRS complex
- <2 to 2.5 mm tall
- Usually rounded and upright

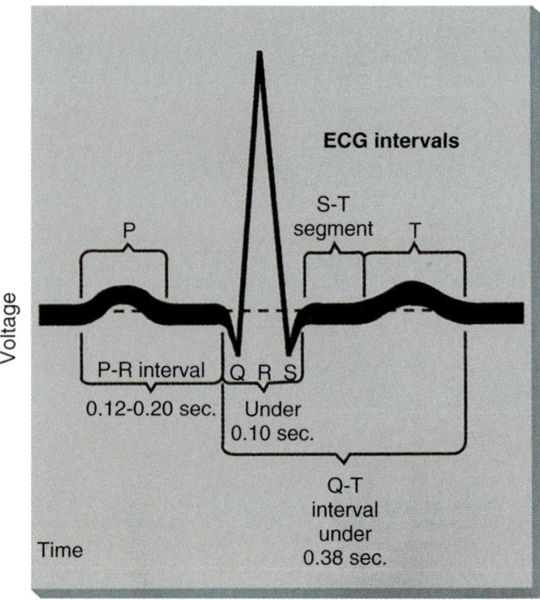

■ **Figure B-9** Electrocardiogram segments and intervals: PR interval, QRS duration, ST segment, QT interval. (From Aehlert B: ECGs made easy, ed 3, St Louis, 2006, Mosby.)

The Normal QRS Complex

- Represents ventricular depolarization
- Normal ≤0.12 second in duration
- Configuration varies based upon the lead chosen.

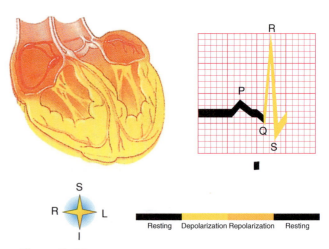

■ **Figure B-10** The QRS complex represents ventricular depolarization. (From Aehlert B: ECGs made easy, ed 3, St Louis, 2006, Mosby.)

The Normal T wave

- Represents ventricular repolarization
- Peak of the T wave represents the start of the relative refractory period.
- Normal height:
  - ≤5 mm in limb leads
  - ≤10 mm in precordial leads
- Upright in most leads (may be negative in aVR)

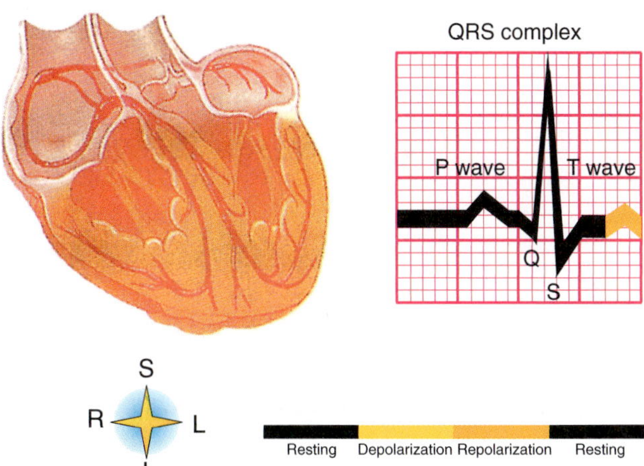

■ **Figure B-11** The T wave represents ventricular repolarization. (From Aehlert B: ECGs made easy, ed 3, St Louis, 2006, Mosby.)

The Normal ST Segment

- Represents interval between ventricular depolarization and ventricular repolarization
- Normally isoelectric

Overall Approach to Interpretation

- First, determine precisely what is on the ECG recording.
  - Descriptive analysis/report
- Then correlate to clinical situation.
  - Clinical impression/meaning

Use a System

- Right patient, properly done
- Rate and rhythm
- Intervals
- Axis
- Voltage (hypertrophy)
- Ischemic changes
- Other findings

Right Patient, Properly Done

- Check name
- Check for unusual axis/morphology

These are suggestive of dextrocardia or limb lead reversal (latter much more common):

- Negative P wave in lead II
- P, QRS, and T all negative in lead I
- Upright QRS in lead aVR

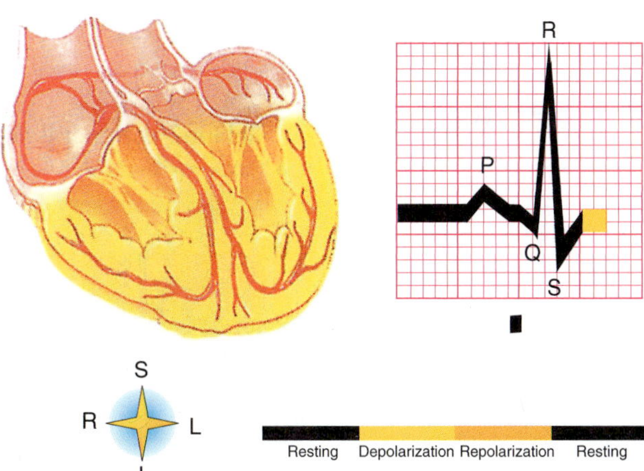

■ **Figure B-12** The ST segment represents the early part of repolarization of the right and left ventricles. (From Aehlert B: ECGs made easy, ed 3, St Louis, 2006, Mosby.)

ECG Dextrocardia

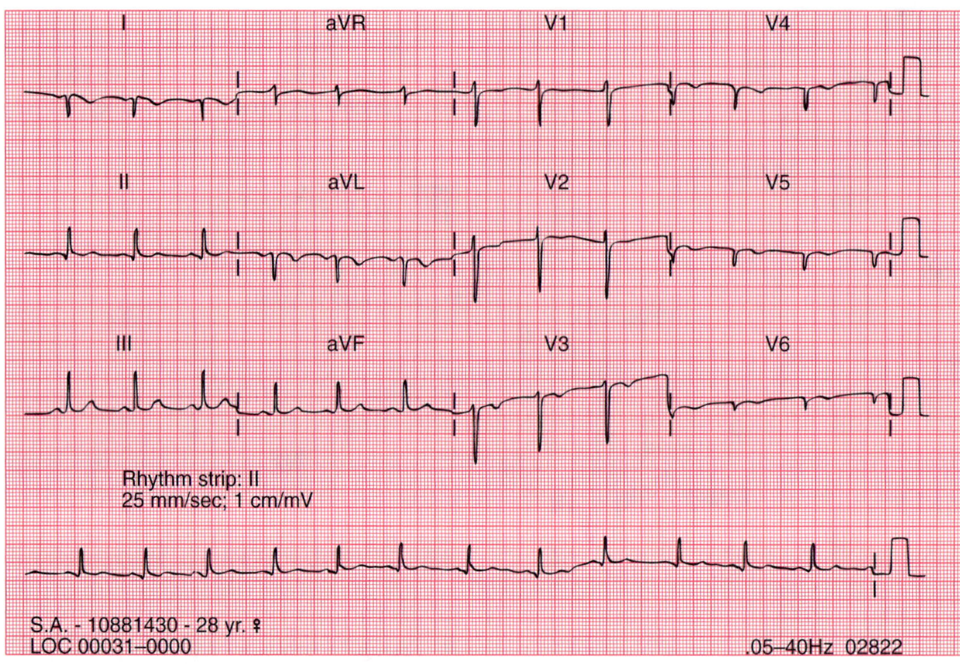

■ **Figure B-13** Example of dextrocardia. Negative QRS wave on lead I and negative P, QRS, and T waves on leads I and aVL. Isoelectric aVR. Negative QRS and T waves in all precordial leads. (From Rakel RE: Textbook of family medicine, ed 7, Philadelphia, 2007, Saunders.)

Rate

- Regular or irregular:
  - Count number of complexes in 6-second strip, and multiply by 10
- Only if regular:

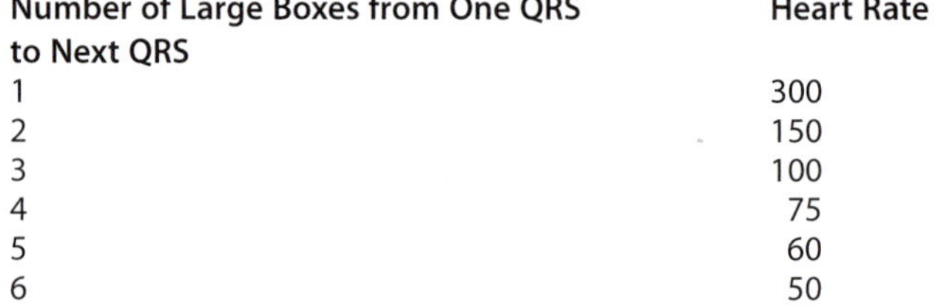

Number of Large Boxes from One QRS to Next QRS	Heart Rate
1	300
2	150
3	100
4	75
5	60
6	50

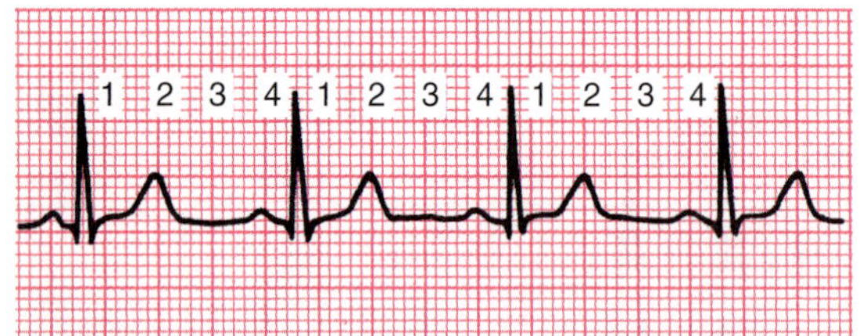

■ **Figure B-14** Heart rate (beats per minute [bpm]) can be measured by counting the number of large (0.2-sec) time boxes between two successive QRS complexes and dividing 300 by this number. In this example, the heart rate is calculated as 300 ÷ 4 = 75 bpm. If the QRS is 1 large box apart, the heart rate is 300; if 2 larges boxes apart, the heart rate is 150. If the QRS complexes are 3 large boxes apart, the heart rate is 100; 4 large boxes apart, the heart rate is 75; 5 large boxes apart, the heart rate is 60; 6 large boxes apart, the heart rate is 50. (From Goldberger AL: Clinical electrocardiography: a simplified approach, ed 7, St Louis, 2006, Mosby.)

Rhythm

- QRS pattern: regular, regularly irregular, irregularly irregular?
- Relation between P and QRS
- Same or variable?
  - QRS after every P?
  - P before every QRS?

Sinus Rhythms

- Normal sinus rhythm (NSR) = rate 60-100
- Sinus tachycardia if >100
- Sinus bradycardia if <60
- Sinus arrhythmia—irregularity associated with respiration

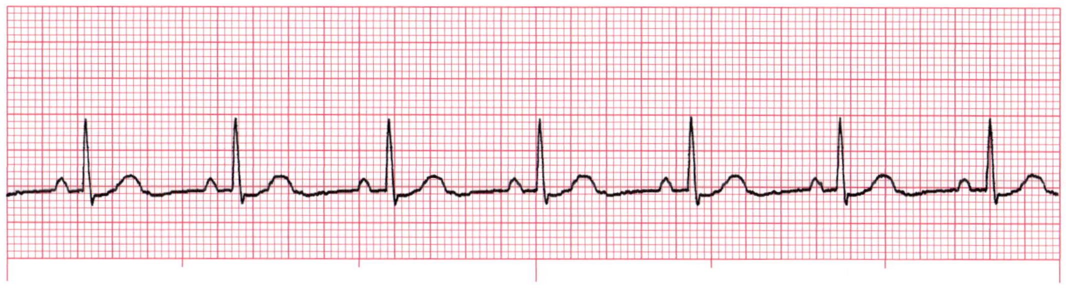

■ **Figure B-15** Sinus rhythm at 70 bpm. (From Aehlert B: ECGs made easy, ed 3, St Louis, 2006, Mosby.)

Dysrhythmias

- Atrial/supraventricular
  - Atrial fibrillation and flutter
  - Wandering atrial pacemaker/multifocal atrial tachycardia (MFAT)
  - Paroxysmal atrial tachycardia (PAT)
  - Atrioventricular nodal reentry tachycardia (AVNRT; most "SVT" is this)
- AV conduction blocks
  - 1st
  - 2nd (type I and II)
  - 3rd (complete)
- Ventricular
  - Idioventricular
  - Ventricular tachycardia
  - Ventricular fibrillation

The Conduction System

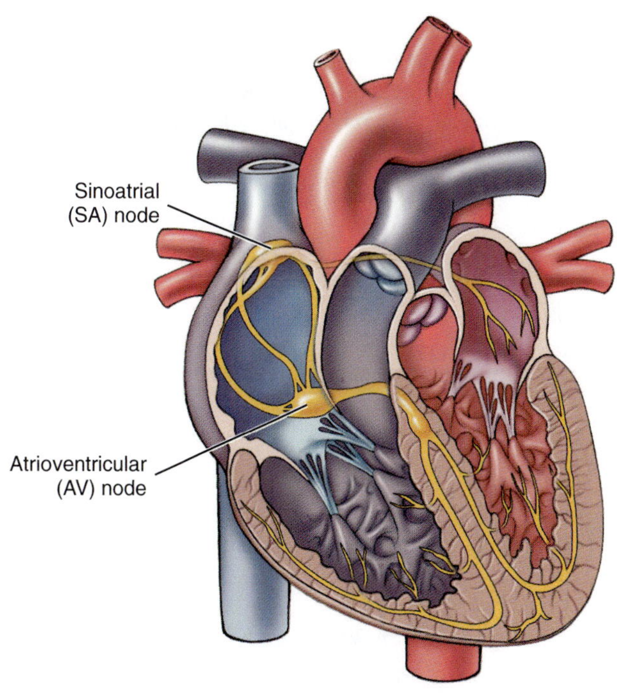

■ **Figure B-16** The cardiac conduction system. (From Aehlert B: ECGs made easy, ed 3, St Louis, 2006, Mosby.)

Atrial Fibrillation

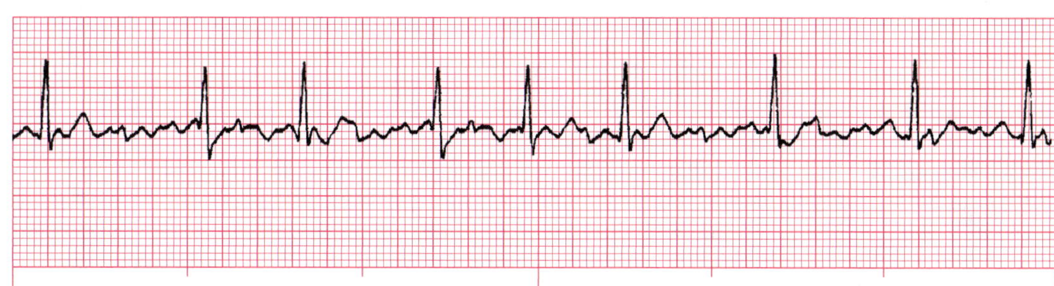

■ **Figure B-17** Atrial fibrillation with a ventricular response of 67 to 120 bpm. (From Aehlert B: ECGs made easy, ed 3, St Louis, 2006, Mosby.)

Atrial Fibrillation

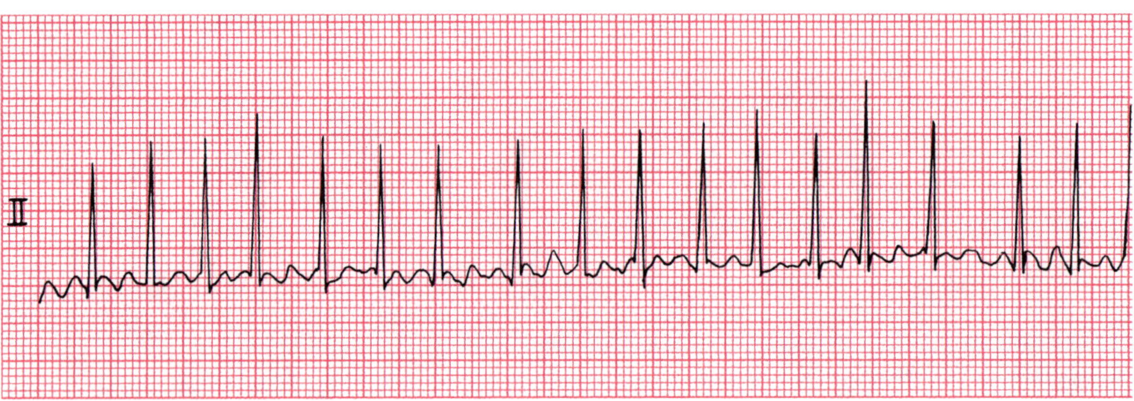

■ **Figure B-18** Atrial fibrillation with a rapid ventricular response. This patient has hyperthyroidism. (The commonly used term *rapid atrial fibrillation* is actually a misnomer, because "rapid" is intended to refer to the ventricular rate rather than the atrial rate. The same is true for the term *slow atrial fibrillation.*) The atrial fibrillation waves here have a "coarse" appearance. (From Goldberger AL: Clinical electrocardiography: a simplified approach, ed 7, St Louis, 2007, Mosby.)

Atrial Flutter

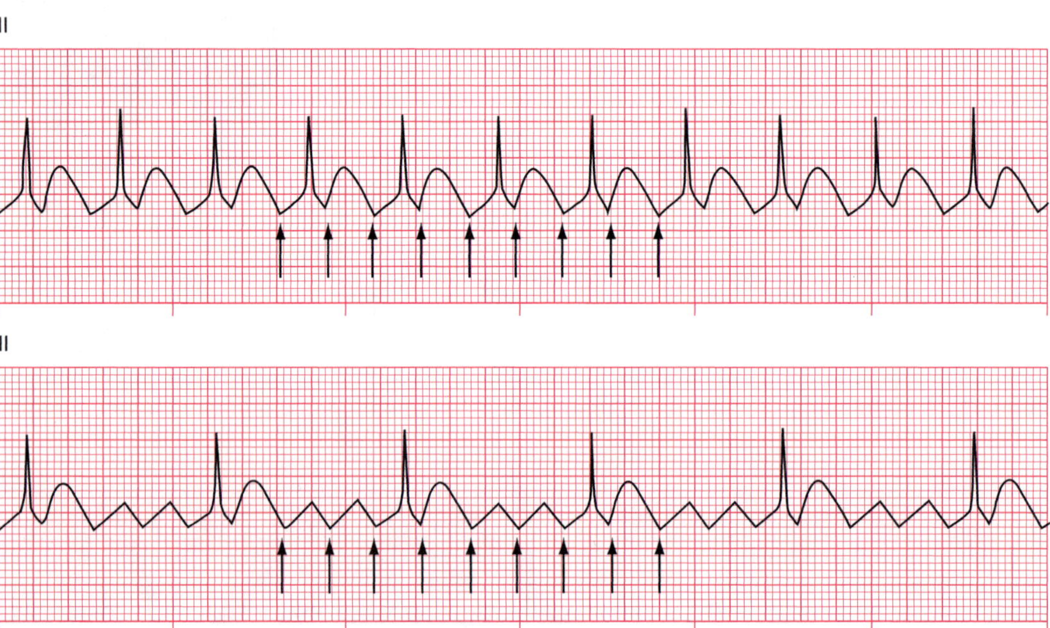

■ **Figure B-19** Atrial flutter. **A,** Atrial flutter with 2:1 conduction (atrial rate = 300 bpm, ventricular rate = 150 bpm). Flutter activity *(arrows)* appears as negative deflections that precede and immediately follow each QRS complex. **B,** Atrial flutter with 4:1 conduction (atrial rate = 300 bpm, ventricular rate = 75 bpm). As you can see, it is much easier to identify the sawtooth pattern of the flutter waves *(arrows)* with the slower ventricular rate. (From Aehlert B: ECGs made easy, ed 3, St Louis, 2006, Mosby.)

Atrial Flutter (2:1 Conduction)

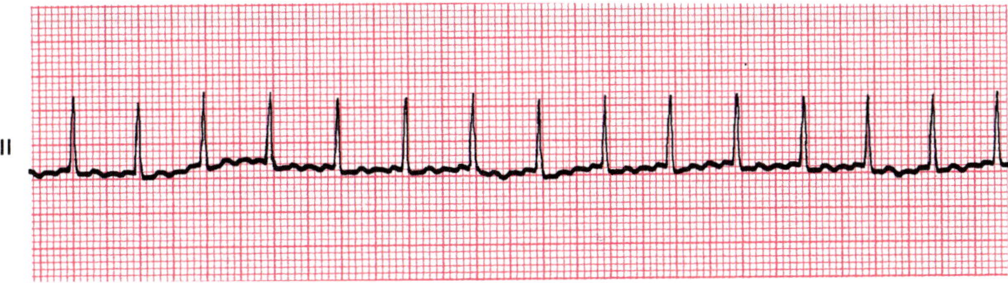

■ **Figure B-20** Atrial flutter with 2:1 conduction. (From Goldberger AL: Clinical electrocardiography: a simplified approach, ed 7, St Louis, 2007, Mosby.)

Wandering Atrial Pacemaker/ Multifocal Atrial Tachycardia (MFAT)

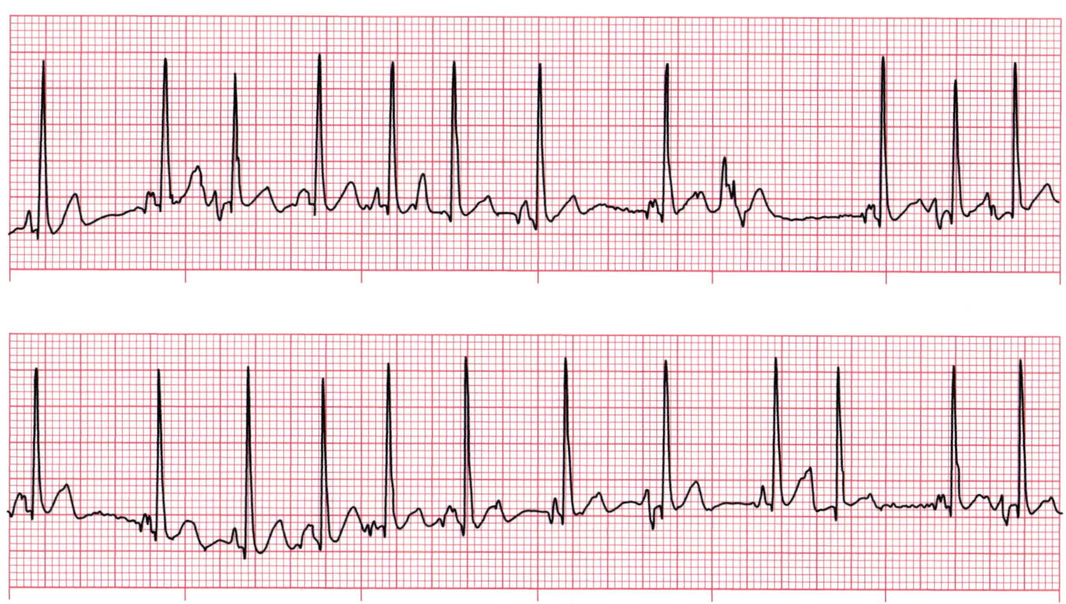

■ **Figure B-21** Multifocal atrial tachycardia (MAT), also known as *chaotic atrial tachycardia.* Premature atrial complexes (PACs) occur at varying cycle lengths and with differing shapes. (From Aehlert B: ECGs made easy, ed 3, St Louis, 2006, Mosby.)

Paroxysmal Atrial Tachycardia

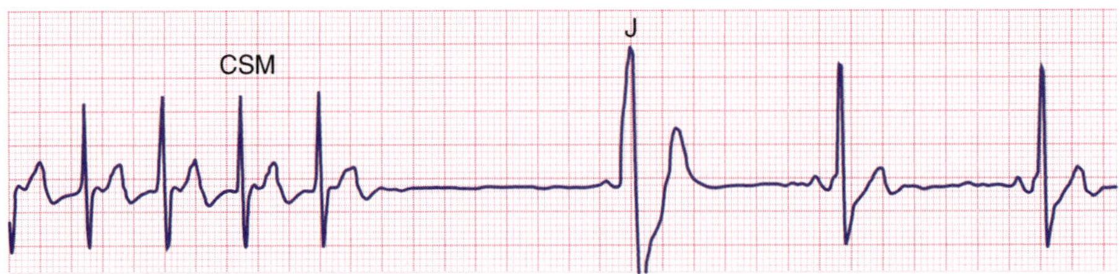

■ **Figure B-22** Paroxysmal atrial tachycardia. Carotid sinus massage may abolish the dysrhythmia and result in a period of sinus suppression with a junctional (J) escape beat. Prolonged periods of asystole may produce anxiety in the physician who is waiting for the resumption of a sinus pacemaker. (From Silverman ME: Recognition and treatment of arrhythmias. In Schwartz GR, Safar P, Stone JH, et al, editors: Principles and practice of emergency medicine, vol 2, Philadelphia, 1978, Saunders. Reproduced by permission.)

Atrioventricular Nodal Reentry Tachycardia

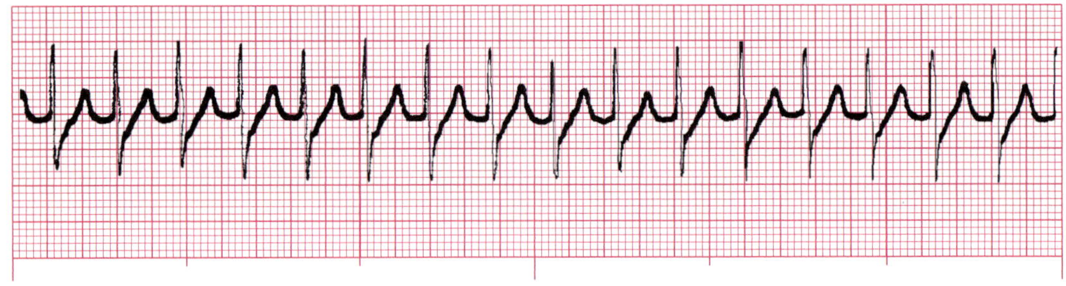

■ **Figure B-23** Atrioventricular nodal reentrant tachycardia (AVNRT). (From Aehlert B: ECGs made easy, ed 3, St Louis, 2006, Mosby.)

- AVNRT is most common specific form of supraventricular tachycardia (SVT).
- Reentry circuit forms, involving the AV node as part of the electrical pathway.
- There may be retrograde P waves (inverted), but these are often hidden in the QRS complex.

Reentry Mechanism

- Alpha arm has longer refractory period and so does not conduct the premature beat.
- Beta arm has shorter refractory so conducts the beat but has slower conduction time.
- By the time impulse gets to juncture of the two arms, alpha tract is repolarized and can conduct retrograde, setting up the reentry circuit or reentry loop.
- Impulses are conducted from the circuit to both ventricles and atria.

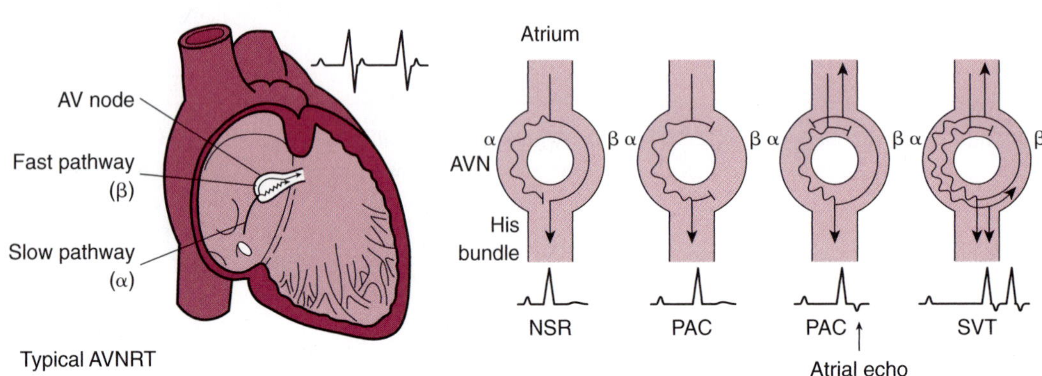

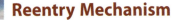

■ **Figure B-24** Schematic for SVT due to AV nodal reentry. *AV,* Atrioventricular node; *NSR,* normal sinus rhythm; *PAC,* premature atrial complex; *SVT,* supraventricular tachycardia. (From Aehlert B: ECGs made easy, ed 3, St Louis, 2006, Mosby.)

PR Interval

- Normal = 0.12 to 0.20 second
- Short = preexcitation syndrome (e.g., Wolff-Parkinson-White)
- Long = conduction system disease, defines first-degree AV block

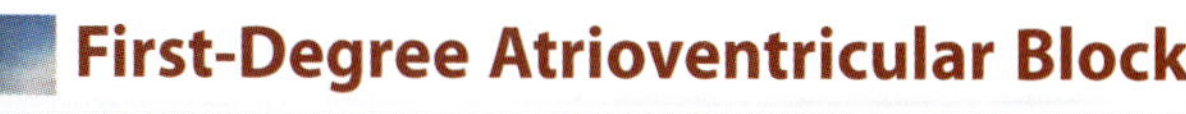

First-Degree Atrioventricular Block

First-Degree AV Block

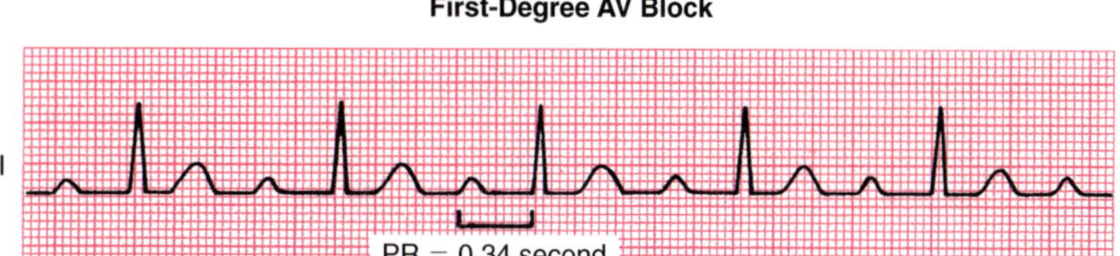

Figure B-25 With first-degree AV block, the PR interval is uniformly prolonged beyond 0.2 second with each beat. (From Goldberger AL: Clinical electrocardiography: a simplified approach, ed 7, St Louis, 2007, Mosby.)

Sinus Bradycardia with First-Degree Atrioventricular Block

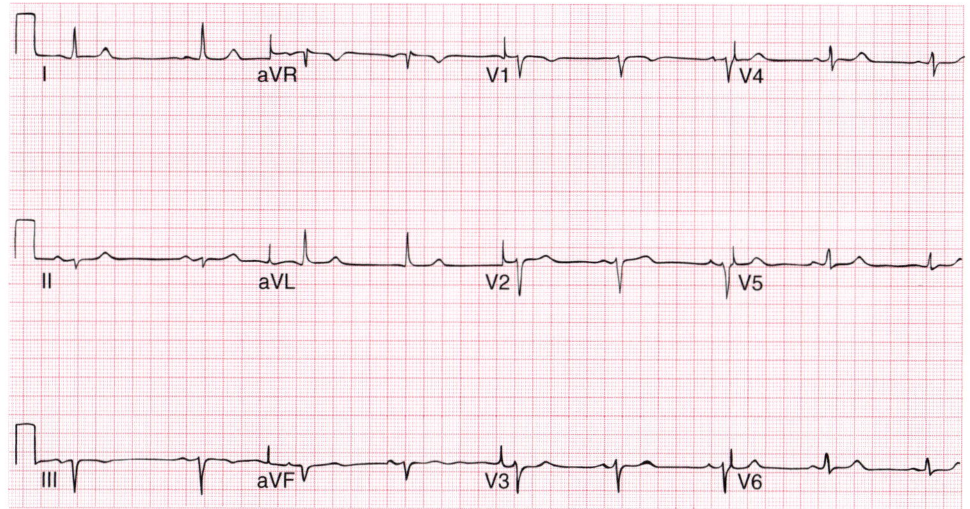

Figure B-26 Sinus bradycardia. (From Marx JA, Hockberger RS, Walls RM, et al: Rosen's emergency medicine, ed 7, St Louis, 2010, Mosby.)

Second-Degree Atrioventricular Block Type I (Wenckebach)

Mobitz Type I (Wenckebach) Second-Degree AV Block

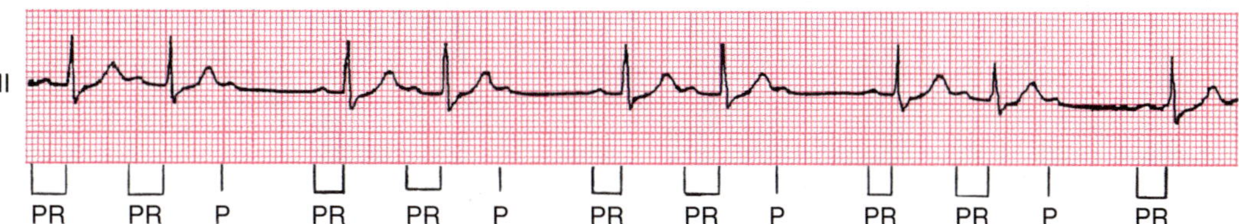

Figure B-27 Notice the progressive increase in PR intervals, with the third sinus P wave in each sequence not followed by a QRS complex. Mobitz type I (Wenckebach) block produces a characteristically syncopated rhythm with grouping of the QRS complexes (group beating). (From Goldberger AL: Clinical electrocardiography: a simplified approach, ed 7, St Louis, 2007, Mosby.)

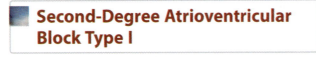

Second-Degree Atrioventricular Block Type I

Mobitz Type I (Wenckebach) Second-Degree AV Block

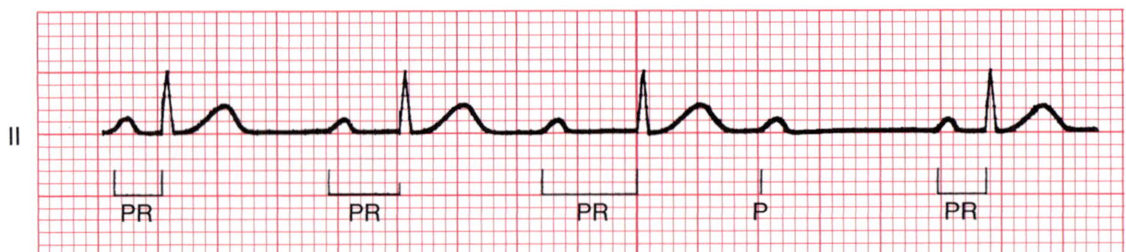

■ **Figure B-28** The PR interval lengthens progressively with successive beats until one sinus P wave is not conducted at all. Then the cycle repeats itself. Notice that the PR interval after the nonconducted P wave is shorter than the PR interval of the beat just before it. (From Goldberger AL: Clinical electrocardiography: a simplified approach, ed 7, St Louis, 2007, Mosby.)

Second-Degree Atrioventricular Block 2:1

- NOTE: cannot determine if type I or II
- If QRS narrow and PR prolonged, more likely type I (delay usually in AV node and more likely reversible)
- Type II usually below AV node and less likely reversible

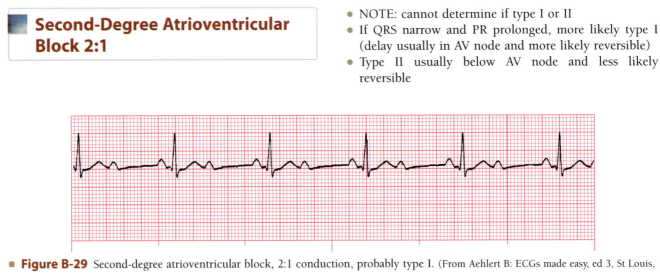

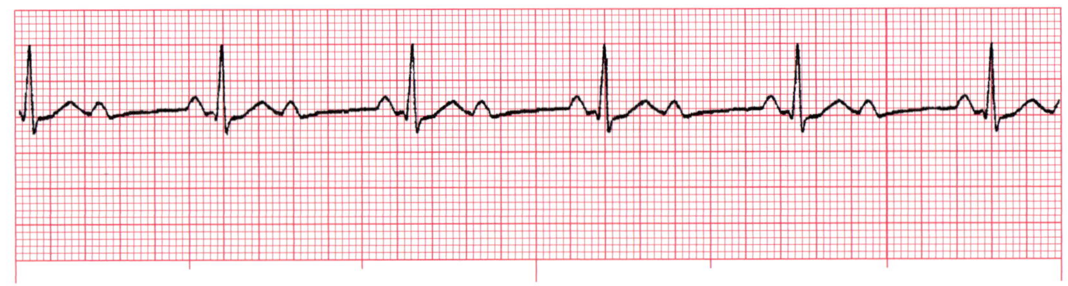

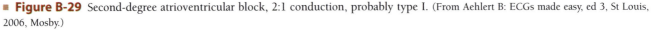

■ **Figure B-29** Second-degree atrioventricular block, 2:1 conduction, probably type I. (From Aehlert B: ECGs made easy, ed 3, St Louis, 2006, Mosby.)

Second-Degree Atrioventricular Block Type II

- Must have at least two consecutive beats with same PR interval, then P wave with dropped QRS
- Block is almost always in the bundle branches, so QRS often wide (as opposed to narrow QRS in type I)

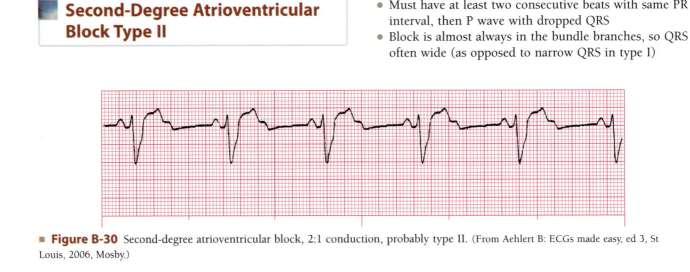

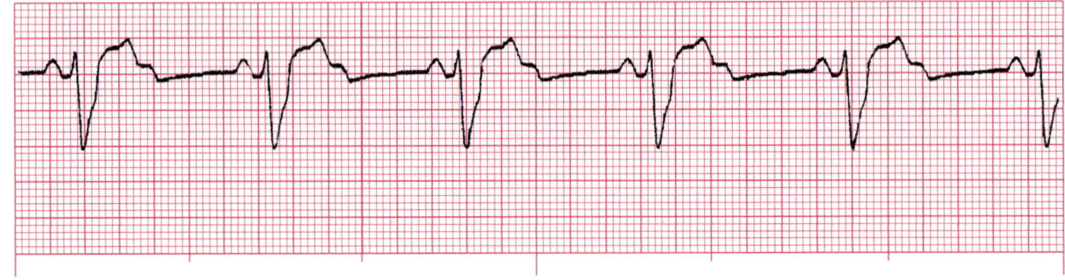

■ **Figure B-30** Second-degree atrioventricular block, 2:1 conduction, probably type II. (From Aehlert B: ECGs made easy, ed 3, St Louis, 2006, Mosby.)

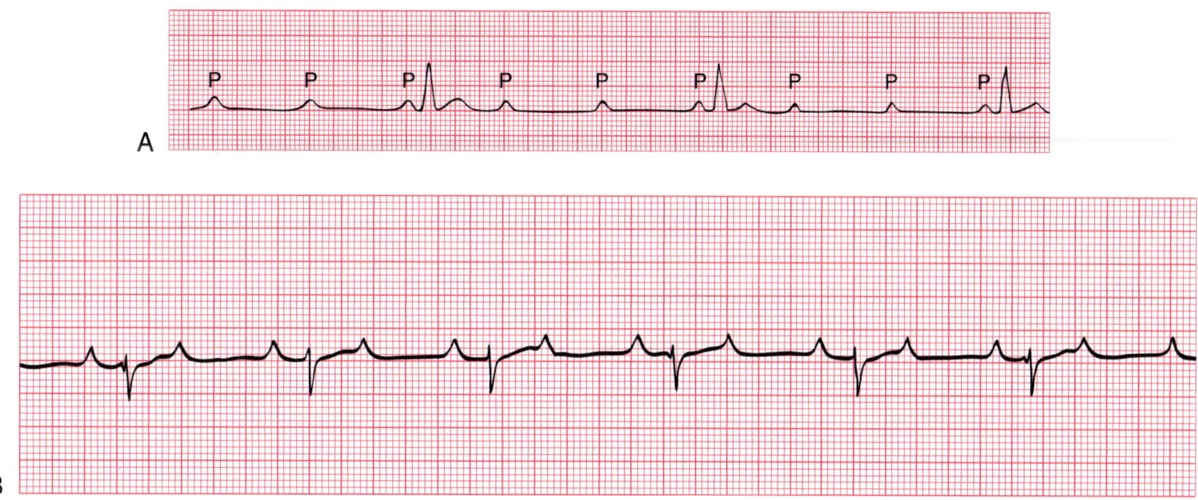

■ **Figure B-31** **A**, Second-degree atrioventricular (AV) block, type II. In this example, 3:1 conduction is seen. **B**, Second-degree AV block with 2:1 conduction. From the rhythm strip alone, it is difficult to categorize this as type I or II block. (From Marx JA, Hockberger RS, Walls RM, et al: Rosen's emergency medicine, ed 7, St Louis, 2010, Mosby.)

Third-Degree Atrioventricular Block (Complete)

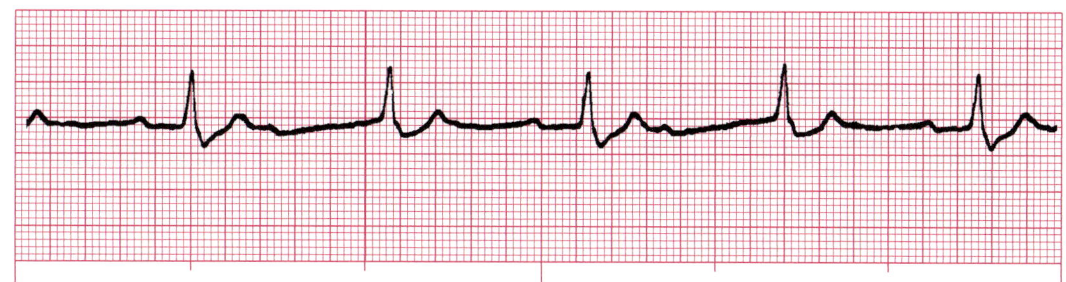

■ **Figure B-32** Complete atrioventricular block with a junctional escape pacemaker (QRS 0.08 to 0.10 sec). (From Aehlert B: ECGs made easy, ed 3, St Louis, 2006, Mosby.)

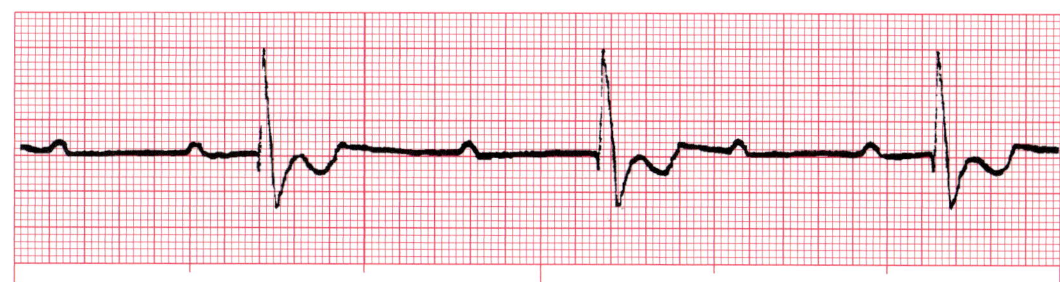

■ **Figure B-33** Complete atrioventricular block with a ventricular escape pacemaker (QRS 0.12 to 0.14 sec). (From Aehlert B: ECGs made easy, ed 3, St Louis, 2006, Mosby.)

Third-Degree Atrioventricular Block

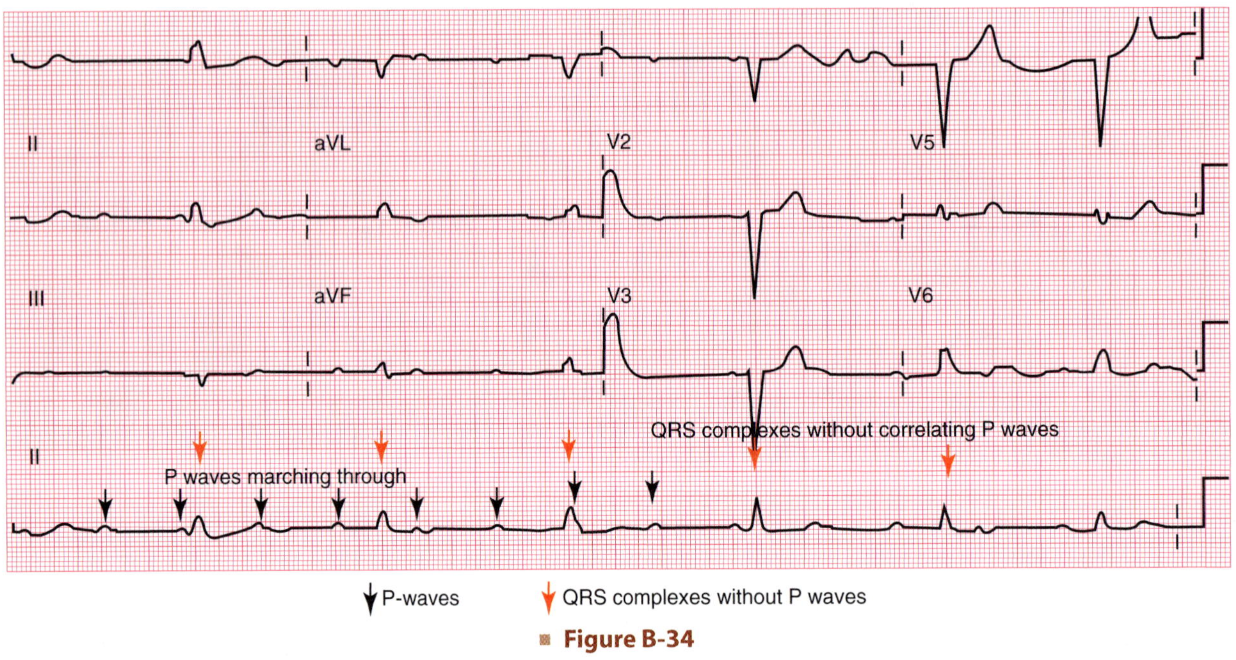

■ **Figure B-34**

NOTES:

- ECG: note P waves and QRS are regular pattern but not in synchrony
  If QRS is narrow, likely junctional escape; if wide QRS, likely distal to AV node.
  - If QRS narrow, may respond to atropine, but typically this rhythm does not respond to atropine and pacing is required if patient is hemodynamically compromised.
- Clinical: treatment based on patient symptoms/condition (hypotension, chest pain, mental status changes)
  - Patients will often need a permanent pacemaker.

Ventricular Tachycardia

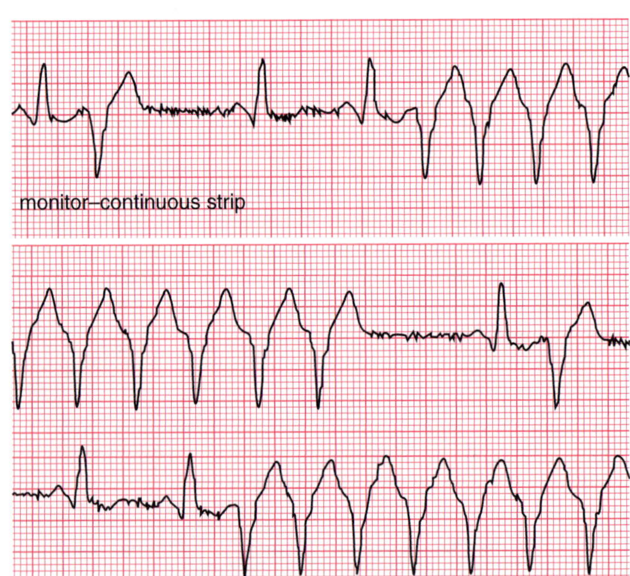

■ **Figure B-35** Ventricular tachycardia. (From Goldberger E: Treatment of cardiac emergencies, ed 5, St Louis, 1990, Mosby.)

Ventricular Tachycardia (Monomorphic)

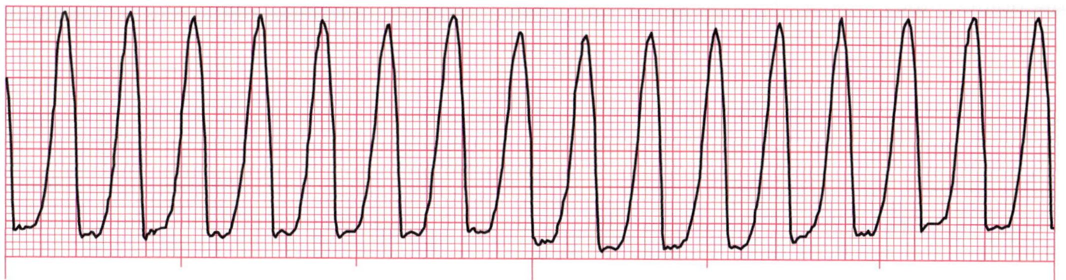

■ **Figure B-36** Monomorphic ventricular tachycardia. (From Aehlert B: ECGs made easy, ed 3, St Louis, 2006, Mosby.)

Ventricular Tachycardia (Polymorphic)

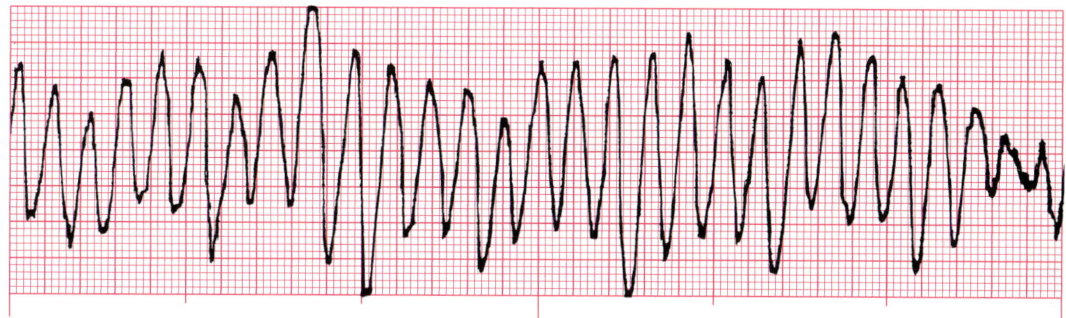

■ **Figure B-37** Polymorphic ventricular tachycardia. This rhythm strip is from a 77-year-old man 3 days post myocardial infarction (MI). His chief complaint at the onset of this episode was chest pain. He had a past medical history of a previous MI and an abdominal aortic aneurysm repair. The patient was given lidocaine and defibrillated several times without success. Laboratory work revealed a serum potassium (K^+) level of 2.0. IV K^+ was administered, and the patient converted to a sinus rhythm with the next defibrillation. (From Aehlert B: ECGs made easy, ed 3, St Louis, 2006, Mosby.)

Ventricular Fibrillation

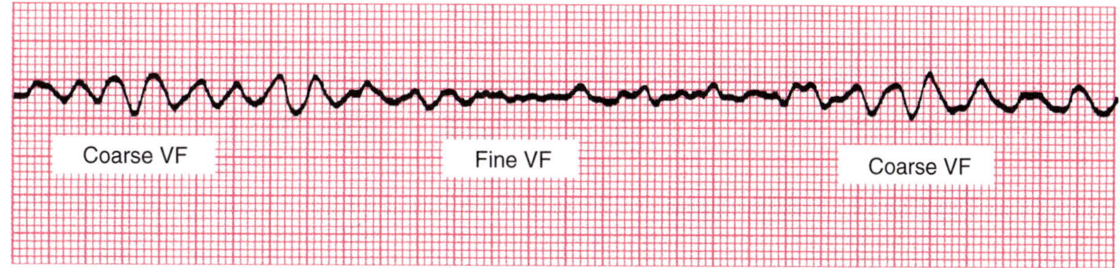

■ **Figure B-38** Ventricular fibrillation (VF) may produce both coarse and fine waves. Immediate defibrillation should be performed. (From Goldberger AL: Clinical electrocardiography: a simplified approach, ed 7, St Louis, 2007, Mosby.)

QRS Duration

- Normal = 0.08 to 0.12 second
- Right bundle branch block (RBBB)
- Left bundle branch block (LBBB)
- Nonspecific intraventricular conduction delay

Right Bundle Branch Block

- QRS >/= 120 msec
- R prime (R′) in V_1
- Wide terminal S in I and V_6

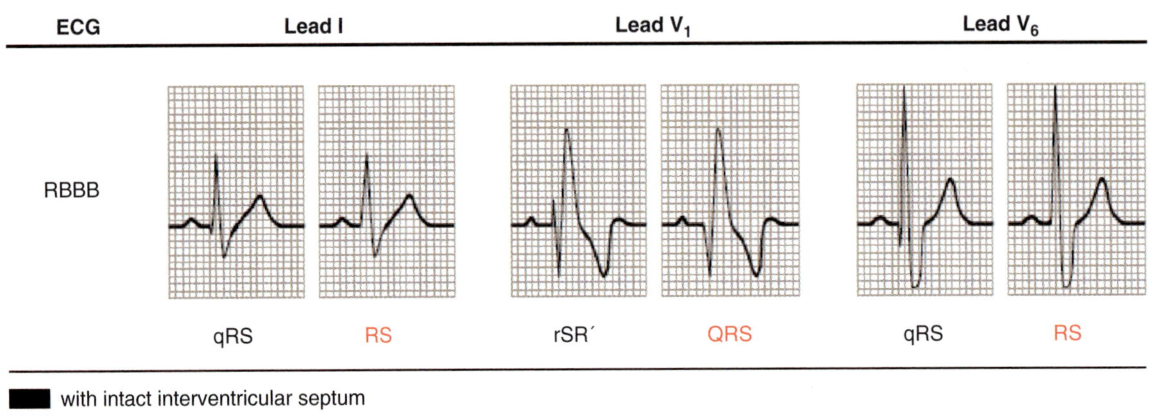

■ **Figure B-39** Black = With intact interventricular septum; Red = Without intact interventricular septum. (From Huszar R: Basic dysrhythmias: interpretation and management, ed 3, St Louis, 2007, Mosby.)

Right Bundle Branch Block

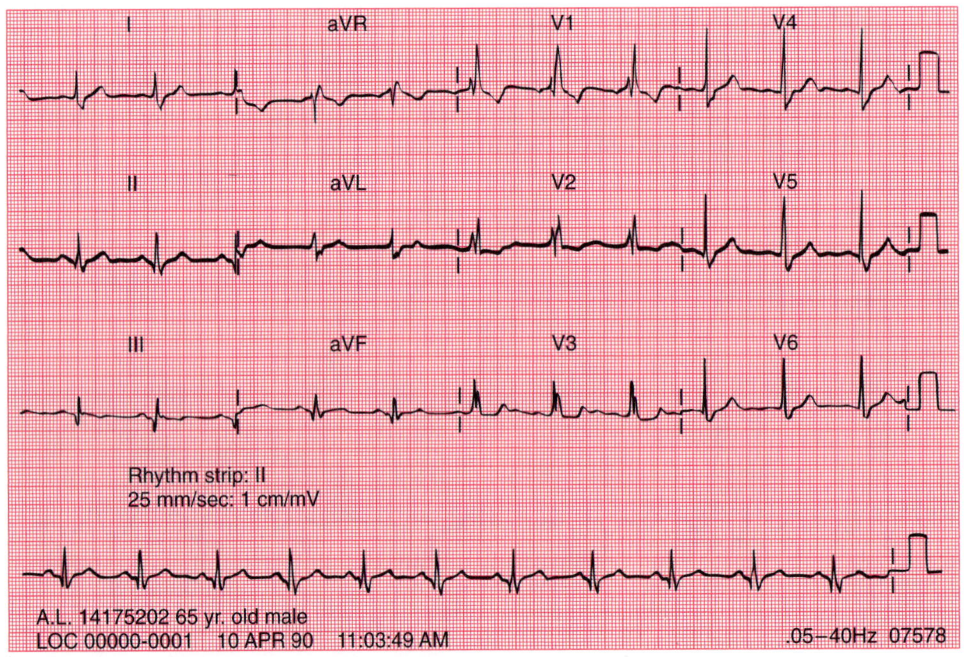

■ **Figure B-40** Example of right bundle branch block. Axis of QRS wave, +60 degrees. Axis of T wave, +30 degrees. Slurred terminal portion of QRS wave in the frontal plane. There is an R-R′ pattern in V_1, a notched QRS wave in V_2 and V_3, and slurring of the terminal portion of the QRS wave in V_6. (From Rakel RE: Textbook of family medicine, ed 7, Philadelphia, 2006, Saunders.)

Left Bundle Branch Block

- QRS >/= 120 msec
- QRS predominantly negative in V_1
- QRS upright in I and V_6
  - No Q (unless infarct)

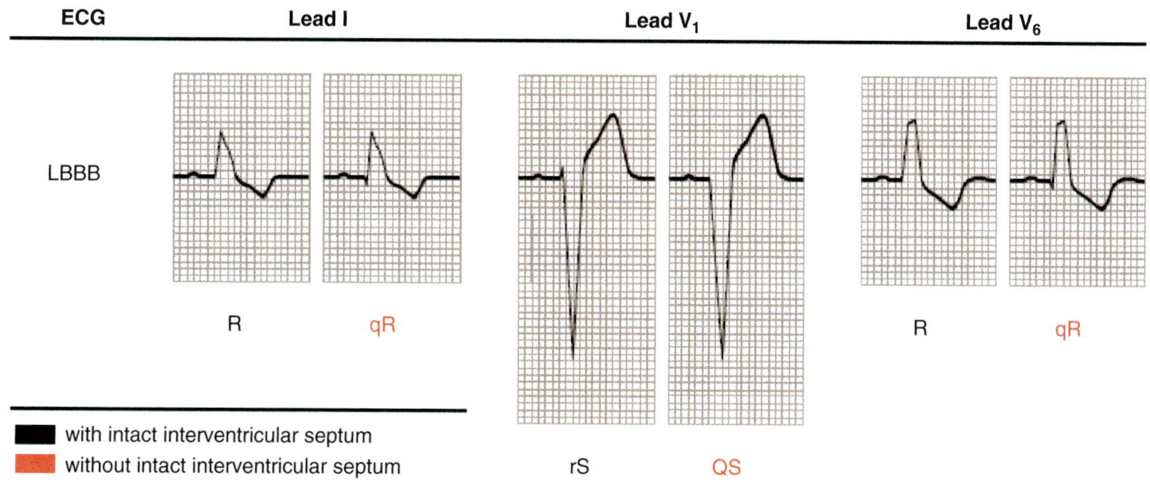

Figure B-41 Black = With intact interventricular septum; Red = Without intact interventricular septum. (From Huszar R: Basic dysrhythmias: interpretation and management, ed 3, St Louis, 2007, Mosby.

- Late depolarization of left ventricle leads to late lateral and posterior positive forces.
- The "normal" ST-T waves in LBBB should be oriented opposite to the direction of the terminal QRS forces. That is, in leads with terminal R or R′ forces, the ST-T should be downward; in leads with terminal S forces, the ST-T should be upward. If the ST-T waves are in the *same direction* as the terminal QRS forces, they should be labeled *primary ST-T wave abnormalities.* In the above ECG, the ST-T waves are "normal" for LBBB; that is, they are *secondary* to the change in the ventricular depolarization sequence.

Left Bundle Branch Block

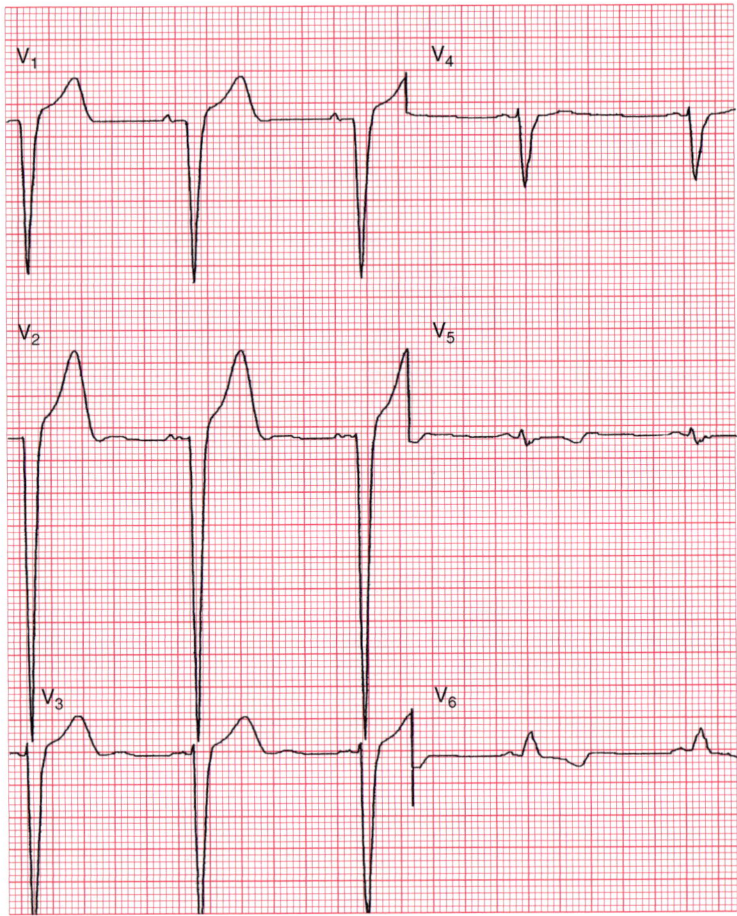

■ **Figure B-42** Poor R wave progression in V_1 through V_4; QRS < 0.12 seconds: left bundle branch block. (From Aehlert B: ECGs made easy, ed 3, St Louis, 2006, Mosby.)

QT Interval

- QTc = corrected for HR:

$$QTc = \frac{QT}{\sqrt{RR}}$$

- Normal QTc is < 0.44 second
  - Slight variation by age and gender
- Prolonged QTc: risk for ventricular fibrillation

Axis

- Frontal plane, based on limb leads
- Normal = 0 to 90 degrees
- Leftward = −1 to −90
- Rightward = 90 to 180
- Indeterminate = 180 to 270

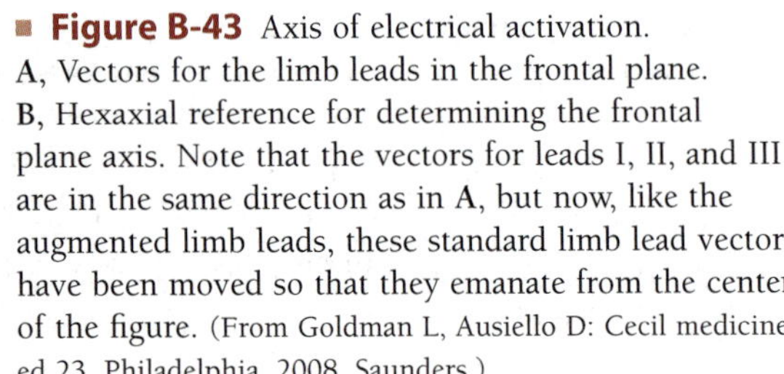

■ **Figure B-43** Axis of electrical activation. **A**, Vectors for the limb leads in the frontal plane. **B**, Hexaxial reference for determining the frontal plane axis. Note that the vectors for leads I, II, and III are in the same direction as in **A**, but now, like the augmented limb leads, these standard limb lead vectors have been moved so that they emanate from the center of the figure. (From Goldman L, Ausiello D: Cecil medicine, ed 23, Philadelphia, 2008, Saunders.)

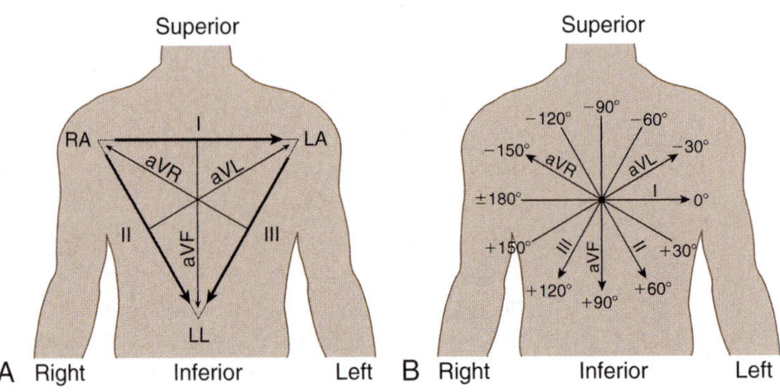

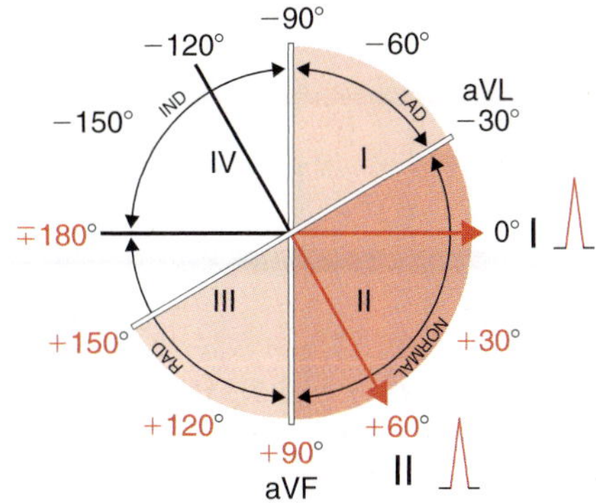

■ **Figure B-44** Axis. (From Huszar R: Basic dysrhythmias: interpretation and management, ed 3, St Louis, 2007, Mosby.)

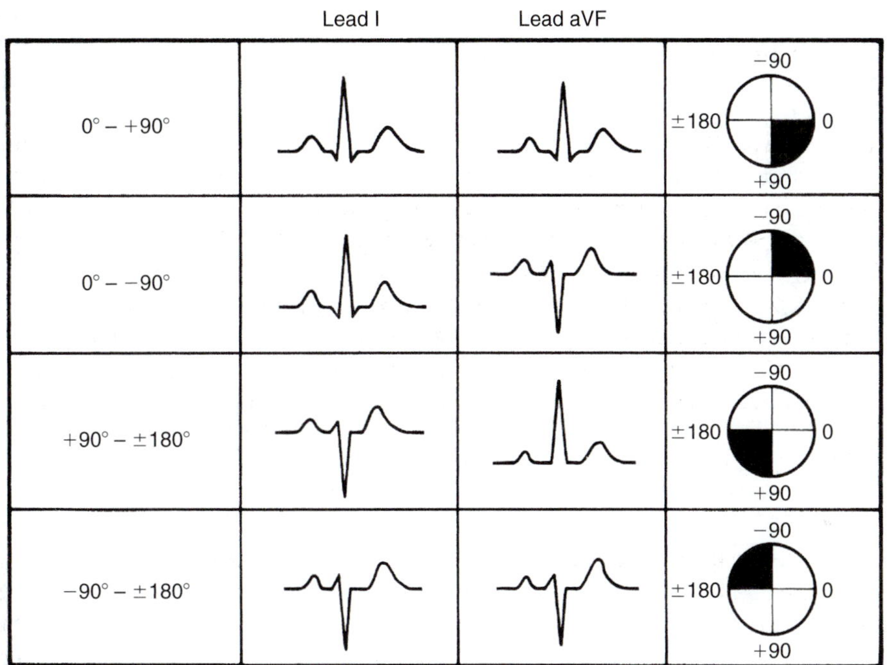

■ **Figure B-45** Locating quadrants of mean QRS axis from leads I and aVF. (From Park MK, Guntheroth WG: How to read pediatric ECGs, ed 4, Philadelphia, Saunders, 2006, p 17.)

Voltage (Hypertrophy)

- Left ventricular (LV) hypertrophy
  - R in aVL > 12 mm
  - S in V_1 or 2 + R in V_5 or 6 > 35 mm
  - LV "strain" pattern common
- Right atrial hypertrophy
  - Tall P in II
- Left atrial hypertrophy
  - Wide P in II and negative P in V_1

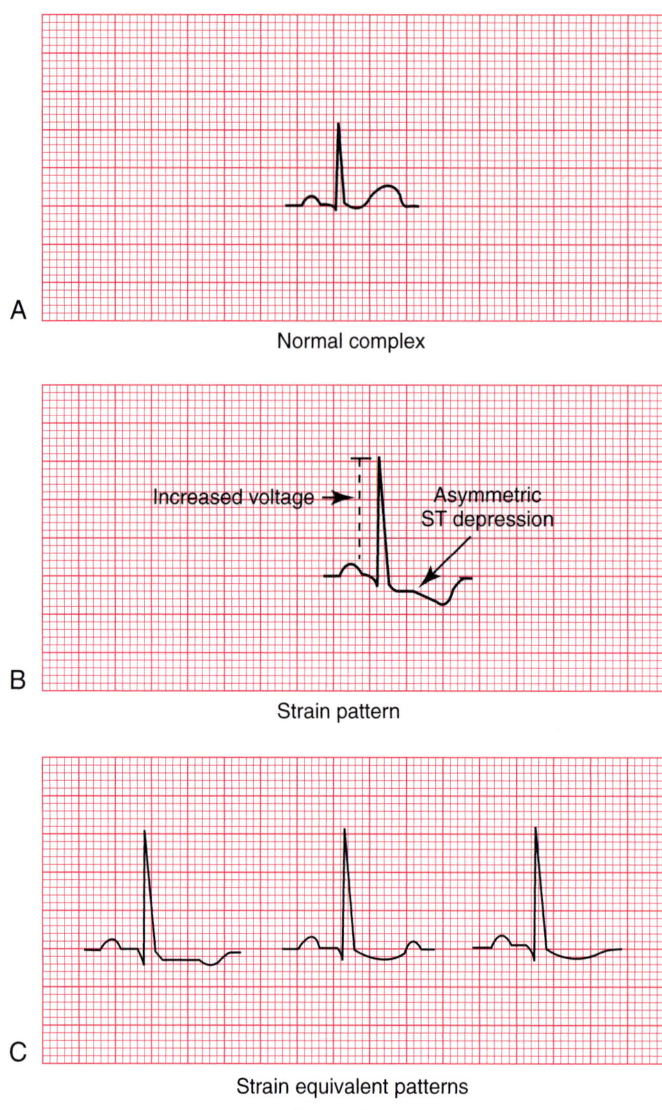

■ **Figure B-46**

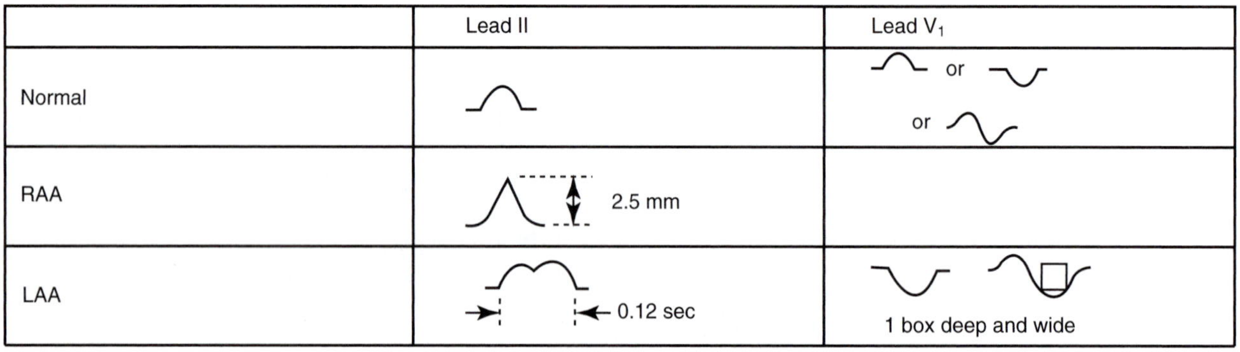

	Lead II	Lead V_1
Normal		or or
RAA	2.5 mm	
LAA	0.12 sec	1 box deep and wide

■ **Figure B-47** P-wave morphologies.

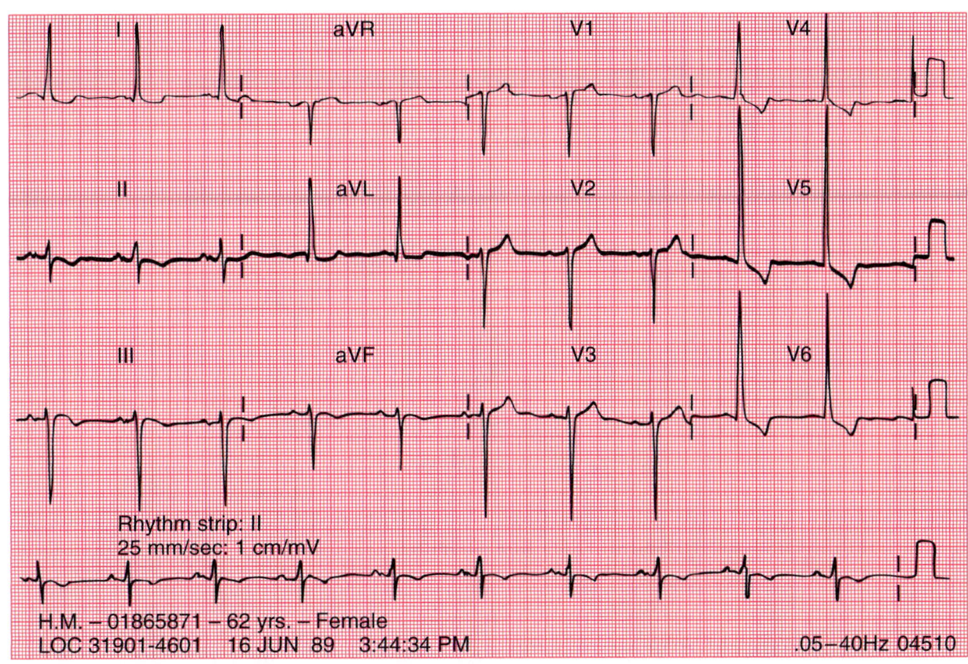

■ **Figure B-48** Example of left ventricular hypertrophy with left ventricular strain. Axis of QRS wave, −30 degrees in the frontal plane. Axis of T wave, −120 degrees. The precordial leads show $S_1 + R_5 = 5.5$ mV. Abnormal negative T waves on V_4, V_5, and V_6. Also, P-mitrale. (From Rakel RE: Textbook of family medicine, ed 7, Philadelphia, 2006, Saunders.)

Acute Ischemia/Infarction

- Ischemia
  - ST depression in arterial territory
  - T wave
- Infarction (ST elevation myocardial infarction [STEMI])
  - Progression over time:
    - T-wave peaking
    - ST elevation in arterial territory (>1 mm limb leads, > 2 mm V leads)
    - T-wave inversion and Q-wave formation

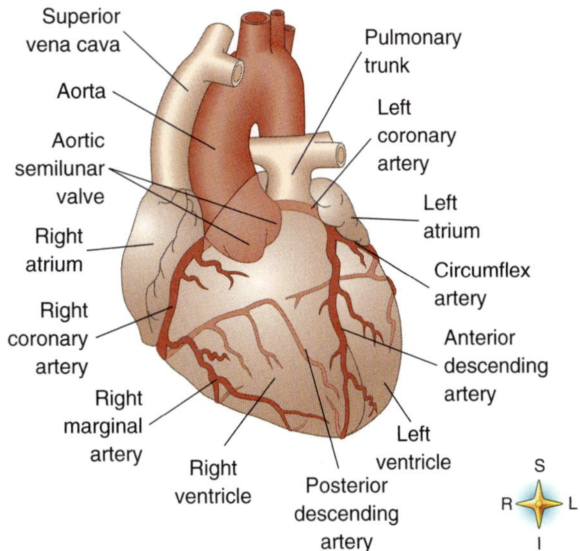

■ **Figure B-49** Anterior view of the coronary circulation. (From Aehlert B: ECGs made easy, ed 3, St Louis, 2006, Mosby.)

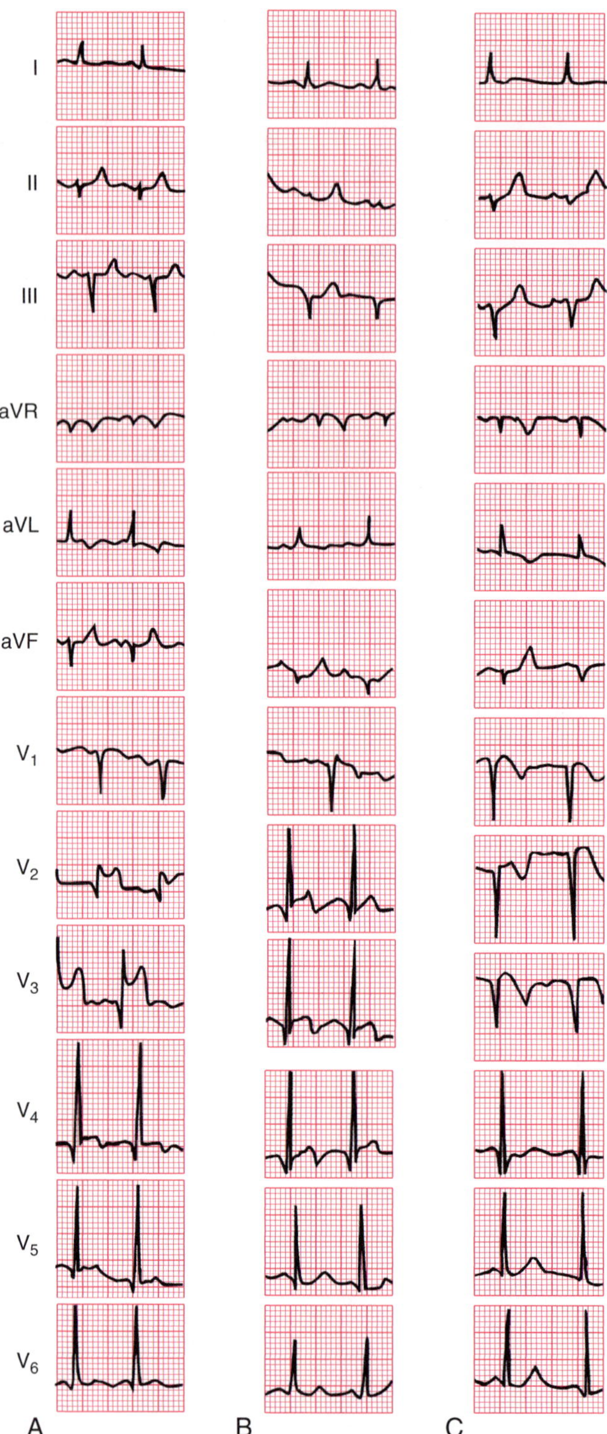

Figure B-50 Evolutionary changes in anteroseptal myocardial infarction reflected in leads V_2 to V_4. **A**, At admission, hyperacute phase is reflected by ST-segment elevation. **B**, At 24 hours. **C**, At 48 hours, there are abnormal (pathologic) Q waves. (From Aehlert B: ECGs made easy, ed 3, St Louis, 2006, Mosby.)

Vascular Territories

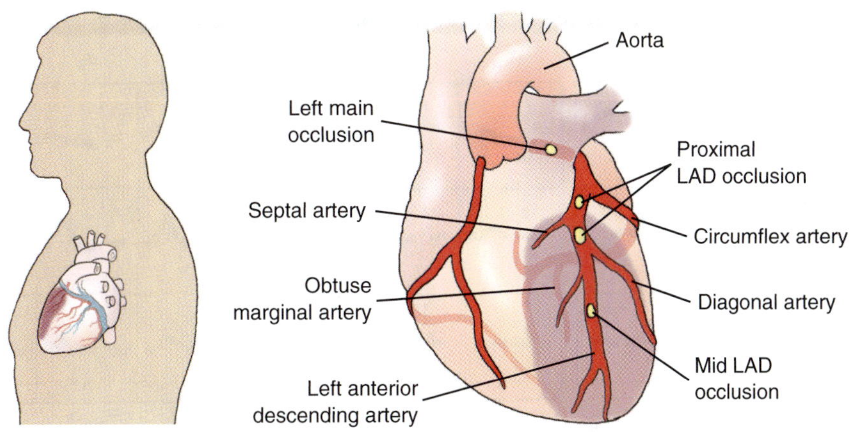

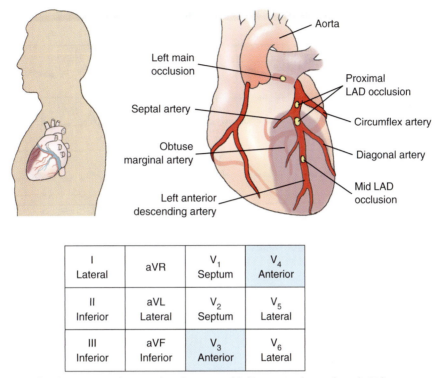

I Lateral	aVR	V_1 Septum	V_4 Anterior
II Inferior	aVL Lateral	V_2 Septum	V_5 Lateral
III Inferior	aVF Inferior	V_3 Anterior	V_6 Lateral

■ **Figure B-51** Anterior wall infarction. Occlusion of midportion of left anterior descending (LAD) artery results in an anterior infarction. Proximal occlusion of LAD may become an anteroseptal infarction if the septal branch is involved or an anterolateral infarction if the marginal branch is involved. If occlusion occurs proximal to both septal and diagonal branches, an extensive anterior infarction (anteroseptal-lateral MI) will result. (From Aehlert B: ECGs made easy, ed 3, St Louis, 2006, Mosby.)

Acute Ischemia

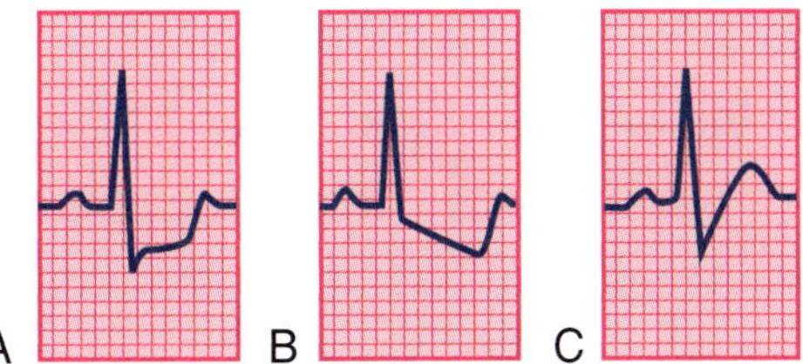

■ **Figure B-52** Horizontal ST depression (A) and down-sloping (B) ST depression—indicative of myocardial ischemia. Up-sloping ST depression (C) may be a normal finding. (From Miller RD, Eriksson LI, Fleisher LA, et al: Miller's anesthesia, ed 7, New York, 2010, Churchill Livingstone.)

Inferior Infarction

ECG Sequence with Inferior Wall Q-Wave Infarction

I II III aV_R aV_L aV_F V_2 V_4 V_6

A

B

C

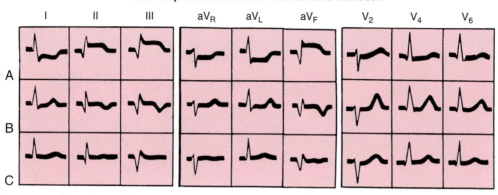

■ **Figure B-53** A, Acute phase of an inferior wall myocardial infarction: ST elevations and new Q waves. B, Evolving phase: deep T-wave inversions. C, Resolving phase: partial or complete regression of ST-T changes (and sometimes of Q waves). In A and B, note reciprocal ST-T changes in anterior leads (I, aVL, and V_2). (From Goldberger AL: Clinical electrocardiography: a simplified approach, ed 7, St Louis, 2007, Mosby.)

Acute Myocardial Infarction: Inferior Wall & Right Ventricle

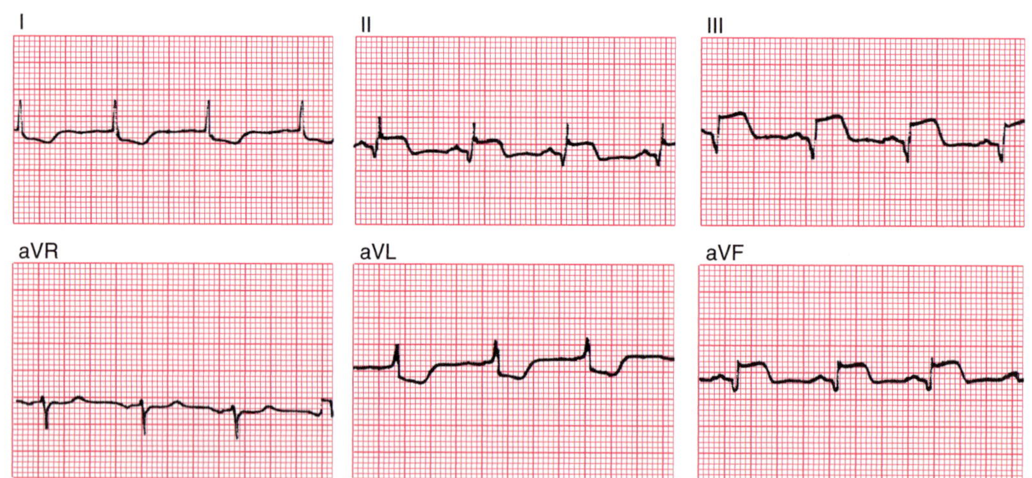

■ **Figure B-54** Acute inferior wall infarction. Note ST-segment elevation in leads II, III, and aVF and reciprocal ST depression in leads I and aVL. Abnormal Q waves are also present in leads II, III, and aVF. (From Aehlert B: ECGs made easy, ed 3, St Louis, 2006, Mosby.)

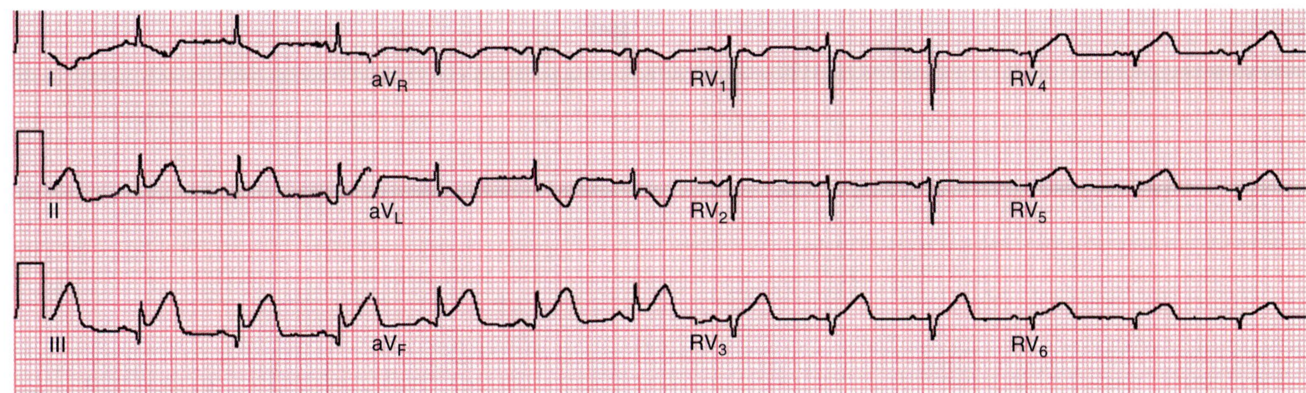

■ **Figure B-55** Right ventricular infarction demonstrated with right-sided precordial leads (V_1R to V_6R). ST-segment elevation of inferior acute myocardial infarction is present, as is reciprocal ST-segment depression in leads I and aVL. Precordial leads are right-sided chest leads, as might be inferred from the relatively low voltage. ST-segment elevation is noted in leads V_3R to V_6R, consistent with right ventricular infarction. (From Marx JA, Hockberger RS, Walls RM, et al: Rosen's emergency medicine, ed 7, St Louis, 2010, Mosby.)

NOTES:
Scenario: 66-year-old woman with indigestion and neck and back pain

Hyperacute ST-segment elevation is seen in leads II, III, and aVF (inferior location); ST depression is seen in leads $V_{1\text{-}2}$ (an expression of posterior wall injury). Right precordial leads V_1R to V_6R illustrate right ventricular infarction when ST-segment elevation occurs in V_3R or adjacent right precordial leads. Reciprocal ST-segment depression is seen in leads I and aVL.

Clinical: high risk for hypotension with nitroglycerin; be prepared to give IV fluids.

Diagnosis/treatment: standard STEMI—primary goal is rapid reperfusion.

Anterior Infarction

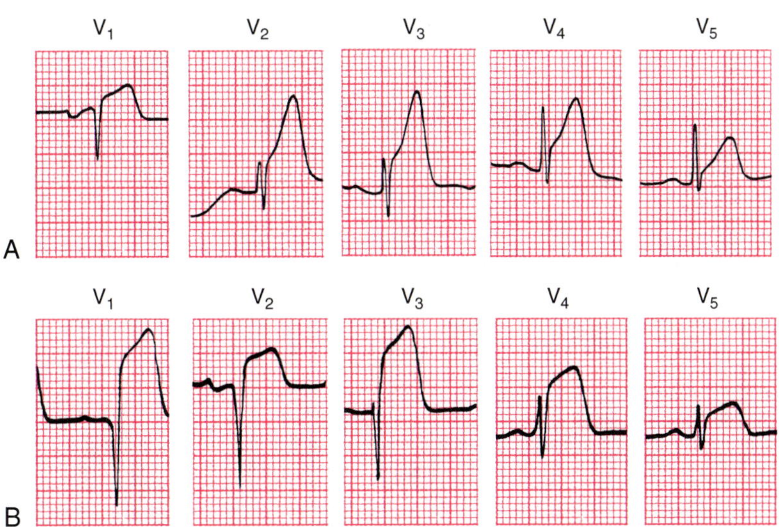

■ **Figure B-56** Chest leads from patient with acute anterior wall infarction. **A**, In earliest phase of infarction, tall positive (hyperacute) T waves are seen in leads V_2 to V_5. **B**, Several hours later, marked ST-segment elevation is present in same leads (current of injury pattern), and abnormal Q waves are seen in leads in V_1 and V_2. (From Goldberger AL: Clinical electrocardiography: a simplified approach, ed 7, St Louis, 2007, Mosby.)

Posterior Wall Myocardial Infarction

- Leads $V_{1\text{-}3}$ have tall, wide R wave and ST depression (mirror image of anterior wall myocardial infarction [AWMI])
- Often associated with IWMI (as in this ECG)

Posterior Wall Myocardial Infarction

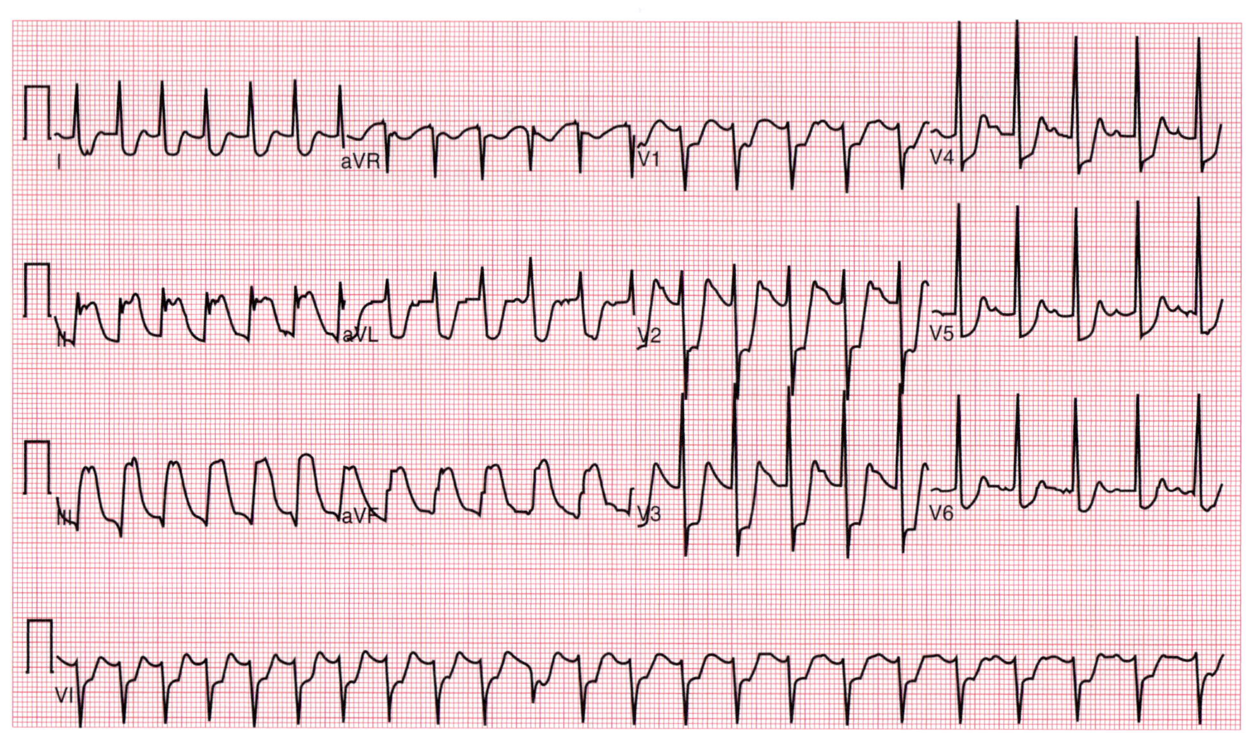

Figure B-57 Electrocardiographic tracing shows an acute inferoposterior myocardial infarction. (From Goldman L, Ausiello D: Cecil medicine, ed 23, Philadelphia, 2008, Saunders.)

Other Findings

• PR depression/QT elevation	Pericarditis
• QRS morphology	
• J or Osborne waves	Hypothermia
• ST segments	
• J point elevation	Early repolarization
• Diffuse elevations	Pericarditis
• Nonspecific depressions	
• T and U waves	Electrolytes

Acute Pericarditis

25 mm/s
10 mm/mV
100 Hz
Pgm 010C/v78
Cart: 2
Tech. : 40

Med:
Age: Ht: Wt:
Sex: M Race: Cauc
Loc: 2 Room: 225
Option: 40
Vent. rate 79 BPM
PR interval 152 ms
QRS duration 88 ms
QT/QTc 372/421 ms
P–R–T axes 63 55 47

Normal sinus rhythm with marked sinus arrhythmia
Acute pericarditis
Abnormal ECG

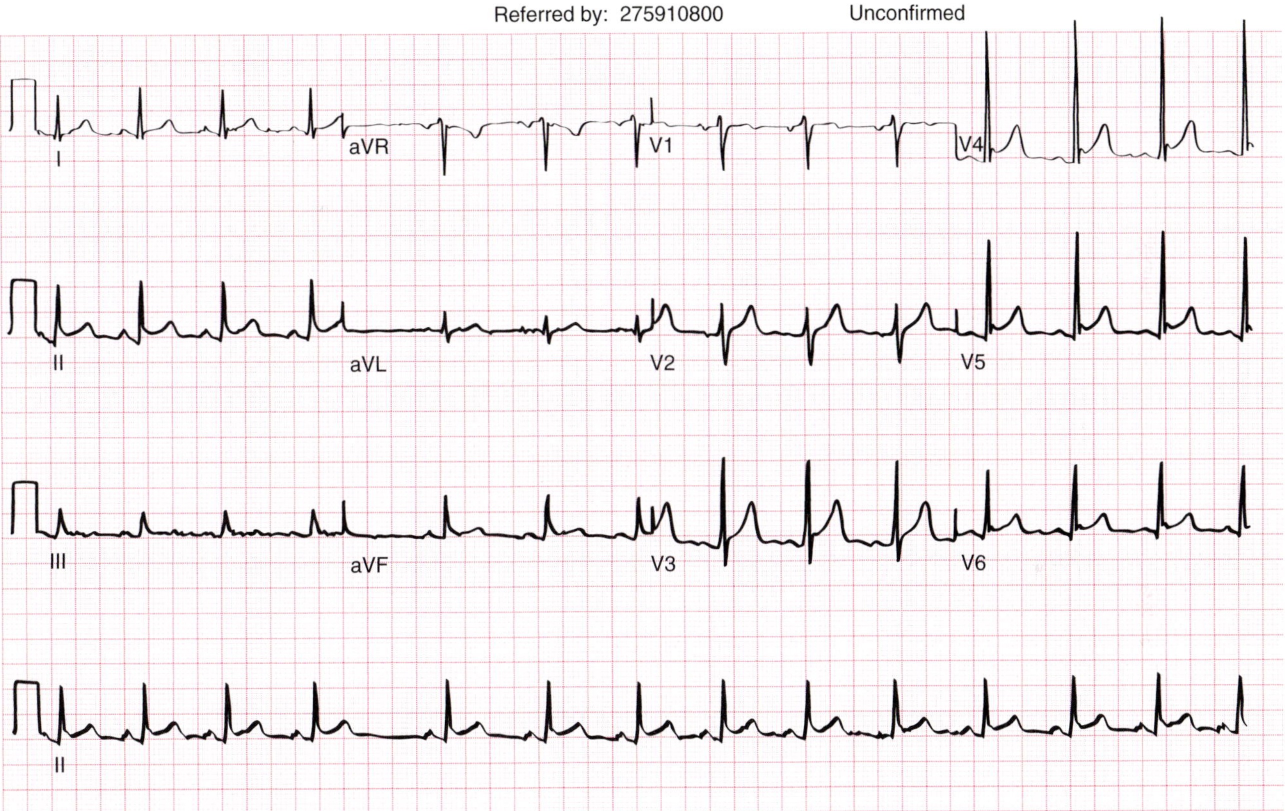

■ **Figure B-58** Electrocardiogram showing acute pericarditis. (Courtesy Ohio Chapter of the American College of Emergency Physicians.)

Electronic Ventricular Pacemaker

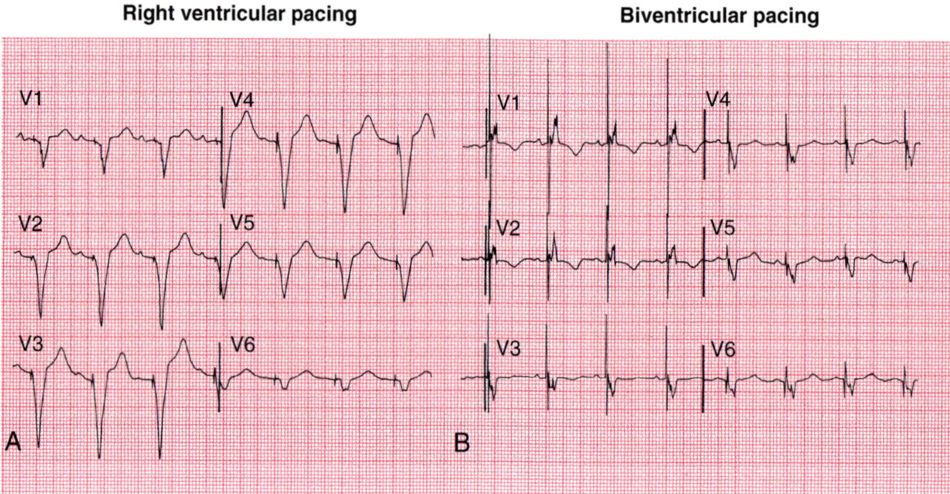

■ **Figure B-59** Right ventricular and biventricular pacing. **A**, Patient with heart failure who had a standard dual chamber (right atrial and right ventricular) pacemaker. **B**, To improve cardiac function, pacemaker was upgraded to a biventricular (BiV) device. Note that during right ventricular pacing (**A**), electrocardiogram shows a left bundle branch block morphology. Preceding sinus P waves are sensed by the atrial lead. In contrast, during biventricular pacing (**B**), QRS complexes show a right bundle branch block morphology. Also, QRS duration is somewhat shorter during biventricular pacing, owing to cardiac resynchronization effects of pacing ventricles in a nearly simultaneous fashion. (From Goldberger AL: Clinical electrocardiography: a simplified approach, ed 7, St Louis, 2007, Mosby.)

Hypothermia

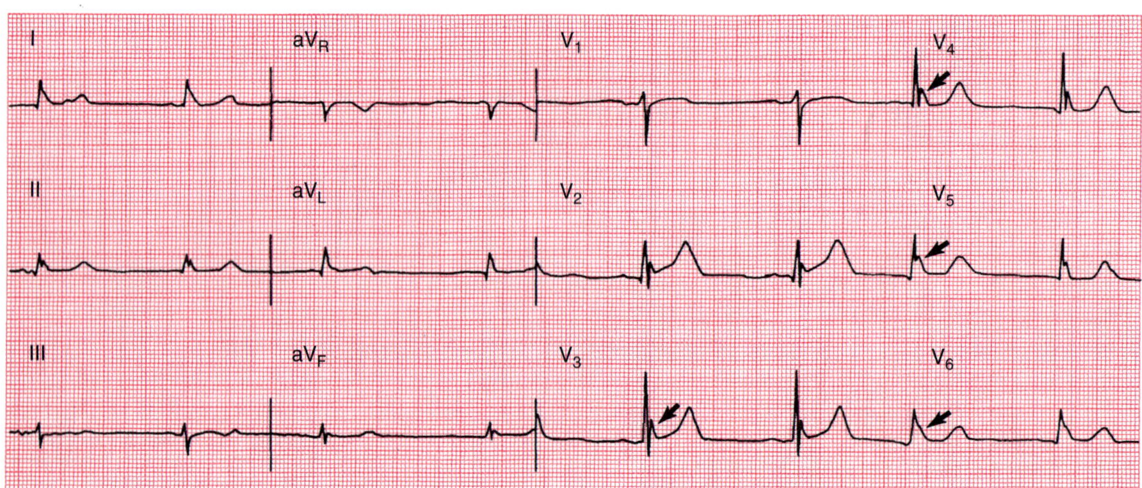

■ **Figure B-60** Systemic hypothermia is associated with a distinctive bulging of the J point (very beginning of the ST segment). The prominent J waves *(arrows)* with hypothermia are referred to as *Osborne waves*. (From Goldberger AL: Clinical electrocardiography: a simplified approach, ed 7, St Louis, 2007, Mosby.)

- The following are characteristic of ECG changes in the hypothermic patient:
  - J waves (Osborne waves)—pathognomonic of hypothermia; terminal notching of QRS—here best seen in II, V_4, and V_5
  - PR prolongation
  - QRS widening
  - QT prolongation
- These rhythm abnormalities are common:
  - Atrial fibrillation
  - Ventricular tachycardia
  - Ventricular fibrillation
  - Electromechanical dissociation
  - Asystole

Hyperkalemia

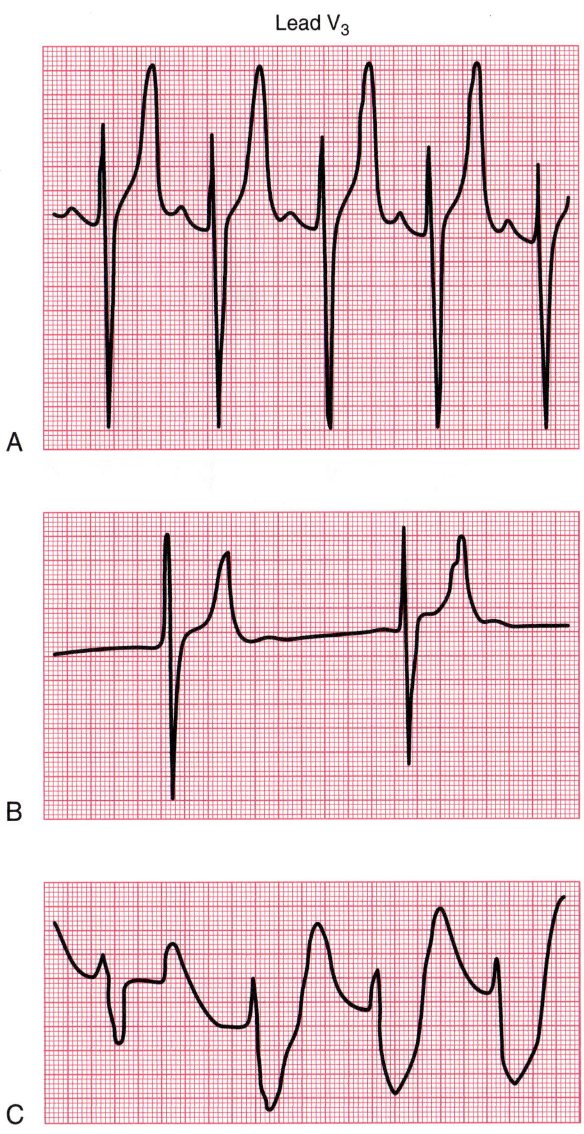

Figure B-61 Effects of progressive hyperkalemia on the electrocardiogram. All illustrations are from lead V_3. **A**, Serum potassium concentration ($[K^+]$) = 6.8 mEq/L; note peaked T waves together with normal sinus rhythm. **B**, Serum $[K^+]$ = 8.9 mEq/L; note peaked T waves and absent P waves. **C**, Serum $[K^+]$ = >8.9 mEq/L; note classic sine wave with absent P waves, marked prolongation of QRS complex, and peaked T waves. (From Goldman L, Ausiello D: Cecil medicine, ed 23, Philadelphia, 2008, Saunders.)

- Marked widening of the QRS duration combined with tall, peaked T waves are suggestive of advanced hyperkalemia. Note the absence of P waves, suggesting a junctional rhythm, but in hyperkalemia, the atrial muscle may be paralyzed while still in sinus rhythm. The sinus impulse conducts to the AV node through internodal tracts without activating the atrial muscle.
- Later stage will lead to more widening of all components, leading to "sine-wave" appearance.
- Angiotensin-converting enzyme (ACE) inhibitors and nonsteroidal antiinflammatory drugs (NSAIDs) as well as other drugs can cause hyperkalemia.

Brugada Syndrome

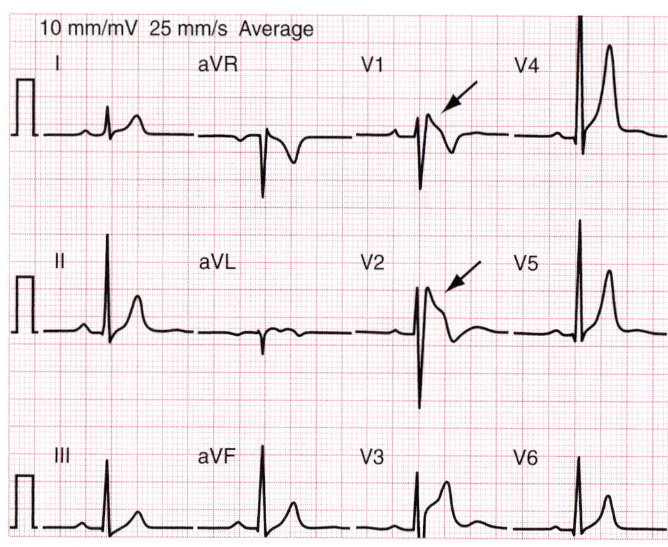

■ **Figure B-62** Brugada syndrome, with ST elevation in V_{1-2}. The ST elevation is coved *(upper, A)* or "saddle back" *(lower, B)* and may be transient. (From Marx JA, Hockberger RS, Walls, RM, et al: Rosen's emergency medicine, ed 7, St Louis, 2010, Mosby.)

- ECG findings of Brugada pattern: pseudo-RBBB and persistent ST-segment elevation in leads V_1 to V_3
- Diagnosis of Brugada syndrome requires typical ECG plus one of the following:
  - Documented ventricular fibrillation
  - Self-terminating polymorphic ventricular tachycardia (VT)
  - Family history of sudden cardiac death at < 45 years
  - Type I ST-segment elevation in family members
  - Electrophysiologic inducibility of VT
  - Unexplained syncope suggestive of a tachyarrhythmia
  - Nocturnal agonal respiration
- Treatment is implantable cardioverter-defibrillator (ICD) if associated with survivor of cardiac arrest (SCA), syncope, VF, or other high-risk factor.

Accessory Pathways

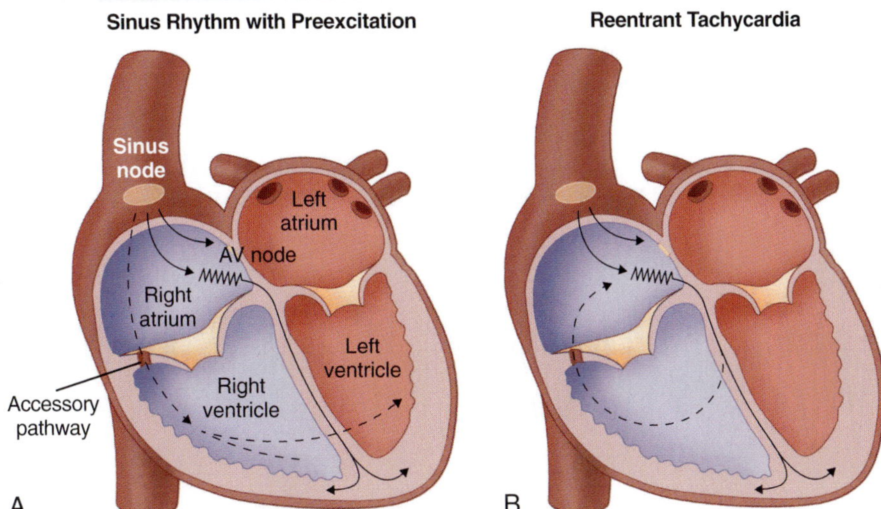

■ **Figure B-63** Accessory pathway in sinus rhythm and in orthodromic reentrant tachycardia. (From Basson CT: A molecular basis for Wolff-Parkinson-White syndrome. N Engl J Med 344:1861, 2001. Copyright © 2001 Massachusetts Medical Society. All rights reserved.)

- A number of AV accessory pathways resulting in preexcitation syndromes have been identified:
  - The muscular AV fiber (AVF), which is also called the *Kent bundle*, traverses the AV annulus and is responsible for most cases of Wolff-Parkinson-White syndrome.
  - Proposed pathways responsible for the Lown-Ganong-Levine syndrome or enhanced AV nodal conduction include an intranodal bypass tract (INBT) and atrionodal tracts (ANT), also known as *James fibers*.
  - Traditionally, the etiology for a Mahaim fiber tachycardia was thought to result from a nodoventricular (NVF) and fasciculoventricular (FVF) fiber. However, the true etiology is likely an atriofascicular fiber (AFF) that arises from the right atrium close to the annulus, inserting into the apical part of the right ventricle close to a fascicular branch of the right bundle branch.

Wolff-Parkinson-White (WPW) Syndrome

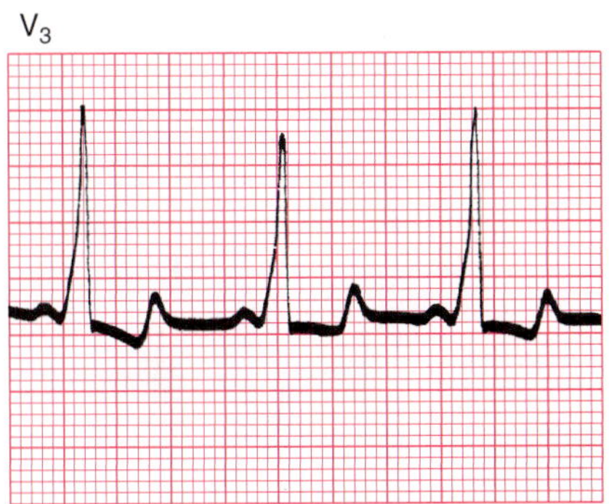

■ **Figure B-64** Lead V_3. Typical Wolff-Parkinson-White pattern showing short PR interval, delta wave, wide QRS complex, and secondary ST and T-wave changes. (From Aehlert B: ECGs made easy, ed 3, St Louis, 2006, Mosby.)

- Clinical: predisposes to tachyarrhythmias because cardiac conduction can bypass normal AV node via Kent fibers and set up orthodromic (narrow QRS) or retrodromic (wide QRS) reentry circuit; if AF occurs can lead to very rapid ventricular rate.
- Treatment of acute tachyarrhythmia: orthodromic: standard drugs for SVT/rate control of AV node
- Antidromic: procainamide; avoid drugs that inhibit AV node.
- Definitive treatment of WPW with arrhythmia is ablation.

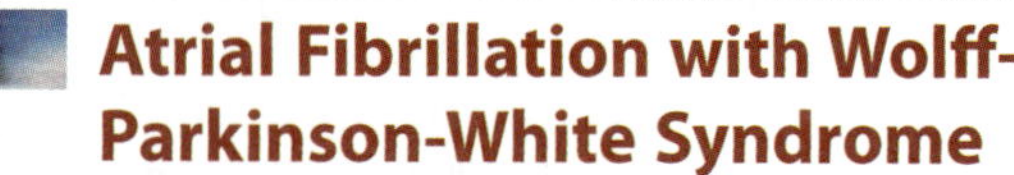

Atrial Fibrillation with Wolff-Parkinson-White Syndrome

Atrial Fibrillation and Wolff-Parkinson-White Syndrome

II

I aVR V1 V4

A

II aVL V2 V5

III aVF V3 V6

B

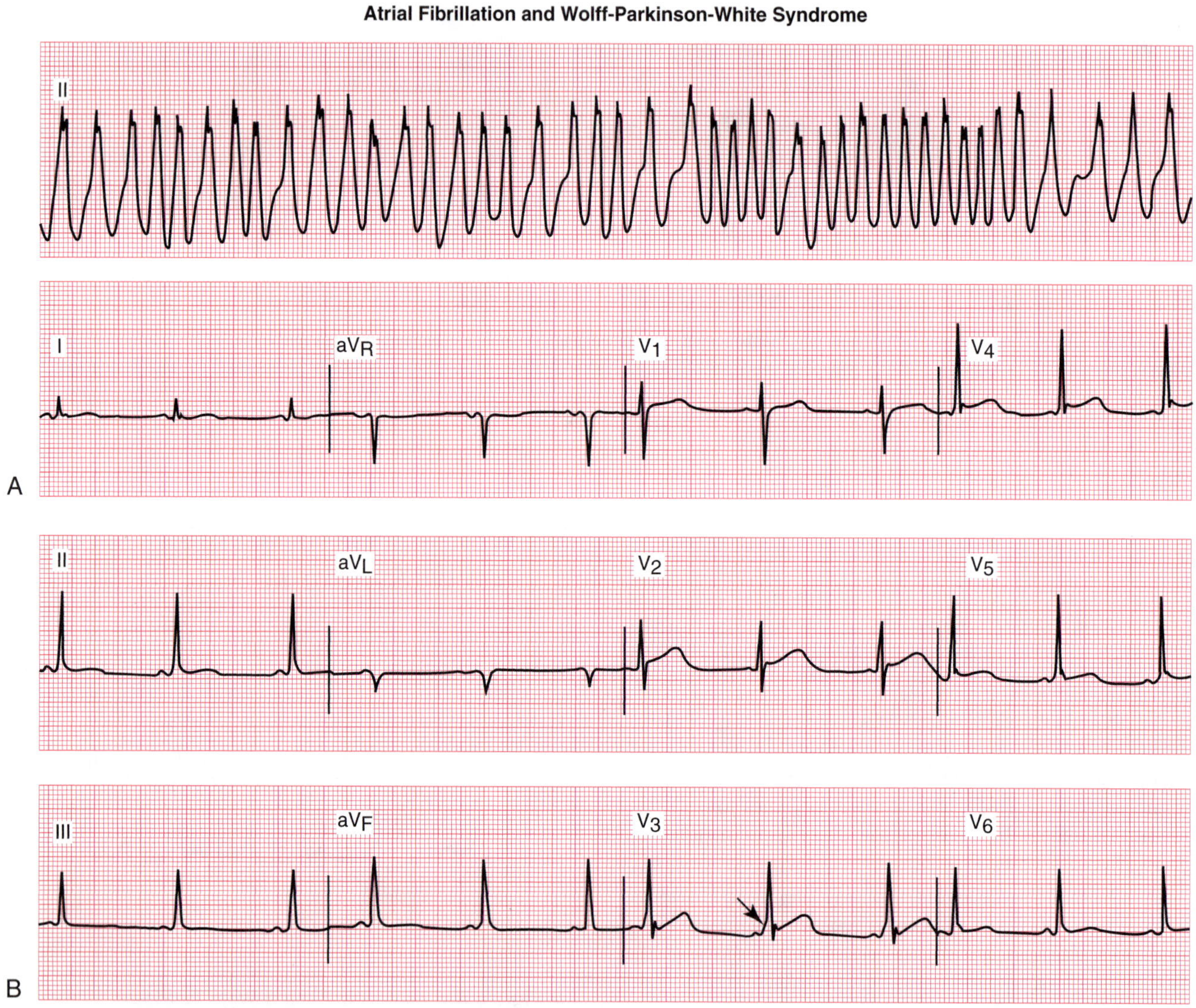

■ **Figure B-65** **A,** Atrial fibrillation with Wolff-Parkinson-White preexcitation syndrome may lead to a wide-complex tachycardia that has a very rapid rate. Note that some R-R intervals are less than 0.20 second. Irregularity is due to underlying atrial fibrillation. **B,** After arrhythmia has been converted to sinus rhythm, classic triad of Wolff-Parkinson-White syndrome is visible but subtle: relatively short PR interval, wide QRS complex, and delta wave (*arrow* in lead V_3). (From Goldberger AL: Clinical electrocardiography: a simplified approach, ed 7, St Louis, 2007, Mosby.)

APPENDIX C

Normal Laboratory Values

PART I Hematology

		Conventional Units	SI Units*
Acid hemolysis test (Ham)		No hemolysis	No hemolysis
Alkaline phosphatase, leukocyte		Total score 14–100	Total score 14–100
Cell counts			
Erythrocytes			
Males		4.6–6.2 million/mm^3	4.6–6.2 × 10^{12}/L
Females		4.2–5.4 million/mm^3	4.2–5.4 × 10^{12}/L
Children (varies with age)		4.5–5.1 million/mm^3	4.5–5.1 × 10^{12}/L
Leukocytes			
Total		4500–11,000 mm^3	4.5–11.0 × 10^9/L
Differential	*Percentage*	*Absolute*	*Absolute*
Myelocytes	0	0/mm^3	0/L
Band neutrophils	3–5	150–400/mm^3	150–400 × 10^6/L
Segmented neutrophils	54–62	3000–5800/mm^3	3000–5800 × 10^6/L
Lymphocytes	25–33	1500–3000/mm^3	1500–3000 × 10^6/L
Monocytes	3–7	300–500/mm^3	300–500 × 10^6/L
Eosinophils	1–3	50–250/mm^3	50–250 × 10^6/L
Basophils	0–1	15–50/mm^3	15–50 × 10^6/L
Platelets		150,000–400,000/mm^3	150–400 × 10^9/L
Reticulocytes		25,000–75,000/mm^3 (0.5%–1.5% of erythrocytes)	25–75 × 10^9/L
Coagulation tests			
Bleeding time (template)		2.75–8.0 min	2.75–8.0 min
Coagulation time (glass tubes)		5–15 min	5–15 min
D-Dimer		<0.5 mcg/mL	<0.5 mg/L
Factor VIII and other coagulation factors		50%–150% of normal	0.5–1.5 of normal
Fibrin split products (Thrombo-Welco test)		<10 mcg/mL	<10 mg/L
Fibrinogen		200–400 mg/dL	2.0–4.0 g/L
Partial thromboplastin time (PTT)		20–35 sec	20–35 sec
Prothrombin time (PT)		12.0–14.0 sec	12.0–14.0 sec
Coombs' test			
Direct		Negative	Negative
Indirect		Negative	Negative
Corpuscular values of erythrocytes			
Mean corpuscular hemoglobin (MCH)		26–34 pg/cell	26–34 pg/cell
Mean corpuscular volume (MCV)		80–96 micrometer^3	80–96 fL
Mean corpuscular hemoglobin concentration (MCHC)		32–36 g/dL	320–360 g/L
Erythrocyte sedimentation rate (ESR)			
Wintrobe			
Males		0–5 mm/h	0–5 mm/h
Females		0–15 mm/h	0–15 mm/h
Westergren			
Males		0–15 mm/h	0–15 mm/h
Females		0–20 mm/h	0–20 mm/h
		20–165 mg/dL	0.20–1.65 g/L
Haptoglobin		26–185 mg/dL	260–1850 mg/L

Continued

PART I Hematology—*Cont'd*

	Conventional Units	SI Units*
Hematocrit		
Males	40–54 mL/dL	0.40–0.54 volume fraction
Females	37–47 mL/dL	0.37–0.47 volume fraction
Newborns	49–54 mL/dL	0.49–0.54 volume fraction
Children (varies with age)	35–49 mL/dL	0.35–0.49 volume fraction
Hemoglobin		
Males	14.0–18.0 g/dL	2.17–2.79 mmol/L
Females	12.0–16.0 g/dL	1.86–2.48 mmol/L
Newborns	16.5–19.5 g/dL	2.56–3.02 mmol/L
Children (varies with age)	11.2–16.5 g/dL	1.74–2.56 mmol/L
Hemoglobin, fetal	<1% of total	<0.01 of total
Hemoglobin A_{1c}	3%–5% of total	0.03–0.05 of total
Hemoglobin A_2	1.5%–3.0% of total	0.015–0.03 of total
Hemoglobin, plasma	0.0–5.0 mg/dL	0–0.8 micromole/L
Methemoglobin	30–130 mg/dL	4.7–20 micromole/L

*Le Système International d'Unités (International System of Units).

PART II Blood Chemistry

	Conventional Units	SI Units*
Alanine aminotransferase (ALT, SGPT), serum	1–45 U/L	1–45 U/L
Aspartate aminotransferase (AST, SGOT), serum	1–36 U/L	1–36 U/L
Base excess, arterial blood, calculated	0 ± 2 mEq/L	0 ± 2 mmol/L
Beta-carotene, serum	60–260 mcg/dL	1.1–8.6 micromole/L
Bicarbonate		
Venous plasma	23–29 mEq/L	23–39 mmol/L
Arterial blood	18–23 mEq/L	18–23 mmol/L
Bile acids, serum	0.3–3.0 mg/dL	3–30 mg/L
Bilirubin, serum		
Conjugated	0.1–0.4 mg/dL	1.7–6.8 micromole/L
Total	0.3–1.1 mg/dL	5.1–19 micromole/L
Calcium, serum	9.0–11.0 mg/dL	2.25–2.75 mmol/L
Calcium, ionized, serum	4.25–5.25 mg/dL	1.05–1.30 mmol/L
Carbon dioxide, total, serum or plasma	24–30 mEq/L	24–30 mmol/L
Carbon dioxide tension (PCO_2), blood	35–45 mm HG	35–45 mm HG
Ceruloplasmin, serum	23–44 mg/dL	230–440 mg/L
Chloride, serum or plasma	96–106 mEq/L	96–106 mmol/L
Cholesterol, serum or EDTA plasma		
Desirable range	<200 mg/dL	<5.18 mmol/L
LDL cholesterol (optimal)	<100 mg/dL	<1000 mg/L
HDL cholesterol (optimal)	≥60 mg/dL	≥600 mg/L
Copper	70–140 mcg/dL	11–22 micromole/L
Corticotropin (ACTH), plasma, 8:00 AM	10–80 pg/mL	2–18 pmol/L
Cortisol, plasma		
8:00 AM	6–23 mcg/dL	170–635 nmol/L
4:00 PM	3–15 mcg/dL	82–413 nmol/L
10:00 PM	<50% of 8:00 AM value	<0.5 of 8:00 AM value
Creatine, serum		
Males	0.2–0.5 mg/dL	15–40 micromole/L
Females	0.3–0.9 mg/dL	25–70 micromole/L
Creatine kinase (CK), serum		
Males	55–170 U/L	55–170 U/L
Females	30–135 U/L	30–135 U/L
Creatine kinase MB isoenzyme, serum	0–4.7 ng/mL	0–4.7 mcg/L
Creatinine, serum	0.6–1.2 mg/dL	50–110 micromole/L

For some procedures the reference values may vary depending on the method used.

PART II Blood Chemistry—*Cont'd*

	Conventional Units	SI Units*
Estradiol-17-beta, adult		
Males	10–65 pg/mL	35–240 pmol/L
Females		
Follicular phase	30–100 pg/mL	110–370 pmol/L
Ovulatory phase	200–400 pg/mL	730–1470 pmol/L
Luteal phase	50–140 pg/mL	180–510 pmol/L
Ferritin, serum	20–200 ng/mL	20–200 mcg/L
Fibrinogen, plasma	200–400 mg/dL	2.0–4.0 g/L
Folate, serum	1.8–9.0 ng/mL	4.1–20.4 nmol/L
Erythrocytes	150–450 ng/mL	340–1020 nmol/L
Follicle-stimulating hormone (FSH), plasma		
Males	4–25 mU/mL	4–25 U/L
Females	4–30 mU/mL	4–30 U/L
Postmenopausal	40–250 mU/mL	40–250 U/L
Gamma-glutamyltransferase (GGT), serum	5–40 U/L	5–40 U/L
Gastrin, fasting, serum	0–110 pg/mL	0–110 ng/L
Glucose, fasting, plasma or serum	70–115 mg/dL	3.9–6.4 mmol/L
Growth hormone (hGH), plasma, adult, fasting	0–6 ng/mL	0–6 mcg/L
Haptoglobin, serum	20–165 mg/dL	0.20–1.65 g/L
Insulin, fasting, plasma	5–25 microU/mL	36–179 pmol/L
Iron, serum	75–175 mcg/dL	13–31 micromole/L
Iron-binding capacity, serum		
Total	250–410 mcg/dL	45–73 micromole/L
Saturation	20%–55%	0.20–0.55
Lactate		
Venous whole blood	5.0–20.0 mg/dL	0.6–2.2 mmol/L
Arterial whole blood	5.0–15.0 mg/dL	0.6–1.7 mmol/L
Lactate dehydrogenase (LDH), serum	110–220 U/L	110–220 U/L
Lipase, serum	10–140 U/L	10–140 U/L
Lutropin (LH), serum		
Males	1–9 U/L	1–9 U/L
Females		
Follicular phase	2–10 U/L	2–10 U/L
Midcycle peak	15–65 U/L	15–65 U/L
Luteal phase	1–12 U/L	1–12 U/L
Postmenopausal	12–65 U/L	12–65 U/L
Magnesium, serum	1.8–3.0 mg/dL	0.75–1.25 mmol/L
Osmolality	286–295 mOsm/kg water	285–295 mmol/kg water
Oxygen, blood, arterial, room air		
Partial pressure (Pao_2)	80–100 mm Hg	80–100 mm Hg
Saturation (Sao_2)	95%–98%	95%–98%
pH, arterial blood	7.35–7.45	7.35–7.45
Phosphate, inorganic, serum		
Adult	3.0–4.5 mg/dL	1.0–1.5 mmol/L
Child	4.0–7.0 mg/dL	1.3–2.3 mmol/L
Potassium		
Serum	3.5–5.0 mEq/L	3.5–5.0 mmol/L
Plasma	3.5–4.5 mEq/L	3.5–4.5 mmol/L
Progesterone, serum, adult		
Males	0.0–0.4 ng/mL	0.0–1.3 mmol/L
Females		
Follicular phase	0.1–1.5 ng/mL	0.3–4.8 mmol/L
Luteal phase	2.5–28.0 ng/mL	8.0–89.0 mmol/L
Prolactin, serum		
Males	1.0–15.0 ng/mL	1.0–15.0 mcg/L
Females	1.0–20.0 ng/mL	1.0–20.0 mcg/L
Protein, serum, electrophoresis		
Total	6.0–8.0 g/dL	60–80 g/L
Albumin	3.5–5.5 g/dL	35–55 g/L
$Alpha_1$ globulin	0.2–0.4 g/dL	2–4 g/L
$Alpha_2$ globulin	0.5–0.9 g/dL	5–9 g/L
Beta globulin	0.6–1.1 g/dL	6–11 g/L
Gamma globulin	0.7–1.7 g/dL	7–15 g/L

Continued

PART II Blood Chemistry—*Cont'd*

	Conventional Units	SI Units*
Pyruvate, blood	0.3–0.9 g/dL	0.03–0.10 mmol/L
Rheumatoid factor	0.0–30.0 IU/mL	0.0–30.0 kIU/mL
Sodium, serum or plasma	135–145 mEq/L	135–145 mmol/L
Testosterone, plasma		
Males, adult	300–1200 ng/dL	10.4–41.6 nmol/L
Females, adult	20–75 ng/dL	0.7–2.6 nmol/L
Pregnant females	40–200 ng/dL	1.4–6.9 nmol/L
Thyroglobulin	3–42 ng/mL	3–42 mcg/L
Thyrotropin (hTSH), serum	0.4–4.8 microIU/mL	0.4–4.8 mIU/L
Thyrotropin-releasing hormone (TRH)	5–60 pg/mL	5–60 ng/L
Thyroxine, free (FT_4), serum	0.9–2.1 ng/dL	12–27 pmol/L
Thyroxine (T_4), serum	4.5–12.0 mcg/dL	58–154 nmol/L
Thyroxine-binding globulin (TBG)	15.0–34.0 mcg/mL	15.0–34.0 mg/L
Transferrin	250–430 mg/dL	2.5–4.3 g/L
Triglycerides, serum, after 12-hour fast	40–150 mg/dL	0.4–1.5 g/L
Triiodothyronine (T_3), serum	70–190 ng/dL	1.1–2.9 nmol/L
Triiodothyronine uptake, resin (T_3RU)	25%–38% uptake	0.25–0.38 uptake
Urate		
Males	2.5–8.0 mg/dL	150–480 micromole/L
Females	2.2–7.0 mg/dL	130–420 micromole/L
Urea, serum or plasma	24–49 mg/dL	4.0–8.2 nmol/L
Urea nitrogen, serum or plasma	11–23 mg/dL	8.0–16.4 nmol/L
Viscosity, serum	1.4–1.8 times water	1.4–1.8 times water
Vitamin A, serum	20–80 mcg/dL	0.70–2.80 micromole/L
Vitamin B_{12}, serum	180–900 pg/mL	133–664 pmol/L

*Le Système International d'Unités (International System of Units).
IU, International unit; *U,* unit.

PART III Urine Chemistry

	Conventional Units	SI Units*
Acetone and acetoacetate, qualitative	Negative	Negative
Albumin		
Qualitative	Negative	Negative
Quantitative	10–100 mg/24 h	0.15–1.5 micromole/day
Aldosterone	3–20 mcg/24 h	8.3–55 nmol/day
Delta-aminolevulinic acid (delta-ALA)	1.3–7.0 mg/24 h	10–53 micromole/day
Amylase	<17 U/h	<17 U/h
Amylase/creatinine clearance ratio	0.01–0.04	0.01–0.04
Bilirubin, qualitative	Negative	Negative
Calcium (regular diet)	<250 mg/24 h	<6.3 mmol/day
Catecholamines		
Epinephrine	<10 mcg/24 h	<55 nmol/day
Norepinephrine	<100 mcg/24 h	<590 nmol/day
Total free catecholamines	4–126 mcg/24 h	24–745 nmol/day
Total metanephrines	0.1–1.6 mg/24 h	0.5–8.1 micromole/day
Chloride (varies with intake)	110–250 mEq/24 h	110–250 mmol/day
Copper	0–50 mcg/24 h	0.0–0.80 micromole/day
Cortisol, free	10–100 mcg/24 h	27.6–276 nmol/day
Creatine		
Males	0–40 mg/24 h	0.0–0.30 mmol/day
Females	0–80 mg/24 h	0.0–0.60 mmol/day
Creatinine	15–25 mg/kg/24 h	0.13–0.22 mmol/kg/day
Creatinine clearance (endogenous)		
Males	110–150 mL/min/1.73 m^2	110–150 mL/min/1.73 m^2
Females	105–132 mL/min/1.73 m^2	105–132 mL/min/1.73 m^2
Cystine or cysteine	Negative	Negative

For some procedures the reference values may vary depending on the method used.

PART III Urine Chemistry—*Cont'd*

	Conventional Units	SI Units*
Dehydroepiandrosterone		
Males	0.2–2.0 mg/24 h	0.7–6.9 micromole/day
Females	0.2–1.8 mg/24 h	0.7–6.2 micromole/day
Estrogens, total		
Males	4–25 mcg/24 h	14–90 nmol/day
Females	5–100 mcg/24 h	18–360 nmol/day
Glucose (as reducing substance)	<250 mg/24 h	<250 mg/day
Hemoglobin and myoglobin, qualitative	Negative	Negative
Homogentisic acid, qualitative	Negative	Negative
17-Hydroxycorticosteroids		
Males	3–9 mg/24 h	8.3–25 micromole/day
Females	2–8 mg/24 h	5.5–22 micromole/day
5-Hydroxyindoleacetic acid		
Qualitative	Negative	Negative
Quantitative	2–6 mg/24 h	10–31 micromole/day
17-Ketogenic steroids		
Males	5–23 mg/24 h	17–80 micromole/day
Females	3–15 mg/24 h	10–52 micromole/day
17-Ketosteroids		
Males	8–22 mg/24 h	28–76 micromole/day
Females	6–15 mg/24 h	21–52 micromole/day
Magnesium	6–10 mEq/24 h	3–5 mmol/day
Metanephrines	0.05–1.2 ng/mg creatinine	0.03–0.70 mmol/mmol creatinine
Osmolality	38–1400 mOsm/kg water	38–1400 mOsm/kg water
pH	4.6–8.0	4.6–8.0
Phenylpyruvic acid, qualitative	Negative	Negative
Phosphate	0.4–1.3 g/24 h	13–42 mmol/day
Porphobilinogen		
Qualitative	Negative	Negative
Quantitative	<2.0 mg/24 h	<9 micromole/day
Porphyrins		
Coproporphyrin	50–250 mcg/24 h	77–380 nmol/day
Uroporphyrin	10–30 mcg/24 h	12–36 nmol/day
Potassium	25–125 mEq/24 h	25–125 mmol/day
Pregnanediol		
Males	0.0–1.9 mg/24 h	0.0–6.0 micromole/day
Females		
Proliferative phase	0.0–2.6 mg/24 h	0.0–8.0 micromole/day
Luteal phase	2.6–10.6 mg/24 h	8–33 micromole/day
Postmenopausal	0.2–1 mg/24 h	0.6–3.1 micromole/day
Pregnanetriol	0.0–2.5 mg/24 h	0.0–7.4 micromole/day
Protein, total		
Qualitative	Negative	Negative
Quantitative	10–150 mg/24 h	10–150 mg/day
Protein/creatinine ratio	<0.2	<0.2
Sodium (regular diet)	60–260 mEq/24 h	60–260 mmol/day
Specific gravity	1.003–1.030	1.003–1.030
Random specimen	1.003–1.030	1.003–1.030
24-hour collection	1.015–1.025	1.015–1.025
Urate (regular diet)	250–750 mg/24 h	1.5–4.4 mmol/day
Urobilinogen	0.5–4.0 mg/24 h	0.6–6.8 micromole/day
Vanillylmandelic acid (VMA)	1–8 mg/24 h	5–40 micromole/24 h

*Le Système International d'Unités (International System of Units).

Adapted from O'Toole MT, editor: Miller-Keane encyclopedia and dictionary of medicine, nursing, and allied health, ed 6, Philadelphia, 1997, Saunders, pp 1843–1845, 1847–1848.

APPENDIX

D Rapid Sequence Intubation

Assessment

The textbooks and educators make it sound so simple: "You should assess and manage the ABCs." You read the literature and value the information that says airway assessment and management are important. These statements are easy to write, easy to read, but many times very difficult to do.

Assessment of Airway

"Look, listen, and feel" really don't have much to do with airway assessment. Those three assessment parameters are best saved for the breathing assessment. Assessment of airway begins with your across-the-room (or across-the-scene) evaluation of the patient.

From across the room, the patient should look up at you and have no unusual airway noises. If not, a quick primary assessment needs to be performed at the patient's side for two reasons: airway patency and airway protection (consciousness).

The airway assessment within the primary survey mandates that you determine the patient's consciousness. Is he awake now? Can this patient protect his airway? Will I need to perform airway maneuvers on the patient now or in the next few minutes to protect his airway?

When determining airway patency, look inside the mouth. Are there secretions, blood, vomitus, loose teeth, or other debris within the orifice that I need to suction? Of all airway tools, the most important are your gloved hands and a good suction device.

In the world of critical care transport, many of our patients have already had airway devices inserted. Once you assess the mouth for debris, move your assessment onto the foreign devices within the upper airway. If the patient already has an adjunct in place, evaluate that device for patency and effectiveness. Will you need to upgrade this device? The old adage is, "If it ain't broke, don't fix it." The decision as to whether or not to change from one airway device to another will be discussed later in this section.

A reminder: airway management in the trauma patient always includes a neutral spine position for the patient; the patient's ear canal should be in a straight line with the sternal notch. Provide neutral inline immobilization devices according to your protocols. Spineboards may be applied prior to transport.

Cough and Airway Assessment

The presence of sputum with cough complicates the ability of the patient to maintain a patent airway. Cystic fibrosis, bronchiectasis, pulmonary abscess, and pulmonary carcinoma all produce purulent sputum. The volume and texture of the sputum may affect airway clearance. The thicker the secretions, the more difficult to clear. If the patient's ability to cough is impaired, an alternative plan to maintain a patent airway must exist. The use of vacuum suction to clear the airway, especially an artificial airway, should be available. Oxygen should also be available, as should a bag-mask system in the event of respiratory compromise.

If the patient is unable to produce a spontaneous cough or clear the airway of secretions, airway maintenance becomes a mechanical procedure that requires the use of aseptic (nonintubated patients) or sterile suctioning technique (intubated or tracheotomized patient). In the nonintubated patient, suctioning of the lower airway is best accomplished by the nasotracheal route, but be cautious with blind suction technique; it's possible to cause laryngospasm and surface trauma to the tracheal mucosa. In the intubated patient, suction is more easily accomplished but still requires caution. Hitting the surface of the carina and lower trachea with the tip of the suction catheter can leave "pock marks" on the carina and remove portions of the mucosal wall, interfering with the lungs' natural defenses. The advent of "closed system" suction catheters has greatly reduced the incidence of infection of the lower respiratory tract during ventilation; it also aids in maintaining constant PEEP levels.

Disorder of the Airway and Respiratory System

Threat to Airway or Airway Compromise

Once the patient has been assessed by the critical care team, some decisions will have to be made. Does this patient have a patent airway right now? Can the patient maintain that airway throughout transport? If the patient has an artificial airway, is it working properly, or should we upgrade to a different device?

Maintaining the integrity of the patient's respiratory system and airway are among the most important skills in emergency and critical care situations. In the critical care transport setting, the provider must not only maintain the patient's airway and respiratory status but also anticipate any possible changes during transport, which often entails much longer time periods than in the acute emergency setting. Excellent airway and ventilatory management skills can make all the difference in patient outcomes.

Airway Tools: The Basics

The patient who is unable to maintain his or her own airway (level of consciousness) or has airway obstruction potential should have a definitive airway placed by the local healthcare team or the critical care crew. All agree that a definitive airway is the tracheal tube. Between 1%–3% of your patients will present with what is termed a difficult airway and placement of the tracheal tube becomes difficult, if not impossible.

Whether you place other airway adjuncts as a bridge (temporizing) to intubation or as a rescue from a failed intubation attempt, all of these devices may become important to your success. The organization of these adjuncts will be oriented toward their position above or below the glottis.

A good worker uses tools to manage problems. The critical care transport team's toolbox includes knowledge, good decision making, and the physical tools of the job. This job is at times difficult, so the more tools you have, the better you'll be able to manage the patient's airway. Let's begin with the basic tools of airway management.

Simple Positioning

The head-tilt, chin lift or head-neutral, jaw thrust positions are easy to perform and generally reliable. However, positioning a patient with an unprotected airway flat on his back poses risks for aspiration. Don't forget that the recovery position (side lying) is also good for the medical patient in order to maintain airway patency and prevent aspiration. The problem with relying on position only is that there is no subglottic protection against aspiration in the patient with altered mental status, and one person is usually occupied with airway management only (Figures D-1, D-2, and D-3).

Did You Know?

A relatively new categorization of airways is termed *supraglottic*. This refers to a properly positioned airway adjunct whose final position rests above the glottis. Many new devices on the market are within this category.[7]

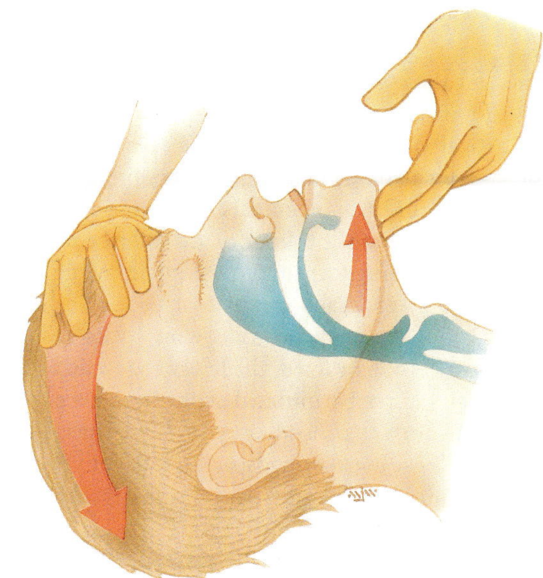

■ **Figure D-1** (From Sanders M: Mosby's paramedic textbook, revised ed 3, St Louis, 2007, Mosby.)

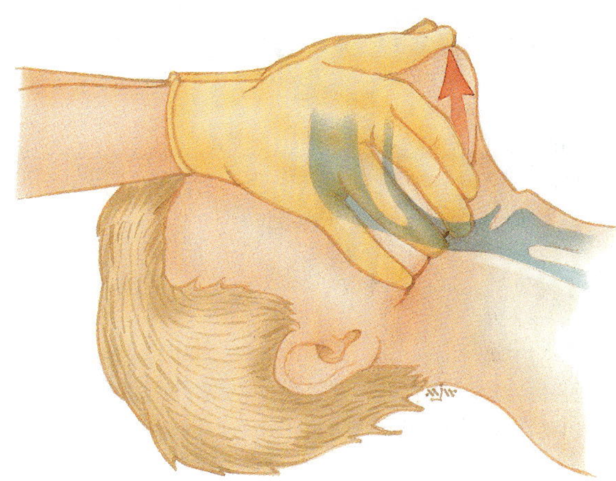

■ **Figure D-2** (From Sanders M: Mosby's paramedic textbook, revised ed 3, St Louis, 2007, Mosby.)

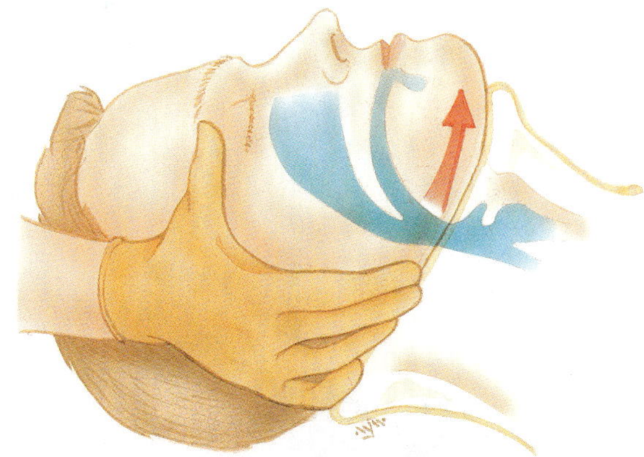

■ **Figure D-3** (From Sanders M: Mosby's paramedic textbook, revised ed 3, St Louis, 2007, Mosby.)

Nasal and Oral Airways

Designed for the conscious/semiconscious patient with an intact gag reflex, the nasal airway has limited indications in the critical care environment. Considered one of the best devices for patients just after extubation, or for those who are in the midst of a generalized seizure, this airway is passed gently along the floor of the lubricated nostril with the distal, slanted opening positioned medially if at all possible. This generally means that the device should be inserted into the right nostril, owing to its design. If the right nostril is obstructed, the left nostril may be used, but insertion should be initiated with the device turned upside down until the distal tip is past the **nasal turbinates**. Nasal bleeding, laryngospasm, and vomiting may occur, especially if the nasal airway chosen is too large or too long for the patient (Figure D-4).

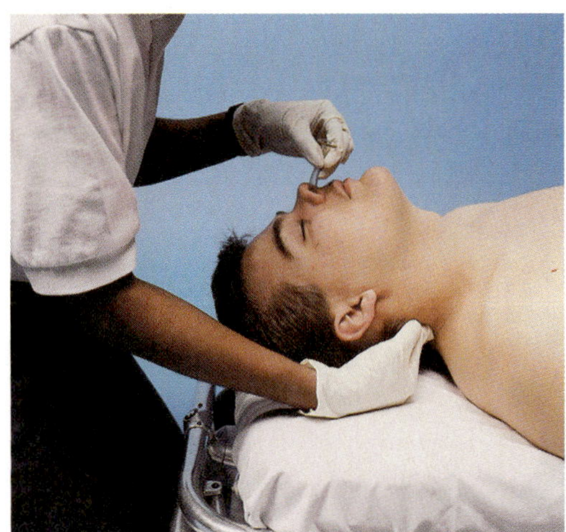

Figure D-4 (From Sanders M: Mosby's paramedic textbook, revised ed 3, St Louis, 2007, Mosby.)

An oral airway is designed to displace the tongue forward in the pharynx and, because of this position, usually stimulates the gag reflex. You should assess for the presence of a gag reflex, along with measuring for correct size prior to use. The distal flange should rest at the level of the central incisors, with the bite block parallel to the hard palate. The two techniques for insertion are shown in Figure D-5. Both techniques are designed to prevent pushing the tongue downward into the pharynx and creating further problems. The other indication for this device is as a protection for the tracheal tube while properly positioned in a biting patient's mouth (bite block; Figure D-5.)

Supraglottic/Extraglottic Airway Devices

Since the development of the first tracheal tube in 1880, airway management has come a long way. The new supraglottic airway devices (now called *extraglottic airway devices*) are being developed at one to two per year, with a scramble in the airway and ventilation industry to decide how to classify and describe all of them. This discussion will be organized into those airway devices that are extraglottic and those that are intraglottic. There will also be information on the valuable tools that allow you to introduce, exchange, or facilitate intubation through the use of stylets or fiberoptic real-time video imaging.

Within the extraglottic category, there are generally nasally and orally inserted devices that are either cuffed or uncuffed. These devices can be divided into cuffed and uncuffed oral laryngeal airways, cuffed and uncuffed nasally inserted laryngopharyngeal airways, and cuffed and uncuffed hypopharyngeal airways. The next section will be devoted to those extraglottic airways that rest in the hypopharynx and can be a bridge or a route to intubation.

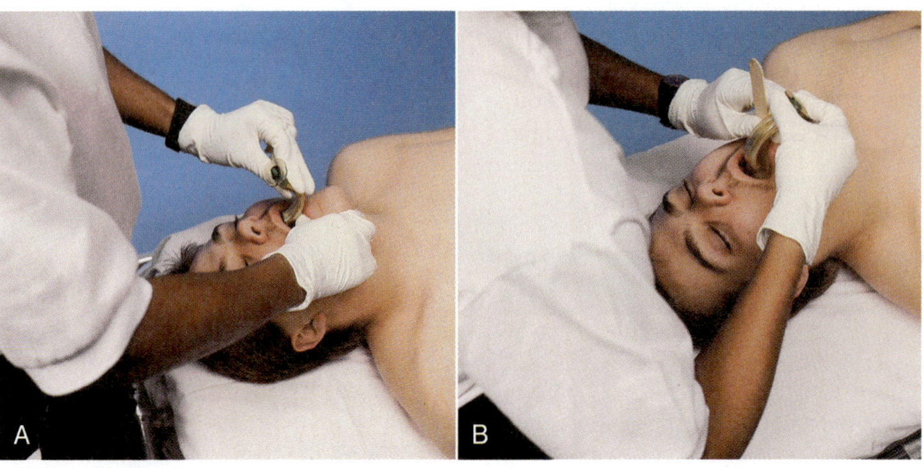

Figure D-5 (From Sanders M: Mosby's paramedic textbook, revised ed 3, St Louis, 2007, Mosby.)

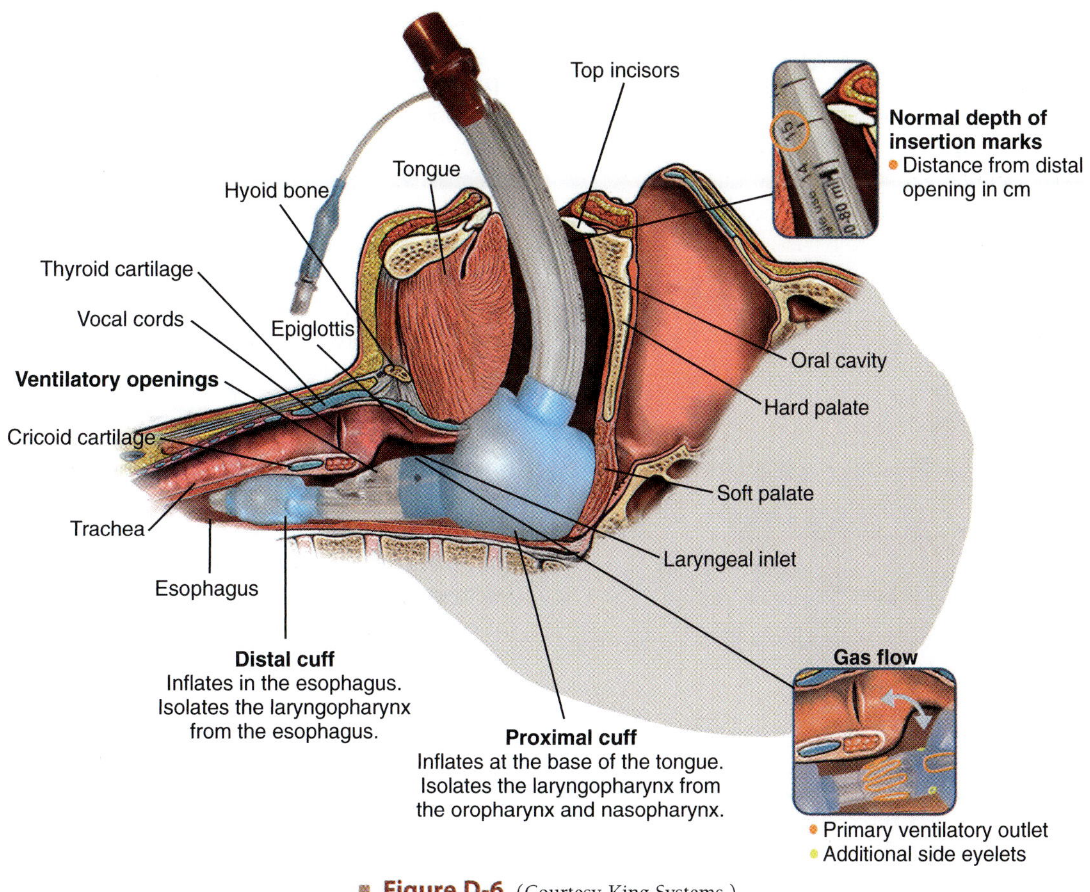

Figure D-6 (Courtesy King Systems.)

Generally, the extraglottic airways are blindly inserted and rest between the base of the tongue and the glottis. Because of this positioning, these devices may allow for aspiration of gastric contents. As stated, they are not the definitive airway but have now become a standard backup in the failed airway protocols.

As you can see in Figure D-6, the extraglottic airway position allows for indirect ventilation. They are relatively easy to insert with just your gloved hands.

The airways are universal in that they have a glottic opening, and this affords you the conduit to indirect intubation. This is accomplished by placing a stylet or exchange catheter through the airway and into the trachea. The extraglottic airway is then removed and an endotracheal tube (ETT) is railroaded over the catheter and into position.

Note that the Esophageal Tracheal Combitube (ETC) is included in the extraglottic airway device category. Developed many years ago as an EMS airway, this is a dual-tube system based on the now outdated esophageal obturator airway. The large latex pharyngeal cuff poses some difficulty, especially while attempting to intubate with an ETT around the device (Figure D-7). Table D-1 lists the common extraglottic airway devices available.

Did You Know?

The term *supraglottic airway* has become very confusing as more and more of these devices occupy various areas in the hypopharynx. Some sit in the infraglottic area, some in both the supra- and infraglottic areas. The new term that is more acceptable for all is *extraglottic*—located outside the glottis.[7]

Intraglottic Airway Devices and Procedures

The art of inserting a soft, curved tracheal tube into a human airway with three separate angles and, on occasion, unique anatomy can be a challenge. The term *tools* was used earlier. While performing endotracheal intubation, you should have as many tools ready for action as possible for such challenges.

There are four principal indications for endotracheal intubation:

1. Airway protection
2. Pulmonary **toilette**
3. Providing positive-pressure ventilation
4. Maintaining oxygenation

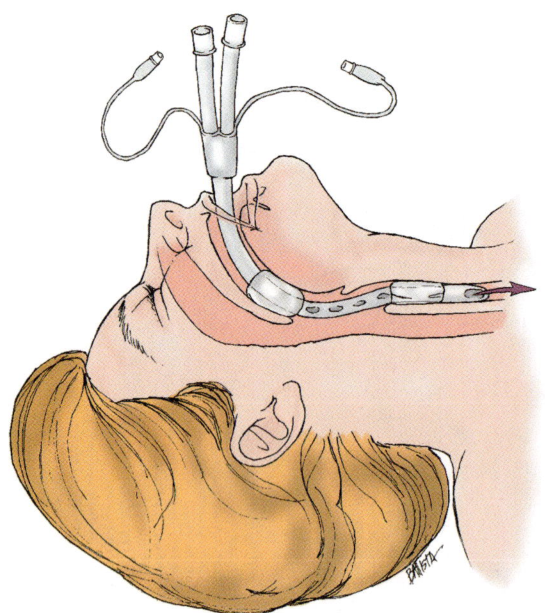

■ **Figure D-7** (From Sanders M: Mosby's paramedic textbook, revised ed 3, St Louis, 2007, Mosby.)

Design standards for ETTs include the inside and outside diameter (ID and OD), distance markers (from the tip), Murphy eye, and **radiopaque** marker. As already noted, ETTs may be cuffed or uncuffed. The purpose of the cuff is to facilitate a seal between the tube and the tracheal wall, preventing aspiration of liquids inferiorly and preventing air leakage in either direction. The cuff also places the tube in the center of the trachea and prevents irritation of the mucosal lining. Uncuffed tubes are designed for pediatric patients in emergency settings, but children who are receiving mechanical ventilation benefit from the cuffed tubes. These cuffs may include special monitoring equipment to measure cuff pressure. Even with special monitoring equipment, cuffs play a role in creating injury to the tracheal wall and should be deflated routinely.

Endotracheal Tube Maintenance The cuff of the endotracheal tube has distinct advantages and disadvantages for the patient. It helps secure the position of the tube, but it may also lead to erosion of the mucosal membrane

TABLE D-1 Extraglottic (Supraglottic) Airway Devices

Device Name/ Manufacturer	Description	Special Features and Clinical Application
LM Classic (LMA North America Inc., San Diego)	Oval inflatable cuff with attached tube connected to PPV Pediatric and adult sizes	Bridge or conduit to intubation for those difficult to intubate and/or ventilate. Exchange catheter may be used through device to railroad tracheal tube into position.
LMA Flexible	LMA cuff to smaller tube that is reinforced	Less kinking of tube and more cuff stability
LMA Unique	Disposable LMA	Same design as the LMA Classic
LMA ProSeal	Modified cuff and two tubes (gastrointestinal [GI], respiratory) with bite block	Second tube for drainage of GI contents; second cuff for better seal. Bridge and route to intubation.
LMA Supreme	Same as LMA ProSeal but disposable version	Disposable version of ProSeal
LMA Fastrach	LMA mask attached to stainless steel curved tube that indicates a reinforced endotracheal tube (ETT)	Facilitates blind or visually guided intubation with larger ETT. Bridge and route to intubation.
LMA CTrach screen and found	Fastrach with built-in fiberoptics; allows for simultaneous view and ventilation during intubation	Used for the patient who has been prescreened and found to be a "difficult airway." Reusable. Bridge and route to intubation.
Soft-Seal Laryngeal Mask (Smiths Medical, Kent, UK)	Similar to LMA but is one piece; cuff is softer with no bars; pediatric and adult sizes	May accommodate a 7.5-mm ETT through fiberoptic bronchoscope (FOB) or video intubation equipment. Bridge and route to intubation
Ambu AuraOnce (Ambu Inc., Glen Burnie, MD)	Disposable, sterile LMA mask with built-in curve; one piece, molded, and no bars. Nondisposable	Facilitates insertion in anatomic position and may avoid mask distortion that can occur with LMA. Bridge and route to intubation.
Ambu Aura 40	Disposable version of AuraOnce	
Air-Q Laryngeal Mask (Cookgas LLC, St. Louis, MO)	Disposable and nondisposable version; hypercurved with unique mask and supplied stylet	Hypercurved design resists kinking; overall larger mask with recessed anterior position; standard ETT insertion allowed through supplied stylet. Bridge and route to intubation.
CobraPLA Perilaryngeal Airway (Engineered Medical Systems, Indianapolis, IN)	Large ID soft tube, cuffed pharyngeal distal end with triangular shape like the head of a cobra. Pediatric and adult sizes.	Disposable large ID tube that allows standard-sized ETTs through tube. Design holds tissue away from grill that abuts aryepiglottic folds and seats on glottis. Bridge and route to intubation.

TABLE D-1 Extraglottic (Supraglottic) Airway Devices—*Cont'd*

Device Name/ Manufacturer	Description	Special Features and Clinical Application
CobraPLUS	Cobra with monitoring capabilities	CobraPLA design with ability to monitor core temperature in all sizes; pediatric sizes allow for distal CO_2
SLIPA Streamlined Liner of the Pharynx Airway (SLIPA Medical LTD., London, UK)	Design similar to LMA Unique, sized by span across thyroid cartilage with no cuff	Hollow mask allows for storage of GI regurgitation (50 mL) to prevent aspiration. Six sizes. Similar to shoe with toe at entrance to esophagus, bridge at base of tongue, heel in nasopharynx.
Esophageal Tracheal Combitube (ETC) (Tyco Healthcare/Mallinckrodt, Pleasanton, CA)	Disposable, double-lumen tube; ETT and esophageal lumen. Large latex pharyngeal cuff: must be over 4 ft tall; two adult sizes	Blindly inserted bridge airway that combines a tracheal tube with the now outdated esophageal obturator airway. Large latex pharyngeal cuff, along with standard distal cuff; eight ventilatory holes rest against glottis. Does provide some protection against GI aspiration.
Elisha Airway Device (EAD) (Elisha Medical Technologies Ltd., Katzrin, Israel)	Molded device that has three channels and allows as large as 8.0 ETT; two cuffs	Allows for ventilation, intubation, and gastric tube insertion through three separate channels. Allows ventilation during intubation.
Chou Airway (Achi Corp., San Jose, CA)	Two-piece adjustable oral airway in adult sizes	Outer tube protects the inner one; inner tube is flexible and creates an open air passage to glottis. Nondisposable.
Intersurgical i-gel™	Noninflatable cuffed extraglottic tube in nondisposable adult sizes. Designed to match perilaryngeal anatomy.	Similar to other devices with gastric channel. Minimizes epiglottic folding that sometimes occurs in LMA. Bridge or route intubation with as large as 8.0 mm ETT.
King Laryngeal-Tracheal Airway LT (King Systems Corp., Noblesville, IN)	Latex-free, single lumen, double cuff design in pediatric and adult sizes	Nondisposable device blindly inserted as a bridge or route to intubation. Mask-free design but similar to LMA ProSeal. Smallest size for those over 12 kg (size 2), with subsequent sizes of 2.5, 3, 4, and 5. Both cuffs inflate with supplied syringe color-coded to tube size. Considered an oropharyngeal tube by the FDA.
King LT-D	Disposable King LT	This is the disposable version of the King LT.
King LT-S	Double-lumen King LT	The second lumen has been placed posterior to the ventilation port and allows gastric access for suction. Similar to LMA ProSEAL. Distal tip has been narrowed to allow for easier insertion.
King LTS-D	Disposable King LT-S only in adult sizes	Disposable version of the King LT-S

and disruption of mucociliary transport. For this reason, pressure within the inflated cuff of the endotracheal tube should be maintained at or below 25 cm H_2O pressure, a level that allows some air to escape yet prevents aspiration from above. Manometers to specifically measure cuff pressure are commercially available, but pressure can be adequately maintained by other means. Two of theses methods include the **maximum occlusion technique** and the **minimum leak technique**. Both techniques are simple, quick, and surprisingly accurate.

Minimum Leak Technique The maximum occlusion technique is performed with a deflated cuff: a slight air leak is tolerated to maintain the health of the tracheal lining. Correct airway size in relation to the inner diameter of the trachea will simplify this process further. If a properly sized tube is chosen, rarely is more than 4–5 mL air required to seal an airway for mechanical ventilation. This becomes vital to the extubated patient, who requires healthy tracheal mucosa to insure adequate cough to protect the airway in the future.

Did You Know?

Injecting 10 to 12 mL of air into the cuff of an endotracheal tube can generate in excess of 90 cm H_2O pressures on surrounding tissue.[9]

Again, adequate cuff pressure is necessary to protect the airway from aspiration. Oral secretions are constantly being produced in response to the presence of the tube because the body reacts to it as a foreign object. These secretions are normally swallowed and managed by the gastrointestinal tract, but in a mechanically ventilated patient, they may pool in the vallecular space or enter the trachea to pool above the vocal cords or the cuff. Pooled secretions carry bacteria from the oral cavity, which pose a threat to the lower airway and lungs. Passive aspiration of these secretions from around the cuff of the endotracheal tube has been linked to **ventilator-associated**

pneumonia (VAP). Roughly 12% of all patients requiring mechanical ventilation will acquire VAP, most often in the first few days. For this reason, mechanically ventilated patients require vigorous oral care and frequent removal of oral secretions from not only the mouth and oropharynx but also from the vallecula and subglottic region. **Before transporting any patient with an advanced airway, it is a good idea to suction the oral cavity and posterior pharynx.**

Tracheostomy Tube Maintenance The same precautions should be taken with tracheostomy tube cuffs as with endotracheal tube cuffs. The cuff should never be deflated while the patient is on mechanical ventilation unless a clinician is present. Some patients may be using a cuffed tube with the cuff deflated for the purpose of communication. Deflating the cuff on smaller-diameter tubes allows air to move through the vocal cords. Other patients may be using an expiratory occlusive valve on the tracheostomy tube, which requires a deflated cuff. The valve is essentially a one-way valve that allows air to enter the trachea through the tracheostomy tube and closes to force air up through the vocal cords and out through the upper airway. The pilot balloon should be in plain view on all patients with cuffed tubes, whether inflated or deflated.

Tracheostomy tubes have several features that bring added challenges to patient care. The most common is the use of the inner cannula—the "tube within a tube." The outer cannula is the tracheostomy tube, whereas the inner cannula is a thin-walled tube, smaller in diameter, that fits inside the tracheostomy tube and locks into place, either by a screw-type mechanism or a snap-lock. The inner cannula is designed to be removed for cleaning without removing the airway. Another feature of the tube is a fenestration. A *fenestration* is an opening on the posterior wall of the tube to allow for the flow of air from the lungs to the upper airway. Fenestrated tubes are usually packaged with one fenestrated cannula, one unfenestrated cannula, and an obturator. The obturator is a blind plug used to insert the tracheostomy tube into the stoma. Fenestrated tubes pose a risk to the tracheal mucosa if left in place for long periods of time, owing to the growth of granuloma into the fenestration. This can cause bleeding, irritation, and stridor. Obstruction of the fenestration by secretions should also be avoided (Table D-2).

TABLE D-2 Checklist for Transporting Critical Patients

Item	Yes	No
1. Endotracheal or tracheostomy tube?	□	□
2. Tube secure and midline?	□	□
3. Oropharynx and distal upper airway clear of secretions?	□	□
4. Cuff pressure acceptable?	□	□
5. Audible leak around cuff?	□	□
6. Breath sounds in all four zones?	□	□
7. Patient awake or sedate?	□	□
For tracheostomy patients:		
8. Tracheostomy tube adaptor free of obstruction?	□	□
9. Speaking valve in place?	□	□
10. If yes to #8, is cuff DEFLATED?	□	□
11. Obturator available?	□	□

Regardless of the type of tube used, tube vigilance during transport cannot be overemphasized. Tubes move. They shift with movement of the patient's head. Think of all the position changes a patient encounters during a simple transport. Check the stability and security of the tube before the initial move, again once the patient is inside the ambulance, prior to exiting the ambulance, and prior to the move to a bed, stretcher, and the like at the receiving facility. Also check tube stability and security at the onset of CPR, after defibrillation, after a seizure, or if the patient becomes agitated at any time. *The best airway protection device is the clinician.* No mechanical device can ever work as well.

Procedure D-1 Suctioning: Endotracheal or Tracheostomy Tube

OVERVIEW

The mere presence of these artificial airways hinders the patient's ability to cough and clear secretions. These tubes may even become completely occluded with thick secretions and create an obstructed airway.

The benefits of suctioning may be outweighed by the potential side effects, including the introduction of pathogens into the respiratory system and the anoxic/apneic period of time required for the suctioning procedure.

Two techniques may be used to suction these devices: open or closed. Open suctioning has many disadvantages that will be discussed. Closed suctioning or in-line suctioning is preferred.

INDICATIONS

- Clear secretions in the artificial airway
- Suspected aspiration of gastric or upper airway secretions
- Facilitate auscultation of adventitious lung sounds over the trachea and bronchi
- When there is an increase in peak airway pressures while on positive pressure ventilation
- Increased coughing, respiratory rate, or both

Procedure D-1 Suctioning: Endotracheal or Tracheostomy Tube—*Cont'd*

- Decrease in oxygenation levels (Pao_2, Sao_2, or Spo_2)
- Sudden onset of respiratory distress
- Obtain samples from the respiratory tree

CONTRAINDICATIONS

- There is no absolute contraindication to suctioning artificial airways.
- In those with high risk for intolerance of suctioning, one must weigh the clinical benefit versus the risk.

COMPLICATIONS ASSOCIATED WITH SUCTIONING

- Respiratory and/or cardiac arrest
- Cardiac dysrhythmias
- Hypertension or hypotension
- Hypoxia
- Increased intracranial pressure
- Bronchospasm
- Pulmonary hemorrhage or bleeding (epithelial denudement; Table D-3)

PROCEDURE—OPEN TECHNIQUE

1. Gather appropriately sized sterile suction catheter, sterile water-soluble lubricant or sterile saline, sterile gloves, and a sterile solution container or basin.
2. Assemble connecting tubing, turn on and test suction unit (100–120 mm Hg). Organize connecting tubing near work surface and keep suction on.
3. Gather bag-mask system with oxygen reservoir, PEEP valve, and connecting tubing.
4. Don facial protection; open suctioning aerosolizes the patient's respiratory secretions.
5. Open sterile catheter onto clean work surface near patient's head. Use the wrapper as your sterile field.
6. Open sterile container, and partially fill with water under sterile technique.
7. Don sterile gloves. Ask for assistance in hyperoxygenating the patient.
8. Using sterile technique, connect catheter to connecting tubing. Suction small amount of water from basin as a test.
9. Insert appropriately sized sterile suction catheter into artificial airway until resistance is met, THEN PULL BACK SLIGHTLY.

Procedure: Hyperoxygen Therapy Prior to/After Suctioning

For at least 30 seconds prior to/after suctioning, hyperoxygenate the patient by:

1. Holding the suction hyperoxygenation button on the ventilator, *or*
2. Increasing the Fio_2 level on the ventilator to 100%, *or*
3. Disconnecting from the ventilator and having an assistant deliver 5 or 6 slow, even breaths to the patient via bag-mask system (15 L O_2, PEEP)

NOTE: Premeasuring depth of insertion of catheter via artificial airway would eliminate trauma to mucous membranes but would suction only the airway, not the patient's respiratory tree.

NOTE: Special catheters are available that can directly suction either the left or right mainstem bronchus. Regular catheters usually enter the right mainstem bronchus.

10. With nondominant hand, occlude suction port while withdrawing and rotating catheter with dominant thumb and forefinger. Apply suction only on the removal phase of this process and only for 10 seconds.
11. Hyperoxygenate patient again. Monitor patient carefully.
12. If secretions remain, you may suction again as indicated in steps 9, 10, and 11. Limit suction attempts to 2–3, then allow patient to rest. Rinse suction catheter between attempts by inserting into sterile water and applying suction.
13. Once lower airways are suctioned and ventilations are resumed to the patient, you may use the same catheter to suction the upper airways (nose and mouth). Once upper airways are suctioned, this catheter is now considered nonsterile and must be discarded.
14. Reposition patient. Reestablish all ventilation parameters. Wash hands. Document the procedure, along with how the patient tolerated it.

TABLE D-3 Guideline for Catheter Size for Endotracheal and Tracheostomy Tube Suctioning*

Patient Age	Endotracheal Tube Size (mm)	Tracheostomy Tube Size (mm, inner diameter)	Suction Catheter Size (French scale [F])
Small child (2–5 years)	4.0–5.0	3.5–4.5	6–8
School-age child (6–12 years)	5.0–6.0	4.5–5.0	8–10
Adolescent to adult	7.0–9.0	5.0–9.0	10–16

*This guide should be used as an estimate only. Actual sizes depend on the size and individual needs of the patient.
From Henneman E, Ellstrom K, St. John RE: Airway management. In AACN protocols for practice: care of the mechanically ventilated patient series, Aliso Viejo, California, American Association of Critical-Care Nurses.

Continued

Procedure D-1 Suctioning: Endotracheal or Tracheostomy Tube—*Cont'd*

NOTE: Instilling sterile saline into the tracheobronchial tree prior to suctioning should not routinely be performed. Instillation of 5 to 10 mL of sterile saline does not thin secretions, may cause hypoxia, and may contribute to the risk of lower-airway infections (see figure).

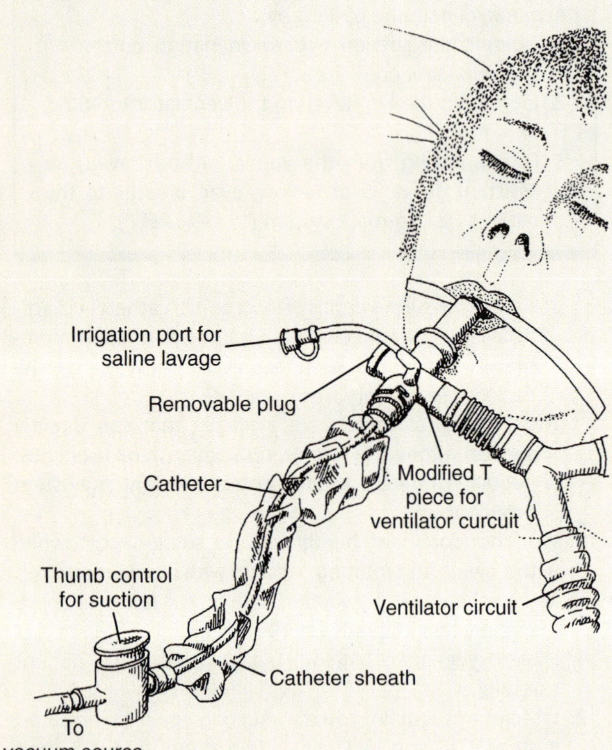

(From Sills JR: Respiratory certification guide, St Louis, 1991, Mosby.)

PROCEDURE—CLOSED TECHNIQUE

1. Wash hands and don Standard Precautions protection.
2. Turn suction to level recommended by manufacturer of closed suction system.
3. Connect suction connecting tubing to closed system port.
4. Hyperoxygenate the patient.
5. Gently, quickly insert the catheter into the artificial airway until resistance is met, THEN PULL BACK SLIGHTLY (with the suction off).
6. Use your nondominant hand to engage suction while your dominant hand withdraws (into sleeve) and rotates catheter between thumb and forefinger. Suction for no more than 10 seconds.
7. Hyperoxygenate the patient. Monitor the patient carefully.
8. You may repeat steps 5, 6, and 7. A total of 2–3 suction passes should be done at any one time.
9. You may open a separate catheter for suctioning the patient's upper airways. Connect separate catheter to connecting tubing and complete procedure.
10. Discard disposable equipment appropriately. Wash hands. Document procedure, including how the patient tolerated it.

NOTE: Some patients do not tolerate suctioning, even with hyperoxygenation therapy. If complications arise:

- Assure that 100% oxygen is being delivered.
- If using open technique, switch to closed technique to avoid removal from ventilator.
- Allow the patient to rest for longer periods of time between suctioning.
- If patient receiving ventilator PEEP, maintain PEEP during suctioning.
- If disconnecting from ventilator to suction, maintain PEEP on bag-mask device.

Procedure D-2 Tracheostomy Tube Care

OVERVIEW

Tracheostomy tubes have a variety of parts with distinct functions that help keep the patient's artificial airway open. The tracheostomy tube is generally smaller in diameter and shorter than an endotracheal tube. Some have a distal cuff to protect against aspiration or air leak while the patient is being mechanically ventilated.

INDICATIONS

- Elective surgical airway when primary is obstructed with lesion or inflammation
- Emergency surgical airway when acute airway obstruction has occurred
- Long-term ventilation therapy (replaces endotracheal tube after 2–3 weeks; see figures).

PARTS TO THE TRACHEOSTOMY TUBE

1. Outer cannula: body of the tube, sometimes with a cuff. (Cuffs not used in children, adult patients with laryngectomies, or when the patient is decannulized.)
2. Neck flange: connected to outer cannula, provides stabilization against the skin of the anterior neck and allows cloth ties to be attached for further securement.
3. Inner cannula: (optional) a clear tube that inserts into the outer cannula and has the standard 15-mm adapter for ventilation attachment.
4. Obturator: blunt-ended, solid stylet used during insertion of the device. These should be kept near the patient in case the tracheostomy has to be reinserted.
5. Pilot balloon: (optional) if the device is cuffed, the pilot balloon operates the same as the cuff on an endotracheal tube.

Procedure D-2 Tracheostomy Tube Care—*Cont'd*

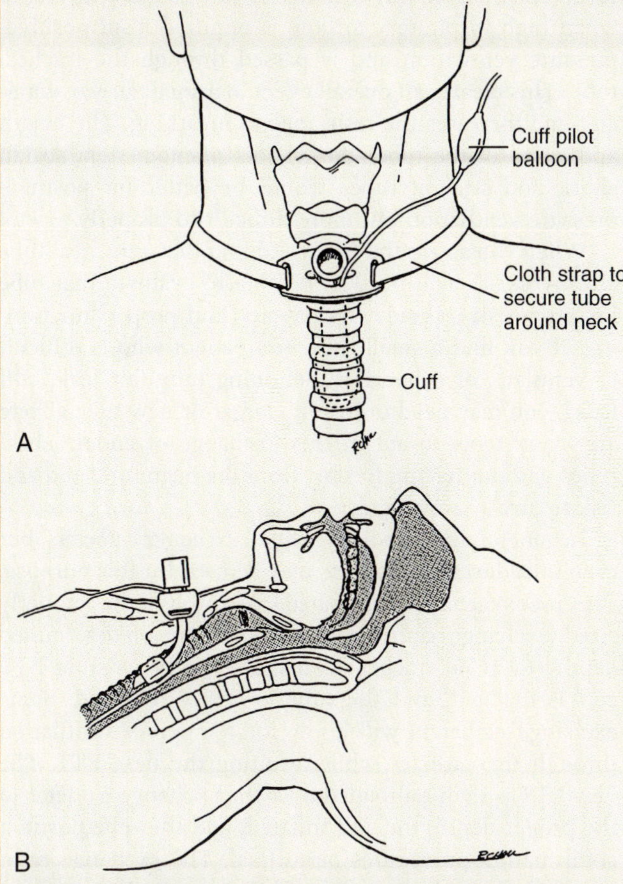

(From Eubanks DH, Bone RC: Comprehensive respiratory care, ed 2, St Louis, 1990, Mosby.)

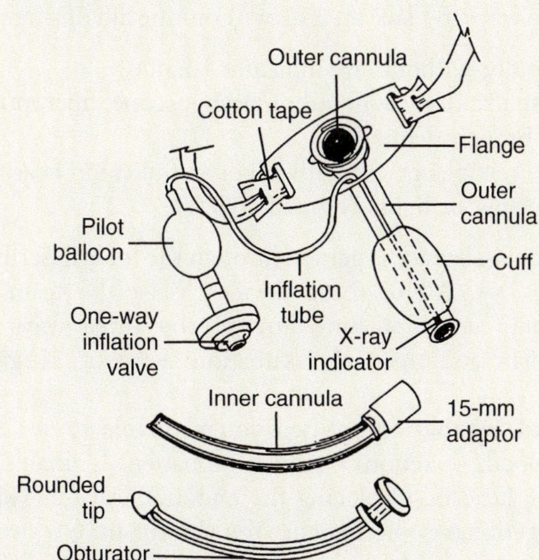

(From Eubanks DH, Bone RC: Comprehensive respiratory care, ed 2, St Louis, 1990, Mosby.)

PROCEDURE

1. Wash hands and don Standard Precautions protection. You should apply facial protection if suctioning or if you anticipate a large amount of secretions and/or the patient is unable to cover stoma while coughing.
2. NEW TIES: Cut twill tape so that length would circle patient's neck twice.
3. Hyperoxygenate and suction patient as needed.
4. Remove soiled dressing and discard appropriately.
5. Discard nonsterile gloves, and wash hands.
6. Prepare sterile field and acquire supplies: sterile saline and hydrogen peroxide solution and container. Mix sterile saline and peroxide into sterile container at a 50:50 mix.
7. Don sterile gloves.
8. Remove inner cannula and place into peroxide/saline solution. You may clean inner cannula with a small sterile brush if necessary.
9. Rinse cleansed inner cannula with sterile saline, reinsert, and lock.

   NOTE: While inner cannula is being cleaned, oxygen and ventilation may be applied to the outer cannula.
10. CLEANSE STOMA. Cleanse stoma site with a sterile saline–impregnated 4 × 4 gauze and then a dry 4 × 4.
11. CLEANSE OUTER CANNULA. Use a sterile saline–impregnated 4 × 4 and cotton swabs to cleanse outer cannula. Pat dry with 4 × 4.
12. Solicit help, and have someone hold the neckplate in place while the old neck ties are released and discarded.

    NOTE: This is especially important if tracheostomy stoma is less than 48 hours old. If the tracheostomy tube is accidentally dislodged, the fresh opening may close.
13. Insert one end of new tie through faceplate and pull until half of length is through the slot. Slide the double tie around the back of the neck and insert through the other slot, looping one end back to original slot. Double square knot on that side.
14. Apply fresh dressing to site.
15. Discard disposable supplies and gloves. Wash hands.
16. Document appearance of stoma site, drainage amount, and color (see figure).

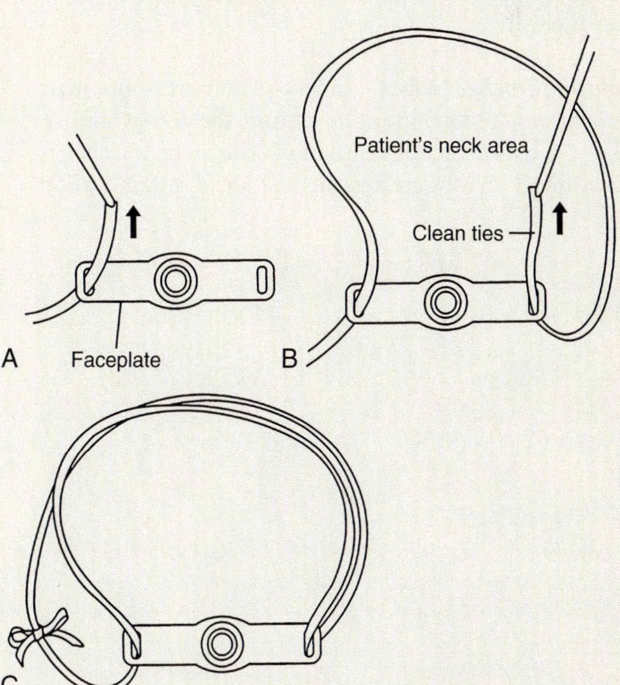

(From AACN procedure manual for critical care, ed 5, St Louis, 2005, Mosby.)

Sizes and Types of Endotracheal Tubes The Magill system of measuring ETT size generally recommends a 7.0 to 7.5 mm ID for females and 8.0 mm ID for males. For children, various formulas have been developed to help us determine the correct size.

Just like the extraglottic devices, there are many types of ETTs designed to meet needs in the operating room, intensive care unit (ICU), and special emergency situations. Single- or double-lumen tubes with flexible tips and nasal, oral, or both nasal and oral routes are available. There are even tubes that are resistant to catching fire in the operating room while lasers are in use. You may encounter some of these unique ETTs as a member of the critical care transport team and should become familiar with their designs.

HI-LO Evac ETT HI-LO Evac ETT (with evacuation lumen) has been designed to prevent ventilator-assisted pneumonia, a deadly **nosocomial** infection commonly acquired in the ICU. It allows for intermittent or continuous evacuation of secretions above the cuff so aspiration of these secretions does not occur and lead to VAP. This same HI-LO has been adapted and named the *Jet Tracheal Tube*. Designed for pediatric **jet ventilation** through the main tube, this has a side lumen for monitoring airway pressures and $PETCO_2$, along with irrigation (Figure D-8).

Double-Lumen ETT The double-lumen ETT (DLT) is designed to provide separate ventilation to each lung. This technique may be adopted to protect one lung or facilitate surgery. DLTs may be further categorized into DLTs that allow ventilation of only one lung while blocking the other. Endobronchial tubes (EBTs), bronchial blockers (BBs), and DLTs are specially designed for thoracic surgery, and some require bronchoscopy to correctly place them.

Replacing Tracheal Tubes In airway and breathing management, you're attempting to protect the airway and recreate the natural act of ventilation. The mere presence of any artificial airway creates thoracic **dead space**, airflow turbulence, and **airway resistance.** Turbulence is increased when high inspiratory airflow is required from positive-pressure ventilation and is passed through the tracheal tube. This creates an overall effect of a small airway diameter and increases the resistance to breathing. The length and curve of the tube adds to this phenomenon, so fat, short, and straight tubes would be better for positive-pressure ventilation but more difficult to properly place.

When you assess the ABCs and find that a tracheal tube already exists, you need to be able to evaluate that tube for proper size, besides its patency and proper functioning. If you find a small tube in a patient who is difficult to ventilate, or a poorly functioning tube (air leak, cuff leak), you may need to insert a larger or new tube. There are many tools to aid in this exchange of endotracheal tubes without having to start from the beginning and add risk to airway management.

In general, these tools are called *exchange catheters*, but even introducers and stylets may be used for this purpose. The preoxygenated, intubated patient has the properly sized exchange catheter inserted to the predetermined depth (to avoid tracheal damage). The preexisting ETT cuff is deflated, and the tube is gently removed. Some exchange catheters will allow for temporary ventilation through the catheter while awaiting the next ETT. The new ETT is then railroaded over the exchange catheter to the proper depth, the cuff inflated, and the tube position confirmation procedures performed. The exchange catheter is then gently removed and the new ETT secured.

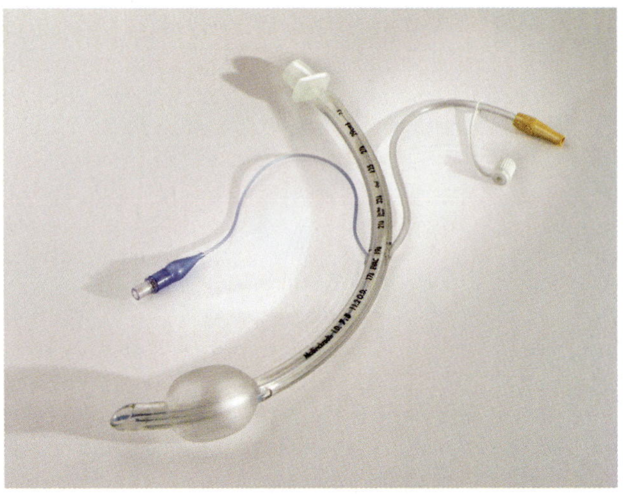

■ **Figure D-8** (Courtesy Mallinckrodt Inc., St Louis.)

Endotracheal Tube Guides and Stylets There are generally three ways to place an ETT without the aid of surgery:

1. Blindly, without any indicator (digital)
2. Visualization (with aid of laryngoscope, fiberoptics, or bronchoscope)
3. Indirect placement with aid of an indicator, hearing, sensing, or lights (lighted stylet)

Intubation assistance is gained through the tools described in Table D-4. All of these devices assist the team in successfully accomplishing any of the three ways to accomplish endotracheal intubation without surgical invasion.

Digital Intubation When you're unable to see the cords (blood, secretions) and/or the patient is unable to move the head/neck, placing the endotracheal tube with your fingers has some benefit. You do not have to overcome the three angles to view the cords. Instead, palpate the epiglottis, and guide the tube into position by feel. The largest obstacle to digital intubation is the presence of a gag reflex and/or a conscious patient. The patient has no choice but to bite down once stimulation to the gag reflex area occurs.

To begin this procedure, you should place a lighted or standard stylet within the ETT and mold the tube into a J or hockey stick configuration. With your knowledge of upper airway anatomy, you know that the epiglottis sits

TABLE D-4 Endotracheal Tube Guides

Name/Manufacturer	Description	Special Features & Clinical Application
Gum Elastic Bougie (Smiths Medical ASD, Keene, NH). Can also be used to railroad endotracheal tube (ETT). Also known as the *Portex Venn Tracheal Tube Introducer.*	Long guide with 35-degree coude tip	Introducer for anterior larynx or those with difficulty opening their mouth; over extraglottic airways properly placed. Either used to directly intubate the trachea or as a stylet to facilitate intubation. If direct, trachea "clicks" are sensed to confirm placement.
Single Use Bougie (Smiths Medical ASD, Keene, NH)	Coude tip with hollow lumen	Used as an introducer that allows for oxygenation and ventilation while placement occurs. Nondisposable.
Parker Flex-It Articulating Tracheal Tube Stylet (Parker Medical, Englewood, CO)	Articulating stylet for both pediatric and adult-sized ETT	Based on the standard stylet design, but with a button at the viewer's end that allows a bougie-like angle at distal end of ETT. Allows for one-handed distal control of ETT; facilitates video intubation, as well.
Frova Intubation Introducer (Cook Critical Care, Bloomington, IN)	Angled distal tip with two side ports; allows for stiff or malleable design	Acts as introducer, stylet, or exchanger in both pediatric and adult sizes, with adaptors that allow ventilation to occur while procedure for intubation continues
Aintree Intubation Catheter; (Cook Critical Care, Bloomington, IN)	Large lumen with angled tip, two side ports and adaptors	Allows for fiberoptic bronchoscope (FOB) during procedure for direct visualization. Also allows for ventilation during procedures; introducer, exchanger, and stylet
Cook and AEC (Adult Exchange Cath.) EF (Extra Firm) lumen	Exchange catheter for double-lumen tubes	Extra-firm catheter made for exchange of double tubes

behind the base of the tongue. Use your dominant first and second fingers to "walk" to the base of the tongue. Use one finger to identify and retract the epiglottis. Angle the preconfigured ETT into the patient's mouth and towards your finger. Once into the entrance of the glottis, use the second finger to trap the tip of the ETT and "drive" it through the glottis. Once engaged, remove your walking fingers, and hold the ETT into position as you alternate short withdrawals of the stylet and advancement of the ETT until properly positioned and the stylet is removed. Confirm placement and secure the device.

Nasotracheal Intubation A secondary route for an endotracheal tube is the nose. Correct placement through the vocal cords can be achieved by either direct visualization in the adult or blindly. No matter the technique, the most common complication is nasal bleeding. These maneuvers are usually more complicated and take longer to accomplish, although one advantage is that oxygenation can be maintained during the procedure by supplementing through the tube.

Because of the unique structure in the area, the endotracheal tube chosen will need to be a half-size smaller than what you would normally choose for the oral route. If available, a special tube with a ringlike apparatus that allows anterior deflection in the tip of the tube should be chosen. Lubricating both the tip of the tube and the patient's chosen nostril will help facilitate movement with less trauma. If time permits, the lubrication can be mixed with 2% lidocaine and 0.25% to 0.5% phenylephrine to provide local anesthetic and help prevent nasal bleeding.

Nasotracheal Intubation via Direct Visualization (Adult) This technique will include use of a laryngoscope and the Magill forceps. Insert the lubricated tube appropriately, then the laryngoscope in a standard manner, with the Magill forceps immediately available. Once the cords are viewed, the forceps may be inserted with your right hand, grasping the tip of the tube in order to direct it anteriorly. Care must be taken to avoid damaging the ETT cuff with the forceps.

Blind Nasotracheal Intubation When direct visualization of the trachea is difficult or impossible (example: teeth clenched), and there is no protocol for rapid sequence intubation (RSI) or vascular access to provide it, this procedure may be helpful. The patient may be seated or supine, but they need to be ventilating themselves well enough to guide your insertion. Once the tube is inserted through the nostril (bevel out, tube at right angle) and into the oropharynx, you should lower your ear over the ETT, listening for breath sounds, and slowly advance the tube while providing cricoid pressure and gaining feedback. Once the tip enters the glottis, a tubular sound is heard, and the patient may cough (described as a bovine cough). To facilitate "hearing" the breath sounds as the guide, a special whistle (teakettle) can be placed over the end of the tube. Another adaptation is to remove the bell from a single-tube stethoscope and insert the distal tube into the ETT.

It may take several attempts to successfully place a tracheal tube through the glottis via the nose. Movement of the patient's head into a flexed position or pulling the mandible forward with the nondominant thumb and forefingers may facilitate movement of the distal tube into position.

Fiberoptic and Video Intubation Bronchoscopes are rigid or flexible devices that aid in the direct visualization of the intraglottic airway for placement of an ETT or for surgical tracheostomy. The flexible types are referred to as **fiberoptic bronchoscopes (FOB)** or flexible fiberoptic bronchoscopes (FFB). FOBs or FFBs are used when intubation via direct laryngoscope is impossible, expected to be a problem, or when a standard intubation attempt has failed. We can expect intubation to be a problem when there are abnormal anatomic features like congenital anomalies, cervical spine abnormalities, **temporomandibular ankylosis**, or a **Mallampati score** of III or IV (described in the RSI section). There are now video-assisted FOBs and FFBs that aid in emergency intubation procedures. The use of these devices is usually restricted by scope of practice to physicians or Certified Respiratory Nurse Anesthetists.

The fiberoptic laryngoscopes that have been entering the healthcare field over the past few years (and newer versions) give the critical care team the advantage of a bronchoscopic view of the airway in a portable device that is well within the scope of practice of the crew. These airway cameras allow for direct laryngoscopy, provide a mechanism to confirm ETT placement, or provide direct visualization when upgrading from extraglottic to intraglottic airway (Figures D-9 and D-10 and Tables D-5 and D-6).

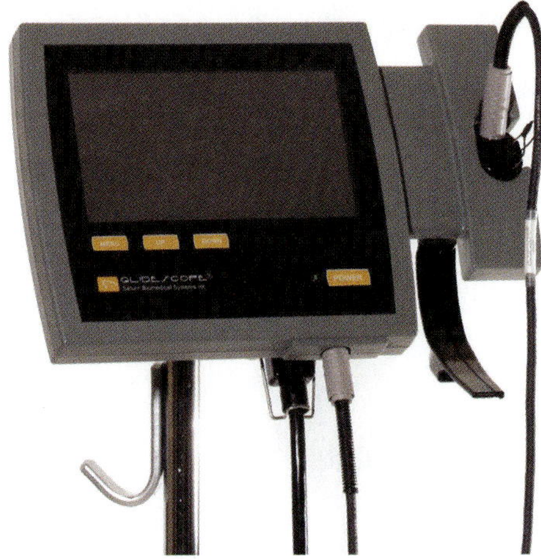

Figure D-9 (Courtesy Verathon Inc.)

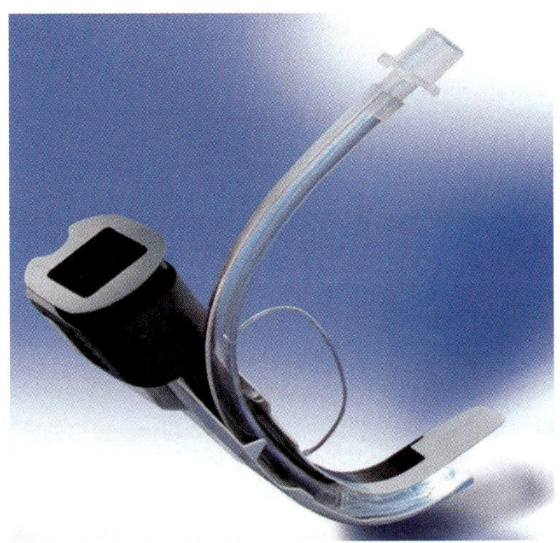

Figure D-10 (Courtesy King Systems.)

Special Airway Techniques

The decision to go beyond direct or fiberoptic visualization of the airways using extraglottic or intraglottic devices is usually situated in a highly stressful, extremely difficult airway procedure. The critical care team must have protocols to guide these decisions. The "Difficult Airway

TABLE D-5 Lighted Stylets

Name/Manufacturer	Description	Special Features and Clinical Application
Flexible Airway Scope Tool (FAST)	Flexible stylet with rigid tip	Designed for adult exchange from intubation laryngeal mask airway (LMA) or other extraglottic airways; confirms endotracheal tube placement
FAST Plus (Clarus Medical, Minneapolis, MN)		For nasal intubation
Shikani Optical Stylet (SOS) (Clarus Medical, Minneapolis)	Like the flexible fiberoptic bronchoscope (FFB), but with J-shaped stylet	Used to intubate or with other devices in difficult cases. Portable device with more application in emergency settings. Oxygen insufflation through device allowed; movable tube stop and oxygen port.
Levitan GLS (Clarus Medical, Minneapolis)	Similar to SOS, with no movable tube stop	Adjunct to direct laryngoscopy or similar to SOS
Trachlight Stylet (Laerdal Light Medical AS, Stavanger, Norway)	Wand with three parts for pediatric and adults	Pediatric and adult light wand for intubation, but good application to replace fiberoptic bronchoscope (FOB) in emergency setting. Blind, direct, or indirect visualization for situations where glottis is hard to see or limited head movement.

TABLE D-6 Fiberoptic and Rigid Laryngoscopes

Name/Manufacturer	Description	Special Features and Clinical Application
GlideScope Video Laryngoscopes (GVL) (Verathon Medical, Bothel, WA)	60-degree-angle blade with camera and lightweight; pediatric and adult sizes	Built to military and EMS specifications. Provides real-time visualization of airway. Rechargeable battery. Feeds live information to a small camera.
DCI Video Laryngoscope System (Karl Storz, Tuttlingen, Germany)	Interchangeable blades (Miller or Mac) in larger sizes	Handle has snap-in, wide-angle camera with fiberscopes that allow for more visibility and less head positioning. Good for difficult airways, obese patients, and verifies endotracheal tube (ETT) placement. Intubates, exchanges, and introduces endoscopy.
Viewmax Laryngoscope Blade (Rush Inc, Research Triangle Park, NC)	Optic side port onto Mac blade in adult and pediatric sizes	Prism mounted, gives "fisheye" appearance of cords with Mac view
McGrath Video Laryngoscope (LMA of North America Inc., San Diego, CA)	Portable, wireless laryngoscope with lightweight design and disposable blades	Good for those with limited mouth opening and head movement with anterior airways, obesity. Adjustable blades allow for multiple patient sizes. Portable and lightweight.
Pentax Airway Scope	Wireless video laryngoscope with special suction blade	Similar to the McGrath but with one blade size that allows for suctioning through the blade
Airtraq (Prodol Meditex SA LLC, Vizcaya, Spain)	Disposable optical laryngoscope with an ET guide	For routine and difficult airway management with fiberscope guide. Self-contained unit. Mount the ETT in the device, and guide it in while watching.
Bullard Elite Laryngoscope (Gyrus ACMI, Southborough, MA)	Indirect fiberoptic laryngoscope in pediatric and adult sizes	Allows for oxygen insufflation and suctioning during use. Can be used with standard handle or fiberoptic source. Optical metal stylets may be attached.
UpsherScope Ultra (Mercury Medical, Clearwater, FL)	Indirect rigid fiberoptic laryngoscope in adult sizes	Same as Bullard Elite, but must use the Upsher handle or fiberoptic source

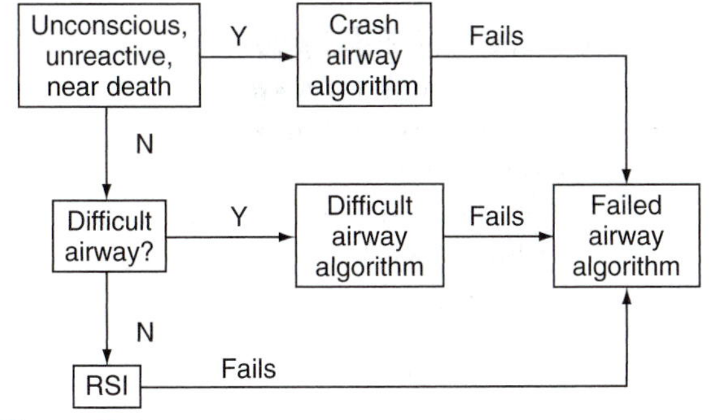

■ **Figure D-11** (From Semonin-Holleran R: Air and surface patient transport principles and practice, ed 3, St Louis, 2005, Mosby.)

Protocol" is defined by the Medical Director of the program but must be well rehearsed by every member of the team. Near the bottom of this decision tree are some special airway techniques, usually categorized as surgical in nature (Figures D-11 to D-15).

Retrograde Intubation

Retrograde intubation may be necessary when you can't ventilate or oxygenate the patient. A large needle is used to gain access to the cricothyroid membrane, and a guidewire is introduced and directed through the needle superiorly. This wire is fed toward the mouth (although it may tend to deviate out the nose). A second person with a Magill forceps assists by grabbing the wire in the pharynx and guiding it out the mouth. The wire is fed through an ETT and facilitated down through the glottis. This is a technique that takes considerable time to perform when you are in a hurry in an emergency, so its use may not always be advantageous.

Cricothyrotomy

Cricothyrotomy may be the final lifesaving procedure in a patient you cannot intubate, ventilate, or oxygenate. There are some commercially designed devices that assist with this procedure.

Needle Cricothyrotomy Needle cricothyrotomy should be performed with a large needle and catheter system. The Cook Emergency Transtracheal Airway Catheter is one example of a non-kinking, large catheter introduced with a needle. Another very simple system is a 14-gauge, 2-inch intravenous (IV) catheter inserted into the cricothyroid membrane with an attached syringe. Once entry into the trachea is obtained, the stylet is removed, and the 15-mm adaptor from a 3-mm ETT can be inserted into the top of the 14-gauge catheter to provide direct ventilation via a bag-mask system. A 14-gauge needle offers no fenestration, so its use is reserved for crisis, short-term therapy.

Percutaneous Cricothyrotomy **Percutaneous cricothyrotomy** may involve the **Seldinger technique**, using a needle to gain access, then subsequent dilation of the opening for catheter entrance. Commercially available products like the Melker Cuffed Emergency Cricothyrotomy Catheter Set by Cook houses a 5.0-mm cuffed airway catheter. QuickTrach (VBM Germany) versions I and II

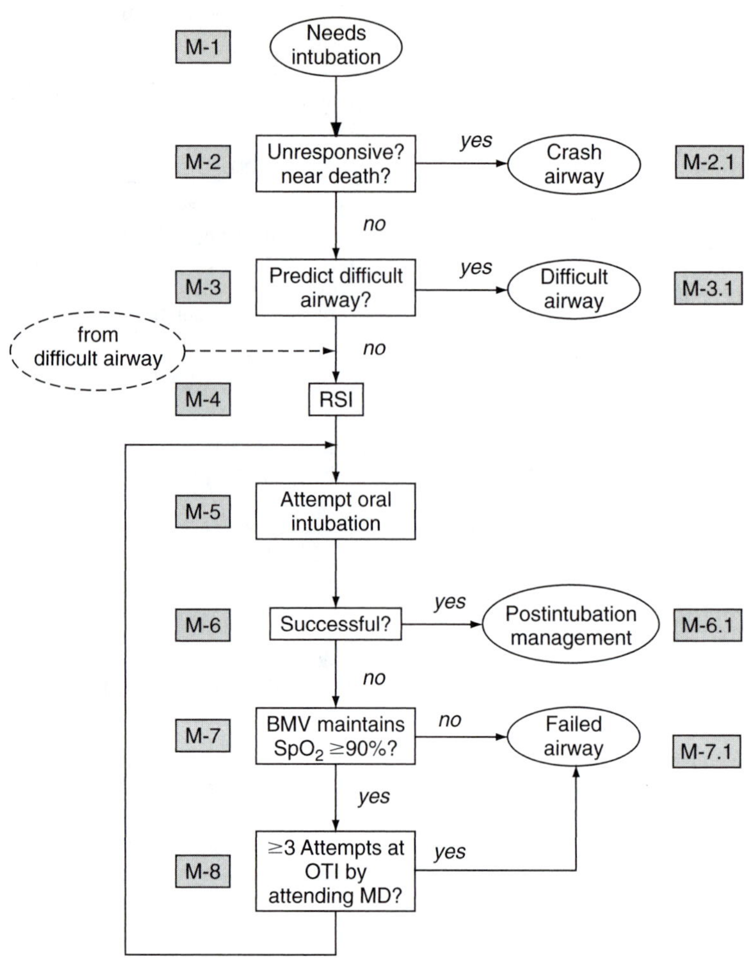

■ **Figure D-12** (From Semonin-Holleran R: Air and surface patient transport principles and practice, ed 3, St Louis, 2005, Mosby.)

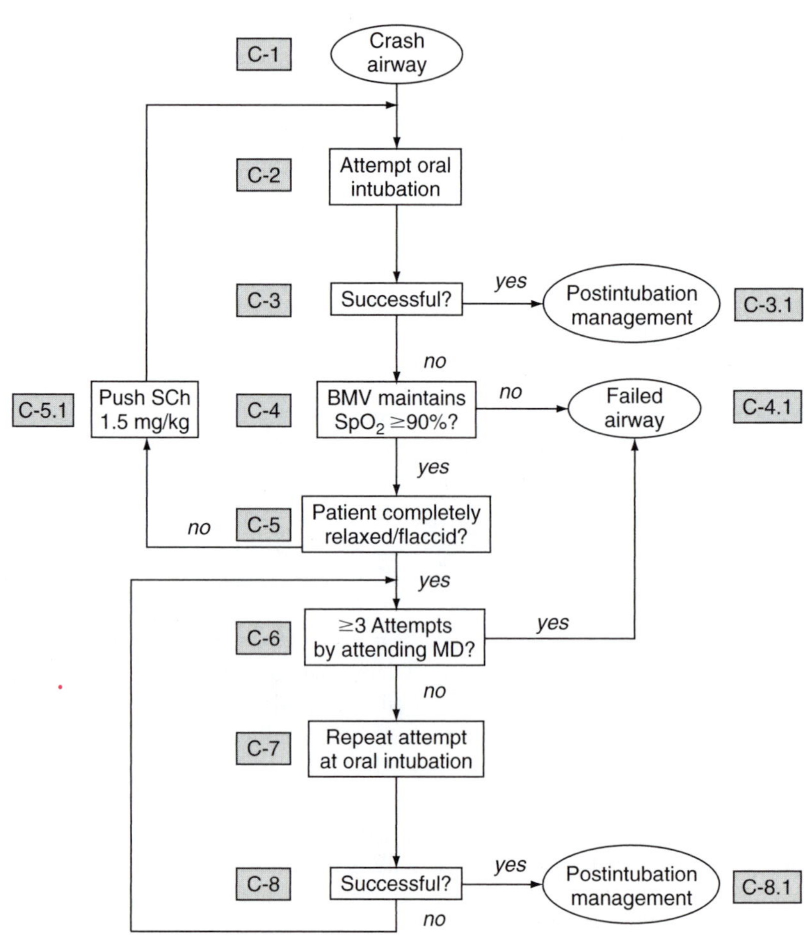

■ **Figure D-13** (From Semonin-Holleran R: Air and surface patient transport principles and practice, ed 3, St Louis, 2005, Mosby.)

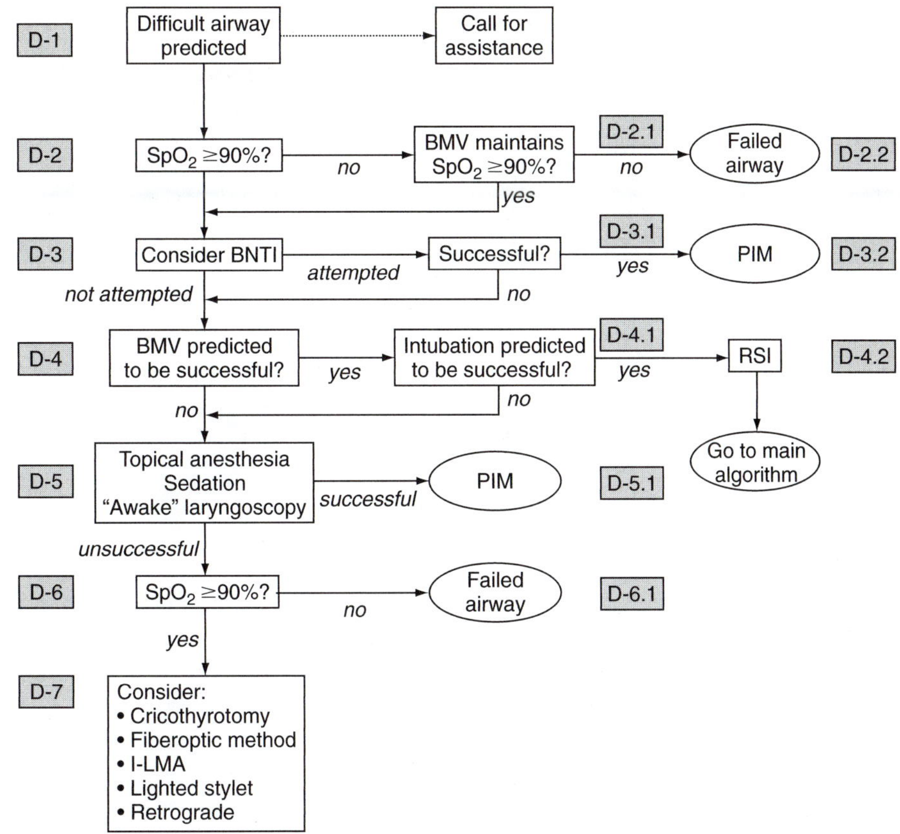

■ **Figure D-14** (From Semonin-Holleran R: Air and surface patient transport principles and practice, ed 3, St Louis, 2005, Mosby.)

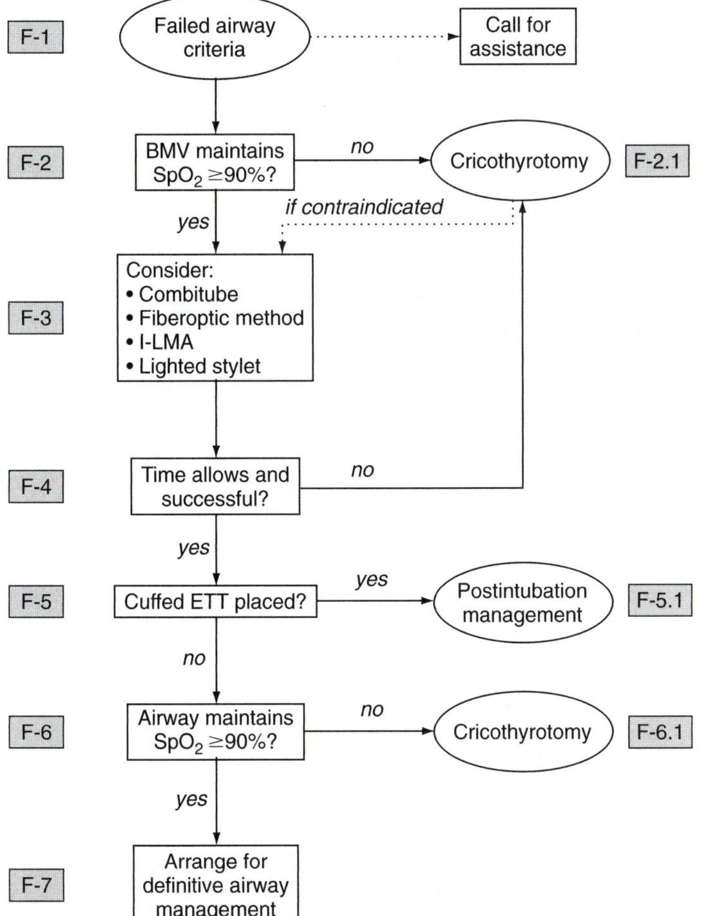

■ **Figure D-15** (From Semonin-Holleran R: Air and surface patient transport principles and practice, ed 3, St Louis, 2005, Mosby.)

provide an uncuffed or cuffed tracheal tube via a large trocar-like needle in both pediatric and adult sizes (Figure D-16).

Surgical Cricothyrotomy Surgical **cricothyrotomy** involves making surgical incisions first through the skin, then through the cricothyroid membrane. A tracheotomy tube or a standard ETT may then be inserted through the opening. This is the fastest surgical technique, especially when no other commercial products are available.

Tracheostomy Emergency **tracheostomy** involves surgical incisions through the skin and into the trachea just beneath the cricoid cartilage. This technique is considered for children younger than 10 years of age or for those with lesions or infections that alter the anatomy of the airway. This technique is reserved for physicians' scope of practice.

Medication-Assisted Intubation

There are many tools now in your kit with which to manage most patients' airways. Which ones your program chooses depends on many issues too numerous to mention but may include cost, familiarity, and preference by the Medical Director. The next part of your overall system of airway management includes the use of medications to facilitate your initial and ongoing airway maneuvers.

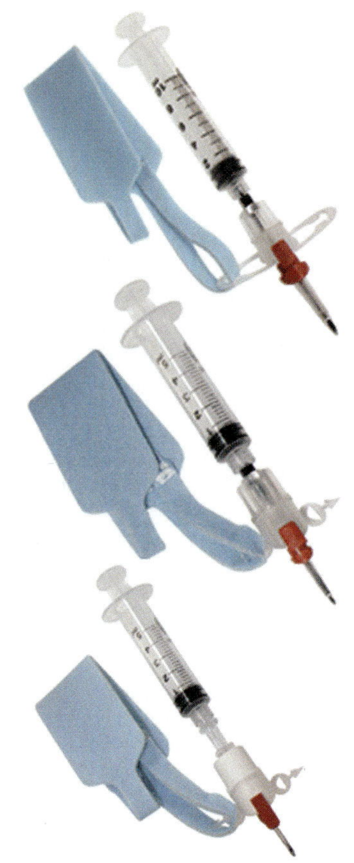

Figure D-16 (Courtesy VBM Medizintechnik GmbH, Germany.)

Procedure D-3 Surgical Airway

OVERVIEW

The creation of an airway via surgical techniques implies that you have tried and have been challenged in providing an airway through "standard" mechanisms. Whether using a needle (percutaneous), a commercial device, or a scalpel (surgical), all techniques will be reviewed here.

INDICATIONS

- A rescue airway when there is complete airway obstruction with failed intubation
- Major facial trauma with inability to intubate or ventilate through the mouth or nose

CONTRAINDICATIONS

- Surgical airway should not be the initial airway management procedure.
- Cricothyrotomy is relatively contraindicated in children younger than 12, owing to the anatomy (percutaneous transtracheal ventilation is recommended).
- Laryngeal or tracheal pathology in the cricothyroid area

CRICOTHYROTOMY—PREPARATION

1. Examine the patient's cricothyroid area for pathology, gain history, and identify landmarks while ventilation is being attempted via bag-mask device.

   Landmarks (refer to figure):

   Identification of the cricothyroid membrane can be done by first identifying the area above the thyroid cartilage (thyrohyoid space) and palpating inferiorly to the thyroid cartilage, then the cricoid ring. Another means of identifying the cricothyroid membrane is to identify the tracheal rings, and move superiorly to first the cricoid ring, then the membrane.
2. Gather and prepare equipment. A "cric kit" should be preassembled and available in your airway kit. This equipment might include a commercial kit or: Betadine skin prep sticks, 4 × 4 gauze sponges, disposable scalpel (#11 blade), 2 Kelly clamps, tracheal hook, cuffed tracheotomy tube (#4 Shiley kit) or 6-mm endotracheal tube (ETT) and syringe. Attach one side of the tie to the flange of the device.

PROCEDURE

1. Cleanse the skin around the cricothyroid membrane with Betadine in a circular fashion to include the thyroid, cricoid, and upper tracheal rings.
2. Provide local anesthetic with 1% lidocaine in the skin over the cricothyroid membrane (if patient awake and time allows).
3. Assemble cricothyrotomy kit onto sterile surface. Don sterile gloves and facial protection.

Procedure D-3 Surgical Airway—*Cont'd*

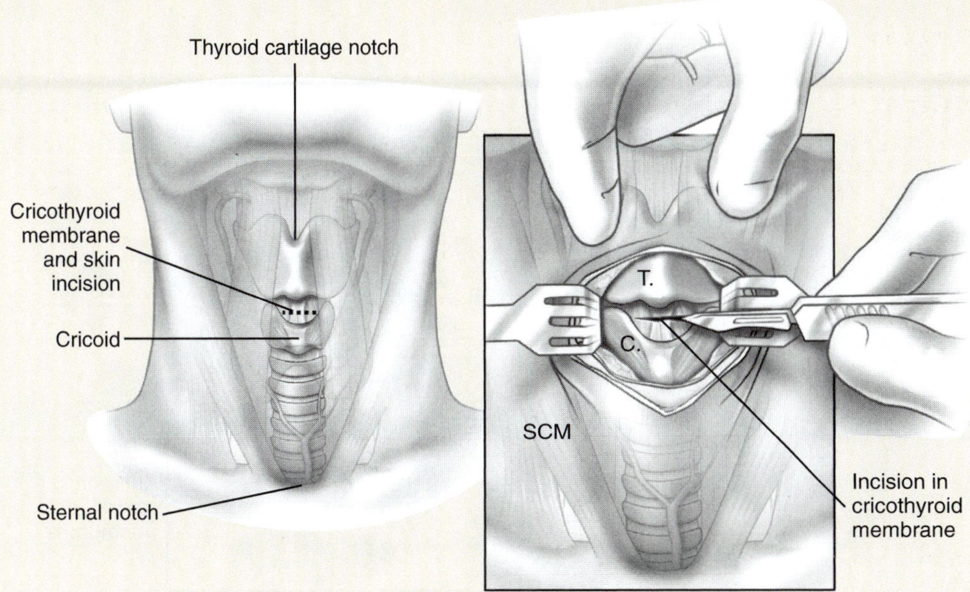

(From Cummings C, Flint P, Harker L, et al: Cummings otolaryngology: head and neck surgery, ed 4, St Louis, 2005, Mosby.)

4. With your nondominant hand, use several digits to immobilize the thyroid cartilage. Keep one finger available to palpate the cricoid ring during procedure.
5. Incise the skin from superior to inferior, with the cricothyroid membrane at the center. This is a midline incision in the superficial skin that extends from the thyroid cartilage to the upper rings of the trachea (see figure).
6. You may use the Kelly forceps to blunt dissect the overlying tissue. Your goal is to be able to directly view the cricothyroid membrane.
7. Once identification of the membrane is seen and palpated, use the scalpel to make a horizontal incision across the lower part of the membrane, approximately 1 cm (see figures).

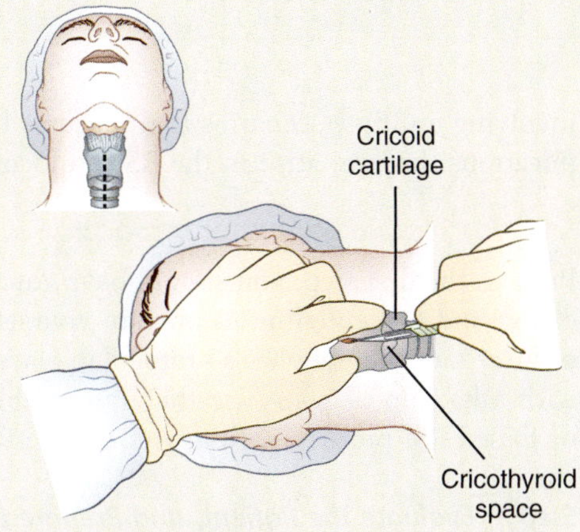

(From Auerbach P: Wilderness medicine, ed 5, St Louis, 2007, Mosby.)

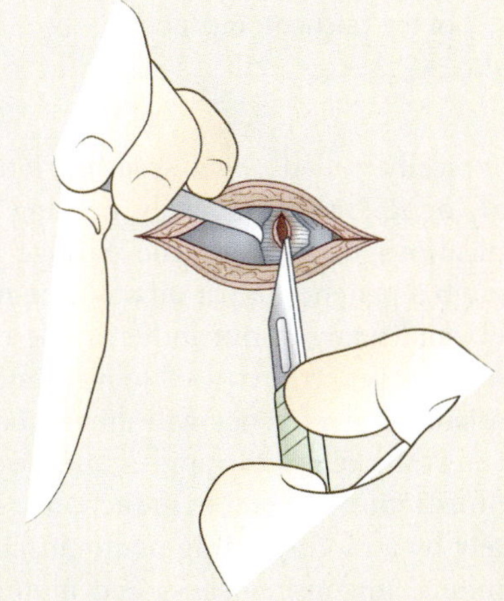

(From Auerbach P: Wilderness medicine, ed 5, St Louis, 2007, Mosby.)

Continued

Procedure D-3 Surgical Airway—*Cont'd*

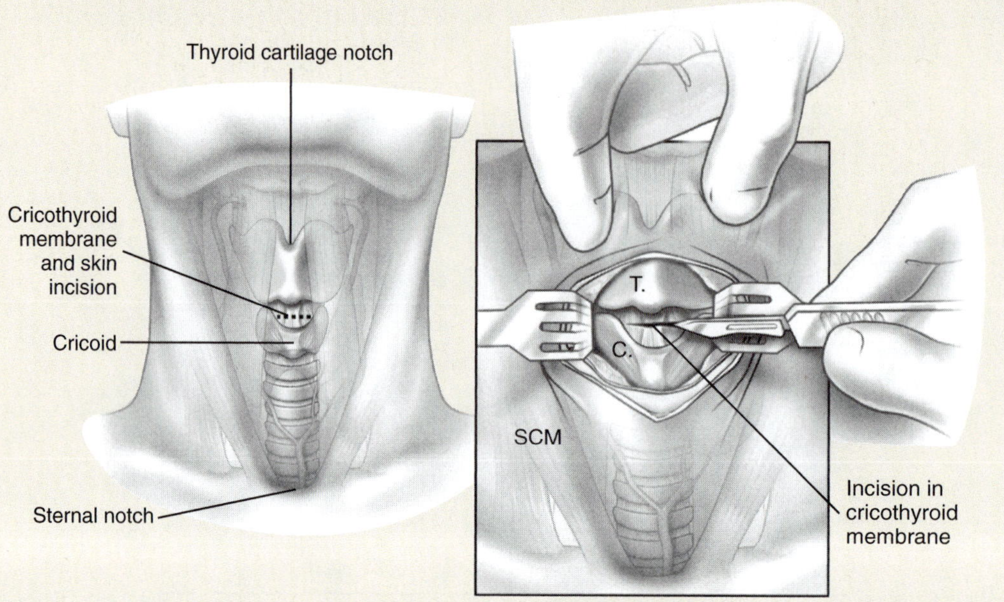

(From Cummings C, Flint P, Harker L, et al: Cummings otolaryngology: head and neck surgery, ed 4, St Louis, 2005, Mosby.)

8. Grasp and retract superiorly the upper margin of the cricothyroid membrane with the tracheal hook (a skin hook will do). An assistant can retract with the hook.
9. Use the Kelly forceps (Trousseau dilator may be used) to identify and widen the opening while inserting the tracheotomy tube within the gap. Insert the tracheotomy tube with the obturator locked in place. Advance this gently and slowly, following the anatomic curve, until the flange is seated on the skin surface. You may also use a second tracheotomy hook on the inferior aspect of the opening to retract from both sides, thus allowing passage of the tracheotomy tube.
10. Once the tracheotomy tube flange is positioned against the skin, inflate the cuff, remove the obturator, and insert the inner cannula. Attach a bag-valve device to this 15-mm adaptor, and gently ventilate while checking for correct position. You may confirm position via the same methods as for ETT.
11. Position the tracheotomy tie around the patient's neck from the prepared, secured side to the other flange of the tube, and tie the opposite side.
12. Continue ventilation and oxygenation.

Typically called *rapid sequence intubation* (or induction), or *RSI*, there is really nothing rapid about using medications to facilitate the passage of a tracheal tube through a patient's upper airway. The name, however, has stuck, and many in our industry use the term to quickly refer to the procedures used to medicate and then intubate a patient. Our reference will mimic that.

Dr. Walls refers to rapid sequence intubation as "the administration of a potent induction agent followed immediately by a rapidly acting neuromuscular blocking agent to induce unconsciousness and motor paralysis for tracheal intubation."[6] There are several steps that can help make this organized procedure successful.

Pre-RSI procedures can actually last months. It includes education to the crew and practice of the techniques and scenarios in the operating room or in simulation labs. Remember, intubation is not just a 30-second skill. You have to be able to make good decisions in simulations involving multiple scenarios that rehearse the many complications that can arise in the RSI protocols.

Standard Rapid Sequence Intubation Process

Prior to the first step, you should have gone through education and credentialing to prepare yourself for this procedure. Your program has a protocol in place for RSI, along with a backup plan in case there are problems (Difficult or Failed RSI protocol). Now you can begin.

Step 1: Evaluate the Patient, and Prepare the Equipment

You've found a patient who needs to be intubated, and you wish to avoid creating pain and complications for him or her. First, assess the patient carefully for signs of a difficult airway. While completing your evaluation, place 90% to 100% oxygen to the patient (discussed shortly).

Assessment of the Patient to Predict a Difficult Airway As part of preparation for RSI, a rapid

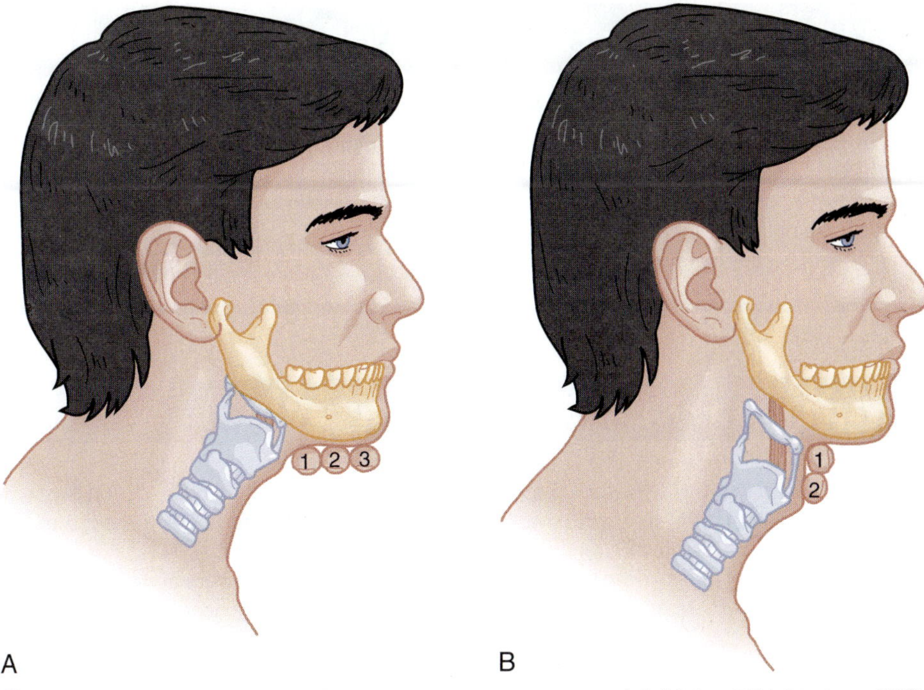

■ **Figure D-17** (From Walls RM, et al: Manual of emergency airway management, Philadelphia, 2004, Lippincott Williams & Wilkins.)

assessment of the patient's anatomy can predict those who may be difficult to ventilate, oxygenate, and intubate. This assessment is integral to making the correct decisions in the RSI protocol (Figures D-17 and D-18).

The assessment continues as you look for airway obstructions and neck mobility. For example, a hematoma or epiglottitis would obstruct the glottis from intubation. If the neck is stiff from disease, aligning the head and neck for intubation would make it a very difficult intubation. Use of fiberoptic scopes or guides can help facilitate intubation in those with limited neck mobility. Box D-1 provides information regarding the Lemon Law evaluation, and Box D-2 provides a recap of the RSI process.

Pre-Procedure Therapy

Step 2: Hyperoxygenate the Patient As soon as the thought of intubation occurs in your management plan for the patient, make sure a high percentage of oxygen is being delivered to them. Think of the lungs as bags full of room air, composed mostly of nitrogen. Your goal is to displace the nitrogen out of the bags, allowing those bags to be a reservoir of oxygen. This reservoir usually allows for longer periods of apnea during the intubation procedure.

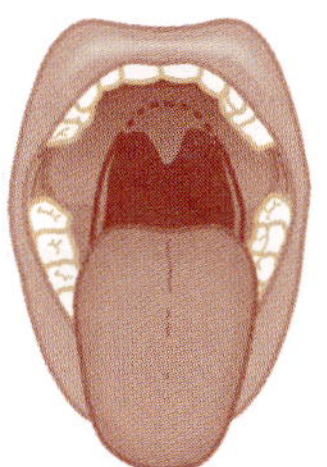

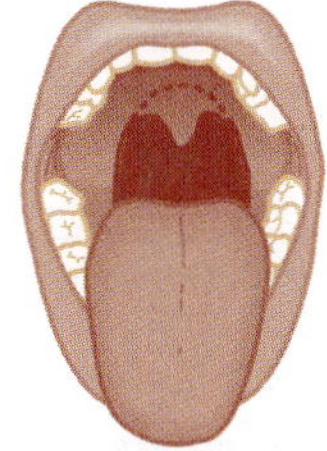

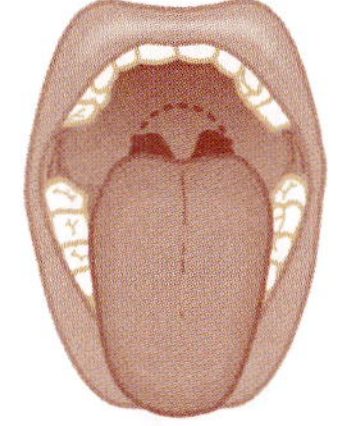

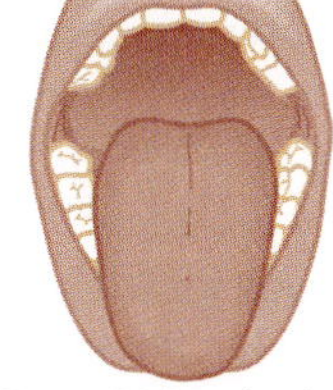

■ **Figure D-18** (From Whitten CE: Anyone can intubate, ed 4, San Diego, 2004, KW Publication.)

Did You Know?

Five minutes of 100% oxygen allows for anywhere from 8 minutes (healthy adult) to 4 minutes (small child) of apnea before desaturation of the hemoglobin to 90% occurs.[6]

Actually providing 100% oxygen to the patient can be a challenge. The nonrebreather mask, with the flowmeter set to deliver enough oxygen to keep the mask's reservoir full, actually delivers about 70% to 75% oxygen to the patient. Using a non-self-inflating bag-mask system (anesthesia bag) with the mask over the patient's mouth and nose would provide an improved percentage of oxygen. If 5 minutes are not available to you, have the patient quickly

BOX D-1 The LEMON Law: An Emergency Evaluation in Preparation for Rapid Sequence Intubation That Helps Predict the Difficult Airway

Look externally: facial hair (hinders mask seal), **cachexia, edentulous mouth**, buck teeth, short "bull" neck, morbid obesity.

Evaluate the 3-3-2 rule (looking at the angles).

Mallampati evaluation (for space in the mouth)

Obstruction? Look for tumors, edema, abscess, epiglottitis, and high cervical spine injury with hematoma.

Neck mobility: Can you move the neck? (Chin to chest?)

From Walls R., et al: Manual of emergency airway management, Philadelphia, 2000, Lippincott Williams & Wilkins.

BOX D-2 Recapping the Rapid Sequence Intubation

Now that you've assessed the patient to see where they fit in the Difficult or Failed Intubation protocol, you should gather equipment in preparation for the procedure:

1. All monitors on the patient. This includes sidestream $ETCO_2$ (if available), pulse oximetry, and 3- or 5-lead cardiac monitor.
2. Your program's recommended airway tools ready. This might include an extraglottic airway and the endotracheal tube (ETT) in the appropriate sizes. The kit includes appropriate syringes for the devices. Check all cuffs. The backup airway must be as ready as the ETT.
3. Laryngoscope and appropriate blade on and checked. Fiberoptics, bougie, guide, or stylet ready. ETT confirmation devices/diagnostics ready. Mechanism to secure ETT is ready.
4. Suction device prepared, turned on, with rigid tip available to your right hand during the intubation procedure. This generally means that the suction is assembled, on, and the rigid tip is placed under the edge of the mattress at the head of the patient.
5. At least one IV (two are better) or IO, and they are functioning. All the drugs chosen have been drawn up and labeled. This includes the induction drugs (initial intubation RSI) and the drugs needed for ongoing sedation and/or paralysis.
6. Bag-mask with oxygen connecting tubing assembled and ready. Ventilator circuit assembled and ventilation parameters dialed in.

Being prepared means there are backup plans and equipment ready to go (lamps, blades, tubes). Good and thorough preparation pays great benefits when the intubation goes smoothly in RSI.

complete 8 full respiratory cycles (as deep as possible) through the anesthesia bag/mask.

Preventilating a patient in preparation for RSI provides positive-pressure ventilation to their esophagus and stomach, thus adding to the risk for regurgitation and subsequent aspiration. If at all possible, avoid positive pressure just to preoxygenate the patient. Box D-3 provides a recap in the RSI sequence.

Are there drugs that should be given to prepare the patient for the actual RSI? Yes, sometimes the RSI process or medications themselves can cause complications in certain types of patients. You need to avoid those complications with pre-RSI therapy.

BOX D-3 Recapping the Rapid Sequence Intubation

You have prepared yourself. You have made the decision to use RSI to intubate your patient. The equipment is prepared, and backup devices and plans are ready. The patient has been receiving 100% oxygen to wash out nitrogen. There are at least two drugs that need to be calculated, drawn up, and prepared for administration: sedation and the drug for paralysis.

Step 3: Pre-Procedure Drugs Many RSI protocols include pretreatment drugs in an attempt to blunt the effects of the paralytics that will be given and/or increase the heart rate. Your Medical Director's protocol for RSI may include several different drugs for these purposes in certain populations of patients. These drugs must be given PRIOR TO the paralytic.

Lidocaine A standard IV dose of lidocaine (1.0 to 1.5 mg/kg) may be given prior to sedation and paralysis to blunt the effects of **depolarizing** paralytics. Given 3 to 5 minutes prior to the RSI drugs, this can decrease bronchospasm and laryngospasm in those with reactive airway disease (asthma). Given to those with increased intracranial pressure (ICP), lidocaine can blunt the rise of ICP during the intubation procedure itself or as the expected side effect of succinylcholine administration (depolarizing drug).

Opiates The use of opioids can diminish the expected sympathetic discharge associated with pain (intubation) and organ pressure rise (depolarizing agent) with RSI. Fentanyl (Sublimaze) is the drug usually chosen because of its short half-life. The standard dose is 0.5 to 50 mcg/kg. Watch for rare but frightening respiratory muscle paralysis (more common in children) with large IV doses of fentanyl. If this occurs, positive-pressure ventilation is used while the sedation and paralytic is quickly given to intubate the patient.

Atropine Succinylcholine (SCh) binds to acetylcholine receptors at the neuromuscular junction with stimulation of some receptors that can create bradycardia, especially in children. Atropine is standard as a pretreatment drug for all children younger than 10 years of age, as kids depend upon heart rate for cardiac output. Atropine may also be given to any patient with relative or absolute bradycardia. The pediatric dose is 0.02 mg/kg IV given approximately 3 minutes prior to SCh.

Once SCh is given, if bradycardia occurs, uptake of atropine may be blocked for a short time, so atropine is given before SCh. The adult dose is 0.5 to 2 mg IV.

Did You Know?

If you must give a second dose of succinylcholine (SCh) in the rapid sequence intubation sequence, the chances of bradycardia are increased dramatically. Just prior to giving a second dose of SCh, atropine should be given no matter what the patient's sinus heart rate at the time.[6]

Defasiculation as Pretreatment Therapy Depolarizing paralytics like SCh create **fasciculations** because of nicotinic acetylcholine receptor stimulation. This is a phenomenon where muscle bundles contract in brief excitatory waves. While this is occurring, many organs suffer from a rise in pressure. In the stomach, this can create passive vomiting (and aspiration), the eye will endure high intraocular pressure, and the brain will suffer from high intracranial pressure. Administering 10% of the dose of a nondepolarizing paralytic just prior to the actual RSI sequence may blunt this affect. This is called **defasciculation**. The defasciculating dose of vecuronium is 0.01 mg/kg, or 0.1 mg/kg of rocuronium. Giving 0.15 mg/kg of SCh can defasciculate, but there is less evidence of its effectiveness versus the rise in ICP or intraocular pressure. Box D-4 provides a recap in the RSI sequence.

Step 4: Sedation and Paralysis The ideal drugs given in the RSI sequence would have a quick onset of action, few side effects, and a short half-life. This would allow spontaneous patient recovery if you cannot ventilate or intubate the patient. Refer to Table D-7 for standard sedation (preanesthesia) drugs and Table D-8 for depolarizing and nondepolarizing paralytics.

Sedation in Rapid Sequence Intubation Quick to act, quick to wear off, with no side effects is the ideal sedation choice for the RSI initial sequence. Beside those

BOX D-4 Recapping the Rapid Sequence Intubation

You have applied 100% oxygen to the patient and have evaluated them for difficult airway. The equipment is set up, and backup devices are nearby. You are following your protocol for the possibility of pre-RSI therapy. (In those <10 years of age, you have given atropine.) The patient now needs to promptly lose consciousness with sedation.

attributes, we want a sedative that provides some analgesia, does not alter cardiac output, and has a reliable reversal agent available, in a very short period of time. Sorry, this agent doesn't exist. In seeking those attributes, however, you should take a look at a quick overview of some of the most commonly used sedatives in your RSI sequence.

Benzodiazepines This type of drug controls the **neuroinhibitor transmitter** and provides analgesia, **anxiolysis**, central muscle relaxation, sedation, anticonvulsant effects, and hypnosis. Certain of these drugs are more amnesic than others, as there are differences in their onset of action. Midazolam (Versed) is the most rapid to act (30 to 60 seconds), but its half-life can be as long as 1 to 2 hours. The dosing of these drugs can be quite a challenge because each patient can have quite a variable response. Generally, the induction dose of midazolam is 0.2 mg/kg IV push, but this also depresses pumping function of the heart and systemic vascular resistance (hypotension). Midazolam is the most commonly used sedative in the RSI sequence, especially for continued sedation and paralysis in transport at doses of 1 to 2.5 mg given IV over 2 minutes, with repeat doses titrated to patient need. Doses as high as 0.3 to 0.35 mg/kg IV are recommended. A continuous IV infusion can be established at 0.02 to 0.10 mg/kg/h (1 to 7 mg/h) and titrated to patient needs.

Etomidate (Amidate) Etomidate is a hypnotic agent that provides quick onset of action (20 to 30 seconds), short duration (7 to 14 minutes) but does not create the hemodynamic instability that Versed can.

The combination of etomidate and SCh in the initial induction of your RSI sequence can blunt the rise in ICP that SCh is infamous for. The recommended dose for induction is 0.3 mg/kg. This drug can create a classic **myoclonic movement** by the patient from stimulation of the brainstem but is often masked by the immediate injection of SCh which causes paralysis. Hiccups and vomiting can occur after administration. If the endotracheal tube is not successfully passed on the first attempt, suction must be available for the unprotected airway. One note of concern stated about this drug is the possibility of decrease in both **cortisol** and **aldosterone** levels with repeated administration. The side effect is avoided if you inject this

TABLE D-7 Intravenously Administered General Anesthetics

Agent	Typical Adult Dose Range for Induction	Onset	Duration	Adverse Effects
BARBITURATE				
thiopental sodium (Pentothal)	3–5 mg/kg	30–60 sec	5–30 min	Respiratory depression Bradycardia Hypotension Paradoxical excitation Confusion Pain at injection site
BENZODIAZEPINE				
midazolam (Versed)	0.5–2 mg slow IV over 2–3 min	1–5 min	Variable, 30 min to 2+ hours	Respiratory depression Hypotension Paradoxical excitation Confusion Pain at injection site
diazepam (Valium)	2–10 mg slow IV over 2–3 min	1–10 min	Variable, with more pronounced "hangover"	
lorazepam (Ativan)	1–4 mg slow IV over 2–5 min	1–10 min	Variable	
OPIOID				
alfentanil (Alfenta)	0.5–75 mcg/kg	Almost immediate	30–60 min	Respiratory depression Bradycardia Hypotension Paradoxical excitation Confusion Nausea/vomiting
fentanyl (Sublimaze)	0.5–50 mcg/kg	Almost immediate	30–60 min	
remifentanil (Ultiva)	0.5–1 mcg/kg	1–3 min	Variable	
sufentanil (Sufenta)	1–30 mcg/kg	1–3 min	Variable	
GENERAL ANESTHETIC				
etomidate (Amidate)	0.2–0.6 mg/kg over 30–60 sec	1 min	3–5 min	Nausea/vomiting Pain at injection site Muscle/eye movements
propofol (Diprivan)	0.5–2.5 mg/kg over 10–60 sec	10–50 sec	3–10 min	Apnea Hypotension Pain at injection site Anaphylaxis
DISSOCIATIVE ANESTHETIC				
ketamine (Ketalar)	1–2 mg/kg	1–2 min	5–15 min	Hypertension Tachycardia ↑ Intracranial pressure Hallucinations Muscle movements Abuse potential

Modified from Lacy CF, et al: Lexi-Comp's drug information handbook, ed 12, Hudson, Ohio, 2004, Lexi-Comp.

drug only once. If you're dealing with a failed airway attempt, consider using another sedative for subsequent attempts. For those patients who would benefit from even a second dose of etomidate (sepsis), consider using methylprednisolone to deter this side effect.

Did You Know?

The most common sedative/paralytic induction agents are etomidate at 0.3 mg/kg and succinylcholine at 1.5 mg/kg IV in quick succession.[6]

Ketamine (Ketalar) The sedation state created by IV administration of ketamine is termed *dissociative anesthesia* because the brain pathways are interrupted before sensory blockade. Just after injection, the heart rate and blood pressure rise and then return to normal within approximately 15 minutes. This may create a rise in ICP, so those patients with hypotension benefit but not when they also have a high ICP. The most sought-after attribute of this drug is its ability to relax bronchial smooth muscle and create bronchodilation, making ketamine the agent of choice for asthma patients. A second attribute is that even though it's considered a sedative, ketamine allows the body to maintain respiratory drive. The induction dose is

TABLE D-8 Neuromuscular Blockers

Agent	Onset (minutes)	Half-Life (minutes)	Duration in Minutes (Bolus Dose)
DEPOLARIZING			
succinylcholine (Anectine)	0.5–1	<1 minute	4–8
NONDEPOLARIZING			
mivacurium (Mivacron)	1.5–3	2	12–20
atracurium (Tracrium)	2–3	20	20–45
cisatracurium (Nimbex)	2–3	20–30	40–60
rocuronium (Zemuron)	1–1.5	60–70	30–60
vecuronium (Norcuron)	2–3	50–80	20–40
doxacurium (Nuromax)	4–6	100–200	100–160
pancuronium (Pavulon)	3–5	100–170	60–100
pipecuronium (Arduan)	3–5	120–180	60–120
tubocurarine	3–5	100–120	60–90

Modified from Lacy CF, et al: Lexi-Comp's drug information handbook, ed 12, Hudson, Ohio, 2004, Lexi-Comp.

1 to 2 mg/kg IV, with an onset of action at 15 to 30 seconds and duration of action about 10 to 15 minutes. After injection, you'll notice an increase in secretions; have suction available. The concomitant use of drying agents like atropine or Robinul may blunt the ketamine "wet effect." The infamous side effect of this drug is hallucinations, but this does not usually apply in an RSI sequence; benzodiazepines are commonly injected for continued sedation and will blunt this affect as well.

Propofol (Diprivan) Propofol is a lipid solution that appears thick and white and is often called "mother's milk." It's also a hypnotic sedative and can diminish cardiac output by depressing pumping function. Propofol has properties that reduce bronchospasm, but it's rarely used in the induction phase of the RSI sequence because of its ability to create hypotension. Its use outside of anesthesiology is restricted to the provider's scope of practice. Propofol is encouraged for continued sedation of intubated patients at 0.2 to 0.6 mcg/kg by IV infusion.

Paralysis in Rapid Sequence Intubation

Neuromuscular Blocking Agents (NMBA) You've already read a brief discussion of some of the effects and side effects of SCh. Now you need to understand the difference between depolarizing and nondepolarizing paralytics. There are generally two classes of muscle relaxants for RSI: **noncompetitive (depolarizing)** and **competitive (nondepolarizing)** neuromuscular blocking agents (NMBAs).

Noncompetitive/Depolarizing Neuromuscular Blocking Agents The only practical drug to list in this category is SCh. Designed to mimic acetylcholine, it blocks the **nicotinic and muscarinic cholinergic receptors**. As long as the patient's body has pseudocholinesterase, this drug will be processed away from the neuromuscular endplates fairly quickly (Figure D-19).

Your Medical Director will commonly choose SCh as your initial RSI paralytic because of its short half-life. The side effects of the drug, however, should make you respect its use. See Appendix E for a synopsis of SCh, along with its adverse effects. Only a small portion of injected SCh actually reaches the neuromuscular junction, so because of that, larger doses are recommended.

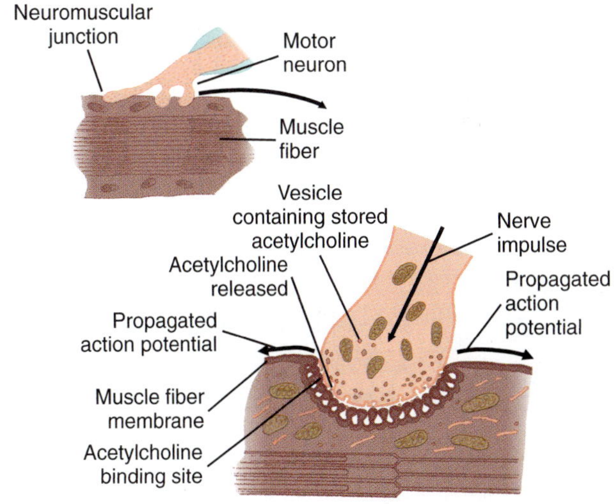

Figure D-19 (From Mosby's dictionary of medicine, nursing & allied health, ed 8, St Louis, 2009, Mosby.)

Competitive/Nondepolarizing Neuromuscular Muscle Relaxants These paralytics compete with or block acetylcholine at the neuromuscular junction. As opposed to SCh, which stimulates this site, creating fasciculations, the nondepolarizing agents do not, and no fasciculations occur. There are two categories within this group of nondepolarizing drugs: aminosteroid and benzylisoquinolinum compounds.

The aminosteroid compounds are the most commonly used in the emergency and transport setting. In general, these drugs have a long time to onset of action (1 to 2 minutes), a longer duration of action (20 to 45 minutes), with fewer side effects than SCh. These agents are given when SCh is contraindicated or during times when a longer duration of action is necessary: continued ventilation during transport.

If they have fewer side effects, why don't we use nondepolarizing agents for RSI? The caution we must exercise when rendering medication-assisted intubation sways our decision making so that we use quick-acting, short-duration drugs when we can because of the chance of failure to ventilate and intubate. Box D-5 provides a recap of the RSI sequence.

Did You Know?

We can hasten the onset of action in nondepolarizing drugs by increasing the dose, but this also lengthens the duration of action of the drug.[6]

Did You Know?

Two separate classes of drugs are routinely administered in rapid sequence intubation: sedatives and paralytics. Neither of these drugs provides pain relief. Please remember to provide analgesia to those patients having pain. They cannot complain (verbally or nonverbally).[9]

BOX D-5 Recapping the Rapid Sequence Intubation

You have evaluated the patient, preoxygenated/hyperoxygenated them, set up and have all equipment checked and ready (including backup devices), have drawn up the appropriate pretreatment, sedative, and paralytic drugs, and have them all clearly identified on the syringe. You are now ready for induction for intubation.

Step 5: Administer Drugs, Position Patient, and Perform Intubation Approximately 3 to 5 minutes prior to the sedative/paralytic drug combination, you have given your pretreatment drugs. Once the personnel are ready, these two drugs are given, usually in rapid succession. Observe the patient for myoclonus or fasciculations. Monitor vital signs, and watch for muscle relaxation and anticipated apnea. Once apnea occurs, don't provide positive-pressure ventilation until after the standard intubation attempt unless the patient suffered from hypoxia. If bag-mask ventilation is necessary, cricoid pressure should be applied and maintained throughout.

Just after the sedative is given, the **Sellick maneuver** or cricothyroid pressure is applied in an attempt to prevent passive regurgitation of GI contents. The assistant's first finger and thumb are positioned on the palpated lateral edges of the cricoid ring, and pressure is applied straight downward. The maneuver depresses the cricoid cartilage ring onto the upper esophagus, collapsing the pathway. Approximately 10 pounds of pressure should be applied until the tracheal tube cuff is inflated AND placement confirmed. The assistant's application of cricoid pressure will prepare for the facilitated view of the cords, discussed shortly.

Did You Know?

In most medical patients, proper positioning of the patient into a sniffing position includes the use of a pillow strategically placed beneath the shoulders, upper back, neck, and head. This helps overcome some of the three angles necessary to view the cords.

Also, the heavier the upper torso of the patient, the higher the upper body should be positioned. Reverse Trendelenburg position may be needed in some morbidly obese patients, and you should step on a footstool, looking over the patient's shoulder.[6]

As you're positioning the laryngoscope blade or fiberoptic device, the assistant should apply a BURP technique to facilitate a central view of the patient's cords. *BURP* refers to applying pressure *b*ackward, *u*pward, (to the patient's) *r*ightward *p*ressure. While the intubator is viewing the cords, they can guide the BURP technique pressure and direction. If the patient has a small mouth cavity, the assistant can use the other hand to retract the right side of the patient's mouth to facilitate both the blade and the approaching ETT, coming from the right side. The ETT is inserted to the proper depth, manually held into position while the stylet or fiberoptic is removed, and the cuff inflated. Positive-pressure ventilation is applied.

If the assistant notices a change in vital signs, the intubation procedure should be stopped and ventilation administered. The next step is listed in your Failed or Difficult Airway protocol. In most cases, this means a second attempt at ET intubation may occur.

Did You Know?

Difficult or Failed Intubation protocols are a step-by-step decision tree that guides the crew through rapid sequence intubation (RSI) should intubation not occur on the first attempt. The backup plans might include an extraglottic airway device as a bridge to a second attempt or a final destination for airway control. Another backup plan is your partner. In a safe system for RSI, both crew members should have strong skills in airway and ventilation management.[6,11]

Step 6: Confirm Placement, and Secure Device There are many ways to confirm ETT placement. Any one procedure for confirmation by itself is not definitive in answering the question: Is that ETT in the correct location? That's why most standards ask you to use two methods of confirmation initially and after each time the patient is moved or might otherwise dislodge the ETT. Of these, many are impractical for the setting of transport.

Notes on ETT Confirmation Procedures

1. Esophageal tube checks may be used as the *initial* means of confirmation in those older than 4 or 5 years of age.
2. Colorimetric end-tidal CO_2 detectors may not change color if perfusion to the lungs and body are compromised. False change in color may occur in the morbidly obese and in those patients who have large amounts of carbonated beverages in the stomach. Disposable devices should only be used for a short period of time as the chemical paper is exposed to air.
3. Chest x-ray (CXR) has become the gold standard for ETT confirmation and is usually done on a daily basis on the mechanically ventilated patient in the ICU. In 12% to 14% of these patients, this diagnostic tool finds malpositioned ETTs. CXR can confirm depth of placement much more reliably than tracheal versus esophageal placement.

There are disadvantages to using CXR to confirm ETT placement:

- Cost
- Radiation of patient
- Time to take and interpret film
- Need for specialized personnel
- Experienced physician to interpret

This means of confirming ETT placement for the critical care team is impractical. The use of B-mode ultrasound can also confirm placement and does so more economically and without radiation and costly time and personnel (if the cuff is inflated with saline).

4. Direct visualization with a laryngoscope or with fiberoptics offers a much more practical method for quick confirmation of ETT placement.
5. $PETCO_2$ should be monitored in all patients mechanically ventilated throughout all transfers. Initial and ongoing monitoring of the end-tidal CO_2 (capnography) also gives us information on ventilation and perfusion.
6. Auscultation of at least three points initially is often the method of choice among transport personnel. Epigastric and bilateral auscultation can identify esophageal tubes versus tracheal tubes and assist in determining depth of placement in adults.
7. Other methods of indirect confirmation include observation of thoracic movement (chest rise and fall) and palpation of tracheal tube in the suprasternal notch. These are less reliable.

All who intubate patients have accidentally placed the tracheal tube in the esophagus. It happens. If looking for mistakes, though, the actual negligent act is when you fail to recognize that the ETT is not in the trachea. Be diligent in monitoring for incorrect placement and displacement of the ETT.

Placement of a commercially prepared product to secure the ETT is the next step. There is evidence that this means of securing the device is better than tape, but there are some things to consider here too. Many ICUs do not use these devices because the plastic piece rests against the patient's mouth and can create irritation and open wounds. Untaping a secured ETT and then applying a commercial device is up to you and your Medical Director. Either way, be careful that the commercial device does not crimp the tube in any way, reducing the ID and thus creating higher airway pressures. Ensure that the centimeter marking at the lip is visible and documented for depth of placement. The addition of a bite block (commercial device or OPA) should be considered if the patient has some control.

Begin the prescribed positive pressure on your ventilator. Monitor vital signs. Box D-6 provides a recap of the RSI procedure.

Step 7: Post Rapid Sequence Intubation Care Evaluate the patient's ABCs. We started this airway management section with that tip and end the medication-assisted intubation section with the same advice. You've applied a series of treatment modalities that may alter all three. Make sure the patient has tolerated the change. Some troublesome signs and their causes are:

1. Bradycardia may be an ominous sign in all patients during and following RSI. Esophageal intubation is one differential that must be ruled out in this case.
2. Hypertension, especially with tachycardia, usually means the patient is awake and not happy with recent events. Administer your ongoing sedation

BOX D-6 Recapping the Rapid Sequence Intubation Procedure Thus Far

You've evaluated your patient for a difficult airway and hyperoxygenated him; you've set up equipment, devices, and medications; pretreatment drugs have been given; the sedative and paralytic have been given. The assistant watches vital signs, applies cricoid pressure, then BURP technique (guided by intubator), then retraction of right side of patient's mouth as you intubate. Tube position confirmed with two methods, then secured.

and paralytic. Reevaluate vital signs once those drugs are in action. Review the side effects of the drugs given. Ketamine is one example of a sedative that can create this situation.

3. Hypotension may be due to positive-pressure ventilation or from the drugs used. Immediately rule out pneumothorax with obstructive shock, and treat if found. In a patient with high airway pressures (asthma, COPD), the sometimes rapid ventilation associated with tube confirmation may have inadvertently created **auto-PEEP**. Once pneumothorax is ruled out, review the patient's history, and provide slow ventilations with reasonable tidal volumes at a 1:3 ratio, monitoring $PETCO_2$ and vital signs. A fluid bolus may help. Vasopressors are rarely needed. Midazolam and propofol may create hypotension.
4. Go to your Difficult or Failed Intubation protocol if airway complications arise.

Administer sedative and nondepolarizing paralytic based on your protocols. It's recommended that you also provide analgesia to the patient. Watch for the recovering patient during the transport through vital signs and onset of spontaneous respirations.

Understanding the half-life of the drugs used will help you organize your management approach during the transport. Be prepared with the next sedative and paralytic BEFORE the next spontaneous breath by the patient. An early sign of recovery from the drugs is a rise in heart rate and blood pressure. As you begin to see this sign, correlate with the expected recovery from the drugs given, and begin to prepare for additional doses. The use of nerve

TABLE D-9 Rapid Sequence Intubation Quick Guide

Time	"Zero" –5 to –8 minutes	"Zero" –2 to –3 minutes	"Zero" –2 minutes	"Zero"	"Zero" +45 to +60 seconds	Post Intubation
Preparation	Prepare equipment, suction, 100% oxygen	Premedications and defasciculating agent	Sedation Apply Sellick's maneuver	Paralyze	Intubate patient	Confirm placement, release Sellick, secure tube.
Routine rapid sequence intubation (RSI), including head injury and patients with normal or elevated blood pressure	Evaluate anatomy, decide backup, prepare and label medications, hyperoxygenate.	Atropine: Pediatric: 0.02 mg/kg Adult: 1 mg Lidocaine, 1.5 mg/kg Norcuron, 0.1 mg/kg	Versed, 0.05–0.1 mg/kg; or Etomidate, 0.3 mg/kg	Succinylcholine, 1.5 mg/kg	WAIT FOR PARALYSIS Intubate patient	Determine continued paralysis AND sedation.
Routine RSI borderline or hypotensive patients	Evaluate anatomy, decide backup, prepare and label medications, hyperoxygenate.	Atropine: Pediatric: 0.02 mg/kg Adult: 1 mg Lidocaine, 1.5 mg/kg Norcuron, 0.1 mg/kg	Versed, 0.05–0.1 mg/kg; or Etomidate, 0.015 mg/kg	Succinylcholine, 1.5 mg/kg	WAIT FOR PARALYSIS Intubate patient	Determine continued paralysis AND sedation.
Non-Sux RSI	Evaluate anatomy, decide backup, prepare and label medications, hyperoxygenate.	Atropine: Pediatric: 0.02 mg/kg Adult: 1 mg Lidocaine, 1.5 mg/kg	Versed, 0.05–0.1 mg/kg; or Etomidate, 0.3 mg/kg Norcuron, 0.1 mg/kg; or Rocuronium, 1.2 mg/kg (first dose, then 0.6 mg/kg) for continued paralysis	Norcuron, 0.1 mg/kg; or Rocuronium, 1.2 mg/kg	WAIT FOR PARALYSIS Intubate patient	Determine continued paralysis AND sedation.

Courtesy Lee Ridge, Paramedic Specialist, FP-C.

BOX D-7 Suggested Contents of Your CCP Airway Toolkit

Nasal and oral airways
Laryngoscope handles
A range of blades from size 0-5 in both straight and curved
Extra batteries and lamps
Lubricant
Fiberoptic laryngoscope/viewer
Stylet
Bougie
Tube exchanger or catheter
Extraglottic airway in all sizes, with appropriate syringe (if needed)
12-mL syringes
All sizes of endotracheal tubes
Rigid tonsil tip suction device and connecting tube
Commercial endotracheal tube (ETT) holder
1-inch tape
Tube confirmation devices
Percutaneous cricothyrotomy kit or scalpel, tracheostomy tube, skin hook or trach hook, and Kelly forceps

stimulators can also help gauge patient recovery from paralytics. Use of noninvasive bispectral monitoring (BIS) of brain waves may be used to monitor the patient's level of sedation. The $PETCO_2$ waveform can also give clues as to when neuromuscular blockade is wearing off. Called the "curare cleft," this dip in the CO_2 waveform plateau indicates spontaneous respirations. The deeper the cleft, the less neuromuscular blockade is still active.

Administering paralytics without sedation is very bad practice and deemed unethical. The patient should always benefit from the actions of the sedative while paralytics are used (Table D-9).

Box D-7 provides suggestions for tools your CCP Airway Toolkit should contain.

Airway assessment and management can be quite a challenge. The team needs to be prepared through a great knowledge base, good protocols, skills practice, and then scenario management to sort through the many "what if's" of airway management.

REFERENCES

1. Sinha PK, Misra S: Supraglottic airway devices other than laryngeal mask airway and its prototypes, Indian J Anaesth 49(4):281–292, 2005.
2. Vaida S, Gaitini D, Ben-David B, et al: A new supraglottic airway, the elisha airway device: a preliminary study, Anesth Analg 99:124–127, 2004.
3. Miller D, Camporata L: Advantages of ProSeal™ and SLIPA™ airways over tracheal tubes for gynecological laparoscopies, Can J Anesth 53(2):188–193, 2006.
4. Greenberg RS, Kay NH: Cuffed oropharyngeal airway (COPA) as an adjunct to fibreoptic tracheal intubation, Br J of Anesth 82(3):395–398, 1999.
5. Hagberg C: Current concepts in the management of the difficult airway; 52nd Annual Refresher Course Lectures from the Clinical Updates and Basic Science Reviews, October, 2001; Annual Meeting of the American Society of Anesthesiologists, ©American Society of Anesthesiologists, Inc.
6. Walls RM, et al: Manual of emergency airway management: companion manual to the national emergency airway management course, Philadelphia, 2000, Lippincott Williams & Wilkins.
7. Hagberg C: Current Concepts in the management of the difficult airway, Anesthesiology News, New York, May 2007, McMahon Publishing.
8. Wiegand D, Carlson K, editors: AACN procedure manual for critical care, ed 5, St. Louis, 2005, Elsevier.
9. Hoffman RJ, et al: High endotracheal tube cuff pressure is typical in endotracheally intubated emergency department patients, Ann Emerg Med 48(4):58, 2006.
10. McKenry ll, et al: Mosby's pharmacology in nursing, ed 22, St. Louis, 2006, Mosby.
11. The University of Iowa Hospitals' EMSLRC: Critical care paramedic curriculum, Iowa City, IA, 1996, University of Iowa.

APPENDIX

E Drug Profiles

 Abciximab (ReoPro)

Classification: GP IIb/IIIa inhibitor

Action: Prevents the aggregation of platelets by inhibiting the integrin GP IIb/IIIa receptor.

Indications: Unstable angina/non–ST elevation myocardial infarction (UA/NSTEMI) patients undergoing planned or emergent percutaneous coronary intervention (PCI).

Adverse Effects: Bleeding from the GI tract, internal bleeding, intracranial hemorrhage, hypotension, stroke, anaphylactic shock.

Contraindications: Bleeding from any source, severe uncontrolled hypertension, surgery or trauma within the previous 6 weeks, stroke within the previous 30 days, renal failure, thrombocytopenia, intracranial mass.

Dosage:

UA/NSTEMI with planned PCI within 24 hours:

- 0.25 mg/kg IV, IO (10 to 60 minutes prior to procedure), then 0.125 mcg/kg/min IV, IO infusion for 18 to 24 hours.

PCI only:

- 0.25 mg/kg IV, IO, then 0.125 mcg/kg/min to a maximum of 10 mcg/min IV, IO infusion.

Special Considerations: Pregnancy Category C.

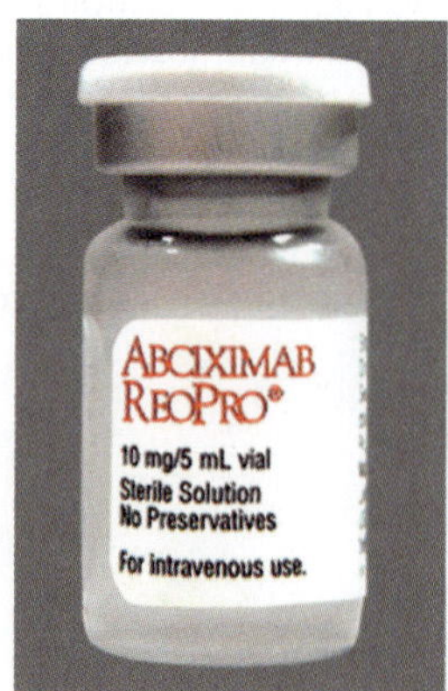

 Acetaminophen (Tylenol, Abenol, Atasol)

Classification: Analgesic

Action: Inhibits prostaglandin synthesis in the central and peripheral nervous system. Although exact mechanisms are unknown, the antiinflammatory effects are minimal. This drug reduces fever via action in the hypothalamus but is less effective than ibuprofen at reducing fever in children.

Indications: Mild to moderate pain and commonly used in the treatment of fever.

Adverse Effects: Overdose is often fatal secondary to liver toxicity and must be treated as a medical emergency. Blood dyscrasias (including hemolytic anemia) and renal dysfunction are rare but possible.

Contraindications: Not to be used with known sensitivity to the drug.

Dosage:

- Adults: (>12 years): 650 to 1000 mg every 4 to 6 hours, not to exceed 4000 mg/day.
- Pediatric:
  - Children < 2 years: Not to be used without physician advice.
  - Children 2 to 12 years: 10 to 15 mg/kg every 4 to 6 hours, maximum of 50 to 75 mg/kg/day.

Special Considerations: Pregnancy Category B. This drug does pass in breast milk. Acetaminophen is contained within the drugs Percocet and Vicodin, along with 200 other prescription and over-the-counter medications.

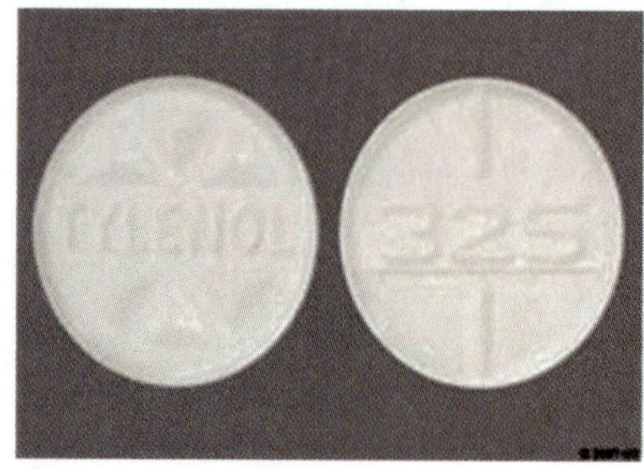

Abbreviations used in this appendix: *CHF,* Congestive heart failure; *CNS,* central nervous system; *COPD,* chronic obstructive pulmonary disease; *ECG,* electrocardiogram; *ET,* endotracheal; *FDA,* U.S. Food and Drug Administration; *GI,* gastrointestinal; *IM,* intramuscular; *IO,* intraosseous; *IV,* intravenous; *MDI,* measured dose inhaler; *MI,* myocardial infarction; *PO,* per os (oral); *SQ,* subcutaneous.

Activated Charcoal

Classification: Antidote, adsorbent

Action: When certain chemicals and toxins are in proximity to the activated charcoal, the chemical will attach to the surface of the charcoal and become trapped.

Indications: Toxic ingestion

Adverse Effects: Nausea/vomiting, constipation, or diarrhea. If aspirated into the lungs, charcoal can induce a potentially fatal form of pneumonitis.

Contraindications: Ingestion of acids, alkalis, ethanol, methanol, cyanide, ferrous sulfate or other iron salts, lithium; coma; GI obstruction.

Dosage:

- Adult: 25 to 100 g/dose.
- Pediatric: 1 to 2 g/kg.

Special Considerations: Pregnancy Category C.

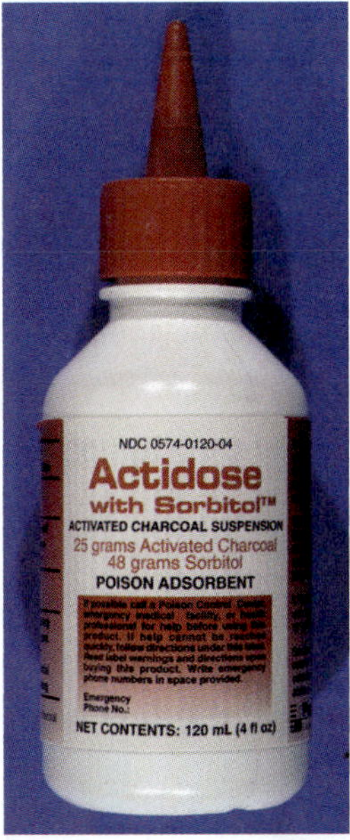

Adenosine (Adenocard)

Classification: Antiarrhythmic

Action: Slows the conduction of electrical impulses at the AV node.

Indications: Stable reentry supraventricular tachycardia (SVT). Does not convert atrial fibrillation (AF), atrial flutter, or ventricular tachycardia (VT).

Adverse Effects: Common adverse reactions are generally mild and short lived: sense of impending doom, complaints of flushing, chest pressure, throat tightness, numbness. Patients will have a brief episode of asystole after administration.

Contraindications: Sick sinus syndrome, second- or third-degree heart block, poison-/drug-induced tachycardia, bronchospastic disease.

Dosage: Note: Adenosine should be delivered only by rapid IV bolus with a peripheral IV or directly into a vein, in a location as close to the heart as possible, preferably in the antecubital fossa. Administration of adenosine must be immediately followed by a 10- to 20-mL saline flush, and then the extremity should be elevated.

- Adult: Initial dose 6 mg rapid IV, IO (over a 1- to 3-second period) immediately followed by a 20-mL rapid saline flush. If the first dose does not eliminate the rhythm in 1 to 2 minutes, 12 mg rapid IV, IO, repeat a second time if required.
- Pediatric:
  - Children > 50 kg: Same as adult dosing.
  - Children < 50 kg: Initial dose 0.1 mg/kg IV, IO (max dose: 6 mg) immediately followed by a ≥ 5-mL rapid saline flush; may repeat at 0.2 mg/kg (max dose: 12 mg).

Special Considerations:

- Use with caution in patients with preexisting bronchospasm and those with a history of AF.
- Elderly patients with no history of PSVT should be carefully evaluated for dehydration and rapid sinus tachycardia requiring volume fluid replacement rather than simply treated with adenosine.
- Pregnancy Category C.

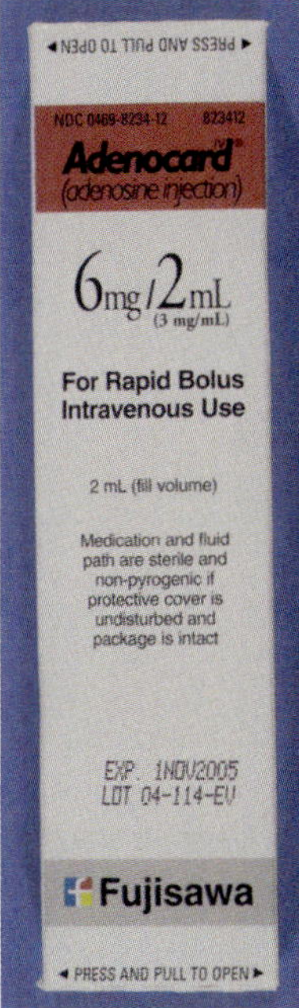

Albuterol (Proventil, Ventolin)

Classification: Bronchodilator, beta agonist

Action: Binds and stimulates $beta_2$ receptors, resulting in relaxation of bronchial smooth muscle.

Indications: Asthma, bronchitis with bronchospasm, and COPD.

Adverse Effects: Hyperglycemia, hypokalemia, palpitations, sinus tachycardia, anxiety, tremor, nausea/vomiting, throat irritation, dry mouth, hypertension, dyspepsia, insomnia, headache, epistaxis, paradoxical bronchospasm.

Contraindications: Angioedema, sensitivity to albuterol or levalbuterol. Use with caution in lactating patients, cardiovascular disorders, cardiac arrhythmias.

Dosage:

Acute bronchospasm:

- Adult:
  - MDI: 4 to 8 puffs every 1 to 4 hours may be required.
  - Nebulizer: 2.5 to 5 mg every 20 minutes for a maximum of three doses. After the initial three doses, escalate the dose or start a continuous nebulization at 10 to 15 mg/hr.
- Pediatric:
  - MDI:
    - 4 years and older: 2 inhalations every 4 to 6 hours; however, in some patients, 1 inhalation every 4 hours is sufficient. More frequent administration or more inhalations are not recommended.
    - Younger than 4 years: Administer by nebulization.
  - Nebulizer:
    - Older than 12 years: The dose for a continuous nebulization is 0.5 mg/kg/hr.
    - Younger than 12 years: 0.15 mg/kg every 20 minutes for a maximum of three doses (maximum 2.5 mg). Alternatively, continuous nebulization at 0.5 mg/kg/hr can be delivered to children younger than 12 years.

Asthma in pregnancy:

- MDI: Two inhalations every 4 hours. In acute exacerbation, start with 2 to 4 puffs every 20 minutes.

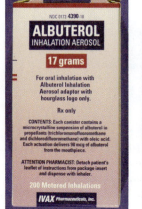

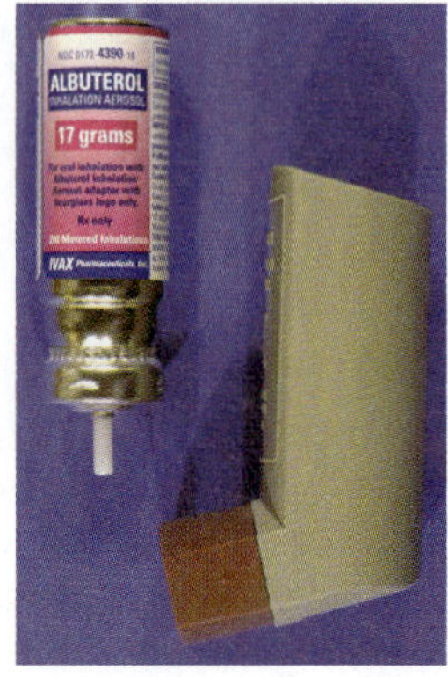

- Nebulizer: 2.5 mg (0.5 mL) by 0.5% nebulization solution. Place 0.5 mL of the albuterol solution in 2.5 mL of sterile normal saline. Flow is regulated to deliver the therapy over a 5- to 20-minute period. In refractory cases, some physicians order 10 mg nebulized over a 60-minute period.

Special Considerations: Pregnancy Category C.

Albuterol/Ipratropium (Combivent)

Classification: Combination bronchodilator

Action: Binds and stimulates $beta_2$ receptors, resulting in relaxation of bronchial smooth muscle, and antagonizes the acetylcholine receptor, producing bronchodilation.

Indications: Second-line treatment (if bronchodilator is ineffective) in COPD or severe acute asthma exacerbations during medical transport.

Adverse Effects: Headache, cough, nausea, arrhythmias, paradoxical acute bronchospasm.

Contraindications: Allergy to soybeans or peanuts; known sensitivity to atropine, albuterol, or their respective derivatives. Used with caution in patients with hypertension, angina, cardiac arrhythmias, tachycardia, cardiovascular disease, congenital long QT syndrome, closed-angle glaucoma.

Dosage:

- Adult: 2 puffs inhaled every 6 hours by MDI, with a maximum daily dose of 12 puffs/day.
- Pediatric: Not recommended for pediatric patients.

Special Considerations: Pregnancy Category C.

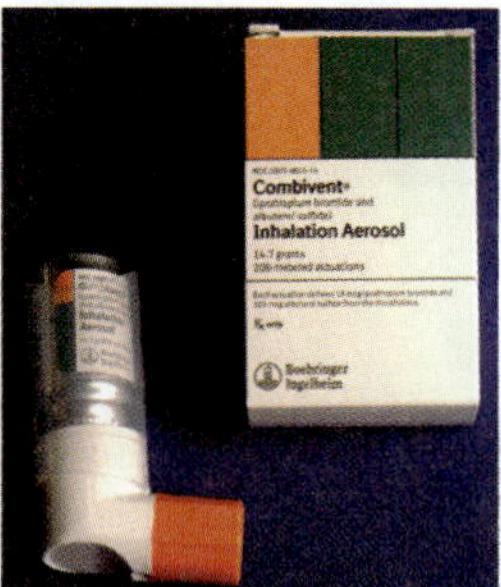

Amiodarone (Cordarone)

Classification: Antiarrhythmic, class III

Action: Acts directly on the myocardium to delay repolarization and increase the duration of the action potential.

Indications: Ventricular arrhythmias; second-line agent for atrial arrhythmias but used with caution in those with heart failure.

Adverse Effects: Burning at the IV site, hypotension, bradycardia.

Contraindications: Sick sinus syndrome, second- and third-degree heart block, cardiogenic shock, when episodes of bradycardia have caused syncope, sensitivity to benzyl alcohol and iodine.

Dosage:

Ventricular fibrillation and pulseless ventricular tachycardia:

- Adult: 300 mg IV, IO. May be followed by one dose of 150 mg in 3 to 5 minutes.
- Pediatric: 5 mg/kg (max dose: 300 mg); may repeat 5 mg/kg IV, IO up to 15 mg/kg.

Relatively stable patients with arrhythmias such as premature ventricular contractions or wide-complex tachycardias with a strong pulse:

- Adult: 150 mg in 100 mL D_5W IV, IO over a 10-minute period; may repeat in 10 minutes up to a maximum dose of 2.2 g over 24 hours.
- Pediatric: 5 mg/kg very slow IV, IO (over 20 to 60 minutes); may repeat in 5-mg/kg doses up to 15 mg/kg (max dose: 300 mg).

Special Considerations: Pregnancy Category D.

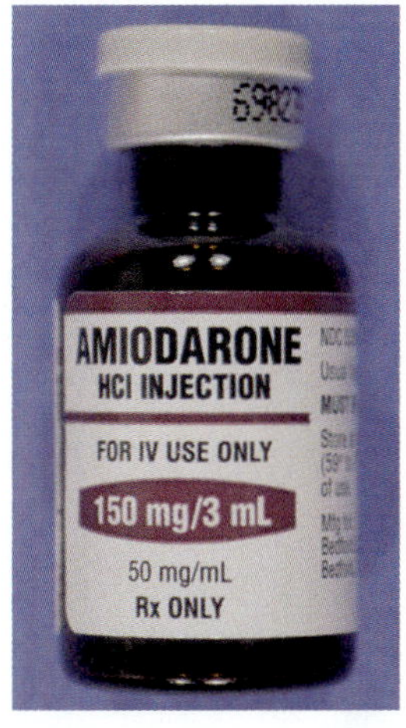

Angiotensin-Converting Enzyme (ACE) Inhibitors: Captopril (Capoten), Enalapril (Vasotec), Lisinopril (Prinivil, Zestril), Ramipril (Altace)

Classification: ACE inhibitor

Action: Blocks the enzyme responsible for the production of angiotensin II, resulting in a decrease in blood pressure.

Indications: Congestive heart failure, hypertension, diabetic nephropathy, post myocardial infarction.

Adverse Effects: Headache, dizziness, fatigue, depression, chest pain, hypotension, palpitations, cough, dyspnea, upper respiratory infection, nausea/vomiting, rash, pruritus, angioedema, renal failure.

Contraindications: Angioedema related to previous treatment with an ACE inhibitor, known sensitivity. Use with caution in aortic stenosis, bilateral renal artery stenosis, hypertrophic obstructive cardiomyopathy, pericardial tamponade, elevated serum potassium levels, acute kidney failure.

Dosage:

- Adult: Medication is administered orally. Dosage is individualized. Enalaprilat (Vasotec), 1.25 mg IV slow every 6 hours.
- Pediatric: Medication is administered orally. Dosage is individualized.

Special Considerations: Pregnancy Category D.

Aspirin, ASA

Classification: Antiplatelet, nonnarcotic analgesic, antipyretic

Action: Prevents the formation of a chemical known as thromboxane A_2, which causes platelets to clump together, or aggregate, and form plugs that cause obstruction or constriction of small coronary arteries.

Indications: Fever, inflammation, angina, acute MI, and patients complaining of pain, pressure, squeezing, or crushing in the chest that may be cardiac in origin.

Adverse Effects: Anaphylaxis, angioedema, bronchospasm, bleeding, stomach irritation, nausea/vomiting.

Contraindications: GI bleeding, active ulcer disease, hemorrhagic stroke, bleeding disorders, children with chickenpox or flulike symptoms, hypersensitivity to nonsteroidal antiinflammatory drugs, and known Samter syndrome (sensitivity syndrome), which includes asthma, nasal polyps, and aspirin sensitivity.

Dosage: Note: "Baby aspirin" 81 mg, standard adult aspirin dose 325 mg.

Myocardial infarction:

- Adult: 160 to 325 mg PO (alternatively, four 81-mg baby aspirin are often given), 300-mg rectal suppository.
- Pediatric: 3 to 5 mg/kg/day to 5 to 10 mg/kg/day given as a single dose.

Pain or fever:

- Adult: 325 to 650 mg PO (1 to 2 adult tablets) every 4 to 6 hours, maximum 4 g/24 hr.
- Pediatric: 40 to 60 mg/kg/day in divided doses every 4 to 6 hours, maximum 4 g/24 hr.

Special Considerations: Aspirin is considered Pregnancy Category D.

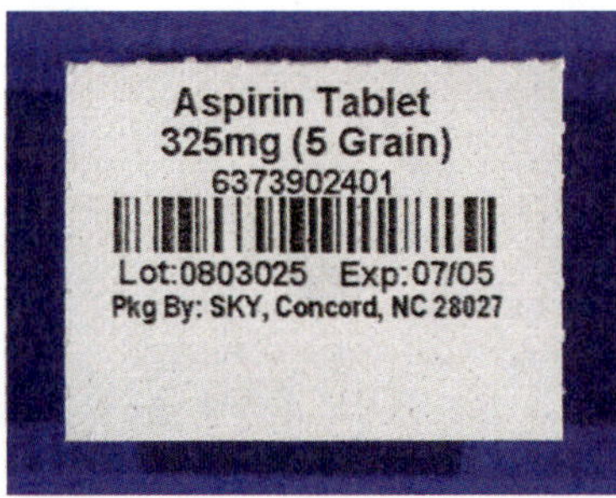

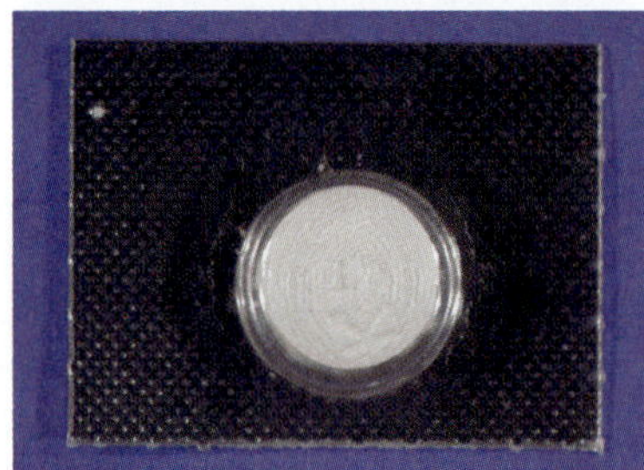

Atenolol (Tenormin)

Classification: Beta-adrenergic, antagonist, antianginal, antihypertensive, class II antiarrhythmic

Action: Inhibits the strength of the heart's contractions and heart rate, resulting in a decrease in cardiac oxygen consumption. Also saturates the beta receptors and inhibits dilation of bronchial smooth muscle ($beta_2$ receptor).

Indications: Acute coronary syndromes (ACS), hypertension, SVT, atrial flutter, AF, migraine prophylaxis.

Adverse Effects: Bradycardia, bronchospasm, hypotension.

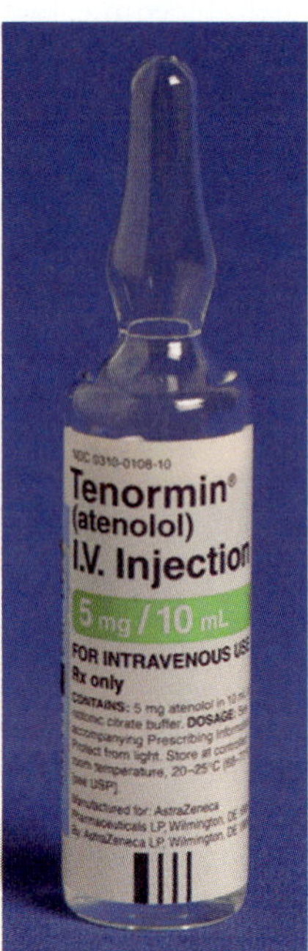

Contraindications: Cardiogenic shock, second- or third-degree atrioventricular (AV) block, severe bradycardia, known sensitivity. Use with caution in hypotension, chronic lung disease (asthma and COPD).

Dosage: ACS:

- Adult: 5 mg IV, IO over a 5-minute period; repeat in 10 minutes.
- Pediatric: Not recommended for pediatric patients.

Special Considerations: Pregnancy Category D.

Atracurium (Tracrium)

Classification: Nondepolarizing neuromuscular blocker

Action: Antagonizes acetylcholine receptors at the motor end plate, producing muscle paralysis.

Indications: Neuromuscular blockade to facilitate ET intubation.

Adverse Effects: Flushing, edema, urticaria, pruritus, bronchospasm and/or wheezing, alterations in heart rate, decrease in blood pressure.

Contraindications: Cardiac disease, electrolyte abnormalities, dehydration, known sensitivity.

Dosage:

- Adult: 0.4 to 0.5 mg/kg IV, IO; repeat with 0.08 to 0.1 mg/kg every 20 to 45 minutes, then every 15 to 25 minutes as needed.
- Pediatric:
  - Older than 2 years: Same as adult dosing.
  - 1 month to 2 years: 0.3 to 0.4 mg/kg IV, IO.

Special Considerations: Do not give by IM injection. Pregnancy Category C.

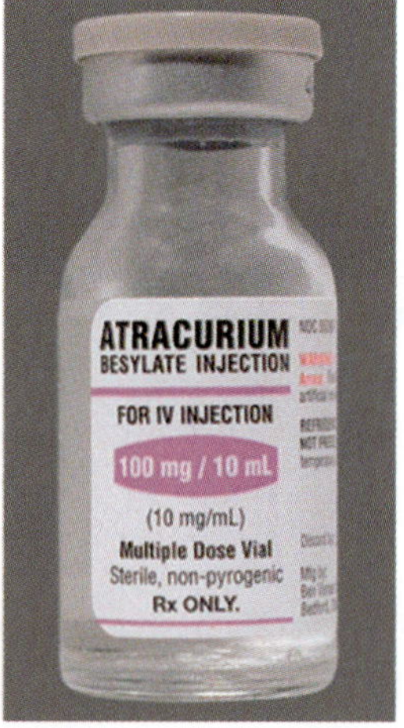

Atropine Sulfate

Classification: Anticholinergic (antimuscarinic)

Action: Competes reversibly with acetylcholine at the site of the muscarinic receptor. Receptors affected (in order from most sensitive to least sensitive) include salivary, bronchial, sweat glands, eye, heart, and GI tract.

Indications: Symptomatic bradycardia, asystole or PEA, nerve agent exposure, organophosphate poisoning.

Adverse Effects: Decreased secretions resulting in dry mouth and hot skin temperature, intense facial flushing, blurred vision or dilation of the pupils with subsequent photophobia, tachycardia, restlessness. Atropine may cause paradoxical bradycardia if the dose administered is too low or if the drug is administered too slowly.

Contraindications: Acute MI, myasthenia gravis, GI obstruction, closed-angle glaucoma, or known sensitivity to atropine, belladonna alkaloids, or sulfites. Will not be effective for infranodal (type II) AV block and new third-degree block with wide QRS complex.

Dosage:

Symptomatic bradycardia:

- Adult: 0.5 mg IV, IO every 3 to 5 minutes to a maximum dose of 3 mg.
- Pediatric: 0.02 mg/kg (minimum 0.1 mg/dose; maximum 0.5 mg/dose) IV, IO, to a total dose of 1 mg.

Asystole/pulseless electrical activity:

- 1 mg IV, IO every 3 to 5 minutes, to a maximum dose of 3 mg. May be administered via ET tube at 2 to 2.5 mg diluted in 5 to 10 mL of water or normal saline.

Nerve agent or organophosphate poisoning:

- Adult: 2 to 4 mg IV, IM; repeat if needed every 20 to 30 minutes until symptoms dissipate. In severe cases, the initial dose can be as large as 2 to 6 mg administered IV. Repeat doses of 2 to 6 mg can be administered IV, IM every 5 to 60 minutes.
- Pediatric: 0.05 mg/kg IV, IM every 10 to 30 minutes as needed until symptoms dissipate.
- Infants <15 lb: 0.05 mg/kg IV, IM every 5 to 20 minutes as needed until symptoms dissipate.

Special Considerations: Half-life 2.5 hours. Pregnancy Category C; possibly unsafe in lactating mothers.

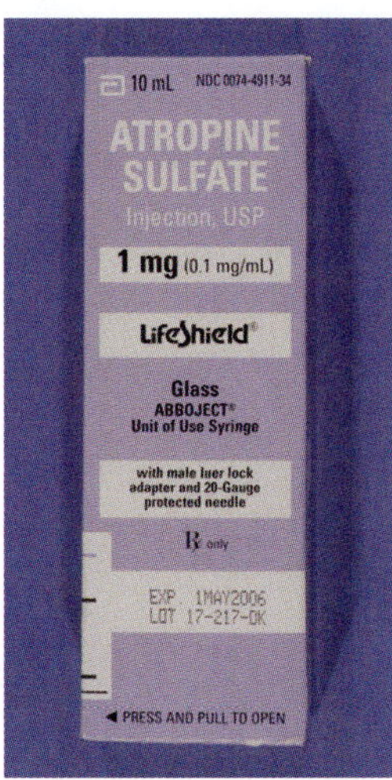

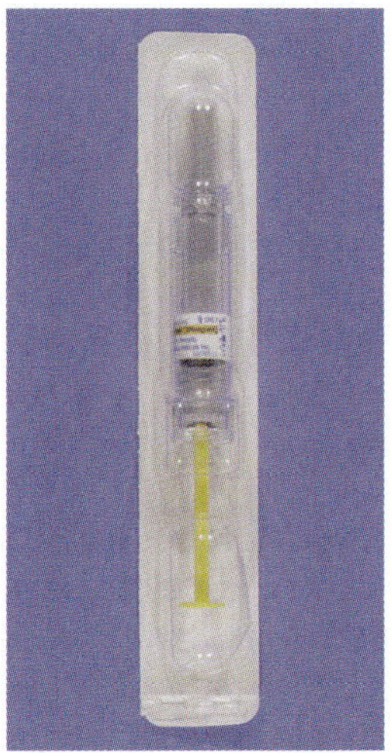

Calcium Gluconate

Classification: Electrolyte solution

Action: Counteracts the toxicity of hyperkalemia by stabilizing the membranes of the cardiac cells, reducing the likelihood of fibrillation.

Indications: Hyperkalemia, hypocalcemia, hypermagnesemia.

Adverse Effects: Soft-tissue necrosis, hypotension, bradycardia (if administered too rapidly).

Contraindications: VF, digitalis toxicity, hypercalcemia.

Dosage: Supplied as 10% solution; therefore each milliliter contains 100 mg of calcium gluconate.

- Adult: 500 to 1000 mg IV, IO administered slowly at a rate of approximately 1 mL/min; maximum dose 200 mg/min IV, IO.
- Pediatric: 60 to 100 mg/kg IV, IO slowly over a 5- to 10-minute period; maximum dose 200 mg/min IV, IO.

Special Considerations: Do not administer by IM or SQ routes, which causes significant tissue necrosis. Pregnancy Category C.

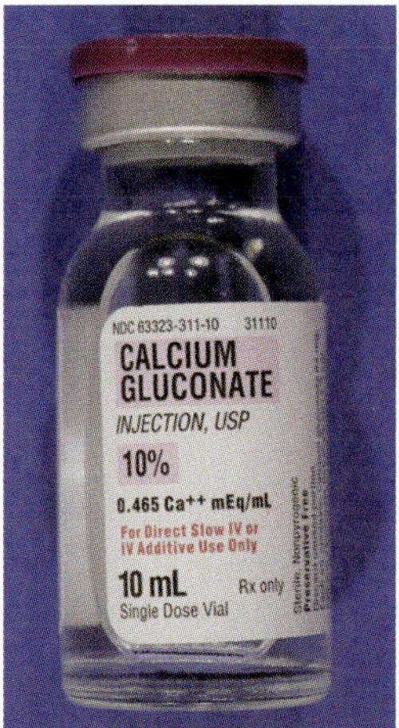

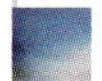

Carbamazepine (Tegretol)

Classification: Anticonvulsant

Action: Decreases the spread of the seizure.

Indications: Partial and generalized tonic-clonic seizures.

Adverse Effects: Dizziness, drowsiness, ataxia, nausea/vomiting, blurred vision, confusion, headache, transient diplopia, visual hallucinations, life-threatening rashes.

Contraindications: AV block, bundle branch block, agranulocytosis, bone marrow suppression, MAOI therapy, hypersensitivity to carbamazepine or tricyclic antidepressants. Use with caution in petit mal, atonic, or myoclonic seizures; liver disease; patients with blood dyscrasia due to drug therapies or blood disorders; patients with a history of cardiac disease; or patients with a history of alcoholism.

Dosage:
- Adult: 200 mg PO every 12 hours.
- Pediatric:
  - 6 to 11 years: 100 mg PO twice daily.
  - Younger than 6 years: 10 to 20 mg/kg/day PO 2 or 3 times per day.

Special Considerations: Pregnancy Category D.

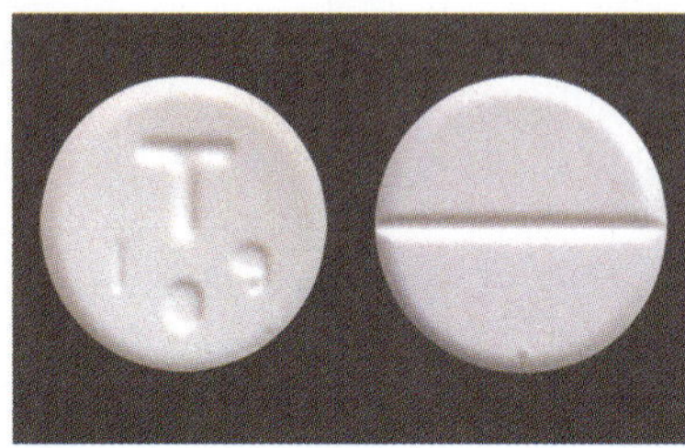

Clopidogrel (Plavix)

Classification: Antiplatelet
Action: Blocks platelet aggregation by antagonizing the GP IIb/IIIa receptors.
Indications: ACS, chronic coronary and vascular disease, ischemic stroke.
Adverse Effects: Nausea, abdominal pain, and hemorrhage.
Contraindications: History of intracranial hemorrhage, GI bleed or trauma, known sensitivity.
Dosage:

Unstable angina pectoris or non–Q wave acute myocardial infarction:
- Adult: Single loading dose of 300 to 600 mg PO followed by a daily dose of 75 mg PO.
- Pediatric: Not recommended for pediatric patients.

Special Considerations: Pregnancy Category B.

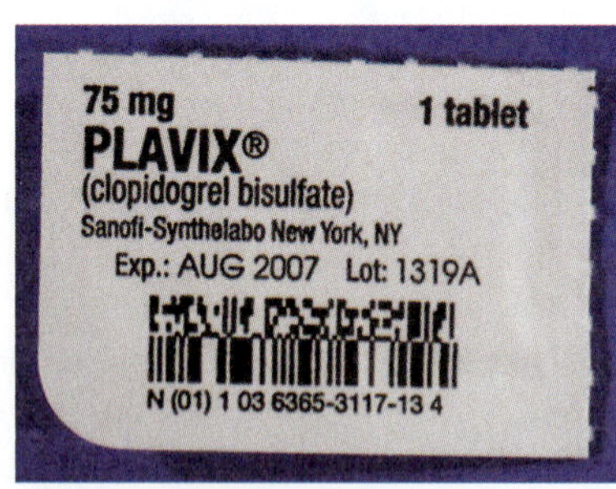

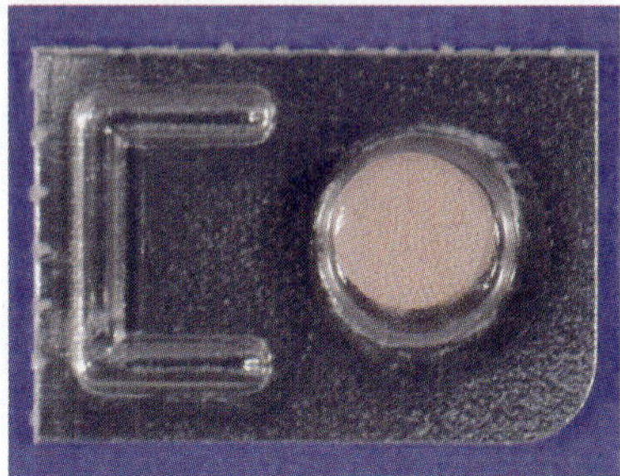

Dexamethasone (Decadron)

Classification: Corticosteroid
Action: Reduces inflammation and immune responses.
Indications: Various inflammatory conditions, adrenal insufficiency, nonresponsive forms of shock.
Adverse Effects: Nausea/vomiting, edema, hypertension, hyperglycemia, immunosuppression.
Contraindications: Fungal infections, known sensitivity.
Dosage:
- Adult: 0.75 to 6 mg/kg/day IV to a maximum dose of 40 mg, depending on indication.
- Pediatric: 0.02 to 0.3 mg/kg IV, IO divided into doses every 6 hours.

Special Considerations: Pregnancy Category C.

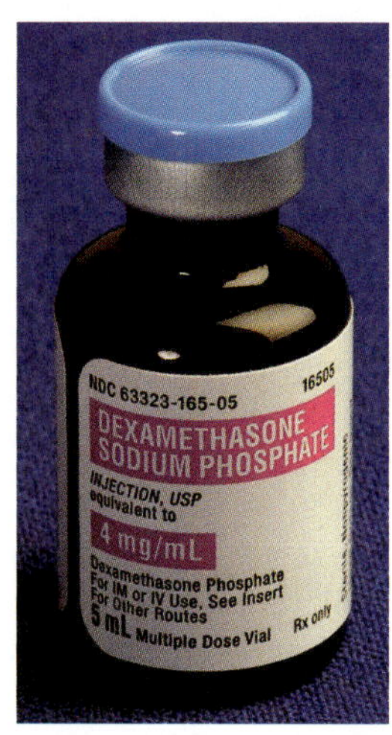

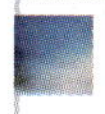

Dextrose (Dextrose 50%, Dextrose 25%, Dextrose 10%)

Classification: Antihypoglycemic
Action: Increases blood glucose concentrations.
Indications: Hypoglycemia
Adverse Effects: Hyperglycemia, warmth, burning from IV infusion. Concentrated solutions may cause pain and thrombosis of the peripheral veins.
Contraindications: Intracranial and intraspinal hemorrhage, delirium tremens, solution is not clear, seals are not intact.
Dosage:

Hyperkalemia:
- Adult: 25 g of dextrose 50% IV, IO.
- Pediatric: 0.5 to 1 g/kg IV, IO.

Hypoglycemia:
- Adult: 10 to 25 g of dextrose 50% IV (20 to 50 mL of dextrose solution).

- Pediatric:
  - >6 months: 2 mL/kg of dextrose 25%.
  - Infants <6 months: 2 to 4 mL/kg of dextrose 10%.

Special Considerations: Pregnancy Category C.

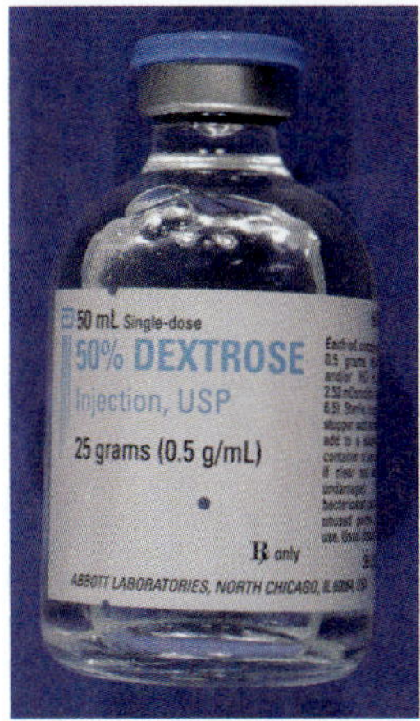

Diazepam (Valium)

Classification: Benzodiazepine, Schedule C-IV

Action: Binds to the benzodiazepine receptor and enhances the effects of GABA. Benzodiazepines act at the level of the limbic, thalamic, and hypothalamic regions of the CNS and can produce any level of CNS depression required (including sedation, skeletal muscle relaxation, and anticonvulsant activity).

Indications: Anxiety, skeletal muscle relaxation, alcohol withdrawal, seizures.

Adverse Effects: Respiratory depression, drowsiness, fatigue, headache, pain at the injection site, confusion, nausea, hypotension, oversedation.

Contraindications: Children younger than 6 months, acute-angle glaucoma, CNS depression, alcohol intoxication, known sensitivity.

Dosage:

Anxiety:

- Adult:
  - Moderate: 2 to 5 mg slow IV, IM.
  - Severe: 5 to 10 mg slow IV, IM (administer no faster than 5 mg/min).
  - Low: Low dosages are often required for elderly or debilitated patients.
- Pediatric: 0.04 to 0.3 mg/kg/dose IV, IM every 4 hours to a maximum dose of 0.6 mg/kg.

Delirium tremens from acute alcohol withdrawal:

- Adult: 10 mg IV

Seizure:

- Adult: 5 to 10 mg slow IV, IO every 10 to 15 minutes; maximum total dose 30 mg.
- Pediatric:
  - IV, IO:
    - 5 years and older: 1 mg over a 3-minute period every 2 to 5 minutes to a maximum total dose of 10 mg.
    - Older than 30 days to younger than 5 years: 0.2 to 0.5 mg over a 3-minute period; may repeat every 2 to 5 minutes to a maximum total dose of 5 mg.
    - Neonate: 0.15 to 0.5 mg/kg/dose given over a 3- to 5-minute period; may repeat every 15 to 30 minutes to a maximum total dose of 2 mg. (Not a first-line agent due to sodium benzoic acid in the injection.)
  - Rectal administration: If vascular access is not obtained, diazepam may be administered rectally to children.
    - 12 years and older: 0.2 mg/kg.
    - 6 to 11 years: 0.3 mg/kg.
    - 2 to 5 years: 0.5 mg/kg.
    - Younger than 2 years: Not recommended.

Special Considerations: Make sure that IV, IO lines are well secured. Extravasation of diazepam causes tissue necrosis. Diazepam is insoluble in water and must be dissolved in propylene glycol. This produces a viscous solution; give slowly to prevent pain on injection. Pregnancy Category D.

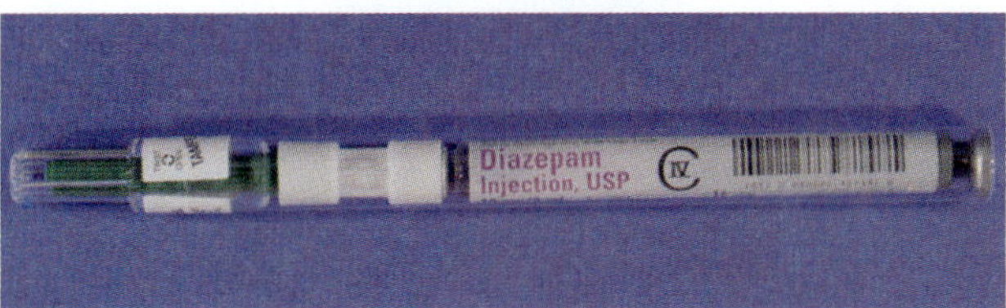

Digoxin (Lanoxin)

Classification: Cardiac glycoside

Action: Inhibits sodium-potassium-adenosine triphosphatase membrane pump, resulting in an increase in calcium inside the heart muscle cell, which causes an increase in the force of contraction of the heart.

Indications: CHF, to control the ventricular rate in chronic AF and atrial flutter, narrow-complex PSVT.

Adverse Effects: Headache, weakness, GI disturbances, arrhythmias, nausea/vomiting, diarrhea, vision disturbances.

Contraindications: Digitalis allergy, VT and VF, heart block, sick sinus syndrome, tachycardia without heart failure, pulse lower than 50 to 60 beats/min, MI, ischemic heart disease, patients with preexcitation AF or atrial flutter (i.e., a delta wave, characteristic of Wolff-Parkinson-White syndrome, visible during normal sinus rhythm), electrolyte imbalances.

Dosage: Dosage is individualized.

Special Considerations: Low levels of serum potassium can lead to digoxin toxicity and bradycardia. Conditions such as administration of steroids or diuretics or vomiting and diarrhea can produce low levels of potassium and subsequent digoxin toxicity. Pregnancy Category C.

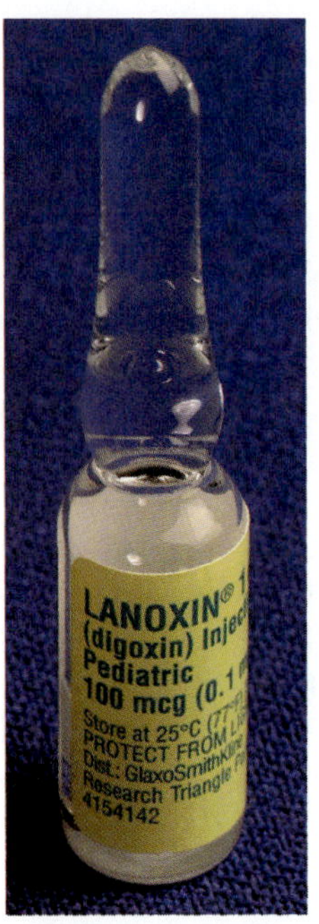

Diltiazem (Cardizem)

Classification: Calcium channel blocker, class IV antiarrhythmic

Action: Blocks calcium from moving into the heart muscle cell, which prolongs the conduction of electrical impulses through the AV node.

Indications: Ventricular rate control in rapid AF.

Adverse Effects: Flushing; headache; bradycardia; hypotension; heart block; myocardial depression; severe AV block; and, at high doses, cardiac arrest.

Contraindications: Hypotension, heart block, heart failure.

Dosage:

- Adult: Optimum dose is 0.25 mg/kg IV, IO over a 2-minute period to control rapid AF; 20 mg is a reasonable dose for the average adult patient. A second, higher dose of 0.35 mg/kg IV, IO (25 mg is a typical second dose) may be administered over a 2-minute period if rate control is not obtained with the lower dose. For continued reduction in heart rate, a continuous infusion can be started at a dose range of 5 to 15 mg/hr.
- Pediatric: Not recommended for pediatric patients.

Special Considerations: Use with extreme caution in patients who are taking beta-blockers because these two drug classes potentiate each other's effects and toxicities. Use reduced dosage and/or slow rate of infusion. Patients with a history of heart failure and heart block are at a higher risk for toxicity. Pregnancy Category C.

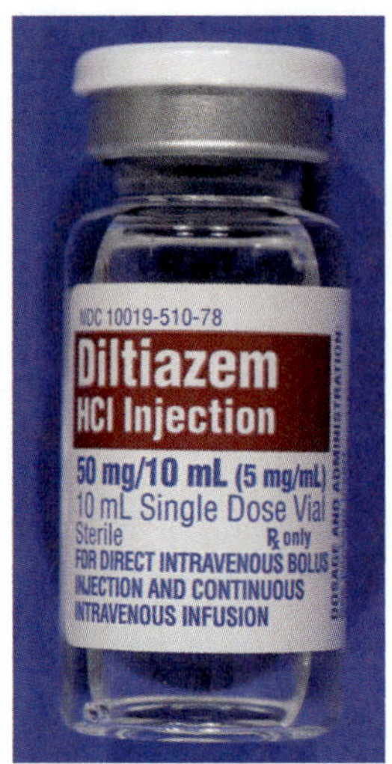

Diphenhydramine Hydrochloride (Benadryl)

Classification: Antihistamine

Action: Binds and blocks H_1 histamine receptors.

Indications: Anaphylactic reactions

Adverse Effects: Drowsiness, dizziness, headache, excitable state (children), wheezing, thickening of bronchial secretions, chest tightness, palpitations, hypotension, blurred vision, dry mouth, nausea/vomiting, diarrhea.

Contraindications: Acute asthma, which thickens secretions; patients with cardiac histories; known sensitivity.

Dosage:

- Adult: 25 to 50 mg IV, IO, IM.
- Pediatric: 2 to 12 years: 1 to 1.25 mg/kg IV, IO, IM.

Special Considerations: Pregnancy Category B.

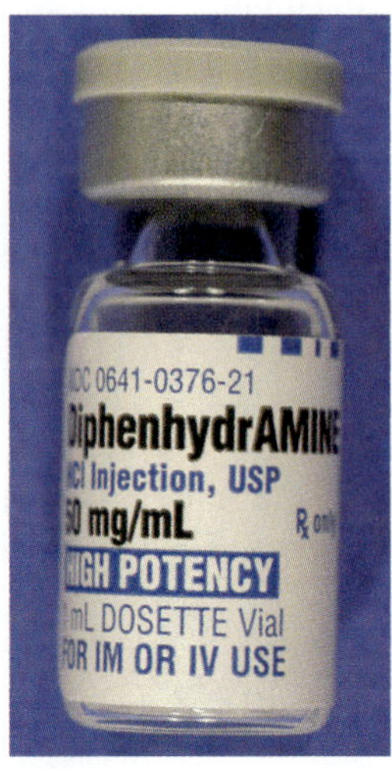

Dobutamine (Dobutrex)

Classification: Adrenergic agent

Action: Acts primarily as an agonist at $beta_1$ adrenergic receptors with minor $beta_2$ and $alpha_1$ effects. Consequently, dobutamine increases myocardial contractility and stroke volume with minor chronotropic effects, resulting in increased cardiac output.

Indications: CHF, cardiogenic shock.

Adverse Effects: Tachycardia, PVCs, hypertension, hypotension, palpitations, arrhythmias.

Contraindications: Suspected or known poisoning/drug-induced shock, systolic blood pressure <100 mm Hg with signs of shock, idiopathic hypertrophic subaortic stenosis, known sensitivity (including sulfites). Use with caution in hypertension, recent MI, arrhythmias, hypovolemia.

Dosage:

- Adult: 2 to 20 mcg/kg/min IV, IO. At doses >20 mcg/kg/min, increases of heart rate of >10% may induce or exacerbate myocardial ischemia.
- Pediatric: Same as adult dosing.

Special Considerations: Half-life 2 minutes. Pregnancy Category B.

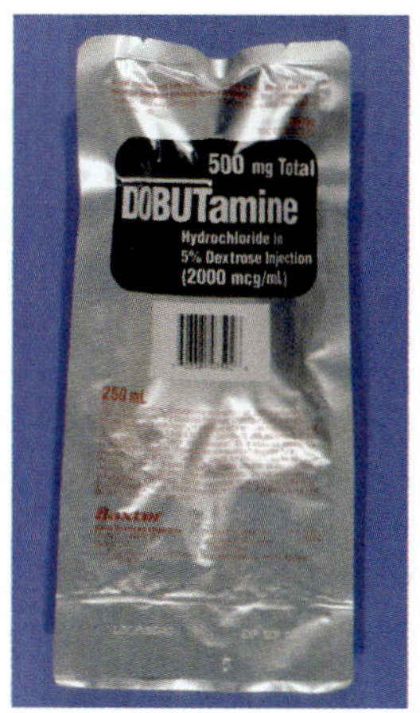

Dolasetron (Anzemet)

Classification: Antiemetic

Action: Prevents/reduces nausea/vomiting by binding and blocking a receptor for the brain chemical serotonin.

Indications: Prevent and treat nausea/vomiting.

Adverse Effects: Headache, fatigue, diarrhea, dizziness, abdominal pain, hypotension, hypertension, ECG changes (prolonged PR and QT intervals, widened QRS), bradycardia, tachycardia, syncope.

Contraindications: Known sensitivity. Use with caution in hypokalemia, hypomagnesemia, cardiac arrhythmias.

Dosage:

- Adult: 12.5 mg IV, IO.
- Pediatric: 2 to 16 years: 0.35 mg/kg IV, IO (max dose: 12.5 mg).

Special Considerations: Pregnancy Category B.

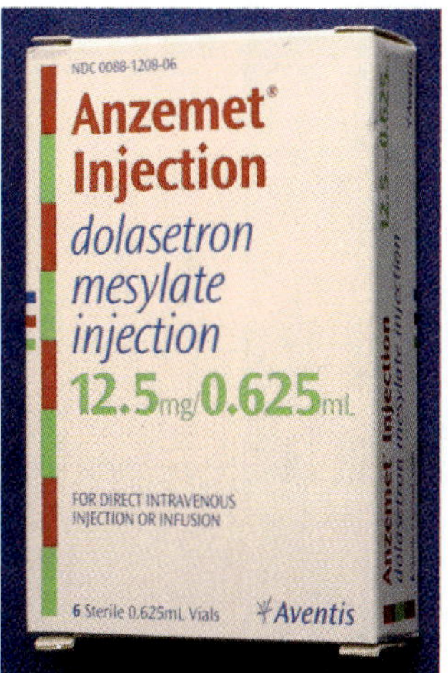

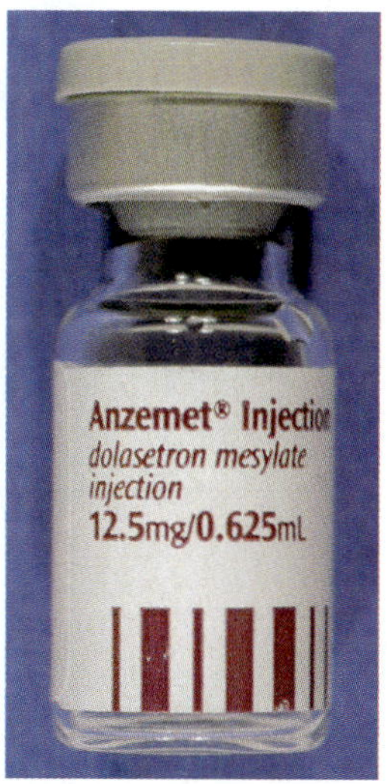

Dopamine (Intropin)

Classification: Adrenergic agonist, inotropic, vasopressor

Action: Stimulates alpha- and beta-adrenergic receptors. At moderate doses (2 to 10 mcg/kg/min), dopamine stimulates $beta_1$ receptors, resulting in inotropy and increased cardiac output while maintaining dopaminergic-induced vasodilatory effects. At high doses (>10 mcg/kg/min), alpha-adrenergic agonism predominates, and increased peripheral vascular resistance and vasoconstriction result.

Indications: Hypotension and decreased cardiac output associated with cardiogenic shock and septic shock, hypotension after return of spontaneous circulation following cardiac arrest, symptomatic bradycardia unresponsive to atropine.

Adverse Effects: Tachycardia, arrhythmias, skin and soft-tissue necrosis, severe hypertension from excessive vasoconstriction, angina, dyspnea, headache, nausea/vomiting.

Contraindications: Pheochromocytoma, VF, VT, or other ventricular arrhythmias, known sensitivity (including sulfites). Correct any hypovolemia with volume fluid replacement before administering dopamine.

Dosage:

- Adult: 2 to 20 mcg/kg/min IV, IO infusion. Starting dose 5 mcg/kg/min; may gradually increase the infusion by 5 to 10 mcg/kg/min to desired effect. Cardiac dose is usually 5 to 10 mcg/kg/min; vasopressor dose is usually 10 to 20 mcg/kg/min. Little benefit is gained beyond 20 mcg/kg/min.
- Pediatric: Same as adult dosing.

Special Considerations: Half-life 2 minutes. Pregnancy Category C.

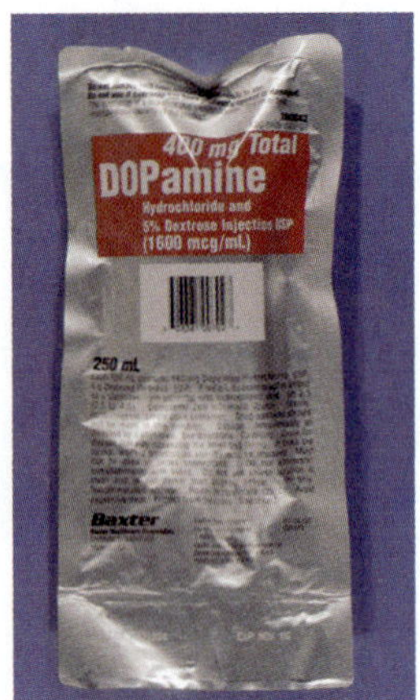

 Enoxaparin (Lovenox, Klexane)

Classification: Parenteral anticoagulant

Action: Isolated from standard heparin, this is a low-molecular-weight form which has a longer duration of action. It blocks factors Xa and IIa, with overall reduction of thrombin.

Indications: Prophylaxis and treatment of venous thrombosis or pulmonary embolus. Prophylaxis for any patient at risk for venous thrombosis event, especially those with procedures that may inhibit lower-extremity movement, and those with arrhythmia or venous thrombosis associated with acute coronary syndrome or unstable angina.

Adverse Effects: Pain at injection site. Increased risk of bleeding in tissues and organs. Thrombocytopenia.

Contraindications: In those with sensitivity to the drug (multidose formulation), heparin, or pork products. Known hypersensitivity to benzyl alcohol. Contraindicated in active major bleeding or in those with thrombocytopenia.

Dosage: For prophylaxis, 30 mg SQ every 12 hours or 40 mg SQ per day for 1 to 2 weeks. For treatment, 1 mg/kg every 12 hours or 1.5 mg/kg/day. In acute coronary syndrome, 1 mg/kg every 12 hours for 2 to 8 days.

Special Considerations: Efficacy of this drug may be reduced in obese patients, and dosage will need to be increased. There is an increased risk for bleeding in those with renal failure, and dosages should be reduced. This drug has been rated Pregnancy Category B for use in all trimesters of pregnancy. Therapy may be guided by antifactor Xa levels, but APTT, PT/INR laboratory analysis is not helpful.

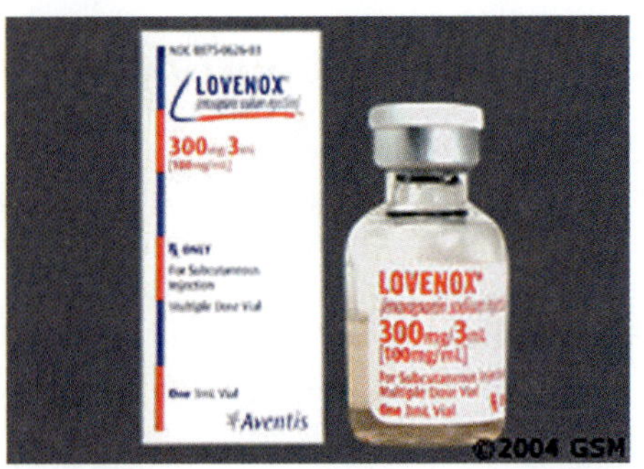

 Epinephrine

Classification: Adrenergic agent, inotropic

Action: Binds strongly with both alpha and beta receptors, producing increased blood pressure, increased heart rate, bronchodilation.

Indications: Bronchospasm, allergic and anaphylactic reactions, restoration of cardiac activity in cardiac arrest.

Adverse Effects: Anxiety, headache, cardiac arrhythmias, hypertension, nervousness, tremors, chest pain, nausea/vomiting.

Contraindications: Arrhythmias other than VF, asystole, PEA; cardiovascular disease; hypertension; cerebrovascular disease; shock secondary to causes other than anaphylactic shock; closed-angle glaucoma; diabetes; pregnant women in active labor; known sensitivity to epinephrine or sulfites.

Dosage:

Cardiac arrest:

- Adult: 1 mg (1:10,000 solution) IV, IO; may repeat every 3 to 5 minutes.
- Pediatric: 0.01 mg/kg (1:10,000 solution) IV, IO; repeat every 3 to 5 minutes as needed (max dose: 1 mg).

Symptomatic bradycardia:

- Adult: 1 mcg/min (1:10,000 solution) as a continuous IV infusion; usual dosage range: 2 to 10 mcg/min IV; titrate to effect.
- Pediatric: 0.01 mg/kg (1:10,000 solution) IV, IO; may repeat every 3 to 5 minutes (max dose: 1 mg). If giving epinephrine by ET tube, administer 0.1 mg/kg.

Asthma attacks and certain allergic reactions:

- Adult: 0.3 to 0.5 mg (1:1000 solution) IM or SQ; may repeat every 10 to 15 minutes (max dose: 1 mg).
- Pediatric: 0.01 mg/kg (1:1000 solution) IM or SQ (max dose: 0.5 mg).

Anaphylactic shock:

- Adult: 0.1 to 0.3 mg (1:10,000 solution) IV slowly over 5 minutes, or IV infusion of 1 to 4 mcg/min, titrated to effect.

- Pediatric: Continuous IV infusion rate of 0.1 to 1 mcg/kg/min (1:10,000 solution); titrate to response.

Special Considerations: Half-life 1 minute. Pregnancy Category C.

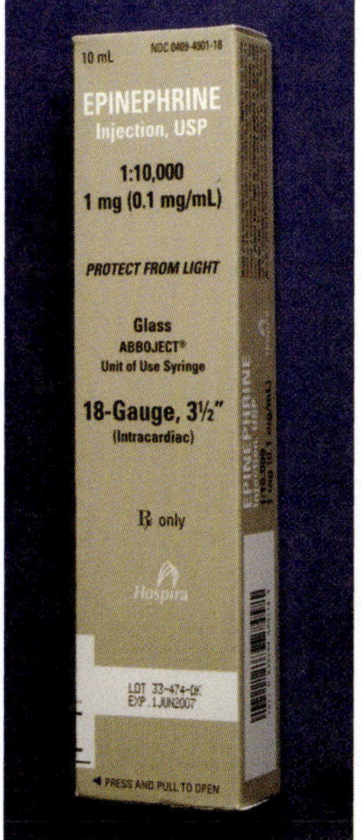

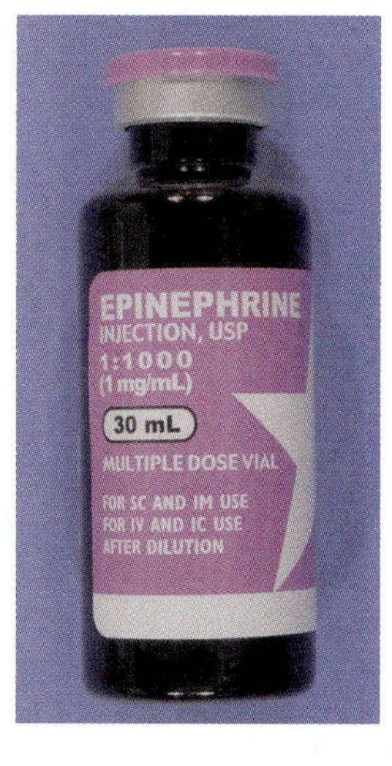

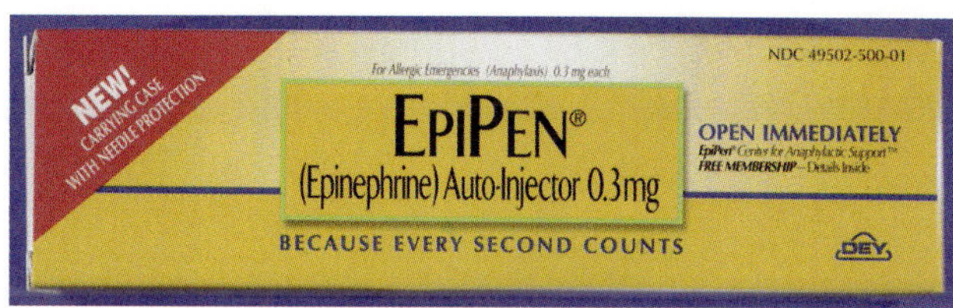

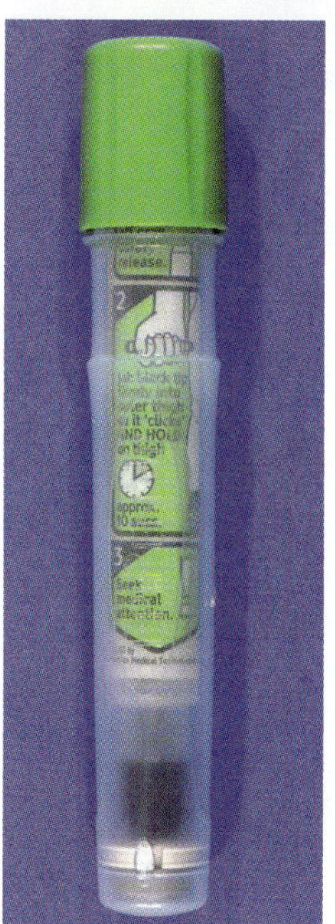

Epinephrine Autoinjectors (EpiPen, EpiPen Jr)

Classification: Adrenergic agonist, inotropic

Action: Binds strongly with both alpha and beta receptors, producing increased blood pressure, increased heart rate, bronchodilation.

Indications: Anaphylactic shock, certain allergic reactions, asthma attacks.

Adverse Effects: Headaches, nervousness, tremors, arrhythmias, hypertension, chest pain, nausea/vomiting.

Contraindications: Arrhythmias other than VF, asystole, PEA; cardiovascular disease; hypertension; cerebrovascular disease; shock secondary to causes other than anaphylactic shock; closed-angle glaucoma; diabetes; pregnant women in active labor; known sensitivity to epinephrine or sulfites.

Dosage:

- Adult: An EpiPen contains 0.3 mg epinephrine to be administered IM into the anterolateral thigh area.
- Pediatric: For children weighing > 30 kg, an EpiPen Jr delivers 0.15 mg IM.

Special Considerations: Half-life 1 minute. Pregnancy Category C.

Eptifibatide (Integrilin)

Classification: GP IIb/IIIa inhibitor

Action: Prevents the aggregation of platelets by binding to the GP IIb/IIIa receptor.

Indications: UA/NSTEMI—to manage medically and for those undergoing PCI.

Adverse Effects: Bleeding from the GI tract, internal bleeding, intracranial hemorrhage, hypotension, stroke, anaphylactic shock.

Contraindications: Bleeding from any source, severe uncontrolled hypertension, surgery or trauma within the previous 6 weeks, stroke within the previous 30 days, renal failure, thrombocytopenia.

Dosage:

- Adult: Loading dose: 180 mcg/kg IV, IO (max dose: 22.6 mg) over 1 to 2 minutes, then 2 mcg/kg/min IV, IO infusion (max dose: 15 mg/hr). Dose is decreased with renal impairment.
- Pediatric: No current dosing recommendations exist for pediatric patients.

Special Considerations: Half-life approximately 90 to 120 minutes. Pregnancy Category B.

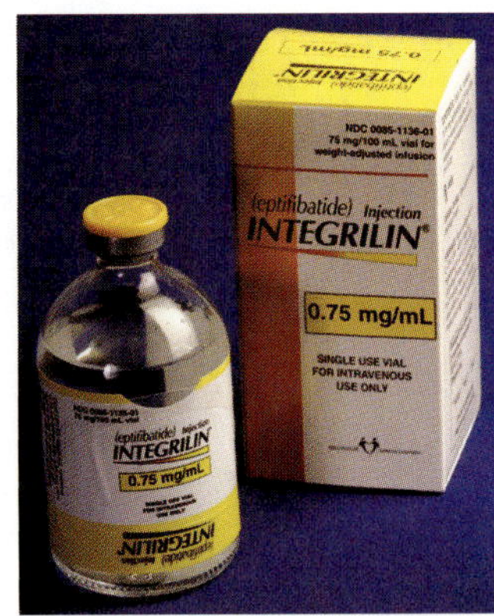

Esmolol (Brevibloc)

Classification: Beta-adrenergic antagonist, class II antiarrhythmic

Action: Inhibits the strength of the heart's contractions, as well as heart rate, resulting in a decrease in cardiac oxygen consumption.

Indications: ACS, MI, acute hypertension, supraventricular tachyarrhythmias, thyrotoxicosis.

Adverse Effects: Hypotension, sinus bradycardia, AV block, cardiac arrest, nausea/vomiting, hypoglycemia, injection site reaction.

Contraindications: Acute bronchospasm, COPD, second- or third-degree heart block, bradycardia, cardiogenic shock, pulmonary edema, sick sinus syndrome, known sensitivity. Use with caution in patients with pheochromocytoma, Prinzmetal's angina, cerebrovascular disease, stroke, poorly controlled diabetes mellitus, hyperthyroidism, thyrotoxicosis, renal disease.

Dosage:

- Adult: 500 mcg/kg (0.5 mg/kg) IV, IO over a 1-minute period, followed by a 50-mcg/kg/min (0.05 mg/kg) infusion over a 4-minute period (maximum total: 200 mcg/kg). If patient response is inadequate, administer a second bolus 500 mcg/kg (0.5 mg/kg) over a 1-minute period, and then increase infusion to 100 mcg/kg/min. Maximum infusion rate: 300 mcg/kg/min.
- Pediatric: Not approved for pediatric patients.

Special Considerations: Half-life 5 to 9 minutes. Any adverse effects caused by administration of esmolol are brief because of the drug's short half-life. Resolution of effects usually within 10 to 20 minutes. Pregnancy Category C.

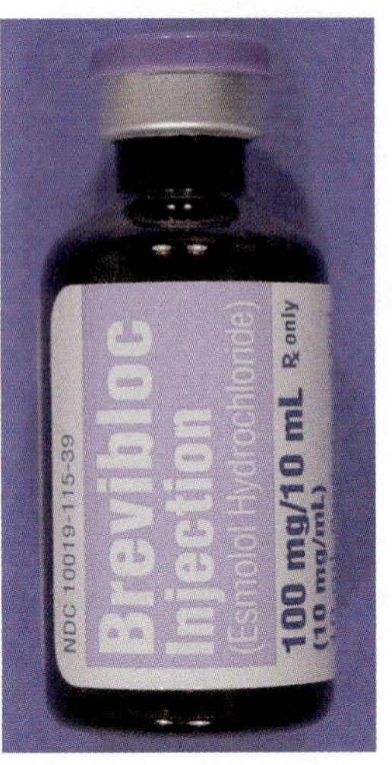

Etomidate (Amidate)

Classification: Hypnotic, anesthesia induction agent

Action: Although the exact mechanism is unknown, etomidate appears to have GABA-like effects.

Indications: Induction for rapid sequence intubation and pharmacologic-assisted intubation, induction of anesthesia.

Adverse Effects: Hypotension, respiratory depression, pain at the site of injection, temporary involuntary muscle movements, frequent nausea/vomiting on emergence, adrenal insufficiency, hyperventilation, hypoventilation, apnea of short duration, hiccups, laryngospasm, snoring, tachypnea, hypertension, cardiac arrhythmias.

Contraindications: Known sensitivity. Use in pregnancy only if the potential benefits justify the potential risk to the fetus. Do not use during labor, and avoid in nursing mothers.

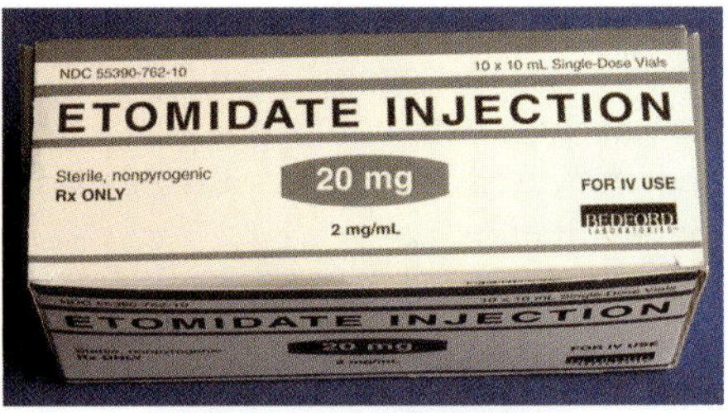

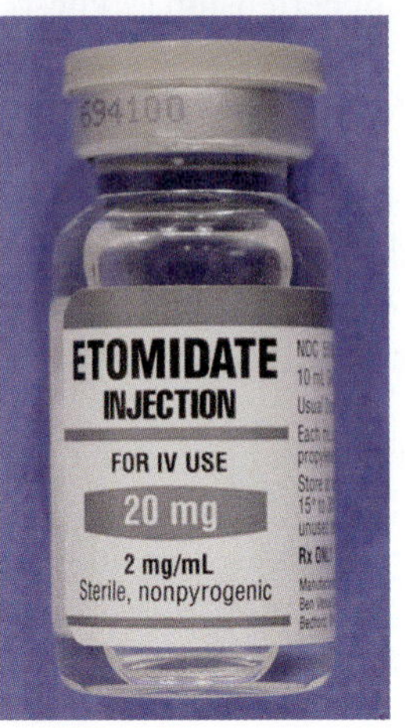

Dosage:
- Adult: 0.3 mg/kg slow IV, IO (over 30 to 60 seconds). A typical adult intubating dose of etomidate is 20 mg slow IV. Consider less (e.g., 10 mg) in the elderly or patients with cardiac conditions.
- Pediatric: Use with extreme caution in those pediatric patients in septic shock.
  - Older than 10 years: Same as adult dosing.
  - Younger than 10 years: Safety has not been established.

Special Considerations: Etomidate is used to prepare a patient for orotracheal intubation. Both personnel and equipment must be present to manage the patient's airway before administration. Pregnancy Category C.

Felbamate (Felbatol)

Classification: Anticonvulsant

Action: Although the mechanism of action is not known, it is believed that felbamate antagonizes the effects of glycine, increases the seizure threshold in absence seizures, and prevents the spread of generalized tonic-clonic and partial seizures.

Indications: Partial seizures with and without generalization in epileptic adults; partial and generalized seizures associated with Lennox-Gastaut syndrome in children.

Adverse Effects: Nausea/vomiting, suicidal ideation and behavior, depression, insomnia, dyspepsia, upper respiratory tract infection, fatigue, headache, constipation, diarrhea, rhinitis, anxiety, aplastic anemia.

Contraindications: Blood dyscrasias, hepatic disease, known sensitivity to carbamates.

Dosage: Should be individualized based on condition.

Special Considerations: Pregnancy Category C.

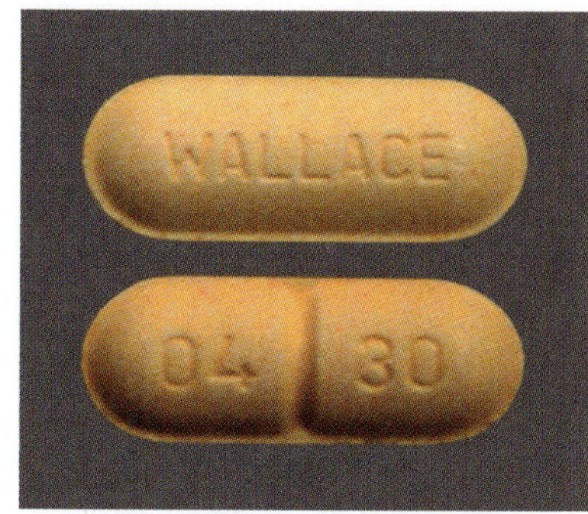

Fentanyl Citrate (Sublimaze)

Classification: Narcotic analgesic, Schedule C-II

Action: Binds to opiate receptors, producing analgesia and euphoria.

Indications: Pain

Adverse Effects: Respiratory depression, apnea, hypotension, nausea/vomiting, dizziness, sedation, euphoria, sinus bradycardia, sinus tachycardia, palpitations, hypertension, diaphoresis, syncope, pain at injection site.

Contraindications: Known sensitivity. Use with caution in traumatic brain injury, respiratory depression.

Dosage: Note: Dosage should be individualized.
- Adult: 50 to 100 mcg/dose (0.05 to 0.1 mg) IM or slow IV, IO (administered over 1 to 2 minutes).
- Pediatric: 1 to 2 mcg/kg IM or slow IV, IO (administered over 1 to 2 minutes).

Special Considerations: Pregnancy Category B.

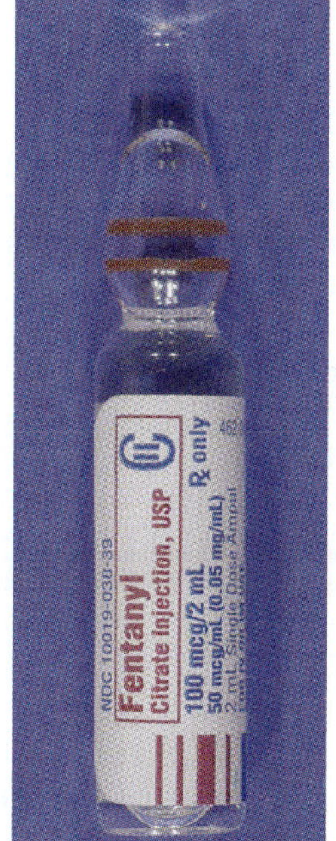

Fibrinolytics: Tissue Plasminogen Activator (tPA), Streptokinase (Streptase, Kabikinase), Reteplase (Retavase), Tenecteplase (TNKase)

Classification: Thrombolytic agent

Action: Dissolves thrombi plugs in the coronary arteries and reestablishes blood flow.

Indications: ST-segment elevation (≥1 mm in two or more contiguous leads), new or presumed new left bundle branch block.

Adverse Effects: Bleeding, intracranial hemorrhage, stroke, cardiac arrhythmias, hypotension, bruising.

Contraindications: ST-segment depression, cardiogenic shock, recent (within 10 days) major surgery, cerebrovascular disease, recent (within 10 days) GI bleeding, recent trauma, hypertension (systolic blood pressure

≥180 mm Hg or diastolic blood pressure ≥110 mm Hg), high likelihood of left heart thrombus, acute pericarditis, subacute bacterial endocarditis, severe renal or liver failure with bleeding complications, significant liver dysfunction, diabetic hemorrhagic retinopathy, septic thrombophlebitis, advanced age (>75 years), patients taking warfarin (Coumadin).

Dosage: Dosing per medical direction.

Special Considerations: Pregnancy Category C.

Flumazenil (Romazicon)

Classification: Benzodiazepine receptor antagonist, antidote

Action: Competes with benzodiazepines for binding at the benzodiazepine receptor, reverses the sedative effects of benzodiazepines.

Indication: Benzodiazepine oversedation

Adverse Effects: Resedation, seizures, dizziness, pain at injection site, nausea/vomiting, diaphoresis, headache, visual impairment.

Contraindications: Cyclic antidepressant overdose; life-threatening conditions that require treatment with benzodiazepines, such as status epilepticus and intracranial hypertension; known sensitivity to flumazenil or benzodiazepines. Use with caution where there is the possibility of unrecognized benzodiazepine dependence and in patients who have a history of substance abuse or who are known substance abusers.

Dosage:

- Adult: Initial dose is 0.2 mg IV, IO over a 15-second period. If the desired effect is not observed after 45 seconds, administer a second 0.2-mg dose, again over a 15-second period. Doses can be repeated a total of 4 times until a total dose of 1 mg has been administered.
- Pediatric: Children older than 1 year, 0.01 mg/kg IV, IO given over a 15-second period. May repeat in 45 seconds and then every minute to a maximum cumulative dose of 0.05 mg/kg or 1 mg, whichever is the lower dose.

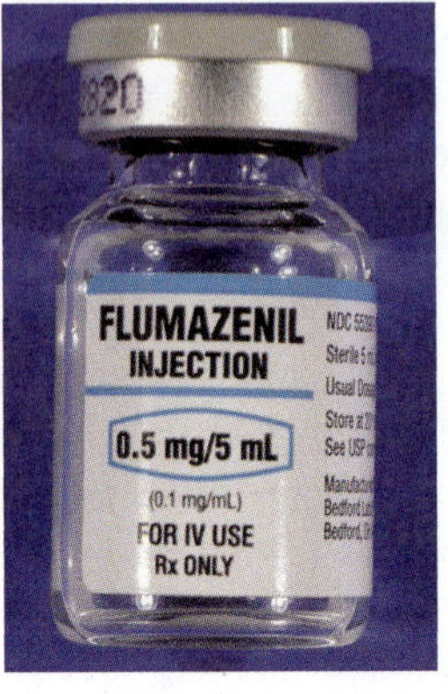

Special Considerations: Monitor for signs of hypoventilation and hypoxia for approximately 2 hours. If the half-life of the benzodiazepine is longer than flumazenil, an additional dose may be needed. May precipitate withdrawal symptoms in patients dependent on benzodiazepines. Flumazenil has not been shown to benefit patients who have overdosed on multiple drugs. Pregnancy Category C.

Fosphenytoin (Cerebyx)

Classification: Anticonvulsant

Action: Alters the movement of sodium and calcium into nervous tissue and prevents the spread of seizure activity.

Indications: Partial and generalized seizures, status epilepticus, seizure prophylaxis.

Adverse Effects: Fosphenytoin can cause several adverse effects often related to drug dose, including sedation, nystagmus, tremors, ataxia, hypertension, dysarthria, gingival hypertrophy, hirsutism, and facial coarsening. Too-rapid administration can cause hypotension.

Contraindications: Bradycardia, bundle branch blocks, agranulocytosis, Adams-Stokes syndrome, hydantoin hypersensitivity.

Dosage: The dose and concentration of fosphenytoin are expressed in PE to simplify the conversion between phenytoin and fosphenytoin.

- Adult: The usual loading dose of fosphenytoin is 10 to 20 mg PE/kg IV, not to exceed 150 mg PE/min IV rate.
- Pediatric: The usual loading dose of fosphenytoin is 10 to 20 mg PE/kg IV, not to exceed 3 mg PE/kg/min (max dose: 150 mg PE/min) IV rate.

Special Considerations: Pregnancy Category D. Compatible with breast-feeding.

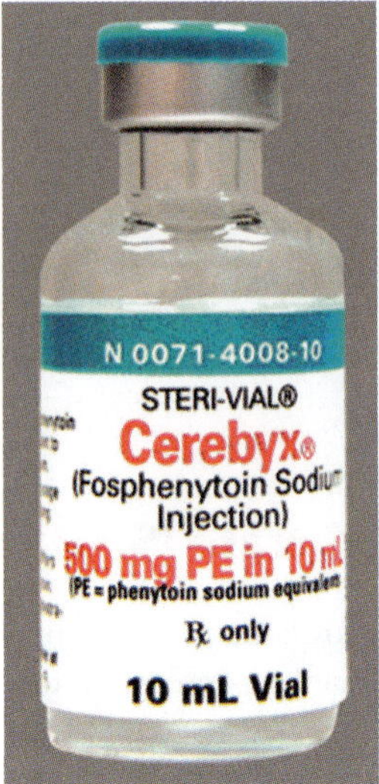

Furosemide (Lasix)

Classification: Loop diuretic

Action: Inhibits the absorption of the sodium and chloride ions and water in the loop of Henle, as well as the convoluted tubule of the nephron. This results in decreased absorption of water and increased production of urine.

Indications: Pulmonary edema, CHF, hypertensive emergency.

Adverse Effects: Vertigo, dizziness, weakness, orthostatic hypotension, hypokalemia, thrombophlebitis. Patients with anuria, severe renal failure, untreated hepatic coma, increasing azotemia, and electrolyte depletion can develop life-threatening consequences.

Contraindications: Known sensitivity to sulfonamides or furosemide.

Dosage:

Congestive heart failure and pulmonary edema:

- Adult: 40 mg IV, IO administered slowly over a 1- to 2-minute period. If a satisfactory response is not achieved within 1 hour, an additional dose of 80 mg can be given. A maximum single IV dose is 160 to 200 mg.
- Pediatric: 1 mg/kg IV, IO, or IM. If the response is not satisfactory, an additional dose of 2 mg/kg may be administered no sooner than 2 hours after the first dose.

Hypertensive emergency:

- Adult: 40 to 80 mg IV, IO.
- Pediatric: 1 mg/kg IV or IM.

Special Considerations: Onset of action for IV, IO administration occurs within 5 minutes and will peak within 30 minutes. Furosemide is a diuretic, so the patient will likely have urinary urgency. Be prepared to help the patient void. Pregnancy Category C.

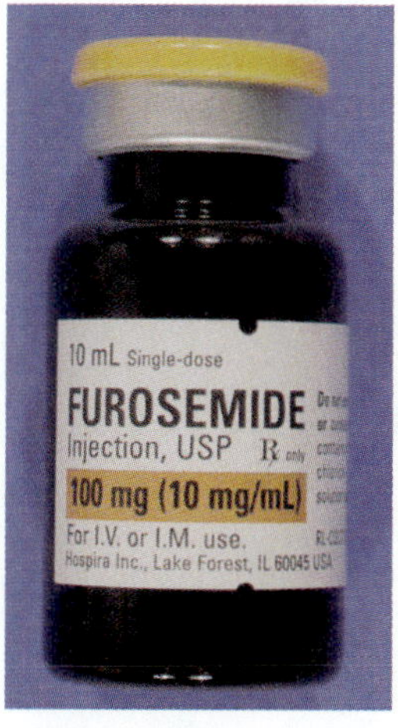

Glucagon

Classification: Hormone

Action: Converts glycogen to glucose.

Indications: Hypoglycemia, beta-blocker overdose.

Adverse Effects: Nausea/vomiting, rebound hyperglycemia, hypotension, sinus tachycardia.

Contraindications: Pheochromocytoma, insulinoma, known sensitivity.

Dosage:

Hypoglycemia:

- Adult: 1 mg IM, IV, IO, or SQ.
- Pediatric (<20 kg): 0.5 mg IM, IV, IO, or SQ.

Beta-blocker overdose:

- Adult: 5 to 10 mg IV, IO over a 1-minute period, followed by a second dose of 10 mg IV if the symptoms of bradycardia and hypotension recur. (Note that this dose is much higher than the dose required to treat hypoglycemia.)
- Pediatric: For patients weighing < 20 kg, the dose is 0.5 mg.

Special Considerations: Pregnancy Category B.

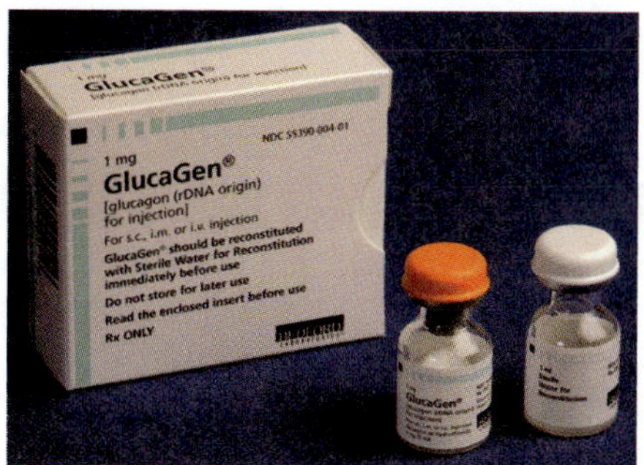

Haloperidol (Haldol)

Classification: Antipsychotic agent

Action: Selectively blocks postsynaptic dopamine receptors.

Indications: Psychotic disorders, agitation.

Adverse Effects: Extrapyramidal symptoms, drowsiness, tardive dyskinesia, hypotension, hypertension, VT, sinus tachycardia, QT prolongation, torsades de pointes.

Contraindications: Depressed mental status, Parkinson's disease.

Dosage:

- Adult:
  - Mild agitation: 0.5 to 2 mg PO or IM.
  - Moderate agitation: 5 to 10 mg PO or IM.
  - Severe agitation: 10 mg PO or IM.
- Pediatric: Not recommended for pediatric patients.

Special Considerations: Pregnancy Category C.

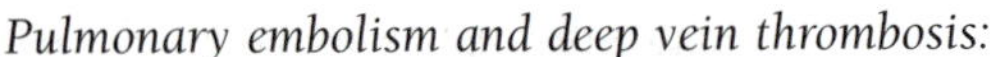

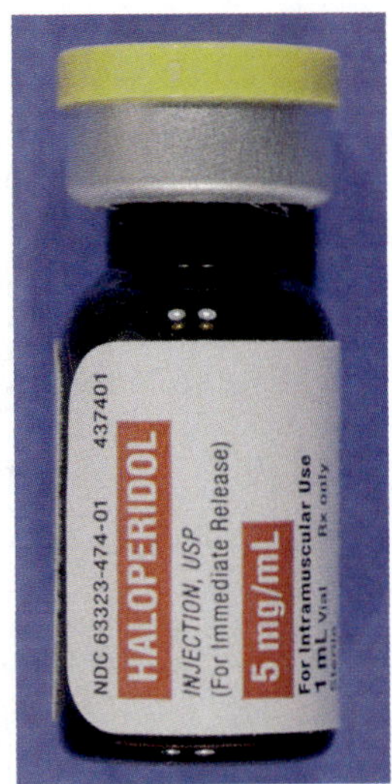

Heparin (Unfractionated Heparin)

Classification: Anticoagulant thus preventing clot deposition in the coronary arteries.

Indications: ACS, acute pulmonary embolism, deep venous thrombosis.

Adverse Effects: Bleeding, thrombocytopenia, allergic reactions.

Contraindications: Predisposition to bleeding, aortic aneurysm, peptic ulceration; known sensitivity or history of heparin-induced thrombocytopenia, severe thrombocytopenia, sulfite sensitivity.

Dosage:

Cardiac indications:

- Adult: 60 U/kg IV (max 4000 units), followed by 12 U/kg/hr (max 1000 units). Once in the hospital, additional dosing is determined based on laboratory blood tests.
- Pediatric: 75 U/kg followed by 20 U/kg/hr.

Pulmonary embolism and deep vein thrombosis:

- Adult: 80 U/kg IV, followed by 18 U/kg/hr.
- Pediatric: 75 U/kg IV followed by 20 U/kg/hr.

Special Considerations: Half-life approximately 90 minutes. Pregnancy Category C.

Hetastarch (Hespan)

Classification: Volume expander, colloid

Action: Causes water to move from interstitial spaces, thereby increasing the oncotic pressure within the intravascular space.

Indications: Hypovolemia when volume must be increased only in the intravascular compartment.

Adverse Effects: Anaphylactic reactions, CHF, pulmonary edema, cardiac arrhythmias, cardiac arrest, severe hypotension, pruritus, edema, platelet dysfunction, bleeding complications, dilution of the serum proteins responsible for the formation of blood clots, nausea/vomiting.

Contraindications: Bleeding disorders, intracranial bleeding, CHF, pulmonary edema, renal failure, thrombocytopenia or other coagulopathy (e.g., hemophilia), known sensitivity to hetastarch or corn.

Dosage: Note: The dosage of hetastarch required is determined by the clinical situation and the severity of the hypovolemia.

- Adult: 500 to 1000 mL IV, IO; more than 1500 mL of hetastarch typically is not administered because of concerns that larger doses can interfere with platelet function and promote bleeding.
- Pediatric: 10 mL/kg per dose IV; the total daily dosage should not exceed 20 mL/kg. Safety of this drug in the pediatric population has not been established.

Special Considerations: Pregnancy Category C.

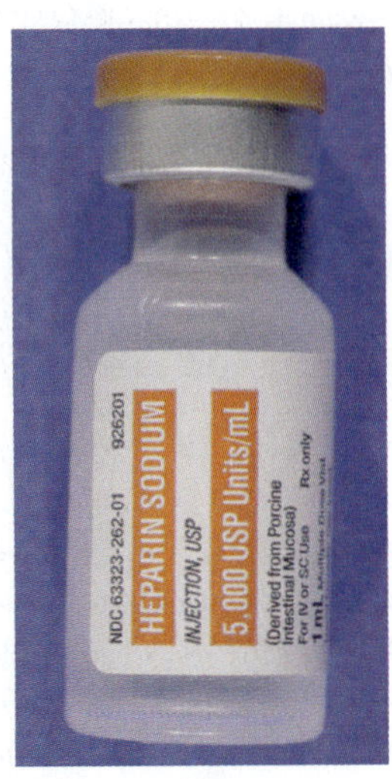

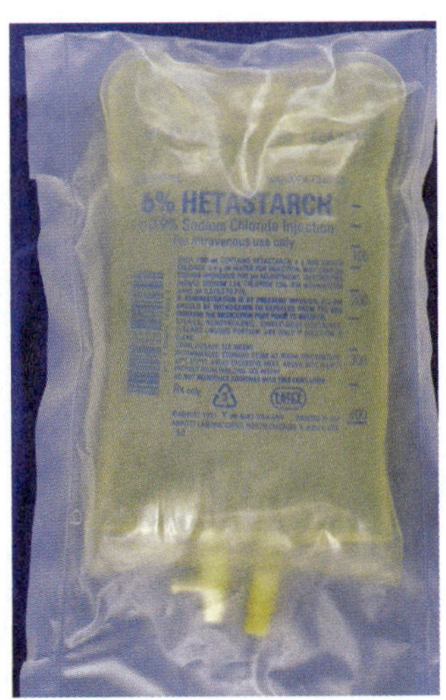

HMG Coenzyme A Statins: Atorvastatin (Lipitor), Fluvastatin (Lescol), Lovastatin (Mevacor), Pravastatin (Pravachol), Rosuvastatin (Crestor), Simvastatin (Zocor)

Classification: HMG coenzyme A statins

Action: Reduces the level of circulating total cholesterol, LDL cholesterol, and serum triglycerides; reduces the incidence of reinfarction, recurrent angina, rehospitalization, and stroke when initiated within a few days after onset of ACS.

Indications: Acute coronary syndromes/acute myocardial infarction prophylaxis, hypercholesterolemia, hyperlipoproteinemia, hypertriglyceridemia, stroke prophylaxis.

Adverse Effects: Constipation, flatulence, dyspepsia, abdominal pain, infection, headache, flulike symptoms, back pain, allergic reaction, asthenia, diarrhea, sinusitis, pharyngitis, rash, arthralgia, nausea/vomiting, myopathy, myasthenia, renal failure, rhabdomyolysis, chest pain, bronchitis, rhinitis, insomnia.

Contraindications: Active hepatic disease, pregnancy, breast-feeding, rhabdomyolysis.

Dosage:

- Adult: Medication is administered orally. Dosage is individualized.
- Pediatric: Safe use has not been established.

Special Considerations: Pregnancy Category X.

Hydralazine (Apresoline)

Classification: Antihypertensive agent, vasodilator

Action: Directly dilates the peripheral blood vessels.

Indications: Hypertension associated with preeclampsia and eclampsia, hypertensive crisis.

Adverse Effects: Headache, angina, flushing, palpitations, reflex tachycardia, anorexia, nausea/vomiting, diarrhea, hypotension, syncope, peripheral vasodilation, peripheral edema, fluid retention, paresthesias.

Contraindications: Patients taking diazoxide or MAOIs, coronary artery disease, stroke, angina, dissecting aortic aneurysm, mitral valve and rheumatic heart diseases.

Dosage:

Preeclampsia and eclampsia:

- Adult: 5 to 10 mg IV, IO. Repeat every 20 to 30 minutes until systolic blood pressure of 90 to 105 mm Hg is attained.

Acute hypertension not associated with preeclampsia:

- Adult: 10 to 20 mg IV, IO, or IM.
- Pediatric:
    - 1 month to 12 years: 0.1 to 0.5 mg/kg IV, IO, or IM (max: 20 mg/dose).

Special Considerations: Pregnancy Category C.

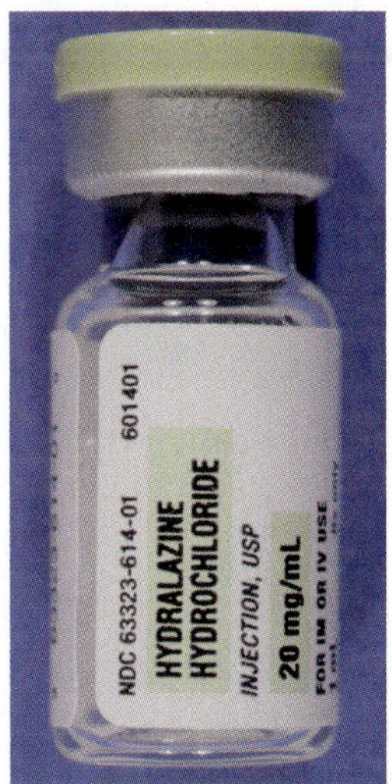

Hydrocortisone Sodium Succinate (Cortef, Solu-Cortef)

Classification: Corticosteroid

Action: Reduces inflammation by multiple mechanisms. As a steroid, it replaces the steroids that are lacking in adrenal insufficiency.

Indications: Adrenal insufficiency, allergic reactions, anaphylaxis, asthma, COPD.

Adverse Effects: Leukocytosis, hyperglycemia, increased infection, decreased wound healing.

Contraindications: Cushing's syndrome, known sensitivity to benzyl alcohol. Use with caution in diabetes, hypertension, CHF, known systemic fungal infection, renal disease, idiopathic thrombocytopenia, psychosis, seizure disorder, GI disease, glaucoma, known sensitivity.

Dosage:

Anaphylactic shock:

- Adult: 100 to 500 mg IV, IO, or IM.
- Pediatric: 2 to 4 mg/kg/day IV, IO, or IM (max: 500 mg).

Adrenal insufficiency:

- Adult: 100 to 500 mg IV, IO, or IM.
- Pediatric: 1 to 2 mg/kg IV, IO, or IM.

Asthma and chronic obstructive pulmonary disease (COPD):

- Adult: 100 to 500 mg IV, IO, IM.
- Pediatric: 1 mg/kg IV, IO. The dose may be reduced for infants and children, but it is governed more by the severity of the condition and response of the patient than by age or body weight. Dose should not be less than 25 mg daily.

Special Considerations: Pregnancy Category C.

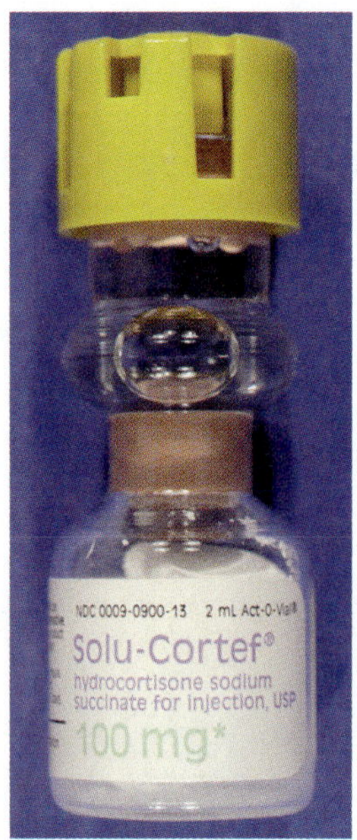

Hydroxocobalamin (Cyanokit)

Classification: Chelates cyanide

Action: Cobalt ion chelates cyanide. Cobalt is a precursor to cyanocobalamin (vitamin B_{12}). Binds with cyanide to form cyanocobalamin (B_{12}) and is excreted in the urine. The Cyanokit preparation is a large dose of B_{12}.

Indications: Cyanide toxicity

Adverse Effects: Anaphylaxis, moderate hypertension, headache, cutaneous rash, red urine and skin.

Contraindications: Known sensitivity to vitamin B_{12}.

Dosage: 5 grams diluted in 100 mL NS, given IV over 15 minutes. Repeat dose if transient or incomplete response. 70 mg/kg for children.

Special Considerations: Hydroxocobalamin (HCO) interferes with colorimetric assays in laboratory analysis. It causes chromaturia and creates reddening of the skin over several days.

Hydromorphone (Dilaudid)

Classification: Analgesic

Action: Blocks the mu receptors to treat pain. Suppresses cough and respiratory centers in the medulla and brainstem.

Indications: For the relief of moderate to severe pain

Adverse Effects: Respiratory depression and hypotension.

Contraindications: Contraindicated in those hypersensitive to Dilaudid, those with respiratory depression (especially if no resuscitative equipment available), and those with status asthmaticus. Should not be used for obstetric analgesia.

Dosage: 1 to 2 mg every 4 to 6 hours subcutaneously or intramuscularly. If given IV, 1 to 2 mg slowly (over 2 to 3 minutes). Hydromorphone HCl-HP (high potency) is only given to those patients who are already receiving opiates for pain relief. Opiate-naïve patients' starting dose should be 0.3 to 0.75 mg. 1.3 mg of this drug is equivalent to 10 mg of morphine.

Special Considerations: Severe hypotension may occur, especially in those with hypovolemia. Doses should be individualized to each patient, reduced in the elderly, those with impaired liver, kidney or pulmonary function. Orthostatic hypotension may occur.

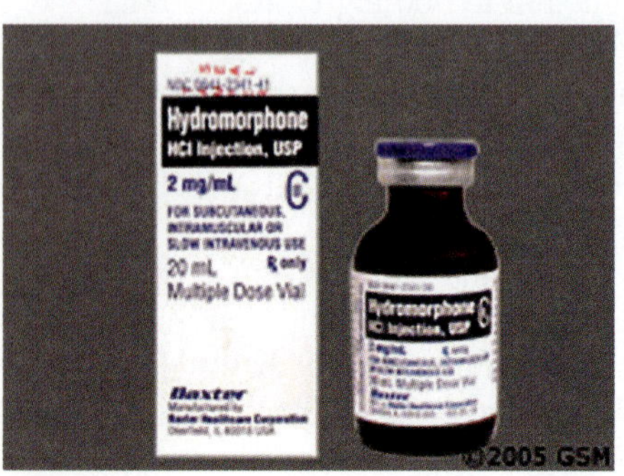

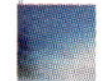

Ibuprofen

Classification: Nonsteroidal antiinflammatory drug (NSAID)

Action: Inhibits prostaglandin synthesis by inhibiting cyclooxygenase (COX) isoenzymes, resulting in analgesic, antipyretic, and antiinflammatory effects.

Indications: Mild to moderate pain, fever, osteoarthritis, rheumatoid arthritis.

Adverse Effects: Anorexia, nausea/vomiting, epigastric/abdominal pain, dyspepsia, constipation, diarrhea, gastritis, melena, flatulence, headache, dizziness.

Contraindications: Sensitivity to NSAID or salicylate. Use with caution in asthma, hepatic disease, renal disease, congestive heart failure, hypertension, cardiac disease, cardiomyopathy, cardiac arrhythmias, significant coronary artery disease, peripheral vascular disease, cerebrovascular disease, fluid retention, or edema.

Dosage:

Mild to moderate pain:

- Adult: 400 mg PO every 4 hours as needed, not to exceed 3200 mg per day.
- Pediatric: 6 months to 12 years: 5 to 10 mg/kg PO every 6 to 8 hours as needed, not to exceed 40 mg/kg/day.

Fever:

- Adult: 200 to 400 mg PO every 4 to 6 hours as needed, not to exceed 3200 mg per day.
- Pediatric: 6 months to 12 years: 5 mg/kg PO if baseline temperature is less than 102.5°F, or 10 mg/kg PO if baseline temperature is greater than 102.5°F (max dose: 40 mg/kg/day).

Osteoarthritis or rheumatoid arthritis:

- Adult: 400 to 800 mg PO 3 to 4 times per day, not to exceed 3200 mg/day.

- Pediatric: 1 to 12 years: 30 to 40 mg/kg/day PO in 3 to 4 divided doses, not to exceed 50 mg/kg/day.

Special Considerations: Pregnancy Category C for trimesters 1 and 2, Category D for the 3rd trimester.

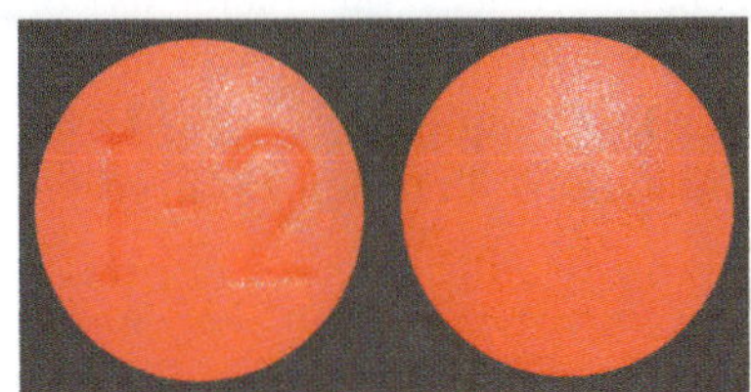

Insulin, Regular (Humulin R, Novolin R)

Classification: Hormone

Action: Binds to a receptor on the membrane of cells and facilitates the transport of glucose into cells.

Indications: Hyperglycemia, insulin-dependent diabetes mellitus, hyperkalemia.

Adverse Effects: Hypoglycemia, tachycardia, palpitations, diaphoresis, anxiety, confusion, blurred vision, weakness, depression, seizures, coma, insulin shock, hypokalemia.

Contraindications: Hypoglycemia, known sensitivity.

Dosage:

Diabetic ketoacidosis:

- Adult: 0.1 Unit/kg IV, IO, or SQ. Because of poor perfusion of the peripheral tissues, SQ administration is much less effective than the IV, IO route. IV, IO insulin has a very short half-life; therefore IV, IO insulin without an infusion is not that effective. The rate for an insulin infusion is 0.05 to 0.1 Unit/kg/hr IV, IO. When dosing insulin, use a U-100 insulin syringe to measure and deliver the insulin. The time from administration to action, as well as the duration of action, varies greatly among different individuals, as well as at different times in the same individual.

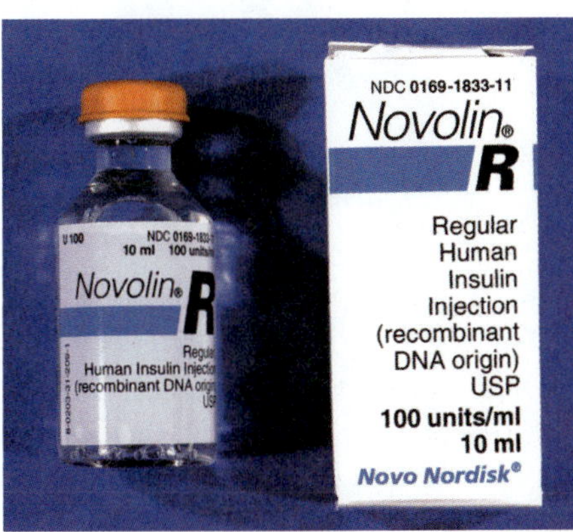

Hyperkalemia:

- Adult: 10 Units IV, IO of regular insulin (Insulin R), co-administered with 50 mL of dextrose 50% over 5 minutes.
- Pediatric: 0.1 Unit/kg Insulin R IV, IO.

Special Considerations: Only regular insulin can be given IV, IO. Pregnancy Category B.

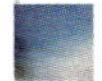

Ipratropium Bromide (Atrovent)

Classification: Bronchodilator, anticholinergic

Action: Antagonizes the acetylcholine receptor on bronchial smooth muscle, producing bronchodilation.

Indications: Asthma, bronchospasm associated with COPD.

Adverse Effects: Paradoxical acute bronchospasm, cough, throat irritation, headache, dizziness, dry mouth, palpitations.

Contraindications: Closed-angle glaucoma, bladder neck obstruction, prostatic hypertrophy, known sensitivity including peanuts or soybeans and atropine or atropine derivatives.

Dosage:

MDI:

- Adult: 2 to 3 puffs every 4 to 6 hours, with no more than 12 inhalations per day or closer than 4 hours apart.
- Pediatric:
  - Older than 12 years: 2 to 3 puffs inhaled every 6 to 8 hours. Maximum of 12 puffs/day.
  - 5 to 12 years: 1 to 2 puffs inhaled every 6 to 8 hours. Maximum of 8 puffs/day.

Nebulization:

- Adult: 0.5 mg every 6 to 8 hours.
- Pediatric: 5 to 14 years: 0.25 to 0.5 mg every 20 minutes for 3 doses as needed.

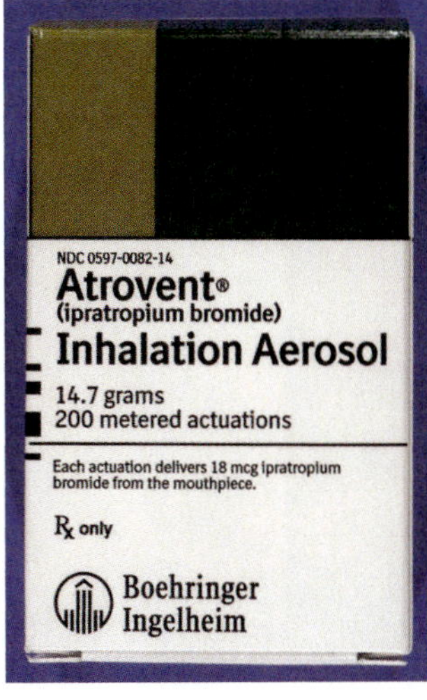

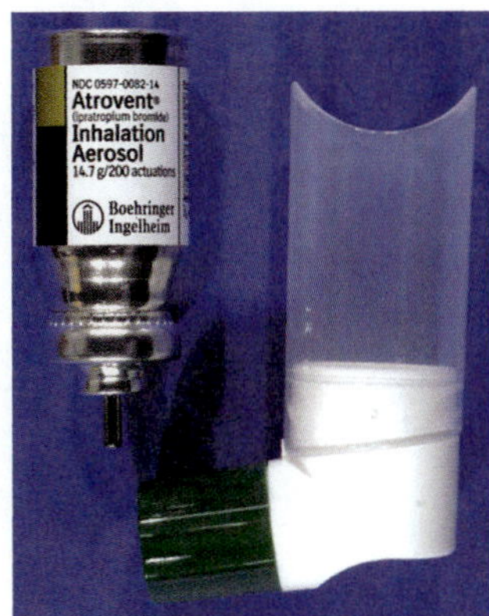

Special Considerations: Ipratropium bromide is not typically used as a sole medication in the treatment of acute exacerbation of asthma. Ipratropium bromide is commonly administered after a beta agonist. Care should be taken to not allow the aerosol spray (especially in the MDI) to come into contact with the eyes. This can cause temporary blurring of vision that resolves without intervention within 4 hours. Pregnancy Category B.

Ketamine (Ketalar)

Classification: General anesthetic

Action: Produces a state of anesthesia while maintaining airway reflexes, heart rate, and blood pressure.

Indications: Pain and as anesthesia for procedures of short duration.

Adverse Effects: Emergence phenomena, hypertension and sinus tachycardia, hypotension and sinus bradycardia, other cardiac arrhythmias (rare), respiratory depression, apnea, laryngospasms and other forms of airway obstruction (rare), tonic and clonic movements, vomiting.

Contraindications: Patients in whom a significant elevation in blood pressure would be hazardous (hypertension, stroke, head trauma, increased intracranial mass or bleeding, MI). Use with caution in patients with increased ICP or increased intraocular pressure (glaucoma) and patients with hypovolemia, dehydration, or cardiac disease (especially angina and CHF).

Dosage: Administer slowly over a period of 60 seconds.

IV, IO:

- Adult: 1 to 4.5 mg/kg IV, IO. 1 to 2 mg/kg produces anesthesia usually within 30 seconds that typically lasts 5 to 10 minutes.
- Pediatric: 0.5 to 2 mg IV, IO over a 1-minute period.

IM:

- Adult: 6.5 to 13 mg/kg IM. 10 mg/kg IM is capable of producing anesthesia within 3 to 4 minutes with an effect typically lasting 12 to 25 minutes. In adults, concomitant administration of 5 to 15 mg of diazepam reduces the incidence of emergence phenomena.
- Pediatric: 3 to 7 mg IM.

Special Considerations: Pregnancy Category C.

Ketorolac (Toradol)

Classification: NSAID

Action: Inhibits the production of prostaglandins in inflamed tissue, which decreases the responsiveness of pain receptors.

Indications: Moderately severe acute pain.

Adverse Effects: Headache, drowsiness, dizziness, abdominal pain, dyspepsia, nausea/vomiting, diarrhea.

Contraindications: Patients with a history of peptic ulcer disease or GI bleed, patients with renal insufficiency, hypovolemic patients, pregnancy (third trimester), nursing mothers, allergy to aspirin or other NSAIDs, stroke or suspected stroke or head trauma, need for major surgery in the immediate or near future (i.e., within 7 days).

Dosage: Note: The following dosage regimen applies to single-dose administration only. IV, IO administration should occur over a period of at least 15 seconds.

- Adult:
  - Younger than 65 years or <50 kg: 30 mg IV, IO or 60 mg IM.
  - Older than 65 years: 15 mg IV, IO or 30 mg IM.
- Pediatric: 0.5 mg/kg IV, IO to a maximum dose of 15 mg, or 1 mg/kg IM to a maximum dose of 30 mg.

Special Considerations: Pregnancy Category C first and second trimesters; Category D in third trimester.

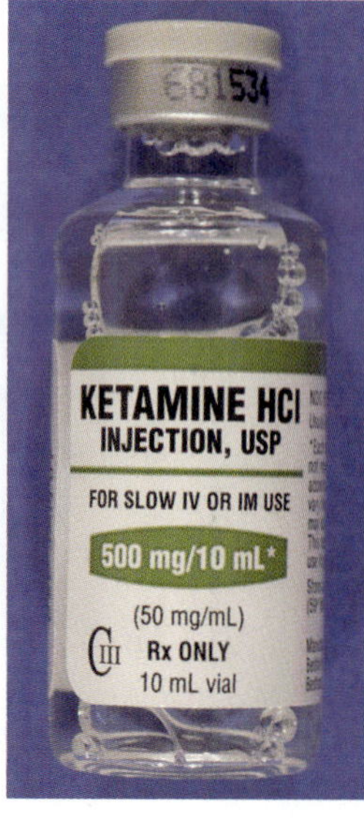

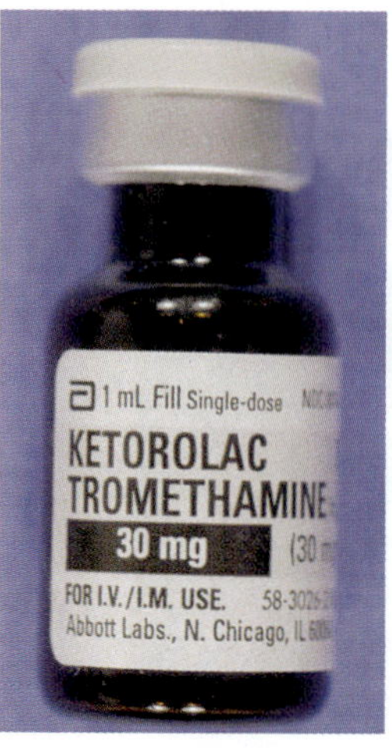

Labetalol (Normodyne, Trandate)

Classification: Beta-adrenergic antagonist, antianginal, antihypertensive

Action: Binds with both the $beta_1$ and $beta_2$ receptors and $alpha_1$ receptors in vascular smooth muscle. Inhibits the strength of the heart's contractions as well as heart rate. This results in a decrease in cardiac oxygen consumption.

Indications: ACS, SVT, severe hypertension.

Adverse Effects: Usually mild and transient; hypotensive symptoms, nausea/vomiting, bronchospasm, arrhythmia, bradycardia, AV block.

Contraindications: Hypotension, cardiogenic shock, acute pulmonary edema, heart failure, severe bradycardia, sick sinus syndrome, second- or third-degree heart block, asthma or acute bronchospasm, cocaine-induced ACS, known sensitivity. Use caution in pheochromocytoma, cerebrovascular disease or stroke, poorly controlled diabetes, with hepatic disease. Use with caution at lowest effective dose in chronic lung disease.

Dosage:

Cardiac indications (Note: Monitor blood pressure and heart rate closely during administration):

- Adult: 20 mg IV, IO over a 1- to 2-minute period. May repeat every 10 minutes to a maximum dose of 300 mg or give initial bolus and then follow with infusion at 2 to 8 mg/min.
- Pediatric: 0.4 to 1 mg/kg/hr to a maximum dosage of 3 mg/kg/hr.

Severe hypertension:

- Adult: Initial dose is 20 mg IV, IO slow infusion over a 2-minute period. After the initial dose, blood pressure should be checked every 5 minutes. Repeat doses can be given at 10-minute intervals. The second dose should be 40 mg IV, IO, and subsequent doses should be 80 mg IV, IO, to a maximum total dose of 300 mg. The effect on blood pressure typically will occur within 5 minutes from the time of administration. Alternatively, may be administered via IV infusion at 2 mg/min to a total maximum dose of 300 mg.

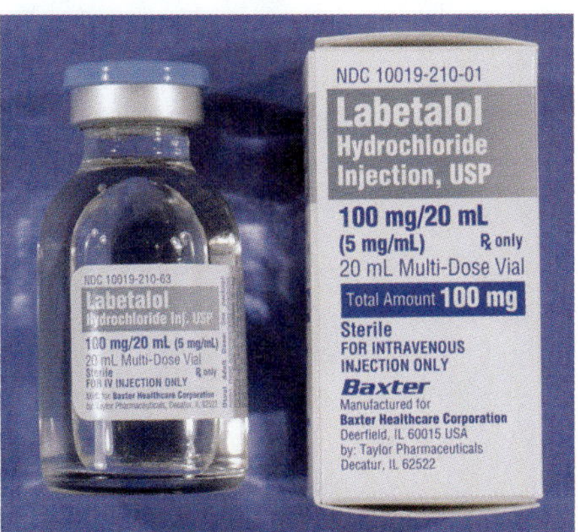

- Pediatric: 0.4 to 1 mg/kg/hr IV, IO infusion with a maximum dose of 3 mg/kg/hr.

Special Considerations: Pregnancy Category C.

Lamotrigine (Lamictal)

Classification: Anticonvulsant, antimanic agent

Action: The exact mechanism of action has not been determined. Studies suggest lamotrigine stabilizes neuronal membranes by acting at voltage-sensitive sodium channels, thereby decreasing presynaptic release of glutamate and aspartate, resulting in decreased seizure activity.

Indications: Seizures, bipolar disorders.

Adverse Effects: Headache, dizziness, nausea/vomiting, ataxia, diplopia.

Contraindications: Known sensitivity.

Dosage:

- Adult: Medication is administered orally. Dosage is individualized.
- Pediatric: Medication is administered orally. Dosage is individualized.

Special Considerations: Pregnancy Category C.

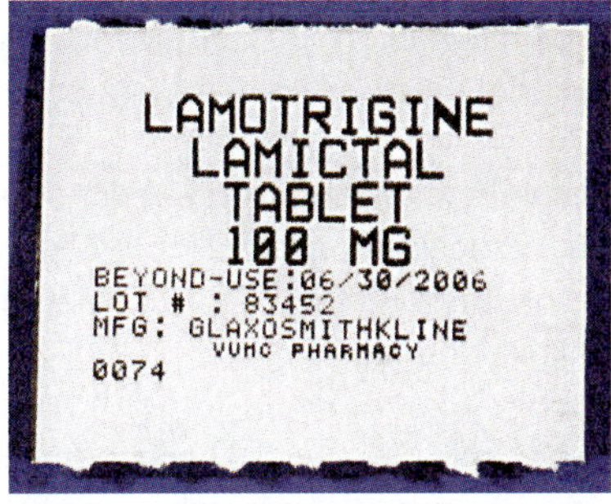

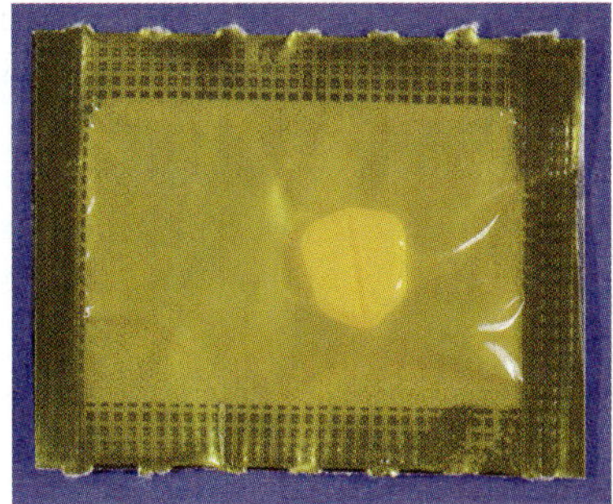

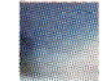

Levalbuterol (Xopenex)

Classification: Beta agonist

Action: Stimulates $beta_2$ receptors, resulting in relaxation of the smooth muscle in the lungs, uterus, and vasculature that supply skeletal muscle.

Indications: Acute bronchospasm or bronchospasm prophylaxis in patient with asthma.

Adverse Effects: Hyperglycemia, hypokalemia, palpitations, sinus tachycardia, anxiety, tremor, nausea/

vomiting, throat irritation, hypertension, dyspepsia, insomnia, headache.

Contraindications: Angioedema, sensitivity to albuterol or levalbuterol. Use with caution in lactating patients, cardiovascular disorders, cardiac arrhythmias. Do not use in patients taking phenothiazines; may cause prolonged QT interval and cardiac arrhythmias. Also avoid use in patients receiving beta$_2$-blockers (sotalol); may decrease bronchodilating effects and cause bronchospasm, prolonged QT interval, and cardiac arrhythmias.

Dosage:

MDI:

- Adult: 2 inhalations every 4 to 6 hours. In some patients, 1 inhalation may be sufficient. For acute exacerbations, 4 to 8 inhalations every 20 minutes up to 4 hours, then every 1 to 4 hours as needed.
- Pediatric:
  - 4 to 12 years: 2 inhalations every 4 to 6 hours. In some patients, 1 inhalation may be sufficient. For acute exacerbations, 4 to 8 inhalations every 20 minutes for 3 doses, then 1 to 4 inhalations every 1 to 4 hours as needed.
  - Younger than 4 years: Safe and effective use has not been established. For acute exacerbations, 2 to 4 inhalations holding a valved holding chamber and face mask every 20 minutes for 3 doses, then 2 to 4 inhalations every 1 to 4 hours as needed.

Nebulizer:

- Adult: Usually, 0.63 mg 3 times/every 6 to 8 hours. For acute exacerbations, 1.25 to 2.5 mg every 20 minutes for 3 doses, then 1.25 to 5 mg every 1 to 4 hours as needed.
- Pediatric:
  - 5 to 11 years: Usually, 0.31 mg 3 times/day, up to 0.63 mg. For acute exacerbations, 0.075 mg/kg (1.25 mg minimum) every 20 minutes for 3 doses, then 0.075 to 0.15 mg/kg (5 mg maximum) every 1 to 4 hours as needed.
  - Younger than 5 years: Safe and effective use has not been established. For acute exacerbations, 0.31 to 1.25 mg every 4 to 6 hours for 3 doses, then as needed.

Special Considerations: Pregnancy Category C.

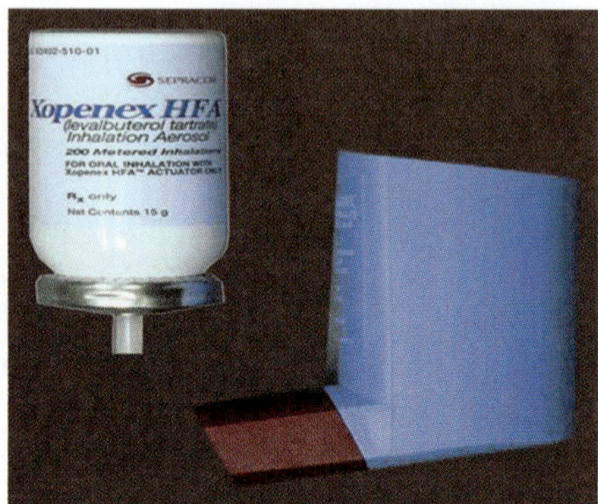

Levetiracetam (Keppra)

Classification: Anticonvulsant, antiepilepsy drug

Action: Mechanism of action unknown but seems to interact with known substances that inhibit excitatory neurotransmission.

Indications: For treatment of partial-onset seizures in adults and indicated as adjunctive therapy in the treatment of myoclonic seizures in adults and adolescents 12 years of age and older with juvenile myoclonic epilepsy. Keppra is indicated as adjunctive therapy in the treatment of primary generalized tonic-clonic seizures in adults and children 6 years of age and older with idiopathic generalized epilepsy.

Adverse Effects: Sedation, headache, muscle weakness, bone marrow suppression, hallucinations, psychosis, and increased risk for infection.

Contraindications: This product should not be administered to patients who have previously exhibited hypersensitivity to levetiracetam or any of the inactive ingredients in Keppra tablets or oral solution.

Dosage: Typical adult dose orally from 500 to 2000 mg twice daily, adjusted for renal insufficiency. Keppra injection is for intravenous use only and must be diluted prior to administration, supplied in a single-use vial of 500 mg/5 mL. Dilute prescribed dose in 100 mL of a compatible diluent, and infuse over 15 minutes. Treatment should be initiated with a daily dose of 1000 mg/day, given as twice-daily dosing (500 mg BID). Additional dosing increments may be given (1000 mg/day additional every 2 weeks) to a maximum recommended daily dose of 3000 mg.

Special Considerations: If used in combination with phenytoin, may increase blood levels of both drugs.

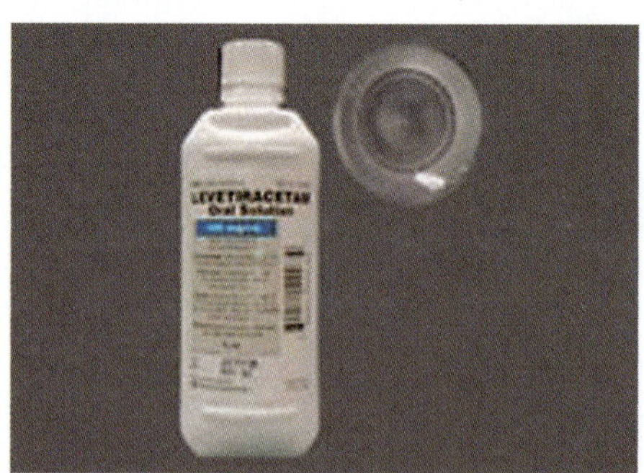

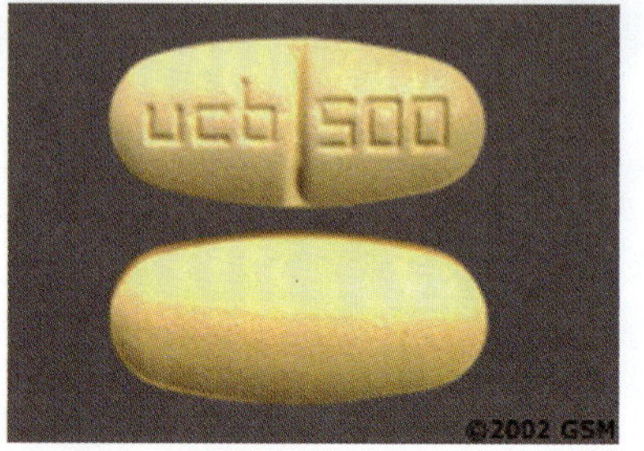

Lidocaine (Xylocaine)

Classification: Antiarrhythmic, class IB

Action: Blocks sodium channels, increasing the recovery period after repolarization; suppresses automaticity in the His-Purkinje system and depolarization in the ventricles.

Indications: Ventricular arrhythmias, when amiodarone is not available: cardiac arrest from VF/VT, stable monomorphic VT with preserved ventricular function, stable polymorphic VT with normal baseline QT interval and preserved left ventricular function (when ischemia and electrolyte imbalance are treated), stable polymorphic VT with baseline QT prolongation suggestive of torsades de pointes.

Adverse Effects: Toxicity (signs may include anxiety, apprehension, euphoria, nervousness, disorientation, dizziness, blurred vision, facial paresthesias, tremors, hearing disturbances, slurred speech, seizures, sinus bradycardia), seizures without warning, cardiac arrhythmias, hypotension, cardiac arrest, pain at injection site.

Contraindications: AV block; bleeding; thrombocytopenia; known sensitivity to lidocaine, sulfite, or paraben. Use with caution in bradycardia, hypovolemia, cardiogenic shock, Adams-Stokes syndrome, Wolff-Parkinson-White syndrome.

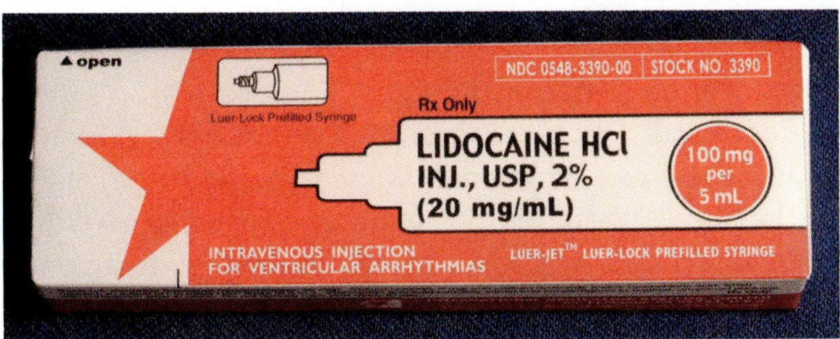

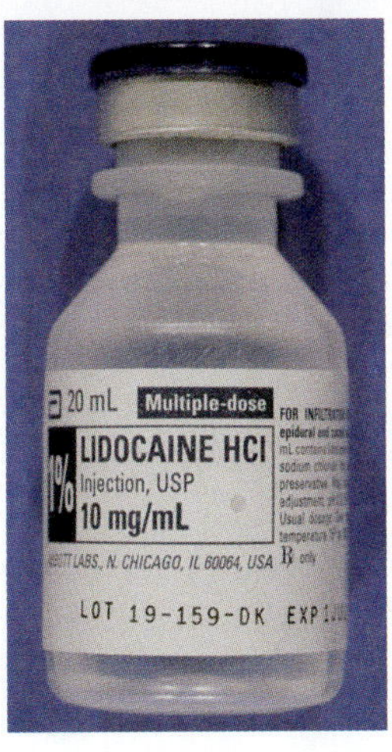

Dosage:

Pulseless ventricular tachycardia and ventricular fibrillation:

- Adult IV, IO: 1 to 1.5 mg/kg IV, IO; may repeat at half the original dose (0.5-0.75 mg/kg) every 5 to 10 minutes to a maximum dose of 3 mg/kg. If a maintenance infusion is warranted, the rate is 1 to 4 mg/min.
- Adult ET tube: 2 to 10 mg/kg ET tube, diluted in 10 mL normal saline or sterile distilled water.
- Pediatric IV, IO: 1 mg/kg IV, IO (maximum: 100 mg). If a maintenance infusion is warranted, the rate is 20 to 50 mcg/kg/min.
- Pediatric ET tube: 2 to 3 mg/kg ET tube, followed by a 5-mL flush of normal saline.

Perfusing ventricular rhythms:

- Adult: 0.5 to 0.75 mg/kg IV, IO (up to 1 to 1.5 mg/kg may be used). Repeat 0.5 to 0.75 mg/kg every 5 to 10 minutes to a maximum total dose of 3 mg/kg. A maintenance infusion of 1 to 4 mg/min (30 to 50 mcg/kg/min) is acceptable.
- Pediatric: 1 mg/kg IV, IO. May repeat every 5 to 10 minutes to a maximum dose of 3 mg/kg. Maintenance infusion rate is 20 to 50 mcg/kg/min.

Special Considerations: Half-life approximately 90 minutes. Pregnancy Category B.

Lorazepam (Ativan)

Classification: Benzodiazepine; Schedule C-IV

Action: Binds to the benzodiazepine receptor and enhances the effects of the brain chemical GABA, an inhibitory transmitter, and may result in a state of sedation, hypnosis, skeletal muscle relaxation, anticonvulsant activity, coma.

Indications: Preprocedure sedation induction, anxiety, status epilepticus.

Adverse Effects: Headache, drowsiness, ataxia, dizziness, amnesia, depression, dysarthria, euphoria, syncope, fatigue, tremor, vertigo, respiratory depression.

Contraindications: Known sensitivity to lorazepam, benzodiazepines, polyethylene glycol, propylene glycol, or benzyl alcohol; COPD; sleep apnea (except while being mechanically ventilated); shock; coma; acute narrow-angle glaucoma.

Dosage: Note: IV, IO lorazepam must be administered slowly.

Analgesia and sedation:

- Adult: 2 mg or 0.044 mg/kg IV, IO, whichever is smaller, up to 2 mg. This dosage will provide adequate sedation in most patients and should not be exceeded in patients older than 50 years.
- Pediatric: 0.05 mg/kg IV, IO. Each dose should not exceed 2 mg IV, IO.

Seizures:

- Adult: 4 mg IV, IO given over 2 to 5 minutes; may repeat in 10 to 15 minutes (max total dose: 8 mg in a 12-hour period).
- Pediatric: 0.05 to 0.1 mg/kg IV to a maximum of 4 mg in one dose. Repeat twice at intervals of 15 to 20 minutes if needed.

Special Considerations: Be prepared to support the patient's airway and ventilation. Pregnancy Category D.

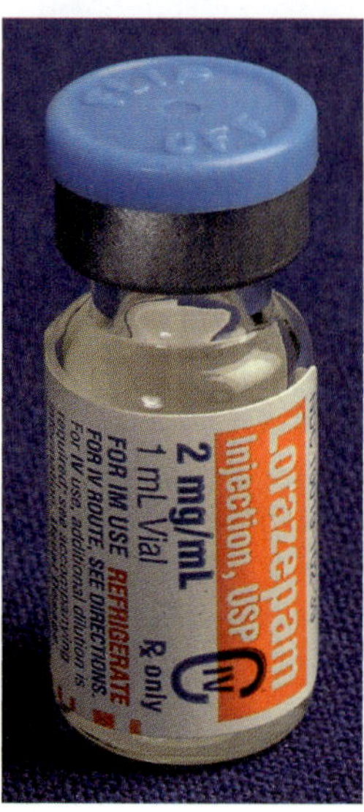

Magnesium Sulfate

Classification: Electrolyte, tocolytic, mineral

Action: Required for normal physiologic functioning. Magnesium is a cofactor in neurochemical transmission and muscular excitability. Magnesium sulfate controls seizures by blocking peripheral neuromuscular transmission. Magnesium is also a peripheral vasodilator and an inhibitor of platelet function.

Indications: Torsades de pointes, cardiac arrhythmias associated with hypomagnesemia, eclampsia and seizure prophylaxis in preeclampsia, status asthmaticus.

Adverse Effects: Magnesium toxicity (signs include flushing, diaphoresis, hypotension, muscle paralysis, weakness, hypothermia, and cardiac, CNS, or respiratory depression).

Contraindications: AV block, GI obstruction. Use with caution in renal impairment.

Dosage:

Pulseless ventricular fibrillation/ventricular tachycardia with torsades de pointes or hypomagnesemia:

- Adult: 1 to 2 g in 10 mL D_5W IV, IO administered over 5 to 10 minutes.
- Pediatric: 25 to 50 mg/kg IV, IO over 10 to 20 minutes; may administer faster for torsades de pointes (max single dose: 2 g).

Torsades de pointes with a pulse or cardiac arrhythmias with hypomagnesemia:

- Adult: 1 to 2 g in 50 to 100 mL D_5W IV, IO administered over 5 to 60 minutes. Follow with 0.5 to 1 g/hr IV, IO titrated to control torsades de pointes.
- Pediatric: 25 to 50 mg/kg IV, IO over 10 to 20 minutes (max single dose: 2 g).

Eclampsia and seizure prophylaxis in preeclampsia:

- Adult: 4 to 6 g IV, IO over 20 to 30 minutes, followed by an infusion of 1 to 2 g/hr.

Status asthmaticus:

- Adult: 1 to 2 g slow IV, IO (over 20 minutes).
- Pediatric: 25 to 50 mg/kg (diluted in D_5W) slow IV, IO (over 10 to 20 minutes) up to 2 g.

Special Considerations: Pregnancy Category A.

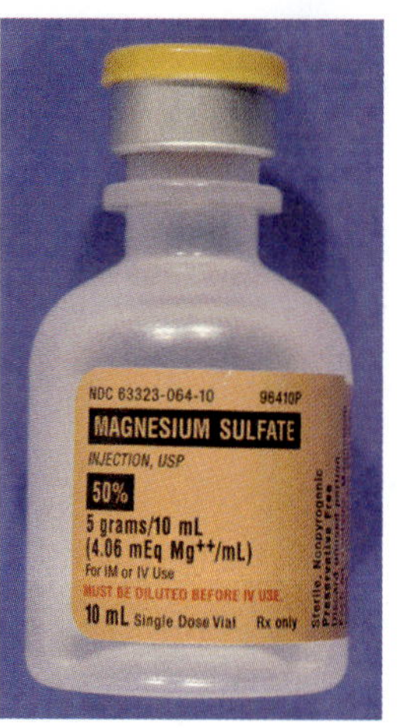

Mannitol (Osmitrol)

Classification: Osmotic diuretic

Action: Facilitates the flow of fluid out of tissues (including the brain) and into interstitial fluid and blood, thereby dehydrating the brain and reducing swelling. Reabsorption by the kidney is minimal, consequently increasing urine output.

Indications: Increased ICP.

Adverse Effects: Pulmonary edema, headache, blurred vision, dizziness, seizures, hypovolemia, nausea/vomiting, diarrhea, electrolyte imbalances, hypotension, sinus tachycardia, PVCs, angina, phlebitis.

Contraindications: Active intracranial bleeding, CHF, pulmonary edema, severe dehydration. Use with caution in hypovolemia, renal failure.

Dosage:

- Adult: 0.25 to 2 g/kg IV, IO, over 30 to 60 minutes, followed by 0.25 to 1 g/kg administered every 4 hours.
- Pediatric: 1 to 2 g/kg IV, IO, over 30 to 60 minutes, followed by 0.25 to 1 g/kg every 4 hours.

Special Considerations: Mannitol should not be given in the same IV, IO line as blood. Pregnancy Category C.

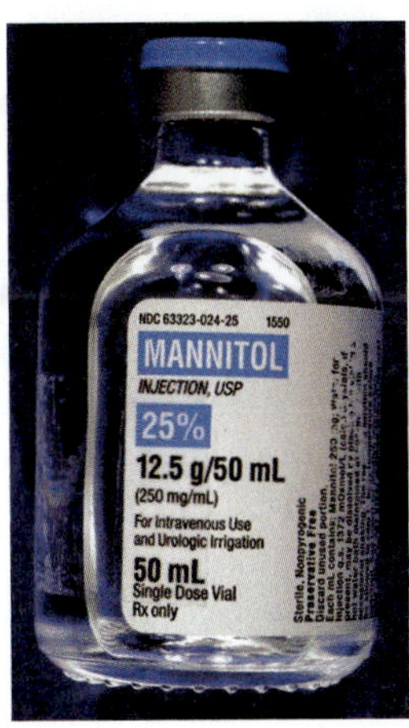

Methylprednisolone Sodium Succinate (Solu-Medrol)

Classification: Corticosteroid
Action: Reduces inflammation by multiple mechanisms.
Indications: Anaphylaxis, asthma, COPD.
Adverse Effects: Depression, euphoria, headache, restlessness, hypertension, bradycardia, nausea/vomiting, swelling, diarrhea, weakness, fluid retention, paresthesias.
Contraindications: Cushing's syndrome, fungal infection, measles, varicella, known sensitivity (including sulfites). Use with caution in active infections, renal disease, penetrating spinal cord injury, hypertension, seizures, CHF.
Dosage:

Asthma and COPD:

- Adult: 40 to 80 mg IV.
- Pediatric: 1 mg/kg (up to 60 mg) IV, IO per day in two divided doses.

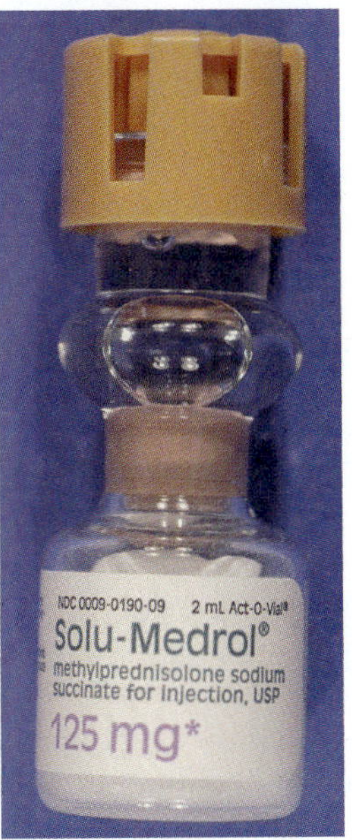

Anaphylactic shock:

- Adult: 1 to 2 mg/kg/dose, then 0.5 to 1 mg/kg every 6 hours.
- Pediatric: Same as adult dosing.

Blunt spinal cord injury:

- Adult: 30 mg/kg IV, IO over a period of 15 minutes, then 45 minutes later, begin an infusion to run for the remaining 23 hours at a dose of 5.4 mg/kg/hr.
- Pediatric: Same as adult dosing.

Special Considerations: May mask signs and symptoms of infection. Pregnancy Category C.

Metoprolol (Lopressor, Toprol XL)

Classification: Beta-adrenergic antagonist, antianginal, antihypertensive, class II antiarrhythmic
Action: Inhibits the strength of the heart's contractions, as well as heart rate. This results in a decrease in cardiac oxygen consumption. Also saturates the beta receptors and inhibits dilation of bronchial smooth muscle ($beta_2$ receptor).
Indications: ACS, hypertension, SVT, atrial flutter, AF, thyrotoxicosis.
Adverse Effects: Tiredness, dizziness, diarrhea, heart block, bradycardia, bronchospasm, drop in blood pressure.
Contraindications: Cardiogenic shock, AV block, bradycardia, known sensitivity. Use with caution in hypotension, chronic lung disease (asthma and COPD).
Dosage:

Cardiac indications:

- Adult: 5 mg slow IV, IO over a 5-minute period; repeat at 5-minute intervals up to a total of three infusions totaling 15 mg IV, IO.

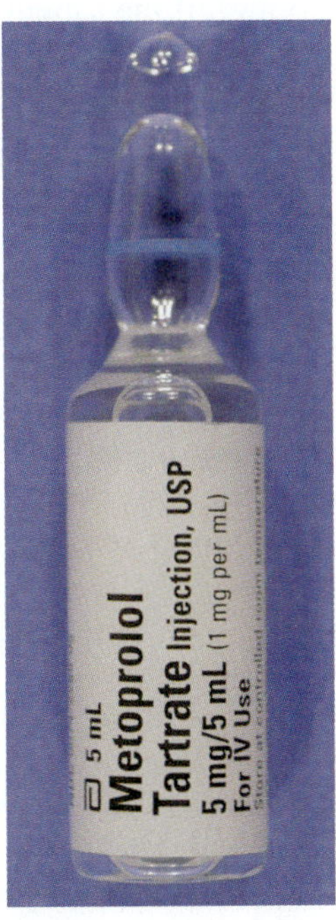

- Pediatric: Not recommended for pediatric patients; no studies available.

Special Considerations: Blood pressure, heart rate, and ECG should be monitored carefully. Use with caution in patients with asthma. Pregnancy Category C.

Midazolam (Versed)

Classification: Benzodiazepine, Schedule C-IV

Action: Binds to the benzodiazepine receptor and enhances the effects of the brain chemical (neurotransmitter) GABA. Benzodiazepines act at the level of the limbic, thalamic, and hypothalamic regions of the CNS to produce short-acting CNS depression (including sedation, skeletal muscle relaxation, and anticonvulsant activity).

Indications: Sedation, anxiety, skeletal muscle relaxation.

Adverse Effects: Respiratory depression, respiratory arrest, hypotension, nausea/vomiting, headache, hiccups, cardiac arrest.

Contraindications: Acute-angle glaucoma, pregnant women, known sensitivity.

Dosage:

Sedation (Note: The dose of midazolam must be individualized. Every dose should be administered slowly over a period of 2 minutes. Allow an additional 2 minutes to evaluate the clinical effect of the dose given):

- Adult:
  - Healthy and younger than 60 years: Some patients require as little as 1 mg IV, IO. No more than 2.5 mg should be given over a 2-minute interval. If additional sedation is required, continue to administer small increments over 2-minute periods (max dose: 5 mg). If the patient also has received a narcotic, he or she will typically require 30% less midazolam than the same patient not given the narcotic.
  - 60 years and older and debilitated or chronically ill patients: This group of patients has a higher risk of hypoventilation, airway obstruction, and apnea. The peak clinical effect can take longer, so dose increments should be smaller, and the rate of injection should be slower. Some patients require a dose as small as 1 mg IV, IO, and no more than 1.5 mg should be given over a 2-minute period. If additional sedation is required, additional midazolam should be given at a rate of no more than 1 mg over a 2-minute period (max dose: 3.5 mg). If the patient also has received a narcotic, he or she will typically require 50% less midazolam than the same patient not given the narcotic.
  - Continuous infusion: Continuous infusions can be required for prolonged transport of intubated, critically ill, and injured patients. After an initial bolus dose, the adult patient will require a maintenance infusion dose of 0.02 to 0.1 mg/kg/hr (1 to 7 mg/hr).
- Pediatric (weight-based): Pediatric patients typically require higher doses of midazolam than adults on the basis of weight (in mg/kg). Younger pediatric patients (<6 years) require higher doses (in mg/kg) than older pediatric patients. Midazolam takes approximately 3 minutes to reach peak effect; wait at least 2 minutes to determine effectiveness of drug and need for additional dosing.
  - 12 to 16 years: Same as adult dosing. Some patients in this age group require a higher dose than that used in adults, but rarely does a patient require more than 10 mg.
  - 6 to 12 years: 0.025 to 0.05 mg/kg IV, IO up to a total dose of 0.4 mg/kg. Exceeding 10 mg as total dose usually is not necessary.
  - 6 months to 5 years: 0.05 to 0.1 mg/kg IV, IO up to a total dose of 0.6 mg/kg. Exceeding 6 mg as total dose usually is not necessary.
  - Younger than 6 months: Dosing recommendations for this age group are unclear. Because this age group is especially vulnerable to airway obstruction and hypoventilation, use small increments with frequent clinical evaluation. Dose: 0.05 to 0.1 mg/kg IV, IO.

Special Considerations: Patients receiving midazolam require frequent monitoring of vital signs and pulse oximetry. Be prepared to support patient's airway and ventilation. Pregnancy Category D.

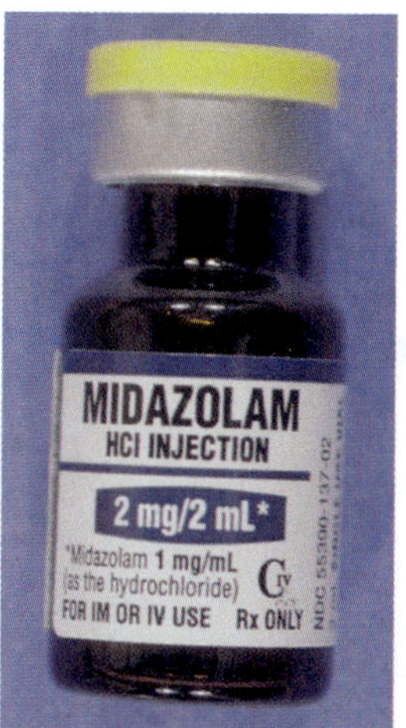

Milrinone (Primacor)

Classification: Inotropic

Action: Milrinone is a positive inotropic drug and vasodilator with minimal chronotropic effect. Milrinone inhibits an enzyme, cAMP phosphodiesterase, which results in an increase in the concentration of calcium inside the cardiac cell. The result is improvement in diastolic function and myocardial contractility.

Indications: Cardiogenic shock, CHF.

Adverse Effects: Cardiac arrhythmias, nausea/vomiting, hypotension.

Contraindications: Valvular heart disease, known sensitivity.

Dosage:

- Adult: 50 mcg/kg IV, IO over a period of 10 minutes, followed by an infusion of 0.375 to 0.5 mcg/kg/min (max dose: 0.75 mcg/kg/min).
- Pediatric: 50 mcg/kg IV or IO over 10 minutes, followed by 0.5 to 1 mcg/kg/min.

Special Considerations: Pregnancy Category C.

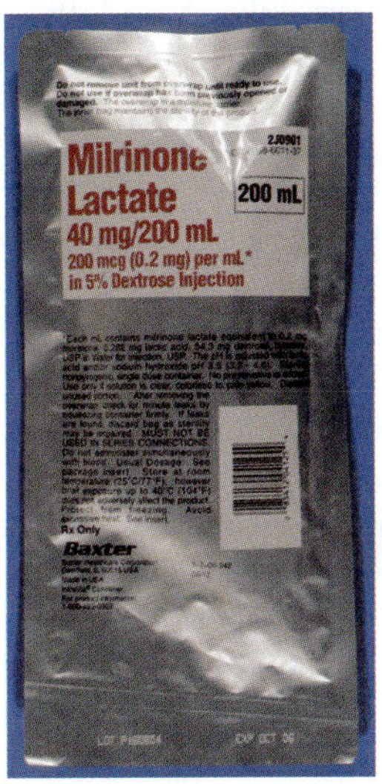

Morphine Sulfate

Classification: Opiate agonist, Schedule C-II

Action: Binds with opioid receptors. Morphine is capable of inducing hypotension by depression of the vasomotor centers of the brain, as well as release of the chemical histamine. In the management of angina, morphine reduces stimulation of the sympathic nervous system caused by pain and anxiety. Reduction of sympathetic stimulation reduces heart rate, cardiac work, and myocardial oxygen consumption.

Indications: Moderate to severe pain, including chest pain associated with ACS, CHF, pulmonary edema.

Adverse Effects: Respiratory depression, hypotension, nausea/vomiting, dizziness, lightheadedness, sedation, diaphoresis, euphoria, dysphoria, worsening of bradycardia and heart block in some patients with acute inferior wall MI, seizures, cardiac arrest, anaphylactoid reactions.

Contraindications: Respiratory depression, shock, known sensitivity. Use with caution in hypotension, acute bronchial asthma, respiratory insufficiency, head trauma.

Dosage:

Pain:

- Adult: 2 to 10 mg IV, IO, IM, or SQ administered slowly over a period of several minutes. The dose is the same whether administered IV, IO, IM, or SQ.
- Pediatric:
  - 6 months to 12 years: 0.05 to 0.1 mg/kg IV, IO, IM, or SQ.
  - Younger than 6 months: 0.1 mg/kg IV, IO, IM, or SQ.

Chest pain associated with acute coronary syndromes, congestive heart failure, and pulmonary edema:

- Administer small doses, and reevaluate the patient. Large doses may lead to respiratory depression and worsen the patient's hypoxia.
- Adult: 2 to 4 mg slow IV, IO over a 1- to 5-minute period with increments of 2 to 8 mg repeated every 5 to 15 minutes until patient relieved of chest pain.
- Pediatric: 0.1 mg/kg/dose IV, IO.

Special Considerations: Monitor vital signs and pulse oximetry closely. Be prepared to support patient's airway and ventilations. Overdose should be treated with naloxone. Pregnancy Category C.

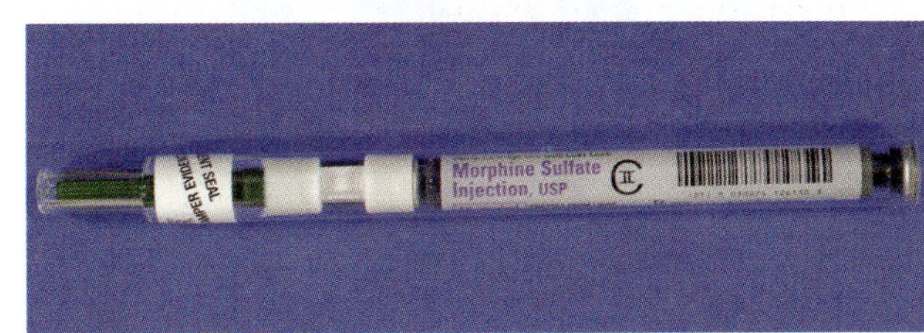

Naloxone (Narcan)

Classification: Opioid antagonist

Action: Binds the opioid receptor and blocks the effect of narcotics.

Indications: Narcotic overdoses, reversal of narcotics used for procedure-related anesthesia.

Adverse Effects: Nausea/vomiting, restlessness, diaphoresis, tachycardia, hypertension, tremulousness, seizures, cardiac arrest, narcotic withdrawal. Patients who have gone from a state of somnolence from a narcotic overdose to wide awake may become combative.

Contraindications: Known sensitivity to naloxone, nalmefene, or naltrexone. Use with caution in patients with supraventricular arrhythmias or other cardiac disease, head trauma, brain tumor.

Dosage:

- Adult: 0.4 to 2 mg IV, IO, ET, IM, or SQ. Alternatively, administer 2 mg intranasally. Higher doses (10 to 20 mg) may be required for overdoses of synthetic narcotics. A repeat dose of one third to two thirds the original dose is often necessary.
- Pediatric:
  - 5 years or older or weight > 20 kg: 2 mg IV, IO, ET, IM, or SQ.
  - Younger than 5 years or weight < 20 kg: 0.1 mg/kg IV, IO, ET, IM, or SQ; may repeat every 2 to 3 minutes.

Special Considerations: Pregnancy Category C.

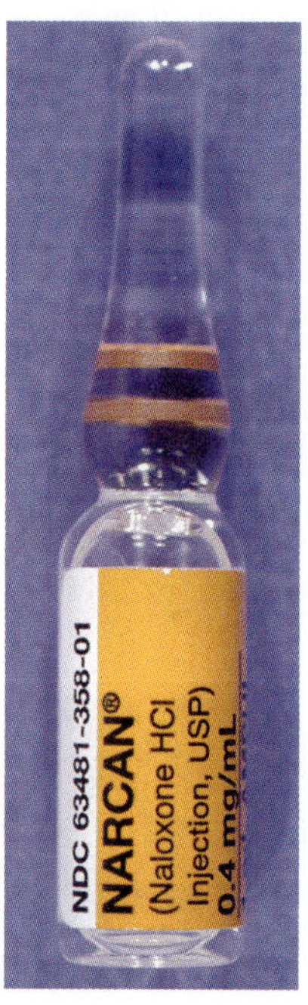

Nicardipine (Cardene)

Classification: Calcium channel blocker

Action: Blocks calcium movement into the smooth muscle of the blood vessel walls, causing vasodilation.

Indications: Hypertension

Adverse Effects: Edema, headaches, flushing, sinus tachycardia, hypotension.

Contraindications: Aortic stenosis, hypotension, known sensitivity. Use with caution in heart failure, cardiac conduction abnormalities, cerebrovascular disease, depressed AV node conduction.

Dosage:

- Adult: 5 mg/hr IV, IO; may increase by 2.5 mg/hr every 5 to 15 minutes (max dose: 15 mg/hr). Once the patient has achieved the desired blood pressure, decrease infusion to a maintenance dose of 5 mg/hr.
- Pediatric: 1 to 7 mcg/kg/min IV, IO infusion.

Special Considerations: Pregnancy Category C.

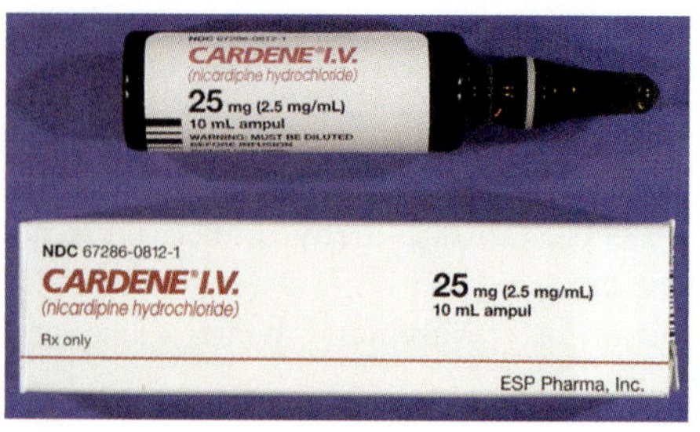

Nitroglycerin (Nitrolingual, NitroQuick, Nitro-Dur)

Classification: Antianginal agent

Action: Relaxes vascular smooth muscle, thereby dilating peripheral arteries and veins. This causes pooling of venous blood and decreased venous return to the heart, which decreases preload. Nitroglycerin also reduces left ventricular systolic wall tension, which decreases afterload.

Indications: Angina, ongoing ischemic chest discomfort, hypertension, myocardial ischemia associated with cocaine intoxication.

Adverse Effects: Headache, hypotension, bradycardia, lightheadedness, flushing, cardiovascular collapse, methemoglobinemia.

Contraindications: Hypotension, severe bradycardia or tachycardia, increased intracranial pressure (ICP), intracranial bleeding, patients taking any medications for erectile dysfunction (such as sildenafil [Viagra], tadalafil [Cialis], or vardenafil [Levitra]), known sensitivity to nitrates. Use with caution in anemia, closed-angle glaucoma, hypotension, postural hypotension, uncorrected hypovolemia.

Dosage:

- Adult:
  - Sublingual tablets: 1 tablet (0.3-0.4 mg) at 5-minute intervals to a maximum of 3 doses.
  - Translingual spray: 1 (0.4 mg) spray at 5-minute intervals to a maximum of 3 sprays.
  - Ointment: 2% topical (Nitro-Bid ointment): Apply 1 to 2 inches of paste over the chest wall, cover with transparent wrap, and secure with tape.
  - IV:
    - Starting dose: 12.5 to 25 mcg
    - Infusion: 5 mcg/min; may increase rate by 5 to 10 mcg/min every 5 to 10 minutes as needed. Endpoints of dose titration for nitroglycerin include a drop in the blood pressure of 10%, relief of chest pain, and return of ST segment to normal on a 12-lead ECG.
- Pediatric IV infusion: The initial pediatric infusion is 0.25 to 0.5 mcg/kg/min IV, IO titrated by 0.5 to 1 mcg/kg/min every 20 to 60 minutes. Usual required dose is 1 to 3 mcg/kg/min to a maximum dose of 5 mcg/kg/min.

Special Considerations: Administration of nitroglycerin to a patient with right ventricular MI can result in hypotension. Pregnancy Category C.

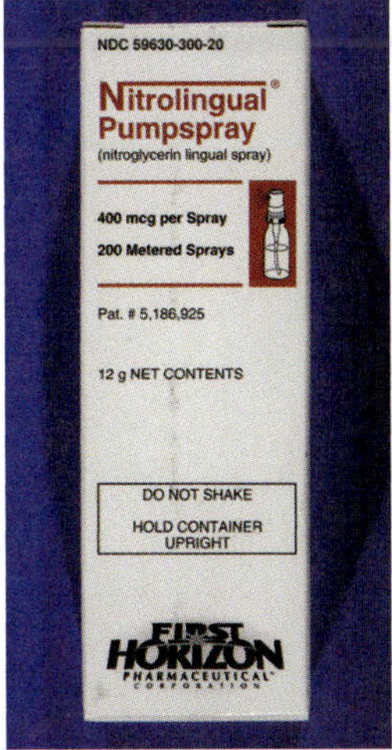

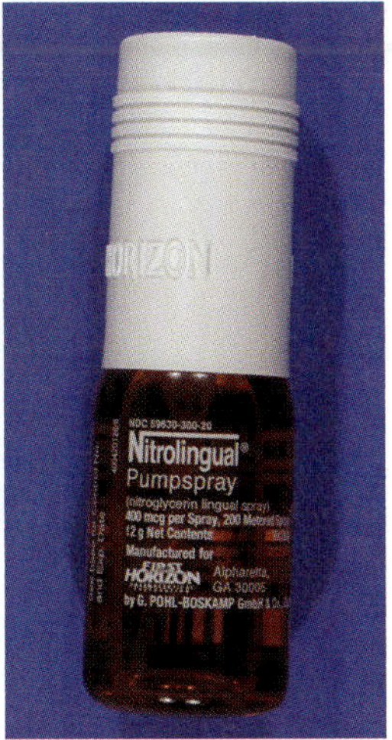

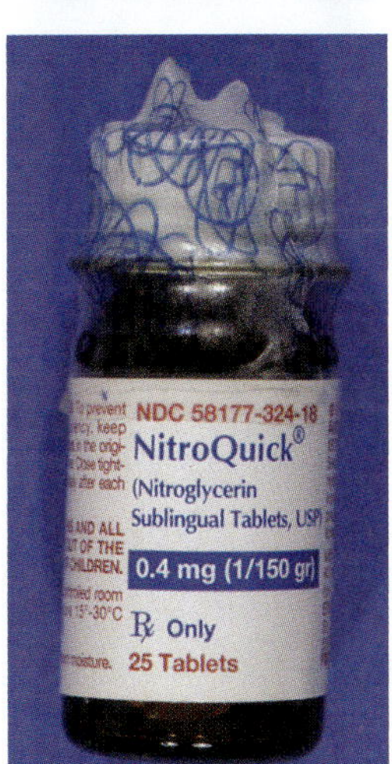

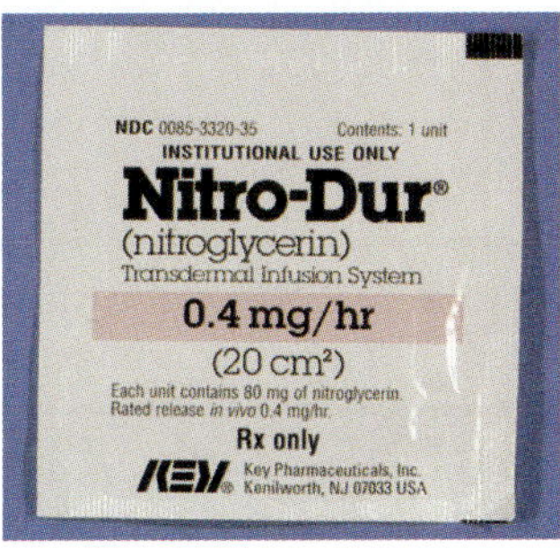

Nitrous Oxide

Classification: Inorganic gas, inhaled anesthetic

Action: Exact mechanism is unknown.

Indications: Mild to severe pain.

Adverse Effects: Delirium, hypoxia, respiratory depression, nausea/vomiting.

Contraindications: Use with caution in head trauma, increased ICP, pneumothorax, bowel obstruction, patients with COPD who require a hypoxic respiratory drive, hypovolemia.

Dosage: Inhaled: 20% to 50% concentration mixed with oxygen.

Special Considerations: Ensure the safety of healthcare professionals. Use only with a scavenger gas system to ensure that unused gas is collected, or scavenged, and that providers are not exposed to significant levels of the agent; always administer with oxygen. Pregnancy Category not noted.

Norepinephrine (Levophed)

Classification: Adrenergic agonist, inotropic, vasopressor

Action: Norepinephrine is an alpha$_1$, alpha$_2$, and beta$_1$ agonist. Alpha-mediated peripheral vasoconstriction is the predominant clinical result of administration, resulting in increasing blood pressure and coronary blood flow. Beta-adrenergic action produces inotropic stimulation of the heart and dilates the coronary arteries.

Indications: Cardiogenic shock, septic shock, severe hypotension.

Adverse Effects: Dizziness, anxiety, cardiac arrhythmias, dyspnea, exacerbation of asthma.

Contraindications: Patients taking MAOIs, tricyclic antidepressants, known sensitivity and hypovolemia.

Dosage:

- Adult: Add 4 mg to 250 mL of D_5W or D_5NS, but not normal saline alone. In cardiogenic shock: 8 to 12 mcg/min. 0.5 to 1 mcg/min as IV, IO, titrated to maintain systolic blood pressure >80 mm Hg. Maintenance dose at 2 to 4 mcg/min. Refractory shock may require doses as high as 30 mcg/min.
- Pediatric: 0.05 to 0.3 mcg/kg/min IV, IO infusion, to a maximum dose of 2 mcg/m^2/min.

Special Considerations: Do not administer in same IV line as alkaline solutions. Large peripheral vein preferred if IV. Half-life 1 minute. Pregnancy Category C.

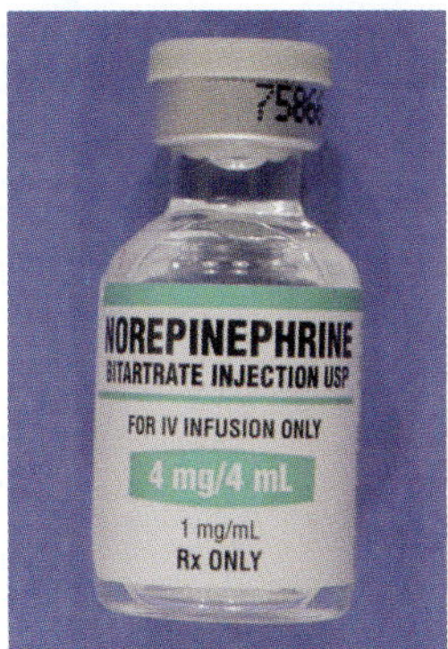

Ondansetron Hydrochloride (Zofran)

Classification: Antiemetic

Action: Blocks serotonin 5-HT3 receptors with reduction of vagus nerve activity.

Indications: For the prevention of chemotherapy and radiation-induced nausea and vomiting and for prevention of postoperative nausea and vomiting.

Adverse Effects: Include fever, headache, constipation, diarrhea, and (rarely) anaphylaxis, chest pain, and bronchospasm.

Contraindications: Hypersensitivity to ondansetron, other selective 5-HT3 antagonists, or any component of the formulation

Dosage: Oral dosage forms should be given 30 minutes prior to chemotherapy; 1 to 2 hours before radiotherapy; 1 hour prior to the induction of anesthesia. Orally disintegrating 8-mg tablets: do not remove from blister until needed. Peel backing off the blister, do not push tablet through. Using dry hands, place tablet on tongue and allow to dissolve. Swallow with saliva. 4 mg IM undiluted. IVPB, dilute into 50 mL D_5W or NS and infuse over 15 to 30 minutes. IV push in a single dose, given over 2 to 5 minutes undiluted. Single maximum daily dose of parenteral ondansetron is 8 mg.

Special Considerations: Teratogenic effects were not observed in animal studies, but considered Pregnancy Category B by FDA. Use of ondansetron for the treatment of nausea and vomiting of pregnancy (NVP) has been evaluated. Additional studies are needed to determine safety to the fetus, particularly during the first trimester. Based on preliminary data, use is generally reserved for severe NVP (hyperemesis gravidarum) or when conventional treatments are not effective.

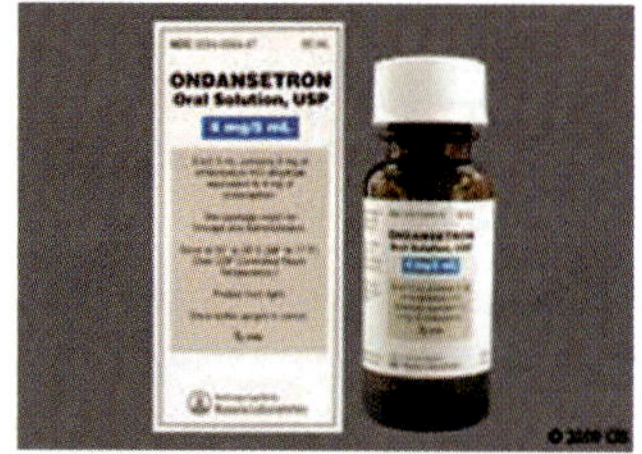

 Oxygen

Classification: Elemental gas

Action: Facilitates cellular energy metabolism.

Indications: Hypoxia, ischemic chest pain, respiratory distress, suspected carbon monoxide poisoning, traumatic injuries, shock.

Adverse Effects: High concentrations can cause decreased level of consciousness and respiratory depression in patients with chronic carbon dioxide retention or chronic lung disease.

Contraindications: Known paraquat poisoning.

Dosage:

Low-concentration oxygen:

- A dose of 1 to 4 L/min by a nasal cannula is appropriate.

High-concentration oxygen:

- A dose of 10 to 15 L/min via nonrebreather mask is appropriate.

Special Considerations: Pregnancy Category A.

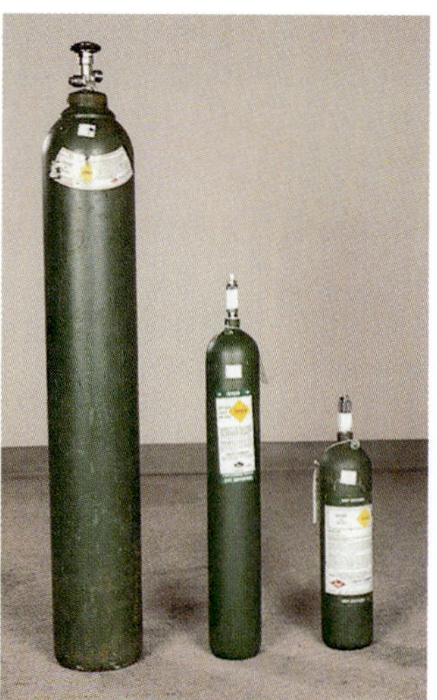

Pancuronium (Pavulon)

Classification: Nondepolarizing neuromuscular blocker

Action: Antagonizes acetylcholine at the motor end plate, producing skeletal muscle paralysis.

Indications: To induce neuromuscular blockade for the facilitation of ET intubation.

Adverse Effects: Muscle paralysis, apnea, dyspnea, respiratory depression, cutaneous flushing, sinus tachycardia.

Contraindications: Known sensitivity to bromides. Use with caution in heart disease, renal disease.

Dosage:

- Adult: 0.06 to 0.1 mg/kg IV, IO; repeat dosing is 0.01 mg/kg every 25 to 60 minutes.
- Pediatric: Same as adult dosing.

Special Considerations: Pregnancy Category C.

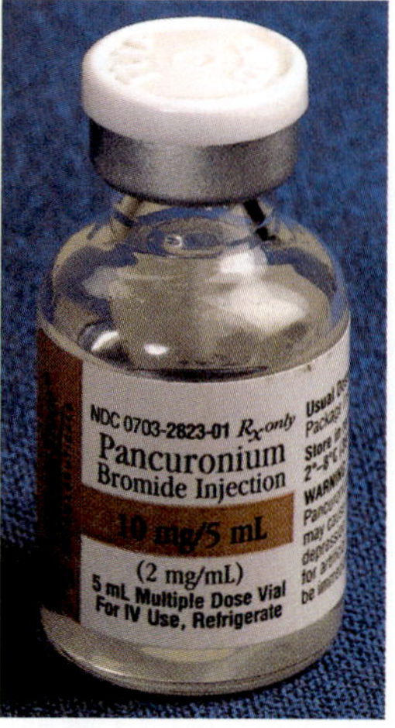

Phenobarbital (Luminal)

Classification: Anticonvulsant, barbiturate, Schedule C-IV

Action: Depresses seizure activity in the cortex, thalamus, and limbic system; increases threshold for electrical stimulation of motor cortex; produces state of sedation.

Indications: Seizures

Adverse Effects: Depression, agitation, respiratory depression, accelerated metabolism of several other medications.

Contraindications: Porphyria, agranulocytosis, known sensitivity to barbiturates. Use with caution with liver dysfunction and respiratory dysfunction.

Dosage:

- Adult: 15 to 18 mg/kg IV, IO; infuse at a rate not faster than 100 mg/min.
- Pediatric: 15 to 20 mg/kg IV, IO; infuse at a rate not faster than 2 mg/kg/min.

Special Considerations: Be prepared to manage the patient's airway. Pregnancy Category D.

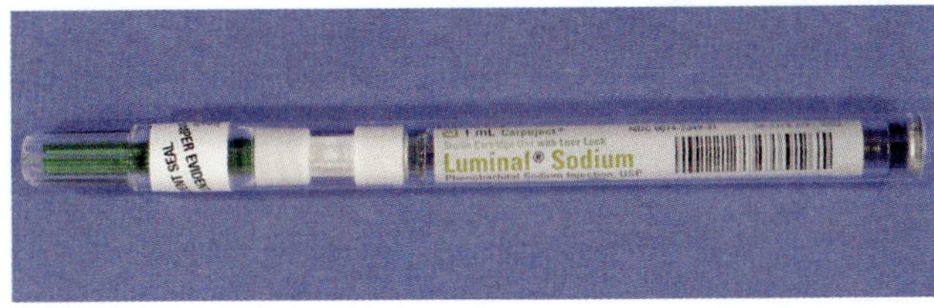

Phentolamine (Regitine)

Classification: Alpha antagonist, antihypertensive

Action: Blocks alpha-adrenergic receptors, causing vasodilation.

Indications: Hypertensive emergencies and hypertension caused by pheochromocytoma, cocaine-induced vasospasm of the coronary arteries.

Adverse Effects: Sinus tachycardia, angina, dizziness, orthostatic hypotension, prolonged hypotensive episodes, nausea/vomiting, diarrhea, weakness, flushing, nasal congestion.

Contraindications: Known sensitivity. Use with caution in acute MI, angina, coronary insufficiency, evidence suggestive of coronary artery disease, peptic ulcer disease.

Dosage:

Hypertensive crisis:

- Adult: 5 mg IV, IO, or IM.
- Pediatric: 1 mg IV or IM for prophylactic treatment of patients with pheochromocytoma and are undergoing surgery.

Cocaine-induced vasospasm:

- Adult: 1 mg every 7 minutes IV, IO or IM.
- Pediatric: Not recommended for pediatric patients.

Special Considerations: Pregnancy Category C.

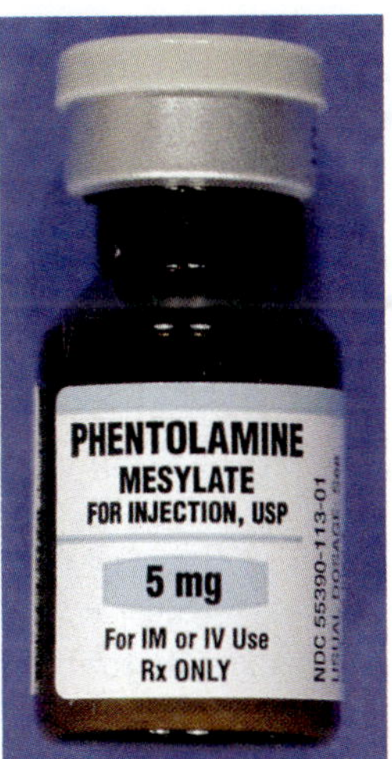

Phenylephrine (Neo-Synephrine)

Classification: Adrenergic agonist

Action: Stimulates the alpha receptors, causing vasoconstriction, which results in increased blood pressure.

Indications: Neurogenic shock, spinal shock, cases of shock in which the patient's heart rate does not need to be increased, drug-induced hypotension.

Adverse Effects: Hypertension, VT, headache, excitability, tremor, MI, exacerbation of asthma, cardiac arrhythmias, reflex bradycardia, soft tissue necrosis.

Contraindications: Acute MI, angina, cardiac arrhythmias, severe hypertension, coronary artery disease, pheochromocytoma, narrow-angle glaucoma, cardiomyopathy, MAOI therapy, known sensitivity to phenylephrine or sulfites.

Dosage:

- Adult: 100 to 180 mcg/min IV, IO. Once the blood pressure has been stabilized, the dose can be reduced to 40 to 60 mcg/min.
- Pediatric (2 to 12 years): 5 to 20 mcg/kg IV, IO followed by 0.1 to 0.5 mcg/kg/min IV, IO (max dose: 3 mcg/kg/min IV, IO).

Special Considerations: Pregnancy Category C.

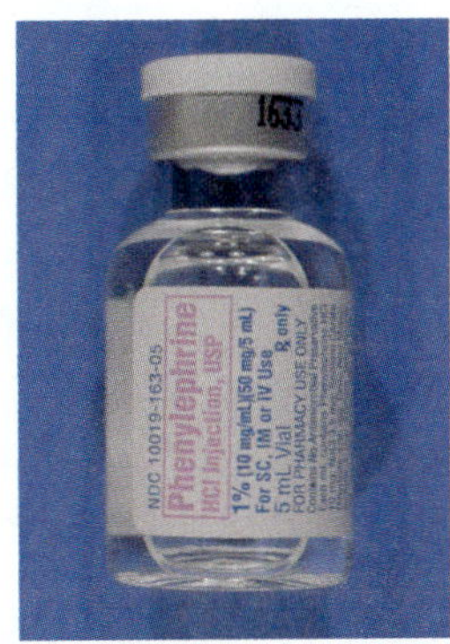

Phenytoin (Dilantin)

Classification: Anticonvulsant

Action: Depresses seizures by affecting the movement of sodium and calcium into neural tissue.

Indications: Generalized tonic-clonic seizures.

Adverse Effects: Nausea/vomiting, depression of cardiac conduction, sedation, nystagmus, tremors, ataxia, dysarthria, gingival hypertrophy, hirsutism, facial coarsening, hypotension.

Contraindications: Sinus bradycardia, sinoatrial block, second- and third-degree heart block, Adams-Stokes syndrome, known sensitivity to hydantoins.

Dosage:

- Adult: 15 to 20 mg/kg IV, IO should be administered slowly at a rate not exceeding 50 mg/min. (This requires approximately 20 minutes in a 70-kg patient.)
- Pediatric: 15 to 20 mg/kg IV, IO, administered at a rate of 1 to 3 mg/kg/min.

Special Considerations: Continuously monitor the ECG and blood pressure during administration. Pregnancy Category D.

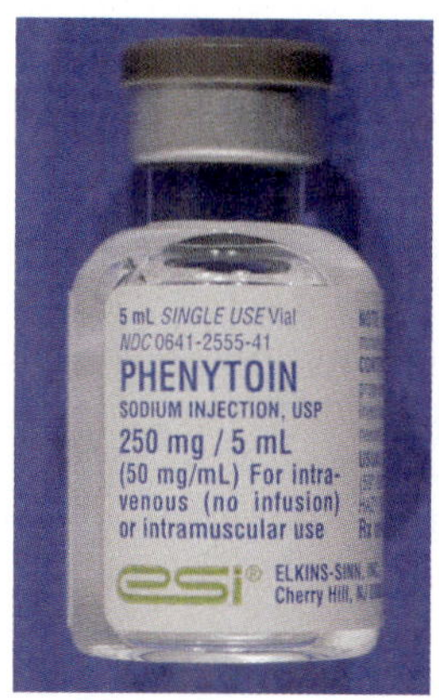

Potassium Chloride

Classification: Electrolyte replacement

Action: Replaces potassium. Slight alterations in extracellular potassium levels can cause serious alterations in both cardiac and nervous function.

Indications: Hypokalemia

Adverse Effects: Hyperkalemia; AV block; cardiac arrest; GI bleeding, obstruction, or perforation; tissue necrosis if the infusion infiltrates into the soft tissues.

Contraindications: Use with caution in patients with cardiac arrhythmias, renal failure, muscle cramps, severe tissue trauma.

Dosage:

- Adult: Dosage must be individualized according to patient serum potassium concentration.
- Pediatric: Dosage must be individualized according to patient serum potassium concentration.

Special Considerations: Pregnancy Category C.

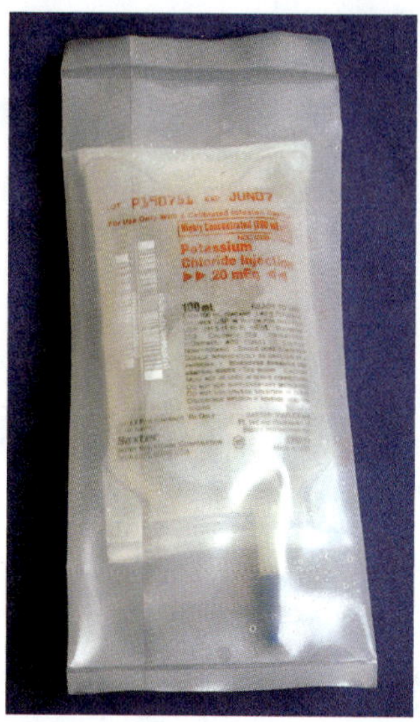

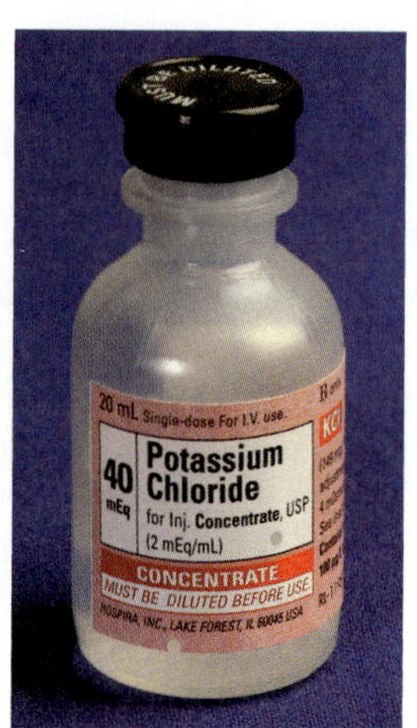

Pralidoxime (2-PAM, Protopam)

Classification: Cholinergic agonist, antidote

Action: Reactivates cholinesterase.

Indications: Toxicity from nerve agents (organophosphates) having cholinesterase activity, myasthenia gravis.

Adverse Effects: Dizziness, blurred vision, diplopia, hyperventilation, laryngospasm, nausea/vomiting, sinus tachycardia.

Contraindications: Myasthenia gravis, and inability to control the airway. Use with caution in those with renal failure.

Dosage:

- Adult: 1 to 2 g (dilute in 100 mL normal saline) over a 15- to 30-minute period. If this is not practical or if pulmonary edema is present, the dose should be given slowly (≥5 minutes) by IV as a 5% solution in water.
    - Autoinjector: Pralidoxime is also available as an autoinjector that delivers 600 mg IM. Repeat doses can be given every 15 minutes to a total of three doses (1800 mg). Pralidoxime autoinjector is not recommended for pediatric patients.
- Pediatric: 20 to 50 mg/kg IV, IO over a 10-minute period.

Special Considerations: Pregnancy Category C.

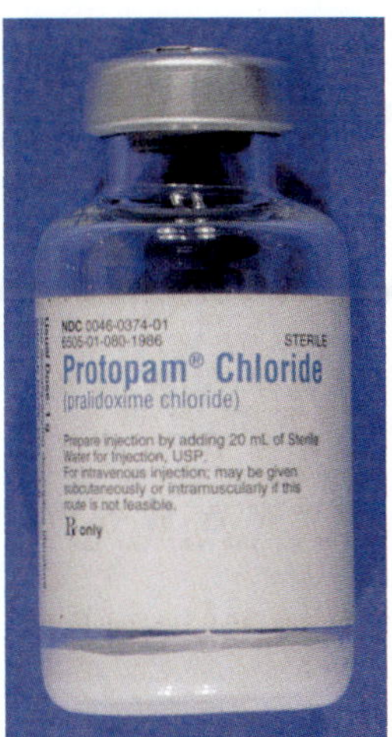

Prednisone

Classification: Corticosteroid
Action: Reduces inflammation.
Indications: Inflammatory conditions, such as asthma with bronchospasm.
Adverse Effects: Many adverse effects of steroid use are not related to short-term use but typically are seen with long-term use and during withdrawal.
Contraindications: Known sensitivity. Adverse effects in Cushing's syndrome. Use with caution in those with fungal infections, measles, varicella.
Dosage:

- Adult: Dosage must be individualized.
- Pediatric: Dosage must be individualized.

Special Considerations: Pregnancy Category not rated by FDA.

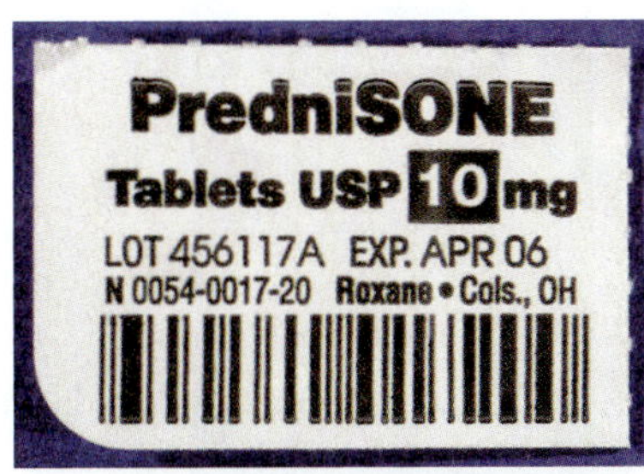

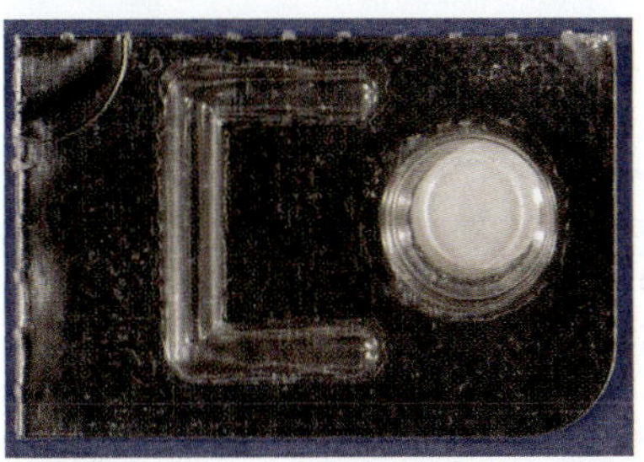

Promethazine (Phenergan)

Classification: Antiemetic, antihistamine
Action: Decreases nausea and vomiting by antagonizing H_1 receptors.
Indications: Nausea/vomiting.
Adverse Effects: Paradoxical excitation in children and elderly patients, CNS depression.
Contraindications: Altered level of consciousness, jaundice, bone marrow suppression, known sensitivity. Use with caution in seizure disorder.
Dosage:

- Adult: 12.5 to 25 mg IV, IO, or IM.
- Pediatric:
  - 2 years and older: 0.25 to 1 mg/kg IV, IO, IM (maximum rate of IV, IO administration is 25 mg/min).

Special Considerations: Pregnancy Category C.

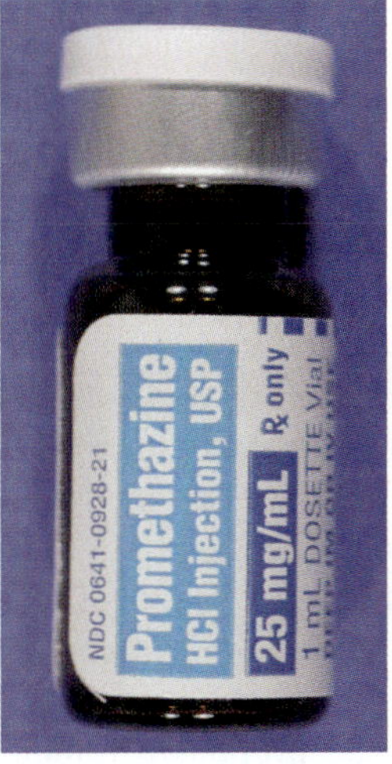

Propofol (Diprivan)

Classification: Anesthetic
Action: Produces rapid and brief state of general anesthesia.
Indications: Anesthesia induction.
Adverse Effects: Apnea, cardiac arrhythmias, asystole, hypotension, hypertension, pain at injection site.
Contraindications: Hypovolemia, known sensitivity (including soybean oil, eggs).
Dosage: A general induction dose used to produce a state of unconsciousness rapidly is 1.5 mg/kg IV, IO.

After the induction bolus, the patient must be given intermittent boluses or a maintenance infusion. For an average adult, an intermittent dose is 20 to 50 mg as needed. Alternatively, a propofol infusion may be ordered. Maintenance of anesthesia with a propofol infusion can be achieved by the following protocols:

Patient Group	Dosage	Rate of Administration (10 mg/mL)
Healthy adults <55 years	2 to 2.5 mg/kg IV, IO	40 mg every 10 seconds
Elderly or debilitated patients	1 to 1.5 mg/kg IV, IO	20 mg every 10 seconds
Cardiac patients	0.5 to 1.5 mg/kg IV, IO	20 mg every 10 seconds
Patients with head injuries	1 to 2 mg/kg IV, IO	20 mg every 10 seconds

Pediatric (3 to 16 years) for procedural sedation	0.5 mg/kg every 3 to 5 minutes IV, IO
Pediatric (3 to 16 years) induction for anesthesia	2.5 to 3.5 mg/kg IV or IO over 20 to 30 minutes

- Adult patients: 25 to 75 mcg/kg/min IV, IO.
- Elderly, debilitated, or head-injured patients: Use approximately 80% of the normal adult dose.
- Pediatric: 125 to 300 mcg/kg/min IV, IO.

Special Considerations: Propofol should be administered only by personnel trained and equipped to manage the patient's airway and provide mechanical ventilation. In elderly and debilitated patients, avoid rapid administration to prevent hypotension, apnea, airway obstruction, and/or oxygen desaturation. Continue to monitor the patient's oxygenation and vital signs and try to limit use of propofol to patients who are intubated. Propofol should not be administered through the same IV catheter as blood or plasma. Pain can occur at the site of injection, which can be minimized by use of larger veins, slower rates of administration, and administration of 1 mL 1% lidocaine before propofol administration. Propofol is listed as a Pregnancy Category B; however, propofol should be avoided in pregnant women because it crosses the placenta and can cause neonatal depression.

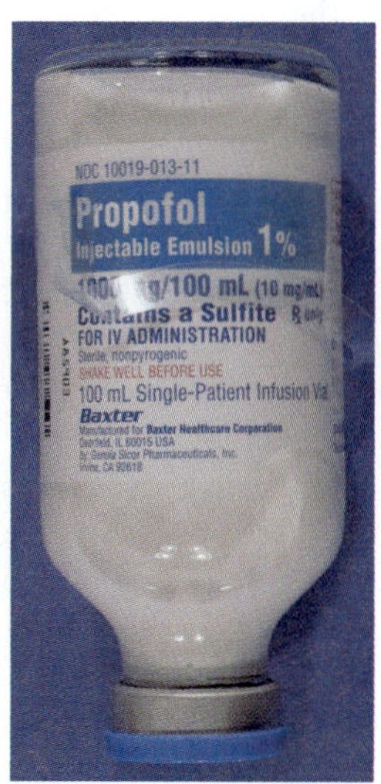

Racemic Epinephrine/Racepinephrine (MicroNefrin S2)

Classification: Bronchodilator, adrenergic agent

Action: Stimulates both alpha and beta receptors, causing vasoconstriction, reduced mucosal edema, and bronchodilation.

Indications: Bronchial asthma, croup.

Adverse Effects: Anxiety, dizziness, headache, tremor, palpitations, tachycardia, cardiac arrhythmias, hypertension, nausea/vomiting.

Contraindications: Glaucoma, elderly, cardiac disease, hypertension, thyroid disease, diabetes, known sensitivity to sulfites.

Dosage:

- Adult: Add 0.5 mL to nebulizer; for hand-bulb nebulizer, administer 1 to 3 inhalations; for jet nebulizer, add 3 mL of diluent, swirl the nebulizer and administer for 15 minutes.
- Pediatric:
  - Older than 4 years: Same as adult dosing.
  - Younger than 4 years: Safe and effective use has not been demonstrated.

Special Considerations: Monitor blood pressure, heart rate, and cardiac rhythm for changes. Onset of action is 1 to 5 minutes. Pregnancy Category C.

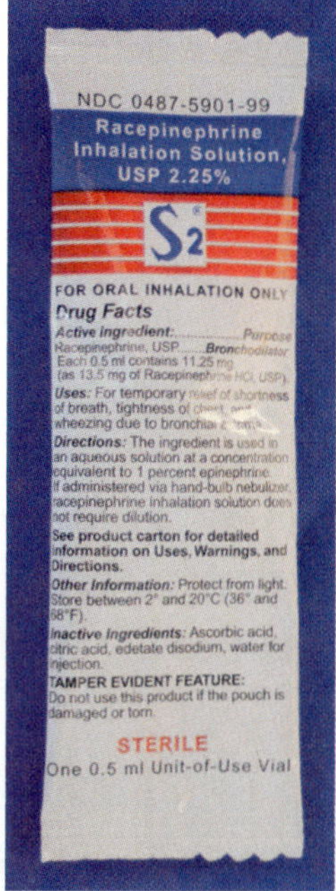

Rocuronium (Zemuron)

Classification: Neuromuscular blocker, nondepolarizing

Action: Antagonizes acetylcholine at the motor end plate, producing skeletal muscle paralysis.

Indications: To induce neuromuscular blockade for the facilitation of ET intubation.

Adverse Effects: Muscle paralysis, apnea, dyspnea, respiratory depression, sinus tachycardia, urticaria.

Contraindications: Known sensitivity to bromides. Use with caution in heart disease, liver disease.

Dosage:

- Adult: 0.6 to 1.2 mg/kg IV, IO.
- Pediatric (older than 3 months): 0.6 to 1.2 mg/kg IV, IO.

Special Considerations: Onset of action is 1 to 1.6 minutes. Duration of action is 22 to 94 minutes. Pregnancy Category C.

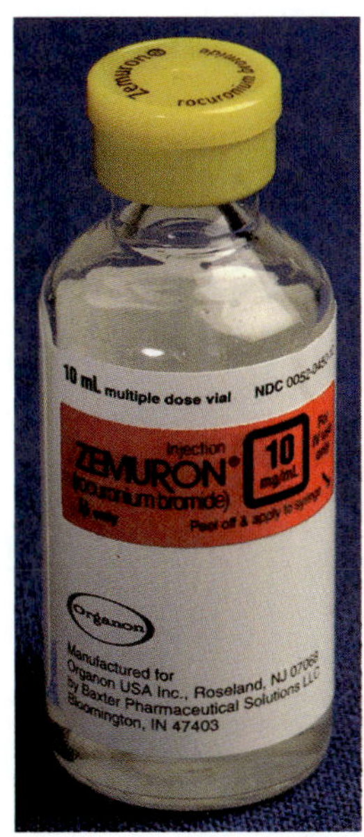

Sodium Bicarbonate

Classification: Electrolyte replacement

Action: Counteracts existing acidosis.

Indications: Acidosis, drug intoxications (e.g., barbiturates, salicylates, methyl alcohol).

Adverse Effects: Metabolic alkalosis, hypernatremia, injection site reaction, sodium and fluid retention, peripheral edema.

Contraindications: Metabolic alkalosis.

Dosage:

Metabolic acidosis during cardiac arrest:

- Adult: 1 mEq/kg slow IV, IO; may repeat at 0.5 mEq/kg in 10 minutes.
- Pediatric: Same as adult dosing.

Metabolic acidosis not associated with cardiac arrest:

- Adult: Dosage should be individualized.
- Pediatric: Dosage should be individualized.

Special Considerations: Do not administer into an IV, IO line in which another medication is being given. Because of the high concentration of sodium within each ampule of sodium bicarbonate, use with caution in patients with CHF and renal disease. Pregnancy Category C.

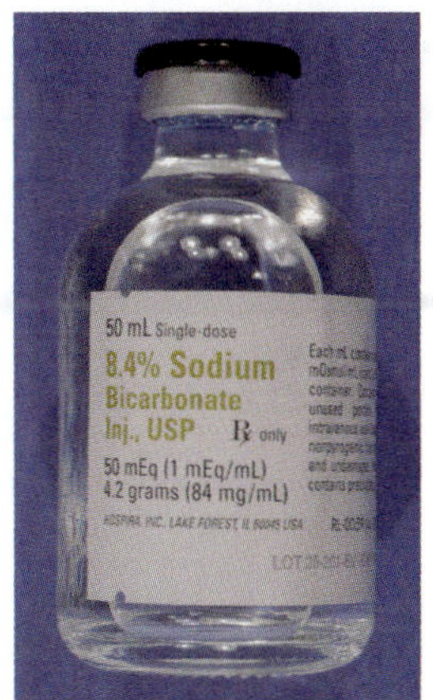

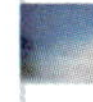

Sodium Nitroprusside (Nipride, Nitropress)

Classification: Antihypertensive agent

Action: Causes direct relaxation of both arteries and veins.

Indications: Hypertensive emergencies.

Adverse Effects: Cyanide toxicity, nausea/vomiting, dizziness, headache, restlessness, abdominal pain, methemoglobinemia.

Contraindications: Hypotension, increased ICP, cerebrovascular disease, coronary artery disease, hepatic disease, renal disease, pulmonary disease.

Dosage:

- Adult: 0.3 to 10 mcg/kg/min IV, IO. Titrate to desired blood pressure.
- Pediatric: Same as adult dosing.

Special Considerations: Nitroprusside will break down when exposed to ultraviolet light. Therefore the infusion should be shielded from light by wrapping the bag with aluminum foil. Pregnancy Category C.

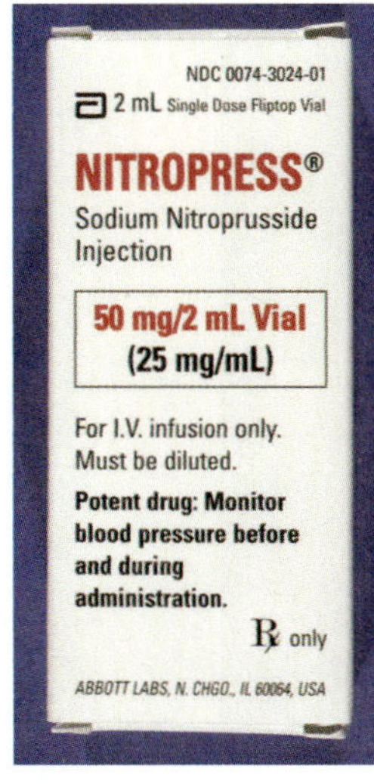

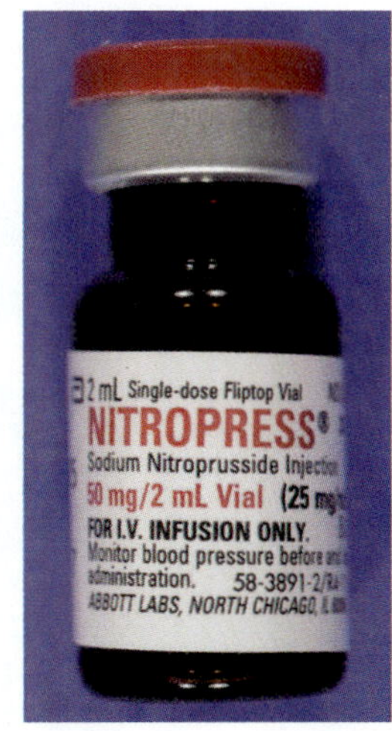

Succinylcholine (Anectine)

Classification: Neuromuscular blocker, depolarizing

Action: Competes with the acetylcholine receptor of the motor end plate on the muscle cell, resulting in muscle paralysis.

Indications: To induce neuromuscular blockade for the facilitation of ET intubation.

Adverse Effects: Anaphylactoid reactions, respiratory depression, apnea, bronchospasm, cardiac arrhythmias, malignant hyperthermia, hypertension, hypotension, muscle fasciculation, postprocedure muscle pain, hypersalivation, rash.

Contraindications: Malignant hyperthermia, burns, trauma. Use with caution in children, cardiac disease, hepatic disease, renal disease, peptic ulcer disease, cholinesterase-inhibitor toxicity, pseudocholinesterase deficiency, digitalis toxicity, glaucoma, hyperkalemia, hypothermia, rhabdomyolysis, myasthenia gravis.

Dosage:

- Adult:
    - IV: 0.6 mg/kg IV, IO (range 0.3 to 1.1 mg/kg).
    - IM: 3 to 4 mg/kg (max dose: 150 mg).
- Pediatric:
    - IV:
        - Adolescents and older children: 1 mg/kg IV, IO.
        - Small children and infants: 2 mg/kg IV, IO.
    - IM: 3 to 4 mg/kg (max dose: 150 mg).

Special Considerations:

- IV administration results in neuromuscular blockade in 0.5 to 1 minute. IM administration results in neuromuscular blockade in 2 to 3 minutes.
- IV administration in infants and children can potentially result in profound bradycardia and, in some cases, asystole. The incidence of bradycardia is greater after the second dose. The occurrence of bradycardia can be reduced with the pretreatment of atropine.

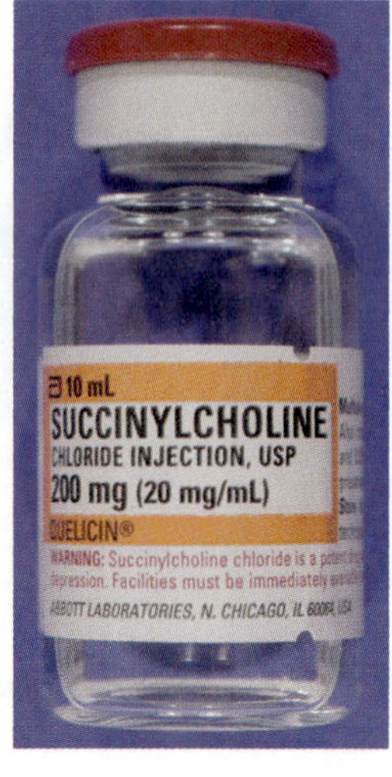

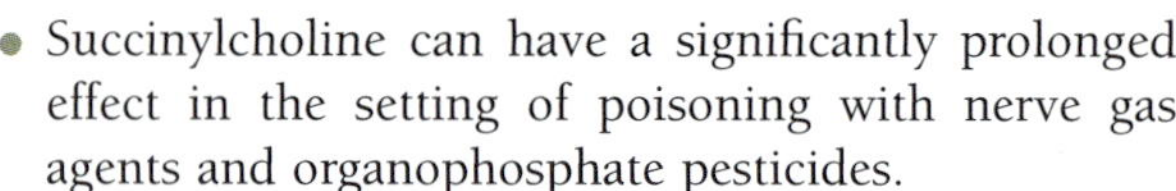

- Succinylcholine can have a significantly prolonged effect in the setting of poisoning with nerve gas agents and organophosphate pesticides.
- Pregnancy Category C.

Terbutaline (Brethine)

Classification: Adrenergic agonist

Action: Stimulates the beta$_2$ receptor, producing relaxation of bronchial smooth muscle and bronchodilation.

Indications: Prevention and reversal of bronchospasm.

Adverse Effects: Cardiac arrhythmias, arrhythmia exacerbation, angina, anxiety, headache, tremor, palpitations, dizziness.

Contraindications: Known sensitivity to sympathomimetics. Use with caution in hypertension, cardiac disease, cardiac arrhythmias, diabetes, elderly, MAOI therapy, pheochromocytoma, thyrotoxicosis, seizure disorder.

Dosage:

- Adult: 0.25 mg SQ. The dose may be repeated in 15 to 30 minutes. Do not exceed 0.5 mg in 4 hours. The usual site for the SQ injection is the lateral deltoid.
- Pediatric: 0.01 mg/kg SQ every 20 minutes for 3 doses.

Special Considerations: Pregnancy Category B.

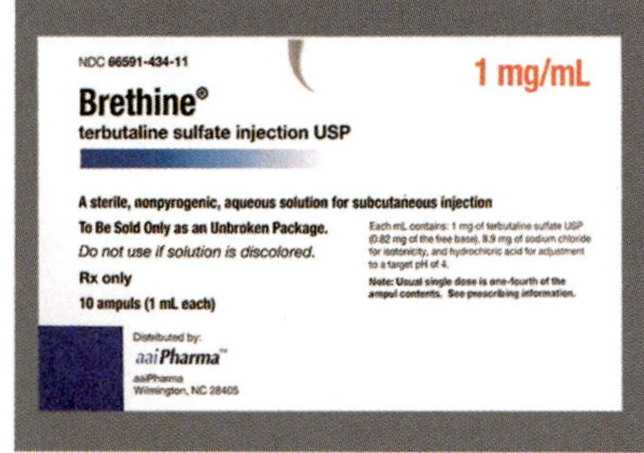

Thiamine (Vitamin B$_1$)

Classification: Vitamin B$_1$

Action: Thiamine combines with adenosine triphosphate to produce thiamine diphosphate, which acts as a coenzyme in carbohydrate metabolism.

Indications: Wernicke-Korsakoff syndrome, beriberi, nutritional supplementation.

Adverse Effects: Itching, rash, pain at injection site.

Contraindications: Known sensitivity.

Dosage:

Wernicke-Korsakoff syndrome:

- Adult: 100 mg IV, IO slow.
- Pediatric: 10 to 25 mg IV or IO slow.

Special Considerations: Pregnancy Category A.

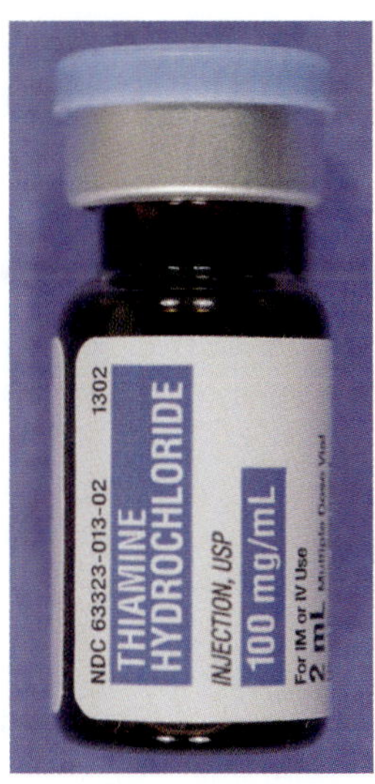

Tirofiban (Aggrastat)

Classification: GP IIb/IIIa inhibitor

Action: Prevents the aggregation of platelets by binding to the GP IIb/IIIa receptor.

Indications: UA/NSTEMI—to manage medically and for those undergoing percutaneous coronary intervention.

Adverse Effects: Bleeding from the GI tract, internal bleeding, intracranial hemorrhage, hypotension, stroke, anaphylactic shock.

Contraindications: Bleeding from any source, severe uncontrolled hypertension, surgery or trauma within the previous 6 weeks, stroke within the previous 30 days, renal failure, thrombocytopenia.

Dosage: 0.4 mcg/kg/min IV, IO for 30 minutes, then 0.1 mcg/kg/min IV, IO infusion for 12 to 24 hours.

Special Considerations: Half-life approximately 2 hours. Pregnancy Category B.

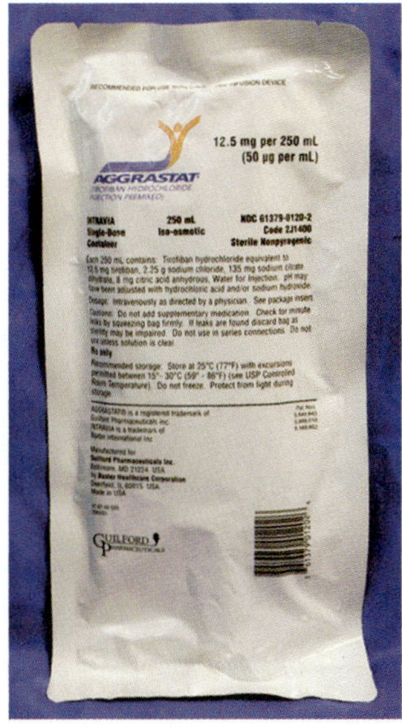

Valproic Acid (Depakote)

Classification: Anticonvulsant, antimanic

Action: Although the exact mechanism of action is unknown, it is suggested that valproic acid increases brain concentrations of GABA.

Indications: Seizures, mood disorders.

Adverse Effects: Tremor, transient hair loss, weight gain, weight loss.

Contraindications: Liver disease.

Dosage: Dosing is individualized.

Special Considerations: Although generally well tolerated, valproic acid does require regular monitoring of blood levels to ensure maintenance of therapeutic levels while minimizing adverse drug reactions. Pregnancy Category D.

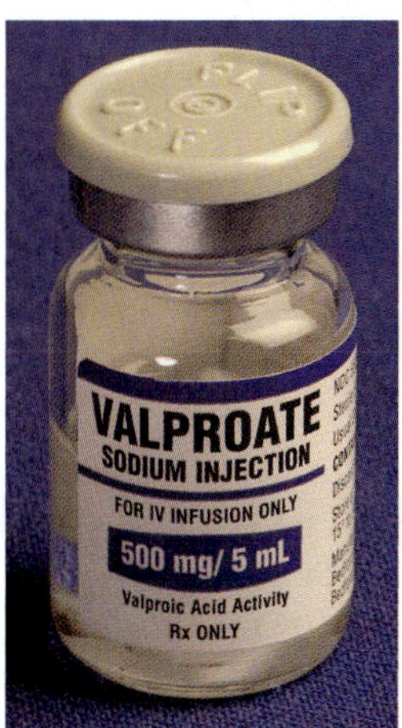

Vasopressin

Classification: Nonadrenergic vasoconstrictor

Action: Vasopressin causes vasoconstriction independent of adrenergic receptors or neural innervation.

Indications: Adult shock-refractory VF or pulseless VT, asystole, PEA, vasodilatory shock.

Adverse Effects: Cardiac ischemia, angina.

Contraindications: Responsive patients with cardiac disease.

Dosage:

- Adult: 40 U IV, IO may replace either the first or second dose of epinephrine. May be given ET, but the optimal dose is not known.

Special Considerations: Pregnancy Category C.

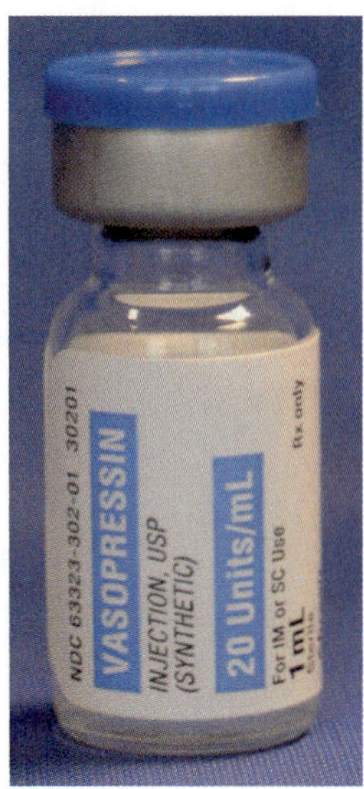

Vecuronium (Norcuron)

Classification: Neuromuscular blocker, nondepolarizing

Action: Antagonizes acetylcholine at the motor end plate, producing skeletal muscle paralysis.

Indications: To induce neuromuscular blockade for the facilitation of ET intubation.

Adverse Effects: Muscle paralysis, apnea, dyspnea, respiratory depression, sinus tachycardia, urticaria.

Contraindications: Known sensitivity to bromides. Use with caution in heart disease, liver disease.

Dosage:

- Adult: 0.08 to 0.1 mg/kg IV, IO.
- Pediatric: Dosage is individualized.

Special Considerations: Pregnancy Category C.

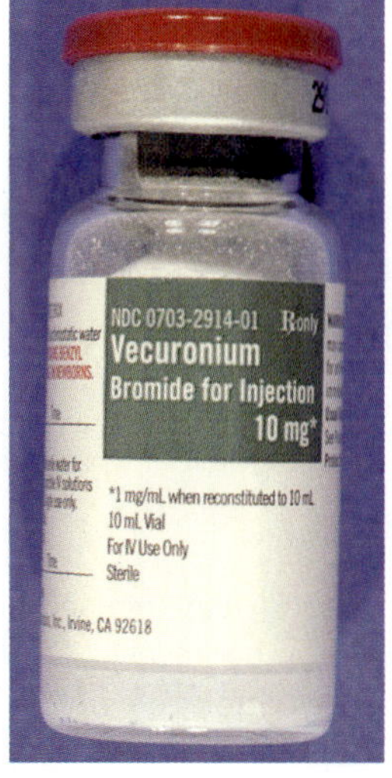

Verapamil (Isoptin)

Classification: Calcium channel blocker; class IV antiarrhythmic

Action: Blocks calcium from moving into the heart muscle cell, which prolongs the conduction of electrical impulses through the AV node. Also dilates arteries.

Indications: Atrial fibrillation, hypertension, PSVT, PSVT prophylaxis.

Adverse Effects: Sinus bradycardia; first-, second-, or third-degree AV block; congestive heart failure; reflex sinus tachycardia; transient asystole; AV block; hypotension.

Contraindications: Second- or third-degree AV block (except in patients with a functioning artificial pacemaker); hypotension (systolic pressure <90 mm Hg) or cardiogenic shock; sick sinus syndrome (except in patients with a functioning artificial pacemaker); Wolff-Parkinson-White syndrome; Lown-Ganong-Levine syndrome; severe left ventricular dysfunction; known sensitivity to verapamil or any component of the formulation; atrial flutter or fibrillation and an accessory bypass tract (WPW, Lown-Ganong-Levine syndrome); in infants younger than 1 yr.

Dosage:

- Adult: 5 to 10 mg IV, IO over 2 minutes (3 minutes in elderly patients). May repeat at 5 to 10 mg every 15 to 30 minutes to a maximum dose of 30 mg.
- Pediatric:
  - Children 1 to 16 years: 0.1 mg/kg IV, IO (maximum 5 mg/dose) over 2 minutes. May repeat in 30 minutes to a maximum dose of 10 mg.
  - Infants younger than 1 year: Not recommended.

Special Considerations: Pregnancy Category C.

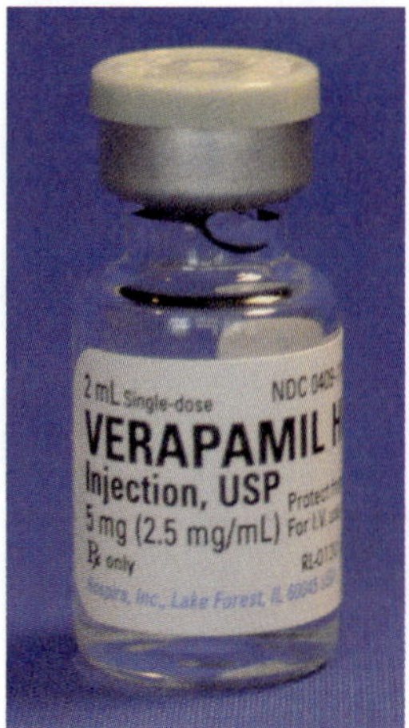

Warfarin (Coumadin)

Classification: Anticoagulant

Action: Inhibits vitamin K-dependent coagulation factors, including factors II, VII, IX, and X and anticoagulant proteins C and S. Interferes with clotting factor synthesis.

Indications: Prophylaxis or treatment of venous thrombosis and pulmonary embolus or any thromboembolic complication associated with atrial fibrillation or cardiac valve replacement. May be used to reduce risk of death associated with recurrent MI, thromboembolic events like stroke, or systemic embolization after MI.

Adverse Effects: Hemorrhage or necrosis in any tissue or organ.

Contraindications: If the hazard of hemorrhage is greater than the potential benefits of anticoagulation therapy (conditions such as pregnancy, surgery, bleeding tendencies, etc.)

Dosage: Initially, an oral dose of 2 to 5 mg/day, with maintenance at 2 to 10 mg/day, individualized to the patient and guided by periodic lab analysis of PT/INR with a goal of 2 to 3, depending on the condition.

Special Considerations: The narrow therapeutic range for this drug can be affected by other drugs and foods rich in vitamin K. Periodic lab analysis must be done to monitor the PT/INR. Pregnancy Category X.

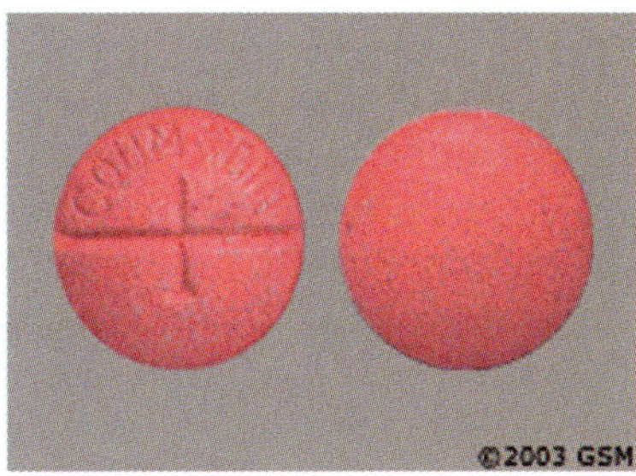

APPENDIX F

Chapter Review Answers

Chapter 1

1. a. Pattern recognition along with the cardinal presentation, history, and physical exam, evaluation of diagnostic findings, and good critical thinking skills all contribute to effective, efficient diagnosis and management of medical patients. (Objective 9)
2. b. Healthcare providers in all environments and situations must remain vigilant in identifying potential safety issues for both the patient and provider. Securing the dog in a kennel away from the patient and providers eliminates that threat. The schizophrenic patient may be temporarily calmed but remains at high risk of outbursts. An armed fugitive is a danger, even though they have left the scene. Prehospital providers should never separate themselves or be placed in a situation where communication, patient care, or escape is difficult. Assistance should be obtained to deal with the angry family member. (Objective 1)
3. d. Prehospital and in-hospital areas that involve patients and their families should be continually assessed for environmental concerns such as comfort and temperature, assistive equipment, and lifting and moving issues. Assistive devices like walkers, oxygen concentrators, and dentures indicate perfusion and nutrition/dehydration issues. All providers should use their sense of smell, vision, hearing, and touch when assessing the environment and patient. (Objective 2)
4. a. This initial diagnosis is based on your global patient assessment and general impression. As additional historical, physical exam, and diagnostic findings are obtained, you'll rule out and rule in various possible differential diagnoses until a working diagnosis is determined. (Objective 4)
5. b. While pulse oximetry may be useful, obtaining end-tidal CO_2 measurement and a 12-lead ECG are not essential treatment interventions with this critical patient. Seizure activity utilizes significant adenosine triphosphate (ATP) energy and glucose, so obtaining a baseline blood glucose level is essential. (Objective 6)
6. Dysuria is the most significant associated complaint relative to the left flank pain complaint. Fever, changes in appetite, and syncope would be key symptoms in complaints of dyspnea, abdominal pain, or alterations in mentation. (Objective 5)
7. c. Restating and summarizing the discussion is essential to clarity and decreases the likelihood of misinterpreting information during verbal communication, especially when a shared language is not spoken. Written documentation should include statements made by the patient, noting they were interpreted by a third party. (Objective 8)
8. d. Once you're safe to evaluate the patient, you must next form a general impression and take a primary survey to determine whether the patient's presentation identifies a life threat, potential life threat, or non–life threat. If a life threat is identified, immediate interventions would be initiated. (Objective 7)
9. d. In the secondary survey, obtaining historical, physical exam, and diagnostic information and initiating treatment interventions are based on the emergent or nonemergent status of the patient. These assessment components are dynamic and don't necessarily follow a rigid format. (Objective 5)
10. c. *Clinical decision making* is the ability to integrate diagnostic data and assessment findings with experience and evidence-based recommendations to diagnose and treat the patient to improve outcomes. The cardinal presentation is the most significant presenting symptom or patient complaint. The AMLS Pathway is a framework for using an assessment-based approach to patient care.

Chapter 2

1. c. Answer *c* is correct because the patient responds after a normal event with appropriate answers; this patient would need to be evaluated for continued drowsiness. Answer *a* is incorrect because repetitive questions suggest altered mental status and a disruption of short-term memory. Answer *b* is incorrect because deep pain is required to elicit a response of localizing pain; this is indicative of altered mental status. Answer *d* is incorrect because the patient is demonstrating auditory hallucinations, a disturbance of perception. Care should be taken with this person, as the behavior may be unpredictable and unsafe. (Objective 1)
2. b. Only the Cincinnati Prehospital Stroke Scale assesses cranial nerves. Cranial nerve VII (facial

nerve) is evaluated when the patient is asked to smile or show his teeth. (Objective 2)

3. a. The best answer is *a* because it rules in or out trauma as a possible cause. Confirming the presence of allergies is important but not likely a factor that assists with the differential diagnosis in this setting. Although it's important to confirm the patient is compliant with his medications, missing one dose of either of these medications is unlikely to cause a syncopal incident. The onset of Alzheimer's is useful information, but it's not vital in generating an initial differential diagnosis. (Objective 5)
4. d. The best answer is *d* because this patient is showing signs and symptoms of a possible stroke. It would be best to transfer the patient to a stroke center or a facility with specialized neurologic and vascular capabilities. (Objective 9)
5. a. The abnormal gaze and pupil size are strong indicators of an intracerebral hemorrhage. Migraines tend to cause disturbances in vision but not changes in gaze or pupil size. The key findings for intracerebral bleeds or hemorrhage are alteration in vital signs (hypertension, pulse and respiration changes), altered LOC, stiff neck or headache, focal neurologic deficits (weakness, gaze preference/deviation of the eyes), difficulty with gait and fine motor control, nausea, vomiting, dizziness or vertigo, or abnormal eye movements. Migraine headaches are severe, recurrent headaches accompanied by incapacitating neurologic symptoms such as cognitive or visual disturbances, dizziness, nausea, and vomiting. The headache may be either unilateral or bilateral. The eyes usually do not deviate, but the patient may complain of photophobia, flashing lights, phonophobia, or zigzagging lines in the visual field. Migraines tend to occur in younger people, but intracerebral bleeds can occur in any age group. (Objective 4)
6. b. A patient with an end-tidal CO_2 should have ventilations assisted to bring $ETCO_2$ readings down to 40 mm Hg. Supplemental oxygen should be applied to return the oxygen saturations to at least 95%. Simply adding oxygen may increase the O_2 sats, but if this doesn't improve them, ventilatory assistance may be necessary. If a patient with a Glasgow Coma Score of 10 is ventilating and oxygenating adequately, assisting ventilations is not required. A patient with an elevated blood sugar may be acidotic due to diabetic ketoacidosis, and ventilation may be used, but an elevated blood sugar in itself is not a reason for ventilation. (Objective 6)
7. d. A stiff neck in the presence of sudden onset of an explosive headache is consistent with a subarachnoid bleed. The stiff neck is associated with irritation of the meninges from the bleeding. (Objective 3)
8. d. A pupil that's dilated, fixed, or slow to respond on the same side of the injury may indicate herniation due to increased intracranial pressure. The classic symptoms of an increasing herniation are coma, fixed and dilated pupil, and decerebrate posturing. (Objective 7)
9. b. *Proprioception* is information that comes to the brain from the body to help determine where the body is in space. She may still be able to feel but can't identify the position of her thumb. (Objective 2)
10. b. Inserting a nasopharyngeal airway is the best answer, since this patient is likely to recover his level of consciousness. The nasal airway will help maintain his airway, but more invasive techniques are not indicated at this time. He doesn't need intubation at present. Placing him in a supine position puts him at risk for aspiration and potentially increases the difficulty of managing his airway. He's breathing and has adequate oxygen saturation, so ventilation is unnecessary at this time. (Objective 8)

Chapter 3

1. a. *Ventilation* is movement of air into and out of the lungs. Airway swelling and bronchoconstriction related to anaphylaxis can obstruct airflow and impair ventilation. (Objective 1)
2. d. Fatigue is an indication of respiratory failure. All other signs may be present during an asthma attack without respiratory failure. (Objective 3)
3. a. Pulmonary edema is more likely to present with a sudden onset, no fever, and bilateral lung findings. Status asthmaticus is more likely to include generalized wheezes and no fever. Pneumothorax is characterized by sudden onset and absent breath sounds; fever is unlikely. (Objective 4)
4. a. Capnography assesses carbon dioxide levels, which measures ventilation. Carbon monoxide detectors measure carboxyhemoglobin levels in the blood. Chest x-ray assesses structural changes in the lung. Oxygen saturation measures oxygen levels in the blood. These levels may decline with a severe decline in ventilation, but this occurs slowly. (Objective 5)
5. c. Fever and swelling do not accompany FBAO. The jaw is not swollen in tonsillitis. Laryngotracheobronchitis (croup) is found in children. (Objective 4)
6. c. Tobacco use is strongly associated with spontaneous pneumothorax. (Objective 2)
7. b. Right heart failure can develop as a consequence of each of these disease processes. (Objective 3)
8. a. This indicates respiratory failure. (Objective 8)
9. c. Guillain-Barré syndrome is a respiratory disease caused by a dysfunction of the nervous system. The loss of nerve impulses to the muscles that control respiration diminish the tidal volume. Many patients have compromised immune systems. This results in an opportune condition for bacteria to grow, resulting in respiratory infections. (Objective 8)

10. a. The risk of barotrauma increases as PEEP and tidal volume increase. (Objective 9)

Chapter 4

1. d. A pulse pressure decline from 42 to 32 indicates a decrease in cardiac output. (Objective 4.)
2. c. The anterior pituitary releases antidiuretic hormone (ADH), also known as *vasopressin*. This is one of the mechanisms that causes vasoconstriction. (Objective 2)
3. d. The inflammation causes fluid loss. (Objective 3)
4. b. Bradycardia, hypotension, and normal skin color and temperature are anticipated below the level of the injury. Even though his blood pressure is borderline, his pulse pressure is narrow. This is inconsistent with neurogenic shock. (Objective 6)
5. b. If the body temperature increases, oxygen demand will increase. Likewise, if the patient becomes hypothermic and shivers to compensate, oxygen demand will increase. (Objective 7)
6. c. Lactic acid is a byproduct of anaerobic metabolism. (Objective 5)
7. b. Patients in the third trimester of pregnancy are at risk for pulmonary embolism, which is a cause of obstructive shock. (Objective 10)
8. c. All the other interventions are appropriate, but epinephrine is the highest priority. (Objective 7)
9. d. Clopidogrel (Plavix) is an antiplatelet agent. (Objective 10)
10. a. Blood return to the heart from the inferior and superior venae cavae is obstructed. This leads to decreased preload and consequently decreased cardiac output. (Objective 2)

Chapter 5

1. c. Clot formation in the vessels causes diminished blood flow through the pulmonary circulation. Blood flow is also redirected, impacting the lungs and causing dyspnea, hypoxia, and an increase in respiratory rate. (Objective 1)
2. a. The chronic alcoholic is at risk for forceful vomiting. This type of vomiting places the patient at risk for acute rupture of the esophagus, known as *Boerhaave's syndrome*. Mediastinitis, sepsis, and shock are frequent signs of this syndrome. Swallowing often aggravates the pain. *Cholecystitis* refers to inflammation of the gallbladder and presents with right shoulder pain. Esophageal varices typically present with dull pain and are related to portal hypertension, often associated with cirrhosis. *Pleurisy* is inflammation of the lining of the lungs and/or chest wall. Typical presentations have sharp pain on inhalation. (Objective 1)
3. c. Left ventricular failure leads to congestion in the pulmonary vessels, causing crackles. Hypertension is often an underlying etiology. Orthopnea occurs during rest or sleep and results in greater tidal volume and air exchange in a tripod or upright position. Reactive airway disease results from inflammation and constriction of the airways, such as in asthma. This presents with wheezing rather than crackles. (Objective 1)
4. d. The renal arteries are off to the side of the abdominal aorta. If these arteries are blocked, this can lead to hypertension. This causes renin to be released and an increase in blood pressure to continue to perfuse the kidneys. (Objective 1)
5. a. Fluid accumulation caused by cancerous lesions and tissue destruction and fluid leakage due to chest radiation therapy put the 55-year-old patient at the highest risk for pericardial tamponade. (Objective 1)
6. a. Nitroglycerin will dilate coronary arteries, thus decreasing preload. It may be necessary to increase the fluid volume to increase right ventricular filling pressures. (Objective 1)
7. a. Nitroglycerin is administered to decrease the pain of ischemia. It can be administered if the systolic blood pressure is 90 mm Hg or above. (Objective 4)
8. d. Chest discomfort, hypotension, and clear lung fields are typical presentations of pulmonary embolism. (Objective 5)
9. b. Benzodiazepines such as lorazepam will reduce the anxiety caused by the pain and cocaine. (Objective 4)
10. d. Involvement of more than one coronary vascular area is typical of pericarditis and rarely happens in a myocardial infarction. (Objective 5)

Chapter 6

1. c. Trousseau's sign, a carpal pedal spasm in response to the inflation of a blood pressure cuff, along with hypocalcemia, bradycardia, and malnutrition are seen in hypoparathyroidism. Congestive heart failure, myxedema, hyponatremia, and hypoglycemia are seen in hypothyroidism. Addison's disease, as seen in adrenal insufficiency and lack of cortisol production, presents with hypoglycemia, hypotension, hyperkalemia, hyponatremia, and emaciation. Cushing's disease, which results in an excess of the production of cortisol, results in hyperglycemia, obesity, hypertension, and electrolyte imbalances. (Objective 4)
2. c. Exophthalmos (protrusion of the eyeball) is a common presentation in hyperthyroidism. In this patient, resultant dehydration from excessive sweat and diarrhea requires aggressive IV therapy. Amiodarone can cause autoimmune destruction of the thyroid gland. Aspirin is associated with decreased protein binding of thyroid hormones and increased unbinding of T_3 and T_4. (Objective 10)

3. b. Dry, yellow skin, hypotension, bradycardia, and low blood sugar are typical presentations of myxedema related to hypothyroidism. Chvostek's sign, hyperactive reflexes, and exophthalmus are symptoms of hyperthyroidism. (Objective 4)
4. d. Typical clinical findings of Addison's disease are hyponatremia, hypoglycemia, and hyperkalemia. The adrenal glands are unable to produce sufficient amounts of corticosteroids to meet the body's demand, so administration of steroids is necessary. If blood glucose levels are low, it may be appropriate to administer glucose. (Objective 4)
5. a. The metabolic alkalosis associated with Cushing's syndrome causes hypernatremia, hypocalcemia, hypertension, and hyperglycemia. Typical presentations are obesity and facial puffiness, often referred to as a *moon face*. A high blood glucose reading is common. (Objective 4)
6. a. Central nervous system dysfunction, tachycardia, confusion, and secretion of epinephrine are typical presentations in hypoglycemia. Patients experiencing hypoglycemia may have a medical history of hypopituitarism and diminished growth hormone secretion. Insulin production decreases. (Objective 3)
7. c. Hyperglycemia which results in fluid shifts that cause dehydration, abdominal pain, and metabolic acidosis requires fluid replacement with IV therapy. Performing a 12-lead ECG provides important diagnostic information, as cardiac dysrhythmias may occur. (Objective 5)
8. d. Acute metabolic acidosis, as seen in prolonged cardiac-arrest resuscitation, may require the administration of sodium bicarbonate. (Objective 6)
9. a. The patient's cardinal presentation of facial twitching (as seen in Chvostek's sign), general weakness, and seizures can signify hypocalcemia. Hypercalcemia can result from thiazide diuretics, hyperthyroidism, adrenal insufficiency, and hyperparathyroidism. Hyperkalemia is often seen in Addison's disease, renal failure, rhabdomyolysis, and digitalis toxicities. Hyponatremia results from hyperglycemia, CHF, excessive sweating, and Addison's disease. (Objective 3)
10. c. This patient suffers from moderate hypothermia; rewarming is appropriate. Atropine, epinephrine, and TCP would be contraindicated in tachycardic dysrhythmias. (Objective 6)

Chapter 7

1. d. The vagus nerve plays a role in GI stimulation. It also exerts parasympathetic stimulation on the SA node and AV node in the heart. (Objective 1)
2. a. Visceral pain in the periumbilical area often relates to the appendix, small bowel, or cecum. (Objective 2)
3. b. Jaundice occurs in patients who have excessive bilirubin. This is often seen in advanced hepatitis. (Objective 3)
4. c. The patient has signs of impending shock. Fluid resuscitation has the highest priority. (Objective 6)
5. c. The sudden onset of illness may indicate allergic reaction. The patient should be carefully questioned about allergies and the foods she ate. (Objective 6)
6. a. Severe right upper quadrant pain that increases with a deep breath suggests gallbladder or liver disease. (Objective 2)
7. c. Esophageal varices are more common in chronic alcoholics. Eating disorders can cause severe vomiting that may precipitate a Mallory-Weiss tear. (Objective 5)
8. c. Visual observation and and physical exam indicate fluid loss. Immediate treatment would be IV therapy with normal saline. (Objective 6)
9. b. Cullen's sign is an indicator of hemorrhagic pancreatitis. (Objective 8)
10. c. Famotidine (Pepcid) is prescribed for stomach and duodenal ulcers to decrease pain and heal inflammation. (Objective 7)

Chapter 8

1. d. The Department of Health ensures the federal regulations are implemented and monitored at the state level. The U.S. Food and Drug Administration (FDA) ensures the safety of prescription medications and over-the-counter drugs and medical devices. The Centers for Disease Control and Prevention (CDC) monitors epidemiology on the international level and is responsible for tracking and improving outcomes related to infectious disease. The Occupational Safety & Health Administration (OSHA) specifies personal protective equipment (PPE) for professionals and oversees compliance, inspection, tracking of exposure, and postexposure reports of airborne and bloodborne pathogens. (Objective 2)
2. a. During the latent stage of a disease, the infection is inactive but may still be communicable. The incubation period ranges from hours to years, during which the pathogen may be reproducing but not causing signs or symptoms. The communicable period comprises the period when the infection can be spread to another person. The disease period begins with the onset of symptoms or disruption of normal body function. (Objective 1)
3. c. An *exposure incident* is specific eye, mouth, other mucous membrane, nonintact skin, or parenteral contact with blood or other potentially infectious materials that results from the performance of a healthcare worker's duties. (Objective 1)
4. a. *Cellular immunity* is a direct attack on pathogens by lymphocytes and other cells. *Autoimmunity* is an

abnormal immune response against the body's own proteins or tissue. (Objective 4)

5. c. Hepatitis A is typically found in the feces of infected people. It replicates in the liver but doesn't damage the liver. Unlike other hepatitis infections, HAV is not transmitted by droplets, airborne, or bloodborne routes. (Objective 6)
6. d. There is no immunization or postexposure prophylaxis to protect against hepatitis C. (Objective 7)
7. c. The rash related to viral meningitis is red and flat. (Objective 8)
8. d. Rubeola is associated with many complications. (Objective 9)
9. d. Immediate reporting is essential for prompt source-patient testing and prophylaxis administration. Refer to agency and local protocols for direction. (Objective 10)
10. d. *Pertussis* is a bacterial infection characterized by a whooping cough or spasmodic, paroxysmal coughing phases. (Objective 8)

Chapter 9

1. a. This is consistent with the sympathomimetic toxidrome. (Objective 2)
2. b. The material safety data sheet (MSDS) is a comprehensive reference for hazardous materials. It includes information on routes of entry, health effects, first aid, firefighter measures, handling, storage, exposures, and the chemical and physical properties of hazardous substances. (Objective 9)
3. d. The digitalis-like properties of this plant cause bradycardia. (Objective 3)
4. d. Benadryl overdose signs and symptoms include dry mouth, fever, ringing in the ears, sleepiness, blurred vision, large pupils, and the potential for seizures. (Objective 4)
5. c. Metabolic acidosis related to metformin is associated with high mortality. (Objective 4)
6. b. Anticholinergic drugs cause ataxia, decreased production of mucus, dry mouth, and perspiration. Cholinergic medications cause an increase of secretions in the saliva, tears, and digestive acids. Sympathomimetics are used in decongestants to decrease histamine responses. (Objective 2)
7. a. *Clostridium botulinum* is a nerve toxin. (Objective 8)
8. b. Pinpoint pupils are consistent with opiate toxidrome. Establishing adequate ventilation is the first priority. (Objective 2)
9. a. Tricyclic antidepressant overdose causes that characteristic ECG change with tachycardia. (Objective 4)
10. d. Do not enter until appropriate authorities deem it safe. (Objective 9)

GLOSSARY

A

abscess (peritonsillar) An abscess in which a superficial soft-tissue infection progresses to create pockets of purulence in the submucosal space adjacent to the tonsils. This abscess and its accompanying inflammation cause the uvula to deviate to the opposing side.

acidosis An abnormal increase in the hydrogen ion concentration in the blood, resulting from an accumulation of an acid or the loss of a base, indicated by a blood pH below the normal range

acute coronary syndrome (ACS) An umbrella term that covers any group of clinical symptoms consistent with acute myocardial ischemia (chest pain due to insufficient blood supply to the heart muscle that results from coronary artery disease). ACS covers clinical conditions ranging from unstable angina to ST-segment elevated myocardial infarction (STEMI) and non–ST-segment elevated myocardial infarction (NSTEMI).

acute myocardial infarction (AMI) Commonly known as a *heart attack*, AMI occurs when the blood supply to part of the heart is interrupted, causing heart cells to die. This is most commonly due to blockage of a coronary artery following the rupture of plaque within the wall of an artery. The resulting ischemia and decreased supply of oxygen, if left untreated, can cause damage and/or death of heart muscle tissue.

Addison's disease An endocrine disease caused by a deficiency of corticosteroid hormones produced by the adrenal cortex. The disease is characterized by nausea, vomiting, abdominal pain, and tanning of the skin.

adrenal crisis An endocrine emergency caused by a deficiency of corticosteroid hormones produced by the adrenal cortex. The disease is characterized by nausea, vomiting, abdominal pain, hypotension, hyperkalemia, and hyponatremia.

Advanced Medical Life Support (AMLS) Assessment Pathway A dependable framework to support the reduction of morbidity and mortality by using an assessment-based approach to determine a differential diagnosis and effectively manage a broad range of medical emergencies

aerobic metabolism The process in which glucose is converted into energy in the presence of oxygen

afterload The force resisting shortening after the muscle is stimulated to contract. In the intact heart, it's the pressure against which the ventricle ejects blood, as measured by the stress acting on the ventricular wall following the onset of contraction. Afterload is determined largely by the peripheral vascular resistance and by the physical characteristics of and blood volume in the arterial system. It's often estimated by determining systolic arterial pressure.

ALI/ARDS Acute lung injury/acute respiratory distress syndrome, a systemic disease that causes lung failure

altered mental status Any behavior that departs from what's normal for a given patient

Amyotrophic lateral sclerosis (ALS) A disease characterized by degeneration of the upper and lower motor neurons; causes voluntary muscles to weaken or atrophy

anaerobic metabolism A process in which when denied oxygen, cells can generate small amounts of energy but release excessive acids as byproducts, especially lactic and carbonic acids

analeptic A substance that quickens the activity of the central nervous system by increasing the rate of neuronal discharge or blocking an inhibitory neurotransmitter

angina, stable Symptoms of chest pain, shortness of breath, or other equivalent symptom, that occurs predictably with exertion then resolves with rest. This suggests the presence of a fixed coronary lesion that prevents adequate perfusion with increased demand.

angioedema A disorder characterized by a sudden swelling, usually of a head or neck structure such as the lip (especially the lower lip), earlobes, tongue, or uvula

antibodies Immunoglobulins produced by lymphocytes in response to bacteria, viruses, or other antigenic substances

antiemetic A substance that prevents or alleviates nausea and vomiting

antigens Substances, usually proteins, the body recognizes as foreign; can evoke an immune response

apneustic center An area located in the pons, this center regulates the depth of respiration.

assessment-based patient management Using the patient's cardinal presentation and historical, diagnostic, and physical exam findings in addition to your own critical thinking skills as a healthcare professional to diagnose and treat a patient

ataxia An unsteady or altered gait due to brain dysfunction, often of the cerebellum, which controls coordination

atelectasis Alveolar collapse

B

biological agent Disease-causing pathogen or toxin that may be used as a weapon to cause disease or injury to humans

blood agents Chemicals absorbed into the body through the action of breathing, skin absorption, or ingestion

blood pressure The tension exerted by blood on the arterial walls, calculated using the following equation: Blood pressure = Flow × Resistance

bloodborne pathogens Pathogenic microorganisms that are transmitted via human blood and cause disease in humans; some examples include hepatitis B virus (HBV) and human immunodeficiency virus (HIV).

C

cardiac cycle A complete cardiac movement or heartbeat. The period from the beginning of one heartbeat to the beginning of the next; diastolic and systolic movement, with the interval in between.

cardiac output (CO) The effective volume of blood expelled by either ventricle of the heart per unit of time (usually volume per minute); equal to the stroke volume multiplied by the heart rate (SV × HR = CO)

cardiac tamponade Also known as *pericardial tamponade*, this is an emergency condition in which fluid accumulates in the pericardium (the sac in which the heart is enclosed). If the amount of fluid increases slowly (such as in hypothyroidism), the pericardial sac can expand to contain a liter or more of fluid prior to tamponade occurring. If the fluid increases rapidly (as may occur after trauma or myocardial rupture), as little as 100 mL can cause tamponade.

cardinal presentation Patient's prime presenting sign or symptom; often the patient's chief complaint, but it may be an objective finding such as unconsciousness or choking.

cerebrospinal fluid A transparent, slightly yellowish fluid that acts as a shock absorber for the brain

cerebrovascular accident (CVA) Another term for stroke

chemoreceptors Chemical receptors that sense changes in the composition of blood and body fluids. The primary chemical changes registered by chemoreceptors are those involving levels of hydrogen (H^+), carbon dioxide (CO_2), and oxygen (O_2).

choking agent (pulmonary agent) An industrial chemical used as a weapon to kill those who inhale the vapor or gas; results in asphyxiation due to lung damage

clinical decision making The ability to integrate diagnostic data and assessment findings with experience and evidence-based recommendations to make decisions regarding the most appropriate treatment outcomes

clinical reasoning The second conceptual component underpinning the AMLS assessment pathway, which combines good judgment with clinical experience to make accurate diagnoses and initiate proper treatment. This process assumes the provider has a strong foundation of clinical knowledge.

cold zone (green zone) A support zone for general triage, stabilization, and management of illness or injuries. Patients and uncontaminated personnel are given access to this zone. However, healthcare personnel must wear protective clothing while in the green zone and properly discard it in predetermined areas on exiting.

communicable diseases Any disease either directly transmitted from one person or animal to another by contact with excreta or other discharges from the body, or indirectly by means of substances or inanimate objects (e.g., contaminated drinking glasses, toys, water) or vectors such as flies, mosquitoes, ticks, or other insects

contaminated, contamination A condition of being soiled, stained, touched, or otherwise exposed to harmful agents, making an object potentially unsafe for use as intended or without barrier techniques. An example is entry of infectious or toxic materials into a previously clean or sterile environment.

D

decontamination The process of removing foreign material such as blood, body fluids, or radioactivity. It does not eliminate microorganisms but is a necessary step preceding disinfection or sterilization.

delirium an acute mental disorder characterized by confusion, disorientation, restlessness, clouding of consciousness, incoherence, fear, anxiety, excitement, and often illusions.

diabetic ketoacidosis An acute endocrine emergency caused by a lack of insulin. The condition is characterized by an elevated blood glucose level, ketone production, metabolic acidosis, dehydration, nausea, vomiting, abdominal pain, and tachypnea.

differential diagnosis The underlying etiology and possible causes of the patient's cardinal presentation

dirty bomb A conventional explosive device used to disperse radiologic agents

Disaster Medical Assistance Team (DMAT) Field-deployable hospital teams, including physicians, nurses, emergency medical technicians, and other medical and nonmedical support personnel

disseminated intravascular coagulation A pathologic form of coagulation that is diffuse rather than localized, as would be the case in normal coagulation. The process damages rather than protects the area involved, and several clotting factors are consumed to such an extent that generalized bleeding or clotting may occur. Also known as *diffuse intravascular coagulation*.

E

embolus A clot or plaque that forms in the circulatory system elsewhere than in an artery, breaks off, and obstructs blood flow when it becomes lodged in a smaller artery

emergency decontamination Process of decontaminating people exposed to and potentially contaminated with hazardous materials by rapidly removing the contamination to reduce their exposure and save lives, with secondary regard for completeness of decontamination

end-tidal CO_2 monitoring Analysis of exhaled gases for carbon dioxide (CO_2); a useful method of assessing a patient's ventilatory status

epidemic A disease that affects a significantly large number of people at the same time and spreads rapidly through a demographic segment of the human population

epidemiology The study of the determinants of disease events in populations

exposure incident A state of being in the presence of or subjected to a force or influence (e.g., viral exposure, heat exposure)

expressive aphasia Inability to speak secondary to a neurologic insult

F

first impression Before physical or verbal contact with the patient, the healthcare provider's visual, auditory, and olfactory observations of the patient's presentation that provide information regarding a "sick or not sick" patient, early identification and management of life-threats, and potential differential diagnoses. This assessment follows the initial observation.

fulminant Describes a sudden, intense occurrence that creates a hazardous environment

fulminant hepatic failure A rare condition that occurs when hepatitis progresses to hepatic necrosis (death of the liver cells); classic symptoms include anorexia, vomiting, jaundice, abdominal pain, and asterixis or flapping.

G

gait disturbance An altered gait pattern that may be caused by an injury to or pathology of the brain, spine, legs, feet, or inner ear

gas exchange The process in which oxygen from the atmosphere is taken up by circulating blood cells, and carbon dioxide from the bloodstream is released to the atmosphere

gastrointestinal (GI) Pertaining to the organs of the GI tract. The GI tract links the organs involved in the consumption, processing, and elimination of nutrients; it begins at the mouth, moves to the esophagus, travels through the chest cavity into the abdomen, and terminates in the pelvic girdle at the rectum.

gastrointestinal decontamination Any attempt to limit absorption or hasten elimination of a toxin from a patient's gastrointestinal tract. Examples include activated charcoal, gastric lavage, and whole-bowel irrigation. While these methods do have a small role in toxicology, their use is not routinely recommended and should be discussed with a poison control center or medical toxicologist.

H

heatstroke A syndrome in which the body loses its ability to regulate temperature, resulting in altered mental status, an elevated core body temperature, and multiorgan failure

hematemesis Vomiting of bright red blood, indicating upper GI bleeding

hematochezia Passage of red blood through the rectum

hemiparesis Unilateral weakness, usually occurring on the opposite side of the body from the stroke

hemiplegia Paralysis on one side of the body

hemorrhagic stroke A stroke that occurs when a diseased or damaged vessel ruptures

history of the present illness (HPI) The most important element of patient assessment. The primary elements of the HPI can be obtained by using the OPQRST and SAMPLER mnemonics.

hospital-acquired infection (HAI)/healthcare-associated infections Infection acquired at least 72 hours after hospitalization; also called *nosocomial infection*

hot zone An area where the hazardous material is located and contamination has occurred. Access to this zone is limited to protect rescuers and patients from further exposure. Specific protective gear worn by trained personnel is required for access.

huffing The act of pouring an inhalant onto a cloth or into a bag and inhaling the substance, usually in an attempt to alter one's mental status

hyperosmolar hyperglycemic nonketotic syndrome An endocrine emergency characterized by a high plasma glucose concentration, absent ketone production, and increased serum osmolality (above 315 mOsm/kg). The syndrome causes severe dehydration, nausea, vomiting, abdominal pain, and tachypnea.

hypoglycemia A plasma glucose concentration of less than 60 mg/dL. This condition is often associated with signs and symptoms such as sweating, cold skin, tachycardia, and altered mental status.

hypothermia Core body temperature below 35°C (95°F). At lower temperatures, hypothermia may induce cardiac arrhythmia and precipitate a decline in mental status.

hypovolemia Abnormally decreased volume of circulating blood in the body; the most common cause is hemorrhage.

I

infectious diseases Any clinically evident communicable disease, or one that can be transmitted from one human being to another or from animal to human by direct or indirect contact

initial observation This visual, auditory, and olfactory observation assists in determining scene or situation safety concerns as well as an overall observation of the patient's cardinal presentation. This process leads to the primary survey.

intoxication The state of being poisoned by a drug or other toxic substance; the state of being inebriated as a result of excessive alcohol consumption

intravascular volume The amount of circulating blood in the vessels

intussusception Prolapse of one segment of the bowel into the lumen of another segment. This kind of intestinal obstruction may involve segments of the small intestine, colon, or terminal ileum and cecum.

ischemia A restriction in oxygen and nutrient delivery to muscle; may be caused by physical obstruction to blood flow, increased demand by the tissues, or hypoxia; leads to damage or dysfunction of tissue

ischemic stroke A stroke that occurs when a thrombus or embolus obstructs a vessel, diminishing blood flow to the brain

K

Korsakoff syndrome The symptoms seen in the late stages of Wernicke's encephalopathy, especially memory loss

L

lethal concentration 50% (LC50) The air concentration of an agent that kills 50% of the exposed animal population; denotes both the concentration and length of exposure time of that population

lethal dose 50% (LD50) The oral or dermal exposure dose that kills 50% of an exposed animal population in 2 weeks.

Lou Gehrig's disease See amyotrophic lateral sclerosis (ALS).

Ludwig's angina A deep-space infection of the anterior neck just below the mandible. The name derives from the sensation of choking and suffocation reported by most patients with this condition.

M

mean arterial pressure (MAP) The average pressure within an artery over a complete cycle of one heartbeat; expressed as: MAP = Diastolic pressure + (1/3 × Pulse pressure)

melena Abnormal black, tarry stool that has a distinctive odor and contains digested blood

methemoglobinemia The presence of methemoglobin in the blood, preventing hemoglobin from carrying and transporting oxygen to the tissues. Hemoglobin is converted to methemoglobin by nitrogen oxides and sulfa drugs.

myxedema Severe hypothyroidism associated with cold intolerance, weight gain, weakness, and declining mental status

N

National Fire Protection Association (NFPA) A national and international voluntary membership organization that promotes improved fire protection and prevention and establishes safeguards against loss of life and property by fire. The NFPA writes and publishes national voluntary consensus standards.

noninvasive positive-pressure ventilation A procedure in which positive pressure is provided through the upper airway by some type of mask or other noninvasive interface

non–ST-segment elevation myocardial infarction (NSTEMI) A type of MI caused by a blocked blood supply that causes non-transmural infarction in an area of the heart. There is no ST-segment elevation on electrocardiogram (ECG) recordings, but other clinical signs of MI are present.

North American Emergency Response Guidebook A book published by the U.S. Government Printing Office that provides a quick reference to hazardous materials emergencies for first responders

nosocomial infection See hospital-acquired infection (HAI).

O

Occupational Safety and Health Administration (OSHA) The U.S. federal agency that regulates worker safety

ophthalmoplegia Abnormal function of the eye muscles

P

packer A person who ingests a large quantity of well-packed drugs for the purpose of smuggling. These carefully prepared packages are less likely to rupture than those ingested by stuffers, but toxicity can be severe if they do because of the large amount of drug present.

pandemic A disease occurring throughout the population of a country, a people, or the world

parenteral Pertaining to treatment other than through the digestive system

perfusion The act of pouring over or through, especially the passage of a fluid through the vessels of a specific organ

pericarditis A condition in which the tissue surrounding the heart (pericardium) becomes inflamed. This can be caused by several factors but is often related to a viral infection. If cardiac dysfunction or signs of congestive heart failure (CHF) are present, this suggests a more serious myocarditis or involvement of the heart muscle.

pharmacokinetics The absorption, distribution, metabolism, and excretion of medications

placards Diamond-shaped signs placed on containers to identify hazardous materials

pleura A thin membrane that surrounds and protects the lungs (visceral pleura) and lines the chest cavity (parietal pleura)

pneumotaxic center An area located in the pons, this center generally controls the rate and pattern of respiration.

preload The mechanical state of the heart at the end of diastole, the magnitude of the maximal (end-diastolic) ventricular volume or the end-diastolic pressure stretching the ventricles. In isolated cardiac muscle, the force stretching the resting muscle to a given length prior to contraction. In the intact heart, the stress on the ventricular wall at the end of diastole, determined largely by the venous return, total blood volume and its distribution, and atrial activity.

primary survey The process of initially assessing the airway, breathing, circulation, and perfusion status to identify and manage life-threatening conditions and establish priorities for further assessment, treatment, and transport

prodromal Early symptoms that mark the onset of a disease

proprioception Information that comes to the brain from the body to determine where the body is in space

psychosis Any major mental disorder characterized by a gross impairment in reality testing. The affected individual incorrectly evaluates the accuracy of perceptions and thoughts and makes incorrect references about external reality. Psychosis is often characterized by regressive behavior, inappropriate mood and affect, and diminished impulse control. Symptoms include hallucinations and delusions.

pulmonary embolism The sudden blockage of a pulmonary artery by a blood clot, often from a deep vein in the legs or pelvis. The embolus travels to the lung artery, where it becomes lodged and can cause tachycardia, hypoxia, and hypotension.

pulse pressure The difference between the systolic and diastolic blood pressure, calculated by subtracting diastolic blood pressure from systolic blood pressure. Normal pulse pressure is 30 to 40 mm Hg. When this difference begins to narrow, it may be a sign of a cardiac tamponade.

pulsus paradoxus An exaggeration of the normal inspiratory decrease in systolic blood pressure. It's defined by an inspiratory fall of systolic blood pressure of greater than 10 mm Hg.

R

radioactive Giving off radiation as the result of the disintegration of atomic nuclei

referred pain Pain felt at a site different from that of an injured or diseased organ or body part

respiration The reciprocal passage of oxygen into the blood and carbon dioxide into the alveoli

respiratory failure A disorder in which the lungs become unable to perform their basic task of gas exchange, the transfer of oxygen from inhaled air into the blood and the transfer of carbon dioxide from the blood into exhaled air

retrovirus Any of a family of ribonucleic acid (RNA) viruses containing the enzyme reverse transcriptase in the virion. Examples of retroviruses include human immunodeficiency virus (HIV1, HIV2) and human T-cell lymphotropic virus (HTLV).

S

secondary survey An in-depth evaluation of the patient's history, physical exam, vital signs, and diagnostic information used to identify additional emergent and nonemergent conditions and modify differential diagnoses and management strategies

shock A condition of profound hemodynamic and metabolic disturbance characterized by failure of the circulatory system to maintain adequate perfusion of vital organs. It may result from inadequate blood volume, cardiac function, or vasomotor tone.

signs Objective evidence that can be observed, felt, seen, heard, touched, or smelled by a healthcare professional

somatic (parietal) pain Generally well-localized pain caused by an irritation of the nerve fibers in the parietal peritoneum or other deep tissues, such as those of the musculoskeletal system. Physical findings include sharp, discrete, localized pain accompanied by tenderness to palpation, guarding of the affected area, and rebound tenderness.

symptoms The *S* in the SAMPLER mnemonic; the patient's subjective perceptions of what he or she feels (e.g., nausea) or has experienced (e.g., a sensation of seeing flashing lights)

systemic vascular resistance The resistance of blood flow through a vessel; determined by the diameter of the vessel

Standard on Hazardous Waste Operations and Emergency Response (HAZWOPER) (CFR 1910.120) Occupational Safety and Health Administration (OSHA) and Environmental Protection Agency (EPA) regulation intended to protect the safety of employees who respond to emergency incidents related to storage and disposal of hazardous materials

Standard Precautions Guidelines recommended by the Centers for Disease Control and Prevention (CDC) for reducing the risk of transmission of bloodborne and other pathogens in hospitals. Standard precautions apply to (1) blood; (2) all body fluids, secretions, and excretions except sweat, regardless of whether or not they contain blood; (3) nonintact skin; and (4) mucous membranes.

stroke Sometimes called a *brain attack* or *cerebral vascular accident (CVA)*, a stroke is a brain injury that occurs when blood flow to the brain is obstructed or interrupted, causing brain cells to die.

stroke volume The amount of blood ejected by the left ventricle at each heartbeat. Amount varies with age, sex, and exercise. Also called *systolic discharge*.

ST-segment elevation myocardial infarction (STEMI) A type of myocardial infarction (MI) caused by a blocked blood supply that causes transmural infarction in an area of the heart. These attacks carry a substantial risk of death and disability and call for a quick response by a STEMI system geared for reperfusion therapy.

stuffer A person who hastily ingests small packets of poorly packaged drugs to avoid apprehension and drug confiscation. The dose is much lower than that seen with packers, but the likelihood of toxicity is much greater because the packages, meant for distribution, are likely to open in the patient's stomach or bowel.

surge capacity The ability to expand care on the basis of a sudden mass-casualty incident. This capacity should be addressed in any emergency management plan.

T

tension pneumothorax A life-threatening condition that results from progressive worsening of a simple pneumothorax, the accumulation of air under pressure in the pleural space. This can lead to progressive restriction of venous return, leading to decreased preload, then systemic hypotension.

therapeutic communication A communication process in which the healthcare provider uses effective communication skills to obtain information about the patient and their condition. Includes using the four E's: engagement, empathy, education, and enlistment.

thoracentesis A procedure to remove fluid or air from the pleural space

thoracic duct Located in the left upper thorax, the thoracic duct is the largest lymph vessel in the body. It returns to the venae cavae the excess fluid not collected by the veins from the lower extremities and abdomen.

thoracostomy A procedure in which a tube may be connected to a Heimlich valve, a one-way valve that lets air escape but not enter the pleural space

thrombus A blood clot or a cholesterol plaque that forms in an artery, occluding blood flow

thyroid storm An endocrine emergency characterized by hyperfunction of the thyroid gland. This disorder is associated with fever, tachycardia, nervousness, altered mental status, and hemodynamic instability.

thyrotoxicosis A condition of excessively elevated thyroid hormone levels; signs and symptoms are tachycardia, tremor, weight loss, and high-output heart failure.

toxidrome A specific syndrome-like group of symptoms associated with exposure to a given poison

tweaker A methamphetamine user who is in a dangerous phase of the addictive cycle. These people can be extremely violent and are easily startled by loud noises and bright lights.

U

ultrasound Also called *sonography* or *diagnostic medical sonography*, this is an imaging method that uses high-frequency sound waves to produce precise images of structures within the body.

unstable angina (UA) Angina of increased frequency, severity, or occurring with less intensive exertion than the baseline. This suggests the narrowing of a static lesion, causing further limitation of coronary blood flow with increased demand.

V

vesicants Substances capable of causing tissue necrosis when extravasated; also called *blister agents* or *mustard agents*

virulence The power of a microorganism to produce disease

visceral pain Poorly localized pain that occurs when the walls of the hollow organs are stretched, thereby activating the stretch receptors. This kind of pain is characterized by a deep, persistent ache ranging from mild to intolerable and commonly described as cramping, burning, and gnawing.

viscus (pl. viscera) The internal organs enclosed within a body cavity, including the abdominal, thoracic, pelvic, and endocrine organs

volvulus A condition in which the stomach rotates more than 180 degrees; this twisting seals the stomach on both ends, blocking the flow of blood and the passage of fluid and food. The condition is characterized by an acute onset of abdominal pain, severe vomiting, and shock.

W

weakness Any localized loss of neurologic function in part or all of an extremity or on one side of the face

Wernicke's encephalopathy A disorder often caused by deficiency of thiamine (vitamin B_1) and characterized by a triad of symptoms: acute confusion, ataxia, and ophthalmoplegia

working diagnosis The presumed cause of the patient's condition, arrived at by evaluating all assessment information thus far obtained while conducting further diagnostic testing to definitively diagnose the illness

INDEX

A

D

E

I

J

K

L

O

W

X

Y

Z